NUTRITIONAL MANAGEMENT OF RENAL DISEASE

THIRD EDITION

ELSEVIER *science & technology books*

Companion Web Site:

http://booksite.elsevier.com/9780123919342

Nutritional Management of Renal Disease, Third Edition
Joel D. Kopple, Shaul G. Massry, Kamyar Kalantar-Zadeh, *Editors*

Resources for Professors:

- All figures from the book available as both Power Point slides and .jpeg files

 TOOLS FOR ALL YOUR TEACHING NEEDS
textbooks.elsevier.com

ACADEMIC PRESS

NUTRITIONAL MANAGEMENT OF RENAL DISEASE

THIRD EDITION

Edited by

JOEL D. KOPPLE
Division of Nephrology and Hypertension,
Los Angeles Biomedical Research Institute
at Harbor-UCLA Medical Center,
Torrance, California
David Geffen School of Medicine at UCLA
and UCLA Fielding School of Public Health,
Los Angeles, California

SHAUL G MASSRY
Keck School of Medicine,
University of Southern California,
Beverly Hills, California

KAMYAR KALANTAR-ZADEH
Division of Nephrology and Hypertension,
University of California Irvine,
School of Medicine, Orange, California
and UCLA Fielding School of Public Health
Los Angeles, California

AMSTERDAM • BOSTON • HEIDELBERG • LONDON
NEW YORK • OXFORD • PARIS • SAN DIEGO
SAN FRANCISCO • SINGAPORE • SYDNEY • TOKYO
Academic Press is an imprint of Elsevier

ELSEVIER

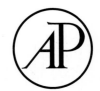

Academic Press is an imprint of Elsevier
32 Jamestown Road, London NW1 7BY, UK
225 Wyman Street, Waltham, MA 02451, USA
525 B Street, Suite 1800, San Diego, CA 92101-4495, USA

First edition 1997
Second edition 2004
Third edition 2013

Notice

No responsibility is assumed by the publisher for any injury and/or damage to persons or property as a matter of products liability, negligence or otherwise, or from any use or operation of any methods, products, instructions or ideas contained in the material herein. Because of rapid advances in the medical sciences, in particular, independent verification of diagnoses and drug dosages should be made

Medicine is an ever-changing field. Standard safety precautions must be followed, but as new research and clinical experience broaden our knowledge, changes in treatment and drug therapy may become necessary or appropriate. Readers are advised to check the most current product information provided by the manufacturer of each drug to be administered to verify the recommended dose, the method and duration of administrations, and contraindications. It is the responsibility of the treating physician, relying on experience and knowledge of the patient, to determine dosages and the best treatment for each individual patient. Neither the publisher nor the authors assume any liability for any injury and/or damage to persons or property arising from this publication.

British Library Cataloguing-in-Publication Data
A catalogue record for this book is available from the British Library

Library of Congress Cataloging-in-Publication Data
A catalog record for this book is available from the Library of Congress

ISBN : 978-0-12-391934-2

For information on all Academic Press publications
visit our website at www.store.elsevier.com

Typeset by TNQ Books and Journals

Printed and bound in United States of America

12 13 14 15   10 9 8 7 6 5 4 3 2 1

Working together to grow
libraries in developing countries

www.elsevier.com | www.bookaid.org | www.sabre.org

ELSEVIER   BOOK AID International   Sabre Foundation

Joel D. Kopple

To my wife: Madelynn Kopple
To our children: David and Robin Kopple, Michael and Yael Kopple,
Deborah and Yury Nedelin, and Joshua and Calanit Kopple
To our grandchildren: Ellis, Tabitha and Maxwell Kopple,
Levi and Liora Kopple, Elisheva, Chavah and Isaac Nedelin,
and Yeshaya and Eliyahu Kopple
and to Jeffrey Alan Kopple

Shaul G. Massry

To my wife: Meira Massry
To our children: Efrat and Ram Cogan, Dr. Guy G. Massry,
Yael and Geoffrey Rendon and Drs Dina and Kenneth Grudko
To our grandchildren: Raef and Emma Cogan, Alexis Massry,
Maya and Joseph Rendon and Sam and Ava Grudko

Kamyar Kalantar-Zadeh

To my wife: Dr Grace-Hyunjoo Lee
To our children: Sara-Soojung, Diana-Sunhee and Hannah-Soyeon Kalantar

Contents

List of Contributors

Marcin Adamczak MD, Department of Nephrology, Endocrinology and Metabolic Disease, Medical University of Silesia, Katowice, Poland

T. Alp Ikizler MD, Department of Medicine, Division of Nephrology, Vanderbilt University, Medical Center, Nashville, TN, USA

James L. Bailey PhD, Renal Division, Department of Medicine, Emory University School of Medicine, Atlanta, GA, USA

Radhakrishna Baliga MD, Department of Pediatrics, University of Mississippi Medical Center, Jackson, Mississippi, USA

Rinaldo Bellomo MD, FRACP, FCICM, Department of Intensive Care, Austin Hospital, Melbourne, Australia

J. Bikhchandani, Creighton University Medical Center, Department of Surgery, Omaha, Nebraska, USA

George L. Blackburn MD, PhD, FACS, Center for the Study of Nutrition Medicine, Department of Surgery, Beth Israel Deaconess Medical Center, Boston, MA, USA

David A. Bushinsky MD, University of Rochester School of Medicine, Rochester, NY, USA

Vito M. Campese MD, Division of Nephrology, Keck School of Medicine, University of Southern California, Los Angeles, CA, USA

Noel J. Cano MD, PhD, Centre Hospitalier Universitaire de Clermont-Ferrand, Université d'Auvergne, Unité de Nutrition Humaine, INRA, CRNH Auvergne, Clermont-Ferrand, France

Juan Jesús Carrero PhD Pharm, PhD Med, Division of Renal Medicine, Karolinska Institutet, Stockholm, Sweden

Steve Chadban BMed(Hons), PhD, FRACP, Royal Prince Alfred Hospital and University of Sydney, New South Wales, Australia

Vimal Chadha MD, Department of Pediatrics, University of Missouri-Kansas City School of Medicine, Kansas City, MO, USA

Maria Chan BSc(Hons), MNutrDiet, AdvAPD, The St George Hospital and University of New South Wales, New South Wales, Australia

Alex Chang MD, Loyola University Medical Center, Department of Medicine, Division of Nephrology and Hypertension, Maywood, IL, USA

Charles Chazot MD, NephroCare Tassin-Charcot, Sainte Foy Les Lyon, France

Michal Chmielewski MD, PhD, Divisions of Baxter Novum and Renal Medicine, Karolinska Institutet, Karolinska University Hospital Huddinge, Stockholm, Sweden and Medical University of Gdansk, Department of Nephrology, Transplantology and Internal Medicine, Gdansk, Poland

Marta Christov MD, PhD, Division of Endocrinology, Massachusetts General Hospital and Department of Medicine, Harvard Medical School, Boston, MA, USA

Horng-Ruey Chua MBBS, MMed, MRCP, Division of Nephrology, University Medicine Cluster, National University Hospital, National University Health System, Singapore

Lydia Chwastiak MD, MPH, Yale University School of Medicine, Connecticut Mental Health Center, New Haven, CT, USA

Burl R. Don MD, FASN, Department of Internal Medicine, Division of Nephrology, University of California, Davis, USA

Wilfred Druml MD, Department of Medicine III, Division of Nephrology, Medical University of Vienna, Vienna, Austria

Ramanath Dukkipati MD, Division of Nephrology and Hypertension, Harbor-UCLA Medical Center, Torrance, CA, USA

Bo Feldt-Rasmussen MD, DMSc, Department of Nephrology, Rigshospitalet, University of Copenhagen, Denmark

Frederic Finkelstein MD, Yale University School of Medicine, New Haven, CT, USA

R.A. Forse, Creighton University Medical Center, Department of Surgery, Omaha, Nebraska, USA

Denis Fouque MD, PhD, Department of Nephrology, Hôpital E. Herriot, Université de Lyon, Lyon, France

Harold A. Franch PhD, Renal Division, Department of Medicine, Emory University School of Medicine, Atlanta, GA, USA and Research Service, Atlanta Veterans Affairs Medical Center, Decatur, GA, USA

Pranav S. Garimella MD, MPH, Tufts University School of Medicine, Tufts Medical Center, Boston, MA, USA

Marvin Grieff MD, University of Rochester School of Medicine, Rochester, NY, USA

Orlando M. Gutiérrez MD, MMSc, Division of Nephrology, Department of Medicine, School of Medicine and Department of Epidemiology, School of Public Health, University of Alabama at Birmingham, Birmingham, AL, USA

Nabil Haddad MD, The Ohio State University Medical Center, Department of Internal Medicine, Columbus, OH, USA

Lee A. Hebert MD, The Ohio State University Medical Center, Department of Internal Medicine, Columbus, OH, USA

Olof Heimbürger MD, PhD, Divisions of Baxter Novum and Renal Medicine, Karolinska Institutet, Karolinska University Hospital Huddinge, Stockholm, Sweden

Raimund Hirschberg MD, UCLA, Division of Nephrology and Hypertension, Harbor-UCLA Medical Center, Torrance, CA, USA

Jessica Houston BS, MT, Division of Nephrology and Hypertension, University of Miami Miller School of Medicine, Miami, FL, USA

Tamara Isakova MD, MMSc, Division of Nephrology and Hypertension, University of Miami Miller School of Medicine, Miami, FL, USA

Sirin Jiwakanon MD, Hatyai Hospital, Hatyai, Songkhla, Thailand and Los Angeles Biomedical Research Institute at Harbor-UCLA, Torrance, CA, USA

George A. Kaysen MD, PhD, FASN, FAHA, Department of Internal Medicine, Division of Nephrology, University of California, Davis, USA

Csaba P. Kovesdy MD, University of Tennessee Health Science Center, Memphis TN, USA

Holly Kramer MD, MPH, Loyola University Medical Center, Department of Medicine, Division of Nephrology and Hypertension and Department of Preventive Medicine and Epidemiology, Maywood, IL, USA

Kiyoshi Kurokawa MD, MACP, National Graduate Institute for Policy Studies, Minato-ku, Tokyo, Japan

Daniel Landau MD, Department of Pediatrics, Soroka Medical Center, Ben Gurion University, Beer Sheva, Israel

Yinan Li MD, Division of Nephrology and Hypertension, Los Angeles Biomedical Research Institute at Harbor-UCLA, Torrance, CA, USA

Bengt Lindholm MD, PhD, Divisions of Baxter Novum and Renal Medicine, Karolinska Institutet, Karolinska University Hospital Huddinge, Stockholm, Sweden

Greta Magerowski BA, Center for the Study of Nutrition Medicine, Department of Surgery, Beth Israel Deaconess Medical Center, Boston, MA, USA

Kevin J. Martin MB, BCh, Division of Nephrology, Saint Louis University, St. Louis, Missouri, USA

Cathi J. Martin RD, Department of Medicine, Division of Nephrology, Vanderbilt University, Medical Center, Nashville, TN, USA

Steve Martino PhD, Yale University School of Medicine, VA Connecticut Healthcare System, West Haven, CT, USA

Rajnish Mehrotra MD, Division of Nephrology and Hypertension, Harbor-UCLA Medical Center, Torrance, CA, USA and David Geffen School of Medicine at UCLA, Los Angeles, CA, USA and Section Head, Nephrology, Harborview Medical Center, University of Washington, Seattle

Michal L. Melamed MD, MHS, Albert Einstein College of Medicine/Montefiore Medical Center, Bronx, NY, USA

William E. Mitch MD, Baylor College of Medicine, Nephrology Division, Department of Medicine, Houston, TX, USA

Toshio Miyata MD, PhD, Director, United Centers for Advanced Research and Translational Medicine (ART), Tohoku University School of Medicine, Aoba-ku, Sendai, Japan

Alessio Molfino MD, PhD, Department of Internal Medicine, Division of Nephrology, University of California, Davis, USA and Clinical Nutrition, Department of Internal Medicine, University of Rome "Tor Vergata", Rome, Italy and Department of Clinical Medicine, Sapienza University of Rome, Rome, Italy

Toshimitsu Niwa MD, PhD, Department of Advanced Medicine for Uremia, Nagoya University Graduate School of Medicine, Showa-ku, Nagoya, Japan

Lara B. Pupim MD, Department of Medicine, Division of Nephrology, Vanderbilt University, Medical Center, Nashville, TN, USA

Ralph Rabkin MD, Department Medicine/Nephrology, Stanford University, Stanford, CA, USA and Research Service, Veterans Affairs Palo Alto Health Care System, Palo Alto, CA, USA

Dominic Raj MD, Professor of Medicine and of Biochemistry and Genetics and of Epidemiology and Biostatistics Chief, Division of Renal Diseases and Hypertension, The George Washington University, Washington DC, USA

Mohan Rajapurkar MD, Department of Nephrology, Muljibhai Patel Urological Hospital, Nadiad, Gujarat, India

Samia Raju MD, Professor of Medicine and of Biochemistry and Genetics and of Epidemiology and Biostatistics Chief, Division of Nephrology, Keck School of Medicine, University of Southern California, Los Angeles, CA, USA

Eberhard Ritz MD, Nierenzentrum, Heidelberg, Germany

Mark J. Sarnak MD MS, Tufts University School of Medicine, Tufts Medical Center, Boston, MA, USA

Sudhir V. Shah MD, FACP, Department of Internal Medicine, Division of Nephrology, UAMS College of Medicine, Little Rock; and John L. McClellan Memorial Veterans Hospital, Central Arkansas Veterans Healthcare System, AR, USA

Rosemarie Shim MD, The Ohio State University Medical Center, Department of Internal Medicine, Columbus, OH, USA

Robert Stanton MD, Harvard Medical School, Joslin Diabetes Center, Boston, MA, USA

Alison l. Steiber PhD, RD, LD, Department of Nutrition, School of Medicine, Case Western Reserve University, Cleveland, OH, USA

Peter Stenvinkel MD, PhD, Divisions of Baxter Novum and Renal Medicine, Karolinska Institutet, Karolinska University Hospital Huddinge, Stockholm, Sweden

Hillel Sternlicht MD, Albert Einstein College of Medicine/Montefiore Medical Center, Bronx, NY, USA

Thomas W. Storer Ph.D., Adjunct Professor of Medicine, Director, Exercise Physiology, Research Laboratory, Boston University School of Medicine, Boston, MA, USA

Sundararaman Swaminathan MD, Division of Nephrology, Department of Internal Medicine, University of Arkansas for Medical Sciences and Renal Section, Medicine Service, Central Arkansas Veterans Healthcare System, Little Rock, Arkansas, USA

Ravi Thadhani MD, MPH, Division of Nephrology, Massachusetts General Hospital and Department of Medicine, Harvard Medical School, Boston, MA, USA

Nosratola D. Vaziri MD, MACP, Division of Nephrology and Hypertension, Departments of Medicine, Physiology and Biophysics, University of California, Irvine, CA, USA

Manuel Velasquez MD, Division of Renal Diseases and Hypertension, The George Washington University, Washington DC, USA

Alexandra Voinescu MD, Division of Nephrology, Saint Louis University, St. Louis, Missouri, USA

Bradley A. Warady MD, Department of Pediatrics, University of Missouri-Kansas City School of Medicine, Kansas City, MO, USA

Daniel E. Weiner MD MS, Tufts University School of Medicine, Tufts Medical Center, Boston, MA, USA

Andrzej Wiecek MD, Department of Nephrology, Endocrinology and Metabolic Disease, Medical University of Silesia, Katowice, Poland

Mark E. Williams MD, FACP, FASN, Joslin Diabetes Center, Department of Medicine, Harvard Medical School, Boston, MA, USA

Maria Wing PhD, Division of Renal Diseases and Hypertension, The George Washington University, Washington DC, USA

Myles Wolf MD, MMSc, Division of Nephrology and Hypertension, University of Miami Miller School of Medicine, Miami, FL, USA

B. Workeneh MD, Baylor College of Medicine, Nephrology Division, Department of Medicine, Houston, TX, USA

Min Zhang MD, Division of Nephrology, Tianjin Union Medical Center, Tianjin, China

Preface

We are pleased to present the Third Edition of Nutritional Management of Renal Disease. Since the first edition of this book was published in 1996, the field of nutrition in renal disease has changed dramatically. This can be observed simply by documenting the changes that have occurred in the table of contents of the current publication as compared to the first edition and second edition (published in 2004). Among the key changes in this field is the growth of evidence concerning the importance of inflammatory, oxidative and carbonyl stress, and the dramatic increase in the prevalence and severity of obesity and its adverse clinical consequences, not only in economically more developed countries but also in the developing world. Therapeutic strategies for the treatment of obesity have increased apace, and there is now exciting evidence for benefits in the treatment of obesity by medical and especially surgical interventions with regard to the prevention and, in some circumstances, the treatment of chronic kidney disease. Chronic renal replacement therapy has become much more widespread worldwide since the 1990s, and there has been a corresponding growth in information concerning the nutritional management of people receiving these treatments. Similarly, there have been exciting developments concerning methods for retarding progression of chronic renal disease, including prevention of acidemia, phosphorus control, reduction of potentially toxic metabolites of tryptophan, regulation of serum lipids and a revisiting of the therapeutic role of low protein diets.

Three chapters address the pathogenesis, methods of detection and adverse events associated with protein-energy wasting. Other chapters discuss the relationship between high dietary intakes or serum levels of phosphorus or calcium and adverse cardiovascular events and mortality and also the role of phosphorus in the rate of progression of chronic kidney disease. The role of the phosphotonin, FGF-23, in phosphorus regulation in kidney disease is discussed. The increased emphasis on healthy lifestyles for chronic kidney disease patients, including exercise training, is reviewed. The many other chapters include discussions of nutritional management of maintenance hemodialysis, chronic peritoneal dialysis, renal transplantation, children with chronic kidney disease, acute kidney insufficiency, anemia, continuous renal replacement therapy and urinary tract stones, uremic toxicity, hypertension and nutrition, alternative medicine and the kidney, anorexia and appetite stimulants, oral and enteral supplements, intradialytic, intraperitoneal and hemodialytic nutrition, treatment with anabolic hormones, drug nutrient interactions in kidney disease, effect of nutrition on renal function in people without renal disease and motivating kidney disease patients to dietary adherence. Three chapters discuss basic information concerning protein, carbohydrate and lipid metabolism in kidney disease and kidney failure. Three chapters review macrominerals, trace elements or vitamins in kidney disease and kidney failure.

As editors, we tried to select experts to author each of the chapters, and it is our judgment that we have entirely succeeded. We express our deep gratitude to the chapter authors for the scholarliness and diligence with which they have researched, developed and formulated their concepts.

A major effort was made to render this book more readable. We have attempted to organize this book so that each chapter can stand by itself and provide a comprehensive review of the assigned subject matter. On the other hand topics in chapters are frequently cross-referenced to other chapters where relevant information is discussed. Finally, we would like to thank the publishers, and particularly Mara Conner and Megan Wickline, for their unfailing support and patience.

It is our hope that this book will serve both as a scholarly resource concerning the many aspects of the field of nutrition and metabolism in renal disease as well as a practical guide to the medical and surgical management of the clinical manifestations of these disorders.

Joel D. Kopple
Shaul G. Massry
Kamyar Kalantar-Zadeh

1

The Influence of Kidney Disease on Protein and Amino Acid Metabolism

B. Workeneh, William E. Mitch

Baylor College of Medicine, Nephrology Division, Department of Medicine, Houston, TX, USA

INTRODUCTION

Epidemic analyses reveal that chronic kidney disease (CKD) is associated with defects in many metabolic processes. It should not be surprising therefore, that among the defects are abnormalities in protein and amino acid metabolism. In this chapter, we will identify specific abnormalities in protein and amino acid metabolism and will discuss interventions to stop or attenuate the loss of protein stores that occurs in patients with CKD. Besides the intellectual satisfaction of learning how CKD stimulates the loss of body weight and influences the "intracellular milieu", we believe that understanding mechanisms which underlie metabolic abnormalities in protein and amino acids is the first step towards devising strategies to block or ameliorate such defects. For example, after the protein and amino acid catabolism caused by acid accumulation were uncovered, investigators demonstrated the salutary effects of correcting acidosis in CKD patients (Table 1.1) [1–4]. Not only does treating metabolic acidosis suppress the protein wasting stimulated by CKD but it was recently reported that correcting acidosis in CKD patients can even slow their loss of kidney function [5].

Another example of the relevance of abnormal protein metabolism to the care of patients with CKD arises from the familiar relationship between low values of serum albumin and mortality in dialysis patients. The low values of serum albumin have generally been attributed to eating an inadequate diet, i.e., were suffering from malnutrition [6]. This diagnosis is erroneous for the following reasons. First, if protein malnutrition was the cause of defects in protein stores, then low values of serum albumin should be corrected by simply altering the diet. Although careful attention to the diet is absolutely required, there should be additional strategies

directed at inhibiting processes causing muscle wasting. Ikizler and colleagues measured protein synthesis and degradation in fasting hemodialysis patients using standard techniques of labeled amino acid turnover [7]. Specifically, they measured the components of protein metabolism before, during and at 2 hours after completing the dialysis treatment. At all three points, protein degradation exceeded protein synthesis suggesting that the dialysis procedure can activate metabolic pathways that stimulate the loss of body protein stores. Subsequently, the investigators tested the influence of providing intravenous parenteral nutrition (IDPN) during hemodialysis and making the same measurements [8]. When given during dialysis, the IDPN supplement improved both protein synthesis and degradation but at two hours after dialysis there was a persistent increase in protein degradation. Thus, abnormalities in protein metabolism were not eliminated by simply infusing amino acids and calories during dialysis. In a third evaluation, the investigators compared the responses associated with administration of IDPN to those induced by an oral nutritional supplement given during hemodialysis. Protein balance improved with both IDPN and the oral supplement. At two hours after completing dialysis, whole body protein balance was still negative, though forearm muscle protein balance was improved [9]. These careful studies indicate that dialysis must activate or stimulate catabolic pathways in CKD patients, increasing the risk of muscle protein wasting. In addition, the results indicate that the unidentified, catabolic pathways are not "turned off" by increasing dietary constituents. Others report similar conclusions: in a randomized, controlled trial, IDPN was given to hemodialysis patients and compared to results obtained in patients not receiving a dietary supplement [10]. After two years, the supplement had improved the serum

TABLE 1.1   Evidence that Metabolic Acidosis Induces Protein and Amino Acid Catabolism in Normal Infants and Children, as well as, CKD Patients

Subjects Investigated	Measurements of Effectiveness	Outcome of Trial
Infants [131]	Low birth weight, acidotic infants were given $NaHCO_3$ or $NaCl$	$NaHCO_3$ supplement improved growth
Children [132] with CKD	Children with CKD had protein degradation measured	Protein loss was ~ 2-fold higher when HCO_3 was < 16 mM compared to > 22.6 mM
Normal adults [126]	Induced acidosis and measured amino acid and protein metabolism	Acidosis increased amino acid and protein degradation
Normal adults [133]	Induced acidosis and measured nitrogen balance and albumin synthesis	Acidosis induced negative nitrogen balance and suppressed albumin synthesis
Chronic kidney disease [134]	Nitrogen balance before and after treatment of acidosis	$NaHCO_3$ improved nitrogen balance
Chronic kidney disease [5]	Two years $NaHCO_3$ therapy vs. standard care	Slowed loss of creatinine clearance and improved nutritional status
Chronic kidney disease [81]	Essential amino acid and protein degradation before and after treatment of acidosis	$NaHCO_3$ suppressed amino acid and protein degradation
Chronic kidney disease [135]	Muscle protein degradation and degree of acidosis	Proteolysis was proportional to acidosis and blood cortisol
Chronic kidney disease [136]	Nitrogen balance before and after treatment of acidosis	$NaHCO_3$ reduced urea production and nitrogen balance
Hemodialysis [137]	Protein degradation before and after treatment of acidosis	$NaHCO_3$ decreased protein degradation
Hemodialysis [138]	Serum albumin before and after treatment of acidosis	$NaHCO_3$ increased serum albumin
CAPD [139]	Protein degradation before and after treatment of acidosis	$NaHCO_3$ decreased protein degradation
CAPD [45]	Weight and muscle gain before and after treatment of acidosis	Raising dialysis buffer increased weight and muscle mass

concentration of albumin. Unfortunately, the supplement did not improve mortality, body mass index, laboratory markers of nutritional status or the rate of hospitalization. Taken together, these reports suggest that correcting metabolic abnormalities induced by CKD or at least blunting their physiologic influence should be explored because new therapies need to be developed to counteract catabolic responses.

CKD INTERRUPTS THE COMPONENTS OF PROTEIN METABOLISM

Proteins in all tissues are continually "turning over" (i.e., being degraded and replaced by new synthesis). This concept was introduced as early as 1939 when Schoenheimer et al. developed methods for tracking the fate of individual proteins and amino acids labeled with the "heavy" isotope of nitrogen (^{15}N).

When ^{15}N-labeled tyrosine was administered to animals, only ~50% of the label was excreted as the parent form [11]. What happened to the remainder? It was found that the unexcreted amino acids were incorporated into body proteins or converted to other molecules. The magnitude of the dynamic processes of protein synthesis and protein degradation is not small. Estimates of protein turnover in adults indicate they degrade and resynthesize roughly 3–5% of body proteins daily and this occurs at measured rates of 3.5 to 4.5 g protein/kg/day [12]. This rate of protein metabolism is equivalent to a breaking down and rebuilding 1 to 1.5 kg of muscle/day (assuming that 20% of muscle weight is protein). From this perspective, it is obvious that the processes of protein breakdown must be highly selective because a degraded protein is irreversibly lost, terminating its actions. The selectivity of protein breakdown is not achieved by a method in which each protein is degraded by its specific protease. Instead, it appears that different conditions or stimuli result in activation of specific proteases to eliminate the substrate protein. As will be detailed, the principal protease in all cells is the ubiquitin-proteasome system (UPS). It is activated by different stimuli and it degrades a large variety of individual proteins or sets of proteins.

In response to CKD, there is an imbalance between protein synthesis and degradation resulting in net loss of protein stores, including that in the major store of protein in the body, skeletal muscle. This loss of protein stores contributes to the excessive frequency of morbidity and mortality in patients with CKD. For example, epidemiologic and clinical reports document that muscle wasting increases the risk of morbidity and mortality in CKD as it does in other catabolic conditions including heart failure, cancer and aging [13–15]. These catabolic conditions cause a specific loss of the contractile proteins that comprise about {2/3} of the protein in muscle and loss of these proteins is largely responsible for the disability of patients who experience muscle wasting [16]. Unfortunately, the muscle wasting advances as does the severity of CKD and can accelerate after the initiation of dialysis therapy. Cross-sectional studies have shown the prevalence of muscle wasting is between 40–70% in patients with end-stage renal disease (ESRD); the variability in these studies largely depends on which methods are used to identify an abnormality in protein stores [17]. Loss of protein stores and especially, those in skeletal muscle results in increasing dependency, a low quality of life with a sedentary, inactive lifestyle which jeopardizes the cardiovascular health of CKD patients [18]. Besides the body weight loss from a decrease in muscle mass, a progressive loss of protein stores includes proteins that regulate metabolism and cellular renewal, further jeopardizing health. Unfortunately, muscle wasting of patients with CKD is often underappreciated and can be insidious and slowly progressive in some patients.

DEFINING MUSCLE WASTING

A major problem in assigning cause–effect relationships for the muscle wasting present in CKD (or other catabolic conditions) is the lack of consensus surrounding definitions of muscle wasting. In large part, the confusion arises because of difficulties encountered in measuring protein stores reliably. In 2008, the International Society of Renal Nutrition and Metabolism proposed that low values of serum albumin, prealbumin and cholesterol plus abnormalities in body weight and anthropometry could identify patients with CKD who have lost protein stores [19]. They also suggested a new descriptive term, protein-energy wasting or PEW, as a method of classifying such patients [19]. The

new term was believed to be needed to avoid confusion associated when malnutrition is used as a diagnosis. Specifically, CKD patients with a low serum albumin are frequently categorized as being malnourished but this diagnosis is incorrect since malnutrition is defined as abnormalities due to an inadequate diet or an unbalanced one. As pointed out earlier, if malnutrition was the cause of a low serum albumin and loss of protein stores, then both abnormalities should be corrected by simply changing the diet. Unfortunately, changing the diet rarely reverses the loss of protein stores in patients with CKD. Other popular diagnoses of lost protein stores in CKD patients were discarded because they were imprecise. For example, sarcopenia was discarded because it generally describes the loss of muscle mass associated with aging while cachexia was discarded because it implies a more severe state of protein depletion. A report from another Consensus Conference concluded that the term, cachexia, should be reserved for patients suffering from a complex metabolic syndrome initiated by illnesses or conditions that cause loss of muscle with or without loss of fat mass [20]. Specifically, it was recommended that a diagnosis of cachexia should be based on a 5% loss of edema-free body weight within 12 months and that there should be anthropometric evidence of muscle wasting plus evidence of inflammation and hypoalbuminemia. These characteristics would generally apply only to patients with CKD that is complicated by other illnesses.

A difficulty in diagnosing the magnitude of lost protein stores lies in measuring the losses accurately. For example, anthropometric determination of body composition is prone to intra- and inter-observer errors leading to variations in estimates of fat and fat-free mass of up to 5%. If anthropometry is required, it is recommended that a single observer make the measurements and that measurements should document changes in body composition over time rather than a cross-sectional evaluation based on a single estimate. Other problems in determining body composition in patients with CKD include the potential dangers of radiologic techniques based on contrast media (iodinated compounds or gadolinium) since both are potentially nephrotoxic; iodinated compounds used as contrast agents can cause loss of residual renal function while the use of gadolinium carries the risk of inducing nephrogenic systemic fibrosis) [21]. There also is a cost problem since estimating muscle mass (the major storehouse of protein) by computerized tomography (CT) or magnetic resonance imaging (MRI) are expensive. Although less expensive, estimates of lean body mass from bioelectric impedance and/or dual energy X-ray absorptiometry (DEXA) are of limited value because they do not readily distinguish between fluid and tissues and patients with CKD can have excess extracellular fluid making interpretation of changes in lean body mass questionable [17]. All of these problems can be avoided by determining body composition by measuring isotopes of potassium and nitrogen, using whole-body counters [17,22]. This measurement is noninvasive and accurate. However, the technique is only available at a few sites in the world.

MECHANISMS OF MUSCLE WASTING

How are proteins degraded within cells including muscle cells? Over the past decade, a great deal has been learned about the pathophysiology of muscle wasting. There are at least four major proteolytic pathways contributing to the loss of muscle protein in CKD. The four pathways are: lysosome-mediated protein degradation; intracellular proteolysis by calcium activated proteases (calpains); ATP-dependent proteases (the UPS is the major process in this category); and poorly understood proteases that do not require energy to break down cellular proteins [12].

In all cells, including muscle, the UPS is the major proteolytic system that degrades proteins. There is abundant evidence that CKD and its complications as well as other catabolic conditions will stimulate the UPS to breakdown muscle proteins causing muscle wasting. For example, the protein breakdown in isolated muscles of rodents with CKD is blocked by inhibitors of the proteasome [23]. Similar responses occur in a model of acute diabetes [24]. Secondly, there is transcription of a similar set of genes when protein degradation is increased in different models of muscle wasting (e.g., CKD, diabetes, starvation and cancer). These results suggest that conditions causing muscle wasting include a coordinated,

multigene response [25]. Since such a large amount of protein is degraded each day and since different proteins not only form the structure of muscle but also regulate cell processes that initiate or conclude gene transcription or metabolic pathways that are rapidly turned on or off, the UPS must exert exquisite specificity for the proteins it degrades. From this perspective, it is not surprising that the muscle atrophy occurring in response to catabolic conditions involves selective degradation of contractile proteins. This is possible because the proteolysis in these conditions is largely determined by the cell's content of two E3 ubiquitin ligases, atrogin-1/MAFbx and MuRF-1 (see below). Expression of these enzymes in muscle is correlated with the rate of muscle protein degradation and their absence suppresses the muscle atrophy that occurs in response to denervation [26].

THE UBIQUITIN-PROTEASOME SYSTEM

The UPS initiates two multistep biochemical reactions: first, it "tags" proteins destined for degradation by conjugating them to ubiquitin (Ub), a member of the heat-shock protein family (Figure 1.1). Secondly, the Ub-tagged protein is degraded by the 26S proteasome [12,27]. The process of Ub-conjugation begins with the ATP dependent activation of Ub by a single E1 isoform (Ub-activating enzyme). The activated Ub then interacts with one of 20–40 isoforms of the E2 Ub-carrier proteins, providing a degree of specificity to the identification of proteins to be degraded breakdown an E2 Ub-carrier protein interacts with only a limited variety of substrate proteins. The more restrictive reaction is catalyzed by E3 ubiquitin ligases. There are

THE UBIQUITIN-PROTEASOME PATHWAY

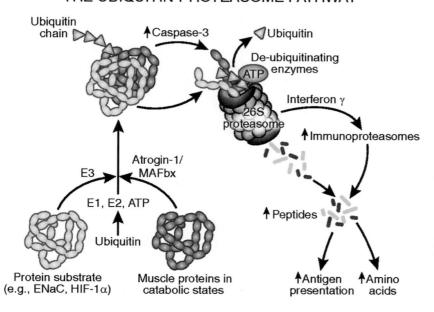

FIGURE 1.1   The UPS degrades protein. Proteins destined for degradation are conjugated to Ub by an ATP-dependent process involving three enzymes: E1, E2 and E3. Selectivity of the protein substrates for degradation principally depends on the E3 ubiquitin ligases. Once a chain of 5 Ubs is attached to the protein substrate, the complex can be recognized by the 26S proteasome. This particle releases Ubs, unfolds the substrate protein and injects it into the central pore of the 26S proteasome. In this channel, the protein is degraded to peptides which are released. Peptidases in the cytoplasm converted to amino acids. Under special conditions, peptides released are joined with the MCH class 1 molecules, becoming antigens. (Figure from Lecker, S.H. and Mitch, W.E. Proteolysis by the Ubiquitin-Proteasome System and Kidney Disease, Journal of the American Society of Nephrology, volume 22, pages 821–824, 2011). This figure is reproduced in color in the color plate section.

more than 1000 of these E3, Ub ligases and each recognizes only a specific protein substrate (or possibly, a class of proteins). Thus, a specific E3 Ub ligase activated it recognizes the protein to be degraded and transfers Ub to lysines in the substrate protein or to lysines in Ub. The latter reaction is repeated until activated Ubs are transferred to from a chain of 4–5 Ubs is attached to the protein. This Ub chain can then be recognized by the 26S proteasome, a very large organelle consisting of >60 proteins that are organized into two particles, a 20S, barrel-shaped particle and 19S regulatory particles present at either or both ends of the 20S particle. Both particles have distinct activities. The 19S particle is capable of recognizing the polyubiquitin chain. In the presence of ATP, the 19S particle cleaves Ubs from the substrate protein so they can presumably be recycled. In addition, the 19S particle unfolds the protein and translocates it into the 20S particle where it is degraded to peptides. The peptides are converted to amino acids by cytosolic peptidases [27]. The importance of these reactions is underscored by the awarding of the 2004 Nobel Prize in Chemistry to Avram Hershko, Aaron Ciechanover and Irwin Rose (http://nobelprize.org/chemistry/laureates/2004/) as discoverers of Ub and its biochemical role in protein degradation.

Both the conjugation of Ub to substrate proteins and the degradation of Ub-conjugated proteins are accelerated in muscle wasting conditions. This is a complex process but considering the multiple steps required for the conjugation of Ub to a substrate protein and then its degradation, it is not surprising that there is increased expression of key contributors to this process in muscle. These participants are recognized by increases in mRNAs of the components, including Ub, subunits of the 26S proteasomes, and two E3 Ub-ligases, Atrogin-1 (also known as MAFbx) and MuRF-1. These E3 Ub-ligases are critical for the breakdown of muscle proteins and their expression increases dramatically (8–20 fold) in rodent models of muscle wasting conditions [28–31].

It has been shown that in cultured muscle cells, the content of Atrogin-1 mRNA correlates closely with rates of protein breakdown providing evidence of their importance [26]. Consequently, understanding how Atrogin-1 and MuRF1 are activated is important for understanding regulation of protein metabolism. Two factors have been identified: the forkhead transcription factors (FoxO); and the inflammation-associated transcription factor, NFκB. To date, it is established that in conditions associated with impairment in insulin and IGF-1 signaling pathways such as CKD, diabetes, excess angiotensin II and inflammation, there is activation of FoxO transcription factors and these result from decreased phosphorylation of FoxOs. Dephosphorylated FoxOs can translocate to the nucleus to increase transcription of Atrogin-1 (and other genes). In response to inflammation, there is activation of NFκB which translocates to the nucleus to increase the transcription of the MuRF1, E3 Ub ligase and mediators of inflammation [27,33].

SYNERGISM OF PROTEOLYTIC PATHWAYS CAUSES MUSCLE WASTING IN CKD

In response to progressive loss of kidney function, muscle protein synthesis decreases somewhat but the more prominent response is the stimulation of protein degradation in muscle [3,34]. In addition to the critical role of the UPS, there is participation of other proteases in causing muscle atrophy. The participation of other proteases is necessary because the UPS readily degrades individual proteins in muscle, including actin, myosin, troponin or tropomyosin but it exhibits only limited proteolytic activity when these proteins are present in complexes. This means that other proteases must initially cleave the muscle proteins that are present in complexes in order to produce substrates for the UPS [35]. In certain conditions including diabetes, excess angiotensin II and inflammation plus CKD, we have found that the protease which performs this initial cleavage of proteins is caspase-3. These findings emphasize how CKD stimulates muscle proteolysis by activating a coordinated, multistep process. Specifically, a two stage process is stimulated by specific signals (i.e., impaired insulin/IGF-1 signaling, glucocorticoids, inflammation, etc.) to cause muscle wasting. First, there is activation of the UPS and caspase-3. The latter performs an initial cleavage of the complex structure of actomyosin and myofibrils to produce substrates for the UPS. Second, there are higher levels of mRNAs encoding certain components of the UPS. Using this finding as an index of muscle wasting, it has been demonstrated that accelerated muscle wasting in CKD involves cellular mechanisms that are similar to those causing muscle wasting in other catabolic conditions, such as cancer cachexia, starvation, insulin deficiency or resistance and or sepsis [12,27]. In fact, there are changes in the expression of about 100 atrophy-related genes called atrogenes in catabolic conditions [23–25,25,36]. These results indicate that there is a common transcriptional program with multiple transcriptional factors which change in a coordinated fashion to cause loss of muscle mass [27].

The role of caspase-3 was initially uncovered in cultured muscle cells when it was found that activated caspase-3 is able to cleave actomyosin, producing protein fragments that are rapidly degraded by the UPS. In addition to uncovering an initial role for caspase-3 in the breakdown of muscle protein, we found that the proteolytic action of caspase-3 leaves a "footprint", a 14 kD C-terminal fragment of actin. The 14 kD actin fragment was most easily detected in the insoluble fraction of muscle; it was rarely present in the soluble fraction of muscle, presumably because the UPS rapidly degrades the 14 kD actin fragment [30].

The role of caspase-3 extended beyond experiments in rodent models of catabolic conditions. For example, the 14 kD actin fragment was found to be increased in muscle biopsies of patients with CKD or following burn injury or with severe osteoarthritis and muscle wasting. Regarding the influence of kidney disease, patients being treated by hemodialysis were studied before and again after many weeks of exercise training at each dialysis session. Compared to values in muscles of normal adults, the 14 kD actin fragment was increased compared to results obtained in muscles of normal adults. Interestingly, the level of the 14 kD actin fragment was statistically reduced in patients who completed a multiweek exercise program of "bicycling" to increase their endurance [37]. Positive results were also obtained in two other conditions. In patients undergoing hip replacement surgery for osteoarthritis, the level of the 14 kD actin fragment in muscle was highly correlated (r = 0.78) with the measured rate of protein degradation obtained simultaneously by evaluating the turnover of labeled amino acids. Finally, the level of the 14 kD actin fragment was high in muscles of the unburned limbs of patients who were hospitalized following a major burn injury. Thus, the 14 kD actin fragment density responded to therapy directed at reducing muscle wasting and it correlated with the measured rate of protein degradation measured when the biopsy was obtained. These results in addition to the results from patients who had muscle atrophy when hospitalized for a burn injury suggest that this actin fragment might serve as a biomarker of accelerated muscle protein degradation. Additional results with larger numbers of patients are needed to address this possibility.

The interrelationships of the UPS and caspase-3 to mediate protein degradation in muscle continue to unfold. Recently, we found that the increase in caspase-3 activity which occurs in catabolic conditions also influences the activity of proteasome-mediated proteolysis in muscle. Initially, it was demonstrated that caspase-3 actually increases the measured activity of the 26S proteasome. This response was linked to cleavage of specific subunits of the 19S particle of the proteasome suggesting that alteration of the specific subunits apparently opens the entrance to the 20S proteasome, permitting substrate proteins to enter the proteasome where they are degraded [38]. In summary, in rodent models and in patients responding to catabolic conditions, caspase-3 exerts two functions that increase muscle protein

degradation: [1] caspase-3 performs an initial cleavage of complexes of muscle proteins, providing substrates for degradation by the UPS; and [2] it stimulates proteolytic activity of the proteasome. These properties exert a "feed-forward" stimulation of muscle proteins when caspase-3 is activated.

The calpains have also been suggested as a protease that can initially cleave myofibrillar proteins to provide substrates for degradation by the UPS. Calpains are calcium-dependent, cysteine proteases that are active in muscular dystrophy or sepsis-induced muscle wasting [39,40]. Their role in the digestion of muscle proteins in other conditions is unclear; the muscle wasting induced by CKD or conditions characterized by impaired insulin/IGF-1 signaling is not blocked by inhibition of calpain activity [23,30].

PROTEOLYTIC ACTIVITIES PRESENT IN MUSCLES OF PATIENTS

In humans, evidence for the participation of specific proteolytic pathways in causing muscle wasting is based mainly on the finding of increased expression of mRNAs encoding Ub and proteasome subunits or evidence of proteolytic activity (e.g., the 14 kD actin fragment) in muscle biopsies. Increased levels of mRNAs encoding Ub or subunits of the proteasome provide evidence for UPS activity in muscles of patients with trauma, cancer, CKD or sepsis [41—44]. For example, patients being treated by chronic ambulatory peritoneal dialysis (CAPD), participated in a year-long, randomized trial to examine the influence of correcting metabolic acidosis [45]. In the patients who were treated to raise serum bicarbonate values there was an increase in body weight and muscle mass plus fewer hospitalizations. Using a similar protocol but for only 4 weeks, we found that correction of metabolic acidosis led to decreased levels of Ub mRNA in muscles [41]. Thus, catabolic conditions can stimulate evidence of UPS-mediated activities in muscles of CKD patients. Alternatively, there is evidence that caspase-3 is activated in muscles of patients who have accelerated protein degradation caused by CKD, severe burn injury or surgery for osteoarthritis [37].

FACTORS TRIGGERING MUSCLE WASTING IN CKD AND OTHER CATABOLIC STATES

Certain CKD-induced complications function to stimulate muscle wasting independently of CKD. Metabolic acidosis is a specific example of this phenomenon. Two factors account for the development of acidosis, the amounts of dietary protein generate more acid while the degree of renal insufficiency limits the excretion of acid generated. Specifically, an excess in dietary protein increases the intake of sulphur-containing amino acids plus phosphorylated proteins and lipids. These substrates are metabolized to sulphuric and phosphoric acids. In the absence of kidney disease, these acids are excreted but as renal function declines, they accumulate and are buffered by bicarbonate, intracellular buffers and bone. This is relevant because metabolic acidosis has been demonstrated to stimulate protein losses in normal infants, children, adults as well as patients with CKD or ESRD being treated by hemo- or peritoneal dialysis (Table 1.1). Recently, the scope of problems associated with metabolic acidosis has extended beyond protein; there are reports that correcting metabolic acidosis can slow the loss of kidney function [5,46].

Besides metabolic acidosis, the complications of CKD that stimulate muscle wasting include impaired intracellular signaling responses to insulin or IGF-1, increased angiotensin II levels, and/or inflammation [18,23,24,47]. A recent report emphasized that new techniques could be brought to bear on these problems. Hung et al. reported that an IL-1 receptor antagonist markedly suppressed circulating levels of inflammatory cytokines. This could provide a means of determining if these cytokines per se are responsible for causing protein wasting. What is not known is whether these complications act synergistically to activate protein wasting in rodent models or in patients? This is relevant because there is a supportive role for glucocorticoids in mediating muscle protein losses. This was uncovered when it was demonstrated that metabolic acidosis will stimulate muscle protein breakdown but only when there is a physiologic increase in glucocorticoid production [1,29,48,49]. Likewise, an increase in glucocorticoids is required in the muscle protein degradation that occurs in models of diabetes, high levels of angiotensin II or sepsis [36,47,50]. Why are glucocorticoids necessary but not sufficient for the activation of muscle protein degradation by the UPS? The answer to this question depends on the ability of glucocorticoids to decrease metabolic responses to insulin or IGF-1. Specifically, glucocorticoids decrease the activation of the phosphatidylinositol 3-kinase/Akt (PI3K/Akt) signaling pathway, resulting in reduced production of the active product, phosphadidylinositol-3,4,5 phosphate leading to decreased phosphorylation and activity of the serine/threonine kinase, Akt [29,51]. A reduced p-Akt level exerts two adverse responses: first, it decreases the phosphorylation of the downstream kinases, mTOR and S6 kinase to suppress protein synthesis. Second, it stimulates protein degradation in muscle. The latter occurs because a decrease in p-Akt leads to reduced phosphorylation of the forkhead family of transcription factors, FoxOs. These dephosphorylated products are therefore, able to migrate into the nucleus where they stimulate the transcription of the muscle-specific E3 Ub ligases, Atrogin-1 and MuRF-1. Increased levels of these enzymes enhances muscle protein degradation by the UPS [29,32,52].

A low p-Akt also activates another protease, caspase-3. This response is due to stimulation of the pro-apoptotic factor, Bax, which migrates to mitochondria leading to release of cytochrome C. The increase in cytosolic cytochrome C increases caspase-3 activity and this in turn, leads to two responses: [1] an increase in substrates for degradation in the UPS; and [2] stimulation of the proteolytic activity of the proteasome [29,38].

The search for a mechanism that explains why a physiologic level of glucocorticoids is required for the activation of muscle protein degradation was initiated by reports indicating that glucocorticoids were required in the following models of adrenalectomized rodents: [1] treatment with NH_4Cl to induce metabolic acidosis; [2] rendered insulin-deficient after streptozotocin treatment; [3] subjected to food deprivation; [4] treated with angiotensin II; or [5] treated to produce sepsis. In each case, there was no acceleration of muscle protein degradation unless the adrenalectomized rodents were also given a physiological dose of glucocorticoids [36,54]. The biochemical basis for this glucocorticoid requirement was recently solved [55]. We showed that the physiologic dose of glucocorticoids are required for the suppression of the phosphorylation of Akt and that a decrease in p-Akt leads to activation of caspase-3 and the UPS as well as increased expression of Atrogin-1. This nongenomic mechanism depends on the activated glucocorticoid receptor interfering with the activation of insulin/IGF-1 signaling and ultimately, a decrease in phosphorylated Akt. In contrast, the mechanisms by which pharmacologic doses of glucocorticoids increase the transcription of Atrogin-1 and activation of the UPS is not known because the promoter of Atrogin-1 does not contain glucocorticoid receptor-related sequences.

Recent reports have identified another contributor that participates in CKD-induced muscle wasting, namely abnormal function of satellite cells. These cells are located under the basal lamina of myofibrils and function as muscle "stem" cells. Specifically, when muscles are injured or when muscle mass is low, satellite cells proliferate and then differentiate into myofibrils to increase the number and size of myofibrils [56]. IGF-1 is a major regulator of satellite cell responses and it is not surprising that CKD impairs the proliferation and differentiation of satellite cells since CKD impairs IGF-1 intracellular signaling [31,57].

MYOSTATIN AND THE REGULATION OF MUSCLE PROTEIN WASTING

Myostatin is a member of the transforming growth factor-β (TGF-β family of secreted proteins) but unlike TGF-β myostatin is predominantly expressed in skeletal muscle (low levels are present in cardiac muscle and adipose tissues). In skeletal muscle, the myostatin precursor, prepromyostatin, is cleaved to promyostatin, which functions to produce an inactive, "latent complex". Myostatin is released from this complex and then can bind to a high-affinity, type-2 activin receptor (ActRIIB) present on muscle membranes [58]. Activation of this receptor leads to phosphorylation of SMAD transcription factors that regulate gene transcription. Notably, other TGF-β family members (e.g., activin A) can bind to ActRIIB and stimulate the same intracellular signaling pathway (Figure 1.2).

There is abundant genetic evidence that myostatin plays a pivotal role in regulating skeletal muscle mass and function. For example, deletion of the myostatin gene in mice causes a dramatic increase in the sizes and number of skeletal muscle fibers [46]. Besides mouse phenotypes, cattle, sheep, dogs and a human bearing a loss-of-function myostatin mutation will exhibit an enormous increase in muscle mass [59–61]. These myostatin mutations can influence athletic performance: whippet dogs bearing a single copy of the myostatin mutation are among the fastest dogs in racing [60]. But, whippets bearing two copies of the same mutation are characterized by so much muscle, they win no races. Likewise, myostatin polymorphism in elite thoroughbred horses suggests these horses have a decided advantage in terms of swiftness [62]. Since myostatin deficiency does produce muscle hypertrophy and can improve physical performance, muscle wasting might be blocked by manipulating myostatin and this could be the basis for a therapeutic strategy.

MYOSTATIN IN MUSCLE INCREASES IN CATABOLIC CONDITIONS

In skeletal muscles, the myostatin protein and its signaling pathway are increased in muscle wasting conditions, including aging, responses to prolonged bed rest, AIDS, kidney failure or heart failure [63–66]. Likewise, in models of cancer cachexia, glucocorticoid administration, mechanical unloading and space flight there are high levels of myostatin in muscle [58,67–69].

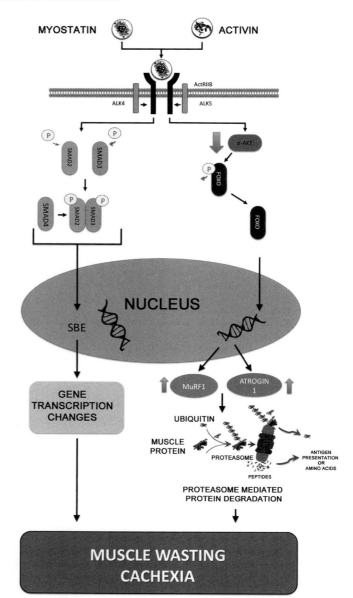

FIGURE 1.2 Myostatin and activin signaling in muscle. Myostatin or activin bind to type IIB activin receptor (ActRIIB) on muscle membranes and when it becomes a dimmer, there is recruitment and activation of the type I activin receptor transmembrane kinase (ALK4 or ALK5). The kinases initiate intracellular signaling cascades: Smad2 and Smad3 become phosphorylated to form a heterodimer and recruit Smad4 into a complex that translocates into the nucleus to bind Smad Binding Element which regulates transcription of downstream response genes. On the right, forkhead transcription factors (FoxO) are dephosphorylated, enter the nucleus and activate the transcription of atrophy-specific E3 ligases MuRF1 and Atrogin1. These E3 ubiquitin ligases provide the specificity that leads to degradation of muscle contractile proteins by the proteasome. (Figure from *Issues in Dialysis*, Edited by Stephen Z. Fadem, Nova Science Publishers, Inc., New York, 2012, page 157, Figure 2). This figure is reproduced in color in the color plate section.

Activin A can interact with the muscle myostatin receptor in response to cancer and in mice given either myostatin or activin A there was almost a 30% decrease in muscle mass [58,58,70]. Could these responses be manipulated to block muscle wasting?

BENEFICIAL RESPONSES FROM BLOCKING MYOSTATIN IN MODELS OF MUSCLE CATABOLISM

As many as 80% of patients with advanced cancers develop muscle wasting and 25% of cancer-related deaths are ascribed to cachexia; this emphasizes the clinical importance of muscle wasting. The major mechanism causing loss of muscle mass is accelerated protein degradation by caspase-3 and the UPS, initiated by hormones or cytokines that impair p-Akt signaling (see above). Blocking this pathway by administering an ActRIIB decoy receptor protected mice from the muscle wasting that is induced by cancers as varied as those from colon-26 carcinoma to gonadal tumors. Importantly, the treatment also produced a significant increase in survival. The reversal of muscle losses occurred even though there was no suppression of circulating levels of TNF-α, IL-1β and IL-6 in the colon-26 carcinoma model [58]. This suggests that the presence of inflammation would not negate the beneficial responses to blocking myostatin and its signaling pathways in muscle.

BLOCKING MYOSTATIN CAN SUPPRESS CKD-INDUCED MUSCLE WASTING

As discussed, CKD produces metabolic responses that are present in certain other catabolic disorders, including muscle protein wasting plus an increase in circulating markers of inflammation and in glucocorticoid production as well as impaired insulin/IGF-1 signaling. The latter includes reduced levels of p-Akt, increased expression of Atrogin-1/MAFbx and activation of protein degradation by caspase-3 and the UPS. Since the muscle level of myostatin is increased by CKD, Zhang et al. evaluated how blocking myostatin would influence muscle wasting in a mouse model of CKD [65]. Mice with CKD and BUN values >80 mg/dL were paired for both BUN levels and weight and pair-fed for 4 weeks. One mouse in each of the paired CKD mice received subcutaneous injections every other day of an anti-myostatin peptibody (a genetically engineered myostatin-neutralizing peptide fused to Fc) while the paired mouse was injected with the diluent. Treatment with the peptibody suppressed the level of myostatin in muscle, reversed the loss of body weight and increased muscle weights. The mechanisms that prevented muscle atrophy included an increase in the rate of protein synthesis and a decrease in protein

degradation plus improvements in satellite cell functions.

Notably, myostatin inhibition in CKD mice decreased circulating levels of inflammatory cytokines and especially, IL-6. The latter was especially interesting because our earlier results had demonstrated that an increase in IL-6 and the acute phase protein, serum amyloid A acted synergistically to impair intracellular IGF-1 signaling [71]. The resulting decrease in p-AKt in muscles led to accelerated protein degradation. Notably, treatment with the antimyostatin peptibody corrected these responses and blocked the CKD-induced muscle catabolism. Finally, it was shown that treatment of cultured muscle cells with TNF-α raised myostatin production in the muscle cells. But, treatment of muscle cells with myostatin increased the production of IL-6. The antimyostatin peptibody blocked these responses, providing a mechanism to explain how an increase in circulating inflammatory markers can cause muscle protein wasting.

CKD CHANGES THE CONCENTRATIONS OF CERTAIN AMINO ACIDS

Fasting patients with CKD have many abnormalities of plasma amino acid concentrations. These include an increase in 3-methylhistidine and 1-methylhistidine, apparently caused by reduced renal clearance of these methylated amino acids. In fasting patients with CKD, plasma valine is usually low as are leucine and isoleucine but to a more modest extent. These results indicate that CKD changes the metabolism of branched-chain amino acids (BCAA). Garibotto et al. have reported that similar differences in BCAA concentrations occur after a meal [72–75]. At least two mechanisms contribute to low levels of BCAA in patients with CKD. A low protein intake can contribute to the plasma levels while decreased gastrointestinal absorption plays a minor role [76]. Unfortunately, the contribution of the diet to changes in plasma amino acids is unpredictable because results from rats with experimental CKD indicate that those fed an excess of protein had the most abnormal BCAA in blood [77]. The second mechanism for low levels of BCAA is metabolic acidosis because it stimulates the acceleration of BCAA catabolism. All three BCAA are irreversibly decarboxylated by branched-chain ketoacid dehydrogenase or BCKAD, and several factors, including metabolic acidosis and glucocorticoids, stimulate its activity in skeletal muscle [2,79]. In patients with CKD as well, acidosis is associated with accelerated catabolism of BCAA and there is a correlation between plasma bicarbonate levels and the free valine content in skeletal muscle of hemodialysis patients [80–82]. In the latter report, it was demonstrated that correction of metabolic acidosis led to increased levels of all three BCAA in the muscle of hemodialysis patients [82].

Other abnormalities in plasma amino acids include an increased citrulline concentration, attributable to impaired conversion of citrulline to arginine by the diseased kidney. However, measurements made in cells or in rats with experimental CKD indicate that the mechanism underlying high citrulline levels is more complex [83]. Besides citrulline, there are unexplained increases in cystine, homocysteine, and aspartate; a decrease in tyrosine (reflecting impaired hydroxylation of phenylalanine) and a high glycine level plus a low or low-normal level of serine. The latter could be related to diminished production of serine from glycine by the diseased kidney [84]. Threonine and lysine concentrations are low for unknown reasons. Overall, the levels of essential amino acids, with some exceptions, tend to be reduced in plasma, whereas some of the nonessential amino acids tend to be increased. The decrease in the levels of essential amino acids is reminiscent of the pattern present in patients with protein malnutrition. But, these abnormalities occur in CKD patients even when they are eating an adequate diet and they persist after a large meal of meat [74,85]. These responses indicate that the low levels are due to CKD-induced changes in amino acid metabolism. Indeed, it has been shown that the low levels of BCAA, the decreased ratios of essential/ nonessential and valine/glycine as well as the degree of the increase in plasma levels of cystine, citrulline, and methylhistidines concentrations are all correlated with GFR, consistent with the proposed metabolic defects which are caused by CKD. There is growing evidence that the concentrations of sulphur-containing amino acids (i.e., methionine, cysteine, cystine, taurine and homocysteine (see below)) are very abnormal in uremic patients, but the mechanisms accounting for these abnormalities have not been defined [86]. This is relevant because CKD patients can have very high levels of homocysteine which is associated with atherosclerosis (see below).

Another abnormality is due to changes in the disposal of amino acids: after an intravenous infusion of amino acids into hemodialysis subjects, the removal of valine and phenylalanine were found to be subnormal, while histidine removal was increased [87]. It is not known whether these measurements contribute to the high plasma levels of histamine found in uremic patients (especially those with pruritus) [88].

In general, the severity in the changes in plasma amino acid concentrations is correlated with the degree of renal insufficiency and the degree of uremic symptoms [89]. The degree of abnormalities tends to worsen with an inadequate protein intake (e.g., there is a direct correlation between the valine/glycine ratio and protein

intake). However, there are other problems since the distribution of amino acids between cells and extracellular fluid are abnormal except for values measured in erythrocytes or the cerebrospinal fluid [72,90—93]. In skeletal muscle, Bergstrom and associates measured the intracellular concentration of amino acids in nondialyzed CKD patients and found abnormalities that differ somewhat from those seen in plasma [94]. Specifically, BCAA levels in muscle were subnormal; ornithine was low as was the levels of histidine, threonine, lysine and arginine. In another evaluation of control and undialyzed CKD patients, it was reported that the BCAA in muscle biopsy specimens were almost normal at least in patients who had little or no metabolic acidosis. It was concluded that the levels should not be as found in muscle samples from acidotic, dialysis patients [80,95].

Metabolites of amino acids, including those that contain sulphur as well as a number of small peptides and amines (including polyamines, guanidines, and other nitrogenous compounds), accumulate in the blood [96,97]. Abnormalities in such metabolites of amino acids are not reviewed because the genesis of these abnormalities is largely unknown and there is no specific therapy for them. Generally, their concentrations decrease when protein intake is reduced and urea appearance falls.

Arginine

Arginine has the potential to influence many physiologic processes because it is the substrate for nitric oxide synthesis. For example, L-arginine supplements reportedly prevent the development of hypertension nephrosclerosis in the salt-sensitive Dahl/Rapp strain of rats [98]. In rats with diabetic nephropathy, dietary supplements of arginine ameliorated the nephropathy and reduced the renal hypertrophy induced by a high-protein diet [99;100]. Finally, arginine supplements improved renal function in rats with bilateral ureteral obstruction or puromycin aminonucleoside-induced nephrosis after only 3 days [101]. Possibly, angiotensin II and nitric oxide in these conditions are working in opposite directions since rats with ablative nephropathy had a reduction in the excretion of nitrates plus nitrites, changes that were reversed by administration of arginine or captopril; there was no additive benefit when both were administered [102]. A long standing stumbling block to the interpretation of these responses is the problem of the arginine paradox: the beneficial effects of arginine supplements occur even though the intracellular arginine concentration is substantially above the K_m of nitric oxide synthase. A solution to this problem was recently reported by Erez et al [103]. They found that intracellular nitric oxide synthase is in a complex with argininosuccinic lyase suggesting that the production of arginine provides a substrate (i.e., arginine) for nitric oxide synthase. This means that nitric oxide synthase is in a compartment that converts newly formed arginine to nitric oxide.

In normal subjects, oral or intravenous administration of arginine causes a diuresis and lowers blood pressure but changes GFR minimally; these changes can be associated with microalbuminuria [104—107]. In patients with heart failure, 15 g/day of oral arginine was reported to reduce endothelin levels and augment the diuretic response to saline loading [106]. Taken together, supplements of arginine could augment diuretic responses to heart failure or increases in extracellular fluid volume. This has not been rigorously tested.

In contrast to these beneficial suggestions, Narita and associates suggested that the beneficial effects of low-protein diets in renal failure might be attributable to a *reduced* intake of arginine [108,109]. They found that dietary restriction of arginine ameliorated the severity of antithymocyte serum-induced glomerulonephritis [110]. In children with CKD, administration of arginine did not induce improved endothelial function [111]. A possible explanation of these discordant roles of nitric oxide in renal disease may be that iNOS is chronically stimulated by cytokines, whereas acutely responsive cNOS activity may be depressed [112]. Further work will be needed to resolve these contradictory findings concerning the role of dietary arginine in progression of CKD.

Tryptophan

The ketoacid/amino acid supplement employed in the feasibility phase (but not the randomized trial) of the MDRD Study was tryptophan-free [113]. This might be relevant because the ketoacid supplement used in the feasibility phase appeared to slow progression of CKD. Reportedly, there is a correlation between the rate of progression and serum free tryptophan concentration [114,115].

Kaysen et al. reported that a dietary supplement of tryptophan could prevent the development of hypertension and proteinuria in rats with CKD induced by subtotal nephrectomy [116]. This response has not been followed up and a mechanism for the proposed benefit is lacking. Additional experimental studies of tryptophan supplementation and progression should be undertaken but currently, are not available. In contrast to a potential of a positive response with L-tryptophan, Niwa and associates documented that indoxyl sulphate, a tryptophan metabolite, is nephrotoxic [117—119]. Its removal by an orally administered sorbent was found to slow progression of CKD in patients fed a low-protein diet, at least as based on sequential

measurements of serum creatinine. A major problem with linking tryptophan to indoxyl sulphate is that oral tryptophan supplements do not increase indoxyl sulphate levels, instead they cause a significant decrease in the urinary excretion of indoxyl sulphate [120]. Hence, the potential role of diet protein restriction in slowing progression can not be attributed to a lower intake of tryptophan and a reduction in indoxyl sulphate production leading to nephrotoxicity.

Homocysteine

In adults without CKD, homocysteine has been linked to acceleration of the development of atherosclerosis and a high homocysteine level may portend a poor prognosis in patients with coronary artery disease [121,122]. In CKD patients circulating homocysteine is found at high levels but the mechanism for this result is unknown [123]. Presumably, the high circulating levels are linked to abnormalities in the metabolism of sulphur amino acids in CKD patients but the biochemistry of impaired metabolism of sulphur-containing amino acids is unknown [86]. In normal adults, the treatment for accelerated atherosclerosis in association with a high homocysteine level is vitamin B_6 plus folinic acid, but this therapy has been only partially successful in CKD patients [123]. It is possible that this abnormality in amino acid metabolism plus inflammation contributes to the accelerated atherosclerosis occurring in CKD [124].

LINKS BETWEEN AMINO ACID AND PROTEIN METABOLISM

Certain examples suggest that the metabolism of amino acids and proteins in muscle are linked. In one situation, there are parallel changes in the catabolism of protein and amino acids in muscle that are initiated by common metabolic processes. For example, the presence of systemic, metabolic acidosis induces an increase in protein catabolism in muscle via mechanisms that not only stimulate the UPS but also increase in the transcription of genes encoding components of the UPS [23]. The link between protein and amino acid metabolism is that systemic metabolic acidosis also accelerates the catabolism of BCAA in muscle in a parallel fashion. There is increased activity of branched-chain ketoacid dehydrogenase, the rate limiting enzyme in the breakdown of BCAA and there is increased transcription of genes which encode subunits of branched-chain ketoacid dehydrogenase. The result is activation of the enzyme and catabolism of BCAA in muscle [2,78]. Similarities in these responses are linked because they share factors that initiate these responses: the catabolism of protein and BCAA in muscle are both mediated by acidosis and an increase in glucocorticoids [1,125]. This is relevant to CKD because there are parallel increases in protein and BCAA degradation: results from normal adults given ammonium chloride or from CKD patients who develop spontaneous metabolic acidosis indicate there is induction of protein and BCAA catabolism [126,127]. Why this occurs and whether it extends to other amino acids is not known.

Another example of metabolic responses in protein metabolism that are linked to amino acids depends on an inverse relationship between changes in the rates of protein synthesis and degradation and the metabolic responses that are initiated by leucine and its metabolites. In isolated muscles, it was shown that the rate of protein synthesis increased in muscles treated with leucine [128]. In addition, it was found that the rate of protein degradation was suppressed in muscles treated with the degradation of leucine to α-ketoisocaproate. Although it is not clear how changes in amino acids are recognized as signals to change muscle protein metabolism, it is fascinating that there appears to be a type of "cross talk" between the metabolism of amino acids and protein.

A third example involving responses to the metabolism of skeletal muscle was recently uncovered. The finding occurred after normal adults ingested 10 g of essential amino acids. Subsequently, muscle biopsies were obtained and changes in microRNAs were evaluated. The results revealed that ingestion of the essential amino acids led to upregulation of microRNAs that can influence the activity of growth-associated genes in muscle. These growth-associated genes included an increase in the mRNA of MyoD (a transcription factor which can stimulate the proliferation of satellite cells). In addition, there was a suppression of the mRNA of myostatin, a negative regulator of muscle growth. How these changes in gene expression translate into an improvement in muscle mass was not explored. However, the results do indicate that changes in amino acid metabolism can affect protein metabolism in muscle. Since CKD affects both protein and amino acid metabolism, it will be important to understand how these links affect the pathophysiology of nutritional problems present in patients with CKD.

CONCLUSION

Catabolic disorders characterized by muscle protein wasting, increased circulating inflammatory cytokines, increased glucocorticoid production and impaired insulin/IGF-1 signaling increase the risks of morbidity and mortality. Physiologic and molecular mechanisms causing muscle protein wasting have been identified

and to some extent solved. However, the development of reliable therapies that prevent or reverse the muscle atrophy has lagged behind. Recent reports suggest a new era is commencing in which multiple strategies can be used to block muscle wasting in patients with CKD. The group of strategies include correcting metabolic acidosis, preventing the development of inflammation and blocking myostatin signaling in muscle. It must be emphasized, however, that benefits of these strategies will not be realized unless patients are provided with well-planned diets. We emphasize the dietary factors in treating CKD patients because ignoring them will counteract benefits from preventive strategies. Specifically, an excess of dietary protein creates more acid to be excreted by the damaged kidney. If excretion is insufficient, metabolic acidosis will develop to cause muscle wasting [5]. Likewise, if the diet contains an excess of phosphates or salt, bone disease or hypertension will develop. In addition, ignoring these factors can cancel benefits on progression of CKD that are achieved by prescribing inhibitors of the renin-angiotensin-aldosterone system [129,130]. Newer strategies directed at manipulating metabolism of protein and amino acids could be developed into new tools that will benefit CKD patients and provide new tools for the nephrologist to manage complications of CKD. Hopefully, we are no longer stuck at devising new definitions in hopes of quantifying the degree of muscle wasting.

References

[1] May RC, Kelly RA, Mitch WE. Metabolic acidosis stimulates protein degradation in rat muscle by a glucocorticoid-dependent mechanism. J Clin Invest 1986;77:614−21.

[2] May RC, Hara Y, Kelly RA, Block KP, Buse MG, Mitch WE. Branched-chain amino acid metabolism in rat muscle: Abnormal regulation in acidosis. Am J Physiol 1987;252:E712−8.

[3] May RC, Kelly RA, Mitch WE. Mechanisms for defects in muscle protein metabolism in rats with chronic uremia: The influence of metabolic acidosis. J Clin Invest 1987;79:1099−103.

[4] Hara Y, May RC, Kelly RA, Mitch WE. Acidosis, not azotemia, stimulates branched-chain amino acid catabolism in uremic rats. Kidney Int 1987;32:808−14.

[5] de Brito-Ashurst I, Varagunam M, Raftery MJ, Yaqoob MM. Bicarbonate supplementation slows progression of CKD and improves nutritional status. J Am Soc Nephrol 2009 September;20(9):2075−84.

[6] Mitch WE. Malnutrition: a frequent misdiagnosis for hemodialysis patients. J Clin Invest 2002;110:437−9.

[7] Ikizler TA, Pupim LB, Brouillette JR, Levenhagen DK, Farmer K, Hakim RM, et al. Hemodialysis stimulates muscle and whole body protein loss and alters substrate oxidation. Amer J Physiol 2002;282:E107−16.

[8] Pupim LB, Flakoll PJ, Brouillette JR, Levenhagen DK, Hakim RM, Ikizler TA. Intradialytic parenteral nutrition improves protein and energy homeostasis in chronic hemodialysis patients. J Clin Invest 2002;110:483−92.

[9] Pupim LB, Majchrzak KM, Flakoll PJ, Ikizler TA. Intradialytic oral nutrition improves protein homeostasis in chronic hemodialysis patients with deranged nutritional status. J Am Soc Nephrol 2006 November;17(11):3149—57.

[10] Baumeister W, Walz J, Zuhl F, Seemuller E. The proteasome: paradigm of a self-comparmentalizing protease. Cell 1998; 92:367—80.

[11] Schoenheimer R, Ratner S, Rittenberg D. Studies in protein metabolism: VII The metabolism of tyrosine. J Biol Chem 1939 October;127:333—44.

[12] Mitch WE, Goldberg AL. Mechanisms of muscle wasting: The role of the ubiquitin-proteasome system. N Engl J Med 1996;335:1897—905.

[13] Kestenbaum B, Sampson JN, Rudser KD, Patterson DJ, Seliger SL, Young B, et al. Serum phosphate levels and mortality risk among people with chronic kidney disease. J Am Soc Nephrol 2005 February;16(2):520—8.

[14] Huang CX, Tighiouart H, Beddhu S, Cheung AK, Dwyer JT, Eknoyan G, et al. Both low muscle mass and low fat are associated with higher all-cause mortality in hemodialysis patients. Kidney Int 2010 April;77(7):624—9.

[15] Kotler DP. Cachexia. Ann Intern Med 2000;133:622—34.

[16] Clarke BA, Drujan D, Willis MS, Murphy LO, Corpina RA, Burova E, et al. The E3 Ligase MuRF1 degrades myosin heavy chain protein in dexamethasone-treated skeletal muscle. Cell Metab 2007 November;6(5):376—85.

[17] Ellis KJ. Human body composition: in vivo methods. Physiol Rev 2000 April;80(2):649—80.

[18] Stenvinkel P, Heimburger O, Paultre F, Diczfalusy U, Wang T, Berglund L, et al. Strong association between malnutrition, inflammation and atherosclerosis in chronic kidney failure. Kidney Int 1999;55:1899—911.

[19] Fouque D, Kalantar-Zadeh K, Kopple JD, Cano N, Chauveau P, Cuppari L, et al. A proposed nomenclature and diagnostic criteria for protein—energy wasting in acute and chronic kidney disease. Kidney Int 2008 May 9;73:391—8.

[20] Evans WJ, Morley JE, Argiles J, Bales C, Baracos V, Guttridge D, et al. Cachexia: a new definition. Clin Nutr 2008 December;27(6): 793—9.

[21] Agarwal R, Brunelli SM, Williams K, Mitchell MD, Feldman HI, Umscheid CA. Gadolinium-based contrast agents and nephrogenic systemic fibrosis: a systematic review and meta-analysis. Nephrol Dial Transplant 2009;24:856—63.

[22] Arora P, Strauss BJ, Borovnicar D, Stroud D, Atkins RC, Kerr PG. Total body nitrogen predicts long-term mortality in haemodialysis patients — a single-centre experience. Nephrol Dial Transplant 1998 July;13(7):1731—6.

[23] Bailey JL, Wang X, England BK, Price SR, Ding X, Mitch WE. The acidosis of chronic renal failure activates muscle proteolysis in rats by augmenting transcription of genes encoding proteins of the ATP-dependent, ubiquitin-proteasome pathway. J Clin Invest 1996;97:1447—53.

[24] Price SR, Bailey JL, Wang X, Jurkovitz C, England BK, Ding X, et al. Muscle wasting in insulinopenic rats results from activation of the ATP-dependent, ubiquitin-proteasome pathway by a mechanism including gene transcription. J Clin Invest 1996;98:1703—8.

[25] Lecker SH, Jagoe RT, Gomes M, Baracos V, Bailey JL, Price SR, et al. Multiple types of skeletal muscle atrophy involve a common program of changes in gene expression. FASEB J 2004;18:39—51.

[26] Sacheck JM, Ohtsuka A, McLary SC, Goldberg AL. IGF-1 stimulates muscle growth by suppressing protein breakdown and expression of atrophy-related ubiquitin ligases, atrogin-1 and MuRF1. Am J Physiol 2004;287:E591—601.

[27] Lecker SH, Mitch WE. Proteolysis by the ubiquitin-proteasome system and kidney disease. J Am Soc Nephrol 2011 May;22(5): 821—4.

[28] Bodine SC, Latres E, Baumhueter S, Lai VK, Nunez L, Clark BA, et al. Identification of ubiquitin ligases required for skeletal muscle atrophy. Sci 2001;294:1704—8.

[29] Lee SW, Dai G, Hu Z, Wang X, Du J, Mitch WE. Regulation of muscle protein degradation: coordinated control of apoptotic and ubiquitin-proteasome systems by phosphatidylinositol 3 kinase. J Am Soc Nephrol 2004;15:1537—45.

[30] Du J, Wang X, Meireles CL, Bailey JL, Debigare R, Zheng B, et al. Activation of caspase 3 is an initial step triggering muscle proteolysis in catabolic conditions. J Clin Invest 2004;113: 115—23.

[31] Bailey JL, Price SR, Zheng B, Hu Z, Mitch WE. Chronic kidney disease causes defects in signaling through the insulin receptor substrate/phosphatidylinositol 3-kinase/Akt pathway: implications for muscle atroply. J Am Soc Nephrol 2006;17:1388—94.

[32] Sandri M, Sandri C, Gilbert A, Skuck C, Calabria E, Picard A, et al. Foxo transcription factors induce the atrophy-related ubiquitin ligase atrogin-1 and cause skeletal muscle atrophy. Cell 2004;117:399—412.

[33] Cai D, Frantz JD, Tawa NE, Melendez PA, Oh BC, Lidov HG, et al. IKKbeta/NF-kappaB activation causes severe muscle wasting in mice. Cell 2004;119:285—98.

[34] Goodship THJ, Mitch WE, Hoerr RA, Wagner DA, Steinman TI, Young VR. Adaptation to low-protein diets in renal failure: Leucine turnover and nitrogen balance. J Am Soc Nephrol 1990;1:66—75.

[35] Solomon V, Goldberg AL. Importance of the ATP-ubiquitin-proteasome pathway in degradation of soluble and myofibrillar proteins in rabbit muscle extracts. J Biol Chem 1996; 271:26690—7.

[36] Mitch WE, Bailey JL, Wang X, Jurkovitz C, Newby D, Price SR. Evaluation of signals activating ubiquitin-proteasome proteolysis in a model of muscle wasting. Am J Physiol 1999; 276:C1132—8.

[37] Workeneh B, Rondon-Berrios H, Zhang L, Hu Z, Ayehu G, Ferrando A, et al. Development of a diagnostic method for detecting increased muscle protein degradation in patients with catabolic conditions. J Am Soc Nephrol 2006;17:3233—9.

[38] Wang XH, Zhang L, Mitch WE, LeDoux JM, Hu J, Du J. Caspase-3 cleaves specific proteasome subunits in skeletal muscle stimulating proteasome activity. J Biol Chem 2010;285: 3527—32.

[39] Wei W, Fareed MU, Evenson A, Menconi MJ, Yang H, Petkova V, et al. Sepsis stimulates calpain activity in skeletal muscle by decreasing calpastatin activity but does not activate caspase-3. Am J Physiol Regul Integr Comp Physiol 2005 March;288(3):R580—90.

[40] Tidball JG, Spencer MJ. Expression of a calpastatin transgene slows muscle wasting and obviates changes in myosin isoform expression during murine muscle disuse. J Physiol 2002; 545:819—28.

[41] Pickering WP, Price SR, Bircher G, Marinovic AC, Mitch WE, Walls J. Nutrition in CAPD: Serum bicarbonate and the ubiquitin-proteasome system in muscle. Kidney Int 2002; 61:1286—92.

[42] Mansoor O, Beaufrere Y, Boirie Y, Ralliere C, Taillandier D, Aurousseau E, et al. Increased mRNA levels for components of the lysosomal, Ca^{++}-activated and ATP-ubiquitin-dependent proteolytic pathways in skeletal muscle from head trauma patients. Proc Natl Acad Sci USA 1996;93:2714—8.

[43] Tiao G, Hobler S, Wang JJ, Meyer TA, Luchette FA, Fischer JE, et al. Sepsis is associated with increased mRNAs of the

ubiquitin-proteasome proteolytic pathway in human skeletal muscle. J Clin Invest 1997;99:163—8.

[44] Williams AB, Sun X, Fischer JE, Hasselgren P-O. The expression of genes in the ubiquitin-proteasome proteolytic pathway is increased in skeletal muscle from patients with cancer. Surgery 1999;126:744—9.

[45] Stein A, Moorhouse J, Iles-Smith H, Baker R, Johnstone J, James G, et al. Role of an improvement in acid-base status and nutrition in CAPD patients. Kidney Int 1997;52:1089—95.

[46] Mahajan A, Simoni J, Sheather SJ, Broglio KR, Rajab MH, Wesson DE. Daily oral sodium bicarbonate preserves glomerular filtration rate by slowing its decline in early hypertensive nephropathy. Kidney Int 2010 August;78(3):303—9.

[47] Song Y-H, Li Y, Du J, Mitch WE, Rosenthal N, Delafontaine P. Muscle-specific expression of insulin-like growth factor-1 blocks angiotensin II-induced skeletal muscle wasting. J Clin Invest 2005;115:451—8.

[48] Wang XH, Hu Z, Hu JP, Du J, Mitch WE. Insulin resistance accelerates muscle protein degradation: activation of the ubiquitin-proteasome pathway by defects in muscle cell signaling. Endocrin 2006;147:4160—8.

[49] Price SR, England BK, Bailey JL, Van Vreede K, Mitch WE. Acidosis and glucocorticoids concomitantly increase ubiquitin and proteasome subunit mRNAs in rat muscle. Am J Physiol 1994;267:C955—60.

[50] Tiao G, Fagan J, Roegner V, Lieberman M, Wang J-J, Fischer JE, et al. Energy-ubiquitin-dependent muscle proteolysis during sepsis in rats is regulated by glucocorticoids. J Clin Invest 1996;97:339—48.

[51] Bodine SC, Stitt TN, Gonzalez M, Kline WO, Stover GL, Bauerlein R, et al. Akt/mTOR pathway is a crucial regulator of skeletal muscle hypertrophy and can prevent muscle atrophy in vivo. Nature Cell Biology 2001;3:1014—9.

[52] Stitt TN, Drujan D, Clarke BA, Panaro F, Timofeyva Y, Klinenber JR, et al. The IGF-1/PI3K/Akt pathway prevents expression of muscle atrophy-induced ubiquitin ligases by inhibiting FOXO transcription factors. Mol Cell 2004;14: 395—403.

[53] Wing SS, Goldberg AL. Glucocorticoids activate the ATP-ubiquitin-dependent proteolytic system in skeletal muscle during fasting. Am J Physiol 1993;264:E668—76.

[54] Hall-Angeras M, Angeras U, Zamir O, Hasselgren P-O, Fischer JE. Effect of the glucocorticoid receptor antagonist RU 38486 on muscle protein breakdown in sepsis. Surgery 1991;109:468—73.

[55] Hu Z, Wang H, Lee IH, Du J, Mitch WE. Endogenous glucocorticoids and impaired insulin signaling are both required to stimulate muscle wasting under pathophysiological conditions in mice. J Clin Invest 2009;119:7650—9.

[56] Tedesco FS, Dellavalle A, az-Manera J, Messina G, Cossu G. Repairing skeletal muscle: regenerative potential of skeletal muscle stem cells. J Clin Invest 2010 January;120(1):11—9.

[57] Zhang L, Wang XH, Wang H, Hu Z, Du J, Mitch WE. Satellite cell dysfunction and impaired IGF-1 signaling contribute to muscle atrophy in chronic kidney disease. J Am Soc Nephrol 2010;21:419—27.

[58] Zhou X, Wang JL, Lu J, Song Y, Kwak KS, Jiao Q, et al. Reversal of cancer cachexia and muscle wasting by ActRIIB antagonism leads to prolonged survival. Cell 2010 August 20;142(4): 531—43.

[59] McPherron AC, Lee SJ. Double muscling in cattle due to mutations in the myostatin gene. Proc Natl Acad Sci U S A 1997 November 11;94(23):12457—61.

[60] Mosher DS, Quignon P, Bustamante CD, Sutter NB, Mellersh CS, Parker HG, et al. A mutation in the myostatin gene increases muscle mass and enhances racing performance in heterozygote dogs. PLoS Genet 2007 May 25;3(5):e79.

[61] Schuelke M, Wagner KR, Stolz LE, Hubner C, Riebel T, Komen W, et al. Myostatin mutation associated with gross muscle hypertrophy in a child. N Engl J Med 2004 June 24;350(26):2682—8.

[62] Binns MM, Boehler DA, Lambert DH. Identification of the myostatin locus (MSTN) as having a major effect on optimum racing distance in the Thoroughbred horse in the USA. Anim Genet 2010 December;41(Suppl. 2):154—8.

[63] Reardon KA, Davis J, Kapsa RM, Choong P, Byrne E. Myostatin, insulin-like growth factor-1, and leukemia inhibitory factor mRNAs are upregulated in chronic human disuse muscle atrophy. Muscle Nerve 2001;24(7):893—9.

[64] Gonzalez-Cadavid NF, Taylor WE, Yarasheski K, Sinha-Hikim I, Ma K, Ezzat S, et al. Organization of the human myostatin gene and expression in healthy men and HIV-infected men with muscle wasting. Proc Natl Acad Sci U S A 1998 December 8;95(25):14938—43.

[65] Zhang L, Rajan V, Lin E, Hu Z, Han HQ, Zhou X, et al. Pharmacological inhibition of myostatin suppresses systemic inflammation and muscle atrophy in mice with chronic kidney disease. FASEB J 2011 May;25(5):1653—63.

[66] Breitbart A, Uger-Messier M, Molkentin JD, Heineke J. Myostatin from the heart: local and systemic actions in cardiac failure and muscle wasting. Am J Physiol Heart Circ Physiol 2011 June;300(6):H1973—82.

[67] Ma K, Mallidis C, Bhasin S, Mahabadi V, Artaza J, Gonzalez-Cadavid N, et al. Glucocorticoid-induced skeletal muscle atrophy is associated with upregulation of myostatin gene expression. Am J Physiol 2003;285:E363—71.

[68] Carlson CJ, Booth FW, Gordon SE. Skeletal muscle myostatin mRNA expression is fiber-type specific and increases during hindlimb unloading. Am J Physiol 1999 August;277(2 Pt 2): R601—6.

[69] Lalani R, Bhasin S, Byhower F, Tarnuzzer R, Grant M, Shen R, et al. Myostatin and insulin-like growth factor-I and -II expression in the muscle of rats exposed to the microgravity environment of the NeuroLab space shuttle flight. J Endocrinol 2000 December;167(3):417—28.

[70] Zimmers TA, Davies MV, Koniaris LG, Haynes P, Esquela AF, Tomkinson KN, et al. Induction of cachexia in mice by systemically administered myostatin. Sci 2002;296:1486—8.

[71] Zhang L, Du J, Hu Z, Han G, Delafontaine P, Garcia G, et al. IL-6 and serum amyloid A synergy mediates angiotensin II-induced muscle wasting. J Am Soc Nephrol 2009 March; 20(3):604—12.

[72] Alvestrand A, Furst P, Bergstrom J. Plasma and muscle free amino acids in uremia: influence of nutrition with amino acids. Clin Nephrol 1982;18:297—305.

[73] Kopple JD, Swenseid MD. Nitrogen balance and plasma amino acid levels in uremic patients fed an essential amino acid diet. Am J Clin Nutr 1974;27:806—12.

[74] Garibotto G, DeFerrari G, Robaudo C, Saffioti S, Paoletti E, Pontremoli R, et al. Effects of a protein meal on blood amino acid profile in patients with chronic renal failure. Nephron 1993;64:216—25.

[75] Young GA, Keogh JB, Parson FM. Plasma amino acids and protein levels in chronic renal failure and changes caused by oral supplements of essential amino acids. Clin Chim Acta 1975;61:205—13.

[76] DeFerrari G, Garibotto G, Robauso C, Sala MR, Tizianello A. Splanchnic exchange of amino acids after amino acid ingestion in patients with chronic renal insufficiency. Am J Clin Nutr 1988;48:72—83.

[77] Meireles CL, Price SR, Pererira AML, Carvalhaes JTA, Mitch WE. Nutrition and chronic renal failure in rats: What is an optimal dietary protein? J Am Soc Nephrol 1999;10:2367–73.

[78] England BK, Greiber S, Mitch WE, Bowers BA, Herring WJ, McKean MJ, et al. Rat muscle branched-chain ketoacid dehydrogenase activity and mRNAs increase with extracellular acidemia. Am J Physiol 1995;268 (Cell Physiol. 37):C1395–400.

[79] Liao DF, Duff JL, Daum G, Pelech SL, Berk BC. Angiotensin II stimulates MAP kinase kinase kinase activity in vascular smooth muscle cells: Role of Raf. Circ Res 1996;79:1007–14.

[80] Bergstrom J, Alvestrand A, Furst P. Plasma and muscle free amino acids in maintenance hemodialysis patients without protein malnutrition. Kidney Int 1990;38:108–14.

[81] Reaich D, Channon SM, Scrimgeour CM, Daley SE, Wilkinson R, Goodship THJ. Correction of acidosis in humans with CRF decreases protein degradation and amino acid oxidation. Am J Physiol 1993;265:E230–5.

[82] Lofberg E, Wernerman J, Anderstam B, Bergstrom J. Correction of metabolic acidosis in dialysis patients increases branched-chain and total essential amino acid levels in muscle. Clin Nephrol 1997;48:230–7.

[83] Jansen A, Lewis S, Cattell V, Cook HT. Arginase is a major pathway of L-arginine metabolism in nephritic glomeruli. Kidney Int 1992;42:1107–12.

[84] Tizianello A, DeFerrari G, Garibotto G, Gurreri G, Robaudo C. Renal metabolism of amino acids and ammonia in subjects with normal renal function and in patients with chronic renal insufficiency. J Clin Invest 1980;65:1162–73.

[85] Edozien JC. The free amino acids of plasma and urine in kwashiorkor. Clin Sci 1966;31:153–66.

[86] Suliman ME, Anderstam B, Lindholm B, Bergstrom J. Total, free, and protein-bound sulphur amino acids in uremic patients. Nephrol Dial Transpl 1997;12:2332–8.

[87] Druml W, Fischer M, Liebisch B, Lenz K, Roth E. Elimination of amino acids in renal failure. Am J Clin Nutr 1994;60:418–23.

[88] Stockenhuber F, Kurz RW, Sertl K, Grimm G, Balcke P. Increased plasma histamine levels in uraemic pruritus. Clin Sci 1990;79:477–82.

[89] Dalton RN, Chantler C. The relationship between BCAA and alpha-ketoacids in blood in uremia. Kidney Int 1983;24(Suppl. 16):S61–6.

[90] Pechar J, Malek P, Dobersky P, et al. Influence of protein intake and renal function on plasma amino acids in patients with renal impairment and after kidney transplantation. Nutr Metab 1978;22:278–87.

[91] Bergstrom J, Furst P, Noree L-O, Vinnars E. Intracellular free amino acids in muscle tissue of patients with chronic uraemia: Effect of peritoneal dialysis and infusion of essential amino acids. Clin Sci Mol Med 1978;54:51–60.

[92] Pye IF, McGale EHF, Stonier C. Studies of cerebrospinal fluid and plasma amino acids in patients with steady-state chronic renal failure. Clin Chim Acta 1979;92:65–72.

[93] Ganda OP, Aoki TT, Soeldner JS, Morrision RS, Cahill GF. Hormone-fuel concentrations in anephric subjects. J Clin Invest 1976;57:1403–11.

[94] Mitch WE, Fouque D. Nutritional therapy of the uremic patient. In: Brenner BM, editor. The Kidney. 9th ed. Philadelphia: W.B. Saunders; 2010.

[95] Divino Filho JC, Barany P, Stehle P, Furst P, Bergstrom J. Free amino-acid levels simultaneously collected in plasma, muscle and erythrocytes of uraemic patients. Nephrol Dial Transpl 1997;12:2339–48.

[96] Wilcken DEL, Gupta VJ, Reddy SG. Accumulation of sulphur-containing amino acids including cystine-homocystine in patients on maintenance hemodialysis. Clin Sci 1980;58:427–30.

[97] Kelly RA, Mitch WE. Creatinine, uric acid and other nitrogenous waste products: Clinical implication of the imbalance between their production and elimination in uremia. Sem Nephrol 1983;3:286–94.

[98] Chen PY, Sanders PW. L-arginine abrogates salt-sensitive hypertension in Dahl/Rapp rats. J Clin Invest 1991;88:1559–67.

[99] Reyes AA, Purkerson ML, Karl I, Klahr S. Dietary supplementation with L-arginine ameliorates the progression of renal disease in rats with subtotal nephrectomy. Am J Kid Dis 1992;20:168–76.

[100] Reyes AA, Karl IE, Kissane J, Klahr S. L-Arginine administration prevents glomerular hyperfiltration and decreases proteinuria in diabetic rats. J Am Soc Nephrol 1993;4:1039–45.

[101] Reyes AA, Porras BH, Chasalow FI, Klahr S. L-arginine decreases the infiltration of the kidney by macrophages in obstructive nephropathy and puromycin-induced nephrosis. Kidney Int 1994;45:1346–54.

[102] Ashab I, Peer G, Blum M, Wollman Y, Chernihovsky T, Hassner A, et al. Oral administration of L-arginine and captopril in rats prevents chronic renal failure by nitric oxide production. Kidney Int 1995;47:1515–21.

[103] Erez A, Nagamani SC, Shchelochkov OA, Premkumar MH, Campeau PM, Chen Y, et al. Requirement of argininosuccinate lyase for systemic nitric oxide production. Nat Med 2011 December;17(12):1619–26.

[104] Bello E, Caramelo C, Lopez MD, Soldevilla MJ, Gonzalez-Pacheco FR, Rovira A, et al. Induction of microalbuminuria by L-arginine infusion in healthy individuals: an insight into the mechanisms of proteinuria. Am J Kid Dis 1999;33:1018–25.

[105] Higashi Y, Oshima T, Ozono R, Matsuura H, Kambe M, Kajiyma G. Effect of L-arginine infusion on systemic and renal hemodynamics in hypertensive patients. Am J Hyperten 1999;12:8–15.

[106] Watanabe G, Tomiyama H, Doba N. Effects of oral administration of L-arginine on renal function in patients with heart failure. J Hypertension 2000;18:229–34.

[107] Herlitz H, Jungersten LU, Wikstrand J, Widgren BR. Effect of L-arginine influsion in normotensive subjects with and without a family history of hypertension. Kidney Int 1999;56:1838–45.

[108] Narita I, Border WA, Ketteler M, Ruoslahti E, Noble NA. L-arginine may mediate the therapeutic effects of low protein diets. Proc Natl Acad Sci USA 1995;92:4552–6.

[109] Narita I, Border WA, Ketteler M, Noble NA. Nitric oxide mediates immunologic injury to kidney mesangium in experimental glomerulonephritis. Lab Invest 1995;72:17–24.

[110] Ketteler M, Ikegaya N, Brees DK, Border WA, Noble NA. L-arginine metabolism in immune-mediated glomerulonephritis in the rat. Am J Kid Dis 1996;28:878–87.

[111] Bennett-Richards KJ, Kattenhorn M, Donald AE, Oakley GR, Varghese Z, Bruckdorfer KR, et al. Oral L-arginine does not improve endothelial dysfunction in children with chronic renal failure. Kidney Int 2002;62:1372–8.

[112] Blantz RC, Lortie M, Vallon V, Gabbai FB, Parmer RJ, Thomson S. Activities of nitric oxide in normal physiology and uremia. Sem Nephrol 1996;16:144–50.

[113] Teschan PE, Beck GJ, Dwyer JT, Greene T, Klahr S, Levey AS, et al. Effect of a ketoacid-aminoacid-supplemented very low protein diet on the progression of advanced renal disease: A reanalysis of the MDRD Feasibility Study. Clin Nephrol 1998;50:273–83.

[114] Walser M. Progression of chronic renal failure in man. Kidney Int 1990;37:1195–210.

[115] Walser M, Ward L, Hill S. Hypotryptophanemia in patients with chronic renal failure on nutritional therapy. J Am Soc Nephrol 1991;2:247 (Abstract).

[116] Kaysen GA, Kropp J. Dietary tryptophan supplementation prevents proteinuria in the seven-eighths nephrectomized rat. Kidney Int 1983;23:473—9.

[117] Owada P, Nakao M, Koike J, Ujiie K, Tomita K, Shiigai T. Effects of oral adsorbent AST-120 on the progression of chronic renal failure-A randomized controlled study. Kidney Int 1997; 52(Suppl. 63):S188—90.

[118] Miyazaki T, Ise M, Hirata M, Endo K, Ito Y, Seo H, et al. Indoxyl sulfate stimulates renal synthesis of transforming growth factor-beta-1 and progression of renal failure. Kidney Int 1997;52(Suppl. 63):S211—4.

[119] Niwa T, Tsukushi S, Ise M, Miyazaki T, Tsubakihara Y, Owada A, et al. Indoxyl sulfate and progression of renal failure-effects of a low-protein diet and oral sorbent on indoxyl sulfate production in uremic rats and undialyzed uremic patients. Min Elect Metab 1997;23:179—84.

[120] Niwa T, Ise M, Miyazaki T. Progression of glomerular sclerosis in experimental uremic rats by administration of indole, a precursor of indoxyl sulfate. Am J Neph 1994; 14:207—12.

[121] Nygard O, Nordrehaug JE, Refsun H, Ueland PM, Farstad M, Vollset SE. Plasma homocysteine levels and mortality in patients with coronary artery disease. N Engl J Med 1997; 337:230—6.

[122] Selhub J, Jacques PF, Bostom AG, D'Agostino RB, Wilson PW, Belanger AJ, et al. Association between plasma homocysteine concentrations and extracranial carotid-artery stenosis. N Engl J Med 1995;332:286—99.

[123] Bostom AG, Lathrop L. Hyperhomocysteinemia in end-stage renal disease: Prevalence, etiology, and potential relationship to arteriosclerotic outcomes. Kidney Int 1997;52:10—20.

[124] Mezzano D, Pais EO, Aranda E, Panes O, Downey P, Ortiz M, et al. Inflammation not hyperhomocysteinemia is related to oxidative stress and hemostatic and endothelial dysfunction in uremia. Kidney Int 2001;60:1844—50.

[125] Wang X, Jurkovitz C, Price SR. Regulation of branched-chain ketoacid dehydrogenase flux by extracellular pH and gluco-corticoids. Am J Physiol 1997;272:C2031—6.

[126] Reaich D, Channon SM, Scrimgeour CM, Goodship THJ. Ammonium chloride-induced acidosis increases protein breakdown and amino acid oxidation in humans. Am J Physiol 1992;263:E735—9.

[127] Schenker JG, Polishuk WZ. Ovarian hyperstimulation syndrome. Obstet Gynecol 1975;46:23—8.

[128] Mitch WE, Clark AS. Specificity of the effect of leucine and its metabolities on protein degradation in skeletal muscle. Biochem J 1984;222:579—86.

[129] Zoccali C, Ruggenenti P, Perna A, Leonardis D, Tripepi R, Tripepi G, et al. Phosphate May Promote CKD Progression and Attenuate Renoprotective Effect of ACE Inhibition. J Am Soc Nephrol 2011 October;22(10):1923—30.

[130] Vegter S, Perna A, Postma MJ, Navis G, Remuzzi G, Ruggenenti P. Sodium Intake, ACE Inhibition, and Progression to ESRD. J Am Soc Nephrol 2012 January;23(1):165—73.

[131] Kalhoff H, Diekmann L, Kunz C, Stock GJ, Manz F. Alkali therapy versus sodium chloride supplement in low birthweight infants with incipient late metabolic acidosis. Acta Paediatr 1997;86:96—101.

[132] Boirie Y, Broyer M, Gagnadoux MF, Niaudet P, Bresson J-L. Alterations of protein metabolism by metabolic acidosis in children with chronic renal failure. Kidney Int 2000;58:236—41.

[133] Ballmer PE, McNurlan MA, Hulter HN, Anderson SE, Garlick PJ, Krapf R. Chronic metabolic acidosis decreases albumin synthesis and induces negative nitrogen balance in humans. J Clin Invest 1995;95:39—45.

[134] Papadoyannakis NJ, Stefanides CJ, McGeown M. The effect of the correction of metabolic acidosis on nitrogen and protein balance of patients with chronic renal failure. Am J Clin Nutr 1984;40:623—7.

[135] Garibotto G, Russo R, Sofia A, Sala MR, Robaudo C, Moscatelli P, et al. Skeletal muscle protein synthesis and degradation in patients with chronic renal failure. Kidney Int 1994;45:1432—9.

[136] Williams B, Hattersley J, Layward E, Walls J. Metabolic acidosis and skeletal muscle adaptation to low protein diets in chronic uremia. Kidney Int 1991;40:779—86.

[137] Graham KA, Reaich D, Channon SM, Downie S, Goodship THJ. Correction of acidosis in hemodialysis decreases whole-body protein degradation. J Am Soc Nephrol 1997;8:632—7.

[138] Movilli E, Zani R, Carli O, Sangalli L, Pola A, Camerini C, et al. Correction of metabolic acidosis increases serum albumin concentration and decreases kinetically evaluated protein intake in hemodialysis patients: A prospective study. Nephrol Dial Transpl 1998;13:1719—22.

[139] Graham KA, Reaich D, Channon SM, Downie S, Gilmour E, Passlick-Deetjen J, et al. Correction of acidosis in CAPD decreases whole body protein degradation. Kidney Int 1996;49: 1396—400.

2

Carbohydrate Metabolism in Kidney Disease and Kidney Failure

Eberhard Ritz[1], Marcin Adamczak[2], Andrzej Wiecek[2]

[1]Nierenzentrum, Im Neueneimer Feld 162, Heidelberg, Germany, [2]Department of Nephrology, Endocrinology and Metabolic Disease, Medical University of Silesia, Katowice, Poland

INTRODUCTION

In patients with chronic kidney disease (CKD) abnormalities of carbohydrate metabolism are encountered at different levels of the insulin-glucose cascade. The two major defects that underlie glucose intolerance in CKD are resistance to the peripheral action of insulin and impaired insulin secretion. When these two abnormalities are present glucose intolerance ensues [1].

Patients with end-stage renal disease (ESRD) are almost always more or less resistant to the peripheral action of insulin. This is true although the half-life of insulin is prolonged as a consequence of delayed insulin removal by the damaged kidney as well as by extrarenal organs. Consequently plasma insulin concentrations tend to be higher at any given rate of insulin secretion [2,3] (Table 2.1).

INSULIN RESISTANCE

As first reported in detail by Westervelt and Schreiner, using the forearm perfusion technique, peripheral glucose uptake is reduced in CKD [4]. This observation was confirmed by DeFronzo [5] using the gold standard method, i.e. the euglycemic insulin clamp technique, which allows to quantitate the amount of glucose metabolized per unit of insulin [5]. Such peripheral resistance to insulin is seen even in early stages of CKD. Peripheral resistance to insulin is a clinically important parameter, because in CKD it is tightly correlated to increased cardiovascular risk (CV) [6] and to accelerated progression of CKD [7].

Liver and kidney are the major sites of *glucose production* in the fasting state [8,9]. Liver and skeletal muscles are the major sites of peripheral *glucose uptake*.

The available data indicate that usually glucose production by the *liver* is not altered in CKD. Specifically deFronzo [3,5] had documented that baseline hepatic glucose production as well as its suppression by insulin [3,5] are not altered. In addition glucose uptake by the liver, which is small to begin with, is also not affected in CKD [5]. The renal contribution to glucose production has long been grossly underestimated and is quite substantial [10].

The main site of decreased insulin sensitivity is *skeletal muscle*. The defect is not at the level of the insulin receptor: in skeletal muscles of rats with chronic uremia the numbers and affinities of the receptors are normal [11–17] as is insulin receptor kinase activity [17]. The defect is presumably at the postreceptor level. Impaired phosphatidyl-inositol 3-kinase activity (PI3-K) was recently documented, presumably due to an excess of p85 [18]. Consequently in uremia higher levels of insulin will be required to increase glucose uptake by skeletal muscle [11].

There is also information on insulin postreceptor events in CKD and uremia. When the beta chain of the receptor has been phosphorylated, a complex series of interactions follows involving insulin receptor substrate (IRS) as well as numerous cofactors [19,20]. More distal effects (e.g. stimulation of proliferation) are mediated via the mitogen activated protein kinase (MAPK) pathway and the inositol-triphosphate (IP3) pathways. The latter is responsible for the upregulation of the insulin-regulated glucose transporter (GLUT-4). The PI3-K complex is a heterodimer composed of an 85-kDa (p85) regulatory subunit and a 110-kDa (p110) catalytic subunit. The subunits and the p85–p110 complexes are differentially regulated by glucocorticoids [21,22]. Stimulation of p85 expression by glucocorticoid

TABLE 2.1   Abnormalities of Carbohydrate Metabolism in Chronic Kidney Disease

- Usually normal fasting blood glucose, but tendency to spontaneous hypoglycemia
- Fasting hyperinsulinemia with prolonged insulin half-life
- Elevated plasma glucagon and growth hormone concentrations
- Impaired glucose tolerance

treatment leads to reduction of PI3-K activity [23]. This may be relevant, because glucocorticoid synthesis is increased in uremia [24], perhaps explaining the increase of p85 and the suppression of PI3-K activity [18] in the muscle of uremic rats.

In uremia the insulin-dependent glucose uptake is altered. GLUT-4 is unique to muscle and adipose tissue. The abundance of GLUT-4 is similar in muscles of CKD patients and healthy subjects [25]. In the heart of uremic rats, however, we observed (in unpublished studies) diminished insulin-dependent glucose uptake and unchanged total GLUT-4, but reduced GLUT-4 incorporation into the plasma membrane. Carbamylation of proteins is a common finding in uremia. Carbamylation modifies signal transduction and translocation of GLUT-4. Therefore it is of interest that N-carbamoyl-L-asparagine reduces insulin sensitive glucose uptake by interfering with GLUT-4 activity [26].

Peripheral resistance to insulin action is frequently found even in early stages of renal disease and is found in the majority of patients with advanced CKD. The resistance to the peripheral action of insulin is markedly improved, however, after several weeks of hemodialysis (HD) [27–29] and of peritoneal dialysis (PD) [28–30]. Presumably, an unidentified dialyzable uremic "toxin", possibly a protein breakdown product, is involved in the genesis of deranged insulin action. Sera of uremic patients contain a compound that inhibits glucose metabolism by normal rat adipocytes [31]. This compound with a molecular weight of 1 to 2 kDa is specific for uremia, because it is not found in nonuremic patients with insulin resistance. Hippurate accumulates in the blood of patients with CKD and inhibits glucose utilization by rat diaphragm, brain, kidney cortex, and erythrocytes. It may therefore contribute to insulin resistance of patients with CKD [32].

A number of further factors have been identified which are involved in the genesis of insulin resistance in kidney disease and are potential targets for intervention. In HD patients, insulin resistance is ameliorated by treatment with erythropoietin [33,34] or 1,25 dihydroxycholecalciferol (1,25(OH)$_2$D$_3$) [35,36]. In predialysis patients it is also ameliorated by restriction of dietary protein [37–39].

Plasma concentrations of the insulin antagonists glucagon [40,41] and growth hormone [42,43] are frequently elevated in CKD. It has been proposed that these two hormones contribute to insulin resistance. This does not completely explain insulin resistance, however, since dialysis improves insulin sensitivity despite no change in the concentrations of growth hormone and glucagon [44,45].

Metabolic acidosis is frequent in CKD. A causal role in insulin resistance is suggested by the observation that correction of acidosis by bicarbonate improves insulin resistance in animal models as well as in uremic patients [46,47].

A finding with major clinical relevance is the observation that major insulin resistance in uremia is caused by inflammation. The molecular pathways following insulin binding include tyrosine phosphorylation of members of IRS family. This process triggers translocation of GLUT-4 from intracellular stores to the cell membrane [48]. Conversely serine phosphorylation of IRS-1 abrogates the association between IRS-1 and insulin receptor leading to the insulin-resistance [49]. Inflammatory mediators such as tumor necrosis factor-α (TNFα) may activate serine kinases such as c-jun-NH$_2$ — terminal-kinase (JNK) and IκB kinase (IKK) which phosphorylate serine residues of IRS-1 and disrupt insulin signaling [50].

Insulin resistance is involved in the development of the catabolic state of uremia. Muscle catabolism in inflammatory states is mediated by proinflammatory cytokines, e.g. interleukins 1 and 6 (IL-1, IL-6) and TNF-α [51–53]. These cytokines act also on the satiety center [54,55]; this may explain the tight relationship between anorexia and the plasma concentration of the proinflammatory cytokines in HD patients [56,57].

It is known that angiotensin 2 (Ang 2) [58,59] interferes with insulin sensitivity in individuals without kidney disease. That Ang 2 contributes to insulin resistance in CKD is suggested by the observation of Satirapoj that in HD patients Valsartan reduced fasting insulinemia and insulin resistance as assessed by the homeostatic model (HOMA-IR index) [60].

Increased visceral fat is an important risk factor for insulin resistance both in the general population and in CKD. Insulin resistance by HOMA-IR is closely linked to both fat mass and to the body mass index (BMI) in CKD. Ramos [61] documented that even in nonobese, nondiabetic patients with advanced CKD, BMI and adiposity were associated with increased F2-isoprostanes and C-reactive protein (CRP) and negatively correlated with protein thiols. They concluded that adiposity amplifies oxidative stress and inflammation [62].

It has been postulated that resistin, a hormone derived from adipose tissue, is involved in the genesis of insulin resistance [63]. Plasma resistin concentrations are high in CKD patients, probably the result of diminished renal clearance [64]. In CKD, however, no relation was found between insulin sensitivity and plasma resistin concentrations [64].

A sedentary lifestyle causes insulin resistance [65]; conversely, exercise training improves insulin sensitivity and this is true for CKD patients as well [66,67].

INSULIN SECRETION

Insulin secretion by the β cells of the pancreatic islets is a complex process. The β cells are stimulated both by nutrients (glucose, amino acids, fatty acids) and by non-nutrient agents, e.g. hormones and neurotransmitters. The islets use different mechanisms to detect nutrient and non-nutrient stimuli, but insulin secretion uses the same intracellular processes irrespective of whether the β cells are activated by nutrient or non-nutrient secretagogues.

Glucose-induced insulin secretion involves glucose uptake by the β cells, followed by glucose metabolism and production of adenosine triphosphate (ATP). ATP facilitates the closure of ATP-dependent K^+ channels, followed by cell membrane depolarization and subsequent activation of voltage-sensitive Ca^+ channels. As a consequence, calcium enters the islets causing an acute rise in cytosolic Ca^+ concentration thus triggering the secretion of insulin.

A number of studies showed that insulin secretion is impaired in CKD [68–71]. One factor responsible for impaired insulin secretion in CKD is high plasma parathormone (*PTH*) concentrations. Insulin secretion, as assessed by the hyperglycemic clamp technique, is improved when the parathyroid gland is suppressed [72,73]. Using the technique of isolated pancreatic islets the underlying molecular mechanisms have been elegantly demonstrated in subtotally nephrectomized (SNX) rats by Fadda [68]; insulin release triggered by glucose (but not by the alternative agent glyceride-−aldehyde) was diminished in SNX rats and this outcome was almost completely prevented by parathyroidectomy [74,68]. The mechanism underlying PTH induced impairment of insulin secretion is an increase of cytoplasmic Ca^+ concentration in pancreatic beta cells as the result of increased Ca^+ entry, followed by decreased Ca^+ extrusion and the resulting reduction of ATP content. As a result closure of ATP-dependent K^+ channels occurs with consecutive reduction of the glucose induced Ca^+ signal. Glucose-induced insulin secretion is impaired even in rats with normal renal function when they receive daily injections of PTH [74,75].

Apart from glucose, amino acids are stimuli triggering insulin secretion, the most potent being L-leucine [76], and an additional stimulus is K^+ [77]. In CKD such insulin secretion triggered by the alternative stimuli L-leucine [71] or K^+ [69] is also impaired.

Similar to animal experiments, in uremic patients, as well reduced insulin secretion in response to secretagogues is mainly the result of chronic PTH excess. This was documented by Mak et al. [78,79] in HD children, in whom insulin secretion increased after parathyroidectomy [78,79].

$1,25[OH]_2D_3$ affects insulin secretion as well. Islet cells express both vitamin D receptors [80,81] and vitamin D dependent calcium-binding protein [82]. After administration of labeled $1,25(OH)_2D_3$, radioactivity is retrieved in the β cells [83]. Insulin secretion is impaired in vitamin D-deficient rats with normal renal function [84]; the defect is reversed by vitamin D [85]. This may be relevant for CKD, because acute intravenous administration of $1,25(OH)_2D_3$ to dialysis patients, improved the early and late phases of insulin secretion [86].

INSULIN CLEARANCE

The kidney plays an important role in insulin metabolism and clearance. Insulin is filtered by the glomeruli and reabsorbed in the proximal tubule [87]. In normal subjects the renal clearance of insulin is about 200 mL/minute [88]. This value exceeds the glomerular filtration rate (GFR), indicating that in addition peritubular uptake of insulin takes place [89]. It is estimated that 6 to 8 U of endogenous insulin are removed daily by the kidney, accounting for 25% to 40% of the total removal of endogenous insulin. A decrease in the metabolic clearance rate of insulin is demonstrable in patients with GFR < 40 mL/minute; a significant prolongation of the insulin half-life is observed when GFR falls below 20 mL/minute [90]. The endogenous insulin clearance increases remarkably when dialysis treatment is started; presumably this is explained by an increase in insulin removal by liver and muscle.

In patients with CKD, diminished renal [90] and extrarenal (liver and muscles) [91] insulin clearance accounts for fasting hyperinsulinemia. It also accounts for decreased insulin requirements in diabetic patients with impaired renal function.

HYPOGLYCEMIA

With respect to the risk of hypoglycemia in patients with CKD it is important to be aware of the fact that − in contrast to the previous opinion − gluconeogenesis is not restricted to the liver. Recent studies document that the kidney contributes no less than 40% to overall gluconeogenesis [92]. In type 2 diabetic patients overall glucose production is increased by as much as 300%; hepatic and renal gluconeogenesis contribute equally to this increase [93]. This explains presumably the clinical observation that CKD patients, both diabetic and nondiabetic, are particularly prone to develop hypoglycemia [94–97].

In a retrospective cohort analysis comprising 243,222 Veterans Health Administration patients hypoglycemic episodes (< 70 mg/dL) were more frequent in diabetic as well as nondiabetic patients with CKD compared to no CKD; the risk of death within one day after hypoglycemia < 70 mg/dL was markedly elevated [97].

The mechanism underlying spontaneous hypoglycemia in uremic patients is not completely clear. In one such patient, a reduction in hepatic glucose output was found, due to diminished availability of substrate for gluconeogenesis [98]. Nondiabetic HD patients treated with glucose-free dialysate frequently develop hypoglycemia [98]; malnutrition, diminished gluconeogenesis, impaired glycogenolysis and impaired degradation of insulin may all contribute to spontaneous hypoglycemia [96,99].

In diabetic patients with CKD, decreased degradation of the administered insulin may result in higher than expected blood insulin levels. This may potentially precipitate hypoglycemia. Repeated episodes of hypoglycemia are occasionally the first clinical sign drawing attention to the presence impaired renal function. Careful adjustment of the insulin dose is then needed. When diabetic patients with impaired renal function are treated with oral diabetic agents, it is important to consider that some oral antidiabetic agents or their active metabolites are cleared via the kidney and cumulate in CKD patients [100,101]. Appropriate dose adjustment is necessary, but it is often better to switch the patients to insulin.

Consequences of Hyperglycemia and Insulin Resistance

Why is the impairment of glucose metabolism in renal failure clinically relevant? There are good arguments that hyperglycemia and insulin resistance contribute to accelerated atherogenesis in renal failure. Shinohara [6] followed 183 nondiabetic HD patients for more than 5 years. CV deaths by Kaplan–Meier estimation were significantly more frequent in subjects of the top tertile of insulin resistance, assessed using the HOMA-IR technique, compared to the lower tertiles. The adverse effect of insulin resistance on mortality was independent of body mass, hypertension, and dyslipidemia.

Moreover, hyperinsulinemia and insulin-resistance may contribute to hypertension [102] and lipid abnormalities.

Insulin is also an important regulator of lipoprotein lipase activity (LPA). Insulin deficiency or insulin resistance are associated with reduced LPA [103]. Lipoprotein lipase plays a major role in triglyceride removal. In patients with CKD LPA is reduced and this is the major cause of hypertriglyceridemia [104]. Further support for a role of insulin in the genesis of dyslipidemia is provided by the observation that administration of insulin to uremic rats corrects the defect in LPA as well as hypertriglyceridemia [105].

Insulin resistance may also participate in pathogenesis of the malnutrition commonly found in CKD patients [57,106]. In rats with acute renal failure protein degradation is increased in perfused or incubated muscle. This defect is closely related to abnormalities in insulin-dependent carbohydrate metabolism [107]. Insulin deficiency (or resistance) stimulates breakdown of muscle and activates a common proteolytic pathway via the ubiquitin–proteasome system [108,109]. Therefore, insulin resistance may also contribute to increased protein catabolism and malnutrition in CKD patients.

Insulin resistance increases salt sensitivity via increased tubular sodium reabsorption and this contributes to hypertension [110].

An interesting link between excessive fructose ingestion and insulin resistance, metabolic syndrome and kidney disease has recently been proposed by Johnson [111].

CARBOHYDRATE METABOLISM IN PATIENTS WITH RENAL REPLACEMENT THERAPY

Hemodialyzed Patients

The initiation of renal replacement therapy by HD reduces insulin resistance. This was found by Kobayashi [112] in a small study using the hyperinsulinemic euglycemic clamp technique. It has also been shown that the use of high-flux membranes lowers insulin resistance in HD patients compared to treatment with low-flux membranes [113,114]. It is relevant that many uremic patients with diabetes have so called "burnt out" diabetes [115], i.e. hyperglycemia disappeared after weight loss resulting from anorexia. On the other hand in patients with terminal uremia and no known history of type 2 diabetes, but with a pathological oral glucose tolerance test, diabetes may reappear after refeeding following the start of HD treatment. This was seen in 10% of type 2 diabetic patients entering the HD program.

In nondiabetic and particularly diabetic HD patients the blood concentrations of glucose and insulin may be affected by the dialysis procedure and particularly by the dialysate glucose concentration. Blood glucose may be lost into the dialysate downhill a concentration gradient, if the dialysate is glucose free; therefore glucose free dialysate is currently no longer used. Today the usual dialysate glucose concentrations range between 100 mg/dL and 200 mg/dL; the net effect will be lowering of markedly elevated glucose levels and protection against hypoglycemia during dialysis sessions [116]. Plasma insulin levels may also decrease during HD sessions as a result of potential glucose load (depending on dialysate glucose concentration) and of insulin clearance (the rate of loss varying between membranes).

Additional metabolic effects of dialysis include improved insulin sensitivity and potential decrease of counter-regulatory hormones (e.g. growth hormone) etc. In dialyzed diabetic patients signs and symptoms of hyperglycemia may be modified: in addition to the classical signs, i.e. thirst, fluid overload, and severe hyperkalemia, the absence of polyuria precludes volume contraction and may even cause volume expansion or pulmonary edema, particularly in the presence of excessive thirst. Further potential complications of hyperglycemia include increased blood pressure, altered mental status, nausea and gastroparesis etc, but symptoms and signs are frequently nonspecific or lacking.

Hypoglycemic drug therapies require special consideration in diabetic patients with ESRD (see also below). The insulin dose must be reduced, often by as much as half. Rapid-acting insulin analogues are less likely to cause hypoglycemia than regular or long-acting insulin, because their pharmacokinetics are less affected by renal failure [117]. Most oral antidiabetic drugs are contraindicated in CKD stage 5 patients and on dialysis [117—119], but thiazolidinediones (TZDs) and repaglinide are the drugs that can be used in HD patients without modification of the dose.

Peritoneal Dialysis Patients

The initiation of renal replacement therapy by PD reduces insulin resistance as shown by Kobayashi [112]. Interestingly some patients develop new-onset hyperglycemia after the start of PD, presumably as a result of high peritoneal glucose load [120]. Peritoneal dialysis patients tend to have higher fasting glucose, blood HbA1$_c$ and HOMA-IR indices compared to hemodialyzed patients, possibly as the result of high glucose load and weight gain [121,122]. Depending on the dwell time and the exposure to high glucose PD solution, up to 80% or more of glucose in the PD solution is absorbed, accounting for a daily glucose load of up to 100—300 g of glucose [123—125]. The absorption of glucose from the dialysis solution predisposes to hyperinsulinemia, weight gain and insulin resistance. Icodextrin, an osmotically active glucose polymer, can be used as an osmotic agent to substitute for glucose. Clinical studies indicate that reduction of hyperinsulinemia and increased insulin sensitivity can be achieved by long-term use of icodextrin containing PD solutions for overnight exchanges [126,127].

Kidney Transplant Recipients and New-Onset Diabetes after Transplantation (NODAT)

The first description of diabetes mellitus as a complication of kidney transplantation dates back to 1964 [124]. Baseline risks that predispose kidney graft recipients to NODAT include advanced age, obesity, male gender, hepatitis C virus infection, nonwhite ethnicity and family history of diabetes i.e. inherited as well as acquired defects in insulin sensitivity and beta cell function [125,126]. The high incidence of NODAT in predisposed individuals during the first months after transplantation reflects superimposition of new transplant-specific factors upon a predisposing baseline metabolic milieu. The best documented transplantation-specific factors include immunosuppressive agents; e.g. glucocorticoids, calcineurin inhibitors (cyclosporine and particularly tacrolimus), sirolimus, and weight gain after transplantation [125,126] (Table 2.2).

NODAT will become even more frequent in the future given the current pandemic of obesity. Based on ADA (American Diabetes Association) criteria of diabetes mellitus, Cosio [127] reported that one year after transplantation the prevalence of NODAT was 13%. In one of the largest epidemiologic studies of NODAT Kasiske found in 11,659 Medicare beneficiaries with a first kidney transplant a cumulative incidence of NODAT of 9%, 16%, and 24% at 3, 12, and 36 months respectively [128]. Many clinical studies in recipients of kidney and other solid organ transplants showed that NODAT increases the risks of cardiovascular disease, graft failure and death [128—130], e.g. Kasiske showed that after kidney

TABLE 2.2 Risk Factors that Predispose Kidney Graft Recipients to New-onset Diabetes Mellitus after Transplantation (NODAT)

NONMODIFIABLE RISK FACTORS

- advanced age
- male gender
- nonwhite ethnicity
- family history of diabetes
- impaired glucose tolerance before transplantation

MODIFIABLE RISK FACTORS

- overweight and obesity
- posttransplantation weight gain
- hepatitis C virus infection
- cytomegalovirus infection
- immunosuppressive agents
  - glucocorticoids
  - calcineurin inhibitors (cyclosporine and to a greater extent tacrolimus)
  - sirolimus

transplantation NODAT is associated with an increased risk of graft failure (relative risk [RR] 1.63, P < 0.0001) and death-censored graft failure (RR 1.87, P < 0.0001) as well as death when compared with graft recipients without NODAT [128]. The excess mortality is mainly attributable to a higher incidence of CV disease.

The therapy of NODAT includes both nonpharmacological and pharmacological interventions: aggressive lifestyle modification, particularly dietary changes, exercise and weight loss irrespective of whether the patient requires pharmacologic treatment for hyperglycemia or not [125,126,131]. The role of altering immunosuppression in an effort to improve glycemic control in patients with NODAT remains controversial. Matas compared the outcomes in NODAT kidney transplant recipients and concluded that prevention of acute rejection was more important than prevention of NODAT in preserving long-term kidney function [132]; therefore a potential benefit of avoiding or reversing NODAT by a change of immunosuppressants (reducing or discontinuing corticosteroids or calcineurin inhibitors) must be weighed against the risk of precipitating acute or chronic rejection [125,126].

TREATMENT OF DIABETES MELLITUS IN DIABETICS WITH CKD

Target of Treatments

The renal benefit of strict glycemic control was documented by the *Diabetes Control and Complications Trial* in type 1 diabetes [133] and in type 2 diabetes by the *UK Prospective Diabetes Study* [134] and the Kumamoto Study [135] respectively. Subsequently the ADVANCE (*The Action in Diabetes and Vascular Disease*) study documented in subjects with type 2 diabetes that strict glycemic control (mean $HbA1_c$ 6.5%) in comparison with the standard control (mean $HbA1_c$ 7.3%) is associated with a significant reduction in renal events, including onset of or worsening of nephropathy [hazard ratio (HR) 0.79; P = 0.006], new-onset microalbuminuria (HR 0.91; P = 0.02) and development of macroalbuminuria (HR 0.70; P < 0.001) [136].

Blood glucose control is more problematic in diabetic patients with kidney disease. While glucose control is undoubtedly beneficial in early stages of type 1 and type 2 diabetes, one can not extrapolate the very positive renoprotective actions of intensive glucose control to all diabetic patients with CKD or even ESRD. Unfortunately, results of sufficiently large prospective randomized controlled intervention studies are not yet available to answer this issue. In CKD patients the limited information is mainly based on the effect the PROactive study (*Prospective Pioglitazone Clinical Trial in Macrovascular*

Events); in this study patients with type 2 diabetes and CKD (n = 597; 11.6% of the 5154 patients) had a particularly high CV risk and presence of CV disease [137]. The incidence of the combined end point (nonfatal myocardial infarction, stroke and death) was 18.3% in patients with CKD compared with 11.5% in patients without CKD (HR 1.65; P < 0.0001). In addition, all-cause mortality was 10.9% compared to 5.9% (HR 1.86) in those without CKD. At end of the study the $HbA1_c$ difference between pioglitazone and placebo was only 0.5% ($HbA1_c$ 6.9 vs. 7.4%). Presumably the well-documented anti-atherogenic effects of pioglitazone [138] was responsible for CV protection in diabetic patients with CKD.

Among hemodialyzed ESRD patients 5-year survival is much lower in diabetic vs. non-diabetic patients [139]. During the last decade several observational studies [140–144] indicated that the survival of diabetic patients on HD is influenced by the quality of glycemic control. Morioka [140] evaluated the impact of glycemic control on survival in 150 diabetic subjects with ESRD starting HD treatment; during the short follow-up period of 2.8 years, 76% of the patients had died. Compared to those with good glycemic control (HbA1c < 7.5%) mortality was higher in those with poor glycemic control ($HbA1_c \geq$ 7.5%). In a 7-year observational study of 114 diabetic patients on HD Oomichi [141] found that mortality was similar in patients with good $HbA1_c <$ 6.5% and HbA1c > 6.5% < 8.0%, but mortality was significantly higher (HR 2.89; P = 0.01) in those with poor glycemic control ($HbA1_c >$ 8.0%). Hayashino [142] analysed mortality in the large Japanese Dialysis Outcomes and Practice Pattern Study studying 1569 HD patients with diabetes and 3342 patients without diabetes. The mortality was significantly higher in diabetic patients on HD whose $HbA1_c$ was in the fifth quintile ($HbA1_c \geq$ 7.3%), but was not different in the four quintiles with $HbA1_c$ ranging from 5.0 to 7.2% [142]. In contrast to these studies in Asian dialysis populations, no correlation between $HbA1_c$ and survival was found in 24,875 diabetic dialysis patients in the US [145]. The failure to see a beneficial effect of glycemic control may be explained by the underlying differences in the tools used to measure glycemia. Kalantar-Zadeh [143] evaluated 23,618 US diabetic HD patients and assessed survival as a function of $HbA1_c$. He observed that higher $HbA1_c$ values were incrementally associated with higher mortality. Compared with patients with $HbA1_c$ in the range of 5–6%, patients with $HbA1_c >$ 10% had higher hazard ratios for adjusted all-cause and CV death: 1.41 and 1.73 respectively (P < 0.001). Remarkably, this relationship was only seen in patients without anemia, perhaps reflecting the loss of specificity of $HbA1_c$ in patients with reduced erythrocyte survival. In the *German Diabetes and Dialysis Study* (4D study), Drechsler [144] investigated the impact of glycemic control on cardiac and vascular outcomes. During 4 years of follow-up, patients with $HbA1_c > 8.0\%$ or $HbA1_c$ from > 6 to $< 8\%$ had an increased risk of sudden death (HR 1.85 and 2.26, respectively; $P < 0.003$) compared with patients with $HbA1_c < 6.0\%$.

Unfortunately, $HbA1_c$ is not an ideal parameter to assess glycemic control in patients with advanced kidney disease. In chronic renal failure, the lifespan of erythrocytes is shortened, and low $HbA1_c$ values may therefore be artificially low because of shorter exposure of erythrocytes to glycemia. As a result and $HbA1_c$ values should be interpreted with caution in patients with serum creatinine concentrations > 2.5 mg/dL [146]. Inaba [147] and Peacock [148] confirmed that in diabetic HD patients, $HbA1_c$ levels significantly underestimate poor glycemic control, while glycated albumin reflects glycemic control more accurately. Unfortunately, this method is not widely available.

Should all diabetic patients be given the same antidiabetic treatment? Currently, there is a worldwide debate whether all diabetic patients should be treated following the same algorithm as proposed for diabetic patients without CKD. The recent consensus paper advocates a more individualized antidiabetic approach, taking into account pathophysiologic criteria, i.e. insulin resistance or insulin deficiency, comorbidity and risk of hypoglycemia [149].

DRUG MANAGEMENT IN DIABETICS WITH CKD (FIGURE 2.1)

Biguanides

Metformin is the only biguanide currently available. It increases insulin sensitivity by activating hepatic and muscle isoforms of AMPK (adenosine monophosphate-activated protein kinase) [150]. This causes decreased hepatic glucose production and increased glucose utilization. Metformin is the treatment of choice for overweight patients with type 2 diabetes mellitus, because in contrast to other antidiabetic agents its effect on body weight is neutral or even a modest weight loss can be achieved. Additional advantages of metformin therapy include a low risk of hypoglycemia and a minor, but beneficial, effect on abnormal lipid profiles [150]. It is also the only hypoglycemic agent with documented reduction of cardiovascular events [151,152] and reduction of malignancy [153,154].

Metformin is cleared by renal excretion and consequently metformin cumulates in CKD [155]. The most dangerous side effect of metformin is lactic acidosis [150]. Although this complication is generally rare, in the context of renal insufficiency the risk of lactic acidosis is increased for two reasons: on the one hand metformin accumulates and on the other hand the renal clearance of lactate is decreased [150]. According to the manufacturers, metformin should not be administered to type 2 diabetic patients with serum creatinine concentrations of > 1.5 mg/dL in men and > 1.4 mg/dL in women. The degree of renal impairment at which metformin is strictly contraindicated remains controversial [155]: some clinicians argue that metformin is tolerated up to a serum creatinine concentration of 220 mmol/L or 2.5 mg/dL; recent studies even suggested that continuation of metformin may be safe down to a minimum estimated glomerular filtration rate (eGFR) of 30 mL/min [156]. This medication must be strictly avoided in ESRD patients, however.

Sulphonylureas

Sulphonylureas enhance the pancreatic insulin secretion. They partially block ATP-sensitive K^+ channels in

Use of the antidiabetic drugs in CKD patients

FIGURE 2.1 Use of the antidiabetic drugs in chronic kidney disease patients.

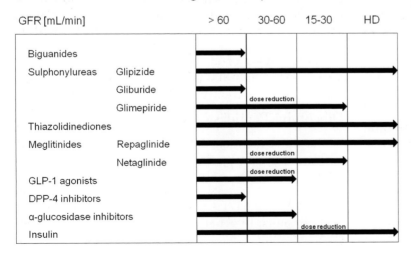

beta cells causing cell membrane depolarization thus opening voltage dependent Ca^{++} channels, increasing intracellular Ca^{++} and thus triggering insulin secretion [157]. As a result of increased plasma insulin concentration weight gain and hypoglycemia are common side effects. The older sulphonylureas are predominantly metabolized in the liver to yield active metabolites which are cleared via the kidney along with unmetabolized drug [117,119]. In patients with kidney dysfunction, accumulation of the parent drug and of metabolites of some sulphonylurea compounds can lead to hypoglycemia. Consequently, these first-generation sulphonylureas should be avoided at least in patients with CKD.

Among the second-generation sulphonylureas (e.g., glipizide, glyburide, and glimepiride), glipizide is preferred because it is metabolized in the liver to inactive metabolites that are eliminated via the kidney [117,158]. Consequently, compared to first generation sulphonylureas, the risk of hypoglycemia in CKD patients is less. Nevertheless because of the remaining risk of hypoglycemia sulphonylureas should be used with caution even in mild to moderate CKD and completely avoided in patients with severe renal impairment [117,119].

Thiazolidinediones

The currently available TZDs, rosiglitazone and pioglitazone, are selective agonists of the peroxisomal proliferator-activated receptor-γ (PPAR-γ) [117,119]. The ligands for these receptors are normally free fatty acids and eicosanoids. By activating PPARγ they inhibit angiogenesis, decrease leptin levels and certain interleukins, while adiponectin levels increase [159]. TZDs act as prandial glucose regulators and improve insulin sensitivity. TZDs are predominantly metabolized and eliminated by the liver [117,119]. Consequently, no dose adjustments are necessary in patients with renal dysfunction [160,161]. A major side effect is sodium retention, particularly in patients with CKD, causing weight gain with reduction of hematocrit, edema and even pulmonary edema, particularly in patients with CV disease [119]. Further side effects include higher fracture rates of distal extremities in women and gastrointestinal side effects [119]. Therefore great caution is advised with PPARγ agonist use in patients with an eGFR less than 30 mL/min [117,119].

Of greatest concern, recent meta-analyses suggest that rosiglitazone treatment leads to an increased risk of myocardial infarctions and heart failure [162,163], while the cardiac risk is decreased by pioglitazone [164]. Since September 2010, the Food and Drug Administration in the USA has restricted the use of rosiglitazone to patients with type 2 diabetes who cannot control their diabetes with other medications, whereas the European Medicines Agency has recommended suspending the marketing authorization of all rosiglitazone-containing medications.

Pioglitazone improved CV outcome in diabetic patients with CKD [165], interfered with progression of diabetic nephropathy in animal models [166] and retards senescence in the kidney [167]. Preliminary data suggesting a link between pioglitazone and bladder cancer are of concern, however [168,169].

Meglitinides

The meglitinides, i.e. repaglinide and netaglinide, are short-acting agents that bind to an ATP dependent K^+ channel on beta-cell membranes (similar but not identical with that occupied by sulphonylurea); the resulting depolarization of pancreatic beta cells causes Ca^{++} influx and increased insulin secretion [170,171]. Side effects of the meglitinides include hypoglycemia and weight gain. One of the significant advantages of meglitinides is the safe administration of these agents in CKD patients, because these drugs are excreted mainly by hepatic clearance [119]. Repaglinide seems to be safer than netaglinide. A minor amount of netaglinide, together with its active metabolite, is excreted in the urine [172]. Therefore in advanced CKD netaglinide treatment still increases the risk of hypoglycemia.

Glucagon-Like Peptide 1 (GLP-1) Agonists

The two main incretins secreted by K cells in the upper small intestine are GLP-1 and glucose-dependent insulinotropic peptide (GIP) [117]. Gut hormones have been shown to play an important role in whole-body glucose homeostasis by suppressing meal-related glucagon secretion, delaying gastric emptying and inducing satiety [172]. As the GLP-1 effect is diminished in type 2 diabetics, administration of exogenous GLP-1s (exenatide, liraglutide) are a rational therapeutic option [173]. However, because GLP-1 is cleared by the kidneys, it is not recommended for patients with an eGFR < 30 mL/min and should be used with caution at eGFR 30–50 mL/min [174]. Since GLP-1 agonists are a new class of agents, long term safety in CKD patients has not been determined.

Dipeptidyl-Peptidase 4 (DPP-4) Inhibitors

The above mentioned incretins, including GLP-1, are rapidly degraded by the enzyme DPP-4. The effort to inhibit this enzyme led to the development of a new class of antiglycemic agents, such as sitagliptin, linagliptin and vildagliptin [171,175]. They pose no intrinsic risk of hypoglycemia. In general DPP-4 inhibitors are not recommended for patients with eGFR <50 mL/min [176].

However, the pharmacokinetics of DPP-4 inhibitors vary among the different agents. Sitagliptin is excreted in the urine. However in one study it was shown that reduced doses of sitagliptin are well tolerated and effective in patients with moderate (eGFR 30–50 mL/min) and even severe (<30 mL/min) CKD [177]. Linagliptin is eliminated via the feces. Results of pharmacokinetic study suggest that no dose adjustment is required for any degree of renal impairment [178,179].

Alpha-Glucosidase Inhibitors

This class of inhibitors of α-glucosidase includes acarbose, miglitol and voglibose. These drugs inhibit the hydrolysis of oligo-, di-, and trisaccharides to glucose and other monosaccharides, thus reducing the postprandial increase of blood glucose [180]. The increased delivery of carbohydrates to the colon frequently causes side effects, e.g. flatulence, bloating, abdominal pain and diarrhea, rendering patient management difficult and reducing compliance [181]. In the context of renal impairment, guidelines do not recommend acarbose in individuals with an eGFR less than 25 mL/min [117,119].

Insulin Treatment in CKD

The use of insulin, human or analogues, is recommended in type 2 diabetic patients with advanced CKD and difficulties in glycemic control. A more theoretical argument is that in these catabolic patients the anabolic effect of insulin is desirable. No clinical evidence is available to decide in advanced CKD the optimal timing for the start of insulin treatment or the initiation of any particular insulin regimen. The start of insulin treatment is usually based on clinical decisions based on individual patient requirements.

In recent years, a number of insulin analogues have been marketed. These newer insulins were developed by modifying the structure of the insulin molecule to alter the pharmacokinetic properties. Based on data from a limited number of small studies, specific insulin analogues are effective and safe in patients with CKD [182,183], but more information is needed.

Major side effects of insulin include weight gain and risk of hypoglycemia. Insulin requirements are often substantially decreased in anorectic patients with ESRD. Dose adjustments are often required to minimize the risk of hypoglycemia, especially with individuals on dialysis [119].

In patients without kidney disease who are given subcutaneous exogenous insulin up to 80% of insulin is cleared by the kidneys. As GFR falls below 20 mL/min, the kidneys are no longer able to efficiently clear insulin resulting in prolonged insulin half-life and an increased potential for hypoglycemia [184]. The American College of Physicians recommended (i) a 25% decrease in the insulin dose when the GFR is decreased to between 50 and 10 mL/min and (ii) a 50% decrease when GFR decreased below 10 mL/min. Additionally, once dialysis is initiated, the insulin resistance seen in ESRD is often improved [185]. Other factors that may contribute to changes of the need for exogenous insulin include reduction in renal gluconeogenesis, uremia-induced anorexia, and weight loss. In fact, one-third of patients with type 2 diabetes no longer require insulin after one year of HD [186]. Therefore, when these patients are treated with insulin, it is imperative to monitor blood glucose concentrations and to adjust the dose as needed in order to avoid hypoglycemia.

There has been much speculation regarding diabetes and increased risk of certain cancers. The hypothesis has been proposed that insulin treatment is the culprit [119,187]. It is difficult, however, to distinguish whether the risk of cancer is increased as the result of insulin use per se or the result of hyperglycemia ("glucose supply" hypothesis) [187].

References

[1] Massry SG, Smogorzewski M. Carbohydrate metabolism in renal failure. In: Kopple JD, Massry SG, editors. Nutritional management of renal disease. Baltimore: Williams and Wilkins; 2007. p. 63–76.

[2] DeFronzo RA, Andres R, Edgar P, et al. Carbohydrate metabolism in uremia: a review. Medicine (Baltimore) 1973;52:469–81.

[3] DeFronzo RA, Alvestrand A, Smith D, et al. Insulin resistance in uremia. J Clin Invest 1981;67:563–8.

[4] Westervelt Jr FB, Schreiner GE. The carbohydrate intolerance of uremic patients. Ann Intern Med 1962;57:266–76.

[5] DeFronzo RA, Alvertrand A. Glucose intolerance in uremia: site and mechanism. Am J Clin Nutr 1980;33:1438–45.

[6] Shinohara K, Shoji T, Emoto M, et al. Insulin resistance as an independent predictor of cardiovascular mortality in patients with end-stage renal disease. J Am Soc Nephrol 2002;13:1894–900.

[7] Becker B, Kronenberg F, Kielstein JT, et al. Renal insulin resistance syndrome, adiponectin and cardiovascular events in patients with kidney disease: the mild and moderate kidney disease study. J Am Soc Nephrol 2005;16:1091–8.

[8] Stumvoll M, Chintalapudi U, Perriello G, et al. Uptake and release of glucose by the human kidney. Postabsorptive rates and responses to epinephrine. J Clin Inves 1995;96:2528–33.

[9] Stumvoll M, Meyer C, Perriello G, et al. Human kidney and liver gluconeogenesis: evidence for organ substrate selectivity. Am J Physiol 1998;274:E817–26.

[10] Meyer C, Stumvoll M, Dostou J, et al. Renal substrate exchange and gluconeogenesis in normal postabsorptive humans. Am J Physiol Endocrinol Metab 2002;282:E428–34.

[11] Smith D, DeFronzo RA. Insulin resistance in uremia mediated by postbinding defects. Kidney Int 1982;22:54–62.

[12] Weisinger J, Contreras NE, Cajias J, et al. Insulin binding and glycolytic activity in erythrocytes from dialyzed and non-dialyzed uremic patients. Nephron 1988;48:190–6.

[13] Taylor R, Heaton A, Hetherington CS, et al. Adipocyte insulin binding and insulin action in chronic renal failure before and

during continuous ambulatory peritoneal dialysis. Metabolism 1986;35:430–5.

[14] Pedersen O, Schmitz O, Hjollund E, et al. Postbinding defects of insulin action in human adipocytes from uremic patients. Kidney Int 1985;27:780–4.

[15] Maloff BL, McCaleb ML, Lockwood DH. Cellular basis of insulin resistance in chronic uremia. Am J Physiol 1983;245:E178–84.

[16] Bak J, Schmitz O, Sorensen SS, et al. Activity of insulin receptor kinase and glycogen synthase in skeletal muscle from patients with chronic renal failure. Acta Endocrinol (Copenhagen) 1989;121:744–50.

[17] Cecchin F, Ittoop O, Sinha MK, et al. Insulin resistance in uremia: insulin receptor kinase activity in liver and muscle from chronic uremic rats. Am J Physiol 1988;254:E394–401.

[18] Bailey JL, Mitch WE. Pathophysiology of uremia. In: Brenner B, editor. The Kidney. 7th ed. Philadelpia: Saunders; 2004. p. 2139–64.

[19] White MF. IRS proteins and the common path to diabetes. Am J Physiol Endocrinol Metab 2002;283:E413–22.

[20] Lee YH, White MF. Insulin receptor substrate proteins and diabetes. Arch Pharm Res 2004;27:361–70.

[21] Folli F, Saad MJ, Kahn CR. Insulin receptor/IRS-1/PI 3-kinase signaling system in corticosteroid-induced insulin resistance. Acta Diabetol 1996;33:185–92.

[22] Rojas FA, Hirata AE, Saad MJ. Regulation of IRS-2 tyrosine phosphorylation in fasting and diabetes. Mol Cell Endocrinol 2001;183:63–9.

[23] Giorgino F, Pedrini MT, Matera L, et al. Specific increase in p85alpha expression in response to dexamethasone is associated with inhibition of insulin-like growth factor-I stimulated phosphatidylinositol 3-kinase activity in cultured muscle cells. J Biol Chem 1997;272:7455–63.

[24] May RC, Kelly RA, Mitch WE. Mechanisms for defects in muscle protein metabolism in rats with chronic uremia: the influence of metabolic acidosis. J Clin Invest 1987;79:1099–103.

[25] Friedman JE, Dohm GL, Elton CW, et al. Muscle insulin resistance in uremic humans: glucose transport, glucose transporters, and insulin receptors. Am J Physiol 1991;261:E87–94.

[26] Kraus LM, Traxinger R, Kraus AP. Uremia and insulin resistance: N-carbamoyl-asparagine decreases insulin-sensitive glucose uptake in rat adipocytes. Kidney Int 2004;65:881–7.

[27] De Fronzo RA, Tobin JD, Rowe JW, et al. Glucose intolerance in uremia: quantification of pancreatic beta cell sensitivity to glucose and tissue sensitivity to insulin. J Clin Invest 1978;62:425–35.

[28] Kobayashi S, Maejima S, Ikeda T, et al. Impact of dialysis therapy on insulin resistance in end-stage renal disease: comparison of haemodialysis and continuous ambulatory peritoneal dialysis. Nephrol Dial Transplant 2000;15:65–70.

[29] Heaton A, Taylor R, Johnston DG, et al. Hepatic and peripheral insulin action in chronic renal failure before and during continuous ambulatory peritoneal dialysis. Clin Sci 1989;77:383–8.

[30] Mak RH. Insulin resistance in uremia: effect of dialysis modality. Pediatr Res 1996;40:304–8.

[31] McCaleb ML, Wish JB, Lockwood DH. Insulin resistance in chronic renal failure. Endocrinol Res 1985;11:113–25.

[32] Dzurik R, Hupkova V, Cernacek P, et al. The isolation of an inhibitor of glucose utilization from the serum of uraemic subjects. Clin Chim Acta 1973;46:77–83.

[33] Spaia S, Pangalos M, Askepidis N, et al. Effect of short-term rHuEPO treatment on insulin resistance in haemodialysis patients. Nephron 2000;84:320–5.

[34] Tuzcu A, Bahceci M, Yilmaz E, et al. The comparison of insulin sensitivity in non-diabetic hemodialysis patients treated with and without recombinant human erythropoietin. Horm Metab Res 2004;36:716–20.

[35] Mak RH. 1,25-Dihydroxyvitamin D_3 corrects insulin and lipid abnormalities in uremia. Kidney Int 1998;53:1353–7.

[36] Kautzky-Willer A, Pacini G, Barnas U, et al. Intravenous calcitriol normalizes insulin sensitivity in uremic patients. Kidney Int 1995;47:200–6.

[37] Gin H, Aparicio M, Potaux L, et al. Low protein and low phosphorus diet in patients with chronic renal failure: influence on glucose tolerance and tissue insulin sensitivity. Metabolism 1987;36:1080–5.

[38] Gin H, Aparicio M, Potaux L, et al. Low-protein, low-phosphorus diet and tissue insulin sensitivity in insulin-dependent diabetic patients with chronic renal failure. Nephron 1991;57:411–5.

[39] Mak R, Turner C, Thompson T, et al. The effect of a low protein diet with amino acid/keto acid supplements on glucose metabolism in children with uremia. J Clin Endocrinol Metab 1986;63:985–9.

[40] Kuku SF, Jaspan JB, Emmanouel DS, et al. Heterogeneity of plasma glucagon-circulating components in normal subjects and patients with chronic renal failure. J Clin Invest 1976;58:742–50.

[41] Emmanouel DS, Jaspan JB, Kuku SF, et al. Pathogenesis and characterization of hyperglucagonemia in the uremic rat. J Clin Invest 1976;58:1266–72.

[42] DeFronzo RA, Tobin J, Boden G, et al. The role of growth hormone in the glucose intolerance of uremia. Acta Diabetol Lat 1979;16:279–86.

[43] Ijaiya K. Pattern of growth hormone response to insulin, arginine and haemodialysis in uraemic children. Eur J Pediatr 1979;131:185–98.

[44] Ross RJ, Goodwin FJ, Houghton BJ, et al. Alteration of pituitary-thyroid function in patients with chronic renal failure treated by haemodialysis or continuous ambulatory peritoneal dialysis. Ann Clin Biochem 1985;22:156–60.

[45] Ramirez G, Bittle PA, Sanders H, et al. The effects of corticotropin and growth hormone releasing hormones on their respective secretory axes in chronic hemodialysis patients before and after correction of anemia with recombinant human erythropoietin. J Clin Endocrinol Metab 1994;78:63–9.

[46] Mak RH. Effect of metabolic acidosis on insulin action and secretion in uremia. Kidney Int 1998;54:603–7.

[47] Kraut JA, Madias NE. Consequences and therapy of the metabolic acidosis of chronic kidney disease. Pediatr Nephrol 2011;26:19–28.

[48] Schenk S, Saberi M, Olefsky JM. Insulin sensitivity: modulation by nutrients and inflammation. J Clin Invest 2008;118:2992–3002.

[49] Gual P, Le Marchand-Brustel Y, Tanti JF. Positive and negative regulation of insulin signaling through IRS-1 phosphorylation. Biochimie 2005;87:99–109.

[50] Rocha VZ, Folco EJ. Inflammatory concepts of obesity. Int J Inflam 2011;2011:529061.

[51] Hotamisligil GS, Murray DL, Choy LN, et al. Tumor necrosis factor alpha inhibits signaling from the insulin receptor. Proc Natl Acad Sci USA 1994;91:4854–8.

[52] Hotamisligil GS. Inflammatory pathways and insulin action. Int J Obes Relat Metab Disord 2003;27:S53–5.

[53] Ikizler TA. Nutrition, inflammation and chronic kidney disease. Curr Opin Nephrol Hypertens 2008;17:162–7.

[54] Chance WT, Fischer JE. Aphagic and adipsic effects of interleukin-1. Brain Res 1991;568:261–4.

[55] Kuhlmann MK, Levin NW. Potential interplay between nutrition and inflammation in dialysis patients. Contrib Nephrol 2008;161:76–82.

[56] Kalantar-Zadeh K, Kopple JD, Humphreys MH, et al. Comparing outcome predictability of markers of malnutrition-inflammation complex syndrome in haemodialysis patients. Nephrol Dial Transplant 2004;19:1507—19.

[57] da Costa JA, Ikizler TA. Inflammation and insulin resistance as novel mechanisms of wasting in chronic dialysis patients. Semin Dial 2009;22:652—7.

[58] Folli F, Kahn CR, Hansen H, et al. Angiotensin II inhibits insulin signaling in aortic smooth muscle cells at multiple levels. A potential role for serine phosphorylation in insulin/angiotensin II crosstalk. J Clin Invest 1997;100:2158—69.

[59] Folli F, Saad MJ, Velloso L, et al. Crosstalk between insulin and angiotensin II signalling systems. Exp Clin Endocrinol Diabetes 1999;107:133—9.

[60] Satirapoj B, Yingwatanadej P, Chaichayanon S, et al. Effect of angiotensin II receptor blockers on insulin resistance in maintenance haemodialysis patients. Nephrology (Carlton) 2007;12: 342—7.

[61] Trirogoff ML, Shintani A, Himmelfarb J, et al. Body mass index and fat mass are the primary correlates of insulin resistance in nondiabetic stage 3-4 chronic kidney disease patients. Am J Clin Nutr 2007;86:1642—8.

[62] Ramos LF, Shintani A, Ikizler TA, et al. Oxidative stress and inflammation are associated with adiposity in moderate to severe CKD. J Am Soc Nephrol 2008;19:593—9.

[63] Rea R, Donnelly R. Resistin: an adipocyte-derived hormone. Has it a role in diabetes and obesity? Diabetes Obes Metab 2004;6:163.

[64] Kielstein JT, Becker B, Graf S, et al. Increased resistin blood levels are not associated with insulin resistance in patients with renal disease. Am J Kidney Dis 2003;42:62—6.

[65] Stuart CA, Shangraw RE, Prince MJ, et al. Bed-rest-induced insulin resistance occurs primarily in muscle. Metabolism 1988;37:802—6.

[66] Goldberg AP, Hagberg J, Delmez JA, et al. The metabolic and psychological effects of exercise training in hemodialysis patients. Am J Clin Nutr 1980;33:1620—8.

[67] Goldberg AP, Hagberg JM, Delmez JA, et al. Metabolic effects of exercise training in hemodialysis patients. Kidney Int 1980;18: 754—61.

[68] Fadda GZ, Hajjar SM, Perna AF, et al. On the mechanism of impaired insulin secretion in chronic renal failure. J Clin Invest 1991;87:255—61.

[69] Fadda GZ, Thanakitcharu P, Comunale R, et al. Impaired potassium-induced insulin secretion in chronic renal failure. Kidney Int 1991;40:413—7.

[70] Nakamura Y, Yoshida T, Kajiyama S, et al. Insulin release from column-perifused isolated islets of uremic rats. Nephron 1985;40:467—9.

[71] Oh HY, Fadda GZ, Smogorzewski M, et al. Abnormal leucine-induced insulin secretion in chronic renal failure. Am J Physiol 1994;267:F853—60.

[72] Mak RH, Bettinelli A, Turner C, et al. The influence of hyperparathyroidism on glucose metabolism in uremia. J Clin Endocrinol Metab 1985;60:229—33.

[73] Mak RH, Turner C, Haycock GB, et al. Secondary hyperparathyroidism and glucose intolerance in children with uremia. Kidney Int 1983;24:S128—33.

[74] Fadda GZ, Akmal M, Premdas FH, et al. Insulin release from pancreatic islets: effects of CRF and excess PTH. Kidney Int 1988;33:1066—72.

[75] Perna AF, Fadda GZ, Zhou XJ, et al. Mechanisms of impaired insulin secretion after chronic excess of parathyroid hormone. Am J Physiol 1990;259:F210—6.

[76] Milner RD. Stimulation of insulin secretion in vitro by essential amino acids. Lancet 1969;1:1075—6.

[77] Oberwetter JM, Boyd 3rd AE. High K$^+$ rapidly stimulates Ca^{2+}-dependent phosphorylation of three protein concomitant with insulin secretion from HIT cells. Diabetes 1987;36:864—71.

[78] Mak RH, Betinelli A, Turner C, et al. The influence of hyperparathyroidism on glucose metabolism in uremia. J Clin Endocrinol Metab 1985;60:229—33.

[79] Mak RH, Turner C, Haycock GB, Chantler C. Secondary hyperparathyroidism and glucose intolerance in children with uremia. Kidney Int 1983;24:S128—33.

[80] Christakos S, Norman AW. Studies on the mode of action of calciferol XXXIX: biochemical characterization of 1,25-dihydroxyvitamin D$_3$ receptors in chick pancreas and kidney cytosol. Endocrinology 1981;108:140—9.

[81] Pike JW. Receptors for 1,25-dihydroxyvitamin D$_3$ in chick pancreas: a partial physical and functional characterization. J Steroid Biochem 1981;16:385—95.

[82] Roth J, Bonner-Weir S, Norman AW, et al. Immunocytochemistry of vitamin D-dependent calcium binding protein in chick pancreas: exclusive localization in β cells. Endocrinology 1982;110:2216—8.

[83] Narbaitz R, Stumpf WE, Sar M. The role of autoradiographic and immunocytochemical techniques in the clarification of sites of metabolism and action of vitamin D. J Histochem Cytochem 1981;29:91—100.

[84] Norman AW, Frankel BJ, Heldt AW, et al. Vitamin D$_3$ deficiency inhibits pancreatic secretion of insulin. Science 1980;209: 823—5.

[85] Cade C, Norman AW. Vitamin D$_3$ improves impaired glucose tolerance and insulin secretion in the vitamin D-deficient rat in vivo. Endocrinology 1986;119:84—90.

[86] Mak RH. Intravenous 1,25-dihydroxycholecalciferol corrects glucose intolerance in hemodialysis patients. Kidney Int 1992;41:1049—54.

[87] Rabkin R, Rubenstein AH, Colwell JA. Glomerular filtration and maximal tubular absorption of insulin (^{125}I). Am J Physiol 1972;223:1093—6.

[88] Rubenstein AH, Mako ME, Horwitz DL. Insulin and the kidney. Nephron 1975;15:306—26.

[89] Rabkin R, Jones J, Kitabchi AE. Insulin extraction from the renal peritubular circulation in the chicken. Endocrinology 1977;101: 1828—33.

[90] Rabkin R, Simon NM, Steiner S, et al. Effect of renal disease on renal uptake and excretion of insulin in man. N Engl J Med 1970;282:182—7.

[91] Rabkin R, Unterhalter SA, Duckworth WC. Effect of prolonged uremia on insulin metabolism by isolated liver and muscle. Kidney Int 1979;16:433—9.

[92] Meyer C, Stumvoll M, Dostou J, et al. Renal substrate exchange gluconeogenesis in normal postabsorptive humans. Am J Physiol 2002;282:E428—34.

[93] Mather A, Pollock C. Glucose handling by the kidney. Kidney Int 2011;79:S1—6.

[94] Garber AJ, Bier DM, Cryer PE, et al. Hypoglycemia in compensated chronic renal insufficiency: substrate limitations of gluconeogenesis. Diabetes 1974;23:982—6.

[95] Nadkarni M, Berns JS, Rudnick MR, et al. Hypoglycemia with hyperinsulinemia in a chronic hemodialysis patient following parathyroidectomy. Nephron 1992;60:100—3.

[96] Arem R. Hypoglycemia associated with renal failure. Endocrinol Metab Clin North Am 1989;18:103—21.

[97] Moen MF, Zhan M, Hsu VD, et al. Frequency of hypoglycemia and its significance in chronic kidney disease. Clin J Am Soc Nephrol 2009;4:1121—7.

[98] Jackson MA, Holland MR, Nicholas J, et al. Occult hypoglycemia caused by hemodialysis. Clin Nephrol 1999;51:242—7.

[99] Takahashi A, Kubota T, Shibahara N, et al. The mechanism of hypoglycemia caused by hemodialysis. Clin Nephrol 2004;62: 362–8.

[100] Gonzalez AR, Khurana RC, Jung Y, et al. Enhanced response to tolbutamide in uremia. Acta Diabetol Lat 1972;9:373–86.

[101] Krepinsky J, Ingram AJ, Clase CM. Prolonged sulfonylurea-induced hypoglycemia in diabetic patients with end-stage renal disease. Am J Kidney Dis 2000;35:500–5.

[102] Ferrannini E, Buzzigoli G, Bonadonna R, et al. Insulin resistance in essential hypertension. N Engl J Med 1987;317:350–7.

[103] Eckel RH, Yost TJ, Jensen DR. Alterations in lipoprotein lipase in insulin resistance. Int J Obes Relat Metab Disord 1995;19: S16–21.

[104] Chan MK, Varghese Z, Moorhead JF. Lipid abnormalities in uremia, dialysis and transplantation. Kidney Int 1981;19: 625–37.

[105] Roullet JB, Lacour B, Drueke T. Partial correction of lipid disturbances by insulin in experimental renal failure. Contrib Nephrol 1986;50:203–10.

[106] Siew ED, Ikizler TA. Insulin resistance and protein energy metabolism in patients with advanced chronic kidney disease. Semin Dial 2010;23:378–82.

[107] May RC, Clark AS, Goheer A, et al. Identification of specific defects in insulin-mediated muscle metabolism in acute uremia. Kidney Int 1985;28:490–5.

[108] Price SR, Bailey JL, Wang X, et al. Muscle wasting in insulino-penic rats results from activation of the ATP-dependent, ubiquitin-proteasome pathway by a mechanism including gene transcription. J Clin Invest 1996;98:1703–8.

[109] Mitch WE. Insights into the abnormalities of chronic renal disease attributed to malnutrition. J Am Soc Nephrol 2002;13: S22–7.

[110] Ritz E. Metabolic syndrome and kidney disease. Blood Purif 2008;26:59–62.

[111] Johnson RJ, Sanchez-Lozada LG, Nakagawa T. The effect of fructose on renal biology and disease. J Am Soc Nephrol 2010; 21:2036–9.

[112] Kobayashi S, Maejima S, Ikeda T, et al. Impact of dialysis therapy on insulin resistance in end-stage renal disease: comparison of haemodialysis and continuous ambulatory peritoneal dialysis. Nephrol Dial Transplant 2000;15:65–70.

[113] Chu PL, Chiu YL, Lin JW, et al. Effects of low- and high-flux dialyzers on oxidative stress and insulin resistance. Blood Purif 2008;26:213–20.

[114] Williams ME. Management of diabetes in dialysis patients. Curr Diab Rep 2009;9:466–72.

[115] Kalantar-Zadeh K, Derose SF, Nicholas S, et al. Burnt-out diabetes: impact of chronic kidney disease progression on the natural course of diabetes mellitus. J Ren Nutr 2009;19: 33–7.

[116] Sharma R, Rosner MH. Glucose in the dialysate: Historical perspective and possible implications? Hemodial Int 2008;12:221–6.

[117] Reilly JB, Berns JS. Selection and dosing of medications for management of diabetes in patients with advanced kidney disease. Semin Dial 2010;23:163–8.

[118] Schernthaner G, Ritz E, Schernthaner GH. Strict glycaemic control in diabetic patients with CKD or ESRD: beneficial or deadly? Nephrol Dial Transplant 2010;25:2044–7.

[119] Sharif A. Current and emerging antiglycaemic pharmacological therapies: the renal perspective. Nephrology (Carlton) 2011;16: 468–75.

[120] Szeto CC, Chow KM, Kwan BC, et al. New-onset hyperglycemia in nondiabetic Chinese patients started on peritoneal dialysis. Am J Kidney Dis 2007;49:524–32.

[121] Tuzcu A, Bahceci M, Yilmaz ME, et al. The determination of insulin sensitivity in hemodialysis and continuous ambulatory peritoneal dialysis in nondiabetic patients with end-stage renal disease. Saudi Med J 2005;26:786–91.

[122] de Moraes TP, Fortes PC, Ribeiro SC, et al. Comparative analysis of lipid and glucose metabolism biomarkers in non-diabetic hemodialysis and peritoneal dialysis patients. J Bras Nefrol 2011;33:173–9.

[123] Lameire N, Matthys E, Matthys E, et al. Effects of long-term CAPD on carbohydrate and lipid metabolism. Clin Nephrol 1988;30(Suppl. 1):53–8.

[124] Wesołowski P, Saracyn M, Nowak Z, et al. Insulin resistance as a novel therapeutic target in patients with chronic kidney disease treated with dialysis. Pol Arch Med Wewn 2010;120: 54–7.

[125] Fortes PC, de Moraes TP, Mendes JG, et al. Insulin resistance and glucose homeostasis in peritoneal dialysis. Perit Dial Int 2009;29:S145–8.

[126] Gürsu EM, Ozdemir A, Yalinbas B, et al. The effect of icodextrin and glucose-containing solutions on insulin resistance in CAPD patients. Clin Nephrol 2006;66:263–8.

[127] Amici G, Orrasch M, Da Rin G, et al. Hyperinsulinism reduction associated with icodextrin treatment in continuous ambulatory peritoneal dialysis patients. Adv Perit Dial 2001; 17:80–3.

[124] Starzl TE, Marchioro TL, Rifkind D, et al. Factors in successful renal transplantation. Surgery 1964;56:296–318.

[125] Bodziak KA, Hricik DE. New-onset diabetes mellitus after solid organ transplantation. Transpl Int 2009;22:519–30.

[126] Bloom RD, Crutchlow MF. New-onset diabetes mellitus in the kidney recipient: diagnosis and management strategies. Clin J Am Soc Nephrol 2008;3:S38–48.

[127] Cosio FG, Kudva Y, van der Velde M, et al. New onset hyperglycemia and diabetes are associated with increased cardiovascular risk after kidney transplantation. Kidney Int 2005;67:2415–21.

[128] Kasiske BL, Snyder JJ, Gilbertson D, et al. Diabetes mellitus after kidney transplantation in the United States. Am J Transplant 2003;3:178–85.

[129] Roth D, Milgrom M, Esquenazi V, et al. Posttransplant hyperglycemia. Increased incidence in cyclosporine-treated renal allograft recipients. Transplantation 1989;47:278–81.

[130] Revanur VK, Jardine AG, Kingsmore DB, et al. Influence of diabetes mellitus on patient and graft survival in recipients of kidney transplantation. Clin Transplant 2001;15:89–94.

[131] Sharif A, Moore R, Baboolal K. Influence of lifestyle modification in renal transplant recipients with postprandial hyperglycemia. Transplantation 2008;85:353–8.

[132] Matas AJ, Gillingham KJ, Humar A, et al. Transplant diabetes mellitus and acute rejection: impact on kidney transplant outcome. Transplantation 2008;85:338–43.

[133] The Diabetes Control and Complications Trial Research Group. The effect of intensive treatment of diabetes on the development and progression of long-term complications in insulin-dependent diabetes mellitus. N Engl J Med 1993;329: 977–86.

[134] UK Prospective Diabetes Study (UKPDS) Group. Intensive blood glucose control with sulphonylureas or insulin compared with conventional treatment and risk of complications in patients with type 2 diabetes (UKPDS 33). Lancet 1998;352:837–53.

[135] Ohkubo Y, Kishikawa H, Araki E, et al. Intensive insulin therapy prevents the progression of diabetic microvascular complications in Japanese patients with non-insulin-dependent diabetes mellitus: a randomized prospective 6-year study. Diabetes Res Clin Pract 1995;28:103–17.

[136] Patel A, MacMahon S, Chalmers J, et al. Intensive blood glucose control and vascular outcomes in patients with type 2 diabetes. N Engl J Med 2008;358:2560—72.

[137] Schneider CA, Ferrannini E, Defronzo R, et al. Effect of pioglitazoneon cardiovascular outcome in diabetes and chronic kidney disease. J Am Soc Nephrol 2008;19:182—7.

[138] Schernthaner G. Pleiotropic effects of thiazolidinediones on traditional and non-traditional atherosclerotic risk factors. Int J Clin Pract 2009;63:912—29.

[139] Nordio M, Limido A, Maggiore U, et al. Survival in patients treated by long-term dialysis compared with the general population. Am J Kidney Dis 2012;59:819—28.

[140] Morioka T, Emoto M, Tabata T, et al. Glycemic control is a predictor of survival for diabetic patients on hemodialysis. Diabetes Care 2001;24:909—13.

[141] Oomichi T, Emoto M, Tabata T, et al. Impact of glycemic control on survival of diabetic patients on chronic regular hemodialysis: a 7-year observational study. Diabetes Care 2006;29:1496—500.

[142] Hayashino Y, Fukuhara S, Akiba T, et al. Diabetes, glycaemic control and mortality risk in patients on haemodialysis: the Japan Dialysis Outcomes and Practice Pattern Study. Diabetologia 2007;50:1170—7.

[143] Kalantar-Zadeh K, Kopple JD, Regidor DL, et al. A1c and survival in maintenance hemodialysis patients. Diabetes Care 2007;30:1049—55.

[144] Drechsler C, Krane V, Ritz E, et al. Glycemic control and cardiovascular events in diabetic hemodialysis patients. Circulation 2009;120:2421—8.

[145] Williams ME, Lacson Jr E, Teng M, et al. Hemodialyzed type I and type II diabetic patients in the US: characteristics, glycemic control, and survival. Kidney Int 2006;70:1503—9.

[146] Schernthaner G, Stummvoll KH, Muller MM. Glycosylated haemoglobinin in chronic renal failure. Lancet 1979;1(8119):774.

[147] Inaba M, Okuno S, Kumeda Y, et al. Glycated albumin is a better glycemic indicator than glycated hemoglobin values in hemodialysis patients with diabetes: effect of anemia and erythropoietin injection. J Am Soc Nephrol 2007;18:896—903.

[148] Peacock TP, Shihabi ZK, Bleyer AJ, et al. Comparison of glycated albumin and hemoglobin A(1c) levels in diabetic subjects on hemodialysis. Kidney Int 2008;73:1062—8.

[149] Schernthaner G, Barnett AH, Betteridge J. Is the ADA/EASD algorithm for the management of type 2 diabetes (January 2009) based on evidence or opinion? A critical analysis. Diabetologia 2010;53:1258—69.

[150] Pilmore HL. Review: metformin: potential benefits and use in chronic kidney disease. Nephrology (Carlton) 2010;15:412—8.

[151] UK Prospective Diabetes Study (UKPDS) Group. Effect of intensive blood glucose control with metformin on complications in overweight patients with type II diabetes (UKPDS34). Lancet 1998;352:854—65.

[152] Holman RR, Paul SK, Bethel MA, et al. 10-year follow-up of intensive glucose control in type 2 diabetes. N Engl J Med 2008;359:1577—89.

[153] Evans JM, Donnelly LA, Emslie-Smith AM, et al. Metformin and reduced risk of cancer in diabetic patients. BMJ 2005;330:1304—5.

[154] Harrower AD. Pharmacokinetics of oral antihyperglycaemic agents in patients with renal insufficiency. Clin Pharmacokinet 1996;31:111—9.

[155] Nye HJ, Herrington WG. Metformin: the safest hypoglycaemic agent in chronic kidney disease? Nephron Clin Pract 2011;118:c380—3.

[156] Bolen S, Feldman L, Vassy J, et al. Systematic review: comparative effectiveness and safety of oral medications for type 2 diabetes mellitus. Ann Intern Med 2007;147:386—99.

[157] Rendell M. The role of sulphonylureas in the management of type 2 diabetes mellitus. Drugs 2004;64:1339—58.

[158] Balant L, Zahnd G, Gorgia A, et al. Pharmacokinetics of glipizide in man: influence of renal insufficiency. Diabetologia 1973;9:331—8.

[159] Boden G, Zhang M. Recent findings concerning thiazolidinediones in the treatment of diabetes. Expert Opin Investig Drugs 2006;15:243—50.

[160] Budde K, Neumayer HH, Fritsche L, et al. The pharmacokinetics of pioglitazone in patients with impaired renal function. Br J Clin Pharmacol 2003;55:368—74.

[161] Chapelsky MC, Thompson-Culkin K, Miller AK, et al. Pharmacokinetics of rosiglitazone in patients with varying degrees of renal insufficiency. J Clin Pharmacol 2003;43:252—9.

[162] Nissen SE, Wolski K. Effect of rosiglitazone on the risk of myocardial infarction and death from cardiovascular causes. N Engl J Med 2007;356:2457—71.

[163] Singh S, Loke YK, Furberg CD. Long-term risk of cardiovascular events with rosiglitazone: A meta-analysis. JAMA 2007;298:1189—95.

[164] Lincoff AM, Wolski K, Nicholls SJ, et al. Pioglitazone and risk of cardiovascular events in patients with type 2 diabetes mellitus: A meta-analysis of randomized trials. JAMA 2007;298:1180—8.

[165] Schneider CA, Ferrannini E, Defronzo R, et al. Effect of pioglitazone on cardiovascular outcome in diabetes and chronic kidney disease. J Am Soc Nephrol 2008;19:182—7.

[166] Ohtomo S, Izuhara Y, Takizawa S, et al. Thiazolidinediones provide better renoprotection than insulin in an obese, hypertensive type II diabetic rat model. Kidney Int 2007;72:1512—9.

[167] Yang HC, Deleuze S, Zuo Y, et al. The PPARgamma agonist pioglitazone ameliorates aging-related progressive renal injury. J Am Soc Nephrol 2009;20:2380—8.

[168] Lewis JD, Ferrara A, Peng T, et al. Risk of bladder cancer among diabetic patients treated with pioglitazone: interim report of a longitudinal cohort study. Diabetes Care 2011;34:916—22.

[169] Piccinni C, Motola D, Marchesini G, et al. Assessing the association of pioglitazone use and bladder cancer through drug adverse event reporting. Diabetes Care 2011;34:1369—71.

[170] Dornhorst A. Insulinotropic meglitinide analogues. Lancet 2001;358:1709—16.

[171] Lotfy M, Singh J, Kalász H, et al. Medicinal chemistry and applications of incretins and DPP-4 inhibitors in the treatment of type 2 diabetes mellitus. Open Med Chem J 2011;5:82—92.

[172] Marbury TC, Ruckle JL, Hatorp V, et al. Pharmacokinetics of repaglinide in subjects with renal impairment. Clin Pharmacol Ther 2000;67:7—15.

[173] Gromada J, Brock B, Schmitz O, Rorsman P. Glucagon-like peptide-1: regulation of insulin secretion and therapeutic potential. Basic Clin Pharmacol Toxicol 2004;95:252—62.

[174] Linnebjerg H, Kothare PA, Park S, et al. Effect of renal impairment on the pharmacokinetics of exenatide. Br J Clin Pharmacol 2007;64:317—27.

[175] Subbarayan S, Kipnes M. Sitagliptin: a review. Expert Opin Pharmacother 2011;12:1613—22.

[176] Herman GA, Stevens C, Van Dyck K, et al. Pharmacokinetics and pharmacodynamics of sitagliptin, an inhibitor of dipeptidyl peptidase IV, in healthy subjects: results from two randomized, double-blind, placebo-controlled studies with single oral doses. Clin Pharmacol Ther 2005;78:675—88.

[177] Bergman AJ, Cote J, Yi B, Marbury T, et al. Effect of renal insufficiency on the pharmacokinetics of sitagliptin, a dipeptidyl peptidase-4 inhibitor. Diabetes Care 2007;30:1862—4.

[178] Barnett AH. Linagliptin: a novel dipeptidyl peptidase 4 inhibitor with a unique place in therapy. adv Ther 2011;28:447—59.

[179] Graefe-Mody U, Friedrich C, Port A, et al. Effect of renal impairment on the pharmacokinetics of the dipeptidyl

peptidase-4 inhibitor linagliptin. Diabetes Obes Metab 2011;13: 939–46.

[180] Yamagishi S, Matsui T, Ueda S, et al. Clinical utility of acarbose, an alpha-glucosidase inhibitor in cardiometabolic disorders. Curr Drug Metab 2009;10:159–63.

[181] Spengler M, Schmitz H, Landen H. Evaluation of the efficacy and tolerability of acarbose in patients with diabetes mellitus: a post-marketing surveillance study. Clin Drug Investig 2005;25:651–9.

[182] Ersoy A, Ersoy C, Altinay T. Insulin analogue usage in a hae-modialysis patient with type 2 diabetes mellitus. Nephrol Dial Transplant 2006;21:553–4.

[183] Czock D, Aisenpreis U, Rasche FM, et al. Pharmacokinetics and pharmacodynamics of lispro-insulin in hemodialysis

patients with diabetes mellitus. Int J Clin Pharmacol Ther 2003; 41:492–7.

[184] O'Mara NB. Agents for the treatment of diabetes mellitus. Semin Dial 2010;23:475–9.

[185] Aronoff GR, Berns JS, Brier ME, et al. Dosing Guidelines for Adults. 4th ed. Philadelphia: American College of Physicians; 1999. Drug prescribing in renal failure; p. 84.

[186] Shrishrimal K, Hart P, Michota F. Managing diabetes in hemo-dialysis patients: observations and recommendations. Cleve Clin J Med 2009;76:649–55.

[187] Johnson JA, Gale EA. Diabetes, insulin use, and cancer risk: are observational studies part of the solution — or part of the problem? Diabetes 2010;59:1129–31.

Altered Lipid Metabolism and Serum Lipids in Kidney Disease and Kidney Failure

Nosratola D. Vaziri

Division of Nephrology and Hypertension, Departments of Medicine, Physiology and Biophysics, University of California, Irvine, California, USA

INTRODUCTION

During the past two decades the burden of chronic kidney disease (CKD) has dramatically increased worldwide, consuming a disproportionate share of the health care resources. CKD is associated with the triad of oxidative stress, inflammation and dyslipidemia which are causally interconnected and form a vicious circuit that drives progression of kidney disease and promotes cardiovascular disease, cachexia-malnutrition syndrome, anemia, and many other complications. This chapter is intended to provide an overview of the features and mechanisms of CKD-associated dyslipidemia, and its role in amplification of inflammation and oxidative stress, disturbance of energy metabolism, progression of renal disease and cardiovascular and other complications.

PLASMA LIPID AND LIPOPROTEIN PROFILE IN CKD/ESRD PATIENTS

Dyslipidemia in patients with non-nephrotic CKD and in ESRD patients maintained on hemodialysis is characterized by hyper-triglyceridemia, elevated plasma concentrations of very low density lipoprotein (VLDL), intermediate density lipoprotein (IDL) and chylomicron remnants, accumulation of oxidized lipids and lipoproteins, low plasma concentration of ApoA1 and HDL cholesterol [1–3]. Unlike patients with heavy proteinuria who have hypercholesterolemia, serum cholesterol and low density lipoprotein (LDL) cholesterol values are frequently within or below the normal limits in hemodialysis-treated ESRD patients and CKD patients without nephrotic proteinuria. In addition LDL in these patients consists of highly atherogenic small-dense particles

which contain abnormal levels of residual triglycerides [3–7]. Finally plasma concentration lipoprotein(a), [Lp(a)] particularly its low molecular variety is elevated and contributes to the risk of cardiovascular events in CKD/ESRD patients [8,9].

Conditions that Modify Lipid Profile in CKD/ESRD

Several conditions significantly modify lipid profile in CKD or ESRD populations. These include dialysis modality (i.e. hemodialysis vs. peritoneal dialysis), lipid-altering drugs (e.g. statins, fibrates, calcineurin inhibitors, steroids, rapamycin, etc.), pre-existing genetic disorders of lipid metabolism, malnutrition and inflammation among others. In addition by acting as a bile acid sequestrant, the commonly prescribed phosphate binding resin, sevelamer, lowers plasma cholesterol concentration. Likewise, inflammation which is a common feature of ESRD, can lower serum total cholesterol and further suppress HDL cholesterol levels. In contrast by simulating nephrotic syndrome [10,11], peritoneal dialysis which results in substantial losses of proteins in the peritoneal dialysate effluent, can significantly increase plasma LDL and total cholesterol concentrations. In addition influx of large quantities of glucose from the peritoneal fluid can further raise plasma triglyceride levels in patients maintained on peritoneal dialysis.

THE NATURE AND MECHANISMS OF CKD-INDUCED LIPID ABNORMALITIES

HDL Metabolism and Function

Normal HDL is a potent antioxidant, anti-inflammatory and anti-atherogenic component of the plasma.

HDL protect against foam cell formation and atherosclerosis by preventing the influx and promoting efflux of cholesterol in the macrophages in the artery wall. The combination of oxidative stress, structurally abnormal LDL, and the over abundance and prolonged plasma residence time of IDL and chylomicron remnants in CKD results in oxidation of LDL, lipoprotein remnants and phospholipids. Once oxidized, these particles stimulate expression of scavenger receptors [e.g. oxidized LDL receptor-1 (LOX-1) and scavenger receptor A-1 (SRA1)] in macrophages and resident cells in the artery wall. The scavenger receptors then engulf these oxidized lipids and lipoproteins, a process that is central to foam cell formation and atherosclerosis.

Normal HDL mitigates influx of lipids and lipoproteins in the macrophages by preventing or reversing lipid peroxidation via its potent anti-oxidant enzymes i.e. paraoxonase-1(PON-1) and glutathione peroxidase (GPX). In addition by raising endothelial production of nitric oxide and inhibiting release of chemokines, normal HDL limits monocyte adhesion and infiltration in the artery wall. Via these actions, normal HDL mitigates foam cell formation by limiting influx of cholesterol and inhibiting monocyte adhesion and infiltration in the artery wall and other tissues.

The other important and well-known mechanism of anti-atherogenic action of HDL is reverse cholesterol transport (RCT) which involves extraction of surplus cholesterol and phospholipids from the lipid laden cells for disposal in the liver. The HDL-mediated RCT involves the following steps: A- binding of nascent, cholesterol ester (CE)-poor HDL to the adenosine triphosphate binding cassette A-1 (ABCA-1) which is the gateway of cholesterol efflux on the surface of the target cell. HDL binding to ABCA-1 triggers de-esterification of intracellular CE leading to release of free cholesterol and its migration to the cell surface and from there to the surface of HDL. B- re-esterification of free cholesterol on the surface of HDL by lecithin cholesterol-acyltransferase (LCAT) which is an essential component of HDL complex. Due to its hydrophobic property CE moves to the core of HDL, a process that by sustaining a favorable concentration gradient maximizes the uptake of cellular cholesterol and maturation of HDL to a CE-rich spherical particle. (C) Once matured, HDL detaches from the cell surface and travels to the liver where it binds to the scavenger receptor-B1 (SR-B1) which is expressed on the hepatocyte and serves as a docking receptor for the mature HDL. Binding to SRB-1 facilitates disposal of the HDL's CE cargo in the liver and clearance of its phospholipid and triglyceride by hepatic lipase. Once emptied, HDL detaches from the hepatocyte and is released in the circulation. In contrast to the CE-rich HDL, CE-poor HDL particles have low affinity for SRB-1 and a high affinity for binding to a novel endocytic receptor (ATP synthase beta) which is expressed on the hepatocytes and mediates removal and degradation of these particles [12].

Effect of CKD on Structure and Function of HDL

As described in a comprehensive review [13], CKD has a profound effect on the concentration, structure and antioxidant, anti-inflammatory and reverse cholesterol transport activities of HDL [14–17]. This is primarily due to: (A) Downregulation of hepatic biosynthesis and reduced plasma level of ApoA-1 which is the main protein component of HDL, the ligand for the HDL's loading and unloading receptors (ABCA1 and SRB-1, respectively), and the principal carrier of HDL's lipid cargo [18–20]. Deficiency of ApoA-1 plays an important part in HDL deficiency and dysfunction in CKD. (B) The other important cause of CKD-associated HDL deficiency and dysfunction is reduced plasma concentration and enzymatic activity of LCAT which is due to its reduced hepatic production in CKD [21,22] and its urinary losses in nephrotic syndrome [23]. The acquired LCAT deficiency in CKD is largely responsible for depressed HDL-mediated RCT, impaired HDL maturation and reduced plasma HDL cholesterol which collectively contributes to the atherogenic diathesis in this population. (C) CKD results in diminished plasma activity and concentration of paraoxonase and glutathione peroxidase [14,16] which contribute to reduction of antioxidant capacity of HDL, thereby limiting its ability to prevent/reverse oxidation of LDL and remnant lipoproteins. Moreover, deficiency of these antioxidant enzymes heightens susceptibility of ApoA-1 to oxidative modification which limits the binding affinity of HDL to ABCA-1 and, thereby, negatively affects RCT [24]. (D) CKD results in diminished anti-inflammatory capacity of HDL [16,17] which normally protects against plaque formation by raising nitric oxide production and inhibiting endothelial cell activation and monocyte adhesion and infiltration. (E) When present, nephrotic proteinuria, results in marked reduction of hepatic HDL docking receptor (SR-B1) protein abundance but not its transcript [19]. This can interfere with the HDL-mediated RCT by limiting the disposal of HDL's cholesterol cargo. The observed reduction in hepatic SRB-1 protein abundance is due to downregulation of the adapter molecule, PDZK1, which is essential for the transport and anchoring of the receptor to the hepatocyte plasma membrane [25]. (F) Deficiency of the hepatic HDL docking receptor is compounded by upregulation of HDL endocytic receptor (Beta ATP synthase) in CKD with, but not without, heavy proteinuria [25,26]. This can contribute to the HDL deficiency by raising its catabolism, (G) oxidative modification of HDL which diminishes its ability to promote cholesterol efflux by limiting its binding affinity for ABCA-1 [24]. And finally, (H) hypo-albuminemia which is common in patients with advanced CKD may contribute to the reduction of HDL cholesterol and plaque formation, since albumin shuttles substantial amounts of free cholesterol from the peripheral tissues to the circulating cholesterol-poor HDL particles [27].

Together the abnormalities of HDL metabolism, structure and function outlined above heavily contribute to the prevailing inflammation and cardiovascular disease in the CKD population. The effects of non-nephrotic CKD or ESRD on HDL metabolism and its adverse consequences are summarized in Figure 3.1.

Effects of CKD on VLDL and Chylomicron Metabolism

VLDL and chylomicrons are triglyceride-rich lipoproteins which deliver endogenous and dietary lipid fuels and construction material to the myocytes, adipocytes and other cell types for production and storage of energy and incorporation in the cellular structures. Metabolism of VLDL and chylomicrons is markedly impaired in CKD. The nascent VLDL particles are assembled in the liver and nascent chylomicrons are packaged in the intestinal cells and released in the circulation. Once released in the circulation the nascent

VLDL and chylomicrons receive Apo E and ApoC from cholesterol-rich HDL-2 particles. Acquisition of ApoE and ApoC is essential for maturation and subsequent clearance of VLD and chylomicrons in the peripheral tissues. However, scarcity of CE-rich HDL (caused by LCAT deficiency) in CKD severely impede this essential process. Normally, chylomicrons and VLDL, bind to the endothelial surface of the capillaries perfusing muscles and adipose tissues via ApoE and activate endothelial-bound lipoprotein lipase via Apo C-2. Once activated, lipoprotein lipase hydrolyses the triglyceride contents of these particles. This leads to release of over 70% of free fatty acid contents of these particles for uptake by myocytes and adipocytes. The particles are then released in the circulation as VLDL remnants also known as IDL and chylomicron remnants. CKD results in significant reduction of lipoprotein lipase abundance and activity in skeletal muscle, adipose tissue and myocardium [28–30]. This is accompanied by downregulation of the endothelium-derived adapter molecule, glycosylphosphatidylinositol-anchored binding protein 1 (GPIHBP1) which plays a critical role in LPL metabolism and function by anchoring LPL on the endothelium and binding chylomicrons [31]. Consequently deficiencies of lipoprotein lipase and its adapter molecule, GPIHBP1, in CKD severely impair metabolism of VLDL and chylomicrons.

CM remnants and a portion of IDL are cleared from the circulation by LDL receptor-related protein (LRP) which is a large multi-functional endocytic receptor expressed in hepatocytes [32]. In an earlier study we found significant downregulation of hepatic LRP in animals with CKD [33]. Given the central role of

Effects of non-nephrotic CKD or ESRD on HDL metabolism

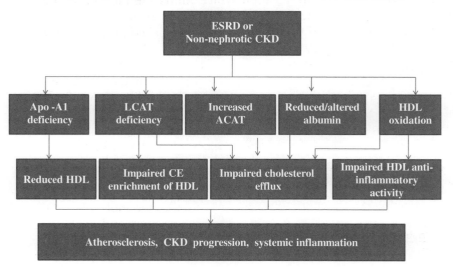

FIGURE 3.1 The non-nephrotic CKD or ESRD results in diminished production and depressed plasma levels of Apo-A1 and LCAT, upregulation of ACAT, reduced plasma concentration and structural modification of albumin, and oxidative modification of HDL. These events lead to reduced HDL cholesterol, impaired antioxidant, anti-inflammatory and reverse cholesterol transport capacities of HDL which collectively promote atherosclerosis, systemic inflammation and CKD progression.

LRP in removing chylomicron remnants, its deficiency contributes to elevated plasma level of these oxidation-prone atherogenic particles in CKD.

Under normal condition the great majority of IDLs are converted to LDL which is a cholesterol ester-rich lipoprotein and is avidly cleared by the liver via LDL receptor. The transformation of IDL to LDL requires removal of triglyceride cargo and cholesterol ester enrichment of IDL. These events are catalyzed by cholesterol ester transfer protein (CETP) and hepatic lipase. CETP-mediates exchange of triglycerides for cholesterol ester between IDL and CE-rich HDL2 particles and hepatic lipase catalyzes hydrolysis of the triglyceride and phospholipid contents of IDL. Although plasma CETP activity and concentration are normal in ESRD [34], the scarcity of CE-rich HDL particles limits the ability of CETP to fulfill its normal function. Moreover, CKD is associated with downregulation of hepatic lipase [35—37] which contributes to accumulation of IDL and formation of CE-poor, triglyceride containing small dense LDL. These abnormal LDL particles are highly oxidation prone and atherogenic and have low binding affinity for LDL receptor. Normally a fraction of VLDL is cleared from the circulation via endocytosis by VLDL receptor which is expressed by myocytes and adipocytes [38]. In an earlier study we found significant downregulation of VLDL receptor expression in the skeletal muscle and adipose tissues in animals with CKD [39,40]. This abnormality can potentially contribute to elevation of plasma VLDL and hypertriglyceridemia and thus compound the effects of lipoprotein lipase, hepatic lipase and LRP

deficiencies and impaired HDL maturation on VLDL and IDL metabolism in CKD. The effect of non-nephrotic CKD or ESRD on metabolism of triglyceride-rich lipoproteins and its adverse consequences are summarized in Figure 3.2.

Effect of CKD on Cholesterol Metabolism

As mentioned above, plasma total cholesterol and LDL cholesterol levels are frequently within or below the normal limits in non-nephrotic CKD patients and ESRD patients receiving hemodialysis therapy. In addition, HMG-CoA reductase expression and activity is normal in the liver of animals with non-nephrotic CKD, induced by subtotal nephrectomy [41]. Moreover hepatic expression of LDL receptor, HDL docking receptor and activity of the cholesterol 7-alpha hydroxylase, the enzyme responsible for conversion of cholesterol to bile acids are normal in these animals [19,42].

Despite having normal or subnormal plasma cholesterol and LDL cholesterol levels and presumably normal cholesterol biosynthesis and cholesterol clearing capacities, the risk of atherosclerosis and cardiovascular disease is greatly increased in CKD patients. In fact, CKD animals exhibit accumulation of cholesterol in the remnant kidney and artery wall [43—45]. This is associated with and driven by oxidation of lipids and lipoproteins, upregulation of scavenger receptor A-1 and oxidized LDL receptor-1 (LOX-1) and acyl-CoA cholesterol acyltransferase (ACAT-1, the enzyme responsible for intracellular

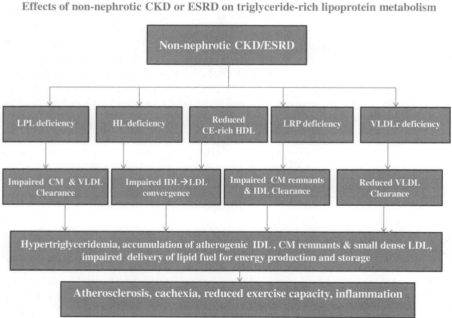

Effects of non-nephrotic CKD or ESRD on triglyceride-rich lipoprotein metabolism

FIGURE 3.2 The non-nephrotic CKD or ESRD results in downregulation of skeletal muscle, adipose tissue and myocardial lipoprotein lipase (LPL) and VLDL receptor (VLDLr), hepatic lipase (HL), LDL receptor related protein (LRP) and marked reduction of plasma cholesterol ester (CE)-rich HDL. Together these abnormalities lead to impaired clearance of chylomicrons and VLDL, accumulation of oxidation-prone atherogenic chylomicron remnants and IDL, formation of small dense LDL, increased plasma triglyceride concentration and reduced delivery of lipid fuel for energy production in myocytes and storage in adipocytes. Accumulation of the atherogenic chylomicron remnants and IDL and formation of small dense LDL promote atherosclerosis and systemic inflammation whereas reduced LPL- and VLDLr-mediated delivery of lipid fuel contributes to cachexia and reduced exercise capacity.

sequestration of cholesterol ester and foam cell formation) in the artery wall and diseased kidney [43–46]. These observations illustrate the critical role of oxidative stress and inflammation as opposed to elevated plasma cholesterol or increased cholesterol biosynthesis as the cause of atherosclerosis in CKD. It is, therefore, not surprising that clinical trials of statins have proven ineffective in lowering the incidence of cardiovascular disease in patients with ESRD maintained on hemodialysis.

When present, nephrotic proteinuria compounds the effect of renal insufficiency by raising cholesterol biosynthesis (upregulation of HMG-CoA reductase) and limiting cholesterol clearance (inducing LDL receptor and HDL docking receptor deficiencies) and, thereby, causing hypercholesterolemia [10,26,47].

THE NATURE AND MECHANISMS OF ADVERSE EFFECTS OF LIPID DISORDERS IN CKD

Alterations of lipid metabolism have far-reaching consequences and contribute to numerous CKD-associated disorders and complications [48,49]. Some of these effects are briefly described below.

Inflammation and Oxidative Stress

As noted above, the CKD-induced constellation of lipoprotein lipase, hepatic lipase and LRP deficiencies and scarcity of cholesterol ester-rich HDL results in extended residence time and accumulation of IDL and chylomicron remnants in the plasma and formation of small dense LDL. The IDL, chylomicron remnants, and small dense LDL particles are exquisitely susceptible to oxidation, a phenomenon which is amplified by the prevailing oxidative stress and HDL deficiency and dysfunction in the CKD population. In fact, plasma concentration of oxidized LDL and lipid peroxidation products is markedly increased in patients and animals with CKD. Oxidized LDL and remnant particles promote inflammation by avidly binding LOX-1, SRA-1 and oxidized phospholipid receptors on monocytes and macrophages, thereby triggering release of proinflammatory cytokines. Riding in the circulating blood these particles can disseminate inflammation throughout the body. Likewise, through lipid peroxidation chain reaction, oxidized lipoproteins can contribute to dissemination and amplification of oxidative stress which is a constant feature of CKD. Accordingly the author believes that dysregulation of lipid metabolism in CKD plays a part in the pathogenesis of systemic inflammation and oxidative stress which are constant features and major mediators of progression of CKD and its cardiovascular and many other complications [49].

Atherosclerosis and Cardiovascular Disease

CKD results in accelerated atherosclerosis and cardiovascular disease which are the main cause of death in this population [50–52]. In addition to the classic atherosclerosis several other conditions contribute to cardiovascular disease in the CKD/ESRD population. These include arteriosclerosis which is marked by stiffening of the arteries, endothelial dysfunction, vascular calcification, myocardial fibrosis, cardiomyocyte/capillary mismatch, dilated cardiomyopathy, and sudden cardiac death [53–56]. These disorders are mediated by hypertension, hypervolemia, phosphate retention, reduced nitric oxide availability (caused by oxidative stress and accumulation of NO synthase inhibitor, asymmetrical dimethylarginine), electrolyte abnormalities, myocardial fibrosis and ischemia (triggering arrhythmias), and drug toxicities among other conditions.

Atherosclerosis in CKD is primarily driven by the prevailing oxidative stress and inflammation as opposed to elevated plasma cholesterol concentration [57]. On the contrary, observational studies have shown an association between low plasma cholesterol and increased risk of cardiovascular and overall mortality in ESRD population [58] and a greater survival in those with higher serum total and LDL cholesterol values [59]. It should be noted however, that the association between higher plasma cholesterol levels with a lower mortality in ESRD patients is most likely related to the cholesterol-lowering action of systemic inflammation as opposed to the salutary effect of high cholesterol concentrations.

Although hypercholesterolemia in patients with familial hypercholesterolemia, chronic nephrotic syndrome, high dietary cholesterol or other causes can lead to atherosclerosis and cardiovascular disease, accelerated atherosclerosis frequently occurs in the absence of hypercholesterolemia in patients with type 2 diabetes and patients with CKD and ESRD [13,60,61]. This is not surprising since relatively small amounts of cholesterol are sufficient to form plaques capable of causing serious cardiovascular events by occluding coronary, cerebral or peripheral arteries. Therefore, disorders that increase influx and/or impair efflux of cholesterol in the macrophages can cause atherosclerosis and cardiovascular disease even when plasma cholesterol is below the normal limits. This is clearly illustrated by the failure of the cholesterol lowering strategies to lower cardiovascular events in the randomized clinical trial of various statin in ESRD patients maintained on hemodialysis [62–64]. The primary mechanism of accelerated atherosclerosis in CKD/ESRD patients is oxidation of small dense LDL, chyomicron remnants and IDL and their avid uptake by macrophages. The increased cholesterol influx is compounded by HDL deficiency and dysfunction which limit reverse cholesterol transport in CKD. Consequently the atherogenic process in highly inflamed patients with CKD proceeds relentlessly regardless of plasma cholesterol level and despite use of cholesterol lowering agents.

Lipotoxicity and its Role in Progression of Kidney Disease

The prevailing oxidative stress in CKD results in accumulation of oxidized lipids and other molecules in the body fluids and tissues [65–67]. Macrophages and mesangial cells in the diseased kidney avidly engulfed oxidized lipids and lipoproteins [68]. Accumulation of lipid in the renal tissue can promote progression of glomerular and tubulo-interstitial lesions in metabolic syndrome [68,69], and in chronic glomerular diseases [70,71]. In fact progression of renal disease in the animals with CKD induced by subtotal nephrectomy is accompanied by heavy accumulation of lipids in the glomeruli and proximal tubular epithelial cells [43] and in the artery wall [44]. Accumulation of lipids in the non-adipose tissues can cause cellular injury and dysfunction [72] as seen in hepatic steatosis and atherosclerosis. Cellular lipid homeostasis is regulated by the balance between influx, efflux, synthesis, and catabolism of lipids. An imbalance in these pathways can result in lipid accumulation in macrophages, mesangial cells, vascular smooth muscle cells and other cell types causing tissue damage. Influx of lipids into macrophages and mesangial cells is mediated by a number of receptors including scavenger receptor class A (SR-AI), class B (CD36) and class E (LOX-1) [73,74]. Lipid accumulation in the wall of aorta and remnant kidney in 5/6 nephrectomized rats is accompanied by marked upregulation of SR-A1 and LOX-1 [43,44], pointing to increased lipid influx in these tissues. Oxidized LDL and inflammatory cytokines stimulate expression of these receptors. This illustrates the causal link between oxidative stress and inflammation with accumulation of lipids in the macrophages and vascular smooth muscle cells in the artery wall and in the macrophages and mesangial cells in the renal tissue in CKD animals.

Development of glomerulosclerosis and progression of kidney disease is invariably associated with proteinuria [75]. Proximal tubular epithelial cells reabsorb filtered proteins including lipid-carrying proteins such as albumin and apolipoprotein A-I via megalin-cubilin complexes expressed on their apical membrane [76,77]. Glomerular proteinuria markedly increases the burden of reabsorbed filtered proteins and their lipid cargo causing expansion of the intracellular lipid pool in proximal tubular epithelial cells. In addition interaction of protein-bound lipids with megalin-cubilin complexes activates several signal transduction pathways which triggers cellular apoptosis and release of proinflammatory and pro-fibrotic mediators and thereby contributes to tubular atrophy, interstitial fibrosis, and inflammation [77]. In fact proteinuria, glomerulosclerosis, tubulo-interstitial fibrosis, inflammation and accumulation of lipids in the proximal tubular epithelial cells in the remnant kidneys of rats 12 weeks after 5/6 nephrectomy was associated with marked upregulation of megalin-cubilin complexes [43]. These findings demonstrate the role of proteinuria in accumulation of lipid in the proximal tubules and the potential lipid-mediated tubular injury and interstitial inflammation and fibrosis.

Studies of the cholesterol efflux pathway in the remnant kidney tissue and artery wall have shown upregulation of ABCA-1 and activation of its upstream transcription factor, liver X receptor (LXR) which is an intracellular sterol-sensing molecule [43,44]. This phenomenon represents the cellular response to elevated cholesterol burden in the arterial and remnant kidney tissues in CKD. The success of the upregulation of cellular cholesterol efflux pathway in unloading of the surplus cholesterol depends on HDL-mediated uptake and disposal of the lipid cargo. However HDL-mediated reverse cholesterol transport is severely impaired in CKD. Several factors contribute to the reduction of HDL-mediated reverse cholesterol transport in CKD. These include diminished hepatic production and plasma concentration of Apo A-I [13,16,17,19], and LCAT [13,21] as well as oxidative modification of HDL [14–17] which can compromise the critical interaction between HDL and ABCA1 transporter [24].

Studies of the de novo lipid biosynthesis have revealed marked suppression of cholesterol production machinery in the diseased kidney [43]. These findings substantiate excessive influx and impaired HDL-mediated efflux as opposed to increased local production as the cause of cholesterol accumulation in the renal tissue. However, fatty acid production machinery is upregulated and PPAR-alpha-driven fatty acid catabolism is suppressed in the diseased kidney [43]. Upregulation of the fatty acid production system in the remnant kidney is driven by activation of carbohydrate response element binding protein (ChREBP) which is an intracellular sensor of glucose. The author believes that activation of ChREBP and consequent increase in fatty acid synthesis in the remnant/diseased kidney is driven by increased filtered glucose load per nephron occasioned by increased single nephron GFR.

Activity of PPAR-alpha which is the master regulator of fatty acids catabolism is markedly reduced in the remnant/diseased kidney. In the normal kidney,

PPAR-alpha is heavily expressed in the proximal tubules and medullary thick ascending limb of loop of Henle and is weakly expressed in mesangial cells [78]. PPAR-alpha regulates expression of genes involved in fatty acid catabolism including liver type fatty acid binding protein (L-FABP) and acyl-CoA oxidase (ACO). These proteins play a critical part in mitochondrial and peroxisomal beta-oxidation of fatty acids. Studies conducted in the author's laboratories [43] revealed significant downregulation of PPAR-alpha activity (nuclear translocation) and its target genes, L-FABP and ACO in the remnant kidneys of rats with CKD. These findings unraveled yet another mechanism that contributes to increased lipid burden and lipotoxicity in the diseased kidney.

Accordingly increased production and depressed catabolism of fatty acids along with heightened influx and impaired efflux of cholesterol and neutral lipids contribute to accumulation of lipids in the diseased kidney. This is accompanied by significant upregulation of the enzyme acyl-CoA cholesterolacyltransferase-1 (ACAT1) which catalyzes esterification of cholesterol and sequestration of cholesterol esters in intracellular vesicles, a process that impedes HDL-mediated cholesterol efflux and leads to foam cell transformation [43]. Earlier studies conducted in the author's laboratories demonstrated that administration of an ACAT inhibitor can ameliorate proteinuria and preserve residual renal function in this model [79] pointing to the role of ACAT in progression of renal disease.

There is little evidence that hyperlipidemia per se can cause kidney disease in the absence of pre-existing renal disease or conditions that cause kidney disease. However when present hyperlipidemia can accelerate progression of preexisting renal disease and amplify the effect of conditions that can induce kidney disease. For instance consumption of a high cholesterol diet augments the development of glomerulosclerosis in rats with unilateral nephrectomy [80]. Similarly, induction of hypercholesterolemia with high-cholesterol diet increases the severity of proteinuria and glomerular lipid deposition in rats with CKD induced by subtotal nephrectomy [81]. Moreover, lipid lowering strategies ameliorate renal injury in several animal models of CKD. For instance administration of lovastatin has been shown to attenuate glomerular injury and albuminuria in Dahl salt-sensitive rats consuming high salt diet [82]. Likewise administration of antihypertensive and cholesterol-lowering agents attenuated severity of histological lesions and the associated proteinuria in rats with nephrotoxic serum nephritis [83]. The salutary effects of lipid lowering interventions in most animal models of CKD is associated with reduction of inflammatory cell infiltration, fibrosis and expression of proinflammatory and pro-fibrotic mediators and consistently observed in different models of renal injury [83—87].

Nutrition and Energy Metabolism

In addition to causing hypertriglyceridemia and contributing to amplification of oxidative stress, inflammation and cardiovascular disease mentioned above, defective clearance of triglyceride-rich lipoproteins leads to impaired energy metabolism, reduced exercise capacity, cachexia and malnutrition syndrome in patients with advanced CKD [49]. By limiting the delivery of lipids to the adipocytes and myocytes, downregulation of lipoprotein lipase and VLDL receptor limits the availability of lipid fuel and construction material to the skeletal muscles and myocardium and adipose tissues in CKD [88]. By necessity this abnormality deprives the skeletal muscle and myocardium from free supplies of lipid fuel and as such can contribute to muscle weakness and myocardial dysfunction. Likewise diminished delivery of fatty acids to the adipose tissue limits the long-term energy storage capacity and contributes to weight loss and cachexia in ESRD patients.

TREATMENT OF CKD-ASSOCIATED DYSLIPIDEMIA

In light of the role of dyslipidemia in progression of CKD and the associated cardiovascular complications, interventions aimed at improving lipid metabolism can be important in the management of patients with CKD. A brief description of the available data on the efficacy of the currently available lipid-modulating drugs in the treatment of CKD-induced dyslipidemia is provided below:

Statins in Primary Prevention of Cardiovascular Disease in ESRD Patients

Three large prospective randomized controlled clinical trials were conducted to address the efficacy of statin therapy in lowering the risk of cardiovascular mortality in ESRD patients maintained on hemo dialysis. The first of these trials was the 4D (Die Deutsche Diabetes Dialyse) study [62] which enrolled 1255 hemodialysis patients with type II diabetes randomized to atorvastatin, 20 mg/day or placebo for 4 years. The study showed no significant reduction of the risk of death from cardiac causes, nonfatal MI and instead revealed a significant increase in the risk of a fatal stroke (95% CI 1.05 to 3.93) in the statin-treated group.

The second large trial termed "An assessment of Survival and Cardiovascular Events (AURORA)" was a double-blind, randomized, placebo-controlled, multi-center trial undertaken to compare the effect of rosuvastatin 10 mg/d versus placebo on cardiovascular morbidity and mortality in ESRD patients maintained on regular hemodialysis treatment [63]. A large number (2776) of patients 50 to 80 years of age on dialysis for at least 3 months were enrolled in this study from 25 countries. The primary end point was major cardiovascular events including fatal and non-fatal myocardial infarction and stroke; the secondary end points included all-cause mortality, revascularization, and death from cardiovascular and non-cardiovascular causes; and the tertiary end points included changes in the baseline lipids and high sensitivity C-reactive protein (hs-CRP). The mean baseline LDL Cholesterol values in the rosuvastatin (100 mg/dL) placebo (99 mg/dL) groups were nearly identical. The mean duration of treatment and the mean length of follow-up were 2.4 and 3.2 years respectively. A total of 1296 patients died and 810 patients discontinued the treatment because of adverse drug reactions or renal transplantation during the study period. The LDL cholesterol concentration fell by approximately 43% and hs-CRP decreased by 11.5% in the rosuvastatin group within the first year of the trial. However, despite marked reduction of cholesterol level in the rosuvastatin-treated group, no significant difference was observed in either mortality or primary or secondary end points between the two groups. Moreover, a significant increased in the rate of fatal hemorrhagic stroke was found in the rosuvastatin-treated patients with diabetes (p = 0.03), confirming the results of the 4D study.

The third and the largest randomized primary prevention statin trial in CKD patients was the Study of Heart and Renal Protection (SHARP) [64]. This study differed from the 4-D and AURORA trials since in addition to the dialysis patients it included a large cohort of CKD patients who did not require dialysis. A total of 9270 patients (3023 ESRD patients on maintenance dialysis and 6247 CKD patients not requiring dialysis) without history of myocardial infarction or coronary revascularization were enrolled in this study. Patients were randomly assigned to receive simvastatin 20 mg/day with or without ezetimibe 10 mg/day or placebo. The median duration of follow-up was 4.9 years. Mean baseline LDL cholesterol levels were 108 mg/dL in the entire group and 100 mg/dL in the dialysis subgroup. It was lowered by 30 mg/dL with simvastatin alone and by 43 mg/dL with simvastatin plus ezetimibe at 1 year.

The study sought to investigate effectiveness of LDL cholesterol reduction on major vascular events and the rate of progression of CKD in as yet dialysis-independent patients. The estimated glomerular filtration rate (eGFR) in the CKD groups averaged 27 mL/min/1.73 m^2. The primary end points were the occurrence of a major atherosclerotic event that included death due to coronary disease, myocardial infarction, non-hemorrhagic stroke, or the need for revascularization procedures.

The study revealed a 17% reduction in major atherosclerotic events [relative risk 0.83; 95% CI 0.74, 0.94; log rank p = 0.002], a 25% reduction in non-hemorrhagic stroke, a 21% reduction in coronary revascularization and trend toward a reduction in nonfatal MI in the entire simvastatin and ezetimibe treated arm. It should be noted however that cholesterol lowering therapy did not significantly reduce either mortality rates or cardiovascular events in the dialysis-dependent ESRD patients enrolled in the SHARP trial. Therefore, the results of the SHARP trial confirmed those of AURORA and 4-D studies and the only reason for the salutary results reported for the entire enrolled population was the fact that the SHARP trial was weighted toward patients with less advanced CKD, in whom the underlying mechanisms of cardiovascular disease is more akin to that in the general population.

Holdaas et al. conducted [89] a multicenter, randomized, placebo-controlled trial in 2102 renal transplant recipients in which participants were randomly assigned to receive fluvastatin or placebo. The primary endpoint included major cardiac events (cardiac death, non-fatal myocardial infarction, or coronary interventions). After an average follow-up of 5 years, fluvastatin significantly reduced serum LDL cholesterol concentration by 32%. Although there were significantly fewer cardiac deaths or non-fatal MI (70 vs. 104, 0.65 [0.48–0.88] p = 0.005) in the fluvastatin group than in the placebo group, the risk reduction for the primary endpoint (risk ratio 0.83 [95% CI 0.64–1.06], p = 0.139) did not reach statistical significance. Likewise the incidence of coronary intervention procedures and other secondary endpoints were not significantly different between the active and placebo-treated groups.

The negative results observed in trials of statins in hemodialysis patients contrast their salutary effects in reducing the risk of cardiovascular events in the general population [90]. As noted above, plasma cholesterol is within or below the normal limits in the majority of ESRD patients maintained on hemodialysis treatment and the atherosclerosis and cardiovascular disease in this population is primarily driven by oxidative stress, inflammation, HDL deficiency and dysfunction, impaired clearance of VLDL and chylomicrons, accumulation of IDL and chylomicron remnants and formation of atherogenic small dense LDL. Since these abnormalities are not amenable to statin therapy, it is not surprising that treatment with these agents does not reduce the risk of cardiovascular disease in this population. However, when present hypercholesterolemia can compound the risk of cardiovascular disease in this population in whom statin therapy can have salutary effects. This supposition was confirmed by a recent post hoc analysis of the 4-D study [91] which demonstrated that atorvastatin significantly reduced the rates of adverse cardiovascular and overall outcomes in patients with the highest quartile of baseline LDL-cholesterol ($\geq$145 mg/dL, 3.76 mmol/L). No such benefit was observed in patients with the other quartiles of LDL-cholesterol at baseline. Consequently statin therapy might be effective in hemodialysis patients with elevated serum LDL cholesterol concentrations.

Statins in Primary Prevention of Cardiovascular Disease in Nondialysis CKD Patients

Data derived from subgroup analysis of the secondary prevention trials have suggested that statins may lower the risk of adverse cardiovascular outcomes in non-dialysis patients with stage I—IV CKD [92,93]. Likewise, meta-analysis of data on 18,176 patients with CKD stages I—IV derived from five different studies, showed a significant reduction (0.81) of the relative risk of all cause mortality with statin therapy [94]. There has been only one prospective randomized trial designed to evaluate efficacy of statins in patients with mild CKD. This study which was called "Prevention of Renal and Vascular End Stage Disease Intervention Trial" (PREVENT IT study) [95] had enrolled 864 patients with microalbuminuria who were randomized to fosinopril 20 mg/day, pravastatin 40 mg/day, or matching placebos and followed for 4 years. The study showed an insignificant reduction in the cardiovascular mortality and hospitalization for cardiovascular morbidity in the pravastatin-treated group. The reason for the disparity in response to statin therapy between the PREVENT IT study and the former two studies is unclear. One possible explanation may be the difference in the magnitude of proteinuria among the study populations. Heavy proteinuria is frequently associated with hypercholesterolemia and increased risk of cardiovascular disease. Hypercholesterolemia in this condition is due to downregulation of hepatic LDL receptor and HDL docking receptor which results in increased hepatic HMG-CoA reductase activity and cholesterol synthesis [11,47,96]. Therefore pharmacological inhibition of HMG-CoA reductase with statins in such cases can have salutary effect. Patients enrolled in the PREVENT IT study had microalbuminuria whereas patients included in the former studies had stage I—IV CKD which usually encompasses a significant subset of patients with significant proteinuria who might

benefit from statin treatment. In this context ESRD patients maintained on chronic peritoneal dialysis experience significant daily losses of proteins in their peritoneal dialysate effluent which can cause hypercholesterolemia simulating nephrotic syndrome in functionally anephric individuals. Unlike the majority of hemodialysis patients who have normal or subnormal plasma cholesterol, peritoneal dialysis patients with hypercholesterolemia may benefit from statin therapy.

Effect of Statins on Progression of Kidney Disease

The available data on the effect of statins on progression of kidney disease are primarily derived from secondary or post-hoc analyses of the secondary prevention studies and a limited number of randomized clinical trials which have directly addressed this issue. The former studies were primarily conducted to determine the effect of statins on cardiovascular outcomes in patients with either pre-existing heart disease or those at high risk of developing cardiac disease. Among these studies, the Heart Protection trial showed a significantly lower rate of decline in GFR in simvastatin-treated compared to placebo-treated groups [97]. The post hoc analysis of data from GREACE (Greek Atorvastatin and Coronary-heart-disease Evaluation) study which compared atorvastatin with usual care in patients with coronary artery disease showed an approximately 5% decline in estimated GFR in untreated patients with dyslipidemia and coronary disease and normal renal function at baseline during the 3-year study period. Treatment with statin prevented the decline in estimated GFR and in fact resulted in an approximately 5% increase in estimated GFR in the treated arm [98]. The salutary effect of statin on renal function was more pronounced in the lower two quartiles of baseline GFR and with higher atorvastatin doses. The subgroup analysis of the CARE trial showed that pravastatin significantly slowed the rate of decline in GFR by 2.5 mL/min/year in patients with GRF below 40 mL/min/1.73 m^2, but not in the study population as a whole [99]. The sub-analysis of data from the "Treatment to New Targets" (TNT) study in patients with coronary heart disease [100] revealed a significant improvement in estimated GFR over the 5-year study period.

As noted above only a few randomized controlled trials (RCTs) have directly explored the impact of statins on renal function. Moreover the majority of these studies were not placebo controlled and were limited in size or duration and used various statins alone or with other lipid-lowering agents. In a meta-analysis of 12 such studies including a total of 362 participants Fried et al concluded that statins may retard progression of renal disease and attenuate proteinuria [101]. Similarly meta-analysis of data from 27 published or unpublished randomized, controlled trials or crossover trials of statins (including close to 40,000 participants) that reported assessment of kidney function showed a significantly slower rate of annual decline in eGFR (1.22 mL/min per year) in the statin-treated participants [102]. The subgroup analysis of the data revealed that the salutary effect of statin therapy was statistically significant in the participants with cardiovascular disease but not in those with glomerulonephritis, diabetic nephropathy or hypertensive kidney disease. In addition to reducing the rate of decline in GFR, statin therapy tended to modestly reduce proteinuria in this population. The efficacy of statin therapy in lowering proteinuria has been demonstrated in meta-analysis of data derived from 50 trials which included large numbers of CKD and transplant patients reported by Strippoli et al. [94] and Douglas and associates [103]. Unlike the other statins rosuvastatin lacks anti-proteinuric effects and can actually increase proteinuria. This is most likely because concentrations of rosuvastatin and its metabolites is elevated in the renal tissue where it can adversely affect the kidney especially when used in high doses as seen in the recently completed "Prospective Evaluation of Proteinuria and Renal Function in diabetic and non-Diabetic Patients with Progressive Renal Disease Trials" (PLANET I and II studies respectively) trials [104]. These Prospective trials were designed to examine the efficacy of 12-month therapy with rosuvastatin (10 mg or 40 mg/day) and atorvastatin (80 mg/day) on progression of renal disease in diabetic and non-diabetic patients with CKD. The studies revealed reduced proteinuria and slower rate of decline in eGFR in atorvastatin-treated group but modest increase in proteinuria and greater decline in eGFR in rosuvastatin-treated arm, particularly in those receiving the higher (40 mg/day) dose. Taken together the available data suggest that with the exception of rosuvastatin, statins can be beneficial in retarding progression of CKD especially in those with significant proteinuria. However these agents should be used with caution as at high doses these agents can have adverse renal and extra-renal consequences. For instance Deslypere and colleagues [105] reported that 10 out of 120 patients receiving a high dose of simvastatin (40 mg/day) developed proteinuria which regressed following discontinuation of the drug and reappeared with its reintroduction. The proteinuric effect seen with rosuvastatin and occasionally with other statins appears to be, at least in part, due to impaired proximal tubular reabsorption of filtered proteins. In fact in vitro studies have shown dose-dependent inhibition of protein uptake by simvastatin, pravastatin and rosuvastatin in cultured human renal proximal tubular epithelial cells [106].

Mechanisms of Protective Effects of Statins in CKD

The salutary effect of statins on progression of kidney disease is mediated by their cholesterol lowering and cholesterol-independent actions. In this context, in vitro and in vivo studies have shown that elevated LDL and oxidized LDL can activate mesangial cells, raise matrix production, stimulate release of chemokines and TGF-β, recruitment of monocytes and their transformation into resident macrophages leading to mesangial matrix expansion, lipid deposition, and foam cell formation [107–110]. These effects are much more intense with the oxidized LDL [111,112] which as noted earlier is significantly increased in patients with CKD.

In addition to their cholesterol lowering properties, statins can confer renal protection by several cholesterol-independent pleiotropic effects via improvement of endothelial function [113], protection of podocyte [114,115], antioxidant and anti-inflammation actions [116,117], reduction of plasminogen activator inhibitor-1 (PAI-1) production [118], suppression of extracellular matrix (ECM) accumulation [119] and inhibition of vascular smooth muscle cells (VSMC), mesangial and monocyte/macrophage proliferation [120–123]. The majority of the cholesterol-independent pleiotropic effects of statins mentioned above are due to reduced production of isoprenoids particularly farnesylpyrophosphate and genarylgenarylpyrophosphate which are the intermediary metabolites of mevalonic acid. Via isoprenylation or prenylation processes, these intermediary metabolites play a critical part in intracellular transport, membrane anchoring, and regulation of the activities of small guanosine triphosphate (GTP) binding proteins such as Ras, Rho, Rac, Rap and Ral [124–129]. These GTP-binding proteins transition between inactive GDP-bound and active GTP-bound forms. As extracellular signals transducers, the GTP-binding proteins regulate many important physiological and pathological functions [130]. The protective effects of statins in kidney disease may be partly due to inhibition of Ras and RhoA [131]. Rac1 which is an important GTP-binding protein plays an essential part in activation of NAD(P)H oxidase. NAD(P)H oxidase is a major source of reactive oxygen species (ROS) in the kidney, vascular tissue and immune cells. Inhibition of Rac1 signaling by statins has been shown to reduce ROS production in albumin-treated proximal tubular epithelial cells and in high glucose-treated aortic endothelial cells [132,133]. In addition to reducing ROS production statins have been shown to raise expression of heme oxygenase-1 (HO-1) which catalyzes degradation of heme and generation of the potent anti-oxidant, bilirubin [134,135]. In addition, statins have been shown to increase glutathione peroxidase activity [136] and reduce LDL oxidation [137]. Thus, by lowering ROS production and raising anti-oxidant capacity, statins can ameliorate oxidative stress.

Another cholesterol-independent mechanism by which statins may slow progression of CKD is their ability to attenuate inflammation. In fact statin therapy has been shown to significantly lower serum C-reactive protein (CRP) which is a proinflammatory and pro-thrombotic mediator. The observed reduction of CRP is partially independent from cholesterol-lowering effects of the drug [138,139]. In addition statins lower the release of proinflammatory cytokines and chemokines, [140,141], inhibit mesangial cell and leukocyte proliferation and macrophage infiltration [142], lower expression of pro-fibrotic mediators [143−147], attenuate expression of leukocyte integrins and endothelial adhesion molecules [148−151]. Besides reducing proinflammatory factors, statins may raise the number of $CD4^+CD25^+$ regulatory T cells (Tregs) which can help to suppress inflammatory response [152].

In the vascular tissue statins upregulate expression and activity of endothelial NO synthase [153], suppress the endothelin system [154,155] and attenuate the effects of angiotensin II by lowering AT1-receptor expression [156] and reducing Ang II-stimulated ROS production by inhibiting Rac1 [157]. In addition by inhibiting PAI-1 production and raising tissue plasminogen activator expression statins can modify the fibrinolytic balance in the vessel wall [158] and thereby lower the risk of cardiovascular events.

As noted above hypercholesterolemia contributes to CKD progression, in part, by damaging the podocytes [169]. Statins have been shown to attenuate podocyte injury in the model of nephrotic syndrome induced by puromycin aminonucleoside which causes podocyte injury and apoptosis [160]. The protective effect of statins in podocytes appears to be mediated by a p21-dependent anti-apoptotic pathway [161]. In fact, statin therapy has been shown to reduce the number of podocytes found in the urine of patients with chronic glomerulonephritis, suggesting diminished podocyte loss and injury by these agents [162].

POTENTIAL ADVERSE EFFECTS OF STATINS

Besides blocking the synthesis of cholesterol, statins block production of important intermediary (e.g. farnesyl-pyrophosphate and geranylgeranyl-pyrophosphates) and alternative (i.e. dolichols and ubiquinone) byproducts of mevalonate pathway. Given the important biological functions of these byproducts, their diminished production can have adverse consequences. For instance ubiquinone (Coenzyme Q10) is critical for mitochondrial electron transport and oxidative phosphorylation and dolichols are involved in production of glycoproteins which are necessary for tissue growth. In addition farnesyl-pyrophosphate and geranylgeranyl-pyrophosphate are necessary for prenylation of proteins which is essential for, intracellular trafficking of newly synthesized proteins between the endoplasmic reticulum and Golgi apparatus, gene transcription and regulation of cell growth. Therefore, by curtailing the availability of these products statins can potentially disturb oxidative phosphorylation, signal transduction, intracellular traffic, gene transcription, and production/regulation of structural proteins [163]. In fact these un-intended effects of statins are responsible for the well-known side effects of statins such as myopathy and liver injury and possibly other less recognized systemic complications. Theoretically the anti-inflammatory/immunosuppressive properties of statins which are beneficial in attenuating systemic inflammation may raise the incidence and severity of microbial infections which are a common cause of morbidity and mortality in advanced CKD. Interestingly large randomized clinical trials of statins in the general population have consistently revealed significant reduction in cardiovascular but not the overall mortality [164−166]. These observations indirectly imply that statins may increase mortality from non-cardiovascular events probably as a result of the cholesterol-independent effects of these agents particularly when used at high doses.

Taken together statins seem to have salutary effects in CKD and ESRD patients with elevated, but not normal serum cholesterol. Among the available statins, those with minimal renal metabolism/excretion are preferable in CKD patients. Given their various side effects, the lowest effective dose should be used in this population.

PPAR-α Agonists

PPAR-α agonists (fibrates) effectively lower serum triglyceride and increase HDL cholesterol concentration. Since HDL deficiency and hypertriglyceridemia are common features of CKD, PPAR-α agonists can be potentially useful in the management of CKD-induced dyslipidemia. A clinical trial of the PPAR-α agonist, gemfibrozil, showed a significant reduction of serum triglyceride, a significant increase in serum HDL cholesterol and lower incidence of coronary death and nonfatal myocardial infarction in patients with mild to moderate CKD and coronary disease and low HDL cholesterol level. The treatment however, did not alter the rate of the decline in kidney function. Instead the drug tended to raise the risk of sustained elevations in serum creatinine in individuals with or without CKD [167,168]. Moreover, the safety and efficacy of these compounds in patients with severe renal disease remains unclear. These concerns have limited the utility of these compounds in the CKD population. Since no dose adjustment is needed for reduced GFR in patients with CKD the National Kidney Foundation clinical practice guidelines (K/DOQI; 2003) recommended gemfibrozil as the fibrate of choice for management of dyslipidemias in patients with kidney disease. The National Lipid Association however, has recommended a 50% reduction in the dose of gemfibrozil for patients with GFR below 60 mL/min/L.73 m^2 and avoidance of all fibrates in patients with GFR less than 30 mL/min/1.73 m^2. Fluvastatin is the only statin whose plasma levels are not increased when combined with gemfibrozil; therefore this combination may be preferred in CKD patients with mixed dyslipidemia [169]. It should be noted that when used concomitantly with statins, fibrates elevate serum level of statins most likely by interfering with the glucuronidation pathway of statin metabolism [170]. The exception is fenofibrate, which does not interfere with statin metabolism. However major dose reduction is necessary when fenofibrate is used in patients with reduced GFR and the drug should be avoided in patients with GFR below 15 mL/min/1.73m^2 [170]. However, in predialysis patients, a combination of fenofibrate, at a dose adjusted according to GFR, with a statin can also be considered.

Niacin

At low doses niacin can raise serum HDL cholesterol and at high doses it can simultaneously increase serum HDL cholesterol and reduce serum LDL, triglyceride and lipoprotein (a) levels. In addition, niacin has antioxidant and anti-inflammatory properties that may further enhance its ability to retard progression of renal disease and atherosclerosis. In fact, animal studies have shown significant attenuation of oxidative stress and lipotoxicity in CKD rats with long-term niacin administration [171,172]. Unfortunately, widespread clinical use of niacin in CKD patients has been limited in part by its poor tolerability. One of the most common side effects of niacin and related compounds is flushing of the skin which is due to prostaglandin-mediated vasodilation and occurs in more than 80% of patients consuming regular crystalline preparations. The flushing can be attenuated by aspirin taken prior to each dose, use of the drug after meals, or use of the extended-release formulation. The other side effects of niacin include hepatotoxicity, hyperuricemia, and

hyperglycemia. Hepatotoxicity which was relatively common with the older generation of sustained-release formulations seems to be uncommon with extended-release niacin. Finally niacin can raise serum glucose level which may be of concern when prescribed for the diabetic patients. However, the glycemic effect of niacin is dose-dependent and is insignificant at low doses.

Experimental Lipid-Modulating Agents

Two new classes of lipid modulating agents targeting HDL have undergone pre-clinical and clinical trials in recent years. CETP inhibitors are among the latest such products that can markedly raise HDL cholesterol concentration. By inhibiting CETP-mediated exchange of cholesterol ester for triglycerides in the circulation these agents significantly elevate HDL cholesterol level. The clinical trial of the first product in this class, torcetrapib, was prematurely halted because contrary to expectations the drug increased the adverse cardiovascular outcomes despite marked increase in plasma HDL [173]. Although this phenomenon was attributed to a slight increase in blood pressure observed in the treated group, I believe that despite markedly raising plasma HDL-cholesterol, CETP inhibitors may worsen cardiovascular outcomes in some patients since the increase in HDL cholesterol in this case is not due to enhanced removal of surplus cholesterol from the artery wall, kidney or other tissues. Rather it is merely due to inhibition of CETP-mediated transfer of cholesterol ester from HDL to IDL/LDL in exchange for triglycerides in the circulation. In fact by limiting the conversion of IDL to LDL and formation of cholesterol ester-rich LDL, inhibition of CETP might lead to accumulation of atherogenic IDL and formation of small dense LDL, events that can accelerate atherosclerosis and intensify inflammation. As noted earlier, CETP is markedly elevated in patients with nephrotic proteinuria. It is conceivable that low doses of CETP inhibitors may have salutary effect in patients with nephrotic syndrome.

The second novel lipid-modulating class of experimental drugs is *ACAT inhibitors*. These drugs inhibit the intracellular enzyme, ACAT which is a key factor in cholesterol metabolism. ACAT catalyzes esterification of free cholesterol to cholesterol ester for incorporation in VLDL in the liver and chylomicrons in the intestine and for sequestration in intracellular vesicles in macrophages, vascular smooth muscle cells and mesangial cells. The latter is the principal step in foam cell formation and an impediment to reverse cholesterol transport which depends on migration of free cholesterol from cytoplasm to plasma membrane for removal by HDL. Increased ACAT activity augments cholesterol synthesis by the liver and impedes HDL-mediated removal of cholesterol in the peripheral tissues. Consequently pharmacological inhibition of ACAT can enhance HDL-mediated reverse cholesterol transport, raise plasma HDL cholesterol and reduce hepatic cholesterol production, events that can have significant protective impact on cardiovascular disease and potentially chronic kidney disease. However increased ACAT activity protects the cholesterol-loaded cells against disruption and death caused by high levels of free cholesterol. This is because due to its amphipathic properties, free cholesterol accumulates in the cellular membranes and when present in excess quantities it compromises the stability and physical properties of cell membranes. Therefore, by raising intracellular free cholesterol in cholesterol loaded cells, ACAT inhibitors can cause disruption of plasma membrane in resident macrophages leading to release of proteolytic enzymes and tissue factor, plaque rupture and thrombosis. In fact due to adverse cardiovascular outcomes a large clinical trial of avasimibe which is a potent ACAT inhibitor, was halted [174]. It is of note that in a series of studies conducted in my laboratories we found a marked increase in ACAT expression and activity in the liver, remnant kidney and arterial wall in animals with nephrotic syndrome [44,175] and chronic renal insufficiency [43,46]. We subsequently found significant improvement in proteinuria, renal function and plasma lipid profile with administration of ACAT inhibitor, avasimibe, in both conditions [79,176]. It is, therefore, conceivable that low doses of ACAT inhibitors might have potential salutary effects on progression of renal disease in patients with nephrotic proteinuria lacking atherosclerosis.

References

[1] Vaziri ND. Dyslipidemia of chronic renal failure: The nature, mechanisms and potential consequences. Am J Physiol, Renal Physiol 2006;290:262—72.

[2] Vaziri ND, Moradi H. Mechanism of dyslipidemia of chronic renal failure. Hemodialysis Int 2006;10:1—7.

[3] Kaysen GA. New insights into lipid metabolism in chronic kidney disease. J Ren Nutr 2011 Jan;21(1):120—3.

[4] O'Neal D, Lee P, Murphy B, Best J. Low-density lipoprotein particle size distribution in end-stage renal disease treated with hemodialysis or peritoneal dialysis. Am J Kidney Dis 1996; 27:84—9.

[5] Rajman I, Harper L, McPake D, et al. Low-density lipoprotein subfraction profiles in chronic renal failure. Nephrol Dial Transplant 1998;13:2281—7.

[6] Attman PO, Samuelsson O, Johansson AC, Moberly JB, Alaupovic P. Dialysis modalities and dyslipidemia. Kidney Int Suppl 2003;84:S110—2.

[7] Deighan CJ, Caslake MJ, McConnell M, Boulton-Jones JM, Packard CJ. Atherogenic lipoprotein phenotype in end-stage renal failure: origin and extent of small dense low-density lipoprotein formation. Am J Kidney Dis 2000;35:852—62.

[8] Kronenberg F, Kuen E, Ritz E, et al. Lipoprotein(a) serum concentrations and apolipoprotein(a) phenotypes in mild and moderate renal failure. J Am Soc Nephrol 2000;11:105—15.

[9] Kronenberg F, Neyer U, Lhotta K, et al. The low molecular weight apo(a) phenotype is an independent predictor for coronary artery disease in hemodialysis patients: a prospective follow-up. J Am Soc Nephrol 1999;10:1027—36.

[10] Vaziri ND, Liang KH. Hepatic HMG-CoA reductase gene expression during the course of puromycin-induced nephrosis. Kidney Int 1995;48:1979—85.

[11] Vaziri ND, Sato T, Liang K. Molecular mechanism of altered cholesterol metabolism in focal glomerulosclerosis. Kidney Int 2003;63:1756—63.

[12] Martinez LO, Jacquet S, Esteve JP, Rolland C, Cabezón E, Champagne E, et al. Ectopic beta-chain of ATP synthase is an apolipoprotein A-I receptor in hepatic HDL endocytosis. Nature 2003;421:75—9.

[13] Vaziri ND, Navab M, Fogelman AM. HDL metabolism and activity in chronic kidney disease. Nature, Reviews Nephrology 2010;6(5):287—96.

[14] Moradi H, Pahl MV, Elahimehr R, Vaziri ND. Impaired antioxidant activity of high-density lipoprotein in chronic kidney disease. Transl Res 2009;153:77—85.

[15] Kalantar-Zadeh K, Kopple JD, Kamranpour N, Fogelman AM, Navab M. HDL-inflammatory index correlates with poor outcome in hemodialysis patients. Kidney Int 2007;72:1149—56.

[16] Vaziri ND, Moradi H, Pahl MV, Fogelman AM, Navab M. In vitro stimulation of HDL anti-inflammatory activity and inhibition of LDL proinflammatory activity in the plasma of patients with end-stage renal disease by an apoA-1 mimetic peptide. Kidney Int 2009;76:437—44.

[17] Vaziri ND, Navab K, Gollapudi P, Moradi H, Pahl MV, Barton CH, et al. Salutary effects of hemodialysis on low-density lipoprotein proinflammatory and high-density lipoprotein anti-inflammatory properties in patient with end-stage renal disease. J Natl Med Assoc 2011;103:524—33.

[18] Attman PO, Alaupovic P. Lipid and apolipoprotein profiles of uremic dyslipoproteinemia — relation to renal function and dialysis. Nephron 1991;57:401—10.

[19] Vaziri ND, Deng G, Liang K. Hepatic HDL receptor, SR-B1 and Apo A-I expression in chronic renal failure. Nephrol Dial Transplant 1999;14:1462—6.

[20] Kamanna VS, et al. Uremic serum subfraction inhibits apolipoprotein A-I production by a human hepatoma cell line. J Am Soc Nephrol 1994;5:193—200.

[21] Vaziri ND, Liang K, Parks JS. Downregulation of hepatic lecithin: cholesterol acyltransferase gene expression in chronic renal failure. Kidney Int 2001;59:2192—6.

[22] Kimura H, Miyazaki R, Suzuki S, Gejyo F, Yoshida H. Cholesteryl ester transfer protein as a protective factor against vascular disease in hemodialysis patients. Am J Kidney Dis 2001; 38:70—6.

[23] Vaziri ND, Liang K, Parks JS. Acquired Lecithin: Cholesterol acyltransferase (LCAT) deficiency in nephrotic syndrome. Am J Physiol (Renal Physiol) 2001;49:F823—9.

[24] Shao B, Oda MN, Oram JF, Heinecke JW. Myeloperoxidase: an inflammatory enzyme for generating dysfunctional high density lipoprotein. Curr Opin Cardiol 2006;21:322—8.

[25] Vaziri ND, Gollapudi p, Han S, Farahmand G, Moradi H. Upregulation of hepatic HDL endocytic receptor and PDZK-1 dependent downregulation of HDL docking receptor in nephrotic syndrome. NDT 2011;103(6):524—33.

[26] Liang K, Vaziri ND. Downregulation of hepatic high-density lipoprotein receptor, SRB—1, in nephrotic syndrome. Kidney Int 1999;56:621—6.

[27] Zhao Y, Marcel YL. Serum albumin is a significant intermediate in cholesterol transfer between cells and lipoproteins. Biochemistry 1996;35:7174—80.

[28] Akmal M, Kasim SE, Soliman AR, Massry SG. Excess parathyroid hormone adversely affects lipid metabolism in chronic renal failure. Kidney Int 1990;37:854—8.

[29] Vaziri ND, Liang K. Downregulation of tissue lipoprotein lipase expression in experimental chronic renal failure. Kidney Int 1996;50:1928—35.

[30] Vaziri ND, Wang XQ, Liang K. Secondary hyperparathyroidism downregulates lipoprotein lipase expression in chronic renal failure. Am J Physiol, Renal Physiol 1997;273: F925—30.

[31] Vaziri ND, Yuan J, Ni Z, Nicholas SB, Norris KC. Lipoprotein lipase deficiency in chronic kidney disease is compounded by downregulation of endothelial GPIHBP1 expression. Clin Exp Nephrol 2012;16(2):238—43.

[32] Herz J, Strickland DK. LRP: a multifunctional scavenger and signaling receptor. J Clin Invest 2001;108:779—84.

[33] Kim C, Vaziri ND. Downregulation of hepatic LDL receptor-related protein (LRP) in chronic renal failure. Kidney Int 2005;67:1028—32.

[34] Pahl MV, Ni Z, Sepassi L, Vaziri ND. Plasma phosphlipid transfer protein, cholesteryl ester transfer protein and lecithin: cholesterol acyltransferase in end-stage E renal disease. NDT 2009;24(8):2541—6.

[35] Klin M, Smogorzewski M, Ni Z, Zhang G, Massry SG. Abnormalities in hepatic lipase in chronic renal failure: role of excess parathyroid hormone. J Clin Invest 1996;97:2167—73.

[36] Liang K, Vaziri ND. Downregulation of hepatic lipase expression in experimental nephrotic syndrome. Kidney Int 1997;51:1933—7.

[37] Sato T, Liang K, Vaziri ND. Protein restriction and AST-120 improve lipoprotein lipase, hepatic lipase and VLDL receptor deficiencies in focal glomerulosclerosis. Kidney Int 2003; 64:1780—6.

[38] Takahashi S, Kawarabayasi Y, Nakai T, et al. Rabbit very low density lipoprotein receptor: A low density lipoprotein receptor like protein with distinct ligand specificity. Proc Natl Acad Sci USA 1992;89:9252—6.

[39] Liang K, Vaziri ND. Acquired VLDL receptor deficiency in experimental nephrosis. Kidney Int 1997;51:1761—5.

[40] Sato T, Liang K, Vaziri ND. Downregulation of lipoprotein lipase and VLDL receptor in rats with focal glomerulosclerosis. Kidney Int 2002;61:157—62.

[41] Liang K, Vaziri ND. Gene expression of LDL receptor, HMG-CoA reductase and cholesterol-7-hydroxylase in chronic renal failure. Nephrol Dial Transplant 1997;12:1381—6.

[42] Liang K, Vaziri ND. Gene expression of LDL receptor, HMG-CoA reductase and cholesterol-7α-hydroxylase in chronic renal failure. Nephrol. Dial. Transplant 1997;12:1381—6.

[43] Kim HJ, Moradi H, Vaziri ND. Renal mass reduction results in accumulation of lipids and dysregulation of lipid regulatory proteins in the remnant kidney. Am J Physiol, Renal Physiol 2009;296(6):F1297—306.

[44] Moradi H, Yuan J, Ni Z, Norris K, Vaziri ND. Reverse cholesterol transport pathway in experimental chronic kidney disease. Am J Nephrol 2009;30:147—54.

[45] Vaziri ND, Bai Y, Yuan J, Said H, Sigala W, Ni Z. ApoA-1 mimetic peptide reverses uremia-induced upregulation of pro-atherogenic pathways in the aorta. Am J Nephrology 2010; 32(3):201—11.

[46] Liang K, Vaziri ND. Upregulation of Acyl-CoA: Cholesterol acyltransferase (ACAT) in chronic renal failure. Am J Physiol: Endocrine and Metab 2002;283:E676—81.

[47] Vaziri ND, Liang K. Down regulation of hepatic LDL receptor expression in experimental nephrosis. Kidney Int 1996;50:887—93.

[48] Vaziri ND. Lipotoxicity and impaired HDL-mediated reverse cholesterol/lipid transport in Chronic Kidney Disease. J Renal Nutrition 2010;20:S35—43.

[49] Vaziri ND, Norris K. Lipid disorders and their relevance to outcomes in Chronic Kidney Disease. Blood Purification 2011;31:189—96.

[50] Lindner A, Charra B, Sherrard DJ, Scribner BH. Accelerated atherosclerosis in prolonged maintenance hemodialysis. N Engl J Med 1974;290:697—701.

[51] Go AS, Chertow GM, Fan D, et al. Chronic kidney disease and the risks of death, cardiovascular events, and hospitalization. N Engl J Med 2004;351:1296—305.

[52] Collins AJ, Foley R, Herzog C, et al. Excerpts from the United States Renal Data System 2007 annual data report. Am J Kidney Dis 2008;51:S1—S320.

[53] Drüeke TB, Massy ZA. Atherosclerosis in CKD: differences from the general population. Nat Rev Nephrol 2010;6:723—35.

[54] Zoccali C, Mallamaci F, Tripepi G. Novel cardiovascular risk factors in end-stage renal disease. J Am Soc Nephrol 2004; 15(Suppl. 1):S77—80.

[55] London GM, Parfrey PS. Cardiac disease in chronic uremia: pathogenesis. Adv Ren Replace Ther 1997;4(3):194—211.

[56] Schwarz U, Buzello M, Ritz E, Stein G, Raabe G, Wiest G, et al. Morphology of coronary atherosclerotic lesions in patients with end-stage renal failure. Nephrol Dial Transplant 2000; 15(2):218—23.

[57] Pecoits-Filho R, Lindholm B, Stenvinkel P. The malnutrition, inflammation, and atherosclerosis (MIA) syndrome — the heart of the matter. Nephrol Dial Transplant 2002;17(Suppl. 11): 28—31.

[58] Liu Y, Coresh J, Eustace JA, et al. Association between cholesterol level and mortality in dialysis patients: role of inflammation and malnutrition. JAMA 2004;291:451—9.

[59] Kilpatrick RD, McAllister CJ, Kovesdy CP, et al. Association between serum lipids and survival in hemodialysis patients and impact of race. J Am Soc Nephrol 2007;18:293—303.

[60] Ansell BJ, et al. Inflammatory/anti-inflammatory properties of high-density lipoprotein distinguish patients from control subjects better than high density lipoprotein cholesterol levels and are favorably affected by simvastatin treatment. Circulation 2003;108:2751—6.

[61] Vaziri ND, Navab M, Fogelman AM. HDL metabolism and activity in chronic kidney disease. Nature, Reviews Nephrology 2010;6:287—96.

[62] Wanner C, Krane V, Marz W, et al. Atorvastatin in patients with type 2 diabetes mellitus undergoing hemodialysis. N Engl J Med 2005;353:238—48.

[63] Fellstrom BC, Jardine AG, Schmieder RE, et al. Rosuvastatin and cardiovascular events in patients undergoing hemodialysis. N Engl J Med 2009;360:1395—407.

[64] Baigent C, Landray MJ, Reith C, et al. The effects of lowering LDL cholesterol with simvastatin plus ezetimibe in patients with chronic kidney disease (Study of Heart and Renal Protection): a randomized placebo-controlled trial. Lancet 2011; 377:2181—92.

[65] Himmelfarb J, Stenvinkel P, Ikizler TA, Hakim R. The elephant in uremia: Oxidant stress as a unifying concept of cardiovascular disease in uremia. Kidney Int 2002;62:1524—38.

[66] Stenvinkel P, Alvestrand A. Inflammation in end-stage renal disease: Sources, consequences, and therapy. Semin Dial 2002;15:329—37.

[67] Vaziri ND. Oxidative stress in chronic renal failure: The nature, mechanism and consequences. Semin Nephrol 2004;24:469—73.

[68] Abrass CK. Cellular lipid metabolism and the role of lipids in progressive renal disease. Am J Nephrol 2004;24:46—53.

[69] Moorhead JF, Chan MK, El-Nahas M, Varghese Z. Lipid nephrotoxicity in chronic progressive glomerular and tubulo-interstitial disease. Lancet 1982;2:1309—11.

[70] Johnson ACM, Yabu JM, Hanson S, Shah VO, Zager RA. Experimental glomerulopathy alters renal cortical cholesterol, SR-B1, ABCA1, and HMG CoA reductase expression. Am J Pathol 2003;163:313—20.

[71] Susztak K, Ciccone E, McCue P, Sharma K, Böttinger EP. Multiple metabolic hits converge on CD36 as novel mediator of tubular epithelial apoptosis in diabetic nephropathy. PloS Med 2005;2:e45.

[72] Schaffer JE. Lipotoxicity: when tissues overeat. Curr Opin Lipidol 2003;14:281—7.

[73] Abrass CK. Cellular lipid metabolism and the role of lipids in progressive renal disease. Am J Nephrol 2004;24:46—53.

[74] Glass CK, Witztum JL. Atherosclerosis: the road ahead. Cell 2001;104:503—16. Li D, Mehta JL. Antisense to LOX-1 inhibits oxidized LDL-mediated upregulation of monocyte chemoattractant protein-1 and monocyte adhesion to human coronary artery endothelial cells. Circulation 101: 2889-2895, 2000.

[75] Remuzzi G, Benigni A, Remuzzi A. Mechanism of progression and regression of renal lesions of chronic nephropathies and diabetes. J Clin Invest 2006;116:228—96.

[76] Moestrup SK, Nielsen LB. The role of the kidney in lipid metabolism. Curr Opin Lipidol 2005;16:301—6.

[77] Baines RJ, Brunskill NJ. The molecular interactions between filtered proteins and proximal tubular cells in proteinuria. Nephron Exp Nephrol 2008;110:e67—71.

[78] Guan Y. Peroxisome proliferator-activated receptor family and its relationship to renal complications of the metabolic syndrome. J Am Soc Nephrol 2004;15:2801—15.

[79] Vaziri ND, Liang K. ACAT inhibition reverses LCAT deficiency and improves plasma HDL in chronic renal failure. Am J Physiol, Renal Physiol 2004;287:F1038—43.

[80] Grone HJ, Walli A, Grone E, Niedmann P, Thiery J, Seidel D, et al. Induction of glomerulosclerosis by dietary lipids. A functional and morphologic study in the rat. Lab Invest 1989;60(3):433—46.

[81] Rayner HC, Ross-Gilbertson VL, Walls J. The role of lipids in the pathogenesis of glomerulosclerosis in the rat following subtotal nephrectomy. Eur J Clin Invest 1990;20(1):97—104.

[82] O'Donnell MP, Kasiske BL, Katz SA, Schmitz PG, Keane WF. Lovastatin but not enalapril reduces glomerular injury in Dahl salt-sensitive rats. Hypertension 1992;20(5):651—8.

[83] Rubin R, Silbiger S, Sablay L, Neugarten J. Combined antihypertensive and lipid-lowering therapy in experimental glomerulonephritis. Hypertension 1994;23(1):92—5.

[84] Zhou MS, Schuman IH, Jaimes EA, Raij L. Renoprotection by statins is linked to a decrease in renal oxidative stress, TGF-beta, and fibronectin with concomitant increase in nitric oxide bioavailability. Am J Physiol Renal Physiol 2008;295(1):F53—9.

[85] Li C, Lim SW, Choi BS, Lee SH, Cha JH, Kim IS, et al. Inhibitory effect of pravastatin on transforming growth factor beta1-inducible gene h3 expression in a rat model of chronic cyclosporine nephropathy. Am J Nephrol 2005;25(6):611—20.

[86] Ota T, Takamura T, Ando H, Nohara E, Yamashita H, Kobayashi K. Preventive effect of cerivastatin on diabetic nephropathy through suppression of glomerular macrophage recruitment in a rat model. Diabetologia 2003;46(6):843—51.

[87] Jandeleit-Dahm K, Cao Z, Cox AJ, Kelly DJ, Gilbert RE, Cooper ME. Role of hyperlipidemia in progressive renal disease: focus on diabetic nephropathy. Kidney Int Suppl 1999;71:S31—6.

[88] Adams G, Vaziri ND. Skeletal muscle dysfunction in chronic renal failure: Effect of exercise. Am J Physiol, Renal Physiol 2006;290:783—91.

[89] Holdaas H, Fellstrom B, Jardine AG, et al. Effect of fluvastatin on cardiac outcomes in renal transplant recipients: a multicentre, randomised, placebo-controlled trial. Lancet 2003;361:2024—31.

[90] Baigent C, Keech A, Kearney PM, Blackwell L, Buck G, Pollicino C, et al. Cholesterol Treatment Trialists' (CTT) Collaborators. Efficacy and safety of cholesterol-lowering treatment: prospective meta-analysis of data from 90,056 participants in 14 randomized trials of statins. Lancet 2005;366: 1267—78.

[91] März W, Genser B, Drechsler C, Krane V, Grammer TB, Ritz E, et al. Wanner C on behalf of the German Diabetes and Dialysis Study Investigators. Atorvastatin and low-density lipoprotein cholesterol in type 2 diabetes mellitus patients on hemodialysis. Clin J Am Soc Nephrol 2011:1316—25.

[92] Tonelli M, Moye L, Sacks FM, Kiberd B, Curhan G. Pravastatin for secondary prevention of cardiovascular events in persons with mild chronic renal insufficiency. Ann Intern Med 2003;138(2):98—104.

[93] Tonelli M, Isles C, Curhan GC, Tonkin A, Pfeffer MA, Shepherd J, et al. Effect of pravastatin on cardiovascular events in people with chronic kidney disease. Circulation 2004; 110(12):1557—63.

[94] Strippoli GF, Navaneethan SD, Johnson DW, Perkovic V, Pellegrini F, Nicolucci A, et al. Effects of statins in patients with chronic kidney disease: meta-analysis and meta-regression of randomised controlled trials. BMJ 2008;336(7645): 645—51.

[95] Asselbergs FW, Diercks GF, Hillege HL, van Boven AJ, Janssen WM, et al. Effects of fosinopril and pravastatin on cardiovascular events in subjects with microalbuminuria. Circulation 2004;110(18):2809—16.

[96] Vaziri ND. Molecular mechanisms of lipid dysregulation in nephrotic syndrome. Kidney Int 2003;63:1964—76.

[97] Collins R, Armitage J, Parish S, Sleigh P, Peto R. Heart Protection Study Collaborative Group. MRC/BHF Heart Protection Study of cholesterol-lowering with simvastatin in 5963 people with diabetes: a randomised placebo-controlled trial. Lancet 2003;361:2005—16.

[98] Athyros VG, Mikhailidis DP, Papageorgiou AA, Symeonidis AN, Pehlivanidis AN, Bouloukos VI, et al. The effect of statins versus untreated dyslipidaemia on renal function in patients with coronary heart disease. A subgroup analysis of the Greek atorvastatin and coronary heart disease evaluation (GREACE) study. J Clin Pathol 2004;57(7):728—34.

[99] Tonelli M, Moye L, Sacks FM, Cole T, Curhan GC. Effect of pravastatin on loss of renal function in people with moderate chronic renal insufficiency and cardiovascular disease. J Am Soc Nephrol 2003;14(6):1605—13.

[100] Shepherd J, Kastelein JJ, Bittner V, Deedwania P, Breazna A, Dobson S, et al. Effect of intensive lipid lowering with atorvastatin on renal function in patients with coronary heart disease: the Treating to New Targets (TNT) study. Clin J Am Soc Nephrol 2007;2(6):1131—9.

[101] Fried LF, Orchard TJ, Kasiske BL. Effect of lipid reduction on the progression of renal disease: a meta-analysis. Kidney Int 2001;59(1):260—9.

[102] Sandhu S, Wiebe N, Fried LF, Tonelli M. Statins for improving renal outcomes: a meta-analysis. J Am Soc Nephrol 2006 Jul;17(7):2006—16.

[103] Douglas K, O'Malley PG, Jackson JL. Meta-analysis: the effect of statins on albuminuria. Ann Intern Med 2006;145(2):117−24.

[104] http://clinicaltrials.gov/ct2/show/NCT00296400?term=planet &rank=1;http://clinicaltrials.gov/ct2/show/NCT00296374? term=planet&rank=2

[105] Deslypere JP, Delanghe J, Vermeulen A. Proteinuria as complication of simvastatin treatment. Lancet 1990;336(8728):1453.

[106] Verhulst A, D'Haese PC, De Broe ME. Inhibitors of HMG-CoA reductase reduce receptor-mediated endocytosis in human kidney proximal tubular cells. J Am Soc Nephrol 2004;15(9): 2249−57.

[107] Coritsidis G, Rifici V, Gupta S, Rie J, Shan ZH, Neugarten J, et al. Preferential binding of oxidized LDL to rat glomeruli in vivo and cultured mesangial cells in vitro. Kidney Int 1991;39(5): 858−66.

[108] Pai R, Kirschenbaum MA, Kamanna VS. Low-density lipoprotein stimulates the expression of macrophage colony-stimulating factor in glomerular mesangial cells. Kidney Int 1995;48(4): 1254−62.

[109] Rovin BH, Tan LC. LDL stimulates mesangial fibronectin production and chemoattractant expression. Kidney Int 1993;43(1):218−25.

[110] Guijarro C, Kasiske BL, Kim Y, O'Donnell MP, Lee HS, Keane WF. Early glomerular changes in rats with dietary-induced hypercholesterolemia. Am J Kidney Dis 1995;26(1):152−61.

[111] Kamanna VS, Pai R, Roh DD, Kirschenbaum MA. Oxidative modification of low-density lipoprotein enhances the murine mesangial cell cytokines associated with monocyte migration, differentiation, and proliferation. Lab Invest 1996;74(6): 1067−79.

[112] Tashiro K, Makita Y, Shike T, Shirato I, Sato T, Cynshi O, et al. Detection of cell death of cultured mouse mesangial cells induced by oxidized low-density lipoprotein. Nephron 1999; 82(1):51−8.

[113] Hernandez-Perera O, Perez-Sala D, Soria E, Lamas S. Involvement of Rho GTPases in the transcriptional inhibition of pre-proendothelin-1 gene expression by simvastatin in vascular endothelial cells. Circ Res 2000;87(7):616−22.

[114] Heusinger-Ribeiro J, Fischer B, Goppelt-Struebe M. Differential effects of simvastatin on mesangial cells. Kidney Int 2004;66(1):187−95.

[115] Shibata S, Nagase M, Fujita T. Fluvastatin ameliorates podocyte injury in proteinuric rats via modulation of excessive Rho signaling. J Am Soc Nephrol 2006;17(3):754−64.

[116] Stoll LL, McCormick ML, Denning GM, Weintraub NL. Antioxidant effects of statins. Drugs Today (Barc) 2004;40(12): 975−90.

[117] Arnaud C, Braunersreuther V, Mach F. Toward immunomodulatory and anti-inflammatory properties of statins. Trends Cardiovasc Med 2005;15(6):202−6.

[118] Mukai Y, Wang CY, Rikitake Y, Liao JK. Phosphatidylinositol 3-kinase/protein kinase Akt negatively regulates plasminogen activator inhibitor type 1 expression in vascular endothelial cells. Am J Physiol Heart Circ Physiol 2007;292(4):H1937−42.

[119] Xu H, Zeng L, Peng H, Chen S, Jones J, Chew TL, et al. HMG-CoA reductase inhibitor simvastatin mitigates VEGF-induced "inside-out" signaling to extracellular matrix by preventing RhoA activation. Am J Physiol Renal Physiol 2006; 291(5):F995−1004.

[120] Khwaja A, Sharpe CC, Noor M, Hendry BM. The role of geranylgeranylated proteins in human mesangial cell proliferation. Kidney Int 2006;70(7):1296−304.

[121] Kramer S, Kron S, Wang-Rosenke Y, Loof T, Khadzhynov D, Morgera S, et al. Rosuvastatin is additive to high-dose candesartan in slowing progression of experimental mesangioproliferative

glomerulosclerosis. Am J Physiol Renal Physiol 2008;294(4): F801−11.

[122] Lee TS, Chau LY. Heme oxygenase-1 mediates the anti-inflammatory effect of interleukin-10 in mice. Nat Med 2002;8(3):240−6.

[123] Yoshimura A, Inui K, Nemoto T, Uda S, Sugenoya Y, Watanabe S, et al. Simvastatin suppresses glomerular cell proliferation and macrophage infiltration in rats with mesangial proliferative nephritis. J Am Soc Nephrol 1998;9(11): 2027−39.

[124] Blanco-Colio LM, Tunon J, Martin-Ventura JL, Egido J. Anti-inflammatory and immunomodulatory effects of statins. Kidney Int 2003;63(1):12−23.

[125] Epstein M, Campese VM. Pleiotropic effects of 3-hydroxy-3-methylglutaryl coenzyme a reductase inhibitors on renal function. Am J Kidney Dis 2005;45(1):2−14.

[126] Konstantinopoulos PA, Karamouzis MV, Papavassiliou AG. Post-translational modifications and regulation of the RAS superfamily of GTPases as anticancer targets. Nat Rev Drug Discov 2007;6(7):541−55.

[127] Konstantinopoulos PA, Papavassiliou AG. Multilevel modulation of the mevalonate and protein-prenylation circuitries as a novel strategy for anticancer therapy. Trends Pharmacol Sci 2007;28(1):6−13.

[128] Van Aelst L, D'Souza-Schorey C. Rho GTPases and signaling networks. Genes Dev 1997;11(18):2295−322.

[129] Wang CY, Liu PY, Liao JK. Pleiotropic effects of statin therapy: molecular mechanisms and clinical results. Trends Mol Med 2008;14(1):37−44.

[130] Burridge K, Wennerberg K. Rho and Rac take center stage. Cell 2004;116(2):167−79.

[131] Gojo A, Utsunomiya K, Taniguchi K, Yokota T, Ishizawa S, Kanazawa Y, et al. The Rho-kinase inhibitor, fasudil, attenuates diabetic nephropathy in streptozotocin-induced diabetic rats. Eur J Pharmacol 2007;568(1−3):242−7.

[132] Whaley-Connell AT, Morris EM, Rehmer N, Yaghoubian JC, Wei Y, Hayden MR, et al. Albumin activation of NAD(P)H oxidase activity is mediated via Rac1 in proximal tubule cells. Am J Nephrol 2007;27(1):15−23.

[133] Vecchione C, Gentile MT, Aretini A, Marino G, Poulet R, Maffei A, et al. A novel mechanism of action for statins against diabetes-induced oxidative stress. Diabetologia 2007;50(4): 874−80.

[134] Grosser N, Erdmann K, Hemmerle A, Berndt G, Hinkelmann U, Smith G, et al. Rosuvastatin upregulates the antioxidant defense protein heme oxygenase-1. Biochem Biophys Res Commun 2004;325(3):871−6.

[135] Lee TS, Chang CC, Zhu Y, Shyy JY. Simvastatin induces heme oxygenase-1: a novel mechanism of vessel protection. Circulation 2004;110(10):1296−302.

[136] Kurusu A, Shou I, Nakamura S, Fukui M, Shirato I, Tomino Y. Effects of the new hydroxy-3-methylglutaryl coenzyme a reductase inhibitor fluvastatin on anti-oxidant enzyme activities and renal function in streptozotocin-induced diabetic rats. Clin Exp Pharmacol Physiol 2000; 27(10):767−70.

[137] Suzumura K, Tanaka K, Yasuhara M, Narita H. Inhibitory effects of fluvastatin and its metabolites on hydrogen peroxide-induced oxidative destruction of hemin and low-density lipoprotein. Biol Pharm Bull 2000;23(7):873−8.

[138] Nawawi H, Osman NS, Yusoff K, Khalid BA. Reduction in serum levels of adhesion molecules, interleukin-6 and C-reactive protein following short-term low-dose atorvastatin treatment in patients with non-familial hypercholesterolemia. Horm Metab Res 2003;35(8):479−85.

[139] Sugiyama M, Ohashi M, Takase H, Sato K, Ueda R, Dohi Y. Effects of atorvastatin on inflammation and oxidative stress. Heart Vessels 2005;20(4):133−6.

[140] Romano M, Diomede L, Sironi M, Massimiliano L, Sottocorno M, Polentarutti N, et al. Inhibition of monocyte chemotactic protein-1 synthesis by statins. Lab Invest 2000; 80(7):1095−100.

[141] Wang HR, Li JJ, Huang CX, Jiang H. Fluvastatin inhibits the expression of tumor necrosis factor-alpha and activation of nuclear factor-kappaB in human endothelial cells stimulated by C-reactive protein. Clin Chim Acta 2005;353(1−2): 53−60.

[142] Pahan K, Sheikh FG, Namboodiri AM, Singh I. Lovastatin and phenylacetate inhibit the induction of nitric oxide synthase and cytokines in rat primary astrocytes, microglia, and macrophages. J Clin Invest 1997;100(11):2671−9.

[143] Kim SI, Han DC, Lee HB. Lovastatin inhibits transforming growth factor-beta1 expression in diabetic rat glomeruli and cultured rat mesangial cells. J Am Soc Nephrol 2000;11(1): 80−7.

[144] Kim SI, Kim HJ, Han DC, Lee HB. Effect of lovastatin on small GTP binding proteins and on TGF-beta1 and fibronectin expression. Kidney Int Suppl 2000;77:S88−92.

[145] Patel S, Mason RM, Suzuki J, Imaizumi A, Kamimura T, Zhang Z. Inhibitory effect of statins on renal epithelial-to-mesenchymal transition. Am J Nephrol 2006;26(4): 381−7.

[146] Yagi S, Aihara K, Ikeda Y, Sumitomo Y, Yoshida S, Ise T, et al. Pitavastatin, an HMG-CoA reductase inhibitor, exerts eNOS-independent protective actions against angiotensin II induced cardiovascular remodeling and renal insufficiency. Circ Res 2008;102(1):68−76.

[147] Weber C, Erl W, Weber KS, Weber PC. HMG-CoA reductase inhibitors decrease CD11b expression and CD11b-dependent adhesion of monocytes to endothelium and reduce increased adhesiveness of monocytes isolated from patients with hypercholesterolemia. J Am Coll Cardiol 1997;30(5):1212−7.

[148] Weitz-Schmidt G, Welzenbach K, Brinkmann V, Kamata T, Kallen J, Bruns C, et al. Statins selectively inhibit leukocyte function antigen-1 by binding to a novel regulatory integrin site. Nat Med 2001;7(6):687−92.

[149] Bernot D, Benoliel AM, Peiretti F, Lopez S, Bonardo B, Bongrand P, et al. Effect of atorvastatin on adhesive phenotype of human endothelial cells activated by tumor necrosis factor alpha. J Cardiovasc Pharmacol 2003;41(2):316−24.

[150] Usui H, Shikata K, Matsuda M, Okada S, Ogawa D, Yamashita T, et al. HMG-CoA reductase inhibitor ameliorates diabetic nephropathy by its pleiotropic effects in rats. Nephrol Dial Transplant 2003;18(2):265−72.

[151] Zapolska-Downar D, Siennicka A, Kaczmarczyk M, Kolodziej B, Naruszewicz M. Simvastatin modulates TNF alpha-induced adhesion molecules expression in human endothelial cells. Life Sci 2004;75(11):1287−302.

[152] Mausner-Fainberg K, Luboshits G, Mor A, Maysel-Auslender S, Rubinstein A, Keren G, et al. The effect of HMG-CoA reductase inhibitors on naturally occurring CD4+CD25+ T cells. Atherosclerosis 2008;197(2):829−39.

[153] Somlyo AV. New roads leading to Ca^{2+} sensitization. Circ Res 2002;91(2):83−4.

[154] Hernandez-Perera O, Perez-Sala D, Soria E, Lamas S. Involvement of Rho GTPases in the transcriptional inhibition of pre-proendothelin-1 gene expression by simvastatin in vascular endothelial cells. Circ Res 2000;87(7):616−22.

[155] Xu CB, Stenman E, Edvinsson L. Reduction of bFGF-induced smooth muscle cell proliferation and endothelin receptor

mRNA expression by mevastatin and atorvastatin. Biochem Pharmacol 2002;64(3):497−505.

[156] Ichiki T, Takeda K, Tokunou T, Iino N, Egashira K, Shimokawa H, et al. Downregulation of angiotensin II type 1 receptor by hydrophobic 3-hydroxy-3-methylglutaryl coenzyme A reductase inhibitors in vascular smooth muscle cells. Arterioscler Thromb Vasc Biol 2001;21(12):1896−901.

[157] Wassmann S, Laufs U, Baumer AT, Muller K, Konkol C, Sauer H, et al. Inhibition of geranylgeranylation reduces angiotensin II-mediated free radical production in vascular smooth muscle cells: involvement of angiotensin AT1 receptor expression and Rac1 GTPase. Mol Pharmacol 2001;59(3): 646−54.

[158] Bourcier T, Libby P. HMG CoA reductase inhibitors reduce plasminogen activator inhibitor-1 expression by human vascular smooth muscle and endothelial cells. Arterioscler Thromb Vasc Biol 2000;20(2):556−62.

[159] Joles JA, Kunter U, Janssen U, Kriz W, Rabelink TJ, Koomans HA, et al. Early mechanisms of renal injury in hypercholesterolemic or hypertriglyceridemic rats. J Am Soc Nephrol 2000;11(4):669−83.

[160] Shibata S, Nagase M, Fujita T. Fluvastatin ameliorates podocyte injury in proteinuric rats via modulation of excessive Rho signaling. J Am Soc Nephrol 2006;17(3):754−64.

[161] Cormack-Aboud FC, Brinkkoetter PT, Pippin JW, Shankland SJ, Durvasula RV. Rosuvastatin protects against podocyte apoptosis in vitro. Nephrol Dial Transplant 2009;24(2):404−12.

[162] Beltowski J, Wójcicka G, Jamroz-Wisniewska A. Adverse Effects of Statins − Mechanisms and Consequences. Current Drug Safety 2009;4:209−28.

[163] Nakamura T, Ushiyama C, Hirokawa K, Osada S, Inoue T, Shimada N, et al. Effect of cerivastatin on proteinuria and urinary podocytes in patients with chronic glomerulonephritis. Nephrol Dial Transplant 2002;17(5):798−802.

[164] Ridker PM, Danielson E, Fonseca FA, et al. Rosuvastatin to prevent vascular events in men and women with elevated C-reactive protein. N Engl J Med 2008;359:2195−207.

[165] Sever PS, Poulter NR, Dahlof B, Wedel H, Beevers G, Caulfield M, et al. The Anglo-Scandinavian Cardiac Outcomes Trial lipid lowering arm: extended observations 2 years after trial closure. Eur Heart J 2008;29:499−508.

[166] Brugts JJ, Yetgin T, Hoeks SE, Gotto AM, Shepherd J, Westendorp RG, et al. The benefits of statins in people without established cardiovascular disease but with cardiovascular risk factors: meta-analysis of randomized controlled trials. BMJ 2009;338:2376−83.

[167] Ponda MP, Barash I. Lipid metabolism in dialysis patients − the story gets more complicated. Seminars in Dialysis 2008;21: 390−4.

[168] Otvos JD, Collins D, Freedman DS. LDL and HDL particle subclasses predict coronary events and are changed favorably by gemfibrozil therapy in the Veterans Affairs HDL Intervention Trial (VA-HIT). Circulation 2006;113:1556−63.

[169] Davidson MH, Armani A, McKenney JM, Jacobson TA. Safety considerations with fibrate therapy. Am J Cardiol 2007;99(6A): 3C−18C.

[170] Jacobson TA, Zimmerman FH. Fibrates in combination with statins in the management of dyslipidemia. J Clin Hypertens (Greenwich) 2006;8(1):35−41. quiz 42-33; "K/DOQI clinical practice guidelines for management of dyslipidemias in patients with kidney disease", 2003.

[171] Cho K, Kim H, Rodriguez-Iturbe B, Vaziri ND. Niacin ameliorates oxidative stress, inflammation, proteinuria, and hypertension in rats with chronic renal failure. Am J Physiol, Renal Physiol 2009;297(1):F106−13.

[172] Cho K, Kim H, Kamanna VS, Vaziri ND. Niacin improves renal lipid metabolism and slows progression in chronic kidney disease. Biochim Biophys ACTA 1800;6—15:2010.

[173] Barter PJ, Caulfield M, Eriksson M, Grundy SM, Kastelein JJ, Komajda M, et al. Effects of torcetrapib in patients at high risk for coronary events. N Engl J Med 2007;357:2109—22.

[174] Tardif JC, Grégoire J, L'Allier PL, Anderson TJ, Bertrand O, Reeves F, et al. Avasimibe and Progression of Lesions on UltraSound (A-PLUS) Investigators. Effects of the acyl coenzyme A:cholesterol acyltransferase inhibitor avasimibe on human atherosclerotic lesions. Circulation 2004;110(21):3372—7.

[175] Vaziri ND, Liang K. Upregulation of acyl-coenzyme A: Cholesterol Acyltransferase (ACAT) in nephrotic syndrome. Kidney Int 2002;61:1769—75.

[176] Vaziri ND, Liang K. Acyl-CoA cholesterol acyltransferase inhibition ameliorates proteinuria, hyperlipidemia, LCAT, SRB-1 and LDL receptor deficiencies in nephrotic syndrome. Circulation 2004;110:419—25.

4

Uremic Toxicity

Michal Chmielewski[1,2], Olof Heimbürger[1], Peter Stenvinkel[1], Bengt Lindholm[1]

[1]Divisions of Baxter Novum and Renal Medicine, Karolinska Institutet, Karolinska University Hospital Huddinge, Stockholm, Sweden [2]Medical University of Gdansk, Department of Nephrology, Transplantology and Internal Medicine, Gdansk, Poland

INTRODUCTION

The state of uremia affects virtually all cells, tissues and organs in the body with consequences for most systems and functions and metabolic, nutritional, hormonal and immune system derangements are therefore prominent features of the uremic syndrome. The word uremia is derived from two ancient Greek words: *ouron* means urine and *haima* means blood; literally, uremia is urine in the blood. Thus, the term uremia implies that accumulation of excretory products such as urea in the blood results in the toxic condition of uremia. However, it is obvious that this definition is too narrow to cover all aspects of the uremic syndrome. A definition that comes closer to reality and emphasizes all aspects of loss of renal cell mass and functions is therefore suggested:

> Uremia is a toxic syndrome caused by severe glomerular insufficiency, associated with disturbances in tubular and endocrine functions of the kidney. It is characterized by retention of toxic metabolites, associated with changes in volume and electrolyte composition of the body fluids and excess or deficiency of various hormones.

The primary event in urine formation is the glomerular ultrafiltration process. The ultrafiltrate is reduced in volume and modified as to composition by the metabolic activity of the tubular cells. The final urine, which is the end-result of these processes contains urea and other nitrogenous metabolites in high concentration, and has an appropriate volume and electrolyte composition to maintain homeostasis. Clearly, the development of the uremic state is primarily the consequence of severe glomerular insufficiency, which is a prerequisite for retention of toxic, nitrogenous metabolites.

The sieving properties of the glomerular filter permit compounds to be filtered and eliminated from the blood.

Consequently, compounds within a very wide molecular weight spectrum are retained in the body fluids in conditions with reduced glomerular filtration, provided that they are not eliminated by other routes.

The fact that end-stage renal disease (ESRD) patients survive if they are treated by maintenance hemodialysis (HD) or peritoneal dialysis (PD) indicates that some of the most important uremic toxins are dialyzable through artificial membranes with a molecular size cut-off less than 10,000 daltons as well as through the peritoneum which has a less well defined dialytic cut-off level allowing dialytic removal also of proteins. On the other hand, the presence of a variety of residual symptoms, and the high mortality in dialysis patients, indicates that toxic compounds accumulating in uremia are either not removed at all, or are insufficiently removed, by standard dialysis [1–3].

Severe glomerular insufficiency is always associated with secondary disturbances in tubular functions, which explains why hyperkalemia and metabolic acidosis are prominent features of uremia. Disturbances in intermediary metabolism due to the loss of metabolizing tubular cells, as well as impaired synthesis of hormones produced by the kidneys such as erythropoietin and calcitriol, and impaired catabolism of peptide hormones are also involved in the symptomatology of the uremic syndrome. It may be impossible to separate such disturbances from direct effects of toxic compounds retained as a consequence of reduced renal function.

UREMIC SYMPTOMS AND SIGNS

Symptoms and signs that are commonly observed in uremia are presented in Table 4.1. Particularly

TABLE 4.1 Uremic Symptoms and Signs

Central Nervous System	Cardiovascular System	Hematologic and Immunologic
Stupor	Pericarditis	Anemia
Coma	Cardiomyopathy	Granulocyte dysfunction
Insomnia	Hypertension	Lymphocyte dysfunction
Tremor	Arteriosclerosis	Immunodeficiency
Asterixis	Heart failure	Infection susceptibility
Myoclonus	Arrythmias	Malignancies
Cramps	Edema-overhydration	Inflammation
Fatigue	Endothelial dysfunction	
Confusion		**Endocrine and metabolic changes**
EEG-changes	**Respiratory system**	Hyperparathyroidism
	Pneumonitis — "uremic lung"	Glucose intolerance
Peripheral nerves	Pulmonary edema	Lipid abnormalities
Numbness, paresthesia		Amino acid disturbances
Restless legs	**Skin**	Oxidative stress
Sensory loss	Dry skin	Malnutrition
Muscle weakness	Pruritus	Hypoalbuminemia
Pareses	Pigmentation	Muscle wasting
Autonomous neuropathy	Bleeding	Growth retardation
Hypotension	Retarded wound healing	Impotence
		Reduced libido
Gastrointestinal tract	**Musculoskeletal system**	**Hypothermia**
Anorexia	Osteodystrophy	
Nausea, vomiting	Osteomalacia	
Hiccup	Pain and fractures	
Stomatitis	Carpal tunnel syndrome	
Gastritis	Amyloidosis	
Parotitis	Myopathy	
Colitis	Muscle weakness and wasting	
Bleeding		
Fetor uremicus		

striking are the *neurological signs* and symptoms including mental changes, fatigue, muscle twitching, stupor, convulsions and coma, as well as symptomatic peripheral neuropathy. The *gastrointestinal symptoms* such as anorexia and vomiting may be associated with stomatitis, glossitis, gastritis, pancreatitis and enterocolitis. *Cardiovascular symptoms* including hypertension, left ventricular hypertrophy and heart failure (disorders closely connected with salt and water retention), pericarditis, cardiac arrhythmias, cardiomyopathy, endothelial dysfunction and atherosclerosis are also common features of the uremic syndrome (Chapter 9).

Other typical changes in fluid and electrolyte balance are hyperkalemia (Chapter 22), metabolic acidosis (Chapter 8), hyperphosphatemia, and disturbances in calcium homeostasis (Chapters 19 and 20). Decreased production and increased destruction of red cells result in anemia (Chapter 25). Impaired hemostasis leads to bleeding from the mucous membranes and in the skin (caused by a defect in platelet aggregation) and fibrinolysis is inhibited as well. Pruritus and hyperpigmentation of the skin in chronic uremia are also frequently encountered.

The immunological response is impaired in uremic patients and the susceptibility to infections may be increased. On the other hand, inflammatory parameters including proinflammatory cytokines are often elevated and may contribute to the Malnutrition, Inflammation and Atherosclerosis (MIA) syndrome which is associated with increased mortality (see section on Proinflammatory cytokines below and Chapters 5 and 17).

Disturbances in calcium and phosphorus metabolism give rise to uremic osteodystrophy causing conditions such as osteomalacia, osteosclerosis, osteitis fibrosa with bone pain, fractures and, in children, retardation of growth (Chapters 19, 20, 21 and 35).

A number of changes in intermediary metabolism are also encountered in uremic patients, including abnormalities in protein and amino acid metabolism (Chapter 1) as well as in carbohydrate (Chapter 2) and lipid metabolism (Chapter 3). Other consequences of renal failure are the loss of endocrine functions of the kidney, insufficient production of erythropoietin contributing to renal anemia (Chapter 25), and lack of active vitamin D (calcitriol) leading to deficient intestinal calcium absorption and osteodystrophy (Chapters 19, 20 and 21). Moreover, the normal kidney has an important role in catabolizing various peptide hormones, and loss of these abilities may lead to endocrine disturbances.

Cell membrane transport is abnormal in uremia. The active sodium efflux is inhibited and the transmembrane potential of skeletal muscle cells is decreased in patients with severe uremia [4,5], signifying inhibition of the electrogenic sodium pump or increased membrane permeability for sodium. This abnormality is reversed by adequate dialysis [6].

In summary, uremia seems to affect practically all organs and tissues of the body; mucous and serous membranes are affected, various transport phenomena in the cell membranes are inhibited and intermediary metabolic processes are impaired. These alterations are responsible for or contribute, directly or indirectly, to the metabolic and nutritional problems in renal disease patients.

TOXIC EFFECTS OF UREMIC PLASMA OR SERUM

Indirect evidence of uremic toxicity has been obtained from bioassay studies in vivo and in vitro, which showed that plasma, serum, ultrafiltrate and dialysate from uremic patients affect numerous biological processes. There are only a few in vivo bioassays of uremic toxicity. Infusion of uremic ultrafiltrate to normal rats results in lowering of intestinal calcitriol receptor number and increased receptor mRNA levels similar to those found in uremic rats [7]. Intraperitoneal administration of a middle molecular fraction from ultrafiltrate obtained at the beginning of the first-dialysis treatment in chronic kidney disease (CKD), and from normal urine, inhibits appetite in the rat [8]. This effect was only obtained for the fraction 1000–5000 Da, which inhibited both sucrose intake and protein intake in a dose dependent manner. These results suggest that toxic compounds in the middle-molecular weight fraction, which are normally excreted in urine, accumulate in the plasma in uremia and suppress food intake. Administration of indoxyl sulfate, a uremic toxin, was shown to promote aortic calcification in hypertensive rats [9].

There is experimental evidence that dialyzable molecules play a role for development of uremic symptoms. In rats with renal failure, uremic encephalopathy quantified by EEG, is attenuated by PD [10]. Progressive loss of nephrons in rats with chronic renal failure may be retarded by PD, suggesting that a circulating uremic toxin is involved in the advancement of glomerulosclerosis [11]. Similarly, tubular injury may be provoked by uremia as shown in experimental studies [12].

There are numerous in vitro studies of uremic toxicity. Uremic sera inhibits in vitro erythropoiesis [13–15], lymphocyte transformation and proliferation [16], natural killer cell activity [17], and mononuclear phagocytes [18]. Platelet-activating factor synthesis is inhibited by uremic ultrafiltrate, and this effect appears to be associated with an inhibition of phospholipase A2 and acetyltransferase activity [19]. Uremic toxins accumulating in the plasma of patients with renal failure not only affect essential neutrophil functions and thereby the unspecific immune response, but also influence neutrophil survival by modulating the rate of apoptotic cell death [20]. Uremic serum reduces inotropy and induces arrhythmias in cultured cardiac myocytes [21]. Plasma from uremic patients depresses nerve-mediated smooth muscle contraction [22].

A variety of metabolic processes in vitro are impaired in the presence of uremic plasma or serum. Glucose utilization and glycolysis are inhibited (Chapters 2 and 31). There is also inhibition of protein synthesis, mitochondrial metabolism, uncoupling of phosphorylation [23], inhibition of fibrinolysis and lipolysis. Production of Apo lipoprotein A-1 is inhibited by uremic serum and its subfractions [24].

Several trans-membrane transport systems in a variety of cells are also inhibited in vitro in the presence of uremic serum or ultrafiltrate. These include transport of sodium in cell membranes [25], calcium in mitochondria [26], erythrocyte membrane calcium pumps [27], uric acid in liver slices [28], hippuric acid derivatives in kidney tissue [29], and amino acids in muscle [30]. The nuclear uptake of calcitriol receptor is inhibited by uremic ultrafiltrate [31], possibly contributing to calcitriol resistance in renal failure patients.

In vitro inhibition of several enzymes has also been reported. Among these are lipoprotein lipase [32], xanthine oxidase [28], phenylalanine hydroxylase [33], Na^+, K^+-ATPase in brain, red cells and aortic strips [34–36], thiopurine methyltransferase [37], delta-amino levulinic acid synthetase [38], and transketolase in red cells [39] and nervous tissue [40], but no inhibition was found in erythrocytes by other investigators [41]. Tranketolase inhibition has been suggested to play a role in peripheral neuropathy of uremia. The effects of uremic serum on trans-membrane transport mechanisms and transport enzymes (Na^+, K^+-ATPase) are of special interest in view of Bricker's [42] hypothesis that a humoral factor, produced as a result of homeostatic adaptation to sodium retention and which decreases tubular sodium reabsorption, might be important in uremia by inhibiting trans-membrane transport in other cells as well.

In conclusion, there is evidence that a variety of clinical disturbances, such as anemia, immunological deficiency, bleeding tendency, disorders of protein, carbohydrate and lipid metabolism, and various membrane transport disturbances may be related to toxins or inhibitors present in plasma or other body fluids in uremic patients. The approximate toxicity of particular uremic toxins is discussed in the following sections of the chapter and depicted in Figure 4.1.

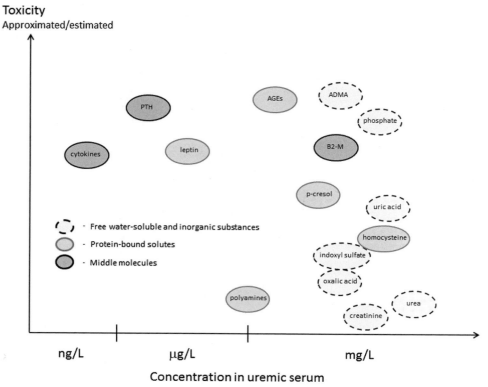

FIGURE 4.1 The estimated toxicity of some particular uremic toxins and classes of toxins with different molecular weights and with different average concentrations in uremic serum. The figure illustrates that the toxicity of a uremic toxin is not strictly related to its molecular weight or to its molar concentration in blood.

DEFINITION OF A UREMIC TOXIN

In order for a substance to be defined as a uremic toxin, a necessary criterion is that it is excreted by the kidney and that it is present in increased concentrations in body fluids and/or tissues in patients with renal failure.

Uremic toxin should fulfill specific conditions [43,44]. These conditions are:

1. The toxin must be chemically identified and characterized.
2. Quantitative analysis of the toxin in biological fluids should be possible.
3. The level of the toxin in biological fluids must be elevated in uremia.
4. A relationship between the level of the toxin in biological fluids and one or more of the manifestations of uremia must be present.
5. A reduction in the level of the toxin in biological fluids must result in the amelioration of the uremic manifestation.
6. Administration of the toxin to achieve levels similar to those observed in uremia must reproduce the uremic manifestation in otherwise normal animals or man (in vitro demonstration of cellular toxicity alone is insufficient to fulfill this criterion).

7. A plausible patho-biological mechanism should be demonstrated to explain the linkage between the toxin and the uremic manifestation.

The ability of an individual toxin to induce or to contribute to uremic symptoms is triggered by the inability of insufficient kidneys to excrete and/or metabolize this toxin. However, it also depends on other factors, as: the rate of synthesis and degradation, the non-renal elimination), the extra- and intracellular distribution, and the presence or absence of compounds that affect the toxin's concentration and/or activity.

Correlations between the appearance of certain uremic signs and the concentration of one or more particular substances in plasma do not prove that a specific substance is responsible since a great number of substances excreted by the kidneys accumulate simultaneously as renal function deteriorates. The identification and quantification of the impact of a potential toxin is therefore difficult. Substances known to be present in raised concentration in patients with uremic signs and symptoms have been given to humans or experimental animals, or added to various tissues, cells or enzymes in vitro to prove whether they exert toxic effects. Many of these experiments are open to criticism since the concentrations used were often much higher than those encountered in the blood of uremic patients.

Another criticism of the in vitro experiments is that they reflect only acute toxicity and, therefore, will be inadequate for assessing chronic toxicity, which occurs in uremia. Even when investigations are performed correctly, with the compound present in concentrations comparable to those found in uremic patients, it may be doubtful if these in vitro effects relate to in vivo toxicity.

It is possible that a number of compounds, each of which present in a concentration too low to be toxic, may act synergistically to produce toxic effects. There is also evidence that when certain compounds, known to accumulate in uremia, are present together in the medium, they may induce in vitro toxic effects that are not found when these compounds are present alone. In normal rats, single doses of cresole, putrescine, methylguanidine and acetoin had no effect on oxygen consumption, but some combinations of these substances reduced oxygen consumption significantly [45]. These studies raise the question of whether testing of some uremic compounds has to be made in a "uremic" environment. Also, most studies on uremic toxins assume their presence in blood, whereas intracellular and local uremic toxin levels are less well investigated. For example, local uremic toxins present in the gastrointestinal tract were found to influence insulin resistance, based on the effects of an oral adsorbent in rats with renal insufficiency [46].

The current understanding of the issue of uremic toxicity allowed for a widely accepted classification of uremic toxins, based on molecular weight and plasma protein-binding characteristics. The molecules have been divided into three major subclasses: (1) small solutes (<500 D) with no known protein binding; (2) solutes with known or likely protein binding; and (3) middle molecules (>500 D). Additionally, a number of inorganic substances, known to exert toxic effects in uremia, have been characterized.

Characteristics forming the basis for this classification, i.e., molecular weight and protein binding, potentially influence the removal pattern of the toxins during dialysis or other methods of extracorporeal elimination.

Currently, well over 100 solutes and compounds have been identified as uremic toxins and this number is growing rapidly. Therefore, the list of some of the currently recognized uremic toxins shown in Table 4.2

TABLE 4.2A Currently Recognized Uremic Retention Solutes [191,254]: Small Water-Soluble Compounds

Small Water-Soluble Compounds		
1-Methyladenosine	Guanidine	Orotidine
1-Methylguanosine	Guanidinoacetate	Oxalate
1-Methylinosine	Guanidinosuccinate	
Phenylacetylglutamine	8-OH-2'Deoxyguanosine	Guanilin
Phenylethylamine		
ADMA[1]	Hypoxanthine	Pseudouridine
α-keto-δ-Guanidinovaleriate	Inosine	SDMA
α-N-Acetylarginine	Malondialdehyde	Sorbitol
Arabinitol	Mannitol	Taurocyamine
Argininic acid	Methylguanidine	Thiocyanate
Benzylalcohol	Myoinositol	Threitol
β-Guanidinopropionate	N2,N2-Dimethylguanosine	Trimethylamine
Creatine	N4-Acetylcytidine	Thymine
Creatinine	N6-Methyladenosine	Uracil
Cytidine	N6-Threonylcarbamoyladenosine	Urea
Dimethylglycine	N-Methyl-2-pyridone-5-carboxamide	Uric acid
Dimethylguanosine	Nitrosodimethylamine	Uridine
Erythritol	Nitrosomethylamine	Xanthine
γ-Guanidinobutyrate	Orotic acid	Xanthosine

[1]ADMA, Asymmetric dimethyl-arginine.

TABLE 4.2B Currently Recognized Uremic Retention Solutes [191,254]: Protein-Bound Compounds

Protein-Bound Compounds		
2-Methoxyresorcinol	Indole-3-acetate	Pentosidine
3-Deoxyglucosone	Indoxyl sulfate	Phenol
CMPF	Kinurenine	Phenylacetic acid
Fructoselysine	Kinurenic acid	p-OH-hippurate
Glyoxal	Melatonin	Putrescine
Hippuric acid	Methylglyoxal	Quinolinic acid
Homocysteine	Nε-Carboxymethyllysine	Spermidine
Hydroquinone	p-Cresol	Spermine

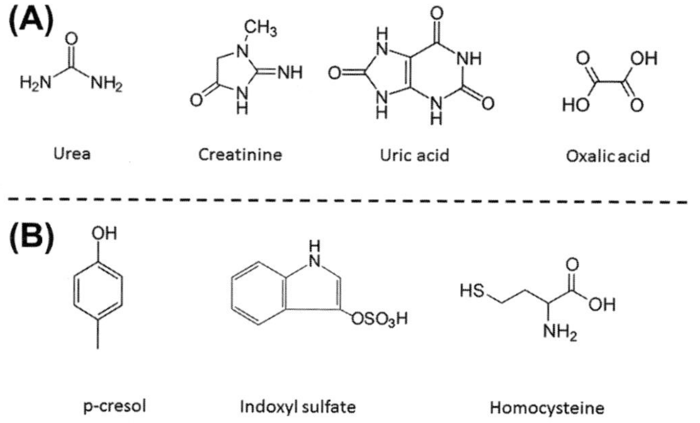

FIGURE 4.2 The structure of some exemplary solutes, belonging either to the class of water-soluble compounds (A) or protein-bound toxins (B).

TABLE 4.2C Currently Recognized Uremic Retention Solutes [191,254]: Middle Molecules

Middle Molecules		
Adiponectin	Dinucleoside polyphosphates	Methionine-enkephalin
Adrenomedullin	DIP I	Motiline
Atrial natriuretic peptide	δ-Sleep-inducing peptide	Neuropeptide Y
β2-Microglobulin	Endothelin	Octopamine
β-Endorphin	Ghrelin	Orexin A
β-Lipotropin	Hepcidin	Parathyroid hormone
Basic fibroblast growth factor	Hyaluronic acid	Retinol binding protein
Calcitonin-gene related peptide	Interleukin-1β	Substance P
Cholecystokinin	Interleukin-6	Tumor necrosis factor α
Clara cell protein	Interleukin-18	Up4A
Complement factor D	κ-Ig Light chain	Uroguanylin
Cystatin C	λ-Ig Light chain	Vasoactive intestinal peptide
Desacylghrelin	Leptin	

is incomplete, as these known compounds most likely will be outnumbered by the quantity of still unidentified solutes. Figure 4.2 shows the structure of some exemplary solutes, belonging either to the class of water-soluble compounds or protein-bound toxins.

IMPACT OF DIALYSIS TREATMENT ON UREMIC TOXICITY

Dialysis patients generally do not exhibit major uremic symptoms, but many patients continue to suffer from residual symptoms and endocrine and metabolic disturbances, as well as morbidity induced by the therapeutic procedures per se, such as cardiovascular instability, enhanced protein catabolism, malnutrition, infection, inflammation, biomaterial incompatibility, and psychological disturbances.

The aim of dialysis treatment is to normalize the volume and composition of the body fluids and remove as efficiently as possible uremic toxins that are of clinical importance. Efficacy of removal by various blood purification modalities is mainly governed by three properties of these substances, molecular size, the degree of plasma protein binding and their inter-compartmental distribution.

Currently, it is acknowledged that the removal of fluid and small soluble solutes is important in preventing short-term or "acute mortality", e.g., related to hyperkalemia. For the long-term outcome, the protein-bound compounds and the middle molecules seem to play a more essential role [47].

Diffusive transport as used in dialysis treatment favors the elimination of small molecular compounds such as urea and creatinine, but larger molecules are also removed, especially when using synthetic high-flux membranes or, peritoneal dialysis as the peritoneal membrane contains pores with larger sizes than pores in low-flux membranes. For elimination of larger molecules, convective transport with high-flux membranes, as used in hemofiltration and hemodiafiltration, is advantageous since larger molecules are eliminated with the same efficacy (clearance) as small molecules up to a molecular size where the sieving properties of the membrane become rate-limiting [48]. Among convective strategies, both post-dilution hemodiafiltration and pre-dilution hemofiltration have been found to be superior to pre-dilution hemodiafiltration in removing middle molecules [49]. Whereas removal of small solutes is flow dependent, the removal of middle and large molecules is time-dependent and can thus be enhanced by increasing the frequency and/or duration of the dialysis sessions [50].

As for *protein-bound toxins*, a larger pore size has little effect on their removal [51]. Post-dilution hemodiafiltration has been found to be better than both pre-dilution hemodiafiltration and pre-dilution hemofiltration [49]. Surprisingly, PD was not found to be effective in eliminating protein-bound uremic toxins, despite considerable trans-peritoneal albumin loss [52,53]. On the other hand, plasma levels of protein-bound solutes tend to be even lower in PD patients, as compared to HD subjects, possibly due to different generation and/or metabolism patterns [54].

A lot of expectations are associated with the ability of adsorptive strategies to eliminate protein-bound compounds. However, more studies are necessary to prove their applicability and advantages in the ESRD population [47].

TOXICITY OF INORGANIC SUBSTANCES IN UREMIA

Homeostatic control of water, inorganic ion and acid base balance is mainly accomplished by the kidneys. When renal function deteriorates, the kidneys are unable to exert full homeostatic control, resulting in disturbances in water and electrolyte metabolism. Water and electrolyte abnormalities contribute to the toxic symptomatology in the majority of uremic patients and, if left unattended, may lead to a fatal outcome. With the advent of improved diagnostic methods, a better understanding of the principles of fluid and electrolyte balance, and more effective therapeutic regimens (ion exchange resins, diuretics, dialysis), currently water and electrolyte disturbances should only rarely be the direct cause of death.

The abnormalities of water and electrolyte metabolism in uremia will be briefly reviewed with emphasis on toxic effects. For a more complete review of the subject, see Chapters 19, 22 and 23.

Water

Water overload may be either approximately isotonic, as in most edematous conditions, or hypotonic, as in water intoxication. A patient with oliguric acute kidney injury is especially prone to develop water intoxication due to excessive water intake, caused by inappropriate thirst or by iatrogenic infusion of an excess of low-electrolyte or electrolyte-free solutions. Water excess in patients with renal failure may produce edema, heart failure and hypertension (see Chapters 9 and 22). In water intoxication a variety of signs and symptoms such as mental confusion, restlessness, twitching, muscle cramps, convulsions and coma may occur. These are probably related to osmotic water transport into the central nervous system, resulting in brain edema.

Sodium

Sodium retention is a cardinal feature of both acute and chronic renal failure and may give rise to hypertension, pulmonary edema, heart failure and peripheral edema (Chapters 9, 22 and 27).

Patients with near-end-stage renal failure can usually maintain sodium homeostasis as fractional sodium reabsorption is decreased in surviving nephrons. This partially compensates for the decrease in glomerular filtration of sodium although the average ability to regulate sodium excretion in relation to the sodium intake is impaired. Several factors have been suggested to contribute to the adaptation of fractional sodium reabsorption in chronic uremia, among them the secretion of a natriuretic hormones may cause general toxic effects on solute transport in the body cells by inhibiting Na^+, K^+-ATPase [42]. Serum samples obtained from HD patients contained substance(s) that inhibited Na, K-ATPase in vitro, and acutely caused alterations in myocyte relaxation and calcium metabolism [55]. This may contribute to the diastolic dysfunction in uremic patients. Sodium overload, found in ESRD patients, has been related to aortic stiffness, a measure of atherosclerosis and cardiovascular risk, as well as to increased oxidative stress, another cardiovascular risk factor [56].

Potassium

In renal insufficiency, failure to excrete potassium may result in hyperkalemia, caused by oral intake or parenteral administration of potassium, or following release of potassium from the tissues during endogenous catabolism. The risk of potassium intoxication is particularly high in patients with acute oliguric post-traumatic renal failure with rapid tissue breakdown; severe hyperkalemia is rarely present when the urinary volumes are adequate, and it is potentiated by metabolic acidosis because potassium moves out of the cells as pH decreases. In addition, several drugs commonly used in ESRD patients may contribute to hyperkalemia such as angiotensin converting enzyme (ACE) inhibitors, ACE receptor blockers, amilorid, and spironolactone.

Progressive hyperkalemia is attended by neuromuscular and cardiovascular disturbances with typical

ECG changes, ultimately leading to bradycardia and cardiac arrest (Chapter 22).

Hydrogen Ions

A common feature of renal failure is metabolic acidosis, resulting from the inability to excrete excess metabolically generated hydrogen ions. Severe and prolonged metabolic acidosis results in major disturbances and a number of fundamental metabolic and physiological processes, causing severe abnormalities in energy and metabolism [57]. Metabolic acidosis in renal failure patients has adverse effects on bone mineral metabolism. It may directly induce dissolution of bone and also alter bone metabolism by stimulating osteoblast-mediated bone resorption, inhibition of osteoblast-mediated bone formation and altering the serum concentrations or biological actions of parathyroid hormone and vitamin D. These effects are discussed more in detail in Chapters 8, 11, 18 and 19 and in review articles [58,59]. Correction of acidosis in HD patients has been shown to forestall the development of hyperparathyroidism-related bone disease [60]. It also seems to be associated with attenuation of the rate of decline of renal function, as shown in experimental and clinical studies [61].

From the nutritional point of view it is of interest that metabolic acidosis is an important stimulus for net protein catabolism, as evident from studies in experimental animals and in humans [62–64]. In rats, protein degradation in muscle is stimulated by metabolic acidosis by mechanisms which require cortisol [65,66]. Experiments in rats with CKD demonstrate that acidosis, rather than uremia per se, appears to enhance muscle protein catabolism [67]. This effect seems to be mediated by the stimulation of skeletal muscle branched-chain keto acid decarboxylation, which increases the catabolism of the branched-chain amino acids (valine, leucine and isoleucine), that are mainly metabolized in muscle tissue [68]. Acidosis stimulates proteolysis in muscle by inducing the transcription of genes encoding for enzymes participating in the ATP-dependent cytosolic ubiquitin-proteasome proteolytic pathway [69].

In non-dialyzed chronic uremic patients, the correction of metabolic acidosis improves the nitrogen balance and reduces urea appearance and muscle proteolysis [70,71]. Studies in normal subjects, using a continuous infusion of 13C-leucine have demonstrated that total body protein breakdown and apparent leucine oxidation are higher during acidosis than during alkalosis [72,73]. In nondialyzed patients with chronic renal failure, the correction of acidosis reduced protein degradation and leucine oxidation [74]. A study in normal subjects demonstrates that metabolic acidosis reduces

the synthesis rate of albumin significantly [75]. The muscle intracellular concentration of valine (one of the branched-chain amino acids) is low in HD patients, and the levels correlate with the pre-dialysis standard bicarbonate level, which varied between 18 and 24 mmol/L, suggesting that even slight and intermittent acidosis may stimulate the catabolism of valine in muscle, resulting in a valine depletion that may potentially limit protein synthesis [76]. Correction of acidosis may prevent acidosis-related protein wasting [64,77,78] and restores low muscle concentration of branched-chain amino acids to normal levels [79]. Indeed, oral sodium bicarbonate in acidotic PD patients led to an improved nutritional status and reduced the risk for hospitalization [80]. This and other experimental and clinical studies lend support to the current guidelines to maintain serum bicarbonate levels at 24 mEq/L or greater in all CKD patients [81].

Phosphate

Phosphate is known to accumulate in patients with renal insufficiency. The plasma concentration rises when the glomerular filtration rate falls below 25% of normal. The role of phosphate retention in causing increased parathyroid activity early in the course of renal failure and its contribution to various clinical and biochemical abnormalities observed in uremic patients is reviewed in Chapters 17, 19 and 20. Restriction of dietary phosphate or removal of phosphate by oral phosphate binders prevents deterioration of renal function in the remnant kidney model of CKD in the rat presumably by prevention of renal calcification [82–84].

A high inorganic phosphate concentration in plasma carries the risk of calcium phosphate deposits in organs and tissues and vascular calcification [85,86]. Although a high phosphate concentration in plasma may reflect high dietary protein intake, a graded independent association between serum phosphate levels and mortality is a constant finding in CKD patients [86–88] (see Chapters 14, 17, 19 and 20).

Magnesium

It is well established that the serum magnesium concentration is raised in most patients with severe renal insufficiency. Magnesium metabolism in CKD is discussed in Chapter 22. Toxic manifestations in the form of vomiting, malaise, hypotension, decreased reflexes, arrhythmias and cardiac arrest have been observed in severe hypermagnesemia after magnesium salt administration to patients with renal failure. However, most observational and interventional studies suggest that higher serum magnesium concentrations in CKD patients may improve survival and slow the progression of vascular calcification [89].

Sulfate

Inorganic sulfate excreted by the kidneys is derived mostly from oxidation of sulfur-containing amino acids. The plasma concentration of sulfate is increased in uremia proportional to acidosis, creatinine and inorganic phosphate concentrations and, inversely proportional, to the glomerular filtration rate [90]. HD patients have increased plasma levels of sulfate which are reduced by the dialysis treatment [91,92].

There is little evidence that sulfate per se is toxic; when sulfate concentration increases, it partly "replaces" the chloride ion in the extracellular fluid. It has been speculated whether sulfate may be involved in the pathogenesis of renal osteodystrophy, possibly by complex formation with calcium in the gut or in plasma [90]. The sweat sulfate concentration is increased in CKD [93], and it has been suggested that unstable calcium sulfate complexes deposited in the skin could be a significant factor in dialysis-related pruritus [93].

Trace Elements

Heavy metals and other trace elements are normal constituents of food and drinking water. Some of them are essential but some can be harmful. In uremic patients accumulation of trace elements has to be expected because of reduced renal excretion. In addition, excessive uptake from dialysis fluid, from dialysis equipment or from medications may occur. High concentrations of aluminum, arsenic, chromium, copper, cobalt, silicon and other trace elements have been observed in uremic plasma and/or tissues. The accumulation and toxicity of trace elements in uremia is discussed in detail in Chapter 23.

FREE WATER-SOLUBLE LOW-MOLECULAR-WEIGHT SOLUTES

Urea

The chemical theory of the pathogenesis of the uremic syndrome begins with Prévost and Dumas [94], who discovered in 1821 that removal of the kidneys leads to a rise in blood urea concentration. However, already in 1831, Richard Bright [95] had questioned the role of urea as a uremic toxin.

Urea is quantitatively the most important end product of nitrogen metabolism in mammals and accounts for about 85% of the urinary nitrogen excretion. The urea concentration increases in the body fluids when glomerular filtration rate is reduced. The blood concentration of urea is, however, also dependent on the nitrogen intake and the balance between endogenous protein synthesis and breakdown. Thus, in conditions of hypercatabolism, e.g. after severe trauma and in sepsis, the urea production rate is grossly increased.

Evidence implicating urea as a toxic substance in uremia was brought forward by a number of investigators who administered urea to experimental animals or to normal subjects. Urea injections shortened the survival of acutely uremic rats [96]. However, it may not be possible to distinguish toxic effects of urea per se from side effects such as dehydration, osmotic diuresis or water shifts between extra- and intracellular fluid.

More relevant are clinical experiments where urea was added to dialysis fluid. Nephrectomized dogs maintained by PD may develop severe toxic symptoms including coma at a blood urea concentration of 370 to 480 mg/dL (62 to 80 mmol/L) [97]. In contrast, dogs whose ureters had been transplanted into the ileum remained virtually free of toxic symptoms, even when the blood urea concentration rose to 800 mg/dL (133 mmol/L) [98]. Dogs subjected to PD against high concentrations of urea 1 g/dL (167 mmol/l) in the dialysis fluid showed shortened survival compared with dogs dialyzed without this addition [99].

Patients with acute kidney injury dialyzed against a solution containing sufficient urea to prevent a change in the blood urea concentration, showed the same degree of clinical improvement in the uremic syndrome during dialysis as patients in whom urea was removed [100]. Chronic uremic patients treated with HD improved despite maintaining the plasma urea concentration in the range 200 to 300 mg/dL (33 to 50 mmol/L) but the hemorrhagic diathesis persisted. At higher concentrations, however, toxic symptoms occurred, such as headache, vomiting and fatigue [101]. In similar experiments in patients with CKD, high concentrations of urea in the blood were associated with malaise, lethargy, pruritus, headache, vomiting and bleeding tendencies [102]. In these patients the lowest plasma concentrations of urea, at which symptoms began to appear, were 200 to 300 mg/dL (33 to 50 mmol/L). When urea loading was stopped, headache and vomiting subsided quickly. Furthermore, addition of urea to the dialysis fluid in uremic subjects caused glucose intolerance [103].

Overall, there is little evidence that high blood urea concentrations per se are harmful in dialysis patients, provided that they are adequately dialyzed. On the contrary, several studies demonstrate that low urea concentrations are associated with reduced survival, presumably because low urea levels reflect a low protein intake, thus being an index of malnutrition [64,104–108].

In a retrospective analysis of laboratory data from more than 12,000 HD patients a low blood urea nitrogen (BUN) level, presumably reflecting a low protein intake, was associated with an increased risk of death, but mortality also increased when BUN was excessively high, presumably as a sign of underdialysis [106].

A large randomized clinical trial in dialysis patients, the HEMO study, revealed no survival benefits associated with greater urea removal [109]. Similarly, difference in the amount of urea removed had no impact on survival in two large trials in patients undergoing continuous ambulatory peritoneal dialysis (CAPD) [110,111].

Urea is widely used for estimating the dose of dialysis based on the removal rate of urea expressed as Kt/V, where K = urea clearance (in milliliters per minute), t = length of dialysis (in minutes), V = distribution volume of urea (in milliliters). A simpler expression of the dose of dialysis for small molecules is the urea reduction rate, i.e., the ratio between pre-dialysis minus post-dialysis concentration and the pre-dialysis concentration of urea [112].

It should be apparent from the foregoing discussion about blood urea levels and clinical outcome in dialysis patients that urea ought to be regarded as a "surrogate molecule" for a uremic toxin. Thus, accumulation of solutes other than urea may correlate better with toxic uremic symptoms and the "residual uremic syndrome" in dialysis patients [113].

Creatinine

Creatinine is together with urea, the most widely known "uremic toxin", and is usually assessed whenever a reduction in kidney function is suspected. This is mainly because creatinine evaluation is cheap, widely accessible and relatively well reflects the renal function. It also forms the basis for estimation of estimated glomerular filtration rate (eGFR) and thus is a major component of all principal eGFR equations.

Creatinine, which is nonenzymatically produced from the creatine pool in skeletal muscle, but is also to some extent generated from exogenous creatine present in meat, is the major *guanidine* compound retained in patients with diminished glomerular filtration rate. Creatinine is routinely determined in plasma or serum as a measure of impairment of renal function and it might be expected that a variety of uremic symptoms correlate with the plasma creatinine level; this does not, however, necessarily imply a causal relationship. In fact, high serum creatinine levels correlate with low mortality in HD patients, presumably because the creatinine generation rate reflects the size of the muscle mass [106]. Creatinine seems to be relatively nontoxic. Large amounts of creatinine have been fed to healthy subjects

without any adverse effects [114,115] and animals also tolerate large doses [116].

Guanidines (Other than Creatinine)

Guanidines in high concentrations inhibit a wide variety of enzymes of biological interest. Guanidine derivatives are potent inhibitors of mitochondrial respiration in vitro [117], and interfere with mitochondrial calcium transport [118]. The first evidence for accumulation of guanidines (other than creatinine) in uremia came in 1915, when Foster [119] extracted a toxic base from uremic blood which, when injected into guinea pigs, caused dyspnea, convulsions, coma and death. Subsequently, this material has been identified as guanidine. Later, numerous studies confirmed that guanidine or guanidine-like compounds are elevated in uremia and hypertension. Guanidino compounds such as methylguanidine and guanidinosuccinic acid are neuroexcitatory agents and may perhaps contribute to the etiology of uremic encephalopathy [120]. Uremic concentrations of guanidine compounds, guanidine-succinate, -proprionate and -butyrate inhibit neutrophil superoxide production in vitro, and this may compromise host defense function [121].

Methylguanidine (MG)

For many years investigators have been interested in the role of methylguanidine (MG) as a uremic toxin. MG is provided by a diet rich in broth or in boiled beef, which contains large amounts of MG formed from the oxidation of creatinine during boiling. Endogenous production of MG occurs by conversion from creatinine and from arginine [122]. Biosynthesis of MG from creatinine takes place in several organs [123]. In rats with renal failure the conversion of MG from creatinine was found to be considerably higher than in normal rats [124]. A low protein diet with essential amino acid supply decreases the serum concentration and urinary excretion of MG in CKD [125] presumably due to decreased turnover of arginine. The increase in urinary excretion of MG in uremia is related to the plasma creatinine concentration, which suggests increased production [126].

There is evidence from tissue determinations in experimental animals, from observations in post-dialysis rebound and from injections of labeled MG, that MG, which is a strongly basic compound, accumulates preferentially in the intracellular fluid compartment [126].

Infusion of MG into dogs caused a syndrome resembling uremia with anorexia, vomiting, diarrhea, pruritus, anemia, altered glucose tolerance, high plasma fibrinogen levels, reduced fibrinolytic activity, defective calcium absorption, stomach and duodenal ulceration, hemorrhage, convulsions and semi-coma [127] MG inhibits the nitric oxide pathway in macrophages [128] and induced relaxation in contraction-stimulated aortic rings [129].

MG was found to elicit proinflammatory effects on leukocytes [130] and to enhance the lipopolysaccharide (LPS)-stimulated intracellular production of TNF-alpha by normal human monocytes. Moreover, the anti-proliferative effect of calcitriol was neutralized in the presence of MG. Finally, after incubation of whole blood in the presence of MG, the *Escherichia coli* stimulated oxidative burst activity of the granulocyte population was found to be significantly inhibited [130]. However, the concentrations of MG used in most studies were considerably higher than those found in uremic sera.

Guanidinosuccinic Acid (GSA)

Guanidinosuccinic acid (GSA) appears in much higher concentrations both in the plasma and urine of uremic patients than in normal plasma and urine, suggesting increased production. GSA also concentrates in cerebrospinal fluid to up to 100 times higher levels than in controls [131,132], reaching levels about 10–20 μmol/L. Low protein diet and essential amino acids diminished the serum concentration and urinary excretion of GSA in CKD [125]. HD removes GSA as well as other guanidine compounds, and this may temporarily decrease the inhibition of erythrocyte transketolase activity in HD patients [133].

Infusion of GSA to normal rats resulted in suppression of calcitriol synthesis at concentrations similar to those present in uremic ultrafiltrate [134]. Behavioral toxicity of intraperitoneally injected GSA was observed in mice resulting in electrocorticographic changes and convulsions [127,135]. Moreover, GSA is suspected to be related to uremic bleeding diathesis [136]. Finally, it has been found to exert an inhibitory effect on the LPS-stimulated intracellular production of TNF-alpha by human monocytes [130].

In conclusion, GSA has been reported to exert a variety of toxic effects in vitro and in vivo, but its role as uremic toxin is still not clear.

Methylated Arginine Metabolites (ADMA, SDMA)

Asymmetric dimethyl-arginine (ADMA), as well as its structural isomer symmetric dimethylarginine (SDMA) were first isolated in 1970 by Kakimoto and Akazawa [137]. Over 20 years later it turned out that patients on HD had higher ADMA levels than controls and that ADMA was able to inhibit nitric oxide (NO) production in vivo and in vitro [138]. It was proposed that ADMA might have a role in hypertension of ESRD patients. Increased concentrations of ADMA have been found also in proteinuric subjects [139]. ADMA levels correlate well with markers of cardiovascular burden such as: dyslipidemia [140], intima-media

thickness of the carotid artery [141] or left ventricular mass [142]. Furthermore, infusion of exogenous ADMA has been found to: increase systemic vascular resistance, elevate mean arterial pressure, reduce cardiac output, augment pulmonary vascular resistance, impair renal blood flow and increase vascular stiffness [143]. Finally, a strong and independent link between ADMA and mortality has been observed, both in the general population as well as in CKD patients [144,145].

On the basis of these studies it has been proposed that ADMA is not only a marker but also a potent mediator of endothelial dysfunction and atherosclerosis [146].

Much less is known about the other methylated arginine metabolite, SDMA. It has been shown to inhibit NO synthesis, although to a much lesser extent than ADMA [147], and to promote production of reactive oxygen species [148]. Current studies demonstrate that SDMA is involved in the inflammatory processes in the course CKD, activating NF-κB and resulting in enhanced expression of IL-6 and TNF-α [149].

Other Guanidines

A number of other guanidine compounds have been found in increased concentrations in serum from uremic patients: guanidine, guanidinobutyric acid, guanidinopropionic acid, taurocyamine, alpha-ketogammaguanidinovaleric acid and homoarginine [131,132].

In a study by Perna et al. [150], the authors demonstrated that guanidine modified albumin structure in such a way that it decreased the protein binding of homocysteine, hence stimulating the release of free, active and potentially damaging homocysteine fraction. Guanidinopropionic acid has been reported to inhibit glucose-6-phosphate dehydrogenase in vitro [151], and also inhibits lymphocyte proliferation [152]. Glycocyamine (and creatinine and creatine) added to post-dialysis uremic plasma has been reported to reduce insulin-binding to its receptors in erythrocytes [153]. High doses of guanidine have been shown to induce alterations in transaminase pattern of liver, kidney and muscle in the rat [154].

Purines

Uric Acid and Other Purine Derivates

Uric acid, the end-product of purine metabolism in primates, is normally excreted in the urine, but to some extent it is also converted by bacteria in the gut. Moderate hyperuricemia frequently occurs early in the course of CKD but becomes marked only in the terminal stage of uremia. Functional adaptation of the residual nephrons in CKD results in increased urate excretion per nephron due to both decreased tubular reabsorption and increased tubular secretion.

Hyperuricemia in advanced renal failure only rarely results in manifest gout unless there is a predisposition to this clinical syndrome. Intravenous infusion of 0.5 to 2 g (3 to 12 mmol) uric acid in normal man raised the serum level as high as 22.4 mg/dL (1.33 mmol/L) without any toxic effects [155]. However, hyperuricemia has been found to be associated with hypertension [156], cardiovascular events [157], stroke [158] as well as metabolic syndrome [159] and diabetes mellitus [160]. Moreover, increased concentration of uric acid has also been shown to be a risk factor for the progression of CKD by some [161], but not all investigators [162].

It has been demonstrated that purine derivates (urate and teophylline) suppress calcitriol synthesis in rats and inhibit receptor binding affinity for DNA [163]. In renal failure patients, treatment with allopurinol suppresses plasma uric acid concentration and increases calcitriol concentrations [164]. These findings suggest that uric acid has a role as a toxin which suppresses synthesis of calcitriol and is involved as factor in renal osteodystrophy.

Increased concentrations of inosine, xantine and hypoxantine have been observed in uremic adults and children [165,166].

Another purine derivative that acts as a uremic toxin, N-methyl-2-pyridone-5-carboxamide (2PY), is one of the end products of nicotinamide-adenine dinucleotide degradation. Its levels have been found to be significantly increased in CKD towards concentrations that are potentially toxic, as 2PY is known to inhibit poly(ADP-ribose) polymerase (PARP-1) activity [167,168].

Pyrimidines

Products of pyrimidine metabolism have also been estimated in uremic plasma. Higher plasma levels of pseudouridine, orotic acid and orotidine have been found in uremic patients than in normals [169–171]. The concentration of pseudouridine was found to be elevated in cerebrospinal fluid of uremic children and it was suggested that elevated pseudouridine might have a role in uremic encephalopathy [166]. Pseudouridine excretion is impaired in renal failure and increased tubular reabsorption contributes to its retention [170]. A fraction isolated from urine which inhibits glucose utilization in vitro in rat diaphragm has been shown to consist of pseudouridine [172].

Polyols

Myoinositol, a member of the vitamin B complex, is a natural constituent of food and is synthesized in muscle, liver, brain and kidneys. The major pathway for myoinositol catabolism require initial oxidation to D-glycuronate in the renal cortex. Patients with renal failure have increased concentrations of myoinositol in plasma, cerebrospinal fluid and cauda equina nerves and increased urinary excretion of myoinositol [173,174] suggesting that the production is increased or catabolism is decreased. Myoinositol has been postulated to contribute to immune dysfunction in CKD [175].

Concentrations of erythritol, mannitol and sorbitol have also been found to be markedly elevated in serum from HD patients [174]. The mannitol concentration in red cells and cerebrospinal fluid is also increased in uremia [176]. A relationship was demonstrated between the increase in sorbitol in cerebrospinal fluid and signs of peripheral neuropathy in non-dialyzed uremic patients [176].

Oxalic Acid

Oxalic acid concentrations are elevated in uremia with plasma concentrations varying in proportion to plasma urea concentrations [177–184]. ESRD patients may develop calcium oxalate kidney stones [185], and calcium oxalate crystal deposits have been found in various organs and tissues, most prominent in myocardium, thyroid gland, kidneys, synovia cartilage, bone, skin, blood vessels and periodontum [186,187].

It is plausible that calcium oxalate microcrystals may be causally related to cardiovascular disease and osteoarthritis of ESRD patients and be a contributing factor to the progression of CKD. Serum calcium oxalate supersaturation is a consequence of oxalate retention rather than increased local production of oxalate in CKD patients [188]. HD reduces the plasma oxalate concentration by about 60% [177,178,182,183]. CAPD and HD patients appear to have about the same plasma oxalate levels [182]. Attempts have been made to reduce serum oxalate in dialysis patients by supplementation of diet with high doses of pyridoxine. The rationale for this being that pyridoxine (vitamin B_6) is the co-enzyme for aminotransferase which catalyzes the transamination of glyoxylate to glycine; if this pathway is impaired, the glyoxylate is oxidized to oxalate. However, the results have been conflicting [179,189,190], and high dose pyridoxine supplementation did not decrease plasma oxalate concentration in a population of HD patients [184].

High doses of ascorbic acid (vitamin C) (800 mg per day) which is a precursor of oxalate causes an elevation of plasma oxalate in HD patients [191], whereas routine supplementation with 100 mg per day has no such effect. Consequently administration of vitamin C should be restricted to doses necessary to correct vitamin C deficiency.

Oxalic acid suppresses replication and migration of human endothelial cells, and inhibits thrombocyte aggregation [192], but it is not known if these findings have any relevance to uremic toxicity in vivo.

PROTEIN-BOUND SOLUTES

This group encompasses compounds with known protein binding or belonging to groups of solutes that are known to be protein bound [193]. Most of these compounds are characterized by a molecular weight of less than 500 Da. However, the removal of these solutes by conventional HD is modest because only the free fraction of the solute is available for diffusion. Moreover, high-flux HD is not effective in decreasing the concentrations of protein-bound uremic retention solutes either [194]. The inability to remove these compounds from ESRD patients is of major concern since the correlation between the concentration of protein-bound uremic retention solutes and clinical outcome is now well documented [195–197]. The importance of residual renal function in the clearance of these compounds has been proven and is now well acknowledged [198].

Homocysteine

In patients with CKD, in whom atherosclerotic complications are a leading cause of death, elevated plasma homocysteine (Hcy) levels occur more frequently than any other conventional risk factors [199]. The prevalence of hyperhomocysteinema is 85–100% among patients with advanced CKD and patients on maintenance dialysis [200–202]. Hyperhomocysteinemia in CKD is associated with various abnormalities in the concentration of other sulfur amino acids and their metabolites, such as elevated plasma levels of s-adenosylmethionine, s-adenosylhomocysteine, cystathionine, cysteine (Cys), cysteinesulfinic acid and inorganic sulfate and glutathione (low levels) and low plasma and muscle taurine levels [203–208].

The mechanisms by which plasma total Hcy levels increase in CKD are not fully understood. Possible causes include accumulation of toxic compounds that inhibit metabolism [209], reduced renal clearance, impaired degradation by the kidneys, deficiencies or altered metabolism of vitamins (B_6, folate, B_{12}) and/or abnormally high requirements for these vitamins [210,211]. Folate is an important determinant of plasma total Hcy, and folate deficiency which is common in uremic patients, may contribute additionally to the high prevalence of hyperhomocysteinemia.

Homocysteine exists in plasma as protein-bound and free forms. More than 70% of plasma total Hcy is protein-bound, with albumin being the main Hcy binding protein [212]. A correlation between plasma total Hcy and serum albumin has been reported in CKD in different studies, and may be related to the high albumin binding of Hcy [200,213–216].

Both retrospective and prospective studies in the general population favor the hypothesis that high Hcy levels promote cardiovascular disease [217]. Similarly, evaluations of the associations between Hcy gene polymorphisms and cardiovascular outcome, using the Mendelian randomization approach, point to the possibility of a causal link [218]. As for CKD subjects, some cross-sectional studies reported higher levels of total Hcy in patients with cardiovascular disease, while other investigators found no difference, or even paradoxically low Hcy concentration [219]. Likewise, many prospective observational studies revealed worse outcome in patients with *lower* total Hcy [219]. Previous studies showed that plasma Hcy was lower in CKD patients with protein-energy wasting (PEW) and with inflammation [200,220,221]. Therefore, it has been suggested that PEW and inflammation might be confounders for the apparent reverse association between total Hcy and clinical outcome [219].

It should be mentioned that another thiol metabolite, S-adenosylhomocysteine (SAH), has been found to be an independent predictor of cardiovascular disease in CKD stage 5 patients [222].

Polyamines

Putrescine, spermidine and spermine are widely distributed in the human body. They are strongly basic, low molecular weight compounds, which appear to be a universal prerequisite for growth [223]. Putrescine, spermidine and spermine are formed in animal tissues, and putrescine is also formed by intestinal bacteria by decarboxylation of lysine and ornithine in the intestine. Free polyamines in plasma, expressed as spermine equivalents, are elevated in children and adult patients with uremia and these elevated concentrations persist following institution of dialysis therapy [224].

The free spermidine concentration is much higher in cells than in plasma. Higher red cell levels of spermidine were found in uremic patients compared to normal controls, whereas the spermine concentrations were not different [225].

Spermine has been identified as an in vitro inhibitor of erythropoiesis in patients with CKD [226,227]. Spermine, spermidine and putrescine exert a significant effect on erythroid colony formation and putrescine inhibits the bioactivity of erythropoietin non-competitively [228]. Moreover, polyamines have been shown to exert inhibitory effects on proliferation and maturation of erythroid precursor cells [15,229]. These data suggest that polyamines are uremic toxins that are involved in the anemia of CKD.

A hypothesis was brought forward that the raised polyamine level in chronic dialysis patients could possibly contribute to accelerated cardiovascular disease, by stimulating proliferation of arterial smooth-muscle cells, a central process in atherogenesis [230].

Indoles

Largely as a result of bacterial action in the gut, tryptophan is deaminated and decarboxylated giving rise to a number of metabolites (tryptamine, indoleacetic acid, skatole, skatoxyl, indole, indoxyl, indican and others). Various indoles have been found in increased concentrations in plasma or in dialysates of uremic patients [231].

Indoxyl sulfate, the most abundant indolic compound in uremic patients, has been linked to increased oxidative stress [232], as well as to inhibition of endothelial regeneration and repair [233]. It also seems to stimulate the progression of experimental glomerulosclerosis [234], and it has been proposed to contribute to cardiovascular disease in the course of CKD through increase in the expression of intercellular adhesion molecule-1 (ICAM-1) and monocyte chemotactic protein-1 (MCP-1) in endothelium [235].

Indoxyl sulfate, which is strongly albumin-bound can be removed by oral adsorbent based on carbon as demonstrated in experimental uremic rats [231,236], as well as in CKD patients [237]. It is also, to some extent, removed by CAPD [238]. However, as for now, there is no proof that decreasing indoxyl sulfate concentration affects renal and/or patient survival [237,239,240].

Concentration of other indoles have been found to be increased in CKD [193]. Similarly to indoxyl sulfate, they are believed to contribute to endothelial dysfunction and to atherosclerosis progression in the course of CKD [241,242].

Phenols

Phenols, phenolic acid and their conjugates have been found in increased concentrations in uremic plasma, cerebrospinal fluid and dialysate, and it has been suggested that they play a primary role in the pathogenesis of the uremic syndrome [243]. They are formed as a result of the deamination, decarboxylation and oxidation of the aromatic amino acids tyrosine and phenylalanine. Some of them are products of bacterial action in the gut. Phenolic compounds are conjugated in the liver with glucuronic or sulfuric acid.

Plasma concentration of several phenolic compounds has been reported to be elevated in renal failure. The major include phenol, p-cresol [244], hippuric acid [245–250], and para-aminohippuric acid [245]. It has also been demonstrated that an oral sorbent decreases

the serum concentration of phenol and cresol in uremic rats [251]. Hippuric acid and para-aminohippuric acid have been suggested as suitable markers of uremic toxicity [245].

Several in vitro studies point to a toxic role of phenols in uremia [252]. However, in a study of the effect of several uremic metabolites on phagocyte reactive species production, only p-cresol had a significant effect at concentrations similar to those in uremic plasma [253]. Moreover, clinical studies demonstrated that p-cresol was related to cardiovascular disease and to mortality in HD patients [196,254]. Such associations were also observed in patients with mild to moderate CKD, where p-cresol turned out to be a predictor of cardiovascular events, independent of GFR and independent of Framingham risk factors [255].

It has to be underlined that although most of the pioneering research on the phenolic compounds has focused on the mother compound p-cresol, it is now well acknowledged that p-cresol is present only at very low concentrations since vast majority of the compound is conjugated to p-cresylsulfate in the intestinal wall and to p-cresylglucuronide in the liver [256]. However, as p-cresol estimations correlate with p-cresylsulfate measurements, it is believed that the results found for p-cresol can be extrapolated to the conjugates as well [257].

Advanced Glycation End Products (AGEs)

Circulating reducing sugars such as glucose react non-enzymatically with proteins (the Maillard reaction) to initiate a posttranscriptional modification process known as advanced glycation [258]. Schiff bases are formed by interaction of the reducing sugar with free amino groups and in the course of days these are rearranged to form Amadori products. Such reversible products are slowly transformed into irregularly cross-linked advanced glycation end products (AGEs), the formation of which have been implicated in the structural and functional alterations of collagen and other long-lived proteins in diabetes and aging [259].

Uremia is associated with increased oxidative stress, resulting in the production of reactive carbonyl compounds which react with protein residues forming AGEs [260].

Indeed, in CKD, AGE concentrations in plasma or serum are significantly increased compared with healthy controls [261]. The major mechanisms include impaired metabolism of reactive carbonyl compounds due to decreased activity of several enzymes, such as: aldose reductase, aldehyde dehydrogenase and glyoxalase [262], together with a reduced clearance of these compounds into the urine [261]. Moreover, the proximal tubule has been identified as the site of catabolism of AGEs, both in vivo and in vitro [263], which contributes to the impaired metabolism of AGEs in CKD.

However, AGE accumulation is not only a consequence of renal failure, but may also contribute to CKD. AGEs have been found to be related to a decrease in the GFR [264]. They are associated with structural renal changes which could lead to CKD progression, followed by a further increase in AGE concentration [261]. Increased AGE concentration could also contribute to cardiovascular disease. The level of serum N^{ε}-carboxymethyllysine (CML) and imidazolone are predictive for left ventricular hypertrophy in ESRD patients [265]. AGEs have been found in atherosclerotic plaques [266] and are thought to be related to vascular calcification in HD patients [267].

Immunochemical studies indicate that tissue AGEs which are being formed *in vivo* appear to contain a common immunological epitope [268,269]. It has been revealed that AGE structures present in the body of uremic patients have immune stimulating properties [270]. AGEs have also been identified in β-2-microglobulin amyloid deposits obtained from dialysis patients (see section on β-2-microglobulin amyloidosis).

Pentosidine, which is one of the members of the AGE group, formed through the Maillard reaction, binds strongly to collagen and other proteins. It accumulates in human tissues with age and its accumulation is enhanced in uremia and diabetes [271−274]. Odetti et al. [274] quantified pentosidine in serum and erythrocytes using HPLC and found moderately elevated serum levels in diabetic patients and very high serum and erythrocyte levels in uremia. It has been suggested that pentosidine may be a molecular marker for the cumulative damage to proteins in diabetes, ageing and uremia [272]. However, the clinical relevance of elevated tissue and plasma levels of pentosidine in renal failure patients is not established.

During PD, AGEs may also form locally in the peritoneal membrane due to reaction with glucose and reactive aldehydes in the form of glucose degradation products (GDPs) present in PD solutions. GDPs are formed during heat sterilization of the PD solution. Although it is generally assumed that glucose and GDPs in the PD solutions mainly have local effects, and not systemic effects, GDPs may contribute to the anorexia caused by PD solutions [275].

The evidence for the associations between increased AGE concentration and mortality in CKD is very limited. Wagner et al. [276] showed higher all-cause mortality for patients with increased serum CML level in a group of 154 long-term HD patients. However, in a prospective study of 232 CKD patients, serum levels of CML, pentosidine and imidazolone were not found to be independent risk factors of cardiovascular end points [277]. Similarly, Schwedler et al. [278] could not show any detrimental influence of increased serum levels of CML on cardiovascular mortality in HD patients; instead, higher AGE levels were associated with improved survival, probably due to better nutritional status. Finally, serum concentration of CML was not an independent cardiovascular, or renal, risk factor in a cohort of 450 patients with diabetic nephropathy [279].

Thus, it seems that serum or plasma concentrations of AGE cannot serve as reliable biomarkers in determining the cardiovascular risk of CKD patients [261]. This may be due to the fact that AGE concentrations are not constant, but fluctuate, as they are affected by various factors, e.g. nutritional sources. In contrast, tissue accumulation of AGEs serves as a long-term memory of AGE formation [261]. Indeed, skin auto-fluorescence, a measure of skin AGEs was found to predict mortality in HD patients [280]. It seems plausible that the tissue accumulation of AGEs is potentially a better predictor of cardiovascular outcome in CKD patients [281].

MIDDLE MOLECULES

Middle molecules (MM) form a class of uremic solutes characterized by their molecular weight exceeding 500 Da. The upper limit of molecular weight has not been strictly defined, although it is generally accepted that it should not exceed 60,000 Da, i.e., the molecules should be filterable through the glomerular basement membrane [193]. Evidence for the existence of peptidic substances with MM characteristics was brought forward by Cristol and co-workers [282] already in 1938. Subsequently, a large number of studies have demonstrated that MM fractions which contain peptides or conjugated amino acids accumulate in plasma or ultrafiltrate from uremic patients [283−289]. Many of the MMs have been shown to be proinflammatory, to generate endothelial dysfunction or smooth muscle cell proliferation, and to interfere in coagulation pathways.

The hypothesis that molecules with a larger molecular size than urea and creatinine might be more toxic than the small solutes stems from observations by Scribner and his group in Seattle that suggested that PD, in spite of less efficiency with regard to dialysis of small molecules, was superior to HD in controlling neuropathy [290], presumably because the peritoneal membrane was more leaky and thus more effective at removing MMs than the HD membranes [291]. The observation that prolongation of dialysis time could arrest or reverse peripheral neuropathy independently of the pre-dialysis values of urea and creatinine also suggested a toxic role of larger molecules than urea and creatinine [292].

These clinical findings formed the basis for the square meter-hour hypothesis [293]. This hypothesis relates the efficiency of dialysis to the numbers of hours of dialysis per week and the active membrane surface area. It was later suggested that the term square meter-hour hypothesis should be changed to MM hypothesis [294].

The most important study up to date evaluating the importance of dialysis time and flux on outcome was the HEMO trial (described above) [109]. Although higher urea removal in the HEMO trial was not associated with improved survival, the post-hoc analyses revealed that mortality was inversely related to the concentration of a major MM, i.e., β2-microglobulin [295].

The MM hypothesis had a great impact on dialyzer and membrane technology and dialysis strategies even before any MMs had been measured in dialysis patients. More permeable membranes were developed in response to the MM hypothesis, and MM removal, assessed in in vitro studies of B_{12} and inulin clearances, was taken into consideration when designing new dialyzers. Some of the advantages of treatment modalities such as hemofiltration, hemodiafiltration, CAPD, and charcoal hemoperfusion have been ascribed to efficient removal of MMs.

Up to now, at least 40 MM have been identified [47]. The vast majority belong to a group of either peptides or cytokines.

Peptides

β2-Microglobulin (β2-M)

β2-microglobulin (β2-M) was first isolated from human urine and characterized by Berggård and Bearn in 1968 [296]. It is a small globular protein with a molecular weight of 11,815 Da. β2-M is present on the plasma membranes of all mammalian cells, except erythrocytes and thrombocytes. It constitutes the light (invariable) chain of the major histocompatibility complex (MHC) (HLA class I). When the HLA-complex is degraded, β2-M is separated from the heavy chain and transferred to the extracellular fluid, a phenomenon called "shedding".

The normal serum concentration of β2-M is 1.0 to 2.5 mg/L. The renal elimination of β2-M is reduced in patients with renal failure; the serum level of β2-M correlates directly with the serum creatinine level and inversely with the GFR. The serum β2-M concentration in dialysis patients can be elevated up to 50-fold, i.e., to about 50 mg/L or more, but if residual renal function is present, the concentration is lower [297–299].

The archetypical MM, β2-M, is capable of forming amyloid in osteoarticular structures in kidney failure patients that undergo chronic HD treatment, leading to, so called, dialysis-related amyloidosis [300,301]. Since 1975, several authors observed an abnormally high incidence of carpal tunnel syndrome (CTS) in chronic HD patients, a complication that is in general only observed after more than 6 years of dialysis and seems to increase with the treatment time. In addition, patients with CTS exhibit signs and symptoms in joints, especially in the shoulder. Destructive arthropathy and bone lesions include generalized arthritis, scapulohumeral periarthritis and arthropathy with joint effusions. The main symptoms include inflammation with stiffness and spontaneous fractures [302]. They are more common in patients who are over 40 years of age on admission for HD, and seem to occur earlier after start of dialysis treatment with increasing age. The incidence of arthropathy is particularly high in centers where patients have been treated for 10 years or more. The percentage of patients who require surgery for CTS increases greatly, from very low for those on HD for less than 8 years, to 50% for those on HD for 14 years and 100% for those on HD for 20 years [298].

Several studies have been conducted in order to identify additional factors that may be of importance for the development of β2-M amyloidosis [1,297,298,303]. Among factors implicated to be of pathophysiological importance are: structural modifications of the β2-M molecule, AGEs, free radicals, cytokines, deposition of iron, calcium and aluminum, and the inflammatory response during HD due to membrane bioincompatibility. The β2-M obtained from amyloid fibrils isolated from connective tissue of HD patients often consists of acidic β2-M, and acidic β2-M from the urine of HD patients, but not β2-M from normal subjects, has brown color and fluorescence, which is characteristic for AGEs formed by the Maillard reaction. The acidic β2-M as well as the amyloid fibrils react with anti-AGE antibody. Niwa et al. [304] reported that AGEs are present both in the amyloid deposits from uremic patients and in infiltrating macrophages surrounding the amyloid deposits.

The major site of breakdown of β2-M is the kidney, where it is filtered in the glomeruli and reabsorbed and degraded in the proximal tubular cells. Extra-renal catabolism contributes only to about 3% of the total elimination of β2-M.

HD membranes of regenerated cellulose (cuprophane) are almost impermeable to β2-M, thus not contributing to its removal by diffusion or convection. Synthetic high-flux membranes for HD, hemofiltration and hemodiafiltration have larger pore-sizes and higher molecular-weight cut-offs and are more efficient and more suitable for removal of larger molecules such as β2-M, especially if used in the hemofiltration mode.

An additional factor contributing to the elimination of β2-M when using such membranes is the adsorption of circulating β2-M onto the membrane [305].

Using the same polysulfone membrane for HD and hemofiltration, it was shown that β2-M was more efficiently removed by convective than by diffusive transport [306–312]. By using a high-flux, biocompatible acrylonitrile membrane for dialysis, about 500 mg of β2-M per week is eliminated [308] – i.e., insufficient amounts compared to the production of β2-M in healthy subjects, which is in the order of about 1500 mg per week. During hemofiltration about 1000 mg/week of β2-M may be eliminated, i.e., still less than the daily production but considerably more than with HD [312], thus being potentially beneficial for preventing or delaying the onset of amyloidosis.

One hundred and forty to 320 mg per week of β2-M are eliminated by CAPD [313] which is more than what is removed by conventional HD. The β2-M plasma levels in CAPD patients have been reported to be about the same in HD patients [310,314] but other reports document lower levels of β2-M in CAPD patients than in patients on conventional HD [315,316]. On the other hand, CAPD removal of β2-M was found to be less substantial than with high-flux HD [52]. When comparing the dialysis modalities it is important to remember that removal via the kidneys, as long as residual renal function is preserved, is of considerable importance [317].

In conclusion, β2-microglobulin has been recognized as the major precursor protein of dialysis-related amyloidosis in long-term dialysis treatment, and it should be recognized as an established uremic toxin.

PTH

Secondary hyperparathyroidism is a constant complication of CKD. The increase in plasma PTH occurs in part as a consequence of phosphate retention, which, by decreasing ionized calcium, stimulates the parathyroid glands to increase PTH-secretion, and, in part, by decreased vitamin D activation, which, in turn, leads to impaired calcium absorption from the gastrointestinal tract.

Disorders of mineral metabolism associated with high PTH concentration lead to high bone turnover, and, in consequence, to osteitis fibrosa. PTH may have several additional toxic effects in uremia, some of which are mediated by increased calcium entry into cells and by exaggerated stimulation of adenosine monophosphate (cAMP) (see Chapter 19). The following uremic manifestations can be induced by excessive plasma levels of PTH: encephalopathy, neuropathy, dialysis dementia, bone disease, aseptic necrosis, soft tissue calcification, soft tissue necrosis, myopathy, pruritus, hypertension, cardiomyopathy

(Chapter 9), carbohydrate intolerance (Chapter 2), hyperlipidemia (Chapter 3), anemia, sexual dysfunction, and protein-energy wasting (Chapter 11).

PTH has attracted attention as a factor that might interfere with blood pressure regulation and cardiovascular function in uremia. Long-term infusion of PTH to normal subjects elicits hypertension [318].

In rats with CKD, parathyroidectomy significantly decreases the blood pressure response to calcium infusion, suggesting that the presence of PTH plays a permissive role for the hypertensive action of hypercalcemia [319].

Hyperparathyroidism is associated with weakness and muscle wasting; but, whether this is a specific effect of PTH, has been debated [320]. Garber found that PTH induces muscle protein breakdown in vitro [321]. However, Wassner and Li did not observe any effect of PTH on glucose uptake, protein synthesis and degradation or amino acid release in rat muscle perfused in vitro either with or without insulin [322]. Proximal muscle weakness and impaired respiratory muscle strength was reported to improve after parathyroidectomy in a uremic patient [323].

The anemia of CKD has also been suggested to be aggravated by hyperparathyroidism. Improvement of anemia has been observed in patients with CKD after parathyroidectomy [324]. It has been reported that PTH inhibits erythropoiesis in vitro, an effect that can be overcome by adding erythropoietin to the medium [325]. Other studies have shown that PTH decreases erythropoiesis directly by causing bone marrow fibrosis [326]. Increased osmotic fragility of erythrocytes and shortened erythrocyte survival have also been reported to be consequences of secondary hyperparathyroidism which might contribute to the anemia of renal failure [327]. However, in a group of patients with varying degrees of renal failure, multivariate analysis showed that plasma PTH itself was not a significant predictor of hematocrit levels or serum inhibition of erythroid progenitor cell growth [328]. Adding PTH or its fragments to the medium had no effect on in vitro erythropoiesis [328]. Similar results have been reported by other investigators [329].

In HD patients, a negative effect of high PTH levels on left ventricular function and cardiac hypertrophy was shown [330,331].

PTH seems to play a role in the glucose intolerance of renal failure. By using clamp techniques it can be demonstrated that parathyroidectomy can prevent glucose intolerance in dogs with CKD without affecting insulin resistance [332], indicating that PTH in CKD interferes with the ability of the beta-cells to augment insulin secretion appropriately in response to the insulin resistant state. In adolescents and young adults, the glucose metabolic rate (hyperglycemic clamp) correlates negatively with the PTH level in plasma but improves after parathyroidectomy, with higher insulin concentrations during hyperglycemia but without any effect on insulin sensitivity [333]. Improved glucose tolerance and insulin secretion without a change in insulin resistance is also seen in uremic children after correction of secondary hyperparathyroidism by phosphate restriction and oral phosphate binders [334].

In conclusion, PTH appears to play a role in mineral disturbances, abnormalities of protein and carbohydrate metabolism, and a variety of other changes seen in uremic patients including anemia. PTH is to be considered as an established uremic toxin.

For a more comprehensive discussion of PTH, the reader is referred to Chapters 19 and 21.

Free Immunoglobulin Light Chains

Immunoglobulin light chains are part of intact immunoglobulins. They contribute to antigen recognition. In CKD, they accumulate in the serum and their concentrations progressively increase with CKD stage [335]. Immunoglobulin light chain deposits in the kidney can aggravate CKD leading to tubule-interstitial lesions and glomerulopathies [336]. Their accumulation in patients with renal failure interferes with essential functions and the apoptotic cell death of neutrophils, and, as a consequence, may contribute to infectious and inflammatory complications which are common in this group of patients [337].

Leptin

Leptin is a 16 kDa peptide, making it a typical representative of the MM group. However, it is protein-bound, and therefore it is included, by some authors, into the family of protein-bound uremic solutes.

The discovery of the *ob* gene product leptin (16 kD) has increased our understanding of the physiological system that regulates eating behavior. This hormone plays a key role in regulating energy intake and energy expenditure, mainly through its action on receptors in the hypothalamus where it inhibits appetite.

Most ESRD patients have inappropriately high leptin levels [338,339], and it is now generally acknowledged that leptin plays an important part in mediating PEW in uremia [340,341]. Serum free leptin levels are elevated whereas serum bound leptin levels remain stable in ESRD patients [342]. Besides regulating appetite, leptin may also play a role in insulin metabolism, sodium handling, hematopoiesis and bone formation in ESRD patients [343].

As the kidneys clear other polypeptide hormones, it seems reasonable to surmise that leptin also accumulates in the case of renal failure due to reduced renal clearance. Indeed, the kidney is the principal site of elimination of circulating leptin in healthy subjects [344]. Moreover, an inverse correlation between leptin and GFR has been demonstrated in patients with various degrees of renal failure [345] and, in rats, bilateral nephrectomy reduces plasma leptin clearance by 80% [346]. Experimental studies in rats show that uptake and degradation of leptin by renal tissue is the main mechanism of elimination [347]. The important role of the kidney in leptin metabolism is further underscored by the fact that renal transplantation normalizes leptin levels [348].

Not all ESRD-patients have elevated leptin levels [349] and some patients have even low leptin levels suggesting that other tissues such as splanchnic organs contribute to leptin removal [350]. Moreover, as ESRD patients have lower leptin mRNA levels than controls, this could suggest that decreased plasma leptin clearance is a part of the efferent feedback loop that down-regulates the expression of the *ob* gene in hyperleptinemic ESRD patients [345]. However, also other factors associated with ESRD, such as hyperinsulinemia and inflammation, may affect leptin levels [351]. It should also be pointed out that female gender and obesity are important factors that affect serum leptin levels also in ESRD patients [343].

Although there is as yet no direct evidence that increased levels of leptin cause anorexia, some indirect evidence suggests that leptin may mediate anorexia in ESRD patients [340,352,353]. Moreover, it has been shown that high levels of serum leptin relative to fat mass might be associated with weight loss in HD patients [354] and increasing serum leptin levels are associated with a loss of lean body mass in CAPD patients [355]. Moreover, leptin has been associated with the elevated secretion of proinflammatory cytokines in the presence of increased fat mass [356]. However, as others found no association between the leptin concentration and recent change in body weight, nutritional status or inflammation in ESRD patients [339,357,358], the question if elevated serum leptin levels cause anorexia is open.

Whereas hyperleptinemia is a common phenomenon in ESRD patients, it is not a ubiquitous finding. Moreover, although some indirect evidence suggests that elevated leptin levels might cause anorexia, not all studies have found such a relationship.

Neuropeptide Y

Neuropeptide Y, a 36-amino acid peptide secreted mainly by the hypothalamus, is a major neurotransmitter promoting increased food intake. Its level has been found to be increased in hypothalamus in experimental models of CKD [359], as well as in plasma of CKD patients [360]. Concentration of neuropeptide Y has been found to be associated with left ventricular hypertrophy [361] and to predict cardiovascular and all-cause mortality in HD patients [362,363].

Dinucleoside Polyphosphates

Similarly to leptin, these vasoregulatory purines and pyrimidines are protein-bound, which makes their classification as MM controversial [364]. Dinucleoside polyphosphates are a group of substances that are involved in the regulation of vascular tone [256]. They also contribute to the proliferation of vascular smooth muscle cells and mesangial cells [365–367]. Finally, they have been shown to directly decrease renal blood flow [364]. In increased concentration, found in CKD subjects, they are believed to contribute to the progression of CKD, to hypertension and to cardiovascular risk [364].

Other

Cystatin C — a 120 amino-acids protein encoded by the CST3 gene and produced by all nucleated cells — is found in virtually all tissues and bodily fluids. While it is used as a biomarker of kidney function, its biological actions including inhibition of lysosomal proteinases of cysteine proteases might contribute to uremic toxicity, and it has been implicated in brain disorders involving amyloid deposition, such as Alzheimer's disease.

Cystatin C has shown a linear association with mortality risk across its entire distribution in a general elderly population [368,369]. Similarly, in CKD, a strong and independent association between cystatin C and all-cause mortality was observed [370]. Cystatin C may provide a more accurate estimate of kidney function than serum creatinine and it appears less sensitive than creatinine to factors other than GFR, particularly muscle mass [371]. However, whether its impact on outcome in CKD reflects only reduced kidney function or whether it has a direct impact on outcome, is currently not known.

Endothelin-1 is regarded as a uremic toxin belonging to the MM group. Its concentration can rise more than 6-fold in CKD subjects [193]. Endothelin-1 has been shown to promote renal fibrosis in experimental models [372], and experimental fibrosis can be prevented with endothelin-1 inhibitors [373,374].

Cytokines

Cytokines are cell-signaling proteins that modify and regulate immunological and inflammatory reactions, contributing to the immunological response of the body. In CKD, especially at the ESRD stage, the concentrations of most cytokines are in general several-fold increased, due to both increased production and decreased removal by renal clearance [375].

Interleukin-6 (IL-6)

Interleukin-6 (IL-6) is a molecule produced by different cells and tissues of the organism. It is involved in the production of acute phase proteins, proliferation of B-lymphocytes and neutrophils. Increased concentration of IL-6 in CKD is mainly a consequence of decreased elimination and increased generation [376]. Both HD and PD have been shown to trigger an increase in plasma IL-6 levels and in IL-6 mRNA expression in blood mononuclear cells [377].

IL-6 has been linked to the progression of carotid atherosclerosis in CKD stage 5 patients [378]. Moreover, it is thought to contribute to anemia in CKD subjects [379]. Finally, IL-6 is thought to be involved in the onset and progression of PEW, through induction of muscle catabolism, increase in lipolysis, and increased energy expenditure, promotion of insulin resistance and suppression of appetite [375].

Tumor Necrosis Factor-α (TNF-α)

TNF-α is an acute phase protein, involved in vascular permeability, increased cytokine production and recruitment of macrophages and neutrophils to the site of infection or inflammation. CKD is associated with a significant increase in TNF-α activity [375]. Increased concentrations of TNF-α have been associated with enhanced catabolism and development of PEW [376,380], as well as with endothelial dysfunction and decreased nitric oxide synthesis [381,382]. Since TNF-α has also been associated to hyperinsulinemia in CKD patients [383], it is not surprising that this cytokine has been classified as uremic toxin.

In conclusion, proinflammatory cytokines, such as IL-6 and TNF-α are elevated in ESRD patients, due to decreased renal clearance, but also due to increased production, especially in dialysis subjects. They are regarded as uremic toxins, although it has not yet been determined whether or not anti-cytokine therapies including removal of cytokines would reduce any specific uremic symptoms.

GENERAL CONCLUSIONS

The emphasis in the quest for the uremic toxins has shifted from small molecular weight inorganic and organic compounds during the 1960s, and before, to MM during the 1970s and PTH and β2-M and other low molecular weight proteins during the 1980s. During the last decades, the research has more and more focused on high molecular weight proteins, protein-bound small molecular weight compounds as well as on alterations in amino acids, peptides and proteins and formation of various end-products such as AGEs.

During the past decades, considerable effort and time have been spent to identify and characterize substances which cause uremic symptoms, and putative uremic toxins have been classified and categorized according to their molecular weight and protein-binding [193,256]. However, in spite of impressive advances within this research during recent years for example within the framework of the European Uremic Toxins (EUTox) Work Group (www.uremic-toxins.org), it remains to be found which compounds cause the most typical and clinically important uremic manifestations, such as anorexia, neurological disturbances and low grade inflammation. Uremia is a syndrome with multi-factorial pathogenesis and we are still far from a complete understanding of all aspects of uremic toxicity. Further research will hopefully elucidate the basic mechanisms involved in uremic toxicity, resulting in the development of improved diagnostic tools, more efficient therapeutic methods to remove uremic toxins or prevent their accumulation. This could have profound clinically significant positive effects including better control of metabolic and nutritional abnormalities in patients with kidney failure.

Acknowledgement

We dedicate this chapter to Jonas Bergstrom and thank him for all his work with earlier versions of this chapter. We the co-authors are grateful for the inspiration and teaching of this truly great nephrologist, scientist, mentor and friend. This chapter is a revised version of earlier chapters on Uremic Toxicity by Jonas Bergstrom et al. in the previous editions of this book which contained a larger number of earlier references.

The work at Baxter Novum is the result of a grant to the Karolinska Institutet from the Baxter Healthcare Corporation. Bengt Lindholm is employed by the Baxter Healthcare Corporation. Peter Stenvinkel is a member of the scientific advisory board of Gambro AB. None of the other authors declare any conflicts of interest.

References

[1] Bergstrom J, Wehle B. Clinical implications of middle and larger molecules. In: Nissenson A, Fine R, Gentile D, editors. Clinical dialysis. Norwalk, CT: Appleton & Lange; 1995. p. 204–34.

[2] Vanholder R, De Smet R. Lameire NH: Redesigning the map of uremic toxins. Contrib Nephrol 2001;(133):42–70.

[3] Horl WH. Uremic toxins: new aspects. J Nephrol 2000;13(Suppl. 3):S83–8.

[4] Cunningham Jr JN, Carter NW, Rector Jr FC, Seldin DW. Resting transmembrane potential difference of skeletal muscle in normal subjects and severely ill patients. J Clin Invest 1971;50(1):49–59.

[5] Bilbrey GL, Carter NW, White MG, Schilling JF, Knochel JP. Potassium deficiency in chronic renal failure. Kidney Int 1973;4(6):423–30.

[6] Cotton JR, Woodard T, Carter NW, Knochel JP. Resting skeletal muscle membrane potential as an index of uremic toxicity.

A proposed new method to assess adequacy of hemodialysis. J Clin Invest 1979;63(3):501–6.

[7] Patel SR, Ke HQ, Hsu CH. Regulation of calcitriol receptor and its mRNA in normal and renal failure rats. Kidney Int 1994;45(4):1020–7.

[8] Anderstam B, Mamoun AH, Sodersten P, Bergstrom J. Middle-sized molecule fractions isolated from uremic ultrafiltrate and normal urine inhibit ingestive behavior in the rat. J Am Soc Nephrol 1996;7(11):2453–60.

[9] Adijiang, A, Higuchi Y, Nishijima F, Shimizu H, Niwa T. Indoxyl sulfate, a uremic toxin, promotes cell senescence in aorta of hypertensive rats. Biochem Biophys Res Commun 399(4):637–41.

[10] Lipman JJ, Lawrence PL, DeBoer DK, et al. Role of dialysable solutes in the mediation of uremic encephalopathy in the rat. Kidney Int 1990;37(3):892–900.

[11] Motojima M, Nishijima F, Ikoma M, et al. Role for "uremic toxin" in the progressive loss of intact nephrons in chronic renal failure. Kidney Int 1991;40(3):461–9.

[12] Palm, F, Nangaku M, Fasching A, et al. Uremia induces abnormal oxygen consumption in tubules and aggravates chronic hypoxia of the kidney via oxidative stress. Am J Physiol Renal Physiol 299(2):F380–6.

[13] Wallner SF, Vautrin RM, Kurnick JE, Ward HP. The effect of serum from patients with chronic renal failure on erythroid colony growth in vitro. J Lab Clin Med 1978;92(3):370–5.

[14] Mitelman M, Levi J, Djaldetti M. Functional activity of uremic erythroblast incubated in autologous and homologous plasma. Blut 1979;38(6):467–71.

[15] Macdougall IC. Role of uremic toxins in exacerbating anemia in renal failure. Kidney Int Suppl 2001;78:S67–72.

[16] Donati D, Degiannis D, Raskova J, Raska Jr K. Uremic serum effects on peripheral blood mononuclear cell and purified T lymphocyte responses. Kidney Int 1992;42(3):681–9.

[17] Asaka M, Iida H, Izumino K, Sasayama S. Depressed natural killer cell activity in uremia. Evidence for immunosuppressive factor in uremic sera. Nephron 1988;49(4):291–5.

[18] Wessel-Aas T. The effect of serum and plasma from haemodialysis patients on human mononuclear phagocytes cultured in vitro. Acta Pathol Microbiol Scand [C] 1981;89(6):345–51.

[19] Wratten ML, Tetta C, De Smet R, et al. Uremic ultrafiltrate inhibits platelet-activating factor synthesis. Blood Purif 1999;17(2-3):134–41.

[20] Cohen G, Rudnicki M, Horl WH. Uremic toxins modulate the spontaneous apoptotic cell death and essential functions of neutrophils. Kidney Int Suppl 2001;78:S48–52.

[21] Weisensee D, Low-Friedrich I, Riehle M, Bereiter-Hahn J, Schoeppe W. In vitro approach to 'uremic cardiomyopathy'. Nephron 1993;65(3):392–400.

[22] Matsumoto A, Yamasaki M, Yonemura K, Tanaka I. Depression of nerve-mediated smooth muscle contractions in vitro by plasma of an anephric rabbit and uremic patients. Jpn J Physiol 1981;31(6):947–56.

[23] Delaporte C, Gros F, Anagnostopoulos T. Inhibitory effects of plasma dialysate on protein synthesis in vitro: influence of dialysis and transplantation. Am J Clin Nutr 1980;33(7):1407–10.

[24] Kamanna VS, Kashyap ML, Pai R, et al. Uremic serum subfraction inhibits apolipoprotein A-I production by a human hepatoma cell line. J Am Soc Nephrol 1994;5(2):193–200.

[25] Kramer HJ, Gospodinov D, Kruck F. Functional and metabolic studies on red blood cell sodium transport in chronic uremia. Nephron 1976;16(5):344–58.

[26] Russell JE, Avioli LV. The effect of chronic uremia on intestinal mitochondrial activity. J Lab Clin Med 1974;84(3):317–26.

[27] Lindner A, Gagne ER, Zingraff J, et al. A circulating inhibitor of the RBC membrane calcium pump in chronic renal failure. Kidney Int 1992;42(6):1328–35.

[28] White AG, Nachev P. Uremic inhibition of purine uptake by rat hepatic slices. Am J Physiol 1975;228(2):436–40.

[29] Orringer EP, Weiss FR, Preuss HG. Azotaemic inhibition of organic anion transport in the kidney of the rat: mechanisms and characteristics. Clin Sci 1971;40(2):159–69.

[30] Cernacek P, Spustova V, Dzurik R. Inhibitor(s) of protein synthesis in uremic serum and urine: partial purification and relationship to amino acid transport. Biochem Med 1982;27(3):305–16.

[31] Patel SR, Ke HQ, Vanholder R, Hsu CH. Inhibition of nuclear uptake of calcitriol receptor by uremic ultrafiltrate. Kidney Int 1994;46(1):129–33.

[32] Yukawa S, Tone Y, Sonobe M, et al. Study on the inhibitory effect of uremic plasma on lipoprotein lipase. Nippon Jinzo Gakkai Shi 1992;34(9):979–85.

[33] Young GA, Parsons FM. Impairment of phenylalanine hydroxylation in chronic renal insufficiency. Clin Sci 1973;45(1):89–97.

[34] Sohn HJ, Stokes GS, Johnston H. An Na, K ATPase inhibitor from ultrafiltrate obtained by hemodialysis of patients with uremia. J Lab Clin Med 1992;120(2):264–71.

[35] Deray G, Pernollet MG, Devynck MA, et al. Plasma digitalislike activity in essential hypertension or end-stage renal disease. Hypertension 1986;8(7):632–8.

[36] Stokes GS, Willcocks D, Monaghan J, Boutagy J, Marwood JF. Measurement of circulating sodium-pump inhibitory activity in uraemia and essential hypertension. J Hypertens Suppl 1986;4(6):S376–8.

[37] Pazmino PA, Sladek SL, Weinshilboum RM. Thiol S-methylation in uremia: erythrocyte enzyme activities and plasma inhibitors. Clin Pharmacol Ther 1980;28(3):356–67.

[38] Yalouris AG, Lyberatos C, Chalevelakis G, et al. Effect of uremic plasma on mouse liver delta-aminolevulinic acid synthetase activity. Clin Physiol Biochem 1986;4(6):368–71.

[39] Kuriyama M, Mizuma A, Yokomine R, Igata A, Otuji Y. Erythrocyte transketolase activity in uremia. Clin Chim Acta 1980;108(2):169–77.

[40] Sterzel RB, Semar M, Lonergan ET, Treser G, Lange K. Relationship of nervous tissue transketolase to the neuropathy in chronic uremia. J Clin Invest 1971;50(11):2295–304.

[41] Warnock LG, Cullum UX, Stouder DA, Stone WJ. Erythrocyte transketolase activity in dialysis patients with neuropathy. Biochem Med 1974;10(4):351–9.

[42] Bricker NS. On the pathogenesis of the uremic state. An exposition of the "trade-off hypothesis". N Engl J Med 1972;286(20):1093–9.

[43] Massry SG. Is parathyroid hormone a uremic toxin? Nephron 1977;19(3):125–30.

[44] Glassock RJ. Uremic toxins: what are they? An integrated overview of pathobiology and classification. J Ren Nutr 2008;18(1):2–6.

[45] Hohenegger M, Vermes M, Esposito R, Giordano C. Effect of some uremic toxins on oxygen consumption of rats in vivo and in vitro. Nephron 1988;48(2):154–8.

[46] Okada K, Takahashi Y, Okawa E, et al. Relationship between insulin resistance and uremic toxins in the gastrointestinal tract. Nephron 2001;88(4):384–6.

[47] Vanholder R, Glorieux G, Van Biesen W. Advantages of new hemodialysis membranes and equipment. Nephron Clin Pract 2010;114(3):c165–72.

[48] Lornoy W, Becaus I, Billiouw JM, et al. On-line haemodiafiltration. Remarkable removal of beta2-microglobulin.

[49] Meert N, Eloot S, Waterloos MA, et al. Effective removal of protein-bound uraemic solutes by different convective strategies: a prospective trial. Nephrol Dial Transplant 2009;24(2):562–70.

[50] Raj DS, Ouwendyk M, Francoeur R. Pierratos A: beta(2)-microglobulin kinetics in nocturnal haemodialysis. Nephrol Dial Transplant 2000;15(1):58–64.

[51] Dhondt A, Vanholder R, Van Biesen W, Lameire N. The removal of uremic toxins. Kidney Int Suppl 2000;76:S47–59.

[52] Evenepoel P, Bammens B, Verbeke K, Vanrenterghem Y. Superior dialytic clearance of beta(2)-microglobulin and p-cresol by high-flux hemodialysis as compared to peritoneal dialysis. Kidney Int 2006;70(4):794–9.

[53] Pham NM, Recht NS, Hostetter TH, Meyer TW. Removal of the protein-bound solutes indican and p-cresol sulfate by peritoneal dialysis. Clin J Am Soc Nephrol 2008;3(1):85–90.

[54] Vanholder R, Meert N, Van Biesen W, et al. Why do patients on peritoneal dialysis have low blood levels of protein-bound solutes? Nat Clin Pract Nephrol 2009;5(3):130–1.

[55] Periyasamy SM, Chen J, Cooney D, et al. Effects of uremic serum on isolated cardiac myocyte calcium cycling and contractile function. Kidney Int 2001;60(6):2367–76.

[56] Ritz E, Dikow R, Morath C, Schwenger V. Salt – a potential "uremic toxin"? Blood Purif 2006;24(1):63–6.

[57] Kopple JD, Kalantar-Zadeh K, Mehrotra R. Risks of chronic metabolic acidosis in patients with chronic kidney disease. Kidney Int Suppl 2005;(95):S21–7.

[58] Bushinsky DA. The contribution of acidosis to renal osteodystrophy. Kidney Int 1995;47(6):1816–32.

[59] Kraut JA. The role of metabolic acidosis in the pathogenesis of renal osteodystrophy. Adv Ren Replace Ther 1995;2(1):40–51.

[60] Lefebvre A, de Vernejoul MC, Gueris J, et al. Optimal correction of acidosis changes progression of dialysis osteodystrophy. Kidney Int 1989;36(6):1112–8.

[61] Yaqoob MM. Acidosis and progression of chronic kidney disease. Curr Opin Nephrol Hypertens 2010;19(5):489–92.

[62] Bergstrom J, Wang T, Lindholm B. Factors contributing to catabolism in end-stage renal disease patients. Miner Electrolyte Metab 1998;24(1):92–101.

[63] Kopple JD. Pathophysiology of protein-energy wasting in chronic renal failure. J Nutr 1999;129(Suppl. 1S):247S–51S.

[64] Lim VS, Kopple JD. Protein metabolism in patients with chronic renal failure: role of uremia and dialysis. Kidney Int 2000;58(1):1–10.

[65] May RC, Kelly RA, Mitch WE. Metabolic acidosis stimulates protein degradation in rat muscle by a glucocorticoid-dependent mechanism. J Clin Invest 1986;77(2):614–21.

[66] May RC, Kelly RA, Mitch WE. Mechanisms for defects in muscle protein metabolism in rats with chronic uremia. J Clin Invest 1987;79:1099–103.

[67] Hara Y, May RC, Kelly RA, Mitch WE. Acidosis, not azotemia, stimulates branched-chain, amino acid catabolism in uremic rats. Kidney Int 1987;32(6):808–14.

[68] May RC, Hara Y, Kelly RA, et al. Branched-chain amino acid metabolism in rat muscle: abnormal regulation in acidosis. Am J Physiol 1987;252(6 Pt 1):E712–8.

[69] Mitch WE, Medina R, Grieber S, et al. Metabolic acidosis stimulates muscle protein degradation by activating the adenosine triphosphate-dependent pathway involving ubiquitin and proteasomes. J Clin Invest 1994;93(5):2127–33.

Long-term clinical observations. Nephrol Dial Transplant 2000;15(Suppl. 1):49–54.

[70] Papadoyannakis NJ, Stefanidis CJ, McGeown M. The effect of the correction of metabolic acidosis on nitrogen and potassium balance of patients with chronic renal failure. Am J Clin Nutr 1984;40(3):623–7.

[71] Williams B, Hattersley J, Layward E, Walls J. Metabolic acidosis and skeletal muscle adaptation to low protein diets in chronic uremia. Kidney Int 1991;40(4):779–86.

[72] Straumann E, Keller U, Kury D, et al. Effect of acute acidosis and alkalosis on leucine kinetics in man. Clin Physiol 1992;12(1):39–51.

[73] Reaich D, Channon SM, Scrimgeour CM, Goodship TH. Ammonium chloride-induced acidosis increases protein breakdown and amino acid oxidation in humans. Am J Physiol 1992;263(4 Pt 1):E735–9.

[74] Reaich D, Channon SM, Scrimgeour CM, et al. Correction of acidosis in humans with CRF decreases protein degradation and amino acid oxidation. Am J Physiol 1993;265(2 Pt 1): E230–5.

[75] Ballmer PE, McNurlan MA, Hulter HN, et al. Chronic metabolic acidosis decreases albumin synthesis and induces negative nitrogen balance in humans. J Clin Invest 1995;95(1):39–45.

[76] Bergström J, Alvestrand A, Fürst P. Plasma and muscle free amino acids in maintenance hemodialysis patients without protein malnutrition. Kidney Int 1990;38:108–14.

[77] Graham KA, Reaich D, Channon SM, et al. Correction of acidosis in CAPD decreases whole body protein degradation. Kidney Int 1996;49(5):1396–400.

[78] Boirie Y, Broyer M, Gagnadoux MF, Niaudet P, Bresson JL. Alterations of protein metabolism by metabolic acidosis in children with chronic renal failure. Kidney Int 2000;58(1): 236–41.

[79] Löfberg E, Wernerman J, Bergström J. Branched-chain amio acids in muscle increase during correction of acidosis in hemodialysis (HD) patients (Abstract). J Am Soc Nephrol 1993:4.

[80] Szeto CC, Wong TY, Chow KM, Leung CB, Li PK. Oral sodium bicarbonate for the treatment of metabolic acidosis in peritoneal dialysis patients: a randomized placebo-control trial. J Am Soc Nephrol 2003;14(8):2119–26.

[81] Chiu YW, Mehrotra R. What should define optimal correction of metabolic acidosis in chronic kidney disease? Semin Dial 2010;23(4):411–4.

[82] Ibels LS, Alfrey AC, Haut L, Huffer WE. Preservation of function in experimental renal disease by dietary restriction of phosphate. N Engl J Med 1978;298(3):122–6.

[83] Loghman-Adham M. Role of phosphate retention in the progression of renal failure. J Lab Clin Med 1993;122(1):16–26.

[84] Nakamura M, Suzuki H, Ohno Y, et al. Oral calcium carbonate administration ameliorates the progression of renal failure in rats with hypertension. Am J Kidney Dis 1995;25(6):910–7.

[85] Braun J, Oldendorf M, Moshage W, et al. Electron beam computed tomography in the evaluation of cardiac calcification in chronic dialysis patients. Am J Kidney Dis 1996;27(3): 394–401.

[86] Goodman WG, Goldin J, Kuizon BD, et al. Coronary-artery calcification in young adults with end-stage renal disease who are undergoing dialysis. N Engl J Med 2000;342(20):1478–83.

[87] Block GA, Hulbert-Shearon TE, Levin NW, Port FK. Association of serum phosphorus and calcium x phosphate product with mortality risk in chronic hemodialysis patients: a national study. Am J Kidney Dis 1998;31(4):607–17.

[88] Kanbay M, Goldsmith D, Akcay A, Covic A. Phosphate – the silent stealthy cardiorenal culprit in all stages of chronic kidney disease: a systematic review. Blood Purif 2009;27(2):220–30.

[89] Spiegel DM. Magnesium in chronic kidney disease: unanswered questions. Blood Purif 2011;31(1-3):172–6.

[90] Michalk D, Klare B, Manz F, Scharer K. Plasma inorganic sulfate in children with chronic renal failure. Clin Nephrol 1981;16(1): 8–12.

[91] Koopman BJ, Jansen G, Wolthers BG, et al. Determination of inorganic sulfate in plasma by reversed-phase chromatography using ultraviolet detection and its application to plasma samples of patients receiving different types of haemodialysis. J Chromatogr 1985;337(2):259–66.

[92] Gutierrez R, Oster JR, Schlessinger FB, et al. Serum sulfate concentration and the anion gap in hemodialysis patients. ASAIO Trans 1991;37(2):92–6.

[93] Cole DE, Boucher MJ. Increased sweat sulfate concentrations in chronic renal failure. Nephron 1986;44(2):92–5.

[94] Prévost JL, Dumas JA. Examen du sang et de son action dans les divers phénomčnes de la vie (Examination of the blood and its action in the different phenomena of life). Ann Chim Phys 1821;23:90.

[95] Bright R. Reports of medical cases, selected with a view of illustrating the symptoms and cure of diseases by reference to morbid anatomy. London: Longman; 1831.

[96] Levine S, Saltzman A. Are urea and creatinine uremic toxins in the rat? Ren Fail 2001;23(1):53–9.

[97] Grollman EF, Grollman A. Toxicity of urea and its role in the pathogenesis of uremia. J Clin Invest 1959;38:749.

[98] Bollman JL, Mann FC. Nitrogenous constituents of blood following transplantation of ureters into different levels of intestine. Proc Soc Exp Biol & Med 1927;24:923.

[99] Gilboe DD, Javid MJ. Breakdown products of urea and uremic syndrome. Proc Soc Exp Biol & Med 1964;115:633.

[100] Merrill JP, Legrain M, Hoigne R. Observations on the role of urea in uremia. Am J Med 1953;14:519.

[101] Johnson. WJ, Hagge WW, Wagoner RD, Dinapoli RP, Rosevear JW. Effects of urea loading in patients with far advanced renal failure. Mayo Clin Proc 1972;47:21.

[102] Hegstrom RM, Murray JS, Pendras JP, Burnell JM, Scribner BH. Two years experience with periodic hemodialysis in the treatment of chronic uremia. Trans Am Soc Artif Intern Organs 1962;8:266.

[103] Hutchings RH, Hegstrom RM, Scribner BH. Two years experience with periodic hemodialysis in the treatment of chronic uremia. Trans Am Soc Artif Intern Organs 1962;8:266.

[104] Degoulet P, Legrain M, Réach I, et al. Mortality risk factors in patients treated by chronic hemodialysis. Nephron 1982;31: 103–10.

[105] Shapiro JI, Argy WP, Rakowski TA, et al. The unsuitability of BUN as a criterion for prescription dialysis. Trans Am Soc Artif Intern Organs 1983;29:129–34.

[106] Lowrie EG, Lew NL. Death risk in hemodialysis patients: the predictive value of commonly measured variables and an evaluation of death rate differences between facilities. Am J Kidney Dis 1990;15(5):458–82.

[107] Bergström J. Nutrition and adequacy of dialysis in hemodialysis patients. Kidney Int 1993;43(Suppl. 41):s261–7.

[108] Acchiardo SR, Moore LW, Latour PA. Malnutrition as a main factor in morbidity and mortality of hemodialysis patients. Kidney Int 1983;24(Suppl. 16):S199–203.

[109] Eknoyan G, Beck GJ, Cheung AK, et al. Effect of dialysis dose and membrane flux in maintenance hemodialysis. N Engl J Med 2002;347(25):2010–9.

[110] Paniagua R, Amato D, Vonesh E, et al. Effects of increased peritoneal clearances on mortality rates in peritoneal dialysis: ADEMEX, a prospective, randomized, controlled trial. J Am Soc Nephrol 2002;13(5):1307–20.

[111] Lo WK, Ho YW, Li CS, et al. Effect of Kt/V on survival and clinical outcome in CAPD patients in a randomized prospective study. Kidney Int 2003;64(2):649–56.

[112] Owen Jr WF, Lew NL, Liu Y, Lowrie EG, Lazarus JM. The urea reduction ratio and serum albumin concentration as predictors of mortality in patients undergoing hemodialysis. N Engl J Med 1993;329(14):1001–6.

[113] Depner TA. Uremic toxicity: urea and beyond. Semin Dial 2001;14(4):246–51.

[114] Rose WC, Dimmitt FW. Experimental studies on creatine and creatinine. VII. The fate of creatine and creatinine when administered to man. J Biol Chem 1916;26:345.

[115] Shannon JA. The renal excretion of creatinine in man. J Clin Invest 1935;14:403.

[116] Mason MF, Resnik H, Mino AS, et al. Mechanism of experimental uremia. Arch Intern Med 1937;60:312.

[117] Davidoff F. Effects of guanidine derivatives on mitochondrial function. I. Phenethylbiguanide inhibition of respiration in mitochondria from guinea pig and rat tissues. J Clin Invest 1968;47(10):2331–43.

[118] Davidoff F. Effects of guanidine derivatives on mitochondrial function. II. Reversal of guanidine-derivative inhibiton by free fatty acids. J Clin Invest 1968;47(10):2344–58.

[119] Foster NB. The isolation of a toxic substance from the blood of uremic patients. Trans Assoc Am Physicians 1915;30:305.

[120] De Deyn PP, D'Hooge R, Van Bogaert PP, Marescau B. Endogenous guanidino compounds as uremic neurotoxins. Kidney Int Suppl 2001;78:S77–83.

[121] Hirayama A, Noronha-Dutra AA, Gordge MP, Neild GH, Hothersall JS. Uremic concentrations of guanidino compounds inhibit neutrophil superoxide production. Kidney Int Suppl 2001;78:S89–92.

[122] Yokozawa T, Fujitsuka N, Oura H. Studies on the precursor of methylguanidine in rats with renal failure. Nephron 1991;58(1):90–4.

[123] Nagase S, Aoyagi K, Narita M, Tojo S. Biosynthesis of methylguanidine in isolated rat hepatocytes and in vivo. Nephron 1985;40(4):470–5.

[124] Yokozawa T, Fujitsuka N, Oura H. Production of methylguanidine from creatinine in normal rats and rats with renal failure. Nephron 1990;56(3):249–54.

[125] Ando A, Orita Y, Nakata K, et al. Effect of low protein diet and surplus of essential amino acids on the serum concentration and the urinary excretion of methylguanidine and guanidinosuccinic acid in chronic renal failure. Nephron 1979;24(4):161–9.

[126] Orita Y, Ando A, Tsubakihara Y, et al. Tissue and blood cell concentration of methylguanidine in rats and patients with chronic renal failure. Nephron 1981;27(1):35–9.

[127] D'Hooge R, Pei YQ, Marescau B, De Deyn PP. Convulsive action and toxicity of uremic guanidino compounds: behavioral assessment and relation to brain concentration in adult mice. J Neurol Sci 1992;112(1-2):96–105.

[128] MacAllister RJ, Whitley GS, Vallance P. Effects of guanidino and uremic compounds on nitric oxide pathways. Kidney Int 1994;45(3):737–42.

[129] Sorrentino R, Sorrentino L, Pinto A. Effect of some products of protein catabolism on the endothelium-dependent and -independent relaxation of rabbit thoracic aorta rings. J Pharmacol Exp Ther 1993;266(2):626–33.

[130] Glorieux GL, Dhondt AW, Jacobs P, et al. In vitro study of the potential role of guanidines in leukocyte functions related to atherogenesis and infection. Kidney Int 2004;65(6):2184–92.

[131] De Deyn PP, Marescau B, Cuykens JJ, et al. Guanidino compounds in serum and cerebrospinal fluid of non-dialyzed patients with renal insufficiency. Clin Chim Acta 1987;167(1):81–8.

[132] Marescau B, De Deyn PP, Qureshi IA, et al. The pathobiochemistry of uremia and hyperargininemia further demonstrates a metabolic relationship between urea and guanidinosuccinic acid. Metabolism 1992;41(9):1021–4.

[133] Pietrzak I, Baczyk K. Erythrocyte transketolase activity and guanidino compounds in hemodialysis patients. Kidney Int Suppl 2001;78:S97–101.

[134] Patel S, Hsu CH. Effect of polyamines, methylguanidine, and guanidinosuccinic acid on calcitriol synthesis. J Lab Clin Med 1990;115(1):69–73.

[135] D'Hooge R, Pei YQ, Marescau B, De Deyn PP. Behavioral toxicity of guanidinosuccinic acid in adult and young mice. Toxicol Lett 1992. 64–65 Spec No: 773-7.

[136] De Deyn PP, Vanholder R, Eloot S, Glorieux G. Guanidino compounds as uremic (neuro)toxins. Semin Dial 2009;22(4):340–5.

[137] Kakimoto Y, Akazawa S. Isolation and identification of N-G, N-G- and N-G, N'-G-dimethyl-arginine, N-epsilon-mono-, di-, and trimethyllysine, and glucosylgalactosyl- and galactosyl-delta-hydroxylysine from human urine. J Biol Chem 1970;245(21):5751–8.

[138] Vallance P, Leone A, Calver A, Collier J, Moncada S. Accumulation of an endogenous inhibitor of nitric oxide synthesis in chronic renal failure. Lancet 1992;339(8793):572–5.

[139] Yilmaz MI, Sonmez A, Saglam M, et al. ADMA levels correlate with proteinuria, secondary amyloidosis, and endothelial dysfunction. J Am Soc Nephrol 2008;19(2):388–95.

[140] Kielstein JT, Zoccali C. Asymmetric dimethylarginine: a novel marker of risk and a potential target for therapy in chronic kidney disease. Curr Opin Nephrol Hypertens 2008;17(6):609–15.

[141] Chirinos JA, David R, Bralley JA, et al. Endogenous nitric oxide synthase inhibitors, arterial hemodynamics, and subclinical vascular disease: the PREVENCION Study. Hypertension 2008;52(6):1051–9.

[142] Zoccali C, Mallamaci F, Maas R, et al. Left ventricular hypertrophy, cardiac remodeling and asymmetric dimethylarginine (ADMA) in hemodialysis patients. Kidney Int 2002;62(1):339–45.

[143] Kielstein JT, Impraim B, Simmel S, et al. Cardiovascular effects of systemic nitric oxide synthase inhibition with asymmetrical dimethylarginine in humans. Circulation 2004;109(2):172–7.

[144] Zocalli C, Bode-Boger SM, Mallamaci F, et al. Plasma concentration of asymmetrical dimethylarginine and mortality in patients with end-stage renal disease: a prospective study. Lancet 2001;358(9299):2113–7.

[145] Meinitzer A, Seelhorst U, Wellnitz B, et al. Asymmetrical dimethylarginine independently predicts total and cardiovascular mortality in individuals with angiographic coronary artery disease (the Ludwigshafen Risk and Cardiovascular Health study). Clin Chem 2007;53(2):273–83.

[146] Kielstein JT, Fliser D, Veldink H. Asymmetric dimethylarginine and symmetric dimethylarginine: axis of evil or useful alliance? Semin Dial 2009;22(4):346–50.

[147] Bode-Boger SM, Scalera F, Kielstein JT, et al. Symmetrical dimethylarginine: a new combined parameter for renal function and extent of coronary artery disease. J Am Soc Nephrol 2006;17(4):1128–34.

[148] Schepers E, Glorieux G, Dhondt A, Leybaert L, Vanholder R. Role of symmetric dimethylarginine in vascular damage by increasing ROS via store-operated calcium influx in monocytes. Nephrol Dial Transplant 2009;24(5):1429–35.

[149] Schepers E, Barreto DV, Liabeuf S, et al. Symmetric Dimethylarginine as a Proinflammatory Agent in Chronic Kidney Disease. Clin J Am Soc Nephrol 2011;6(10):2374–83.

[150] Perna AF, Ingrosso D, Satta E, et al. Plasma protein aspartyl damage is increased in hemodialysis patients: studies on causes and consequences. J Am Soc Nephrol 2004;15(10):2747–54.

[151] Gurreri G, Ghiggeri G, Salvidio G, et al. Effects of hemodialysis on guanidinopropionic acid metabolism. Nephron 1986;42(4):295−7.

[152] Shainkin-Kestenbaum R, Winikoff Y, Dvilansky A, Chaimovitz C, Nathan I. Effect of guanidino-propionic acid on lymphocyte proliferation. Nephron 1986;44(4):295−8.

[153] Rocic B, Breyer D, Granic M, Milutinovic S. The effect of guanidino substances from uremic plasma on insulin binding to erythrocyte receptors in uremia. Horm Metab Res 1991;23(10):490−4.

[154] Ramanjaneyulu PS, Indira K, Rao SV. Guanidine induced alterations in tissue transaminase patterns in the rat. Biochem Mol Biol Int 1993;31(6):1177−80.

[155] Folin O, Berglund H, Deriek C. The uric acid problem. An experimental study of animals and man including gouty subjects. J Biol Chem 1924;60:361.

[156] Masuo K, Kawaguchi H, Mikami H, Ogihara T, Tuck ML. Serum uric acid and plasma norepinephrine concentrations predict subsequent weight gain and blood pressure elevation. Hypertension 2003;42(4):474−80.

[157] Fang J, Alderman MH. Serum uric acid and cardiovascular mortality the NHANES I epidemiologic follow-up study, 1971-1992. National Health and Nutrition Examination Survey. Jama 2000;283(18):2404−10.

[158] Bos MJ, Koudstaal PJ, Hofman A, Witteman JC, Breteler MM. Uric acid is a risk factor for myocardial infarction and stroke: the Rotterdam study. Stroke 2006;37(6):1503−7.

[159] Bo S, Cavallo-Perin P, Gentile L, Repetti E, Pagano G. Hypouricemia and hyperuricemia in type 2 diabetes: two different phenotypes. Eur J Clin Invest 2001;31(4):318−21.

[160] Nakanishi N, Okamoto M, Yoshida H, et al. Serum uric acid and risk for development of hypertension and impaired fasting glucose or Type II diabetes in Japanese male office workers. Eur J Epidemiol 2003;18(6):523−30.

[161] Siu YP, Leung KT, Tong MK, Kwan TH. Use of allopurinol in slowing the progression of renal disease through its ability to lower serum uric acid level. Am J Kidney Dis 2006;47(1):51−9.

[162] Sturm G, Kollerits B, Neyer U, Ritz E, Kronenberg F. Uric acid as a risk factor for progression of non-diabetic chronic kidney disease? The Mild to Moderate Kidney Disease (MMKD) Study. Exp Gerontol 2008;43(4):347−52.

[163] Hsu CH, Patel SR, Young EW, Vanholder R. Effects of purine derivatives on calcitriol metabolism in rats. Am J Physiol 1991;260(4 Pt 2):F596−601.

[164] Vanholder R, Patel S, Hsu CH. Effect of uric acid on plasma levels of 1,25(OH)2D in renal failure. J Am Soc Nephrol 1993;4(4):1035−8.

[165] Severini G, Aliberti LM. Liquid-chromatographic determination of inosine, xanthine, and hypoxanthine in uremic patients receiving hemodialysis treatment. Clin Chem 1987;33(12):2278−80.

[166] Gerrits GP, Monnens LA, De Abreu RA, et al. Disturbances of cerebral purine and pyrimidine metabolism in young children with chronic renal failure. Nephron 1991;58(3):310−4.

[167] Rutkowski B, Swierczynski J, Slominska E, et al. Disturbances of purine nucleotide metabolism in uremia. Semin Nephrol 2004;24(5):479−83.

[168] Rutkowski B, Slominska E, Szolkiewicz M, et al. N-methyl-2-pyridone-5-carboxamide: a novel uremic toxin? Kidney Int Suppl 2003;(84):S19−21.

[169] Schoots AC, Gerlag PG, Mulder AW, Peeters JA, Cramers CA. Liquid-chromatographic profiling of solutes in serum of uremic patients undergoing hemodialysis and chronic ambulatory peritoneal dialysis (CAPD); high concentrations of pseudouridine in CAPD patients. Clin Chem 1988;34(1):91−7.

[170] Dzurik R, Lajdova I, Spustova V, Opatrny Jr K. Pseudouridine excretion in healthy subjects and its accumulation in renal failure. Nephron 1992;61(1):64−7.

[171] Daniewska-Michalska D, Motyl T, Gellert R, et al. Efficiency of hemodialysis of pyrimidine compounds in patients with chronic renal failure. Nephron 1993;64(2):193−7.

[172] Lajdova I, Spustova V, Mikula J, Cernay P, Dzurik R. Isolation of an additional inhibitor of glucose utilization in renal insufficiency: pseudouridine. J Chromatogr 1990;528(1):178−83.

[173] Niwa T, Asada H, Maeda K, et al. Profiling of organic acids and polyols in nerves of uraemic and non-uraemic patients. J Chromatogr 1986;377:15−22.

[174] Niwa T, Tohyama K, Kato Y. Analysis of polyols in uremic serum by liquid chromatography combined with atmospheric pressure chemical ionization mass spectrometry. J Chromatogr 1993;613(1):9−14.

[175] Bartnicki P, Zbrog Z, Baj Z, Tchorzewski H, Luciak M. Myoinositol may be a factor in uremic immune deficiency. Clin Nephrol 1997;47(3):197−201.

[176] Pitkanen E, Bardy A, Pasternack A, Servo C. Plasma, red cell and cerebrospinal fluid concentrations of mannitol and sorbital in patients with severe chronic renal failure. Ann Clin Res 1976;8(6):368−73.

[177] Boer P, van Leersum L, Hene RJ, Mees EJ. Plasma oxalate concentration in chronic renal disease. Am J Kidney Dis 1984;4(2):118−22.

[178] Ramsay AG, Reed RG. Oxalate removal by hemodialysis in end-stage renal disease. Am J Kidney Dis 1984;4(2):123−7.

[179] Morgan SH, Maher ER, Purkiss P, Watts RW, Curtis JR. Oxalate metabolism in end-stage renal disease: the effect of ascorbic acid and pyridoxine. Nephrol Dial Transplant 1988;3(1):28−32.

[180] Prenen JA, Dorhout Mees EJ, Boer P. Plasma oxalate concentration and oxalate distribution volume in patients with normal and decreased renal function. Eur J Clin Invest 1985;15(1):45−9.

[181] Wolthers BG, Meijer S, Tepper T, Hayer M, Elzinga H. The determination of oxalate in haemodialysate and plasma: a means to detect and study "hyperoxaluria" in haemodialysed patients. Clin Sci (Colch) 1986;71(1):41−7.

[182] McConnell KN, Rolton HA, Modi KS, Macdougall AI. Plasma oxalate in patients with chronic renal failure receiving continuous ambulatory peritoneal dialysis or hemodialysis. Am J Kidney Dis 1991;18(4):441−5.

[183] Marangella M, Petrarulo M, Mandolfo S, et al. Plasma profiles and dialysis kinetics of oxalate in patients receiving hemodialysis. Nephron 1992;60(1):74−80.

[184] Costello JF, Sadovnic MC, Smith M, Stolarski C. Effect of vitamin B6 supplementation on plasma oxalate and oxalate removal rate in hemodialysis patients. J Am Soc Nephrol 1992;3(4):1018−24.

[185] Oren A, Husdan H, Cheng PT, et al. Calcium oxalate kidney stones in patients on continuous ambulatory peritoneal dialysis. Kidney Int 1984;25(3):534−8.

[186] Hoffman GS, Schumacher HR, Paul H, et al. Calcium oxalate microcrystalline-associated arthritis in end-stage renal disease. Ann Intern Med 1982;97(1):36−42.

[187] Reginato AJ, Ferreiro Seoane JL, Barbazan Alvarez C, et al. Arthropathy and cutaneous calcinosis in hemodialysis oxalosis. Arthritis Rheum 1986;29(11):1387−96.

[188] Worcester EM, Nakagawa Y, Bushinsky DA, Coe FL. Evidence that serum calcium oxalate supersaturation is a consequence of oxalate retention in patients with chronic renal failure. J Clin Invest 1986;77(6):1888−96.

[189] Balcke P, Schmidt P, Zazgornik J, Kopsa H, Deutsch E. Effect of vitamin B6 administration on elevated plasma oxalic acid levels in haemodialysed patients. Eur J Clin Invest 1982;12(6):481—3.

[190] Tomson CR, Channon SM, Parkinson IS, et al. Effect of pyridoxine supplementation on plasma oxalate concentrations in patients receiving dialysis. Eur J Clin Invest 1989;19(2):201—5.

[191] Ono K. Secondary hyperoxalemia caused by vitamin C supplementation in regular hemodialysis patients. Clin Nephrol 1986;26(5):239—43.

[192] Camici M, Evangelisti L, Raspolli-Galletti M. The effect of oxalic acid on the aggregability of human platelet rich plasma. Prostaglandins Leukot Med 1986;21(1):107—10.

[193] Vanholder R, De Smet R, Glorieux G, et al. Review on uremic toxins: classification, concentration, and interindividual variability. Kidney Int 2003;63(5):1934—43.

[194] Lesaffer G, De Smet R, Lameire N, et al. Intradialytic removal of protein-bound uraemic toxins: role of solute characteristics and of dialyser membrane. Nephrol Dial Transplant 2000;15(1):50—7.

[195] De Smet R, Van Kaer J, Van Vlem B, et al. Toxicity of free p-cresol: a prospective and cross-sectional analysis. Clin Chem 2003;49(3):470—8.

[196] Bammens B, Evenepoel P, Keuleers H, Verbeke K, Vanrenterghem Y. Free serum concentrations of the protein-bound retention solute p-cresol predict mortality in hemodialysis patients. Kidney Int 2006;69(6):1081—7.

[197] Bammens B, Evenepoel P, Verbeke K, Vanrenterghem Y. Removal of middle molecules and protein-bound solutes by peritoneal dialysis and relation with uremic symptoms. Kidney Int 2003;64(6):2238—43.

[198] Marquez IO, Tambra S, Luo FY, et al. Contribution of residual function to removal of protein-bound solutes in hemodialysis. Clin J Am Soc Nephrol 2011;6(2):290—6.

[199] Bostom AG, Lathrop L. Hyperhomocysteinemia in end-stage renal disease: prevalence, etiology, and potential relationship to arteriosclerotic outcomes. Kidney Int 1997;52(1):10—20.

[200] Suliman ME, Qureshi AR, Barany P, et al. Hyperhomocysteinemia, nutritional status, and cardiovascular disease in hemodialysis patients. Kidney Int 2000;57(4):1727—35.

[201] Bostom AG, Shemin D, Lapane KL, et al. High dose-B-vitamin treatment of hyperhomocysteinemia in dialysis patients. Kidney Int 1996;49(1):147—52.

[202] van Guldener C, Janssen MJ, Lambert J, et al. Folic acid treatment of hyperhomocysteinemia in peritoneal dialysis patients: no change in endothelial function after long-term therapy. Perit Dial Int 1998;18(3):282—9.

[203] Perna AF, Ingrosso D, De Santo NG, Galletti P, Zappia V. Mechanism of erythrocyte accumulation of methylation inhibitor S-adenosylhomocysteine in uremia. Kidney Int 1995;47(1):247—53.

[204] Suliman ME, Divino Filho JC, Barany P, et al. Effects of high-dose folic acid and pyridoxine on plasma and erythrocyte sulfur amino acids in hemodialysis patients. J Am Soc Nephrol 1999;10(6):1287—96.

[205] Ross EA, Koo LC, Moberly JB. Low whole blood and erythrocyte levels of glutathione in hemodialysis and peritoneal dialysis patients. Am J Kidney Dis 1997;30(4):489—94.

[206] Ceballos-Picot I, Witko-Sarsat V, Merad-Boudia M, et al. Glutathione antioxidant system as a marker of oxidative stress in chronic renal failure. Free Radic Biol Med 1996;21(6):845—53.

[207] Alvestrand A, Furst P, Bergstrom J. Plasma and muscle free amino acids in uremia: influence of nutrition with amino acids. Clin Nephrol 1982;18(6):297—305.

[208] Bergstrom J, Alvestrand A, Furst P, Lindholm B. Sulphur amino acids in plasma and muscle in patients with chronic renal failure: evidence for taurine depletion. J Intern Med 1989;226(3):189—94.

[209] Suliman M, Anderstam B, Bergström J. Evidence of taurine depleton and accumulation of cysteinsulfinic acid in chronic dialysis patients. Kidney Int 1996;50(1713—1717).

[210] Descombes E, Hanck AB, Fellay G. Water soluble vitamins in chronic hemodialysis patients and need for supplementation. Kidney Int 1993;43(6):1319—28.

[211] Jennette JC, Goldman ID. Inhibition of the membrane transport of folates by anions retained in uremia. J Lab Clin Med 1975;86(5):834—43.

[212] Ueland PM, Refsum H. Plasma homocysteine, a risk factor for vascular disease: plasma levels in health, disease, and drug therapy. J Lab Clin Med 1989;114(5):473—501.

[213] Hultberg B, Andersson A, Sterner G. Plasma homocysteine in renal failure. Clin Nephrol 1993;40(4):230—5.

[214] Suliman ME, Lindholm B, Barany P, Bergstrom J. Hyperhomocysteinemia in chronic renal failure patients: relation to nutritional status and cardiovascular disease. Clin Chem Lab Med 2001;39(8):734—8.

[215] Fodinger M, Mannhalter C, Wolfl G, et al. Mutation (677 C to T) in the methylenetetrahydrofolate reductase gene aggravates hyperhomocysteinemia in hemodialysis patients. Kidney Int 1997;52(2):517—23.

[216] Vychytil A, Fodinger M, Wolfl G, et al. Major determinants of hyperhomocysteinemia in peritoneal dialysis patients. Kidney Int 1998;53(6):1775—82.

[217] Perna AF, Ingrosso D, Violetti E, et al. Hyperhomocysteinemia in uremia—a red flag in a disrupted circuit. Semin Dial 2009;22(4):351—6.

[218] Trabetti E. Homocysteine MTHFR gene polymorphisms, and cardio-cerebrovascular risk. J Appl Genet 2008;49(3):267—82.

[219] Suliman ME, Lindholm B, Barany P, Qureshi AR, Stenvinkel P. Homocysteine-lowering is not a primary target for cardiovascular disease prevention in chronic kidney disease patients. Semin Dial 2007;20(6):523—9.

[220] Suliman ME, Stenvinkel P, Heimburger O, et al. Plasma sulfur amino acids in relation to cardiovascular disease, nutritional status, and diabetes mellitus in patients with chronic renal failure at start of dialysis therapy. Am J Kidney Dis 2002;40(3):480—8.

[221] Suliman ME, Stenvinkel P, Qureshi AR, et al. Hyperhomocysteinemia in relation to plasma free amino acids, biomarkers of inflammation and mortality in patients with chronic kidney disease starting dialysis therapy. Am J Kidney Dis 2004;44(3):455—65.

[222] Valli A, Carrero JJ, Qureshi AR, et al. Elevated serum levels of S-adenosylhomocysteine, but not homocysteine, are associated with cardiovascular disease in stage 5 chronic kidney disease patients. Clin Chim Acta 2008;395(1-2):106—10.

[223] Janne J, Poso H, Raina A. Polyamines in rapid growth and cancer. Biochim Biophys Acta 1978;473(3-4):241—93.

[224] Saito A, Takagi T, Chung TG, Ohta K. Serum levels of polyamines in patients with chronic renal failure. Kidney Int Suppl 1983;16:S234—7.

[225] Swendseid ME, Panaqua M, Kopple JD. Polyamine concentrations in red cells and urine of patients with chronic renal failure. Life Sci 1980;26(7):533—9.

[226] Radtke HW, Rege AB, LaMarche MB, et al. Identification of spermine as an inhibitor of erythropoiesis in patients with chronic renal failure. J Clin Invest 1981;67(6):1623—9.

[227] Galli F, Beninati S, Benedetti S, et al. Polymeric protein-polyamine conjugates: a new class of uremic toxins affecting erythropoiesis. Kidney Int Suppl 2001;78:S73—6.

[228] Kushner D, Beckman B, Nguyen L, et al. Polyamines in the anemia of end-stage renal disease. Kidney Int 1991;39(4):725—32.

[229] Yoshida K, Yoneda T, Kimura S, et al. Polyamines as an inhibitor on erythropoiesis of hemodialysis patients by in vitro bioassay using the fetal mouse liver assay. Ther Apher Dial 2006;10(3): 267–72.

[230] Bagdade JD, Subbaiah PV, Bartos D, Bartos F, Campbell RA. Polyamines: an unrecognised cardiovascular risk factor in chronic dialysis? Lancet 1979;1(8113):412–3.

[231] Niwa T, Ise M. Indoxyl sulfate, a circulating uremic toxin, stimulates the progression of glomerular sclerosis. J Lab Clin Med 1994;124(1):96–104.

[232] Dou L, Jourde-Chiche N, Faure V, et al. The uremic solute indoxyl sulfate induces oxidative stress in endothelial cells. J Thromb Haemost 2007;5(6):1302–8.

[233] Dou L, Bertrand E, Cerini C, et al. The uremic solutes p-cresol and indoxyl sulfate inhibit endothelial proliferation and wound repair. Kidney Int 2004;65(2):442–51.

[234] Niwa T, Ise M, Miyazaki T. Progression of glomerular sclerosis in experimental uremic rats by administration of indole, a precursor of indoxyl sulfate. Am J Nephrol 1994;14(3):207–12.

[235] Tumur Z, Shimizu H, Enomoto A, Miyazaki H, Niwa T. Indoxyl sulfate upregulates expression of ICAM-1 and MCP-1 by oxidative stress-induced NF-kappaB activation. Am J Nephrol 2010;31(5):435–41.

[236] Niwa T, Miyazaki T, Hashimoto N, et al. Suppressed serum and urine levels of indoxyl sulfate by oral sorbent in experimental uremic rats. Am J Nephrol 1992;12(4):201–6.

[237] Schulman G, Agarwal R, Acharya M, et al. A multicenter, randomized, double-blind, placebo-controlled, dose-ranging study of AST-120 (Kremezin) in patients with moderate to severe CKD. Am J Kidney Dis 2006;47(4):565–77.

[238] Niwa T, Yazawa T, Kodama T, et al. Efficient removal of albumin-bound furancarboxylic acid, an inhibitor of erythropoiesis, by continuous ambulatory peritoneal dialysis. Nephron 1990;56(3):241–5.

[239] Shoji T, Wada A, Inoue K, et al. Prospective randomized study evaluating the efficacy of the spherical adsorptive carbon AST-120 in chronic kidney disease patients with moderate decrease in renal function. Nephron Clin Pract 2007;105(3):c99–107.

[240] Akizawa T, Asano Y, Morita S, et al. Effect of a carbonaceous oral adsorbent on the progression of CKD: a multicenter, randomized, controlled trial. Am J Kidney Dis 2009;54(3): 459–67.

[241] Pawlak K, Mysliwiec M, Pawlak D. Kynurenine pathway - a new link between endothelial dysfunction and carotid atherosclerosis in chronic kidney disease patients. Adv Med Sci 2010;55(2):196–203.

[242] Pawlak K, Brzosko S, Mysliwiec M, Pawlak D. Kynurenine, quinolinic acid—the new factors linked to carotid atherosclerosis in patients with end-stage renal disease. Atherosclerosis 2009;204(2):561–6.

[243] Wardle EN, Wilkinson K. Free phenols in chronic renal failure. Clin Nephrol 1976;6(2):361–4.

[244] Niwa T. Phenol and p-cresol accumulated in uremic serum measured by HPLC with fluorescence detection. Clin Chem 1993;39(1):108–11.

[245] Schoots AC, Dijkstra JB, Ringoir SM, Vanholder R, Cramers CA. Are the classical markers sufficient to describe uremic solute accumulation in dialyzed patients? Hippurates reconsidered. Clin Chem 1988;34(6):1022–9.

[246] Zimmerman L, Jornvall H, Bergstrom J. Phenylacetylglutamine and hippuric acid in uremic and healthy subjects. Nephron 1990;55(3):265–71.

[247] Liebich HM, Bubeck JI, Pickert A, Wahl G, Scheiter A. Hippuric acid and 3-carboxy-4-methyl-5-propyl-2-furanpropionic acid in

serum and urine. Analytical approaches and clinical relevance in kidney diseases. J Chromatogr 1990;500:615–27.

[248] Schoots AC, De Vries PM, Thiemann R, et al. Biochemical and neurophysiological parameters in hemodialyzed patients with chronic renal failure. Clin Chim Acta 1989;185(1):91–107.

[249] Vanholder RC, De Smet RV, Ringoir SM. Assessment of urea and other uremic markers for quantification of dialysis efficacy. Clin Chem 1992;38(8 Pt 1):1429–36.

[250] Rutten GA, Schoots AC, Vanholder R, et al. Hexachlorobenzene and 1,1-di(4-chlorophenyl)-2,2-dichloroethene in serum of uremic patients and healthy persons: determination by capillary gas chromatography and electron capture detection. Nephron 1988;48(3):217–21.

[251] Niwa T, Ise M, Miyazaki T, Meada K. Suppressive effect of an oral sorbent on the accumulation of p-cresol in the serum of experimental uremic rats. Nephron 1993;65(1):82–7.

[252] Wardle EN. How toxic are phenols? Kidney Int Suppl 1978;(8):S13–5.

[253] Vanholder R, De Smet R, Waterloos MA, et al. Mechanisms of uremic inhibition of phagocyte reactive species production: characterization of the role of p-cresol. Kidney Int 1995;47(2): 510–7.

[254] Meijers BK, Bammens B, De Moor B, et al. Free p-cresol is associated with cardiovascular disease in hemodialysis patients. Kidney Int 2008;73(10):1174–80.

[255] Meijers BK, Claes K, Bammens B, et al. p-Cresol and cardiovascular risk in mild-to-moderate kidney disease. Clin J Am Soc Nephrol 2010;5(7):1182–9.

[256] Vanholder R, Van Laecke S, Glorieux G. What is new in uremic toxicity? Pediatr Nephrol 2008;23(8):1211–21.

[257] Jourde-Chiche N, Dou L, Cerini C, et al. Protein-bound toxins – update 2009. Semin Dial 2009;22(4):334–9.

[258] Miyata T, Kurokawa K, Van Ypersele De Strihou C. Advanced glycation and lipoxidation end products: role of reactive carbonyl compounds generated during carbohydrate and lipid metabolism. J Am Soc Nephrol 2000;11(9):1744–52.

[259] Brownlee M, Cerami A, Vlassara H. Advanced glycosylation end products in tissue and the biochemical basis of diabetic complications. N Engl J Med 1988;318(20):1315–21.

[260] Miyata T, Sugiyama S, Saito A, Kurokawa K. Reactive carbonyl compounds related uremic toxicity ("carbonyl stress"). Kidney Int Suppl 2001;78:S25–31.

[261] Busch M, Franke S, Ruster C, Wolf G. Advanced glycation end-products and the kidney. Eur J Clin Invest 2010; 40(8):742–55.

[262] Thornalley PJ. Protein and nucleotide damage by glyoxal and methylglyoxal in physiological systems—role in ageing and disease. Drug Metabol Drug Interact 2008;23(1-2):125–50.

[263] Saito A, Takeda T, Sato K, et al. Significance of proximal tubular metabolism of advanced glycation end products in kidney diseases. Ann N Y Acad Sci 2005;1043:637–43.

[264] Semba RD, Ferrucci L, Fink JC, et al. Advanced glycation end products and their circulating receptors and level of kidney function in older community-dwelling women. Am J Kidney Dis 2009;53(1):51–8.

[265] Stein G, Busch M, Muller A, et al. Are advanced glycation end products cardiovascular risk factors in patients with CRF? Am J Kidney Dis 2003;41(3 Suppl. 1):S52–6.

[266] Sakata N, Imanaga Y, Meng J, et al. Increased advanced glycation end products in atherosclerotic lesions of patients with end-stage renal disease. Atherosclerosis 1999;142(1):67–77.

[267] Taki K, Takayama F, Tsuruta Y, Niwa T. Oxidative stress, advanced glycation end product, and coronary artery calcification in hemodialysis patients. Kidney Int 2006;70(1): 218–24.

[268] Makita Z, Vlassara H, Cerami A, Bucala R. Immunochemical detection of advanced glycosylation end products in vivo. J Biol Chem 1992;267(8):5133–8.

[269] Makita Z, Radoff S, Rayfield EJ, et al. Advanced glycosylation end products in patients with diabetic nephropathy. N Engl J Med 1991;325(12):836–42.

[270] Glorieux G, Helling R, Henle T, et al. In vitro evidence for immune activating effect of specific AGE structures retained in uremia. Kidney Int 2004;66(5):1873–80.

[271] Sell DR, Monnier VM. End-stage renal disease and diabetes catalyze the formation of a pentose-derived crosslink from aging human collagen. J Clin Invest 1990;85(2):380–4.

[272] Sell DR, Nagaraj RH, Grandhee SK, et al. Pentosidine: a molecular marker for the cumulative damage to proteins in diabetes, aging, and uremia. Diabetes Metab Rev 1991;7(4):239–51.

[273] Monnier VM, Sell DR, Nagaraj RH, et al. Maillard reaction-mediated molecular damage to extracellular matrix and other tissue proteins in diabetes, aging, and uremia. Diabetes 1992;41(Suppl. 2):36–41.

[274] Odetti P, Fogarty J, Sell DR, Monnier VM. Chromatographic quantitation of plasma and erythrocyte pentosidine in diabetic and uremic subjects. Diabetes 1992;41(2):153–9.

[275] Zheng ZH, Sederholm F, Anderstam B, et al. Acute effects of peritoneal dialysis solutions on appetite in non-uremic rats. Kidney Int 2001;60(6):2392–8.

[276] Wagner Z, Molnar M, Molnar GA, et al. Serum carboxymethyllysine predicts mortality in hemodialysis patients. Am J Kidney Dis 2006;47(2):294–300.

[277] Busch M, Franke S, Muller A, et al. Potential cardiovascular risk factors in chronic kidney disease: AGEs, total homocysteine and metabolites, and the C-reactive protein. Kidney Int 2004;66(1):338–47.

[278] Schwedler SB, Metzger T, Schinzel R, Wanner C. Advanced glycation end products and mortality in hemodialysis patients. Kidney Int 2002;62(1):301–10.

[279] Busch M, Franke S, Wolf G, et al. The advanced glycation end product N(epsilon)-carboxymethyllysine is not a predictor of cardiovascular events and renal outcomes in patients with type 2 diabetic kidney disease and hypertension. Am J Kidney Dis 2006;48(4):571–9.

[280] Meerwaldt R, Hartog JW, Graaff R, et al. Skin autofluorescence, a measure of cumulative metabolic stress and advanced glycation end products, predicts mortality in hemodialysis patients. J Am Soc Nephrol 2005;16(12):3687–93.

[281] Meerwaldt R, Zeebregts CJ, Navis G, et al. Accumulation of advanced glycation end products and chronic complications in ESRD treated by dialysis. Am J Kidney Dis 2009;53(1):138–50.

[282] Cristol PE, jeanbrau E, Monnier P. La polypeptidémie en pathologie rénale. J Med Franc 1938;27:24.

[283] Osada J, Gea T, Sanz C, Millan I, Botella J. Evaluation of dialysis treatment in uremic patients by gel filtration of serum. Clin Chem 1990;36(11). 1906-10.

[284] Zimmerman L, Jornvall H, Bergstrom J, Furst P, Sjovall J. Characterization of middle molecule compounds. Artif Organs 1981;4(Suppl. 4):33–6.

[285] Zimmerman L, Jornvall H, Bergstrom J, Furst P, Sjovall J. Characterization of a double conjugate in uremic body fluids. FEBS Lett 1981;129(2):237–40.

[286] Gallice P, Fournier N, Crevat A, et al. Separation of one uremic middle molecules fraction by high performance liquid chromatography. Kidney Int 1983;23(5):764–6.

[287] Abiko T, Onodera I, Sekino H. Characterization of an acidic tripeptide in neurotoxic dialysate. Chem Pharm Bull (Tokyo) 1980;28(5):1629–33.

[288] McCaleb ML, Izzo MS, Lockwood DH. Characterization and partial purification of a factor from uremic human serum that induces insulin resistance. J Clin Invest 1985;75(2):391–6.

[289] Kaplan B, Gotfried M, Ravid M. Amino acid containing compounds in uremic serum-search for middle molecules by high performance liquid chromatography. Clin Nephrol 1986;26(2):66–71.

[290] Tenckhoff H, Curtis FK. Experience with maintenance peritoneal dialysis in the home. Trans Am Soc Artif Intern Organs 1970;16:90–5.

[291] Scribner BH. Discussion. Trans Am Soc Artif Intern Organs 1965;11:29.

[292] Jebsen RH, Tenckhoff H, Honet JC. Natural history of uremic polyneuropathy and effects of dialysis. N Engl J Med 1967;277(7):327–33.

[293] Babb AL, Popovich RP, Christopher TG, Scribner BH. The genesis of the square meter-hour hypothesis. Trans Am Soc Artif Intern Organs 1971;17:81–91.

[294] Babb AL, Farrell PC, Uvelli DA, Scribner BH. Hemodialyzer evaluation by examination of solute molecular spectra. Trans Am Soc Artif Intern Organs 1972;18(0):98–105. 122.

[295] Cheung AK, Rocco MV, Yan G, et al. Serum beta-2 microglobulin levels predict mortality in dialysis patients: results of the HEMO study. J Am Soc Nephrol 2006;17(2):546–55.

[296] Berggard I, Bearn AG. Isolation and properties of a low molecular weight beta-2-globulin occurring in human biological fluids. J Biol Chem 1968;243(15):4095–103.

[297] Charra B, Calemard E, Laurent G. Chronic renal failure treatment duration and mode: their relevance to the late dialysis periarticular syndrome. Blood Purif 1988;6(2):117–24.

[298] Gejyo F, Homma N, Maruyama H, Arakawa M. Beta 2-microglobulin-related amyloidosis in patients receiving chronic hemodialysis. Contrib Nephrol 1988;68:263–9.

[299] Vanholder R, Glorieux G, De Smet R, Lameire N. New insights in uremic toxins. Kidney Int Suppl 2003;(84):S6–10.

[300] Heegaard NH. beta(2)-microglobulin: from physiology to amyloidosis. Amyloid 2009;16(3):151–73.

[301] Gejyo F, Yamada T, Odani S, et al. A new form of amyloid protein associated with chronic hemodialysis was identified as beta 2-microglobulin. Biochem Biophys Res Commun 1985;129(3):701–6.

[302] Drueke TB. Beta2-microglobulin and amyloidosis. Nephrol Dial Transplant 2000;15(Suppl. 1):17–24.

[303] Drueke T, Touam M, Zingraff J. Dialysis-associated amyloidosis. Adv Ren Replace Ther 1995;2(1):24–39.

[304] Niwa T, Miyazaki S, Katsuzaki T, et al. Immunohistochemical detection of advanced glycation end products in dialysis-related amyloidosis. Kidney Int 1995;48(3):771–8.

[305] Cheung AK, Chenoweth DE, Otsuka D, Henderson LW. Compartmental distribution of complement activation products in artificial kidneys. Kidney Int 1986;30(1):74–80.

[306] Floge J, Granolleras C, Bingel M, et al. Beta 2-microglobulin kinetics during haemodialysis and haemofiltration. Nephrol Dial Transplant 1987;1(4):223–8.

[307] Floege J, Bartsch A, Schulze M, et al. Clearance and synthesis rates of beta 2-microglobulin in patients undergoing hemodialysis and in normal subjects. J Lab Clin Med 1991;118(2):153–65.

[308] Zingraff J, Beyne P, Urena P, et al. Influence of haemodialysis membranes on beta 2-microglobulin kinetics: in vivo and in vitro studies. Nephrol Dial Transplant 1988;3(3):284–90.

[309] Simon P, Cavarle YY, Ang KS, Cam G, Catheline M. Long-term variations of serum beta 2-microglobulin levels in hemodialysed uremics according to permeability and bioincompatibility of dialysis membranes. Blood Purif 1988;6(2):111–6.

[310] Blumberg A, Burgi W. Behavior of beta 2-microglobulin in patients with chronic renal failure undergoing hemodialysis, hemodiafiltration and continuous ambulatory peritoneal dialysis (CAPD). Clin Nephrol 1987;27(5):245–9.

[311] Kaiser JP, Hagemann J, von Herrath D, Schaefer K. Different handling of beta 2-microglobulin during hemodialysis and hemofiltration. Nephron 1988;48(2):132–5.

[312] Floege J, Granolleras C, Deschodt G, et al. High-flux synthetic versus cellulosic membranes for beta 2-microglobulin removal during hemodialysis, hemodiafiltration and hemofiltration. Nephrol Dial Transplant 1989;4(7):653–7.

[313] Sethi D, Murphy CM, Brown EA, Muller BR, Gower PE. Clearance of beta-2-microglobulin using continuous ambulatory peritoneal dialysis. Nephron 1989;52(4):352–5.

[314] Ballardie FW, Kerr DN, Tennent G, Pepys MB. Haemodialysis versus CAPD: equal predisposition to amyloidosis? Lancet 1986;1(8484):795–6.

[315] Tielemans C, Dratwa M, Bergmann P, et al. Continuous ambulatory peritoneal dialysis vs haemodialysis: a lesser risk of amyloidosis? Nephrol Dial Transplant 1988;3(3):291–4.

[316] Sethi D, Brown EA, Gower PE. CAPD, protective against developing dialysis-associated amyloid? Nephron 1988;50(1):85–6.

[317] Vanholder RC, Ringoir SM. Adequacy of dialysis: a critical analysis. Kidney Int 1992;42(3):540–58.

[318] Hulter HN, Melby JC, Peterson JC, Cooke CR. Chronic continuous PTH infusion results in hypertension in normal subjects. J Clin Hypertens 1986;2(4):360–70.

[319] Iseki K, Massry SG, Campese VM. Effects of hypercalcemia and parathyroid hormone on blood pressure in normal and renal-failure rats. Am J Physiol 1986;250(5 Pt 2):F924–9.

[320] Kopple JD, Cianciaruso B, Massry SG. Does parathyroid hormone cause protein wasting? Contrib Nephrol 1980;20:138–48.

[321] Garber AJ. Effects of parathyroid hormone on skeletal muscle protein and amino acid metabolism in the rat. J Clin Invest 1983;71(6):1806–21.

[322] Wassner SJ, Li JB. Lack of an acute effect of parathyroid hormone within skeletal muscle. Int J Pediatr Nephrol 1987;8(1):15–20.

[323] Gomez-Fernandez P, Sanchez Agudo L, Miguel JL, Almaraz M, Vila Dupla MJ. Effect of parathyroidectomy on respiratory muscle strength in uremic myopathy. Am J Nephrol 1987;7(6):466–9.

[324] Szucs J, Mako J, Merey J. Blood requirement and subtotal parathyroidectomy in patients with chronic renal failure treated with hemodialysis. Clin Nephrol 1983;19(3):134–6.

[325] Meytes D, Bogin E, Ma A, Dukes PP, Massry SG. Effect of parathyroid hormone on erythropoiesis. J Clin Invest 1981;67(5):1263–9.

[326] Potasman I, Better OS. The role of secondary hyperparathyroidism in the anemia of chronic renal failure. Nephron 1983;33(4):229–31.

[327] Akmal M, Telfer N, Ansari AN, Massry SG. Erythrocyte survival in chronic renal failure. Role of secondary hyperparathyroidism. J Clin Invest 1985;76(4):1695–8.

[328] McGonigle RJ, Wallin JD, Husserl F, et al. Potential role of parathyroid hormone as an inhibitor of erythropoiesis in the anemia of renal failure. J Lab Clin Med 1984;104(6):1016–26.

[329] Lutton JD, Solangi KB, Ibraham NG, Goodman AI, Levere RD. Inhibition of erythropoiesis in chronic renal failure: the role of parathyroid hormone. Am J Kidney Dis 1984;3(5):380–4.

[330] Drueke T, Fauchet M, Fleury J, et al. Effect of parathyroidectomy on left-ventricular function in haemodialysis patients. Lancet 1980;1(8160):112–4.

[331] London GM, De Vernejoul MC, Fabiani F, et al. Secondary hyperparathyroidism and cardiac hypertrophy in hemodialysis patients. Kidney Int 1987;32(6):900–7.

[332] Akmal M, Massry SG, Goldstein DA, et al. Role of parathyroid hormone in the glucose intolerance of chronic renal failure. J Clin Invest 1985;75(3):1037–44.

[333] Mak RH, Bettinelli A, Turner C, Haycock GB, Chantler C. The influence of hyperparathyroidism on glucose metabolism in uremia. J Clin Endocrinol Metab 1985;60(2):229–33.

[334] Mak RH, Turner C, Haycock GB, Chantler C. Secondary hyperparathyroidism and glucose intolerance in children with uremia. Kidney Int Suppl 1983;16:S128–33.

[335] Hutchison CA, Harding S, Hewins P, et al. Quantitative assessment of serum and urinary polyclonal free light chains in patients with chronic kidney disease. Clin J Am Soc Nephrol 2008;3(6):1684–90.

[336] Cohen G, Horl WH. Free immunoglobulin light chains as a risk factor in renal and extrarenal complications. Semin Dial 2009;22(4):369–72.

[337] Cohen G, Haag-Weber M, Mai B, Deicher R, Horl WH. Effect of immunoglobulin light chains from hemodialysis and continuous ambulatory peritoneal dialysis patients on polymorphonuclear leukocyte functions. J Am Soc Nephrol 1995;6(6):1592–9.

[338] Stenvinkel P, Heimbürger O, Lönnqvist F. Serum leptin concentrations correlate to plasma insulin concentrations independent of body fat content in chronic renal failure. Nephrol Dial Transpl 1997;12:1321–5.

[339] Merabet E, Dagogo-Jack S, Coyne DW, et al. Increased plasma leptin concentrations in end-stage renal disease. J Clin Endocrinol Metab 1997;82:847–50.

[340] Young GA, Woodrow G, Kendall S, et al. Increased plasma leptin/fat ratio in patients with chronic renal failure: a cause of malnutrition. Nephrol Dial Transpl 1997;12:2318–23.

[341] Mak RH, Cheung W. Cachexia in chronic kidney disease: role of inflammation and neuropeptide signaling. Curr Opin Nephrol Hypertens 2007;16(1):27–31.

[342] Widjaja A, Kielstein JT, Horn R, et al. Free serum leptin but not bound leptin concentrations are elevated in patients with end-stage renal disease. Nephrol Dial Transplant 2000;15(6):846–50.

[343] Stenvinkel P. Leptin and its clinical implications in chronic renal failure. Mineral Electrol Metab 1999;25(4–6):298–302.

[344] Sharma K, Considine RV, Michael B, et al. Plasma leptin is partly cleared by the kidney and is elevated in hemodialysis patients. Kidney Int 1997;51(6):1980–5.

[345] Nordfors L, Lonnqvist F, Heimburger O, et al. Low leptin gene expression and hyperleptinemia in chronic renal failure. Kidney Int 1998;54(4):1267–75.

[346] Cumin F, Baum HP, Levens N. Leptin is cleared from the circulation primarily by the kidney. Int J of Obesity 1996;20:1120–6.

[347] Zeng J, Patterson BW, klien S, et al. Whole body leptin kinetics and renal metabolism in vivo. Am J Physiol 1997;273:E1102–6.

[348] Kokot F, Adamczak M, Wiecek A. Plasma leptin concentration in kidney transplant patients at the early posttransplant period. Nephrol Dial Transpl 1998;13:2276–80.

[349] Eggertsen G, Heimburger O, Stenvinkel P, Berglund L. Influence of variation at the apolipoprotein E locus on lipid and lipoprotein levels in CAPD patients. Nephrol Dial Transplant 1997;12(1):141–4.

[350] Garibotti G, Russo R, Franceschini R, et al. Inter-organ leptin exchange in humans. Biochem & Biophys Res Commun 1998;247:504–9.

[351] Stenvinkel P, Heimburger O, Lonnqvist F. Serum leptin concentrations correlate to plasma insulin concentrations

independent of body fat content in chronic renal failure. Nephrol Dial Transplant 1997;12(7):1321—5.

[352] Daschner M, Tönshoff B, Blum WF, et al. Inappropriate elevation of serum leptin levels in children with chronic renal failure. J Am Soc Nephrol 1998;9:1074—9.

[353] Johansen KL, Mulligan K, Tai V, Schambelan M. Leptin, body composition, and indices of malnutrition in patients on diaysis. J Am soc Nephrol 1998;9:1080—4.

[354] Odamaki M, Furuya R, Yoneyama T, et al. Association of the serum leptin concentration with weight loss in chronic hemodialysis patients. Am J Kidney Dis 1999;33:361—8.

[355] Stenvinkel P, Lindholm B, Lönnqvist F, Katzarski K, Heimbürger O. Increases in serum leptin during peritoneal dialysis are associated with inflammation and a decrease in lean body mass. J Am Soc Nephrol 2000;11:1303—9.

[356] Axelsson J, Qureshi AR, Heimburger O, et al. Body fat mass and serum leptin levels influence epoetin sensitivity in patients with ESRD. Am J Kidney Dis 2005;46(4):628—34.

[357] Dagogo-Jack S, Ovalle F, Geary B, Landt M, Coyne DW. Hyperleptinaemia in patients with end-stage renal disease treated by peritoneal dialysis. Perit Dial Int 1998;18:34—40.

[358] Rodriguez-Carmona A, Perez Fontan M, Cordido F, Garcia Falcon T, Garcia-Buela J. Hyperleptinemia is not correlated with markers of protein malnutrition in chronic renal failure. A cross-sectional study in predialysis, peritoneal dialysis and hemodialysis patients. Nephron 2000;86(3):274—80.

[359] Sucajtys-Szulc E, Karbowska J, Kochan Z, et al. Up-regulation of NPY gene expression in hypothalamus of rats with experimental chronic renal failure. Biochim Biophys Acta 2007;1772(1):26—31.

[360] Bald M, Gerigk M, Rascher W. Elevated plasma concentrations of neuropeptide Y in children and adults with chronic and terminal renal failure. Am J Kidney Dis 1997;30(1):23—7.

[361] Zoccali C, Mallamaci F, Tripepi G, et al. Neuropeptide Y, left ventricular mass and function in patients with end stage renal disease. J Hypertens 2003;21(7):1355—62.

[362] Odar-Cederlof I, Ericsson F, Theodorsson E, Kjellstrand CM. Neuropeptide-Y and atrial natriuretic peptide as prognostic markers in patients on hemodialysis. ASAIO J 2003;49(1):74—80.

[363] Zoccali C, Mallamaci F, Tripepi G, et al. Prospective study of neuropeptide y as an adverse cardiovascular risk factor in end-stage renal disease. J Am Soc Nephrol 2003;14(10):2611—7.

[364] Jankowski V, Gunthner T, Herget-Rosenthal S, Zidek W, Jankowski J. Dinucleoside polyphosphates and uremia. Semin Dial 2009;22(4):396—9.

[365] Ogilvie A, Blasius R, Schulze-Lohoff E, Sterzel RB. Adenine dinucleotides: a novel class of signalling molecules. J Auton Pharmacol 1996;16(6):325—8.

[366] Heidenreich S, Tepel M, Schluter H, Harrach B, Zidek W. Regulation of rat mesangial cell growth by diadenosine phosphates. J Clin Invest 1995;95(6):2862—7.

[367] Jankowski J, Hagemann J, Yoon MS, et al. Increased vascular growth in hemodialysis patients induced by platelet-derived diadenosine polyphosphates. Kidney Int 2001;59(3):1134—41.

[368] Shlipak MG, Sarnak MJ, Katz R, et al. Cystatin C and the risk of death and cardiovascular events among elderly persons. N Engl J Med 2005;352(20):2049—60.

[369] Shlipak MG, Wassel Fyr CL, Chertow GM, et al. Cystatin C and mortality risk in the elderly: the health, aging, and body composition study. J Am Soc Nephrol 2006;17(1):254—61.

[370] Menon V, Shlipak MG, Wang X, et al. Cystatin C as a risk factor for outcomes in chronic kidney disease. Ann Intern Med 2007;147(1):19—27.

[371] Madero M, Sarnak MJ. Association of cystatin C with adverse outcomes. Curr Opin Nephrol Hypertens 2009;18(3):258—63.

[372] Seccia TM, Maniero C, Belloni AS, et al. Role of angiotensin II, endothelin-1 and L-type calcium channel in the development of glomerular, tubulointerstitial and perivascular fibrosis. J Hypertens 2008;26(10):2022—9.

[373] Gagliardini E, Corna D, Zoja C, et al. Unlike each drug alone, lisinopril if combined with avosentan promotes regression of renal lesions in experimental diabetes. Am J Physiol Renal Physiol 2009;297(5):F1448—56.

[374] Nagatoya K, Moriyama T, Kawada N, et al. Y-27632 prevents tubulointerstitial fibrosis in mouse kidneys with unilateral ureteral obstruction. Kidney Int 2002;61(5):1684—95.

[375] Carrero JJ, Park SH, Axelsson J, Lindholm B, Stenvinkel P. Cytokines, atherogenesis, and hypercatabolism in chronic kidney disease: a dreadful triad. Semin Dial 2009;22(4):381—6.

[376] Stenvinkel P, Ketteler M, Johnson RJ, et al. IL-10, IL-6, and TNF-alpha: central factors in the altered cytokine network of uremia—the good, the bad, and the ugly. Kidney Int 2005;67(4):1216—33.

[377] Takahashi T, Kubota M, Nakamura T, Ebihara I, Koide H. Interleukin-6 gene expression in peripheral blood mononuclear cells from patients undergoing hemodialysis or continuous ambulatory peritoneal dialysis. Ren Fail 2000;22(3):345—54.

[378] Stenvinkel P, Heimburger O, Jogestrand T. Elevated interleukin-6 predicts progressive carotid artery atherosclerosis in dialysis patients: association with Chlamydia pneumoniae seropositivity. Am J Kidney Dis 2002;39(2):274—82.

[379] Raj DS. Role of interleukin-6 in the anemia of chronic disease. Semin Arthritis Rheum 2009;38(5):382—8.

[380] Mitch WE, Du J, Bailey JL, Price SR. Mechanisms causing muscle proteolysis in uremia: the influence of insulin and cytokines. Miner Electrolyte Metab 1999;25(4-6):216—9.

[381] Wang P, Ba ZF, Chaudry IH. Administration of tumor necrosis factor-alpha in vivo depresses endothelium-dependent relaxation. Am J Physiol 1994;266(6 Pt 2):H2535—41.

[382] Yoshizumi M, Perrella MA, Burnett Jr JC, Lee ME. Tumor necrosis factor downregulates an endothelial nitric oxide synthase mRNA by shortening its half-life. Circ Res 1993;73(1):205—9.

[383] Lai HL, Kartal J, Mitsnefes M. Hyperinsulinemia in pediatric patients with chronic kidney disease: the role of tumor necrosis factor-alpha. Pediatr Nephrol 2007;22(10):1751—6.

5

Inflammation in Chronic Kidney Disease

Juan Jesús Carrero, Peter Stenvinkel

Division of Renal Medicine, Karolinska Institutet, Stockholm, Sweden

GENERAL CONSIDERATIONS

Inflammation (Latin *inflammatio*, to set on fire) represents a complex biological response of vascular tissues to harmful stimuli. Inflammation should, in its initial acute form, be regarded as a protective attempt by the organism to remove the injurious stimuli as well as to initiate the healing process for the tissue. Whereas the acute release of proinflammatory cytokines may have beneficial effects, a chronic low-grade systemic inflammatory activity is, however, likely to be detrimental for the organism. This is the problem faced in the uremic milieu, characterized by a state of persistent low-grade chronic inflammation, and where the persistent effect of causative stimuli leads to functional changes as well as destruction of cells and tissues.

In chronic kidney disease (CKD) and especially in end-stage renal disease (ESRD), the systemic concentrations of both pro- and anti-inflammatory cytokines are multi-fold higher, due to both decreased renal clearance and increased tissue production. Because of this, inflammation is a major characteristic in advanced CKD worldwide according to CRP estimations [1—7]. Reports from the National Health and Nutrition Examination Survey III (NHANES) show that half of the patients with GFR 15—60 mL/min had CRP levels >2.1 mg/L [8]. The European dialysis patient currently has a median CRP of 5 mg/L (Figure 5.1), the American patient slightly higher levels and the Asian dialysis patients substantially lower [1—7]. Via both direct and indirect effects chronic inflammation is an important inducer of the protein-energy wasting (PEW) syndrome. The purpose of this chapter is to describe the physiopathology and implications of these complex inflammatory processes in the context of PEW. At the same time we will discuss applicability of regular CRP monitoring in the clinical setting and possible therapeutic initiatives to tackle this risk factor.

MULTIFACTORIAL CAUSES OF INFLAMMATION IN CHRONIC KIDNEY DISEASE

There are many and varied factors, inherent or not to a reduction in kidney function, that contribute to systemic inflammation, being intercurrent clinical events the most important [9]. Infectious agents and microorganisms are also causative or contributory factors to the inflammatory cascade, being also associated with atherosclerosis progression [10—13]. Reductions in kidney function *per se*, or even small changes in residual renal function (RRF) further seem to impact on "uremic inflammation". It has thus been hypothesized that retention of circulating cytokines [14], advanced glycation end products (AGEs) [15] and pro-oxidants [16] initiate and enhance the proinflammatory milieu when renal function declines. Additional mechanisms by which a failing kidney function may promote inflammation include volume overload, impaired intestinal barrier function with passage of endotoxins, sympathetic overactivity (and/or blunted vagal nerve activity) [17] or chronic inflammatory process associated to periodontitis [18,19].

The HD procedure *per se* can contribute to increased systemic inflammation comprising, among others, the interaction of circulating monocytes with nonbiocompatible membranes [20], blood contact with nonsterile dialysate solution [21], use of unpure dialysate [22—24], the extent of convective transport, and the frequency and duration of dialysis [25,26]. However, the overall contribution of the dialysis procedure is unlikely a major instigator of inflammation because of the high prevalence of inflammation biomarkers in

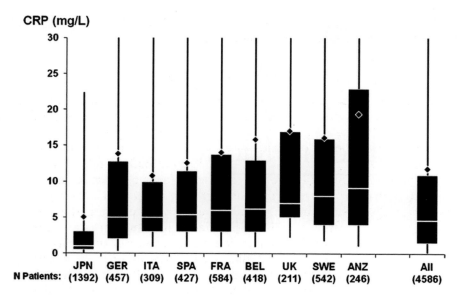

CRP (mg/L)

FIGURE 5.1 Distribution of C-reactive protein (CRP) in different countries from the DOPPS study, restricted to patients on dialysis >90 days in facilities that routinely measure CRP (n = 4586). The top and bottom of the boxes indicate the 25th and 75th percentiles of the distribution. The horizontal line within the box indicates the median (50th percentile), and the diamond indicates the mean. Vertical lines extend to the 5th and 95th percentiles. Reproduced with permission from Clin J Am Soc Nephrol. 2011 Oct;6(10):2452−61.

CKD 5 patients not yet renal replacement therapy [27,28]. Overhydration and volume overload may, via bacterial or endotoxin translocation in patients with severe gut edema, lead to immunoactivation and increased inflammatory cytokine production [29]. Finally, strong interrelations between inflammation, RRF and left ventricular hypertrophy (LVH) have been documented in dialysis patients [4].

Obesity, a common finding in CKD patients, may also contribute to an enhanced inflammatory activity. Both truncal fat mass [30] or abdominal fat deposition [31] have been associated with increased systemic inflammation in dialysis patients. Also in nondialyzed CKD patients, longitudinal variations in abdominal fat are accompanied by parallel changes in systemic inflammation (Figure 5.2). The reasons for this association relate to the capacity of adipocytes and fat-infiltrated macrophages of secreting adipokines, IL-6 or TNF-α into systemic circulation [32,33]. Many adipokines exert further proinflammatory effects [34−36], considering the dramatic effect that loss of RRF has on the clearance of adipokines, the systemic effects of adipokine imbalance in CKD patients may be even greater than in the general population. Furthermore, uremic fat may be overactivated, since proinflammatory genes have been demonstrated to be upregulated in visceral fat from CKD patients as compared to matched controls [37]. As a final remark, we should emphasize that obesity, as a proinflammatory state, may also link to PEW. The concept of obese sarcopenia demonstrated that PEW exists at any BMI categories (underweight, normal and overweight), and that increased CRP or IL-6 levels were a feature of PEW in any given body weight [38]. This may be particularly true for abdominal obesity, which was accompanied by a higher prevalence of malnutrition and

inflammation, while at the same time the patients have lower muscle mass and strength [31].

To finish, studies show that the inflamed uremic phenotype may also be the result of genetic differences, since Asian dialysis patients treated in the USA still have a markedly lower inflammation and lower adjusted relative risk of mortality than Caucasians [39]. Indeed, a substantial genetic heritability (35−40%) has been found for CRP production [40,41], and many studies demonstrate a significant impact of genetic variations on the uremic inflammatory response [42,43]. Some paradoxical racial differences in CKD outcome may be however influenced by uremic inflammation: While in the general population African Americans experience a higher mortality rate than Caucasians, African Americans treated with dialysis

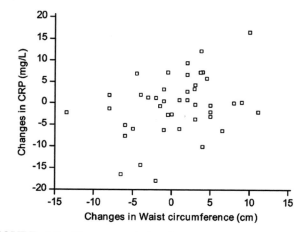

FIGURE 5.2 Direct association between 1-year variations in waist circumference and CRP levels in CKD patients stages 3−4. Reproduced with permission from Nephrol Dial Transplant. 2012;27:1423−8.

typically survive longer than Caucasians [44]. A recent American prospective cohort study of incident dialysis patients observed that the survival advantage among African American dialysis patients was found to only exist in the setting of high levels of inflammation [45]. Thus, racial differences in the presence and response to inflammation may underlie this long-observed survival paradox and may be worthy of further investigation. Lastly and perhaps in connection to this, shortening of telomeres (nucleoprotein complexes protecting the chromosome ends that are involved in chromosome stability and repair) has been associated with an inflamed phenotype and increased mortality in dialysis patients [46].

INFLAMMATION AS A CAUSE OF PROTEIN-ENERGY WASTING

Inflammation is an important contributory component of the complex PEW syndrome, both by direct mechanisms on muscle proteolysis but also indirect ones, impinging upon and magnifying other causes of PEW in a vicious circle. A scheme of presentation of the mechanisms by which inflammation leads to PEW is depicted in Figure 5.3.

Inflammation Leading to Anorexia

Anorexia or loss of appetite is one of the initial steps leading to reduced nutrient intake in CKD, being this issue discussed in more detail in Chapter 38. Cytokines and adipokines are capable of inducing anorexia by influencing meal size, meal duration and frequency. Specific cytokines and adipokines also access the brain acting directly on hypothalamic neurons and/or generating mediators targeting both peripheral and/or brain target sites [47,48]. In fact, inflammation is a common feature accompanying the occurrence of anorexia in clinical studies of dialysis patients [49–52]. In addition, inflammation is also a feature of other pathophysiological processes related to the patient's ability and desire to eat, such as dental problems and incidence of periodontitis [18], alterations and infections in the gastrointestinal tract [53] and hypothalamic resistance to orexigenic adipokines [54]. Also olfactory function is impaired in hemodialysis patients and related with the severity of malnutrition and inflammation [55]. Because inflammation inhibits progenitor cell proliferation and

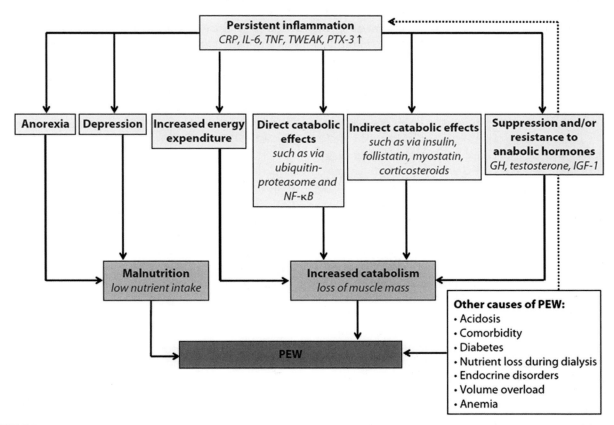

FIGURE 5.3 Proposed mechanistic pathways by which persistent inflammation may promote protein-energy wasting via malnutrition and increased catabolism in patients with CKD. Reproduced with permission from Contrib Nephrol 2011;171:120–6.

olfactory regeneration [56] it can be speculated that persistent uremic inflammation may further impact the patients desire to eat via this pathway.

Inflammation, a Cause of Depression?

Depressive symptoms are more frequent with gradual reduction in renal function and relate to poor outcome and mortality in this and other patient groups [57–59]. Cytokines are thought to be important mediators of brain immune connection and may play an important role in the pathogenesis of depression due to their effect on neurotransmitters and neurohormones [57,60]. In dialysis patients, depressive symptoms seemed to worsen in the presence of increased IL-6 levels [61–63], and 8 weeks of fluoxetine treatment in depressed HD patients decreased serum IL-1β levels [64]. Depression may undeniably link to fatigue [65] and unwillingness to eat [66], contributing in a vicious circle to anorexia, physical inactivity, PEW and worse outcome, all of which have also been attributed, in part, to the effects of systemic inflammation.

Inflammation and Increased Energy Expenditure

Many of the metabolic abnormalities present during the inflammatory response, including fever, elevated oxygen consumption, enhanced lipolysis and fat utilization, increased concentration of catabolic hormones and extensive protein catabolism, consume high quantities of energy and may account for as much as 15% of the daily energy expenditure [67]. The stimulatory effect of inflammation on energy expenditure has been suggested in various studies in nondialysis and dialysis patients, in which CRP, IL-6 and physical activity levels were important determinants of energy expenditure in these populations [4,68–70]. Because increased resting energy expenditure has been associated with high mortality rates and worse nutritional status in dialysis patients [4], the impact of increased energy expenditure on muscle mass and body fat stores needs further evaluation.

Direct Catabolic Effects of Inflammation

One of the main detrimental effects of proinflammatory cytokine activation in ESRD patients is muscle depletion [71]. In animal and human studies, infusion of TNF-α, IL-1 and IL-6 leads to increased muscle protein breakdown [72–74]. Consequently, clinical studies in CKD patients have shown links between inflammatory cytokines and muscle wasting [3,75–77]. A main mechanism of inflammation-induced wasting is via activation of NF-κB and ATP-ubiquitin-dependent proteolytic pathways (leading to cleavage of a characteristic 14 kDa actin fragment)

that cause muscle wasting [78]. As Raj et al. [79] observed ineffective utilization of exogenous amino acids for muscle protein synthesis during HD, they hypothesized that increased skeletal muscle expression of IL-6 further augmented muscle protein catabolism in ESRD. In another study, Boivin et al. [80] reported increased caspase-3 activity (an initial step resulting in loss of muscle protein is activation) and augmented apoptosis in uremic skeletal muscle, which may be due to increased IL-6 stimulation. TNF-α, and IL-6 seems to play important roles in the processes of frailty and uremic wasting [14], however they may not explain the whole picture. Indeed, a recent study in HD patients showed that while semestral variation of IL-6 levels strongly predicted outcome, such IL-6 variation did not associate with body compositional changes in mixed multivariate models [81]. Other proinflammatory mediators that so far received relatively little attention in the nephrological community may concomitantly contribute: IL-15 for instance is an immunoregulatory cytokine that exhibits proinflammatory activity by acting on a wide variety of cell types that, paradoxically, seems to have an anabolic role as the administration of IL-15 to cachectic tumor-bearing animals results in an improvement in the protein wasting process based mainly on the inhibition of protein degradation [82]. Recently, the TNF-related weak inducer of apoptosis (TWEAK) has been implicated in several biological responses including inflammation, angiogenesis, and osteoclastogenesis. As chronic administration of TWEAK resulted in reduced skeletal muscle weight in mice with an associated increase in the activity of ubiquitin–proteasome system and NF-kappaB [83] upregulation of the TWEAK-Fn14 system in the context of uremia may promote PEW [84]. Finally, Zhang et al. [85] demonstrated a previously unrecognized role for serum amyloid A in acting synergistically with IL-6 to impair insulin/IGF-1 signaling by increasing SOCS3 transcription, which results in muscle proteolysis. They proposed that angiotensin II may stimulate an interaction between the liver and skeletal muscle because the liver becomes the major source of both IL-6 and serum amyloid A.

Inflammation and Resistance to Anabolic Pathways

The uremic state is associated with abnormalities in the synthesis and action of many hormones, some of which may further contribute to the PEW syndrome, such as the case of erythropoietin and anemia. One of the most important pro-catabolic hormonal misbalances in CKD is insulin resistance, which in the general population has since long shown intimate links with systemic inflammation [86,87]. Administration of recombinant TNF to cultured cells or to animals impairs insulin action, and obese mice lacking functional TNF or TNF-receptors have improved insulin sensitivity compared with wild types counterparts [88]. In accordance, chronic administration of infliximab (a chimeric of anti TNF antibody) improve insulin resistance [89]. Whereas TNF increases lipolysis [90], which is highly linked to the development of insulin resistance, IL-6 inhibits insulin action both in vitro and in vivo muscle, liver and adipocytes [91]. Thus, decreased insulin sensitivity caused by persistent inflammation can predispose to loss of muscle mass by decreasing the anabolic action of insulin on the skeletal muscle. In fact, in clinical conditions where insulin resistance develops, such as in elderly subjects and in patients with type-2 diabetes mellitus, muscle wasting is often observed. By using stable isotope tracer techniques, Pupim et al. [92] showed that HD-patients with type-2 diabetes had significantly increased skeletal muscle protein breakdown as compared to nondiabetic HD-patients. Also, incident dialysis patients with diabetes mellitus had significantly accelerated loss of lean body mass (LBM) as compared to nondiabetics during the first year of dialysis therapy [93].

Resistance to anabolism by the growth hormone (GH)/Insulin growth factor (IGF)-1 axis may constitute another factor contributing to the loss of strength and muscle mass in CKD. While several clinical studies have reported that GH has a salutary effect on body composition and muscle protein synthesis in CKD patients [94], the responses to GH treatment vary considerably [95]. As inflammation inhibits GH action [96], it can be postulated that the GH response is blunted in uremia. Indeed, Garibotto et al. [97] found that whereas GH forearm perfusion caused a decrease in the negative potassium and protein balance of HD-patients without inflammation no such effect was seen in HD-patients with inflammation. Their finding, thus,

implies that a resistance to pharmacologic doses of GH is not related to uremia *per se* but rather to an increased inflammatory state. In addition, IL-6 administration inhibits IGF-1 secretion, further contributing to the sarcopenic process [98]. Interestingly, recombinant GH replacement therapy in CKD patients in well-designed studies has consistently been linked to improved anabolic function, stimulation of protein synthesis, decrease in urea generation, and improvement in nitrogen balance [99].

Low thyroid hormone levels in CKD patients have traditionally been interpreted either as an acute adaptation aimed at reducing energy expenditure and minimizing protein catabolism or as a chronic maladaptation participating in the wasting syndrome of prolonged critical illness [100]. Recent studies, nevertheless, associate low triiodothyronine levels in CKD stage 5 patients with systemic inflammatory markers (Figure 5.4), endothelial dysfunction and the prediction of all-cause and cardiovascular mortality [101−103]. Interestingly, correction of metabolic acidosis in dialysis patients is able to restore these hormonal derangements [104,105]. Several hypotheses connect the state of subclinical hypothyroidism with low-grade persistent inflammation in uremia [106]. Indeed, interleukin signaling down-regulate the peripheral conversion of total thyroxine (T4) into T3 in both experimental [107] and clinical [108] studies. In HD-patients, inflammation was accompanied by reductions in T3 levels, reverting these to normal as inflammation resolved [106]. It is therefore plausible that low triioodothyronine levels in ESRD represent an intermediate link between inflammation, PEW and mortality. Indeed, a recent study showed in fact that the impact of free T3 on mortality prediction was abrogated after adjustment for CRP and albumin, taken in this study as surrogates of PEW [109].

Prolactin retention in CKD impairs the production of gonadotropic hormones. In men, this translates into

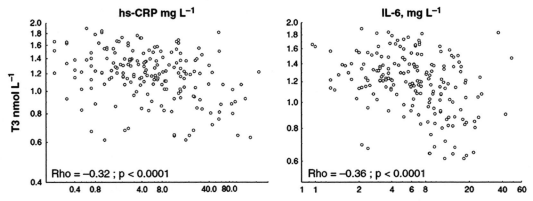

FIGURE 5.4 Strong inverse associations between total triiodothyronine (T3) levels and markers of inflammation (IL-6 and CRP) in euthyroid ESRD patients. Reproduced with permission from J Intern Med 2007 Dec;262(6):690−701.

a high prevalence of testosterone deficiency (male hypogonadism), with women displaying also very low testosterone concentrations [110–113]. Testosterone is a potent anabolic hormone that actively induces muscle protein synthesis [114]. Both muscle mass loss in wasted patients [115] or rapid weight loss during weight reduction regimens [116] have been correlated with testosterone decline. In dialysis and pre-dialysis patients, low testosterone levels were associated with increased mortality risk [117–119], and the observation that adjustment for S-creatinine levels (used as a surrogate marker of muscle mass) abrogated this mortality prediction [117] may indirectly support this pathophysiological mechanism. Androgen therapy in uremic patients (alone or in combination with resistance training) has resulted in significant amelioration of both muscle mass and nutritional status [120,121].

INFLAMMATION AS A CATALYST OF OTHER RISK FACTORS

Persistent low-grade inflammation in CKD may, in addition to putative direct pro-atherogenic and pro-wasting effects, serve as a catalyst and modulate the effects of other risk factors for PEW and CVD [122]. While inflammation may enhance the appearance of PEW, inflammation can also interact with malnutrition and CVD in exacerbating the mortality risk. A Dutch study demonstrated an interaction effect between these risk factors in relation to outcome [123]. The concurrent presence of inflammation, CVD and PEW was associated with a 16 deaths/100 person-years higher mortality rate than expected from the solo effects of these features. Thus, this observation translates epidemiological observations into evidence for the existence of a syndrome of PEW, inflammation and atherosclerotic CVD [124] where the whole is more than its parts [28]. Parekh et al. [125] also reported that while sudden cardiac death was common among ESRD patients, inflammation and malnutrition significantly increased its occurrence independent of traditional cardiovascular risk factors. Specifically, across increasing CRP tertiles cross-classified with decreasing albumin tertiles, an exacerbation of the risk for sudden cardiac death was observed.

OTHER CONSEQUENCES OF INFLAMMATION

There is a wealth of data linking *vascular calcification* with systemic inflammation. TNF can induce mineralization of calcifying vascular cells in vitro [126] and co-culture of these cells with monocyte/macrophages can accelerate mineralization [127]. Receptor activator of NF-kappaB ligand (RANKL) is a membrane-bound or soluble cytokine essential for osteoclast differentiation, whereas the decoy receptor osteoprotegerin (OPG) masks RANKL activity. As both seem to influence the inflammatory component of atherosclerosis [128], it is of interest that OPG upregulates endothelial cell adhesion molecule response to TNF [129]. These findings suggest a mechanism by which OPG may stimulate inflammation in atheroma and thereby promote the progression and complications of atherosclerosis, which would agree with the observed detrimental effects on survival of both increased inflammation and OPG levels in HD-patients [130,131]. On the other hand, vascular calcification, as part of the atherosclerotic process, is due to the deposition in the arterial intima of basic calcium phosphate crystals, similar to those that mineralize bone. It was recently shown that these crystals could interact with and activate human monocyte-derived macrophages, inducing a proinflammatory state via protein kinase C and MAP kinase pathways [132]. This would again imply a vicious circle of inflammation and arterial calcification that could explain the associations between inflammation and outcome in CKD. Finally, the most well studied inhibitor of ossification is fetuin-A. In CKD, low levels of circulating fetuin-A are associated with cardiac valvular calcification, increased cardiovascular burden, increased mortality risk [133–135,136]. Inflammation and PEW may be important causes of a decrease in serum fetuin-A levels in patients with CKD, as it behaves as a negative acute phase reactant [137,138].

MONITORING INFLAMMATION

CRP has in the clinical setting aroused as the prototypic marker of inflammation due to its reliability, low cost and wide availability. The key points to consider when monitoring inflammation in the clinical setting are however the reasons why CRP needs to be measured and the likelihood that diagnostic and therapeutic strategies might change on the basis of these test results. Despite a decade of extensive research on the causes and effects of uremic inflammation, no randomized trials with testing of inflammatory markers as the primary intervention have been performed, nor have cost-effectiveness analyses been completed to assess additional costs or cost savings through the use of such tests. Consequently, the following suggestions about the routine monitoring of inflammatory markers are not evidence-based.

Monitoring of Inflammation for Prognostic Purposes

Prospective epidemiological studies in CKD, dialysis or kidney transplant patients [28,139–147] have all consistently shown that a single measurement of inflammatory biomarkers are independent predictors of poor outcome. There is nevertheless an elevated biological intra- and inter-individual variability for inflammatory mediators in the setting of CKD, even more for the unspecific CRP responses. While a decreased renal function, increased number of co-morbidities, PEW and the uremic environment (oxidative stress, accumulation of AGS, etc.) affect inter-individual inflammatory variability [148], intra-individual variation may be further exacerbated by intercurrent clinical events, type of vascular access, membrane bio-incompatibility, dialysate backflow, endotoxemia and the intermittent presence of dialysis [26,53,149,150]. Volume status, fluid intake and RRF are also associated with this phenomenon [151]. Although it appears essential to understand and to evaluate inflammation in the context of its variability as disease evolves few studies address the consequences of regular monitoring of inflammatory markers on outcome. Of those, it seems apparent that the average of serial measurements of CRP or IL-6 provides a better survival prediction than single measurements [53,152]. Patients with a persistent CRP or IL-6 elevation during a specific time period exhibit worse outcome than those with persistent low levels or those increasing their CRP value [1,153] (Figure 5.5).

At present, there is insufficient evidence to support the regular monitoring of inflammation in the clinic with regards to mortality prediction. The recent study from Bazeley et al. [7] demonstrated however that CRP may have prognostic value beyond that provided by traditional risk factor algorithms (Framingham). The inclusion of CRP in such 1-year mortality prediction model contributed to correctly re-classify 13% of the patients with regards to their risk. Thus, these results can make it possible to create specific algorithms for short-term mortality prediction in CKD patients. Whether this may have prognostic applicability is not yet evident, but such algorithm could represent a decision tool towards the implementation of more aggressive therapeutic approaches in dialysis patients at risk.

Monitoring of Inflammation for Diagnostic Purposes

Probably the most useful indication of CRP monitoring is the screening and detection of underlying inflammatory processes and the assignment of appropriate treatment [154]. Possible underlying inflammatory processes include graft-related or catheter-related infections, peripheral arterial disease, silent coronary ischemia, ulcers, inflammatory bowel disease, malignancies, periodontitis or hepatitis. According to AHA/CDC recommendations, a second CRP measurement taken two weeks after the first might be useful in identifying transient processes while reducing biological variation in usual clinical practice. A careful patient monitoring is warranted as well after these processes are resolved, as it has been reported that during the 30 days following an infection-related hospitalization in dialysis patients, the risk of cardiovascular events increases by 25% [155]. Patients showing CRP elevations over short periods of time should undergo an extensive clinical work-up, whether they exert clinical symptoms or not. Other seemingly valid reasons for performing serial CRP measurements could be to motivate individuals at risk of inflammation to improve their lifestyles (such as smoking cessation, dental care, dietary modification, exercise, weight loss) or to comply with drug therapies. Clearly, persistent CRP elevations or increases in inflammatory biomarkers indicate patients at high risk of dying, and major efforts should be made to address the causes of such elevations.

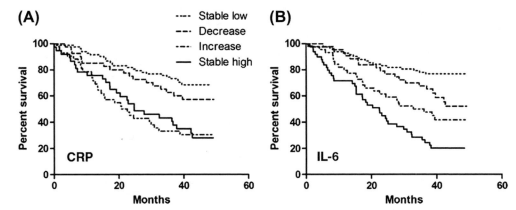

FIGURE 5.5 Persistent elevation of CRP and IL-6 in hemodialysis patients during a 3-month monitoring was associated with increased risk of mortality. Reproduced with permission from Nephrol Dial Transplant 2011 Apr;26(4):1313–8.

TREATMENT OF INFLAMMATION IN CHRONIC KIDNEY DISEASE

No sufficiently powered randomized controlled trials targeting uremic inflammation as a means of improving morbidity and mortality in CKD patients have yet been performed. Nor is there evidence that by improving systemic inflammation nutritional status is restored. Therefore, the following recommendations for treating inflammation in patients with CKD reflect the authors' opinion. Based on the concept that inflammation plays a pivotal role in the development of the uremic phenotype, circulating inflammatory markers have the potential to be primary targets for novel treatments including not only specific anti-inflammatory therapies but also various anti-oxidative and anti-wasting approaches.

When pre-existing complications (including dialysis-related causes) have been excluded as a cause of persistent inflammation, some interventional approaches could be cautiously considered, including strategies to modify physical activity [156], cognitive-behavior [157] and the use of bioactive nutrients with immune properties [158–161].

Certain medications have nonspecific immunomodulatory effects on CKD. For instance, in inflamed patients with moderate CKD rosuvastatin treatment reduced CRP levels and improved both cardiovascular events and all-cause mortality [162]. In contrast, data on the effects of statins on inflammatory biomarkers in ESRD are not that consistent [163,164]. Cholecalciferol supplementation may also have anti-inflammatory properties in CKD patients [165,166]. Sevelamer, which possesses LPS-binding properties, is associated with a reduction in circulating CRP and endotoxin levels as well as amelioration of endothelial dysfunction [167,168]. ACEI/ARBs [169–171], aliskiren (a direct renin inhibitor) [172] or allopurinol [173] have also shown suppressive effects on inflammatory markers. Among the currently available anti-cytokine therapies, etanercept, a TNF-receptor antagonist, was tested targeting uremic persistent inflammation in a small number of patients on HD, primarily aiming at an improvement in nutritional profiles [174]. Forty-four weeks of treatment with etanercept showed positive effects on albumin and prealbumin levels compared to the placebo group with no occurrence of adverse events, while the treatment resulted in a nonsignificant change in CRP and IL-6 [174]. Anakinra, a recombinant human IL-1-receptor antagonist, lowered plasma CRP and IL-6 levels in patients with type-2 diabetes [175]. In a recent small prospective controlled trial [176], 22 patients with markers of inflammation on HD were randomized to anakinra or placebo over four weeks. As those who received treatment showed a 53% reduction in CRP,

40% reduction in IL-6 levels and 23% increase in mean prealbumin further studies are needed to evaluate the impact of such therapy on outcome in this patient group. Finally, it should be recognized that persistent inflammation might impact on drug metabolism as inflammation is able to down-regulate multiple P450 enzymes [177]. Indeed, a recent study showed a strong correlation between CRP levels and CYP3A4 activity (assessed by alprazolam 4-hydroxylation) in a small group of HD-patients [178]. How this may affect the metabolism of commonly-used drugs in CKD deserves further study.

References

[1] Nascimento MM, Pecoits-Filho R, Qureshi AR, Hayashi SY, Manfro RC, Pachaly MA, et al. The prognostic impact of fluctuating levels of C-reactive protein in brazilian haemodialysis patients: A prospective study. Nephrol Dial Transplant 2004;19:2803–9.

[2] Stenvinkel P, Wanner C, Metzger T, Heimburger O, Mallamaci F, Tripepi G, et al. Inflammation and outcome in end-stage renal failure: Does female gender constitute a survival advantage? Kidney Int 2002;62:1791–8.

[3] Kaizu Y, Ohkawa S, Odamaki M, Ikegaya N, Hibi I, Miyaji K, et al. Association between inflammatory mediators and muscle mass in long-term hemodialysis patients. Am J Kidney Dis 2003;42:295–302.

[4] Wang AY, Sea MM, Tang N, Sanderson JE, Lui SF, Li PK, et al. Resting energy expenditure and subsequent mortality risk in peritoneal dialysis patients. J Am Soc Nephrol 2004;15:3134–43.

[5] Muntner P, Hamm LL, Kusek JW, Chen J, Whelton PK, He J. The prevalence of nontraditional risk factors for coronary heart disease in patients with chronic kidney disease. Annals of internal medicine 2004;140:9–17.

[6] Avesani CM, Draibe SA, Kamimura MA, Colugnati FA, Cuppari L. Resting energy expenditure of chronic kidney disease patients: Influence of renal function and subclinical inflammation. Am J Kidney Dis 2004;44:1008–16.

[7] Bazeley J, Bieber B, Li Y, Morgenstern H, de Sequera P, Combe C, et al. C-reactive protein and prediction of 1-year mortality in prevalent hemodialysis patients. Clin J Am Soc Nephrol 2011;6:2452–61.

[8] Eustace JA, Astor B, Muntner PM, Ikizler TA, Coresh J. Prevalence of acidosis and inflammation and their association with low serum albumin in chronic kidney disease. Kidney International 2004;65:1031–40.

[9] van Tellingen A, Grooteman MPC, Schoorl M, Bartels PCM, Schoorl M, van der Ploeg T, et al. Intercurrent clinical events are predicitive of plasma C-reactive protein levels in hemodialysis patients. Kidney Int 2002;62:632–8.

[10] Stenvinkel P, Heimburger O, Jogestrand T. Elevated interleukin-6 predicts progressive carotid artery atherosclerosis in dialysis patients: Association with chlamydia pneumoniae seropositivity. Am J Kidney Dis 2002;39:274–82.

[11] Zoccali C, Mallamaci F, Tripepi G, Parlongo S, Cutrupi S, Benedetto FA, et al. Chlamydia pneumoniae, overall and cardiovascular mortality in end-stage renal disease (ESRD). Kidney Int 2003;64:579–84.

[12] Kato A, Takita T, Furuhashi M, Maruyama Y, Hishida A. Association between seroprevalence of anti-chlamydial antibodies and long-term cardiovascular mortality in chronic hemodialysis patients. Atherosclerosis 2006;188:120–5.

[13] Kim DK, Kim HJ, Han SH, Lee JE, Moon SJ, Kim BS, et al. Chlamydia pneumoniae accompanied by inflammation is associated with the progression of atherosclerosis in CAPD patients: A prospective study for 3 years. Nephrol Dial Transplant 2008;23:1011–8.

[14] Stenvinkel P, Ketteler M, Johnson RJ, Lindholm B, Pecoits-Filho R, Riella M, et al. IL-10, IL-6, and TNF-alpha: Central factors in the altered cytokine network of uremia – the good, the bad, and the ugly. Kidney Int 2005;67:1216–33.

[15] Suliman M, Heimburger O, Barany P, Anderstam B, Pecoits-Filho R, Ayala ER, et al. Plasma pentosidine is associated with inflammation and malnutrition in end-stage renal disease patients starting on dialysis therapy. J Am Soc Nephrol 2003;14:1614–22.

[16] Dounousi E, Papavasiliou E, Makedou A, Ioannou K, Katopodis KP, Tselepis A, et al. Oxidative stress is progressively enhanced with advancing stages of ckd. Am J Kidney Dis 2006;48:752–60.

[17] Borovikova LV, Ivanova S, Zhang M, Yang H, Botchkina GI, Watkins LR, et al. Vagus nerve stimulation attenuates the systemic inflammatory response to endotoxin. Nature 2000;405: 458–62.

[18] Chen LP, Chiang CK, Chan CP, Hung KY, Huang CS. Does periodontitis reflect inflammation and malnutrition status in hemodialysis patients? Am J Kidney Dis 2006;47:815–22.

[19] Buhlin K, Barany P, Heimburger O, Stenvinkel P, Gustafsson A. Oral health and proinflammatory status in end-stage renal disease patients. Oral health & Preventive dentistry 2007;5: 235–44.

[20] Memoli B, Minutolo R, Bisesti V, Postiglione L, Conti A, Marzano L, et al. Changes of serum albumin and C-reactive protein are related to changes of interleukin-6 release by peripheral blood mononuclear cells in hemodialysis patients treated with different membranes. Am J Kidney Dis 2002;39:266–73.

[21] Schindler R, Beck W, Deppisch R, Aussieker M, Wilde A, Gohl H, et al. Short bacterial DNA fragments: Detection in dialysate and induction of cytokines. J Am Soc Nephrol 2004;15:3207–14.

[22] Arizono K, Nomura K, Motoyama T, Matsushita Y, Matsuoka K, Miyazu R, et al. Use of ultrapure dialysate in reduction of chronic inflammation during hemodialysis. Blood Purif 2004; 22(Suppl. 2):26–9.

[23] Schiffl H, Lang SM, Stratakis D, Fischer R. Effects of ultrapure dialysis fluid on nutritional status and inflammatory parameters. Nephrol Dial Transplant 2001;16:1863–9.

[24] Bossola M, Sanguinetti M, Scribano D, Zuppi C, Giungi S, Luciani G, et al. Circulating bacterial-derived DNA fragments and markers of inflammation in chronic hemodialysis patients. Clin J Am Soc Nephrol 2009;4:379–85.

[25] Ayus JC, Mizani MR, Achinger SG, Thadhani R, Go AS, Lee S. Effects of short daily versus conventional hemodialysis on left ventricular hypertrophy and inflammatory markers: A prospective, controlled study. J Am Soc Nephrol 2005;16: 2778–88.

[26] Panichi V, Rizza GM, Taccola D, Paoletti S, Mantuano E, Migliori M, et al. C-reactive protein in patients on chronic hemodialysis with different techniques and different membranes. Biomed Pharmacother 2006;60:14–7.

[27] Barreto DV, Barreto FC, Liabeuf S, Temmar M, Lemke HD, Tribouilloy C, et al. Plasma interleukin-6 is independently associated with mortality in both hemodialysis and pre-dialysis patients with chronic kidney disease. Kidney Int 2010;77:550–6.

[28] Stenvinkel P, Heimburger O, Paultre F, Diczfalusy U, Wang T, Berglund L, et al. Strong association between malnutrition,

inflammation, and atherosclerosis in chronic renal failure. Kidney Int 1999;55:1899–911.

[29] Enia G, Mallamaci F, Benedetto FA, Panuccio V, Parlongo S, Cutrupi S, et al. Long-term capd patients are volume expanded and display more severe left ventricular hypertrophy than haemodialysis patients. Nephrol Dial Transplant 2001;16: 1459–64.

[30] Axelsson J, Qureshi AR, Suliman ME, Honda H, Pecoits-Filho R, Heimbürger O, et al. Truncal fat mass as a contributor to inflammation in end-stage renal disease. Am J Clin Nutr 2004;80:1222–9.

[31] Cordeiro AC, Qureshi AR, Stenvinkel P, Heimburger O, Axelsson J, Barany P, et al. Abdominal fat deposition is associated with increased inflammation, protein-energy wasting and worse outcome in patients undergoing haemodialysis. Nephrol Dial Transplant 2010;25:562–8.

[32] Weisberg SP, McCann D, Desai M, Rosenbaum M, Leibel RL, Ferrante Jr AW. Obesity is associated with macrophage accumulation in adipose tissue. J Clin Invest 2003;112: 1796–808.

[33] Wellen KE, Hotamisligil GS. Obesity-induced inflammatory changes in adipose tissue. J Clin Invest 2003;112:1785–8.

[34] Carrero JJ, Cordeiro AC, Lindholm B, Stenvinkel P. The emerging pleiotrophic role of adipokines in the uremic phenotype. Current Opinion in Nephrology and Hypertension 2010;19:37–42.

[35] Yamamoto T, Carrero JJ, Lindholm B, Stenvinkel P, Axelsson J. Leptin and uremic protein-energy wasting – the axis of eating. Semin Dial 2009;22:387–90.

[36] Maury E, Brichard SM. Adipokine dysregulation, adipose tissue inflammation and metabolic syndrome. Mol Cell Endocrinol 2010;314:1–16.

[37] Witasp A, Carrero JJ, Heimburger O, Lindholm B, Hammarqvist F, Stenvinkel P, et al. Increased expression of proinflammatory genes in abdominal subcutaneous fat in advanced chronic kidney disease patients. J Intern Med 2011;269:410–9.

[38] Honda H, Qureshi AR, Axelsson J, Heimburger O, Suliman ME, Barany P, et al. Obese sarcopenia in patients with end-stage renal disease is associated with inflammation and increased mortality. Am J Clin Nutr 2007;86:633–8.

[39] Wong JS, Port FK, Hulbert-Shearon TE, Carroll CE, Wolfe RA, Agodoa LY, et al. Survival advantage in Asian American end-stage renal disease patients. Kidney Int 1999;55:2515–23.

[40] Pankow JS, Folsom AR, Cushman M, Borecki IB, Hopkins PN, Eckfeldt JH, et al. Familial and genetic determinants of systemic markers of inflammation: The nhlbi family heart study. Atherosclerosis 2001;154:681–9.

[41] Westendorp RG, Langermans JA, Huizinga TW, Verweij CL, Sturk A. Genetic influence on cytokine production in meningococcal disease. Lancet 1997;349:1912–3.

[42] Luttropp K, Stenvinkel P, Carrero JJ, Pecoits-Filho R, Lindholm B, Nordfors L. Understanding the role of genetic polymorphisms in chronic kidney disease. Pediatr Nephrol 2008;23(11):1941–9.

[43] Luttropp K, Lindholm B, Carrero JJ, Glorieux G, Schepers E, Vanholder R, et al. Genetics/genomics in chronic kidney disease – towards personalized medicine? Semin Dial 2009;22: 417–22.

[44] Agodoa L, Eggers P. Racial and ethnic disparities in end-stage kidney failure-survival paradoxes in African-Americans. Semin Dial 2007;20:577–85.

[45] Crews DC, Sozio SM, Liu Y, Coresh J, Powe NR. Inflammation and the paradox of racial differences in dialysis survival. J Am Soc Nephrol 2011;22(12):2279–86.

[46] Carrero JJ, Stenvinkel P, Fellstrom B, Qureshi AR, Lamb K, Heimburger O, et al. Telomere attrition is associated with inflammation, low fetuin-A levels and high mortality in prevalent haemodialysis patients. J Intern Med 2008;263: 302−12.

[47] Plata-Salaman CR. Cytokines and feeding. Int J Obes Relat Metab Disord 2001;25(Suppl. 5):S48−52.

[48] Carrero JJ, Aguilera A, Stenvinkel P, Gil F, Selgas R, Lindholm B. Appetite disorders in uremia. J Ren Nutr 2008;18:107−13.

[49] Carrero JJ, Qureshi AR, Axelsson J, Avesani CM, Suliman ME, Kato S, et al. Comparison of nutritional and inflammatory markers in dialysis patients with reduced appetite. Am J Clin Nutr 2007;85:695−701.

[50] Kalantar-Zadeh K, Block G, McAllister CJ, Humphreys MH, Kopple JD. Appetite and inflammation, nutrition, anemia, and clinical outcome in hemodialysis patients. Am J Clin Nutr 2004;80:299−307.

[51] Bossola M, Luciani G, Giungi S, Tazza L. Anorexia, fatigue, and plasma interleukin-6 levels in chronic hemodialysis patients. Ren Fail 2010;32:1049−54.

[52] Aguilera A, Codoceo R, Selgas R, Garcia P, Picornell M, Diaz C, et al. Anorexigen (TNF-alpha, cholecystokinin) and orexigen (neuropeptide Y) plasma levels in peritoneal dialysis (PD) patients: Their relationship with nutritional parameters. Nephrol Dial Transplant 1998;13:1476−83.

[53] Snaedal S, Heimburger O, Qureshi AR, Danielsson A, Wikstrom B, Fellstrom B, et al. Comorbidity and acute clinical events as determinants of C-reactive protein variation in hemodialysis patients: Implications for patient survival. Am J Kidney Dis 2009;53:1024−33.

[54] Chen K, Li F, Li J, Cai H, Strom S, Bisello A, et al. Induction of leptin resistance through direct interaction of C-reactive protein with leptin. Nature Medicine 2006;12:425−32.

[55] Raff AC, Lieu S, Melamed ML, Quan Z, Ponda M, Meyer TW, et al. Relationship of impaired olfactory function in ESRD to malnutrition and retained uremic molecules. Am J Kidney Dis 2008;52:102−10.

[56] Turner JH, Liang KL, May L, Lane AP. Tumor necrosis factor alpha inhibits olfactory regeneration in a transgenic model of chronic rhinosinusitis-associated olfactory loss. Am J Rhinol Allergy 2010;24:336−40.

[57] Kimmel PL, Peterson RA, Weihs KL, Simmens SJ, Alleyne S, Cruz I, et al. Multiple measurements of depression predict mortality in a longitudinal study of chronic hemodialysis outpatients. Kidney Int 2000;57:2093−8.

[58] Riezebos RK, Nauta KJ, Honig A, Dekker FW, Siegert CE. The association of depressive symptoms with survival in a Dutch cohort of patients with end-stage renal disease. Nephrol Dial Transplant 2010;25:231−6.

[59] Chilcot J, Wellsted D, Vilar E, Farrington K. An association between residual renal function and depression symptoms in haemodialysis patients. Nephron Clin Pract 2009;113:c117−124.

[60] Schiepers OJ, Wichers MC, Maes M. Cytokines and major depression. Prog Neuropsychopharmacol Biol Psychiatry 2005; 29:201−17.

[61] Sonikian M, Metaxaki P, Papavasileiou D, Boufidou F, Nikolaou C, Vlassopoulos D, et al. Effects of interleukin-6 on depression risk in dialysis patients. Am J Nephrol 2010; 31:303−8.

[62] Montinaro V, Iaffaldano GP, Granata S, Porcelli P, Todarello O, Schena FP, et al. Emotional symptoms, quality of life and cytokine profile in hemodialysis patients. Clin Nephrol 2010;73:36−43.

[63] Preljevic VT, Osthus TB, Sandvik L, Bringager CB, Opjordsmoen S, Nordhus IH, et al. Psychiatric disorders, body mass index and C-reactive protein in dialysis patients. Gen Hosp Psychiatry 2011;33:454−61.

[64] Lee SK, Lee HS, Lee TB, Kim DH, Koo JR, Kim YK, et al. The effects of antidepressant treatment on serum cytokines and nutritional status in hemodialysis patients. J Korean Med Sci 2004;19:384−9.

[65] Jhamb M, Argyropoulos C, Steel JL, Plantinga L, Wu AW, Fink NE, et al. Correlates and outcomes of fatigue among incident dialysis patients. Clin J Am Soc Nephrol 2009;4: 1779−86.

[66] Carrero JJ. Identification of patients with eating disorders: Clinical and biochemical signs of appetite loss in dialysis patients. J Ren Nutr 2009;19:10−5.

[67] Buttgereit F, Burmester GR, Brand MD. Bioenergetics of immune functions: Fundamental and therapeutic aspects. Immunol Today 2000;21:192−9.

[68] Utaka S, Avesani CM, Draibe SA, Kamimura MA, Andreoni S, Cuppari L. Inflammation is associated with increased energy expenditure in patients with chronic kidney disease. Am J Clin Nutr 2005;82:801−5.

[69] Mafra D, Deleaval P, Teta D, Cleaud C, Arkouche W, Jolivot A, et al. Influence of inflammation on total energy expenditure in hemodialysis patients. J Ren Nutr 2011;21:387−93.

[70] Kamimura MA, Draibe SA, Dalboni MA, Cendoroglo M, Avesani CM, Manfredi SR, et al. Serum and cellular interleukin-6 in haemodialysis patients: Relationship with energy expenditure. Nephrol Dial Transplant 2007;22:839−44.

[71] Carrero JJ, Chmielewski M, Axelsson J, Snaedal S, Heimburger O, Barany P, et al. Muscle atrophy, inflammation and clinical outcome in incident and prevalent dialysis patients. Clinical Nutrition (Edinburgh, Scotland) 2008;27:557−64.

[72] Delano MJ, Moldawer LL. The origins of cachexia in acute and chronic inflammatory diseases. Nutr Clin Pract 2006; 21:68−81.

[73] Goodman MN. Interleukin-6 induces skeletal muscle protein breakdown in rats. Proc Soc Exp Biol Med 1994;205:182−5.

[74] Strassmann G, Fong M, Kenney JS, Jacob CO. Evidence for the involvement of interleukin 6 in experimental cancer cachexia. The Journal of Clinical Investigation 1992;89:1681−4.

[75] Stenvinkel P, Ketteler M, Johnson RJ, Lindholm B, Pecoits-Filho R, Riella M, et al. Interleukin-10, IL-6 and TNF-a: Important factors in the altered cytokine network of end-stage renal disease − the good, the bad and the ugly. Kidney Int 2005; 67:1216−33.

[76] Kl Johansen, Kaysen GA, Young BS, Hung AM, da Silva M, Chertow GM. Longitudinal study of nutritional status, body composition, and physical function in hemodialysis patients. Am J Clin Nutr 2003;77:842−6.

[77] Stenvinkel P, Lindholm B, Lonnqvist F, Katzarski K, Heimburger O. Increases in serum leptin levels during peritoneal dialysis are associated with inflammation and a decrease in lean body mass. J Am Soc Nephrol 2000;11:1303−9.

[78] Raj DS, Adeniyi O, Dominic EA, Boivin MA, McClelland S, Tzamaloukas AH, et al. Amino acid repletion does not decrease muscle protein catabolism during hemodialysis. American Journal of Physiology. Endocrinology and Metabolism 2007;292:E1534−1542.

[79] Raj DS, Moseley P, Dominic EA, Onime A, Tzamaloukas AH, Boyd A, et al. Interleukin-6 modulates hepatic and muscle protein synthesis during hemodialysis. Kidney International 2008;73:1054−61.

[80] Boivin MA, Battah SI, Dominic EA, Kalantar-Zadeh K, Ferrando A, Tzamaloukas AH, et al. Activation of caspase-3 in the skeletal muscle during haemodialysis. European Journal of Clinical Investigation 2010;40:903−10.

[81] Beberashvili I, Sinuani I, Azar A, Yasur H, Shapiro G, Feldman L, et al. Il-6 levels, nutritional status, and mortality in prevalent hemodialysis patients. Clin J Am Soc Nephrol 2011;6:2253—63.

[82] Argiles JM, Lopez-Soriano FJ, Busquets S. Therapeutic potential of interleukin-15: A myokine involved in muscle wasting and adiposity. Drug Discovery Today 2009;14:208—13.

[83] Dogra C, Changotra H, Wedhas N, Qin X, Wergedal JE, Kumar A. TNF-related weak inducer of apoptosis (tweak) is a potent skeletal muscle-wasting cytokine. Faseb J 2007;21: 1857—69.

[84] Carrero JJ, Ortiz A, Qureshi AR, Martin-Ventura JL, Barany P, Heimburger O, et al. Additive effects of soluble tweak and inflammation on mortality in hemodialysis patients. Clin J Am Soc Nephrol 2009;4:110—8.

[85] Zhang L, Du J, Hu Z, Han G, Delafontaine P, Garcia G, et al. Il-6 and serum amyloid a synergy mediates angiotensin ii-induced muscle wasting. J Am Soc Nephrol 2009;20:604—12.

[86] Haffner SM. The metabolic syndrome: Inflammation, diabetes mellitus, and cardiovascular disease. Am J Cardiol 2006; 97:3A—11A.

[87] Gonzalez AS, Guerrero DB, Soto MB, Diaz SP, Martinez-Olmos M, Vidal O. Metabolic syndrome, insulin resistance and the inflammation markers C-reactive protein and ferritin. Eur J Clin Nutr 2006.

[88] Hotamisligil GS, Shargill NS, Spiegelman BM. Adipose expression of tumor necrosis factor-alpha: Direct role in obesity-linked insulin resistance. Science 1993;259:87—91.

[89] Yazdani-Biuki B, Stelzl H, Brezinschek HP, Hermann J, Mueller T, Krippl P, et al. Improvement of insulin sensitivity in insulin resistant subjects during prolonged treatment with the anti-tnf-alpha antibody infliximab. Eur J Clin Invest 2004; 34:641—2.

[90] Tsigos C, Kyrou I, Chala E, Tsapogas P, Stavridis JC, Raptis SA, et al. Circulating tumor necrosis factor alpha concentrations are higher in abdominal versus peripheral obesity. Metabolism 1999;48:1332—5.

[91] Senn JJ, Klover PJ, Nowak IA, Mooney RA. Interleukin-6 induces cellular insulin resistance in hepatocytes. Diabetes 2002;51:3391—9.

[92] Pupim LB, Flakoll PJ, Majchrzak KM, Aftab Guy DL, Stenvinkel P, Ikizler TA. Increased muscle protein breakdown in chronic hemodialysis patients with type 2 diabetes mellitus. Kidney Int 2005;68:1857—65.

[93] Pupim LB, Heimburger O, Qureshi AR, Ikizler TA, Stenvinkel P. Accelerated lean body mass loss in incident chronic dialysis patients with diabetes mellitus. Kidney Int 2005;68:2368—74.

[94] Pupim LB, Flakoll PJ, Yu C, Ikizler TA. Recombinant human growth hormone improves muscle amino acid uptake and whole-body protein metabolism in chronic hemodialysis patients. Am J Clin Nutr 2005;82:1235—43.

[95] Kotzmann H, Yilmaz N, Lercher P, Riedl M, Schmidt A, Schuster E, et al. Differential effects of growth hormone therapy in malnourished hemodialysis patients. Kidney Int 2001; 60:1578—85.

[96] Cooney RN, Shumate M. The inhibitory effects of interleukin-1 on growth hormone action during catabolic illness. Vitamins and hormones 2006;74:317—40.

[97] Garibotto G, Russo R, Sofia A, Ferone D, Fiorini F, Cappelli V, et al. Effects of uremia and inflammation on growth hormone resistance in patients with chronic kidney diseases. Kidney Int 2008;74:937—45.

[98] Barbieri M, Ferrucci L, Ragno E, Corsi A, Bandinelli S, Bonafe M, et al. Chronic inflammation and the effect of IGF-I on muscle strength and power in older persons. Am J Physiol Endocrinol Metab 2003;284:E481—487.

[99] Feldt-Rasmussen B, Lange M, Sulowicz W, Gafter U, Lai KN, Wiedemann J, et al. Growth hormone treatment during hemodialysis in a randomized trial improves nutrition, quality of life, and cardiovascular risk. J Am Soc Nephrol 2007;18:2161—71.

[100] Vanhorebeek I, Langouche L, Van den Berghe G. Endocrine aspects of acute and prolonged critical illness. Nature clinical practice 2006;2:20—31.

[101] Carrero JJ, Qureshi AR, Axelsson J, Yilmaz MI, Rehnmark S, Witt MR, et al. Clinical and biochemical implications of low thyroid hormone levels (total and free forms) in euthyroid patients with chronic kidney disease. J Intern Med 2007;262:690—701.

[102] Zoccali C, Mallamaci F, Tripepi G, Cutrupi S, Pizzini P. Low triiodothyronine and survival in end-stage renal disease. Kidney Int 2006;70:523—8.

[103] Yilmaz MI, Sonmez A, Karaman M, Ay SA, Saglam M, Yaman H, et al. Low triiodothyronine alters flow-mediated vasodilatation in advanced nondiabetic kidney disease. Am J Nephrol 33:25—32.

[104] Wiederkehr MR, Kalogiros J, Krapf R. Correction of metabolic acidosis improves thyroid and growth hormone axes in haemodialysis patients. Nephrol Dial Transplant 2004;19:1190—7.

[105] Disthabanchong S, Treeruttanawanich A. Oral sodium bicarbonate improves thyroid function in predialysis chronic kidney disease. Am J Nephrol 32:549—56.

[106] Zoccali C, Tripepi G, Cutrupi S, Pizzini P, Mallamaci F. Low triiodothyronine: A new facet of inflammation in end-stage renal disease. J Am Soc Nephrol 2005;16:2789—95.

[107] Torpy DJ, Tsigos C, Lotsikas AJ, Defensor R, Chrousos GP, Papanicolaou DA. Acute and delayed effects of a single-dose injection of interleukin-6 on thyroid function in healthy humans. Metabolism 1998;47:1289—93.

[108] Bartalena L, Brogioni S, Grasso L, Velluzzi F, Martino E. Relationship of the increased serum interleukin-6 concentration to changes of thyroid function in nonthyroidal illness. J Endocrinol Invest 1994;17:269—74.

[109] Ozen KP, Asci G, Gungor O, Carrero JJ, Kircelli F, Tatar E, et al. Nutritional state alters the association between free triiodothyronine levels and mortality in hemodialysis patients. Am J Nephrol 2011;33:305—12.

[110] Carrero JJ, Qureshi AR, Nakashima A, Arver S, Parini P, Lindholm B, et al. Prevalence and clinical implications of testosterone deficiency in men with end-stage renal disease. Nephrol Dial Transplant 2011;26:184—90.

[111] Gungor O, Kircelli F, Carrero JJ, Asci G, Toz H, Tatar E, et al. Endogenous testosterone and mortality in male hemodialysis patients: Is it the result of aging? Clin J Am Soc Nephrol 2010;5:2018—23.

[112] Yilmaz MI, Sonmez A, Qureshi AR, Saglam M, Stenvinkel P, Yaman H, et al. Endogenous testosterone, endothelial dysfunction, and cardiovascular events in men with nondialysis chronic kidney disease. Clin J Am Soc Nephrol 2011;6(7):1617—25.

[113] Carrero JJ, Barany P, Yilmaz MI, Qureshi AR, Sonmez A, Heimburger O, et al. Testosterone deficiency is a cause of anaemia and reduced responsiveness to erythropoiesis-stimulating agents in men with chronic kidney disease 2012; 27(2):709—15.

[114] Iglesias P, Carrero JJ, Diez JJ. Gonadal dysfunction in men with chronic kidney disease: Clinical features, prognostic implications and therapeutic options. Journal of Nephrology J Nephrol 2012;25(1):31—42.

[115] Grinspoon S, Corcoran C, Lee K, Burrows B, Hubbard J, Katznelson L, et al. Loss of lean body and muscle mass correlates with androgen levels in hypogonadal men with acquired

immunodeficiency syndrome and wasting. J Clin Endocrinol Metab 1996;81:4051–8.

[116] Karila TA, Sarkkinen P, Marttinen M, Seppala T, Mero A, Tallroth K. Rapid weight loss decreases serum testosterone. Int J Sports Med 2008;29(11):872–7.

[117] Carrero JJ, Qureshi AR, Parini P, Arver S, Lindholm B, Barany P, et al. Low serum testosterone increases mortality risk among male dialysis patients. J Am Soc Nephrol 2009;20:613–20.

[118] Kyriazis J, Tzanakis I, Stylianou K, Katsipi I, Moisiadis D, Papadaki A, et al. Low serum testosterone, arterial stiffness and mortality in male haemodialysis patients. Nephrol Dial Transplant 2011;26:2971–7.

[119] Haring R, Nauck M, Volzke H, Endlich K, Lendeckel U, Friedrich N, et al. Low serum testosterone is associated with increased mortality in men with stage 3 or greater nephropathy. Am J Nephrol 2011;33:209–17.

[120] Johansen KL, Mulligan K, Schambelan M. Anabolic effects of nandrolone decanoate in patients receiving dialysis: A randomized controlled trial. Jama 1999;281:1275–81.

[121] Johansen KL, Painter PL, Sakkas GK, Gordon P, Doyle J, Shubert T. Effects of resistance exercise training and nandrolone decanoate on body composition and muscle function among patients who receive hemodialysis: A randomized, controlled trial. J Am Soc Nephrol 2006;17:2307–14.

[122] Carrero JJ, Stenvinkel P. Persistent inflammation as a catalyst for other risk factors in chronic kidney disease: A hypothesis proposal. Clin J Am Soc Nephrol 2009;4(Suppl. 1):S49–55.

[123] de Mutsert R, Grootendorst DC, Axelsson J, Boeschoten EW, Krediet RT, Dekker FW. Excess mortality due to interaction between protein-energy wasting, inflammation and cardiovascular disease in chronic dialysis patients. Nephrol Dial Transplant 2008;23:2957–64.

[124] Stenvinkel P, Heimburger O, Lindholm B, Kaysen GA, Bergstrom J. Are there two types of malnutrition in chronic renal failure? Evidence for relationships between malnutrition, inflammation and atherosclerosis (mia syndrome). Nephrol Dial Transplant 2000;15:953–60.

[125] Parekh RS, Plantinga LC, Kao WH, Meoni LA, Jaar BG, Fink NE, et al. The association of sudden cardiac death with inflammation and other traditional risk factors. Kidney Int 2008;74:1335–42.

[126] Tintut Y, Patel J, Parhami F, Demer LL. Tumor necrosis factor-alpha promotes in vitro calcification of vascular cells via the camp pathway. Circulation 2000;102:2636–42.

[127] Tintut Y, Patel J, Territo M, Saini T, Parhami F, Demer LL. Monocyte/macrophage regulation of vascular calcification in vitro. Circulation 2002;105:650–5.

[128] Collin-Osdoby P. Regulation of vascular calcification by osteoclast regulatory factors rankl and osteoprotegerin. Circ Res 2004;95:1046–57.

[129] Mangan SH, Campenhout AV, Rush C, Golledge J. Osteoprotegerin upregulates endothelial cell adhesion molecule response to tumor necrosis factor-alpha associated with induction of angiopoietin-2. Cardiovascular Research 2007;76:494–505.

[130] Morena M, Terrier N, Jaussent I, Leray-Moragues H, Chalabi L, Rivory JP, et al. Plasma osteoprotegerin is associated with mortality in hemodialysis patients. J Am Soc Nephrol 2006;17:262–70.

[131] Matsubara K, Stenvinkel P, Qureshi AR, Carrero JJ, Axelsson J, Heimburger O, et al. Inflammation modifies the association of osteoprotegerin with mortality in chronic kidney disease. J Nephrol 2009;22:774–82.

[132] Nadra I, Mason JC, Philippidis P, Florey O, Smythe CD, McCarthy GM, et al. Proinflammatory activation of macrophages by basic calcium phosphate crystals via protein kinase c

and map kinase pathways: A vicious cycle of inflammation and arterial calcification? Circ Res 2005;96:1248–56.

[133] Ketteler M, Bongartz P, Westenfeld R, Wildberger JE, Mahnken AH, Bohm R, et al. Association of low fetuin-A (AHSG) concentrations in serum with cardiovascular mortality in patients on dialysis: A cross-sectional study. Lancet 2003;361:327–33.

[134] Stenvinkel P, Wang K, Qureshi AR, Axelsson J, Pecoits-Filho R, Gao P, et al. Low fetuin-A levels are associated with cardiovascular death: Impact of variations in the gene encoding fetuin. Kidney Int 2005;67:2383–92.

[135] Hermans MM, Brandenburg V, Ketteler M, Kooman JP, van der Sande FM, Boeschoten EW, et al. Association of serum fetuin-A levels with mortality in dialysis patients. Kidney Int 2007;72:202–7.

[136] Wang AY, Woo J, Lam CW, Wang M, Chan IH, Gao P, et al. Associations of serum fetuin-A with malnutrition, inflammation, atherosclerosis and valvular calcification syndrome and outcome in peritoneal dialysis patients. Nephrol Dial Transplant 2005;20:1676–85.

[137] Gangneux C, Daveau M, Hiron M, Derambure C, Papaconstantinou J, Salier JP. The inflammation-induced down-regulation of plasma fetuin-A (alpha2hs-glycoprotein) in liver results from the loss of interaction between long c/ebp isoforms at two neighbouring binding sites. Nucleic Acids Res 2003;31:5957–70.

[138] Moe SM, Chen NX. Inflammation and vascular calcification. Blood Purif 2005;23:64–71.

[139] Yeun JY, Levine RA, Mantadilok V, Kaysen GA. C-reactive protein predicts all-cause and cardiovascular mortality in hemodialysis patients. Am J Kidney Dis 2000;35(3):469–76.

[140] Zimmermann J, Herrlinger S, Pruy A, Metzger T, Wanner C. Inflammation enhances cardiovascular risk and mortality in hemodialysis patients. Kidney Int 1999;55:648–58.

[141] Iseki K, Tozawa M, Yoshi S, Fukiyama K. Serum C-reactive (CRP) and risk of death in chronic dialysis patients. Nephrol Dial Transpl 1999;14:1956–60.

[142] Bologa RM, Levine DM, Parker TS, Cheigh JS, Serur D, Stenzel KH, et al. Interleukin-6 predicts hypoalbuminemia, hypocholesterolemia, and mortality in hemodialysis patients. Am J Kidney Dis 1998;32:107–14.

[143] Qureshi AR, Alvestrand A, Divino-Filho JC, Gutierrez A, Heimburger O, Lindholm B, et al. Inflammation, malnutrition, and cardiac disease as predictors of mortality in hemodialysis patients. J Am Soc Nephrol 2002;13(Suppl. 1):S28–36.

[144] Varagunam M, Finney H, Trevitt R, Sharples E, McCloskey DJ, Sinnott PJ, et al. Pretransplantation levels of C-reactive protein predict all-cause and cardiovascular mortality, but not graft outcome, in kidney transplant recipients. Am J Kidney Dis 2004;43:502–7.

[145] Noh H, Lee SW, Kang SW, Shin SK, Choi KH, Lee HY, et al. Serum C-reactive protein: A predictor of mortality in continuous ambulatory peritoneal dialysis patients. Nephrol Dial Transpl 1998;18:387–94.

[146] Ducloux D, Bresson-Vautrin C, Kribs M, Abdelfatah A, Chalopin J-M. C-reactive protein and cardiovascular disease in peritoneal dialysis patients. Kidney Int 2002;62:1417–22.

[147] Wang A, Woo J, Wai Kei C, Wang M, Man Sei M, Lui S-F, et al. Is a single time-point C-reactive protein predictive of outcome in peritoneal dialysis patients? J Am Soc Nephrol 2003;14:1871–9.

[148] Landray MJ, Wheeler DC, Lip GY, Newman DJ, Blann AD, McGlynn FJ, et al. Inflammation, endothelial dysfunction, and platelet activation in patients with chronic kidney disease: The chronic renal impairment in Birmingham (CRIB) study. Am J Kidney Dis 2004;43:244–53.

[149] Stigant CE, Djurdjev O, Levin A. C-reactive protein levels in patients on maintenance hemodialysis: Reliability and reflection on the utility of single measurements. Int Urol Nephrol 2005;37:133—40.

[150] Korevaar JC, van Manen JG, Dekker FW, de Waart DR, Boeschoten EW, Krediet RT. Effect of an increase in C-reactive protein level during a hemodialysis session on mortality. J Am Soc Nephrol 2004;15:2916—22.

[151] Ortega O, Rodriguez I, Gracia C, Sanchez M, Lentisco C, Mon C, et al. Strict volume control and longitudinal changes in cardiac biomarker levels in hemodialysis patients. Nephron Clin Pract 2009;113:c96—103.

[152] Rao M, Guo D, Perianayagam MC, Tighiouart H, Jaber BL, Pereira BJ, et al. Plasma interleukin-6 predicts cardiovascular mortality in hemodialysis patients. Am J Kidney Dis 2005; 45:324—33.

[153] den Elzen WP, van Manen JG, Boeschoten EW, Krediet RT, Dekker FW. The effect of single and repeatedly high concentrations of C-reactive protein on cardiovascular and non-cardiovascular mortality in patients starting with dialysis. Nephrol Dial Transplant 2006;21:1588—95.

[154] Meuwese CL, Stenvinkel P, Dekker FW, Carrero JJ. Monitoring of inflammation in patients on dialysis: Forewarned is forearmed. Nat Rev Nephrol 2011;7:166—76.

[155] Ishani A, Collins AJ, Herzog CA, Foley RN. Septicemia, access and cardiovascular disease in dialysis patients: The USRDS wave 2 study. Kidney Int 2005;68:311—8.

[156] Castaneda C, Gordon PL, Parker RC, Uhlin KL, Roubenoff R, Levey AS. Resistance training to reduce the malnutrition-inflammation complex syndrome of chronic kidney disease. Am J Kidney Dis 2004;43:607—16.

[157] Chen HY, Cheng IC, Pan YJ, Chiu YL, Hsu SP, Pai MF, et al. Cognitive-behavioral therapy for sleep disturbance decreases inflammatory cytokines and oxidative stress in hemodialysis patients. Kidney Int 2011;80:415—22.

[158] Bowden RG, Wilson RL, Deike E, Gentile M. Fish oil supplementation lowers C-reactive protein levels independent of triglyceride reduction in patients with end-stage renal disease. Nutr Clin Pract 2009;24:508—12.

[159] Hsu SP, Wu MS, Yang CC, Huang KC, Liou SY, Hsu SM, et al. Chronic green tea extract supplementation reduces hemodialysis-enhanced production of hydrogen peroxide and hypochlorous acid, atherosclerotic factors, and proinflammatory cytokines. Am J Clin Nutr 2007;86:1539—47.

[160] Himmelfarb J, Phinney S, Ikizler TA, Kane J, McMonagle E, Miller G. Gamma-tocopherol and docosahexaenoic acid decrease inflammation in dialysis patients. J Ren Nutr 2007; 17:296—304.

[161] Nascimento MM, Suliman ME, Silva M, Chinaglia T, Marchioro J, Hayashi SY, et al. Effect of oral N-acetylcysteine treatment on plasma inflammatory and oxidative stress markers in peritoneal dialysis patients: A placebo-controlled study. Perit Dial Int 2010;30:336—42.

[162] Ridker PM, MacFadyen J, Cressman M, Glynn RJ. Efficacy of rosuvastatin among men and women with moderate chronic kidney disease and elevated high-sensitivity C-reactive protein: A secondary analysis from the jupiter (justification for the use of statins in prevention — an intervention trial evaluating rosuvastatin) trial. J Am Coll Cardiol 2010;55:1266—73.

[163] Krane V, Winkler K, Drechsler C, Lilienthal J, Marz W, Wanner C. Effect of atorvastatin on inflammation and outcome in patients with type 2 diabetes mellitus on hemodialysis. Kidney Int 2008;74:1461—7.

[164] Fellstrom BC, Jardine AG, Schmieder RE, et al. Rosuvastatin and cardiovascular events in patients undergoing hemodialysis. The New England Journal of Medicine 2009;360:1395—407.

[165] Stubbs JR, Idicula A, Slusser J, Menard R, Quarles LD. Cholecalciferol supplementation alters calcitriol-responsive monocyte proteins and decreases inflammatory cytokines in esrd. J Am Soc Nephrol 2010;21:353—61.

[166] Matias PJ, Jorge C, Ferreira C, Borges M, Aires I, Amaral T, et al. Cholecalciferol supplementation in hemodialysis patients: Effects on mineral metabolism, inflammation, and cardiac dimension parameters. Clin J Am Soc Nephrol 2010;5:905—11.

[167] Stinghen AE, Gonçalves SM, Bucharles S, Branco FS, Gruber B, Hauser AB, et al. Sevelamer decreases systemic inflammation in parallel to a reduction in endotoxemia. Blood Purif 2010;29:352—6.

[168] Caglar K, Yilmaz MI, Saglam M, Cakir E, Acikel C, Eyileten T, et al. Short-term treatment with sevelamer increases serum fetuin-A concentration and improves endothelial dysfunction in chronic kidney disease stage 4 patients. Clin J Am Soc Nephrol 2008;3:61—8.

[169] Yilmaz MI, Axelsson J, Sonmez A, Carrero JJ, Saglam M, Eyileten T, et al. Effect of renin angiotensin system blockade on pentraxin 3 levels in type-2 diabetic patients with proteinuria. Clin J Am Soc Nephrol 2009;4:535—41.

[170] Yilmaz MI, Sonmez A, Ortiz A, Saglam M, Kilic S, Eyileten T, et al. Soluble tweak and ptx3 in nondialysis ckd patients: Impact on endothelial dysfunction and cardiovascular outcomes. Clin J Am Soc Nephrol 2011;6(4):785—92.

[171] Yamamoto D, Takai S, Hirahara I, Kusano E. Captopril directly inhibits matrix metalloproteinase-2 activity in continuous ambulatory peritoneal dialysis therapy. Clin Chim Acta 2010;411:762—4.

[172] Morishita Y, Hanawa S, Chinda J, Iimura O, Tsunematsu S, Kusano E. Effects of aliskiren on blood pressure and the predictive biomarkers for cardiovascular disease in hemodialysis-dependent chronic kidney disease patients with hypertension. Hypertens Res 2011;34(3):308—13.

[173] Goicoechea M, de Vinuesa SG, Verdalles U, Ruiz-Caro C, Ampuero J, Rincón A, et al. Effect of allopurinol in chronic kidney disease progression and cardiovascular risk. Clin J Am Soc Nephrol 2010;5:1388—93.

[174] Don BR, Kim K, Li J, Dwyer T, Alexander F, Kaysen GA. The effect of etanercept on suppression of the systemic inflammatory response in chronic hemodialysis patients. Clin Nephrol 2010;73:431—8.

[175] Larsen CM, Faulenbach M, Vaag A, Vølund A, Ehses JA, Seifert B, et al. Interleukin-1-receptor antagonist in type 2 diabetes mellitus. N Engl J Med 2007;356:1517—26.

[176] Hung AM, Ellis CD, Shintani A, Booker C, Ikizler TA. Il-1β receptor antagonist reduces inflammation in hemodialysis patients. J Am Soc Nephrol 2011;22:437—42.

[177] Morgan ET. Impact of infectious and inflammatory disease on cytochrome p450-mediated drug metabolism and pharmacokinetics. Clin Pharmacol Ther 2009;85:434—8.

[178] Molanaei H, Stenvinkel P, Qureshi AR, Carrero JJ, Heimbürger O, Lindholm B, et al. Metabolism of alprazolam (a marker of cyp3a4) in hemodialysis patients with persistent inflammation. Eur J Clin Pharmacol 2012;68:571—7.

6

Catalytic (Labile) Iron in Kidney Disease

Radhakrishna Baliga[1], Mohan M. Rajapurkar[2], Sudhir V. Shah[3]

[1]Department of Pediatrics, University of Mississippi Medical Center, Jackson, Mississippi, USA

[2]Department of Nephrology, Muljibhai Patel Urological Hospital, Nadiad, Gujarat, India

[3]Department of Internal Medicine, Division of Nephrology, UAMS College of Medicine, Little Rock; and
John L. McClellan Memorial Veterans Hospital, Central Arkansas Veterans Healthcare System, AR, USA

INTRODUCTION

Despite advances in understanding the pathophysiology of acute kidney injury and chronic kidney disease, treatment for kidney disease remains unsatisfactory. In this chapter, we briefly recount the importance of acute kidney injury and chronic kidney disease, then provide a brief description of labile iron, and, finally, summarize the role of labile iron in acute and chronic kidney disease. This focus on iron is particularly relevant because of the availability of iron chelators to potentially provide new therapeutic tools to prevent and/or treat kidney disease.

Several recent studies highlight the clinical relevance of acute kidney injury (AKI). Acute kidney injury has been shown to be an independent risk factor for morbidity and mortality, and even a modest increase in serum creatinine (0.3 mg/dL) is associated with high in-hospital mortality [1]. Recent studies indicate that AKI is an important determinant of post-hospital discharge mortality [2,3] as well as end-stage kidney disease (ESKD) [4,5]. The suggested new definition of AKI and the rationale behind it is detailed in the publication [6] resulting from a consensus conference under the auspices of the Acute Kidney Injury Network (AKIN), in which over 20 global societies representing both nephrologists and intensive care physicians participated.

Chronic kidney disease (CKD) is a global public health problem that affects approximately 10–15% of the adult population [7,8] and is associated with a high prevalence of cardiovascular disease [9] and high economic cost [10]. The expected marked increase in diabetes, the most common cause of CKD; increasing incidence of end-stage kidney disease despite the use of angiotensin receptor blockers (ARBs); and the multiplier effect of CKD on cardiovascular disease, all point to a major challenge facing healthcare systems worldwide.

Despite promising results [11], a phase 3 trial for a novel treatment for diabetic nephropathy was unsuccessful [12]. Thus, there is an urgent need for new therapeutic modalities for halting progression of kidney disease.

DEFINITION OF CATALYTIC (LABILE) IRON AND ITS IMPORTANCE IN TISSUE INJURY

Iron is the most abundant transitional metal in the body. The term "labile iron pool" was proposed in 1946 by Greenberg and Wintrobe [13] and reintroduced by Jacobs in 1977 as a "transient iron pool" to denote a low-molecular-weight pool of weakly chelated iron that passes through the cell. The term "chelatable iron" is also used, as most methodological approaches for detection of this pool of iron ions are based on the use of metal chelators [14]. Critical to iron's importance in biological processes is its ability to cycle reversibly between its ferrous and ferric oxidation states. This precise property, which is essential for its functions, also makes it very dangerous, because free iron can catalyze the formation of free radicals that can damage the cell. **Thus, from a pathophysiological standpoint, the broadest definition of a labile iron pool is that it consists of chemical forms that can participate in redox cycling, and is therefore often referred to as catalytic iron [15].**

Our bodies contain as much as 3 to 5 grams of total iron, but the pool of labile iron that can be measured [15,16] is estimated to be less than 70 to 90 mg. Although the existence of a cellular pool of metabolically labile iron proved controversial, the development of iron-sensitive fluorescent probes has provided much evidence in favor of intracellular labile pools [17]. In most cells iron homeostasis consists of iron uptake, utilization, and storage. The process of iron uptake is carried out by a transferrin receptor (TFR) and the divalent metal transporter 1 (DMT1, also called DCT1; NRAMP2), whereas ferritin is an intracellular iron-sequestering protein. Recent studies are beginning to yield information on the pathways of iron transport, its export from the cell via the divalent iron ion exporter ferroportin 1 [18] and its regulatory mechanisms including hepcidin [19]. Since uptake and storage of iron is carried out by different proteins, the pool of accessible iron ions constitutes a crossroad of metabolic pathways of iron-containing compounds.

Probes for labile iron are comprised of a fluorescent reporter group coupled to a high-affinity iron (II or III) chelator. The fluorophore responds to metal binding by undergoing a change in fluorescence. The most commonly used fluorophores include fluorescein and rhodamine derivatives attached to a chelator (reviewed in [20]). A complementary approach for estimating cellular labile iron is based on metal-driven catalysis of oxidant formation [21]. The advantages of this method are high sensitivity and selectivity for redox-active labile iron. Studies using a variety of methods have begun to define intracellular distribution of labile iron (for reviews see Kruszewski [14] and Esposito [22]).

In vivo, most of the iron is bound to heme or non-heme protein and does not directly catalyze the generation of hydroxyl radicals or a similar oxidant [15]. Catalytic iron can be measured by various assays including the bleomycin-detectable iron assay, which is based on the observation that the anti-tumor antibiotic bleomycin, in the presence of iron salt and a suitable reducing agent, binds to and degrades DNA with the formation of a product that reacts with thiobarbituric acid to form a chromogen. Thus the assay detects iron complexes capable of catalyzing free-radical reactions in biological samples [23,24]. The binding of the bleomycin-iron complex to DNA makes the reaction site-specific and antioxidants rarely interfere. The bleomycin assay detects only "free" iron and not iron bound to specific transport proteins or to enzymes.

The ability of iron to participate in redox cycling makes it potentially hazardous by enabling it to participate in the generation of powerful oxidant species such as hydroxyl radical (metal-catalyzed Haber–Weiss reaction, below) and/or reactive iron–oxygen complexes such as ferryl or perferryl ion [15]. In several systems, the amount of free-radical generation is related to the amount of labile iron present [17].

$$Fe^{3+} + O_2^{\bullet} \longrightarrow Fe^{2+} + O_2$$

$$Fe^{2+} + H_2O_2 \longrightarrow Fe^{3+} + OH^- + OH^{\bullet}$$

$$O_2 + H_2O_2 \qquad\qquad O_2 + OH^- + OH^{\bullet}$$

Iron also has a major role in the initiation and propagation of lipid peroxidation, either by catalyzing the conversion of primary oxygen radicals to hydroxyl radicals or forming a perferryl ion. In addition, iron can directly catalyze lipid peroxidation, the oxidative reaction of polyunsaturated lipids, by removing hydrogen atoms from polyunsaturated fatty acids in the lipid bilayers of organelle membranes [15].

The pathological effects of iron accumulation in tissue in iron-overload states, such as are described in thalassemia patients, are well known. What is new in the field is the recognition that iron plays an important role in the pathophysiology of tissue injury in the absence of systemic iron overload. There appear at least two distinct pathophysiological mechanisms for accumulation of labile or catalytic iron that participate in tissue injury. It is now known that specific defects in cellular iron metabolism and/or an increase in labile iron may be important in several disease processes not associated with iron overload [18,25]. For example, in Friedreich's ataxia, a neuromuscular disorder, the deficiency of the iron-chaperone protein frataxin results in improper processing of iron for heme and iron-sulphur cluster formation, leading to accumulation of iron in the mitochondria [25]. In some other neuromuscular disorders, deficiencies in pantothenate kinase, a key enzyme in coenzyme A synthesis, leads to iron depositions and brain damage [25]. In addition to these specific defects in cellular iron, there is compelling evidence that increased labile iron from several subcellular sources participates in tissue injury in a variety of disease states.

There are two broad lines of evidence for the role of labile iron in disease states: that it is increased in disease states, and that iron chelators provide a protective effect, thus establishing a cause–effect relationship (Table 6.1).

TABLE 6.1 Catalytic (labile) Iron

WHAT IS CATALYTIC IRON?

- A transient iron pool of low-molecular-weight, weakly chelated iron that passes through the cell
- The broadest definition of labile iron pool (LIP) is that it consists of chemical forms that can participate in redox cycling (catalytic iron)
- LIP is less than 3% (70–90 mg) of total cellular iron (3–5 g)

EVIDENCE FOR ITS PARTICIPATION IN DISEASE STATES:

- LIP (catalytic iron) is increased in disease states
- Iron chelators have a protective effect, establishing a cause-effect relationship

CATALYTIC IRON IS A COMMON THEME OF CELLULAR INJURY IN DISEASE STATES OF:

- Acute and chronic kidney disease
- Acute myocardial infarction
- Neurodegenerative disorders

This has been demonstrated in many disease states including acute and chronic kidney disease, acute myocardial infarction, and neurodegenerative disorders [26]. Thus, its role in disease processes appears to be a common theme of cellular injury.

ROLE OF CATALYTIC IRON IN ACUTE KIDNEY INJURY

Catalytic Iron in Myoglobinuric Acute Kidney Injury

During the Battle of Britain, Bywaters and Beall described the first causative association of acute kidney injury with skeletal muscle injury with release of muscle cell contents, including myoglobin, into plasma (rhabdomyolysis) [27]. Since then, the spectrum of etiologies for rhabdomyolysis, myoglobinuria, and renal failure has been expanded with the recognition of both traumatic and nontraumatic causes [28]. The most widely used model of myoglobinuric acute kidney injury is produced by subcutaneous or intramuscular injection of hypertonic glycerol [29].

There is a marked and specific increase in catalytic iron content in myoglobinuric acute kidney injury [30]. An iron chelator provides a protective effect on renal function and is associated with a significant reduction in histological evidence of renal damage [31]. Paller also demonstrated that deferoxamine treatment is protective in three models of myoglobinuric renal injury, namely, hemoglobin-induced nephrotoxicity, glycerol-induced acute kidney injury, and a combined renal ischemia/hemoglobin insult [32]. Similarly, Zager in his studies demonstrated the protective effect of an iron chelator in myohemoglobinuric injury [33]. Taken together, the increase in catalytic iron as well as the histological and functional protective effect of an iron chelator implicates a role for labile iron in glycerol-induced acute kidney injury.

The prevailing dogma is that myoglobin from the muscle serves as an important source of iron in glycerol-induced acute kidney injury. This is not surprising because myoglobin released from injured muscles is rich in heme iron. An alternative or additional potentially rich source of iron is cytochrome P450 (CYP), first described to play a role in reperfusion injury of the lung and kidney [34]. Cytochrome P450 is a heme-containing enzyme that can generate reactive oxygen metabolites during the oxidative metabolism of exogenous and endogenous compounds. Baliga et al. have shown that cytochrome P450 may be a significant source of iron in this model of acute kidney injury [30].

Catalytic Iron in Cisplatin-Induced Nephrotoxicity

Cisplatin is a widely used antineoplastic agent with nephrotoxicity as a major side effect. The underlying mechanism of this nephrotoxicity is still not well known. Baliga et al. have examined the catalytic iron content and the effect of iron chelators in an in vitro model of cisplatin-induced cytotoxicity in LLC-PK$_1$ (renal tubular epithelial) cells and in an in vivo model of cisplatin-induced acute kidney injury in rats [35]. The exposure of LLC-PK$_1$ cells to cisplatin results in a significant increase in catalytic iron released into the medium. Concurrent incubation of LLC-PK$_1$ cells with iron chelators including deferoxamine and 1,10-phenanthroline significantly attenuates cisplatin-induced cytotoxicity as measured by lactate dehydrogenase (LDH) release. Bleomycin-detectable iron content is also markedly increased in the kidney of rats treated with cisplatin. Similarly, administration of deferoxamine in rats provides marked functional (as measured by blood urea nitrogen and creatinine) and histological protection against cisplatin-induced acute kidney injury [35].

Baliga et al. also have shown that cytochrome P450 may serve as a significant source of catalytic iron in cisplatin-induced nephrotoxicity [36]. Utilizing CYP2E1-null (CYP2E1−/−) mice, Liu and Baliga have demonstrated a pivotal role of CYP2E1 in cisplatin-induced nephrotoxicity [37]. Incubation of CYP2E1−/− kidney slices with cisplatin results in a significant decrease in the generation of reactive oxygen metabolites and attenuation of cytotoxicity as compared to that of wild-type mice (CYP2E1+/+). CYP2E1-null mice had marked functional and histological protection against cisplatin-induced renal injury, thus demonstrating the importance of cytochrome P450 2E1 in cisplatin nephrotoxicity. Taken together, these data support a critical role for iron in mediating tissue injury via hydroxyl radical (or a similar oxidant) in this model of nephrotoxicity.

Catalytic Iron in Gentamicin Nephrotoxicity

Nephrotoxicity is a major complication of the use of aminoglycoside antibiotics (including gentamicin), which are widely used in the treatment of Gram-negative infections. The precise mechanism(s) of gentamicin nephrotoxicity remains unknown.

GENTAMICIN-INDUCED MOBILIZATION OF IRON FROM RENAL CORTICAL MITOCHONDRIA

In vivo, most of the iron is bound to heme and nonheme proteins and does not directly catalyze the generation of the hydroxyl radical; the source of iron available to participate in this process is uncertain. Based on the ability of superoxide to release iron from the iron-storage protein ferritin (which normally provides a secure means of storing iron in an inert form), ferritin has been suggested as a possible source of iron for the generation of powerful oxidant species. A source of iron not previously considered is iron-rich mitochondria, which contain heme as well as nonheme iron.

Ueda et al. examined whether gentamicin enhances the release of iron from renal cortical mitochondria and, if so, whether gentamicin induces iron mobilization from mitochondria directly or through generation of hydrogen peroxide [38]. Rat renal mitochondria incubated with gentamicin results in a time- and dose-dependent iron release as measured by the formation of the iron-bathophenanthroline complex FeII(BPS)3. Based on a previous study that gentamicin enhances the generation of hydrogen peroxide by renal cortical mitochondria, Ueda et al. examined whether the effect of gentamicin on iron release is mediated by hydrogen peroxide. Catalase (which decomposes hydrogen peroxide), as well as pyruvate, a potent scavenger of hydrogen peroxide, prevents gentamicin-induced iron mobilization, indicating that gentamicin-induced iron mobilization from mitochondria is mediated by hydrogen peroxide. Direct addition of hydrogen peroxide to mitochondria results in release of iron. These results demonstrate that gentamicin induces the release of iron from mitochondria and that this is mediated through the generation of hydrogen peroxide. These results also indicate that mitochondria should be considered as a potential source of iron for the generation of other oxidant species or initiation of lipid peroxidation in other models of tissue injury.

EVIDENCE SUGGESTING A ROLE FOR IRON IN GENTAMICIN-INDUCED ACUTE RENAL FAILURE IN RATS

In vitro and in vivo studies indicate enhanced generation of hydrogen peroxide and release of iron in response to gentamicin. Most, if not all, of the hydrogen peroxide generated by mitochondria is derived from the dismutation of superoxide. Thus, the enhanced generation of hydrogen peroxide by gentamicin suggests that superoxide anion production is also increased. Superoxide and hydrogen peroxide may interact (with trace metals such as iron as the redox agent) to generate highly reactive and unstable oxidizing species including the hydroxyl radical. Several studies have in fact shown that agents that enhance the generation of hydrogen peroxide and superoxide anion by mitochondria also enhance generation of the hydroxyl radical. Walker et al. demonstrated that hydroxyl radical scavengers and iron chelators provide a marked protective effect on renal function in gentamicin-induced acute renal failure in rats [39]. In addition, histological evidence of damage is markedly reduced by the interventional agents. Studies from other laboratories have provided support for these observations. Administration of superoxide dismutase or the oxidant scavenger dimethylthiourea provided a marked protection against gentamicin-induced impairment of renal function and lipid peroxidation, and dimethylthiourea attenuated tubular damage [40]. In contrast it has been reported that, despite amelioration of gentamicin-induced lipid peroxidation by treatment of the antioxidant diphenyl-phenyenediamine, it failed to prevent nephrotoxicity [41]. However, it was also demonstrated that co-administration of antioxidants vitamin E and selenium is protective against gentamicin-induced nephrotoxicity [42]. It is not clear why the contradictory results are obtained; however, one explanation is that it may be due to the difference in the mechanisms for protective effect of antioxidants. Additional support for a role of iron-catalyzed free-radical generation has been provided by demonstrating that gentamicin-induced generation of hydroxyl radicals is reduced by iron chelators in vitro [43] and iron supplementation enhances gentamicin nephrotoxicity in vivo [44,45]. Taken together, it appears that reactive oxygen metabolites and catalytic iron play an important role in gentamicin nephrotoxicity.

Catalytic Iron in Contrast-Media-Associated Nephrotoxicity

Rajapurkur et al. in a preliminary study have reported that kidney donors undergoing either an intravenous pyelogram or a renal arteriogram have a marked increase in urinary catalytic iron accompanied by evidence of tubular injury as reflected by an increase in urinary alkaline phosphatase and N-acetyl-β-glucosaminidase [46]. Since the effect of labile iron is to increase oxidative stress, it is of interest that there is good experimental evidence for the role of oxidants in contrast-induced acute kidney injury [47–49]. More importantly, in human studies Efrati et al. reported a mean increase of 28% in urinary F2-isoprotane levels after coronary angiography [50]. Drager et al. collected urine samples for urinary F2-isoprostane (a marker of oxidative stress) immediately before and after cardiac catheterization and reported a several-fold increase in urinary isoprostane in the control group after contrast exposure [51].

These human studies indicate an association between catalytic iron and oxidative stress with contrast-induced nephropathy, but they do not establish a cause—effect relationship. Unfortunately, there do not appear to be any satisfactory animal models of contrast-induced acute kidney injury [52]. However, Vari et al., utilizing a model in rabbits that they have developed [53], examined the effect of an iron chelator on renal function. An infusion of contrast media was associated with a significant decrease in creatinine clearance, which was prevented in rabbits pretreated with an iron chelator, suggesting an important role of catalytic iron in this model (Table 6.2) [54].

Catalytic Iron in Ischemia-Reperfusion Injury

Ischemia-reperfusion is an important cause of acute kidney injury. In this section, evidence for the role of labile iron in this injury is reviewed. In addition, we briefly describe the role of labile iron in cardiac ischemia-reperfusion injury to provide supportive evidence for these mechanisms in cellular injury.

Iron has been demonstrated to accumulate in renal proximal tubules following experimental ischemia-reperfusion injury [55]. More importantly, Baliga et al. have shown a marked increase in labile iron after ischemia-reperfusion injury [56], and an iron chelator has been shown to be protective [57,58]. Additional evidence for the role of iron in ischemia-reperfusion injury comes from reports that other types of iron-binding and/or iron-translocating compounds also provide protection against ischemia. The amount of circulating redox-active iron has been shown to increase significantly in an experimental model of ischemia-reperfusion injury, and an infusion of apotransferrin (but not iron-saturated apotransferrin) results in a dose-dependent improvement in renal function following reperfusion [59]. In addition, the recent discovery of neutrophil gelatinase-associated lipocalin (NGAL), which is an important iron-transporting and iron-translocating compound, provides additional evidence for the importance of iron in acute kidney injury [60]. The biology of NGAL is complex and incompletely defined, but it is important in renal development in that it stimulates the epithelial cell phenotype, is proapoptotic, and is an iron-binding and -transporting protein [61]. Furthermore, NGAL is one of the most upregulated genes and proteins in the kidney following ischemic insult [60], and infusion of NGAL protein has

been demonstrated to be protective of renal ischemia-reperfusion injury [61].

During experimental cardiac ischemic injury, there is a 30-fold increase in labile iron [62]. This increase in the cellular labile iron pool is mediated primarily by the release of iron from ferritin and is associated with severe oxidative stress, which in turn further increases levels of cellular labile iron [62–64]. Therapeutically, both deferiprone and deferoxamine have been demonstrated to protect against experimental cardiac ischemia-reperfusion injury [65–67]. Iron loading has been demonstrated to further increase cardiac ischemia-reperfusion injury and again deferoxamine is protective, even in the iron-overloaded state [65]. Although evidence derived from animal models is extremely valuable mechanistically, it is of greater significance that deferoxamine has also been shown to improve outcomes in man following coronary artery bypass graft surgery [68]. Taken together, the body of scientific and clinical data supporting the importance of the role of iron in the pathogenesis of ischemic injury is compelling. The role of catalytic iron and oxidants in acute kidney injury is summarized in Table 6.3.

CATALYTIC IRON IN CHRONIC KIDNEY DISEASE (TABLE 6.3)

Catalytic Iron in Experimental Glomerular Disease

The role of iron has been examined in several models of leukocyte-dependent and -independent models of glomerular disease [69]. The anti-glomerular basement membrane antibody is a well-characterized model of complement- and neutrophil-dependent glomerular injury. In this model in rabbits, Boyce et al. reported that an iron chelator significantly attenuates proteinuria [70]. In addition to proliferative glomerulonephritis, the ability of glomerular cells to generate oxidants suggests that they may act as important mediators of injury in glomerular

TABLE 6.2 Animal Model of Contrast-Induced Nephropathy

	Group 1 Saline Only		Group 2 DFO	
	Pre-	Post-	Pre-	Post-
CCR (mL/min)	8.64 ± 1	$4.96 \pm 1.5^*$	11.6 ± 1.5	10.2 ± 1.6

$P \leq 1$; pre- versus post-contrast infusion.

TABLE 6.3 Catalytic Iron in Kidney Disease

Catalytic Iron and Oxidants in Models of Acute Kidney Injury	
Model	Reference Number
Rhabdomyolysis	[30,31,32,33]
Cisplatin	[35,36,37]
Gentamicin	[38,39,40,42,43,44,45]
Contrast	[46,47,48,49,50,51,54]
Ischemia/reperfusion	[34,55,56,57,58,59,62]

diseases that lack infiltrating leukocytes. An animal model of minimal change disease is induced by a single intravenous injection of puromycin aminonucleoside. Catalytic iron (measured as bleomycin-detectable iron) is markedly increased in glomeruli from nephrotic rats, and an iron chelator prevents an increase in catalytic iron in the glomeruli and provides complete protection against proteinuria, suggesting an important pathogenic role for catalytic iron in this model [71,72].

Baliga et al. have demonstrated that cytochrome treatment of PAN resulted in a marked increase in catalytic iron associated with significant loss of glomerular cytochrome P450 content. Administration of CYP inhibitors significantly prevented injury-induced loss of CYP content and increase in catalytic iron in the glomeruli accompanied by a marked decrease in proteinuria [73]. In an in vitro study using glomerular epithelial cells (GEC), CYP inhibitors also markedly prevented a PAN-induced increase in catalytic iron and hydroxyl radical formation accompanied by significant protection against PAN-induced cytotoxicity. Taken together these data indicate that CYP, a group of heme protein, may serve as a significant source of this catalytic iron. In addition, they have shown with in vivo and in vitro studies that cytochrome P450 2B1, an isozyme present in the glomerulus, is a source of catalytic iron that participates in glomerular injury in this model [74,75].

Passive Heymann nephritis, induced by a single intravenous injection of anti-Fx1A, is a complement-dependent model of glomerular disease that resembles membranous nephropathy in humans. The administration of an iron chelator markedly reduces proteinuria, suggesting the role of labile iron in passive Heymann nephritis [76]. Baliga et al. have shown that feeding an iron-deficient diet provides protection in this model [77].

Role of Iron in Experimental Progressive Kidney Disease

The severity of tubulointerstitial injury is a major determinant of the degree and rate of progression of renal failure. The data supporting the role of iron in models of progressive renal disease consist of demonstration of increased iron in the kidney; enhanced oxidant generation, which provides a mechanism by which iron can be mobilized; and the beneficial effect of iron-deficient diets and iron chelators. Rats with proteinuria have increased iron content in proximal tubular cells, and iron accumulation was the only independent predictor of both functional and structural damage [78]. Similarly, it has been shown that there is a substantial iron accumulation associated with increased cortical malondialdehyde in proximal tubular cells in the remnant kidney, suggesting reactive oxygen species generation. The sources of increased iron in the kidney have not been well-delineated, but Alfrey

et al. have suggested that urinary transferrin provides a potential source of iron [79,80].

Several studies have demonstrated an important role of iron in progressive kidney disease. It was reported that an iron-deficient diet (Figure 6.1) or iron chelators prevent the development of tubulointerstitial disease and renal functional deterioration in nephrotoxic serum nephritis [80,81]. Remuzzi et al. have shown that rats fed an iron-deficient diet have a significant reduction in proteinuria and develop less glomerulosclerosis [82]. An iron chelator significantly reduces iron accumulation and tubular damage in the rat remnant kidney, a model for progressive renal disease [83].

Catalytic Iron in Human Disease

A sufficient body of in vitro and in vivo information exists to postulate that catalytic iron is an important mediator in glomerular pathophysiology and progressive kidney disease. While the collective information on the role of oxidants and iron derived from models of glomerular disease as well as progressive renal failure is impressive, there is little information on the potential role of these mechanisms in human disease. There are many differences between animal models and glomerular disease in humans. For example, the animal model of minimal change disease is a toxic model whereas the mechanism of minimal change disease in humans is not known. Similarly, the anti-Fx1A antibody, which is used for the animal model of membranous nephropathy, has been difficult to demonstrate in human membranous nephropathy. Indeed, the lessons from animal models of acute kidney injury have been disappointing when attempting to translate to human disease. We will summarize the limited information from human studies which lend support that the mechanisms observed in animal models appear to be applicable to human disease.

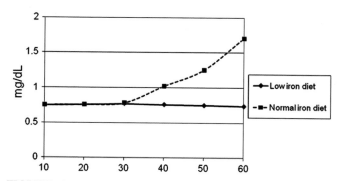

FIGURE 6.1 Effect of a low-iron diet in halting progression of kidney disease. Feeding a low-fat diet to rats with nephrotoxic serum nephritis prevented a rise in serum creatinine and provided histological protection.

CATALYTIC IRON IN DIABETIC NEPHROPATHY

Howard et al. have shown that urinary iron excretion is increased early in the course of diabetic kidney disease in humans [84]. We have compared labile iron in subjects with no renal disease or diabetes to patients with diabetes (Figure 6.2A). Our data demonstrate that patients with overt diabetes have a marked increase in urinary catalytic iron. Similarly, patients with microalbuminuria have a marked and highly significant increase in urinary catalytic iron, indicating that urinary catalytic iron is not merely a reflection of albuminuria. Finally, some patients in the diabetic control group who do not have microalbuminuria have high catalytic iron, leading us to postulate that urinary catalytic iron precedes the onset of microalbuminuria and may predict patients at risk for diabetic nephropathy. Interestingly, recent studies have demonstrated that non-transferrin-bound iron levels are frequently increased in diabetes and have been implicated in a few studies with the vascular complications of diabetes [85].

We conducted a single-center, single-arm, open-label, proof-of-concept study to evaluate the safety and efficacy of the oral iron chelator deferiprone in reducing albuminuria in patients with diabetic nephropathy [86]. Adult patients with a diagnosis of diabetes mellitus and significant abnormal albumin excretion but with serum creatinine levels < 1.2 mg/dL were included in this study. Patients received standard of care and enalapril, which was kept constant throughout the study. Deferiprone was administered in a daily dose of ~50 mg/kg in three divided doses for nine months. The mean age of the 37 patients (21 males and 16 females) was 51.27 ($\pm$ 1.67) years. The blood glucose control measured by HbA1c was not significantly different between the baseline and final visit (P = 0.68). The mean albumin-to-creatinine ratio decreased with treatment of deferiprone as shown in Figure 6.2B. The serum creatinine levels remained stable throughout the course of the study. The calculated mean arterial blood pressure (MAP) declined from a baseline value of 100.78 $\pm$ 1.7 to 97 $\pm$ 0.6 at 3 months (P = 0.2), but remained relatively stable from then on to 6 months (96.24 $\pm$ 0.7; P = 0.6) and 9 months. No clinically significant side effects

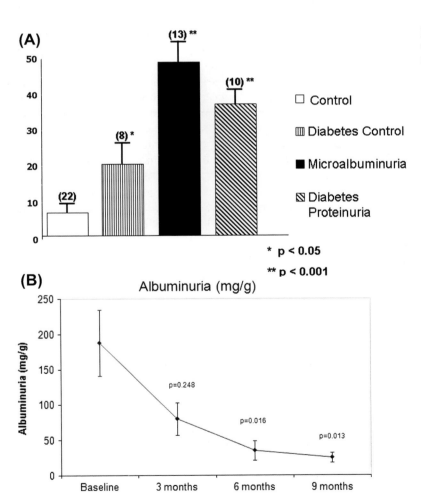

FIGURE 6.2 Urinary catalytic iron in patients with diabetic nephropathy (A) and the effect of the iron chelator deferiprone on proteinuria (B).

were observed. Future randomized, double-blind trials, with careful monitoring of safety issues, may lead to use of a new class of agents for the treatment of diabetic nephropathy.

CATALYTIC IRON IN CHRONIC KIDNEY DISEASE

Nankivell et al. have reported increased iron content in patients with chronic kidney disease [87]. Using the urinary catalytic iron assay described before, we have shown a marked increase in patients who have biopsy-proven glomerulonephritis (Figure 6.3A).

We conducted an open-label, proof-of-concept study in which patients with biopsy-proven glomerulonephritis were treated with deferiprone (50 mg/kg/day), and protein and serum creatinine were obtained 2–6 months after the administration of the iron chelator. As shown in Figure 6.3, Panels B, C, and D, treatment

with the iron chelator significantly decreased the amount of total urinary protein in patients with glomerulonephritis [88]. Serum creatinine was 1.10 ± 0.15 before and 0.90 ± 0.10 (n = 11) at the end of the study period. Our data indicate an increase of catalytic iron in patients with glomerulonephritis and that treatment with an oral iron chelator leads to a reduction in proteinuria.

There is at least one published study in the literature in which the effect of a metal chelator on progressive kidney disease has been examined. Lin et al. have shown that chelation therapy with ethylenediaminetetraacetic acid (EDTA) in patients with chronic renal insufficiency results in a reduced rate of decline in the glomerular filtration rate [89]. The authors attribute the beneficial effect to the chelation of lead, which also participates in the Fenton reaction. However, given the affinity constants for iron and lead, the large experimental evidence for the role of iron in kidney disease, and the demonstrated efficacy of EDTA in enhancing excretion

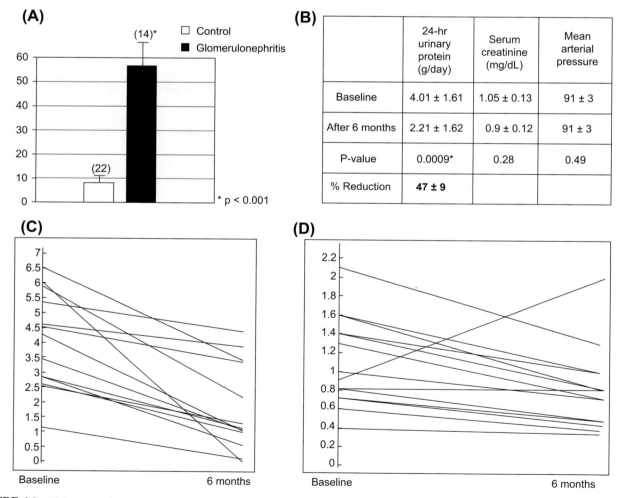

FIGURE 6.3 Urinary catalytic iron in patients with biopsy-proven glomerulonephritis (A); effect of deferiprone on urinary protein and serum creatinine in patients with steroid-resistant glomerulonephritis (B). Panels C and D depict individual patient data.

of urinary iron, we believe that the beneficial effects are more likely to be explained by the chelation of iron rather than lead [90].

CONCLUDING COMMENTS

One has to be cautious in extrapolating results from animal studies to humans. Unfortunately, all clinical trials in acute kidney injury based on animal models have failed. These include trials related to atrial natriuretic peptide [91,92], insulin-like growth factor [93,94], thyroxine [95,96], and furosemide [97,98]. Nonetheless, evidence that labile iron appears to be involved in a variety of models of acute kidney injury suggests that it may be a common mechanism of tissue injury. Additionally, demonstration of an increase in labile iron in humans lends support to the possibility of similar pathophysiological mechanisms in humans. The availability of iron chelators with a favorable side-effect profile for short-term use makes them attractive for randomized clinical trials to evaluate their efficacy and safety in preventing or treating acute kidney injury.

There are several points from animal and human studies related to halting progression with a metal chelator that are worth noting. The observation that a reduction in proteinuria (provided it is not attributable to a fall in GFR) results in slowing progression of kidney disease has been reasonably well-established, only with ACE inhibitors and ARBs. This is in keeping with the data that albumin itself appears to have a significant effect on tubular cells, including enhanced generation of oxidants and activation of the inflammatory response. However, it is conceivable for a therapeutic agent to preserve the tubulointerstitial region by abolishing the consequences of proteinuria or having a direct protective effect on the tubules. In diabetic and nondiabetic CKD, animal and human studies highlight the possibility of a beneficial effect without a reduction in proteinuria. In a recent study, bicarbonate supplementation slowed the rate of progression of renal failure to ESRD without reducing proteinuria [99]. In an open-label trial, pirfenidone was shown to slow the loss of kidney function in patients with focal segmental sclerosis with no reduction in proteinuria [100]. In a model of diabetic nephropathy, pirfenidone was shown to reduce generation of reactive oxidant species and significantly reduce mesangial matrix expansion without affecting albuminuria. In studies by Alfrey, an iron-deficient diet or iron chelator provided both functional and histological protection against progression in a model of nephrotoxic serum kidney disease without affecting proteinuria [79,81]. Similarly, in the study by Lin et al., EDTA provided protection against progression without

reducing urinary protein [89]. Thus, clinical studies targeted toward halting progression should focus not only on short-term studies on proteinuria, but they would have to be of sufficient duration to evaluate the effect on renal function.

The evidence reviewed suggests the possibility of using iron chelators to halt the progression of kidney disease. The long-term use required for chronic kidney disease makes oral iron chelators more attractive than parenteral medications. Currently, two oral iron chelators have been approved for human use in iron overload states: deferasirox and deferiprone. Deferasirox has been shown to have some nephrotoxicity [101] but may nonetheless be potentially beneficial in patients with kidney disease. Deferiprone (1,2-dimethyl-3-hydroxypyridin-4-1, also known as L1) is the most extensively studied oral iron chelator and is approved for treatment of iron overload states in Europe and India. In addition to its suitability for long-term treatment (because of oral administration), it has better tissue penetration compared to deferoxamine. The high-membrane permeability of deferiprone is well documented, as shown by its capacity to access and deplete intracellular iron pools [25]. In addition, a recent study has demonstrated its ability to remove labile iron from nuclei, endosomes, and mitochondria [25]. The major adverse effect reported so far in several thousand patients receiving deferiprone for periods of up to 14 years is transient agranulocytosis in 0.6% of patients. Based on the collective evidence to date, randomized, controlled, double-blind trials may be warranted to evaluate the efficacy and safety of iron chelators to halt progression of chronic kidney disease [102,103].

References

[1] Chertow GM, Burdick E, Honour M, Bonventre JV, Bates DW. Acute kidney injury, mortality, length of stay, and costs in hospitalized patients. J Am Soc Nephrol 2005;16(11): 3365−70.

[2] Lafrance J-P, Miller DR. Acute kidney injury associates with inreased long-term mortality. J Am Soc Nephrol 2010;21: 345−52.

[3] Hobson CE, Yavas S, Segal MS, Schold JD, Tribble CG, Layon AJ, et al. Acute kidney injury is associated with increased long-term mortality after cardiothoracic surgery. Circulation 2009;119:2444−53.

[4] Hsu C. Linking the population epidemiology of acute renal failure, chronic kidney disease and end-stage renal disease. Curr Opin Nephrol Hypertens 2007;16:221−6.

[5] Triverio P-A, Martin P-Y, Romand J, Pugin J, Perneger T, Saudan P. Long-term prognosis after acute kidney injury requiring renal replacement therapy. Nephrol Dial Transplant 2009;24(7):2186−9.

[6] Mehta RL, Kellum JA, Shah SV, Molitoris BA, Ronco C, Warnock DG, et al. Acute Kidney Injury Network (AKIN): Report of an initiative to improve outcomes in acute kidney injury. Crit Care 2007;11(2):R31.

[7] Coresh J, Selvin E, Stevens LA, Manzi J, Kusek JW, Eggers P, et al. Prevalence of chronic kidney disease in the United States. JAMA 2007;298(17):2038–47.

[8] Xue JL, Ma JZ, Louis TA, Collins AJ. Forecast of the number of patients with end-stage renal disease in the United States to the year 2010. J Am Soc Nephrol 2001;12:2753–8.

[9] Sarnak MJ, Levey AS, Schoolwerth AC, Coresh J, Culleton BF, Hamm LL, et al. Kidney disease as a risk factor for development of cardiovascular disease: a statement from the American Heart Association Councils on Kidney in Cardiovascular Disease, High Blood Pressure Research, Clinical Cardiology, and Epidemiology and Prevention. Circulation 2003;108(17): 2154–69.

[10] Szczech LA, Lazar IL. Projecting the United States ESRD population: Issues regarding treatment of patients with ESRD. Kidney Int 2004;66(Suppl. 90):S3–7.

[11] Lambers Heerspink H, Greene T, Lewis JB, Raz I, Rohde RD, Hunsicker LG, et al. Effects of sulodexide in patients with type 2 diabetes and persistent albuminuria. Nephrol Dial Transplant 2007;23(6):1946–54.

[12] Packham DK, Wolfe R, Reutens AT, Berl T, Heerspink HL, Rohde R, et al. R.C. A, Group. ftCS. Sulodexide fails to demonstrate renoprotection in overt type 2 diabetic nephropathy. J Am Soc Nephrol 2011; [Epub ahead of print].

[13] Greenberg GR, Wintrobe WM. A labile iron pool. J Biol Chem. 1946;165:397–8.

[14] Kruszewski M. The role of labile iron pool in cardiovascular diseases. Acta Biochim Pol 2004;51(2):471–80.

[15] Halliwell B, Gutteridge JM. Role of free radicals and catalytic metal ions in human disease: an overview. Methods in Enzymol 1990;186:1–85.

[16] Kakhlon O, Cabantchik ZI. The labile iron pool: characterization, measurement, and participation in celullar processes. Free Rad Biol Med 2002;33(8):1037–46.

[17] Esposito BP, Breuer W, Sirankapracha P, Pootrakul P, Hershko C, Cabantchik I. Labile plasma iron in iron overload: redox activity and susceptibility to chelation. Blood 2003;102(7): 2670–7.

[18] Andrews NC. Forging a field: the golden age of iron biology. Blood 2008;112(2):219–30.

[19] Ganz T, Nemeth E. Hepcidin and disorders of iron metabolism. Annu Rev Med 2011;62:347–60.

[20] Esposito BP, Epsztejn S, Breuer W, Cabantchik ZI. A review of fluorescence methods for assessing labile iron in cells and biological fluids. Analytic Biochemistry 2002;304: 1–18.

[21] Glickstein H, El RB, Shvartsman M, Cabantchik ZI. Intracellular labile iron pools as direct targets of iron chelators: a fluorescence study of chelator action in living cells. Blood 2005;106(9):3242–50.

[22] Esposito BP, Breuer W, Slotki I, Cabantchik ZI. Labile iron in parenteral iron formulations and its potential for generating plasma nontransferrin-bound iron in dialysis patients. Euro J Clin Invest 2002;32(Suppl. 1):42–9.

[23] Gutteridge JMC, Rowley DA, Halliwell B. Superoxide-dependent formation of hydroxyl radicals in the presence of iron salts. Detection of "free" iron in biological systems by using bleomycin-dependent degradation of DNA. Biochem J 1981;199: 263–5.

[24] Gutteridge JMC, Cao W, Chevion M. Bleomycin-detectable iron in brain tissue. Free Rad Res Comm 1991;11(6):317–20.

[25] Sohn YS, Breuer W, Munnich A, Cabantchik ZI. Redistribution of accumulated cell iron: a modality of chelation with therapeutic implications. Blood 2008;111(3):1690–9.

[26] Boddaert N, Le Quan Sang KH, Rötig A, Leroy-Willig A, Gallet S, Brunelle F, et al. Selective iron chelation in Friedreich ataxia: biologic and clinical implications. Blood 2007;110(1): 401–8.

[27] Bywaters EGL, Beall D. Crush injuries with impairment of renal function. Br Med J 1941;1:427–32.

[28] Gabow PA, Kaehny WD, Kelleher SP. The spectrum of rhabdomyolysis. Medicine 1982;61(3):141–52.

[29] Hostetter TH, Wilkes BM, Brenner BM. Renal circulatory and nephron function in experimental acute renal failure. In: Brenner BM, Lazarus JM, editors. Acute renal failure. 1st ed. Vol 1. Philadelphia: W.B. Saunders Company; 1983. p. 99–115.

[30] Baliga R, Zhang Z, Baliga M, Shah SV. Evidence for cytochrome P-450 as a source of catalytic iron in myoglobinuric acute renal failure. Kidney Int 1996;49:362–9.

[31] Shah SV, Walker PD. Evidence suggesting a role for hydroxyl radical in glycerol-induced acute renal failure. Am J Physiol 1988;255(24):F438–43.

[32] Paller MS. Hemoglobin- and myoglobin-induced acute renal failure in rats: role of iron in nephrotoxicity. Am J Physiol 1988;255(24):F539–44.

[33] Zager RA. Combined mannitol and deferoxamine therapy for myohemoglobinuric renal injury and oxidant tubular stress. Mechanistic and therapeutic implications. J Clin Invest 1992;90:711–9.

[34] Paller MS, Jacob HS. Cytochrome P-450 mediates tissue-damaging hydroxyl radical formation during reoxygenation of the kidney. Proc Natl Acad Sci USA 1994;91:7002–6.

[35] Baliga R, Zhang Z, Baliga M, Ueda N, Shah SV. In vitro and in vivo evidence suggesting a role for iron in cisplatin-induced nephrotoxicity. Kidney Int 1998;53:394–401.

[36] Baliga R, Zhang Z, Baliga M, Ueda N, Shah SV. Role of cytochrome P-450 as a source of catalytic iron in cisplatin-induced nephrotoxicity. Kidney Int 1998;54:1562–9.

[37] Liu H, Baliga R. Cytochrome P450 2E1 null mice provide novel protection against cisplatin-induced nephrotoxicity and apoptosis. Kidney Int 2003;63:1687–96.

[38] Ueda N, Guidet B, Shah SV. Gentamicin-induced mobilization of iron from renal cortical mitochondria. American Journal of Physiology 1993;265(34):F435–9.

[39] Walker PD, Shah SV. Evidence suggesting a role for hydroxyl radical in gentamicin-induced acute renal failure in rats. J Clin Invest 1988;81:334–41.

[40] Nakajima T, Hishida A, Kato A. Mechanisms for protective effects of free radical scavengers on gentamicin-mediated nephropathy in rats. Am J Physiol Renal Physiol 1994;266(35): F425–31.

[41] Ramsammy LS, Josepovitz C, Ling KY, Lane BP, Kaloyanides GJ. Effects of diphenyl-phenylenediamine on gentamicin-induced lipid peroxidation and toxicity in rat renal cortex. Journal of Pharmacology and Experimental Therapeutics 1986;238(1):83–8.

[42] Ademuyiwa O, Ngaha EO, Ubah FO. Vitamin E and selenium in gentamicin nephrotoxicity. Human Exp Toxicol 1990;9:281–8.

[43] Yang CL, Du XH, Han YX. Renal cortical mitochondria are the source of oxygen free radicals enhanced by gentamicin. Renal Failure 1995;17(1):21–6.

[44] Kays SE, Crowell WA, Johnson MA. Iron supplementation increases gentamicin nephrotoxicity in rats. J Nutr 1991;121: 1869–75.

[45] Ben Ismail TH, Ali BH, Bashir AA. Influence of iron, deferoxamine and ascorbic acid on gentamicin-induced nephrotoxicity in rats. Gen Pharmacol 1994;25(6):1249–52.

[46] Rajapurkar M, Gang S, Hegde U, Gohel K, Shah SV. Study of urinary catalytic (bleomycin-detectable) iron following radio-contrast exposure in healthy kidney donors [abstract]. J Am Soc Nephrol 2007;18:575A.

[47] Parvez Z, Rahman MA, Moncada R. Contrast media-induced lipid peroxidation in the rat kidney. Invest Radiol 1989;24:697−702.

[48] Bakris GL, Lass N, Gaber AO, Jones JD, Burnett Jr JC. Radio-contrast medium-induced declines in renal function: a role for oxygen free radicals. Am J Physiol 1990;258(Renal Fluid Electrolyte Physiol 27):F115−20.

[49] Yoshioka T, Fogo A, Beckman JK. Reduced activity of antioxidant enzymes underlies contrast media-induced renal injury in volume depletion. Kidney Int 1992;41:1008−15.

[50] Efrati S, Dishy V, Averbukh M, Blatt A, Krakover R, Weisgarten J, et al. The effect of N-acetylcysteine on renal function, nitric oxide, and oxidative stress after angiography. Kidney Int 2003;64(6):2182−7.

[51] Drager LF, Andrade L, Barros De Toledo JF, Laurindo FR, Machado Cesar LA, Seguro AC. Renal effects of N-acetylcysteine in patients at risk for contrast nephropathy: decrease in oxidant stress-mediated renal tubular injury. Nephrol Dial Transplant Jul 2004;19(7):1803−7.

[52] Sandler CM. Contrast-agent-induced acute renal dysfunction − is iodixanol the answer? N Engl J Med 2003;348(6):551−3.

[53] Vari RC, Natarajan LA, Whitescarver SA, Jackson BA, Ott CE. Induction, prevention and mechanisms of contrast media-induced acute renal failure. Kidney Int 1988;33(3):699−707.

[54] Hanss BG, Valencia SH, Shah SV, Vari RC. The iron chelator deferoxamine prevents contrast media induced acute renal failure in the rabbit [abstract]. J Am Soc Nephrol 1990;1(4):612.

[55] Fagoonee S, Gburek J, Hirsch E, Marro S, Moestrup SK, Laurberg JM, et al. Plasma protein haptoglobin modulates renal iron loading. Am J Pathol 2005;166(4):973−83.

[56] Baliga R, Ueda N, Shah SV. Increase in bleomycin-detectable iron in ischaemia/reperfusion injury to rat kidneys. Biochem J 1993;291(3):901−5.

[57] Paller MS, Hedlund BE. Role of iron in postischemic renal injury in the rat. Kidney Int 1988;34:474−80.

[58] Huang H, He Z, Roberts II LJ, Salahudeen AK. Deferoxamine reduces cold-ischemic renal injury in a syngeneic kidney transplant model. Am J Transplant 2003;3:1531−7.

[59] de Vries B, Walter SJ, von Bonsdorff L, Wolfs TG, van Heurn LW, Parkkinen J, et al. Reduction of circulating redox-active iron by apotransferrin protects against renal ischemia-reperfusion injury. Transplantation 2004;77(5):669−75.

[60] Devarajan P. Update on mechanisms of ischemic acute kidney injury. J Am Soc Nephrol 2006;17(6):1503.

[61] Mishra J, Mori K, Ma Q, Kelly C, Yang J, Mitsnefes M, et al. Amelioration of ischemic acute renal injury by neutrophil gelatinase-associated lipocalin. J Am Soc Nephrol 2004;15:3073−82.

[62] Voogd A, Sluiter W, van Eijk HG, Koster JF. Low molecular weight iron and the oxygen paradox in isolated rat hearts. J Clin Invest 1992;90:2050−5.

[63] Nath KA, Norby SM. Reactive oxygen species and acute renal failure. Am J Med 2000;109:555−78.

[64] Kruszewski M. Labile iron pool: the main determinant of cellular response to oxidative stress. Mutat Res 2003;531:81−92.

[65] van der Kraaij AMM, Mostert LJ, van Eijk HG, Koster JF. Iron-load increases the susceptibility of rat hearts to oxygen reperfusion damage. Protection by the antioxidant (+)-cyanidanol-3 and deferoxamine. Circulation 1988;78:442−9.

[66] van der Kraaij AMM, van Eijk HG, Koster JF. Prevention of postischemic cardiac injury by the orally active iron chelator 1,2-dimethyl-3-hydroxy-4-pyridone (L1) and the antioxidant (+)-cyanidanol-3. Circulation 1989;80:158−64.

[67] Nicholson SC, Squier M, Ferguson DJP, Nagy Z, Westaby S, Evans RD. Effect of desferrioxamine cardioplegia on ischemia-reperfusion in isolated rat heart. Ann Thorac Surg 1997;63:1003−11.

[68] Paraskevaidis JA, Iliodromitis EK, Vlahakos D, Tsipras DP, Nikolaidis A, Marathias A, et al. Deferoxamine infusion during coronary artery bypass grafting ameliorates lipid peroxidation and protects the myocardium against reperfusion injury: immediate and long-term significance. Euro Heart J 2005;26(3):263−70.

[69] Shah SV, Baliga R, Fonseca VA, Rajapurkar M. Oxidants in chronic kidney disease. J Am Soc Nephrol 2007;18(1):16−28.

[70] Boyce NW, Holdsworth SR. Hydroxyl radical mediation of immune renal injury by desferrioxamine. Kidney Int 1986;30:813−7.

[71] Ueda N, Baliga R, Shah SV. Role of "catalytic" iron in an animal model of minimal change nephrotic syndrome. Kidney Int 1996;49:370−3.

[72] Thakur V, Walker PD, Shah SV. Evidence suggesting a role for hydroxyl radical in puromycin aminonucleoside-induced proteinuria. Kidney Int 1988;34:494−9.

[73] Liu H, Shah SV, Baliga R. Cytochrome P-450 as a source of catalytic iron in minimal change nephrotic syndrome in rats. Am J Physiol Renal Physiol 2001;280:F88−94.

[74] Liu H, Bigler SA, Henegar JR, Baliga R. Cytochrome P450 2B1 mediates oxidant injury in puromycin-induced nephrotic syndrome. Kidney Int 2002;62(3):868−76.

[75] Tian N, Arany I, Waxman DJ, Baliga R. Cytochrome P450 2B1 gene silencing attenuates puromycin aminonucleoside-induced cytotoxicity to glomerular epithelial cells. Kidney Int 2010;78(2):182−90.

[76] Shah SV. Evidence suggesting a role for hydroxyl radical in passive Heymann nephritis in rats. American Journal of Physiology 1988;254(23):F337−44.

[77] Baliga R, Ueda N, Shah SV. Kidney iron status in passive Heymann nephritis and the effect of iron deficient diet. J Am Soc Nephrol 1996;7:1183−8.

[78] Harris DC, Tay C, Nankivell BJ. Lysosomal iron accumulation and tubular damage in rat puromycin nephrosis and ageing. Clin Exp Pharmacol Physiol 1994;21(2):73−81.

[79] Alfrey AC. Toxicity of tubule fluid iron in the nephrotic syndrome. Am J Physiol 1992;263(32):F637−41.

[80] Cooper MA, Buddington B, Miller NL, Alfrey AC. Urinary iron speciation in nephrotic syndrome. Am J Kidney Dis 1995;25(2):314−9.

[81] Alfrey AC, Froment DH, Hammond WS. Role of iron in the tubulo-interstitial injury in nephrotoxic serum nephritis. Kidney Int 1989;36:753−9.

[82] Remuzzi A, Puntorieri S, Brugnetti B, Bertani T, Remuzzi G. Renoprotective effect of low iron diet and its consequence on glomerular hemodynamics. Kidney Int 1991;39:647−52.

[83] Nankivell BJ, Chen J, Boadle RA, Harris DCH. The role of tubular iron accumulation in the remnant kidney. J Am Soc Nephrol 1994;4:1598−607.

[84] Howard RL, Buddington B, Alfrey AC. Urinary albumin, transferrin and iron excretion in diabetic patients. Kidney Int 1991;40:923−6.

[85] Lee D-H, Liu DY, Jacobs DR, Shin H-R, Song K, Lee I-K, et al. Common presence of non-transferrin-bound iron among patients with type 2 diabetes. Diabetes Care 2006;29:1090−5.

[86] Rajapurkar MM, Alam MG, Bhattacharya A. Novel treatment for diabetic nephropathy [abstract]. J Am Soc Nephrol 2007;18:329A.

[87] Nankivell BJ, Boadle RA, Harris DCH. Iron accumulation in human chronic renal disease. Am J Kidney Dis 1992;20(6):580—4.

[88] Rajapurkar MM, Baliga R, Shah SV. Treatment of patients with glomerulonephritis with an oral iron chelator [abstract]. J Am Soc Nephrol 2007;18:57—58A.

[89] Lin J-L, Lin-Tan D-T, Hsu K-H, Yu C-C. Environmental lead exposure and progression of chronic renal diseases in patients without diabetes. N Engl J Med 2003;348(4):277—86.

[90] Owda AK, Alam MG, Shah SV. Environmental lead exposure and chronic renal disease. N Engl J Med 2003;348(18):1810.

[91] Nakamoto M, Shapiro JI, Shanley PF, Chan L, Schrier RW. In vitro and in vivo protective effect of atriopeptin III on ischemic acute renal failure. J Clin Invest 1987;80(3):698—705.

[92] Allgren RL, Marbury TC, Rahman SN, Weisberg LS, Fenves AZ, Lafayette RA, et al. Anaritide in acute tubular necrosis. N Eng J Med 1997;336(12):828—34.

[93] Ding H, Kopple JD, Cohen A, Hirschberg R. Recombinant human insulin-like growth factor-I accelerates recovery and reduces catabolism in rats with ischemic acute renal failure. J Clin Invest 1993;91:2281—7.

[94] Hirschberg R, Kopple J, Lipsett P, et al. Multicenter clinical trial of recombinant human insulin-like growth factor I in patients with acute renal failure. Kidney Int 1999;55:2423—32.

[95] Siegel NJ, Gaudio KM, Katz LA, Reilly HF, Ardito TA, Hendler FG, et al. Beneficial effect of thyroxin on recovery from toxic acute renal failure. Kidney Int 1984;25:906—11.

[96] Acker CG, Singh AR, Flick RP, Bernadini J, Greenberg A, Johnson JP. A trial of thyroxine in acute renal failure. Kidney Int 2000;57:293—8.

[97] Heyman SN, Brezis M, Greenfeld Z, Rosen S. Protective role of furosemide and saline in radiocontrast-induced acute renal failure in the rat. Am J Kidney Dis 1989;14(5):377—85.

[98] Solomon R, Werner C, Mann D, D'Elia J, Silva P. Effects of saline, mannitol, and furosemide on acute decreases in renal function induced by radiocontrast agents. N Engl J Med 1994;331(21):1416—20.

[99] de Brito-Ashurst I, Varagunam M, Raftery MJ, Yaqoob MM. Bicarbonate supplementation slows progression of CKD and improves nutritional status. J Am Soc Nephrol 2009;20:2075—84.

[100] Cho ME, Smith DC, Branton MH, Penzak SR, Kopp JB. Pirfenidone slows renal function decline in patients with focal segmental glomerulosclerosis. Clin J Am Soc Nephrol 2007;2:906—13.

[101] Cohen AR. New advances in iron chelation therapy. Hematology Am Soc Hematol Educ Program 2006:42—7.

[102] Cohen AR, Galanello R, Piga A, De Sanctis V, Tricta F. Safety and effectiveness of long-term therapy with the oral iron chelator deferiprone. Blood 2003;102(5):1583—7.

[103] Kontoghiorghes GJ, Kolnagou A, Peng C-T, Shah SV, Aessopos A. Safety issues of iron chelation therapy in patients with normal range iron stores including thalassaemia, neurodegenerative, renal and infectious diseases. Exp Opin Drug Saf 2010;9(2):201—6.

Carbonyl Stress in Uremia

Toshio Miyata[1], *Kiyoshi Kurokawa*[2]

[1]Director, United Centers for Advanced Research and Translational Medicine (ART), Tohoku University School of Medicine: Aoba-ku, Sendai, Japan [2]National Graduate Institute for Policy Studies, Minako-ku, Tokyo, Japan

INTRODUCTION

Cardiovascular complications are important factors influencing the mortality of patients undergoing long-term dialysis treatment. Actual cardiovascular mortality in dialysis patients exceeds the expected mortality estimated on the basis of traditional risk factors, suggesting the existence of other unknown factor(s) that accelerate cardiovascular complications in uremia.

The accumulation in uremic circulation of uremic toxins or metabolites has been implicated for the development of atherosclerotic lesions in uremia. The field of uremic toxins has expanded markedly during the last decade. Most studies on uremic toxins have focused on disorders of enzymatic biochemistry. Attention has recently turned to progressive, nonenzymatic biochemistry. In this chapter, we focus on the carbonyl-amine chemistry in uremia, which results in two types of irreversible alterations of proteins: advanced glycation through the Maillard reaction and advanced lipoxidation derived from lipid peroxidation. We discuss chemistry of various reactive carbonyl compounds (RCOs) accumulating in the serum ("carbonyl stress"), their patho-biochemistry particularly in relation to atherosclerosis and, finally, the contribution of nutrition to carbonyl stress.

INCREASED AGE AND OTHER PROTEIN MODIFICATIONS

In addition to the enzymatic glycosylation, a nonenzymatic process is initiated when proteins are exposed to glucose or other carbohydrates. For example, the glycosylated hemoglobin (hemoglobin A1c, HbA_{1c}) is formed in a nonenzymatic glycation pathway by hemoglobin's exposure to plasma glucose. This nonenzymatic process, called Maillard reaction, generates first reversible Schiff base adducts, subsequently more stable Amadori rearrangement products and, eventually, the irreversible advanced glycation end products (AGEs) [1]. The role of AGEs in human pathology was initially highlighted in diabetes with hyperglycemia: AGEs levels are correlated with those of fructoselysine [2], a surrogate marker of prevailing plasma glucose concentration, and also with the severity of diabetic complications [3], a finding supporting their clinical relevance.

Of interest, AGEs accumulate in uremic patients to a much greater extent than in diabetics. Plasma levels of two well-known AGEs, pentosidine [4] and carboxymethyllysine (CML) [5], in hemodialysis patients by far exceed those in normal or diabetic subjects. Other AGE adducts also accumulate in uremia such as glyoxal-lysine dimmer (GOLD), methylglyoxal-lysine dimmer (MOLD), and imidazolone [6,7]. Among dialysis patients, diabetics and nondiabetics had similar plasma pentosidine and CML levels [4,5]. Neither pentosidine nor CML correlated with fructoselysine levels in uremic subjects. It became thus clear that factor(s) other than hyperglycemia are critical for AGE formation in uremia. The fact that over 90% of plasma pentosidine and CML are bound to albumin [4,5], suggest that its accumulation does not result from a decreased renal clearance of AGE modified proteins.

The second approach to irreversible protein modification in uremia derives from studies of lipid metabolism, especially lipid peroxidation. Proteins are modified not only by carbohydrates but also by lipids. For instance, proteins modified by malondialdehyde accumulate in plasma proteins of hemodialysis patients [5]. Malondialdehyde as well as other lipid peroxidation product modified proteins, are called the advanced lipoxidation end products (ALEs) [8].

Uremia is thus characterized by irreversible nonenzymatic protein modifications by AGEs/ALEs. In renal failure patients, lipid peroxidation and advanced glycation of plasma proteins or skin collagens increase in close relation to each other [5,9].

CARBONYL STRESS

Both AGEs and ALEs are formed by carbonyl amine chemistry between protein amino residues and reactive carbonyl compounds (RCOs) [8]. These RCOs are constantly produced during the metabolism of carbohydrates, lipids and amino acids [10−12]. Recent studies confirm the accumulation of various RCOs derived from both carbohydrates and lipids in uremic plasma and suggest that they are indeed precursors of AGEs and ALEs [8,13,14]. The prevailing plasma pentosidine level, for example, is shown to mirror the level of its RCOs precursor [13]. The accumulation in uremic plasma of various RCOs derived from either carbohydrates or lipids as well as the subsequent carbonyl modification of proteins suggest that chronic uremia may be characterized as a state of "carbonyl stress" [14] (Figure 7.1). AGEs/ALEs are therefore not markers of hyperglycemia/hyperlipemia in uremia, but represent carbonyl stress and RCO accumulation.

Two competing but not mutually exclusive hypotheses should be considered to account for the cause of carbonyl stress [14]: an increased generation or a decreased detoxification of RCOs. First, the production of RCOs is increased by oxidative stress. Several reports point to the existence of an increased oxidative stress in uremia [15]. The uremic oxidative stress is further worsened during hemodialysis treatment, i.e., activation of complement and neutrophils, and generation of reactive oxygen species. A causal role of the oxidative stress in AGE and ALE formation is supported by the correlation existing in uremic serum between pentosidine and oxidative markers, such as dehydroascorbate (oxidized ascorbate) [16] and advanced oxidation protein products (AOPP) [17].

However, recent studies have shown that several RCOs derived from nonoxidative chemistry are also raised in uremia, suggesting the simultaneous involvement of nonoxidative chemistry in the genesis of uremic carbonyl stress. For example, the levels of 3-deoxyglucosone [18] and methylglyoxal [19], and of their protein adducts, all of which are formed independently from oxidative reactions, are increased in plasma proteins of hemodialysis patients. Carbonyl stress thus represents much broader derangement in the nonenzymatic biochemistry of both oxidative and nonoxidative reactions.

The alternative hypothesis is therefore proposed: the RCOs rise in uremia is derived from a decreased removal of RCOs. RCOs are detoxified by several enzymatic pathways, such as the glyoxalase pathway [20]. Reduced glutathione (GSH) and nicotinamide adenine dinucleotide phosphate (NAD(P)H) contribute to their activity. RCOs such as methylglyoxal and glyoxal react reversibly with the thiol group of glutathione and are subsequently detoxified by glyoxalases I and II into D-lactate and glutathione. NAD(P)H also replenishes glutathione by increasing the activity of glutathione reductase. Decreased levels of glutathione and NAD(P)

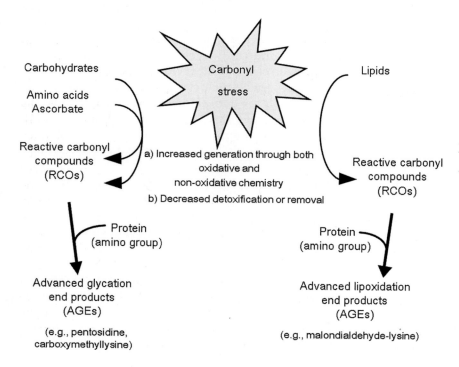

FIGURE 7.1 Carbonyl stress generated in uremia during the metabolism of carbohydrates, lipid, and amino acids. Both advanced glycation end products (AGEs) and advanced lipoxidation end products (ALEs) are formed by carbonyl amine chemistry between protein amino residues and reactive carbonyl compounds (RCOs), which are constantly produced in uremia during the metabolism of carbohydrates, lipids and amino acids either by an increased generation of RCOs through both oxidative and nonoxidative chemistry or by a decreased detoxification or removal of RCOs.

H can therefore result in augmented levels of a wide range of RCOs. It is of interest to know in this context that the glutathione concentration in red blood cells and the serum activity of glutathione-dependent enzymes are significantly reduced in uremia [21].

There has been little evidence that the RCO detoxification mechanism might influence in vivo RCO formation and therefore serum AGE levels. Of note, a patient on hemodialysis has been identified, in whom a deficiency of glyoxalase I was associated with unusually elevated levels of AGEs (pentosidine and CML) and of their precursors [22]. This patient had suffered from recurrent cardiovascular complications despite the absence of significant risk factors. Subsequently, genetic defects of the glyoxalase 1 have been identified in a subpopulation of schizophrenic patients [23]. Despite normal renal function and normoglycemia, these patients are associated with strikingly elevated levels of AGEs, implicating the glyoxalase detoxification system in the actual level of AGEs in vivo.

Mechanism that regulates carbonyl stress is another issue of interest. Superoxide dismutase (SOD) and glutathione peroxidase are antioxidant enzymes involved in the metabolism of hydrogen peroxide which accelerates carbonyl stress [12,24]. It is of note that glutathione peroxidase activities correlated inversely with pentosidine levels in uremic plasma [21]. On the other hand, the plasma extracellular-SOD levels correlated with the pentosidine levels. These data suggest a link of altered redox regulation by antioxidant enzymes to an increased carbonyl stress. Furthermore, recent observation gives a new perspective in the regulation of AGE production by linking it to the prevailing effect of nitric oxide (NO) [25]: NO effectively inhibits the pentosidine generation in vitro. It is best explained by the ability of NO to scavenge carbon-centered radicals and hydroxyl radicals, and consequently to suppress the formation of RCOs and pentosidine. NO might be therefore implicated in the atherogenic and inflammatory effects of carbonyl stress.

CLINICAL CONSEQUENCES OF CARBONYL STRESS

It remains to be demonstrated whether carbonyl stress is the passive result of long-term accumulation of vascular protein modifications or, alternatively, it plays an active role in the pathogenesis of atherosclerosis. Recent studies however support the active contribution of carbonyl stress in the atherogenesis.

The levels of AGEs in arterial tissues are higher in dialysis patients than in normal subjects [26]. Both AGEs/ALEs are detectable by means of immunohistochemical approaches in the fatty streaks and in the thickened neointima of uremic patients [27]. Available evidence suggests that plasma levels of pentosidine is an independent variable of the presence of ischemic heart diseases and hypertension [28], and of left ventricular wall thickness measured by echocardiography in hemodialysis patients [29]. Skin accumulation of AGEs using the autofluorescence reader, a recently developed noninvasive device, showed that the AGE accumulation is an important predictor for arterial stiffening in ESRD subjects [30].

In vitro, AGE and ALE modified proteins initiate a range of cellular responses [31–35], including stimulation of monocyte chemotaxis and apoptosis, secretion of inflammatory cytokines from macrophages, proliferation of vascular smooth muscle cells, stimulation of platelet aggregation, and of vascular endothelial growth factor (VEGF) production from endothelial cells. Independently of their AGE and ALE mediated effects, RCOs also interfere with various cellular functions and induce not only structural but also functional alterations of proteins. For example, exposure in vitro of cultured mesothelial and endothelial cells to methylglyoxal increases mRNA and protein synthesis of VEGF [36]. Repeated intraperitoneal loads of methylglyoxal, given to rats, also increase in vivo the peritoneal membrane expression of VEGF [36]. Noteworthy in this context is the demonstration that, both in long-term peritoneal dialysis patients and in chronic uremic rat model [36,37], an increasing staining for AGEs, CML and pentosidine, is detected in peritoneal arterial walls, together with an augmented VEGF and basic fibroblast growth factor (FGF2) expression.

There are two major pathways, direct and indirect, through which carbonyl stress is sensed by cells and triggers a cascade of intracellular signal transduction. In the indirect pathway, the RCOs first interact with proteins or lipids in the physiological environment surrounding the cells, which then undergo nonenzymatic glycation and lipoxidation resulting in the production of AGEs and ALEs. They bind with the receptor(s) on cell surfaces, e.g., RAGE, thereby initiating intracellular signal transduction [38]. By contrast, the direct pathway works before generation of AGEs and ALEs. The RCOs directly attack target molecules on cell surfaces or inside the cells, which initiate the subsequent signal transduction [39–43]. For example, glyoxal and methylglyoxal possess two reactive carbonyl groups to make protein aggregates by crosslinking, which may amplify the signals for tyrosine phosphorylation of cellular proteins [39]. In another model, the binding of 4-hydroxynonenal, a RCO generated during lipid peroxidation, with epidermal growth factor receptor (EGFR) induces its clustering on the cell surface, thereby activating the mitogen activated protein (MAP) family kinases [40].

In vascular lesions, an increased oxidative stress, together with altered redox regulation and decreased RCO detoxification, may increase carbonyl stress, exacerbate endothelial dysfunction and, eventually, lead to the development of atherosclerosis.

The consequences of carbonyl stress have also been implicated in other complications associated with uremia or long-term dialysis. First, renal failure is associated with resistance to the action of calcitriol (1.25 dihydroxivitamin D) [44], which is partly attributed to the inhibition by unknown uremic toxins of the interaction between the vitamin D receptor and vitamin D response elements [45]. Patel and coworkers [46] demonstrated that RCOs capable of Schiff base formation with lysine residues of the vitamin D receptor inhibit its interaction with the vitamin D response element. Second, dialysis related amyloidosis is a serious bone and joint destruction associated with uremia [47]. Immunohistochemical and chemical analyses have indicated that β2-microglobulin amyloid deposits are modified by carbonyl stress [48–50]. Third, the major problem associated with long-term peritoneal dialysis is the progressive deterioration of the peritoneal membrane structure and function, i.e., ultrafiltration failure, which curtails its use in approximately 50 % of patients within 5 years [51]. Recent studies have cast a new light on its molecular mechanism [52]. During peritoneal dialysis, RCOs resulting both from glucose PD fluid and from uremic circulation enter the peritoneum [53], modify the peritoneal membrane [54], and initiate a number of cellular responses, leading to angiogenesis and vasodilation. The latter may increase the permeability for small solutes and glucose, stimulate glucose reabsorption, and result in faster than normal dissipation of the osmotic gradient across the peritoneal membrane with an eventual loss of ultrafiltration [52].

NUTRITION AND CARBONYL STRESS

The advanced glycation of proteins have been initially unravelled by food and nutrition biochemists. Various kinds of food indeed contain a significant amount of CML and pentosidine [55,56]. Previous studies demonstrated that, although the modification of proteins with AGEs reduces the digestibility of proteins either by gaining resistance to the enzymatic digestion of proteases or by inhibiting digestive enzyme activity [56], a significant proportion of dietary AGEs are absorbed by the gastrointestinal tract into the circulation [57,58]. He et al. demonstrated that ~10% of ingested AGE-modified ovalbumin was absorbed into the rat circulation [58]. Of particular interest is the demonstration of a relationship between

renal function and exogenous or food derived AGE levels in the serum [57]. Synthesized pentosidine was given orally to both normal and uremic rats, and their kinetics in the circulation was investigated. In normal rats, plasma pentosidine rose slightly and transiently to become undetectable at 6 h. By contrast, in rats with 6/7 nephrectomy, plasma pentosidine peaked at 3 h and fell thereafter (calculated biological half-life of 4.08 ± 1.68 h). In bilaterally nephrectomized rats, plasma pentosidine level peaked at 12 h and decreased subsequently (calculated biological half-life of 47.3 ± 10.2 h). The pathological contribution of exogenous or food derived AGEs still remains unknown.

Several lines of evidence have implicated the dietary contribution to the in vivo AGE accumulation. Dietary calorie restriction reduces the accumulation of tissue AGEs without affecting survival of the animals [59,60]. Of note is the recent report by Sell et al. that longitudinal determination of the rates of pentosidine and CML formation predicts the individual longevity in mice, and that calorie restriction retard this rate as compared to ad libitum feeding [61]. Recent study by Uribarri et al. demonstrated that dietary AGEs contribute significantly to the elevated plasma AGE levels in uremic patients [62]. More studies are required to elucidate the contribution of nutrition to the pathophysiology of carbonyl stress and to the eventual cardiovascular associated mortality.

References

[1] Brownlee M, Cerami A, Vlassara H. Advanced glycosylation end products in tissue and the biochemical basis of diabetic complications. N Engl J Med 1988;318:1315–21.

[2] Dyer DG, Dunn JA, Thorpe SR, et al. Accumulation of Maillard reaction products in skin collagen in diabetes and aging. J Clin Invest 1993;91:2463–9.

[3] McCance DR, Dyer DG, Dunn JA, et al. Maillard reaction products and their relation to complications in insulin-dependent diabetes mellitus. J Clin Invest 1993;91:2470–8.

[4] Miyata T, Ueda Y, Shinzato T, et al. Accumulation of albumin-linked and free-form pentosidine in the circulation of uremic patients with end-stage renal failure: Renal implications in the pathophysiology of pentosidine. J Am Soc Nephrol 1996; 7:1198–206.

[5] Miyata T, Fu MX, Kurokawa K, et al. Autoxidation products of both carbohydrates and lipids are increased in uremic plasma: Is there oxidative stress in uremia? Kidney Int 1998;54:1290–5.

[6] Odani H, Shinzato T, Usami J, et al. Imidazolium crosslinks derived from reaction of lysine with glyoxal and methylglyoxal are increased in serum proteins of uremic patients: Evidence for increased oxidative stress in uremia. FEBS Lett 1998;427:381–5.

[7] Takayama F, Aoyama I, Tsukushi S, et al. Immunohistochemical detection of imidazolone and Nε-(carboxymethyl)lysine in aortas of hemodialysis patients. Cell Mol Biol 1998;44:1101–9.

[8] Miyata T, van Ypersele de Strihou C, Kurokawa Kiyoshi, et al. Alterations in non-enzymatic biochemistry in uremia: Origin

and significance of "carbonyl stress" in long-term uremic complications. Kidney Int 1999;55:389–99.

[9] Meng J, Sakata N, Imanaga Y, et al. Evidence for a link between glycoxidation and lipoperoxidation in patients with chronic renal failure. Clin Nephrol 1999;51:280–9.

[10] Wells-Knecht KJ, Zyzak DV, Litchfield JE, et al. Mechanism of autoxidative glycosylation: Identification of glyoxal and arabinose as intermediates in the autoxidative modification of protein by glucose. Biochemistry 1995;34:3702–9.

[11] Esterbauer H, Schuer RJ, Zollner H. Chemistry and biochemistry of 4-hydroxynonenal, malondialdehyde and related aldehyde. Free Radic Biol Med 1991;11:81–128.

[12] Anderson MM, Hazen SL, Hsu FF, et al. Human neutrophils employ the myeloperoxidase-hydrogen peroxide-chloride system to convert hydroxy-amino acids into glycolaldehyde, 2-hydroxypropanol, and acrolein: a mechanism for the generation of highly reactive α-hydroxy and α, β-unsaturated aldehydes by phagocytes at sites of inflammation. J Clin Invest 1997; 99:424–32.

[13] Miyata T, Ueda Y, Yamada Y, et al. Accumulation of carbonyls accelerate the formation of pentosidine, an advanced glycation end product. J Am Soc Nephrol 1998;9:2349–56.

[14] Miyata T, Kurokawa K, van Ypersele de Strihou C. Advanced glycation and lipoxidation end products: Role of reactive carbonyl compounds generated during carbohydrate and lipid metabolism. J Am Soc Nephrol 2000;11:1744–52.

[15] Miyata T, Maeda K, Kurokawa K, et al. Oxidation conspires with glycation to create noxious advanced glycation end products in renal failure. Nephrol Dial Transplant 1997;12:255–8.

[16] Miyata T, Wada Y, Cai Z, et al. Implication of an increased oxidative stress in the formation of advanced glycation end products in patients with end-stage renal failure. Kidney Int 1997;51:1170–81.

[17] Witko-Sarsat V, Friedlander M, Capeillere-Blandin C, et al. Advanced oxidation protein products as a novel marker of oxidative stress in uremia. Kidney Int 1996;49:1304–13.

[18] Niwa T, Takeda N, Miyazaki T, et al. Elevated serum levels of 3 deoxyglucosone, a potent protein-cross-linking intermediate of the maillard reaction, in uremic patients. Nephron 1995; 69:438–43.

[19] Odani H, Shinzato H, Matsumoto Y, et al. Increase in three a, β-dicarbonyl compound levels in human uremic plasma: Specific in vivo determination of intermediates in advanced maillard reaction. Biochem Biophys Res Commun 1999;256:89–93.

[20] Thornalley PJ. Advanced glycation and development of diabetic complications: Unifying the involvement of glucose, methylglyoxal and oxidative stress. Endocrinol Metab 1996; 3:149–66.

[21] Ueda Y, Miyata T, Hashimoto T, et al. Implication of altered redox regulation by antioxidant enzymes in the increased plasma pentosidine, an advanced glycation end product, in uremia. Biochem Biophys Res Commun 1998;245:785–90.

[22] Miyata T, van Ypersele de Strihou C, Imasawa T, et al. Glyoxalase I deficiency is associated with an unusual level of advanced glycation end products in a hemodialysis patient. Kidney Int 2001;60:2351–9.

[23] Arai M, Yuzawa H, Nohara I, et al. Enhanced carbonyl stress in a subpopulation of schizophrenia. Arch Gen Psychiatry 2010; 67:589–97.

[24] Nagai R, Ikeda K, Higashi T, et al. Hydroxyl radical mediates N-epsilon-(carboxymethyl)lysine formation from Amadori products. Biochem Biophys Res Commun 1997;234:167–72.

[25] Asahi K, Ichimori K, Nakazawa H, et al. Nitric oxide inhibits the formation of advanced glycation and products. Kidney Int 2000;58:1780–7.

[26] Makita Z, Radoff S, Rayfield EJ, et al. Advanced glycosylation end products in patients with diabetic nephropathy. N Engl J Med 1991;325:836–42.

[27] Miyata T, Ishikawa S, Asahi K, et al. 2-Isopropylidenehydrazono-4-oxo-thiazolidin-5ylacetanilide (OPB-9195) inhibits the neointima proliferation of rat carotid artery following balloon injury: Role of glycoxidation and lipoxidation reactions in vascular tissue damage. FEBS Letter 1999;445:202–6.

[28] Sugiyama S, Miyata T, Ueda Y, et al. Plasma level of pentosidine, an advanced glycation end product, in diabetic patients. J Am Soc Nephrol 1998;9:1681–8.

[29] Zoccali C, Mallamaci F, Asahia K, et al. Pentosidine, carotid atherosclerosis and alterations in left ventricular geometry in hemodialysis patients. J Nephrol 2001;14:293–8.

[30] Ueno H, Koyama H, Tanaka S, et al. Skin autofluorescence, a marker for advanced glycation end product accumulation, is associated with arterial stiffness in patients with end-stage renal disease. Metabolism 2008;57:1452–7.

[31] Miyata T, Inagi R, Iida Y, et al. Involvement of β2-microglobulin modified with advanced glycation end products in the pathogenesis of hemodialysis-associated amyloidosis: Induction of human monocyte chemotaxis and macrophage secretion of tumor necrosis factor-a and interleukin 1. J Clin Invest 1994; 93:521–8.

[32] Miyata T, Hori O, Zhang JH, et al. The receptor for advanced glycation endproducts mediates the interaction of AGE-β2-microglobulin with human mononuclear phagocytes via an oxidant-sensitive pathway: Implication for the pathogenesis of dialysis-related amyloidosis. J Clin Invest 1997; 98:1088–94.

[33] Hou FF, Miyata T, Boyce J, et al. β2-Microglobulin modified with advanced glycation end products delays monocyte apoptosis and induces differentiation into macrophage-like cells. Kidney Int 2001;59:990–1002.

[34] Miyata T, Iida Y, Wada Y, et al. Monocyte/macrophage response to β2-microglobulin modified with advanced glycation end products. Kidney Int 1996;49:538–50.

[35] Miyata T, Notoya K, Yoshida K, et al. Advanced glycation end products enhance osteoclast-induced bone resorption in cultured mouse unfractionated bone cells and in rats implanted with devitalized bone particles. J Am Soc Nephrol 1997;8: 260–70.

[36] Inagi R, Miyata T, Yamamoto T, et al. Glucose degradation product methylglyoxal enhances the production of vascular endothelial growth factor in peritoneal cells: Role in the pathogenesis of peritoneal membrane dysfunction in peritoneal dialysis. FEBS Lett 1999;463:260–4.

[37] Combet S, Miyata T, Moulin P, et al. Vascular proliferation and enhanced expression of endothelial nitric oxide synthase in human peritoneum exposed to long-term peritoneal dialysis. J Am Soc Nephrol 2000;11:717–28.

[38] Yan SD, Schmidt AM, Anderson GM, et al. Enhanced cellular oxidant stress by the interaction of advanced glycation end products with their receptors/binding proteins. J Biol Chem 1994;269:9889–97.

[39] Ahkand AA, Kato M, Suzuki H, et al. Carbonyl compounds cross-link cellular proteins and activate protein-tyrosine kinase p60[c-src]. J Cellular Biochemistry 1999;72:1–7.

[40] Liu W, Ahkand AA, Kato M, et al. 4-Hydroxynonenal triggers an epidermal growth factor receptor-linked signal pathway for growth inhibition. J Cell Sci 1999;112:2409–17.

[41] Liu W, Kato M, Akhand AA, et al. 4-Hydroxynonenal induces a cellular redox-related activation of the caspase cascade for apoptotic cell death. J Cell Sci 2000;113: 635–41.

[42] Du J, Suzuki H, Nagase F, et al. Methylglyoxal induces apoptosis in Jurkat leukemia T-cells by activating c-Jun N-terminal kinase. J Cell Biochem 2000;77:333–44.

[43] Ahkand AA, Hossain K, Mitsui H, et al. Glyoxal and methylglyoxal trigger distinct signals for MAP family kinases and caspase activation in human endothelial cells. Free Radic Biol Med 2001;31:20–30.

[44] Fukagawa M, Kaname S, Igarashi T, et al. Regulation of parathyroid hormone synthesis in chronic renal failure in rats. Kidney Int 1991;39:874–81.

[45] Patel SR, Ke HQ, Vanholder R, et al. Inhibition of calcitriol receptor binding to vitamin D response elements by uremic toxins. J Clin Invest 1995;96:50–9.

[46] Patel SR, Xu Y, Koenig RJ, et al. Effect of glyoxylate on the function of the calcitriol receptor and vitamin D metabolism. Kidney Int 1997;52:39–44.

[47] Miyata T, Jadoul M, Kurokawa K, et al. β2-Microglobulin in renal disease. J Am Soc Nephrol 1998;9:1723–35.

[48] Miyata T, Oda O, Inagi R, et al. β2-Microglobulin modified with advanced glycation end products is a major component of hemodialysis-associated amyloidosis. J Clin Invest 1993;92:1243–52.

[49] Miyata T, Inagi R, Wada Y, et al. Glycation of human β2-microglobulin in patients with hemodialysis-associated amyloidosis: Identification of the glycated sites. Biochemistry 1994;33:12215–21.

[50] Niwa T, Miyazaki S, Katsuzaki T, et al. Immunohistochemical detection of advanced glycation end products in dialysis-related amyloidosis. Kidney Int 1995;48:771–8.

[51] Krediet RT. The peritoneal membrane in chronic peritoneal dialysis. Kidney Int 1999;55:341–56.

[52] Miyata T, Devuyst O, Kurokawa K, et al. Toward better dialysis compatibility: advances in the biochemistry and pathophysiology of the peritoneal membranes. Kidney Int 2002;61:375–86.

[53] Miyata T, Kurokawa K, van Ypersele de Strihou C. Advanced glycation and lipoxidation end products: Role of reactive carbonyl compounds generated during carbohydrate and lipid metabolism. J Am Soc Nephrol 2000;11:1744–52.

[54] Nakayama M, Kawaguchi Y, Yamada K, et al. Immunohistochemical detection of advanced glycosylation end products in the peritoneum and its possible pathophysiological role in CAPD. Kidney Int 1997;51:182–6.

[55] Erbersdobler HF. Protein reactions during food processing and storage their relevance to human nutrition. Bibl Nutr Dieta 1989;43:140–55.

[56] O'Brien J, Morrissey PA. Nutritional and toxocological aspects of the Maillard browning reaction in foods. Crit Rev Food Sci Nutr 1989;28:211–48.

[57] Miyata T, Ueda Y, Horie K, et al. Renal catabolism of advanced glycation end products: the fate of pentosidine. Kidney Int 1998;53:416–22.

[58] He C, Sabol J, Mitsuhashi T, et al. Inhibition of reactive products by aminoguanidine facilitates renal clearance and reduces tissue sequestration. Diabetes 1999;48:1308–15.

[59] Lingelbach LB, Mitchell AE, Rucker RB, et al. Accumulation of advanced glycation endproducts in aging male Fischer 344 rats during long-term feeding of various dietary carbohydrates. Nutrient Metabolism 2000;130:1247–55.

[60] Teillet L, Verbeke P, Gouraud S, et al. Food restriction prevents advanced glycation end product accumulation and retards kidney aging in lean rats. J Am Son Nephrol 2000;11:1488–97.

[61] Sell DR, Kleinman NR, Monnier VM. Longitudinal determination of skin collagen glycation and glycoxidation rats predicts early death in C57BL/6NNIA mice. FASEB J 2000;14:146–56.

[62] Uribarri J, Peppa M, Cai W, et al. Restriction of dietary glycotoxins reduces excessive advanced glycation end products in renal failure patients. J Am Soc Nephrol 2003;14:728–31.

Effect of Acidemia and Alkalemia on Nutrition and Metabolism

James L. Bailey[1], Harold A. Franch[1,2]

[1]Renal Division, Department of Medicine, Emory University School of Medicine, Atlanta, GA, USA

[2]Research Service, Atlanta Veterans Affairs Medical Center, Decatur, GA, USA

INTRODUCTION

When considering what properties a uremic toxin must have, the ability to cause weight loss, muscle wasting and bone loss are naturally at the top of the list. Loss of lean body mass and bone minerals are hallmarks of uremia, and epidemiologic data suggest that nutritional markers indicating low body mass index or decreased skeletal muscle mass correlate strongly with mortality among dialysis patients [1,2]. Although hydrogen ion is only one of many toxins that contributes to the complications of uremia, it is an established toxin with a demonstrated ability to cause many adverse effects including the promotion of protein catabolism [3]. Treatment of acidemia is associated with improved clinical outcomes [3]. The western diet, rich in acid-producing protein but low in base-producing fruit and vegetables, will produce acidosis whenever renal acid secretion is impaired (e.g., chronic kidney disease (CKD)). Because the body's response to a net acid diet is similar to its response to frank acidemia, interest in the effects of acidemia extend beyond nephrology. Studies in older individuals have shown that supplementing a net acid diet with base is anabolic for both bone and muscle [4,5]. In fact, alkali supplements are considered legal drugs for improvement of athletic performance [6]. In this chapter, we will examine the acute and chronic effects of metabolic acidosis and alkalosis with a focus on the relationship between the chronic response to acidemia and the catabolic effects on bone and muscle. Finally, we will examine the benefits and risks of correction of acidemia on protein and bone metabolism. The role of bicarbonate therapy for slowing progression of CKD is discussed in Chapter 18.

ACUTE RESPONSES TO ACIDOSIS AND ALKALOSIS

Acutely, acidosis and alkalosis affect physiology by donating or accepting protons with the carboxylic acid side chains of proteins providing the source of protons. The change in charge of these side chains alters the function, binding, folding and stability of enzymes, receptors, and transport proteins leading to characteristic acute responses. The body tolerates acute metabolic acidemia readily [7]. For example, the blood pH falls below 7.2 during strenuous exercise without immediate adverse effects. In some ways, acute acidemia in the arterial blood pH 7.2–7.4 range helps the body during exercise or acute illness. Cardiac index generally rises when the pH is reduced but is above 7.2 because the release of catecholamines is mildly stimulated by central sensing mechanisms and because vasodilation increases [8]. Increased tissue oxygen delivery occurs due to this rise in cardiac index, the Bohr effect (shifting oxygen from hemoglobin to tissues), and also the stimulation of the respiratory drive [9]. Because of these effects, recent critical care guidelines for patients with shock and lactic acidosis do not recommend correction of acidosis if the arterial blood pH is above 7.15 [10]. The cardiovascular consequences of more severe acute acidemia are clear from animal studies [7]. Part of the vasodilator response to acidemia is due to reduced effectiveness of catecholamine receptor signaling [11]. Below an arterial pH 7.1, the effects of catecholamine resistance surpass the consequences of the elevation in plasma catecholamines, and cardiac index falls. The incidence of cardiac arrhythmias also rises with severe acidemia, and the arrhythmias are pronounced below a pH of 6.9 [12]. Studies show numerous defects in immune function when the pH is below 6.9, and there is a severe compromise in the responses to infection [13,14]. However, milder acidemia may actually benefit some aspects of immune function: an arterial pH above 7.0 seems to improve certain aspects of immune function, including macrophage cytokine release in response to nitric oxide, while a pH of 6.5 suppresses it [13]. In extremely strenuous competitive sport, there is concern about the adverse effects on exercise performance if the pH falls too low, but whether supplementation with alkali immediately before exercise will improve performance remains unproven.

In contrast, acute metabolic alkalemia appears to be dangerous in the acutely ill medical or surgical patient, and the risk of death rises with increasing arterial blood pH [15,16]. Because metabolic alkalosis is often engendered by life threatening conditions (e.g., heart failure, volume depletion), it is not clear whether the increase in mortality is due to the acute alkalosis itself or to the underlying condition causing the alkalosis. Certainly, metabolic alkalemia decreases tissue oxygen delivery via vasoconstriction and the Bohr effect. Decreased oxygen delivery due to metabolic alkalemia may also contribute to decreased cerebral blood flow resulting in lethargy, confusion and worsening heart failure. In severe cases, coma and seizures may result. The respiratory center can be depressed and alveolar ventilation decreased. However, the most feared complications of acute alkalemia are due to the lowering of ionized calcium levels as a consequence of increased albumin binding [17]. Neuromuscular irritability, which is manifested by muscle twitching, spasm and tetany, is associated with alkalemia and is most likely calcium related. An alkaline pH has been shown to decrease aldosterone release in response to angiotensin II. Myocardial contractility is blunted as is the inotropic response to norepinephrine. As with severe acidemia, arrythmias are also increased. When the pH is greater than 7.75, the fall in ionized calcium is life threatening, and cardiac arrest commonly occurs.

COMPARING EFFECTS OF ACIDEMIA TO THOSE OF STARVATION

The body does not tolerate even small degrees of chronic acidemia without a catabolic response. In fact, epidemiologic studies suggest that consumption of a net acid diet without clinical metabolic acidosis is associated with some of the same catabolic effects. As we will discuss below, acidemia stimulates a variety of specific endocrine and muscle responses that enhance muscle and bone catabolism. Given the strength and sensitivity of the catabolic response to acidemia or acid load, it is worth risking the teleological question: what

is the benefit of this response? Most obviously, the catabolic response to chronic acidemia helps drive the buffering and excretion of excess hydrogen ions [18]. This response is consistent with a net acid diet producing many of the same effects as frank acidemia. The calcium carbonate apatite of bone directly dissolves with acid and hormonal responses accelerate this buffering process. The liberation of amino acids from muscle allows for increased liver glutamine production and net acid secretion in the form of ammonia.

A second benefit of the response to acidemia comes from the role of acidosis from ketone formation in the catabolic response to starvation [19,20] (Figure 8.1). As glycogen stores are depleted during starvation, insulin deficiency triggers a transition in metabolism to ketone body formation [20,21]. The acid formed from the ketone bodies leads to changes in intracellular energy, redox sensing systems and intracellular insulin signaling that contribute to a reduction in basal metabolic rate (BMR) [20,22]. Phosphate from bone and amino acids from solid organs and muscle maintain serum phosphate and amino acid levels. In the absence of ketosis, amino acids are used sparingly for energy; and visceral organs,

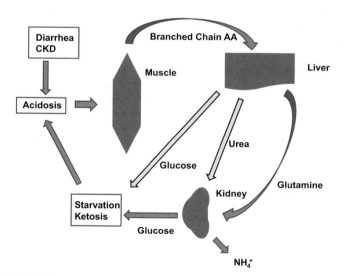

FIGURE 8.1 Starvation and acidemia alter gluconeogenesis from amino acids. In the fed state, excess amino acids are converted to glucose via the urea cycle (yellow). Urea formation has an energetic cost of ~35% of the energy equivalent in the glucose formed. In starvation (blue), ketone formation leads to a mild acidemia enhancing the release of branched chain amino acids from muscle. During acidemia, the liver preferentially converts branched chain amino acids to glutamine which is deaminated in the kidney to produce ammonium and glucose. Glucose production from glutamine is much more energetically favorable than the glucose generated during urea synthesis in the urea cycle making the former process more adaptive in starvation. Metabolic acidemia from other causes activates the same pathways leading to excretion of hydrogen ions via ammonium at the cost of losing amino acids and proteins. This figure is reproduced in color in the color plate section.

not muscle, provide the bulk of the amino acids. Burning amino acids for energy is energetically unfavorable due to the high metabolic cost of urea formation [23]. In contrast, acidity from ketosis stimulates glucose formation from renal deamination of glutamine. Glucose derived from glutamine is energetically favorable because the nitrogen from glutamine is directly secreted by the kidney in the form of ammonium without further metabolism [24]. Thus, the integrated catabolic response to academia allows energy conservation in the production of glucose from branched chain amino acids in starvation.

ENDOCRINE RESPONSES TO ACIDEMIA

Much attention has been given to acid-induced changes in the function of endocrine organs, including the release of cortisol, insulin, thyroxin, insulin-like growth factor (IGF-I), aldosterone, and parathyroid hormone (PTH). In many cases, activation of endocrine responses enhances the ability of bone to buffer or a normal kidney to excrete acid, but the same responses can cause catabolism and contribute to uremic symptoms in the context of renal failure [25]. In addition, other uremic toxins can interact with endocrine mediators. In many cases, acidemia has an additive effect on these endocrine responses. The chronic buffering of acid by bone is also facilitated by a multitude of hormonal changes.

Acidemia increases circulating adrenal cortical hormones [26]. Plasma adrenocorticotropin (ACTH) levels rise after an infusion of inorganic acids, and increased ACTH stimulates the production of both glucocorticoids and aldosterone [27]. There may also be a direct effect of low pH on the adrenal gland to stimulate the release of aldosterone, a response that depends on an increase in intracellular calcium [28]. Since both cortisol and aldosterone increase renal acid excretion in subjects with normal renal function [29,30], the rise in ACTH can be seen as a homeostatic mechanism that acts to raise net acid excretion. Acidemia also appears to lower 11-β hydroxysteroid dehydrogenase activity in aldosterone sensitive cells in the kidney. This prevents destruction of cortisol and allows it to more readily activate the aldosterone receptor [31]. Interestingly, acidemia is not the only cause of elevated glucocorticoid levels in uremia, since adding bicarbonate to the diet to block the development of acidosis in rats with CRF does not normalize glucocorticoid production [32]. This uremia-associated stimulation of glucocorticoid production is a crucial factor that induces abnormalities of calcium and protein metabolism (see below) [33]. Aldosterone may also play a role in uremic complications. With a reduction in glomerular filtration rate,

increases in plasma levels of both endothelin and aldosterone have been reported in human subjects. These increases are ameliorated with the addition of alkali [34]. Reports indicating that spironolactone and eplerenone can help prevent mortality in patients with congestive heart failure suggest that aldosterone might exacerbate some of the cardiovascular complications seen in kidney failure [35]. These and other studies suggest that correction of metabolic acidosis and hydrogen ion retention slows progression of renal disease [36–38]; that adrenal hormones may be involved in this response is discussed in Chapter 18. Although acidemia stimulates production of catecholamines, glucocorticoids, aldosterone, and endothelin, supplementation of the diet of mildly hypertensive patients without kidney disease with potassium chloride is as equally effective at lowering blood pressure as potassium bicarbonate [39]. One possible interpretation of this result is that a net acid diet is not a sufficiently potent stimulant of these mediators to induce a clinically measurable increase in blood pressure in humans with normal renal function.

Acidemia suppresses the clinical actions and cellular signaling stimulated by both insulin and insulin like growth factor-1 (IGF-I) in different ways. Acidemia does not alter islet cell secretion of insulin, but does induce resistance to insulin action in peripheral tissues; reversal of acidemia improves the sensitivity of glucose metabolism to insulin [40]. In contrast, acidemia reduces growth hormone release from the pituitary gland, and this leads to lower levels of IGF-I production.

Metabolic acidemia also suppresses plasma adiponectin levels in subjects ingesting oral ammonium chloride. This is important because adiponectin enhances insulin sensitivity and enhances anti-atherogenic and anti-inflammatory properties [41]. Beyond its suppressive effect on adiponectin, acidemia decreases the elevated plasma leptin levels associated with chronic kidney disease [42]. Taken together, these factors promote protein catabolism, decrease protein synthesis and promote negative nitrogen balance. In the 1999–2000 and 2001–2002 National Health and Nutrition Examination Surveys, insulin sensitivity was estimated by an index based on fasting insulin and triglyceride levels [43]. Lower serum bicarbonate levels and a higher anion gap were found to be independently associated with insulin resistance. However, insulin sensitivity was not measurably improved by bicarbonate supplementation in healthy older subjects despite an increase in muscle strength [44,45]. Again it is possible that a net acid diet is insufficient to induce clinically measurable insulin resistance; frank acidemia may be necessary. Further studies will be needed to define the clinical importance of net acid diets versus frank acidemia on insulin resistance and its synergy with other factors such as obesity, glucocorticoids and uremia.

The response to an infusion of physiological concentrations of growth hormone is very mildly impaired in acidemia, but larger concentrations may completely reverse the effects of acidemia. Two factors appear to blunt the response to administered growth hormone: first, the density of IGF-I receptors in muscle is lowered by acidemia; and second there is a defect in the signaling that results from the binding of IGF-I [46–48]. IGF-I resistance in uremia does not improve with correction of acidemia suggesting that separate mechanisms (possibly including corticosteroids) play a role in IGF-I resistance [49,50]. Administration of super-physiological doses of growth hormone reduces nitrogen losses [51]. IGF-I (like insulin) is a major determinant of amino acid release from skeletal muscle, although part of the beneficial response on nitrogen balance may involve improvement in plasma cortisol and/or aldosterone levels [52]. These studies point out how complex interactions occurring between different endocrine mediators can work together to either exacerbate or relieve the effects of acidemia. Abnormalities in insulin and IGF-I physiology also play an important role in the growth suppression seen in children with acidemia [53].

Acidemia increases the sensitivity of the parathyroid gland to changes in ionized calcium and also stimulates release of parathyroid hormone (PTH) [54]. Parathyroid hormone has long been known to decrease renal net acid secretion by inhibiting renal tubular bicarbonate reabsorption [55]. In patients with normal renal function, acidemia decreases proximal tubular phosphate reabsorption resulting in hypophosphatemia, and this causes a secondary stimulation of 1,25-dihydroxyvitamin D production. The resulting rise in the activity of vitamin D counteracts the direct effects of acidemia on the parathyroid, so that serum PTH concentrations are usually unchanged or even fall slightly with acidemia [56]. In patients with end-stage renal disease, acidemia has almost no effect on phosphate excretion or 1,25 vitamin D production because of the loss of kidney function. Instead, acidemia increases PTH by a direct effect on the parathyroid glands [54,57]. Importantly, correction of acidemia in maintenance hemodialysis patients who have secondary hyperparathyroidism improves the ability of calcium to suppress the parathyroid gland's release of PTH [54]. In patients with moderate chronic kidney disease, correction of metabolic acidemia with sodium bicarbonate has been shown to attenuate the rise in PTH and serum urea nitrogen levels [58].

Similar to uremia, acidemia lowers serum levels of the thyroid hormones, free T3 and T4, and may slightly raise reverse T3 [59,60]. Notwithstanding the altered thyroid function tests, uremic patients are usually clinically euthyroid. Resistance to the effects of TSH occurs within the thyroid gland and is associated with elevated levels of TSH and thyroid releasing hormone. That these alterations in thyroid function are sensitive to acidemia is underscored by their correction with alkali [61]. While the clinical significance of this mild hypothyroid-like response has not been demonstrated in acidemia, it is postulated to play a counterregulatory role minimizing loss of muscle in uremia [62]. There is little or no effect in acidemia of the altered thyroid function on bone. Thus, this response appears to be an exception to the overall paradigm of hormonal alterations contributing to acid-induced catabolism.

CALCIUM METABOLISM

Acids are initially buffered by the bicarbonate system followed by buffering by proteins and bone (Table 8.1). Bone will buffer acid directly, because hydrogen ion exchanges with sodium and potassium in bone mineral. This exchange does not result in an equivalent loss of calcium for every hydrogen ion absorbed [64]. Most acids also interact with the calcium carbonate in bone and release the bound calcium [65]. In respiratory acidosis, the high carbonate concentration in blood (derived from CO_2) prevents bone resorption by this mechanism. Metabolic acidemia also stimulates bone-reabsorbing osteoclasts while simultaneously suppressing the activity of the bone-stimulating osteoblasts [66].

TABLE 8.1   Catabolic Effects of Chronic Metabolic Acidemia on Calcium and Protein Metabolism

---

1. DISSOLUTION OF BONE

a. Direct effect of acid on bone mineral content
b. Increased osteoclast and decreased osteoblast activity
c. Increased plasma glucocorticoids
d. Increased serum parathyroid hormone (acidemia induced increased PTH has clinically apparent adverse effects only in patients with kidney failure)
e. Decreased plasma insulin-like growth factor-I

2. HYPERCALCIURIA AND HYPERPHOSPHATURIA LEADING TO PHOSPHATE AND CALCIUM WASTING

a. Increased filtered load of calcium and phosphorous
b. Decreased tubular reabsorption of calcium and phosphorous

3. PROTEIN LOSS AND MUSCLE WASTING

a. Activation of the ubiquitin-proteasome proteolytic system
  (i) Direct effects of low arterial blood pH
  (ii) Increased plasma glucocorticoids
  (iii) Insulin resistance in non-hepatic organs
b. Activation of branched-chain ketoacid dehydrogenase
  (i) Direct effect of low arterial blood pH
  (ii) Increased plasma glucocorticoids
c. Increased hepatic glutamine synthesis and renal glutamine extraction

The proliferation of osteoblasts and the formation of bone matrix proteins are suppressed at a transcriptional level [57]. This direct effect of acidemia on bone demineralization appears to occur by different mechanisms than those induced by cortisol, PTH, or IGF-I and are additive to those effects. For example, parathyroidectomy does not block the effects of acidemia on bone [57].

In patients who have normal renal function, the mobilization of calcium from bone through the effect of acidemia leads to an increase in renal calcium excretion. If there is a rise in serum calcium resulting from the mobilization of bone calcium, the amount of calcium filtered at the glomerulus increases, but the major effect of acidemia on renal calcium handling is glucocorticoid inhibition of tubular calcium reabsorption. This occurs independently of the level of filtered calcium [18]. Thus, acidemia contributes directly to negative calcium balance by causing dissolution of bone and by raising renal calcium losses. An increased incidence of nephrolithiasis occurs which is compounded by increased proximal tubular reabsorption of citrate [18,67,68]. In patients undergoing radical or partial nephrectomy, preoperative metabolic acidemia has been associated with a higher incidence of nephrolithiasis, osteoporosis and fractures [69].

In patients with CKD and ESRD, the excess calcium which is mobilized from bone in the setting of acidemia remains in the extracellular space and raises the theoretical possibility of ectopic calcification. However, it has long been known that metabolic alkalemia rather than acidemia predisposes to ectopic calcification in uremia [70]. In rats with kidney failure given vitamin D, metabolic acidemia inhibits soft-tissue calcification. In the absence of metabolic acidemia, vitamin D administration to rats with a similar degree of renal failure results in significant calcification in the aorta, stomach and kidney, and higher mortality results [71]. Studies in cultured rat aortas suggest that the decrease in calcium phosphate solubility with alkaline pH, and not secondary hormonal changes, augments vascular calcification [72]. In vivo, the decrease in ionized calcium with alkalemia partly counters the lower solubility of calcium phosphate as pH rises. In normal individuals, metabolic alkalosis is not associated with ectopic calcification, despite a decrease in urinary calcium excretion [73]. The calcium-alkali syndrome (formerly called milk alkali syndrome) results when alkalemia is combined with excessive calcium intake [74,75]. Despite the reduction in the urinary fractional excretion of calcium and the stimulation of citrate excretion in this syndrome, the rise in filtered load of calcium and high urinary pH can lead to nephrocalcinosis and nephrolithiasis. In both CKD and hypercalcemic individuals with normal renal function, alkalemia appears to be a greater risk for ectopic calcification than acidemia.

Although there are no randomized controlled trials in the pediatric population, it is likely that the catabolic effect of acidemia on bone has great clinical importance for the growth of children [76]. Correction of acidemia is recommended before inaugurating growth factor therapy in children with CKD. Acidemia may have particular impact on the chondrocytes in the growth plate [77]. In rats, 14 days of metabolic acidemia reduced new bone formation and this was associated with a specific defect in the height of the hypertrophic zone of the growth plate. Acidemia reduced both cartilage production and bone formation in these rodents.

In summary, correction of acidemia with alkali has been shown to improve bone mineralization and histology in acidotic patients, including those treated by hemodialysis [78]. Still, it has not been documented that reduced fracture rates or other improved clinical outcomes are associated with improved acid-base status in dialysis patients. The major concern with alkali therapy is ectopic calcification, especially in patients with CKD or hypercalcemia. Further studies will be needed to determine how to obtain the benefits of alkali therapy on bone, while minimizing the risks of ectopic calcification.

PROTEIN MALNUTRITION

Experimental studies have revealed integrated mechanisms whereby acid accumulation causes loss of muscle mass. Acid directly stimulates hepatic glutamine production and accelerates muscle protein degradation, leading to release of amino acids that are used to synthesize glutamine in the liver [26]. Moreover, acidemia increases the oxidation of branched-chain amino acids (BCAA) in muscle to provide much of the nitrogen used in the hepatic synthesis of glutamine [79]. The evidence for the latter response is that metabolic acidemia activates the rate limiting enzyme for the irreversible decarboxylation of BCAA, branched-chain ketoacid dehydrogenase (BCKAD) in muscle, and this response accounts for BCAA degradation [79]. Plasma levels of BCAA in rats with kidney failure are low compared to pair-fed, control rats, and these low levels are linked to increased oxidation of BCAA in muscle [80]. The influence of acidemia in initiating and maintaining these processes was proven by adding $NaHCO_3$ to the diet to correct the metabolic acidemia of chronic uremia: both plasma levels of BCAA and the rates of amino acid oxidation in muscle were restored to normal [80]. This response reflects activation of BCKAD activity and occurs in the muscle of acidemic patients. Studies of normal adults confirm that an acid diet results in a 25% stimulation of BCAA decarboxylation [81].

Acidemia has a similar effect in stimulating muscle protein breakdown. In chronically uremic rats, muscle protein degradation is high and correction of the acidemia of CRF reduces protein catabolism to normal levels, but impairment of protein synthesis persists after correction of acidemia [32,82]. Metabolic acidemia overrides the body's normal adaptive responses to a low protein diet that includes a suppression of the oxidation of essential amino acids and the degradation of protein [83]. In non-dialyzed patients, a switch to an isocaloric, low-protein diet decreased skeletal muscle and whole body protein degradation, presumably because the low protein diet reduced acidemia [84]. This has been further highlighted by a study in African American patients with chronic kidney disease, in whom net endogenous acid production was reduced through a decrease in dietary protein intake and increase in intake of fruits and vegetables. Their serum bicarbonate levels rose [85]. Thus, abundant evidence from experimental models and human studies demonstrate that metabolic acidemia accelerates irreversible oxidation of BCAA and degradation of skeletal muscle protein.

There is also evidence that acidemia suppresses albumin synthesis and leads to lower serum albumin levels. When metabolic acidemia was induced in healthy volunteers through the ingestion of ammonium chloride, there was a significant decline in the synthesis rate of albumin as well as serum albumin levels [86]. Consistent with these findings, serum albumin and pre-albumin levels increased significantly in a group of elderly patients when given sufficient alkali to maintain serum bicarbonate levels at 24 mM [87]. Similar findings were observed in randomized studies of stage 4 CKD patients [36], but it has been harder to demonstrate these results in patients with ESRD. Correction of acidemia with alkali has been shown to improve serum albumin levels in some studies of ESRD patients [36,88], but not in others [89]. It appears that the serum albumin-lowering effects of inflammation may contribute to these conflicting results in ESRD patients [90]. When metabolic acidemia was corrected in hemodialysis patients with and without inflammation as measured by C-reactive protein, there was a reduction in protein catabolism as measured by nPNA in both groups. However, the serum albumin levels rose only in those patients with low inflammatory markers as measured by the C-reactive protein.

The mechanisms causing muscle proteolysis involve direct and indirect responses. Regarding the direct effect, when the pH in the media of cultured myocytes is lowered, there is a slight decrease in protein synthesis coupled with an increase in protein degradation. This is compatible with a direct effect of acid causing a change in protein metabolism [91,92]. In uremic rats, however, there must also be an indirect effect, because the pH in muscle measured is normal *in vivo* in the resting state as well as during recovery from acidification [93]. This suggests that other factors must act as signals to increase protein degradation. One of these factors is glucocorticoids, because they are known to be released by acidemia and they directly induce catabolism [26,32]. This was tested in rats, where it was found that adrenalectomy blocks the acidemia-induced stimulus on protein and amino acid catabolism, but adding a physiologic amount of glucocorticoids restores the catabolic influence of acidemia, in vivo [94]. Both acidemia and glucocorticoids are also required to increase the activity of BCKAD and the ubiquitin-proteasome proteolytic system in muscle and cultured myocytes (see below) [92,95].

METABOLIC ACIDEMIA STIMULATES THE UBIQUITIN/PROTEASOME PROTEOLYTIC PATHWAY

In all cells, including skeletal muscle, there are multiple proteolytic systems. These systems include lysosomal proteolytic pathways (microautophagy, microautophagy and chaperone-mediated autophagy), the calcium-activated proteases in the cytoplasm, plus ATP-independent and ATP-dependent cytosolic pathways [96]. The best described ATP-dependent cytosolic pathway is the ubiquitin/proteasome system [96]. In the ubiquitin-proteasome pathway, proteins are targeted for degradation by ATP-dependent conjugation to ubiquitin, a small protein found in all cells. Protein-ubiquitin conjugates are degraded in another ATP-dependent process by the 26S proteasome, a large multi-catalytic, multiple subunit proteolytic complex. The proteasome is found in the nucleus and cytoplasm of all cells [96].

Activation of the ATP-dependent ubiquitin/proteasome pathway in acidemia requires glucocorticoids: the rise in ATP-dependent proteolysis occurring in skeletal muscle of acidemic rats is abolished by adrenalectomy, and restored by physiologic doses of glucocorticoids [26,97]. Interestingly, the response to acidemia includes activation of gene transcription. The abundance of ubiquitin mRNA and mRNAs encoding subunits of the proteasome rises in muscle of rats with chronic kidney failure and acidemia [82]. Studies show that the changes in mRNA require glucocorticoids and are the result of increased gene transcription [82,97]. Moreover, abnormalities in insulin/IGF-I signaling activate muscle protein degradation in the ubiquitin/proteasome system and caspase-3, a protease that breaks down the complex structure of muscle proteins to provide substrates for the ubiquitin/proteasome system (Figure 8.2) [98—100]. Both acidemia and glucocorticoids

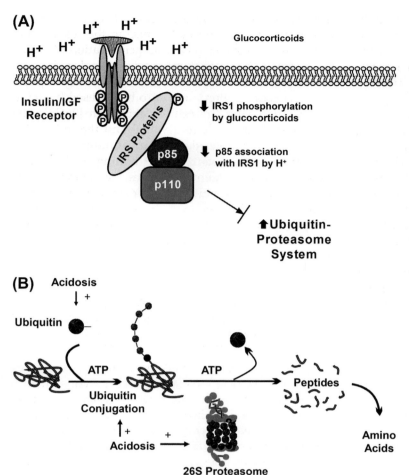

(A)

Glucocorticoids

H+ H+ H+ H+ H+ H+

Insulin/IGF Receptor

IRS Proteins

↓ IRS1 phosphorylation by glucocorticoids

↓ p85 association with IRS1 by H+

p85

p110

↑Ubiquitin-Proteasome System

(B) Acidosis ↓ +

Ubiquitin

ATP

Ubiquitin Conjugation

↑ +

Acidosis + →

26S Proteasome

ATP

Peptides

Amino Acids

FIGURE 8.2 (A) Acidemia and glucocorticoids block insulin and/or insulin-like growth factor-I (IGF-I) signaling to activate the ubiquitin-proteasome system in muscle. Signaling through the insulin or IGF-I receptors normally prevents muscle wasting. Acidemia and glucocorticoids work synergistically to impair signaling through the insulin receptor after the binding of insulin or IGF-I. Glucocorticoids partially reduce the phosphorylation of insulin receptor substrate-I induced by insulin binding, while acidemia blocks recruitment of the phosphoinositide 3-kinase p85 subunit to prevent downstream signaling. Impairing signaling allows activation of the ubiquitin proteasome system. (B) Acidemia stimulates the ubiquitin—proteasome system by affecting multiple steps. Proteins freed from the muscle fibers by caspase 3 are conjugated by ubiquitin. The ubiquitin presents these protein fragments to the proteasome where they are destroyed. Acidemia increases the amount of ubiquitin and proteasomes in cells and also increases the conjugation of protein with ubiquitin. This figure is reproduced in color in the color plate section.

block intracellular signaling induced by the insulin/IGF-1 receptor, but by slightly different mechanisms [100,101]. Glucocorticoids reduce insulin receptor substrate-1 phosphorylation, whereas acidemia has a greater effect on recruitment of the phosphoinositide 3-kinase p85 subunit to prevent downstream signaling. There is strong evidence that both glucocorticoids and a second signal that induces insulin resistance are required for muscle atrophy [102]. These signaling pathways regulate two major proteolytic systems responsible for muscle atrophy: ubiquitin-proteasome and caspase-3. The cleavage of muscle proteins by caspase-3 is a preliminary step required for muscle proteins to be digested by the ubiquitin-proteasome system [103]. Supporting this model, insulin and IGF-I suppress protein degradation in the body, and acidemia induces insulin resistance [49,104]. Rats with insulin-dependent diabetes mellitus also exhibit increased muscle proteolysis via the ubiquitin-proteasome system suggesting that reduced insulin activity could contribute to activation of this important pathway [105]. However, diabetes induces other metabolic interactions that may not be present in acidemia, so the contribution of acidemia to insulin resistance in

uremia and of insulin resistance to protein wasting in acidemia remains to be determined.

There is growing evidence that exercise may ameliorate or reverse problems related to chronic kidney disease. In rat studies, muscle mass can be increased through the use of isometric exercise [106]. In the setting of metabolic acidemia, exercise may transiently worsen the acidemia and may reverse the normal anabolic effects of exercise [107]. Addition of bicarbonate prior to high intensity exercise appears to attenuate the human growth hormone and cortisol response [108]. These findings may have relevance in patients with chronic kidney disease undergoing rehabilitation therapy. The association of acidemia with functional outcomes was examined in the National Health and Nutrition Examination Survey 1999—2002. Serum bicarbonate and gait speed determined from a 20 foot timed walk were measured in over 2500 adults 50 years or older. Lower serum bicarbonate levels were associated with slower gait speed and decreased quadriceps strength in older adults [109]. Further studies are needed to determine the effect of alkali therapy on functional outcomes.

Although acidemia activates the ubiquitin-proteasome system in muscle leading to wasting, the response in the kidney is in the opposite direction. Acidemia suppresses protein breakdown in the renal cortex and in suspensions of isolated tubules [110]. The high ammonia concentrations present in acidemia suppress lysosomal proteolysis in renal tubular cells in culture causing increased accumulation of proteins destroyed in lysosomes [111]. This lysosomal pathway is known as chaperone mediated autophagy [112]. Since chaperone-mediated autophagy controls the half-life of many proteins important for growth, including glycolytic enzymes and the Pax 2 transcription factor, blocking this pathway could contribute to renal tubular hypertrophy and hyperplasia [113]. In vivo, Rabkin and co-workers examined rats fed ammonium chloride and found that there is a decrease in lysosomal cathepsin activity in the renal cortex [114]. Thus, the amino acids that are being lost by muscle are metabolized to ammonia and the latter response provides a stimulus to growth of the kidney [115]. Whether these effects of acidemia on renal lysosomes influence development and progression of renal disease remains to be determined (see Chapter 18 for a discussion of acidemia and the progression of renal failure).

CLINICAL IMPLICATIONS OF ACIDEMIA FOR PROTEIN NUTRITION

How does metabolic acidemia affect nutritional status? It has long been felt that anorexia contributes to protein malnutrition in patients with metabolic acidemia, but it has been difficult to quantify the relative contribution of anorexia to protein malnutrition. On the other hand, there is evidence that excessive protein catabolism is the dominant mechanism for loss of edema-free lean body mass. First, in rats with chronic renal failure, high protein diets were associated with metabolic acidemia, stunted growth, and a lower efficiency of utilization of dietary protein for growth [115]. Second, in poorly growing infants with metabolic acidemia, nitrogen excretion does not correlate with protein intake suggesting that their poor nitrogen balance is due to increased catabolism rather than decreased dietary protein intake [116]. Third, normal adults with experimentally-induced metabolic acidemia who are eating a constant diet exhibit both increased oxidation of the essential branched chain amino acids as well as protein degradation [81]. Fourth, patients undergoing maintenance hemodialysis or continuous ambulatory peritoneal dialysis with acidemia exhibit excessive protein catabolism that can be suppressed when acidemia is corrected with dietary alkali supplements

[117,118]. Fifth, in maintenance hemodialysis patients there is a strong linear correlation between the degree of acidemia measured just before a dialysis treatment and the free valine concentrations measured in biopsied muscle [119]. Treating dialysis patients with sodium bicarbonate raises the levels of branched-chain amino acids in muscle; this strategy will provide more essential amino acids that can be used in the synthesis of muscle protein [120]. Chronic renal failure patients experience a reduction in the severity of acidemia both by taking supplements of sodium bicarbonate and by ingesting low protein diets. Either strategy is effective at promoting protein accrual because both improve nitrogen balance and raise the plasma concentrations of the branched-chain amino acids [84,121].

Taken together, these recent clinical studies support the concept that correcting acidemia is a strategy that will improve protein metabolism in renal failure patients. However, there are significant factors to consider in the measurement of acid/base status in this population. Kirschbaum reported that the standard practice of using distant reference laboratories to measure bicarbonate levels led to falsely low values [122]. Local laboratories also can give falsely low bicarbonate values when the blood or serum sample is left exposed to the air and carbon dioxide escapes [122]. Consequently, decision-making should be based on the entire constellation of clinical data, regardless of the location of the laboratory. Because most cross sectional studies of the effects of acid/base status on nutritional parameters rely on a mixture of data from different laboratories, there is serious concern about their interpretation. For example, it is difficult to evaluate the observation that a single measurement of low pre-dialysis serum bicarbonate may reflect the acid load from a higher protein intake in the particular preceding interdialytic interval, when the researchers do not report the techniques used for measuring serum bicarbonate [123]. Thus, one must take as much care in evaluating the acid/base status of patients described in the medical literature as with one's own patients.

This same concern applies to studies examining acid loading using estimates of the net acid load of the diet. Most epidemiologic studies use the Frasseto formula to estimate net acid excretion (NAE):

$$
\begin{aligned}
&\text{NAE (mEq/day)} \\
&\quad = -10.2 + 54.5 \, (\text{dietary protein (g/day)}/ \\
&\quad\quad\quad\quad\quad \text{potassium (mEq/d)}) \, [124]
\end{aligned}
$$

This formula was verified in populations who ingested most of their protein from meat. Thus, this equation should not be assumed to be accurate for other populations. Furthermore, potassium and protein intake have strong independent effects on health outcomes, possibly confounding interpretation. Studies suggest that an alternative formula, the potential renal acid load (PRAL), may be a more accurate estimate of renal acid excretion, but this formula is seldom used because it requires knowledge of the dietary intake of magnesium, calcium, phosphorous, and potassium [125,126]. Regardless of the formula utilized to estimate the ingested acid load, results from such epidemiologic studies of the estimated acid intake will need to be confirmed by independent methods.

Although it is generally accepted that correction of metabolic acidosis is an important goal in the management of patients with chronic kidney disease, there is no consensus as to what constitutes an optimal correction. For patients with protein-energy wasting, there is loss of somatic and visceral protein stores which is not entirely accounted for by inadequate nutrient intake. Accumulating evidence suggests that an arterial pH closer to the upper limit of the reference range (e.g., a serum bicarbonate concentration of 24–30 mEq/L) may have even greater benefit for this subpopulation [127]. The major concern about such recommendations is the lack of information about the long-term effects of chronic metabolic alkalosis [15]. Given the concern about ectopic calcification with alkalemia, this endpoint will have to be carefully studied in future randomized trials of bicarbonate therapy.

Finally, the similarity between the complications of chronic metabolic acidemia and those of aging suggest there may be a link between acid homoeostatic responses and osteoporosis and protein malnutrition in the geriatric population [18]. The fall in glomerular filtration rate that occurs with aging coupled with a diet that generates a large daily acid load due to the consumption of excess amino and nucleic acids in meat could lead to chronic activation of mechanisms that buffer and excrete acid. This may be especially true for the poor in western countries: they typically consume inadequate amounts of organic bases from fruits and vegetables; this phenomenon may be compounded if they consume excessive protein. The metabolic responses just discussed will not only impair calcium and protein metabolism, but also could result in plasma bicarbonate concentrations that are in the low-normal range [18]. This has been called the "eubicarbonatemic" metabolic acidosis hypothesis, because compensatory and buffering mechanisms keep the serum bicarbonate normal despite an ongoing acid-induced catabolic response. As discussed above, the limited clinical data that are available generally support the eubicarbonatemic metabolic acidosis hypothesis. The hypothesis has been extended to state that net acid diets also cause insulin resistance and

cardiovascular risk, but there are far less data to support this possibility. Further research is needed to examine these questions [128].

In summary, there is abundant evidence from experimental animals, cultured cells, normal adults and patients with kidney disease, that metabolic acidosis is a major cause of abnormalities in calcium and protein metabolism. Although interpretation of serum bicarbonate values is sometimes difficult, and the optimal goals for serum bicarbonate concentrations are not known, the treatment of low serum bicarbonate is straightforward and results in a gain of body weight and muscle mass [129]. For people with advanced chronic kidney disease, the simple acts of restricting dietary protein, increasing fruit and vegetable consumption (before the start of chronic dialysis therapy) or supplementing alkali (before or after the start of dialysis) can powerfully reduce the risk of many of the major complications of uremia.

References

[1] Steinman TI. Serum albumin: its significance in patients with ESRD. Semin Dial 2000;13:404–8.

[2] Fouque D, Kalantar-Zadeh K, Kopple J, et al. A proposed nomenclature and diagnostic criteria for protein-energy wasting in acute and chronic kidney disease. Kidney Int 2008;73:391–8.

[3] Franch HA, Mitch WE. Catabolism in uremia: the impact of metabolic acidosis. J Am Soc Nephrol 1998;9:S78–81.

[4] Frassetto L, Morris RC, Sebastian A. Potassium bicarbonate reduces urinary nitrogen excretion in postmenopausal women. J Clin Endocrinol Metab 1997;82:254–9.

[5] Sebastain A, Harris ST, Ottaway JH, et al. Improved mineral balance and skeletal metabolism in postmenopausal women treated with potassium bicarbonate. N Engl J Med 1994;330: 1776–81.

[6] Riewald S. Using supplementation legally to enhance performance. Strength and Conditioning J 2008;30:39–40.

[7] Kraut JA, Madias NE. Consequences and therapy of the metabolic acidosis of chronic kidney disease. Pediatr Nephrol 2011;26:19–28.

[8] Mitchell JH, Wildenthal K, Johnson Jr RL. The effects of acid-base disturbances on cardiovascular and pulmonary function. Kidney Int 1972;1:375–89.

[9] Hsia CCW. Respiratory function of hemoglobin. N Engl J Med 1998;338:239–47.

[10] Dellinger R, Levy M, Carlet J, et al. Surviving sepsis campaign: International guidelines for management of severe sepsis and septic shock. Intensive Care Medicine 2000;34:17–60.

[11] Marsh JD, Margolis TI, Kim D. Mechanism of diminished contractile response to catecholamines during acidosis. Am J Physiol 1988;254:H20–7.

[12] Orchard CH, Cingolani HE. Acidosis and arrhythmias in cardiac muscle. Cardiovascular Research 1994;28:1312–9.

[13] Kellum J, Song M, Li J. Science review: Extracellular acidosis and the immune response: clinical and physiologic implications. Critical Care 2004;8:331–6.

[14] Lardner A. The effects of extracellular pH on immune function. J Leukoc Biol 2001;69:522–30.

[15] Laski ME, Sabatini S. Metabolic alkalosis, bedside and bench. Semin Nephrol 2006;26:404—21.

[16] Anderson LE, Henrich WL. Alkalemia-associated morbidity and mortality in medical and surgical patients. South Med J 1987;80:729—33.

[17] Luke RG. Metabolic alkalosis: General considerations. In: Gennari FJ, Adrogue HJ, Galla JH, editors. Acid-base disorders and their treatment. Boca Raton: Taylor and Francis Group; 2005. p. 501—18.

[18] Alpern RJ, Sakhaee K. The clinical spectrum of chronic metabolic acidosis: Homeostatic mechansims produce significant morbidity. Am J Kidney Dis 1997;29:291—302.

[19] Golden MH. The development of concepts of malnutrition. J Nutrit 2002;132:2117S—22S.

[20] Shetty PS. Adaptation to low energy intakes: the responses and limits to low intakes in infants, children and adults. Eur J Clin Nutrit 1999;53(Suppl. 1):S14—33.

[21] Finn PF, Dice JF. Proteolytic and lipolytic responses to starvation. Nutrition 2006;22:830—44.

[22] Emery PW. Metabolic changes in malnutrition. Eye 2005;19:1029—34.

[23] Cahill Jr GF. Fuel metabolism in starvation. Ann Rev Nutrit 2006;26:1—22.

[24] Mitch WE, Price SR, May RC, et al. Metabolic consequences of uremia: Extending the concept of adaptive responses to protein metabolism. Am J Kid Dis 1994;23:224—8.

[25] Slatopolsky E, Caglar S, Pennell JP, et al. On the pathogenesis of hyperparathyroidism in chronic experimental renal insufficiency in the dog. J Clin Invest 1971;50:492—9.

[26] May RC, Kelly RA, Mitch WE. Metabolic acidosis stimulates protein degradation in rat muscle by a glucocorticoid-dependent mechanism. J Clin Invest 1986;77:614—21.

[27] Wood CE, Isa A. Intravenous acid infusion stimulates ACTH secretion in sheep. Am J Physiol 1991;260:E154—61.

[28] Kramer RE, Robinson TC, Schneider EG, et al. Direct modulation of basal and angiotensin II-stimulated aldosterone secretion by hydrogen ions. J Endocrinol 2000;166:183—94.

[29] Wilcox CS, Cemerikic DA, Giebisch G. Differential effects of acute mineralo- and glucocorticosteroid administration on renal acid elimination. Kidney Int 1982;21:546—56.

[30] Henger A, Tutt P, Riesen WF, et al. Acid-base and endocrine effects of aldosterone and angiotensin II inhibition in metabolic acidosis in human patients. J Lab Clin Med 2000;136:379—89.

[31] Thompson A, Bailey MA, Michael AE, et al. Effects of changes in dietary intake of sodium and potassium and of metabolic acidosis on 11 beta-hydroxysteroiddehydrogenase activities in rat kidney. Exp Nephrol 2000;8:44—51.

[32] May RC, Kelly RA, Mitch WE. Mechanisms for defects in muscle protein metabolism in rats with chronic uremia: The influence of metabolic acidosis. J Clin Invest 1987;79:1099—103.

[33] Mitch WE, Wilcox CS. Disorders of body fluids, sodium and potassium in chronic renal failure. Am J Med 1982;72:536—50.

[34] Wesson DE, Simoni J, Broglio K. Acid retention accompanies reduced GFR in humans and increases plasma levels of endothelin and aldosterone. Am J Physiol 2011;300:F830—7.

[35] Pitt B, Zannad F, Remme WJ, et al. The effect of spironolactone on morbidity and mortality in patients with severe heart failure. Randomized Aldactone Evaluation Study Investigators. N Eng J Med 1999;34:709—17.

[36] de Brito-Ashurst I, Varagunum M, Raftery M, et al. Bicarbonate supplementation slows progression of CKD and improves nutritional status. J Am Soc Nephrol 2009;20:2075—84.

[37] Greene El, Kren S, Hostetter TH. Role of aldosterone in the remnant kidney model in the rat. J Clin Invest 1996;98:1063—8.

[38] Mahajan A, Simoni J, Sheather SJ, et al. Daily oral sodium bicarbonate preserves glomerular filtration rate by slowing its decline in early hypertensive nephropathy. Kidney Int 2010;78:303—9.

[39] He FJ, Marciniak M, Carney C, et al. Effects of potassium chloride and potassium bicarbonate on endothelial function, cardiovascular risk factors, and bone turnover in mild hypertensives. Hypertension 2010;55:681—8.

[40] Mak RHK. Insulin resistance but IGF-2 sensitivity in chronic renal failure. Am J Physiol 1996;271:F114—9.

[41] Disthabanchong S, Niticharoenpong K, Stitchantrakul W, et al. Metabolic acidosis lowers circulating adiponectin through inhibition of adiponectin gene transcription. Nephrology Dialysis Transplantation 2011;26:592—8.

[42] Kopple JD, Kalantar-Zadeh K, Mehrotra R. Risks of chronic metabolic acidosis in patients with chronic kidney disease. Kidney Int 95:S21-S27

[43] Farwell WR, Taylor EN. Serum bicarbonate, anion gap and insulin resistance in the National Health and Nutrition Examination Survey. Diabetic Medicine 2008;25:798—804.

[44] Dawson-Hughes B, Castaneda-Sceppa C, Harris S, et al. Impact of supplementation with bicarbonate on lower-extremity muscle performance in older men and women. Osteoporosis Int 2010;21:1171—9.

[45] Harris S, Dawson-Hughes B. No effect of bicarbonate treatment on insulin sensitivity and glucose control in non-diabetic older adults. Endocrine 2010;38:221—6.

[46] Ding H, Gao X-L, Hirschberg R, et al. Impaired actions of insulin-like growth factor-1 on protein synthesis and degradation in skeletal muscle of rats with chronic renal failure: Evidence for a postreceptor defect. J Clin Invest 1996;97:1064—75.

[47] Ordonez FA, Santos F, Martinez V, et al. Resistance to growth hormone and insulin-like growth factor-I in acidotic rats. Pediatr Nephrol 2000;14:720—5.

[48] Ding H, Qing DP, Kopple JD. IGF-1 resistance in chronic renal failure: current evidence and possible mechanisms. Kidney Int Suppl 1997;62:S45—7.

[49] Bereket A, Wilson TA, Kolasa AJ, et al. Regulation of the insulin-like growth factor system by acute acidosis. Endocrinology 1996;137:2238—45.

[50] Brungger M, Hulter HN, Krapf R. Effect of chronic metabolic acidosis on the growth hormone/IGF endocrine axis: New cause of growth hormone insensitivity in humans. Kidney Int 1997;51:216—21.

[51] Mahlbacher K, Sicuro A, Gerber H, et al. Growth hormone corrects acidosis-induced renal nitrogen wasting and renal phosphate depletion and attenuates renal magnesium wasating in humans. Metab Clin Exp 1999;48:763—70.

[52] Sicuro A, Mahlbacher K, Hulter HN, et al. Effect of growth hormone on renal and systemic acid-base homeostasis in humans. Am J Physiol 1998;274(4 Pt 2):F650—F567.

[53] Hanna JD, Krieg Jr RJ, Scheinman JI, et al. Effects of uremia on growth in children. Semin Nephrol 1996;16:230—41.

[54] Graham KA, Reaich D, Channon SM, et al. Correction of acidosis in hemodialysis patients increases the sensitivity of the parathyroid glands to calcium. J Am Soc Nephrol 1997;8:627—31.

[55] Arruda JA, Nascimento L, Westenfelder C, et al. Effect of parathyroid hormone on urinary acidification. Am J Physiol 1977;232:F429—33.

[56] Krapf R, Vetsch R, Vetsch W, et al. Chronic metabolic acidosis increases the serum concentration of 1,25-hydroxyvitamin D in humans by stimulating its production rate. J Clin Invest 1992;90:2456—63.

[57] Bushinski DA, Frick KK. The effects of acid on bone. Curr Opin Nephrol Hypertens 2000;9:369—79.

[58] Mathur RP, Dash SC, Gupta N, et al. Effects of correction of metabolic acidosis on blood urea and bone metabolism in patients with mild to moderate chronic kidney disease: a prospective randomized single blind controlled trial. Renal Failure 2006;28:1—5.

[59] Brungger M, Hulter HN, Krapf R. Effects of chronic metabolic acidosis on thyroid hormone homeostasis in humans. Am J Physiol 1997;272:F648—53.

[60] Kaptein EM, Feinstein EI, Nicoloff JT, et al. Serum reverse triiodothyronine and thyroxine kinetics in patients with chronic renal failure. J Clin Endocrinol Metab 1983;57:181—9.

[61] Disthabanchong S, Treeruttanawanich A. Oral sodium bicarbonate improves thyroid function in predialysis chronic kidney disease. Am J Nephrol 2010;32:549—56.

[62] Lim VS, Tsalikian E, Flanigan MJ. Augmentation of protein degradation by L-triiodothyronine in uremia. Metabolism 1989;38:1210—5.

[63] Kraut JA. Disturbances of acid-base balance and bone disease in end-stage renal disease. Semin Dial 2000;13:261—6.

[64] Bushinsky DA, Chabala JM, Gavrilov KL, et al. Effects of in vivo metabolic acidosis on midcortical bone ion composition. Am J Physiol 1999;277:F813—9.

[65] Bushinky DA. The contribution of acidosis to renal osteodystrophy. Kidney Int 1995;47:1816—32.

[66] Bushinsky DA. Bone disease in moderate renal failure. Cause, nature and prevention. Annu Rev Med 1997;48:167—76.

[67] Melnick JZ, Srere PA, Elshourbagy NA, et al. Adenosine triphosphate citrate lyase mediates hypocitraturia in rats. J Clin Invest 1981;67:553—62.

[68] Pak CY, Britton F, Peterson R, et al. Ambulatory evaluation of nephrolithiasis. Classification, clinical presentation and diagnostic criteria. Am J Med 1980;69:19—30.

[69] Bagrodia A, Mehrazin R, Bazzi WM, et al. Comparison of rates and risk factors for development of osteoporosis and fractures after radical or partial nephrectomy. Urology 2011; 78:614—9.

[70] Parfitt AM. Soft-tissue calcification in uremia. Arch Intern Med 1969;124:544—56.

[71] Mendoza FJ, Lopez I, Montes de Oca A, et al. Metabolic acidosis inhibits soft tissue calcification in uremic rats. Kidney Int 2008;73:407—14.

[72] Lomaashvili K, Garg P, O'Neill WC. Chemical and hormonal determinants of vascular calcification in vitro. Kidney Int 2006;69:1464—70.

[73] Sutton RA, Wong NL, Dirks JH. Effects of metabolic acidosis and alkalosis on sodium and calcium transport in the dog kidney. Kidney Int 1979;15:520—33.

[74] Medarov BI. Milk-alkali syndrome. Mayo Clin Proc 2009;84: 261—7.

[75] Patel AM, Goldfarb S. Got calcium? Welcome to the calcium-alkali syndrome. J Am Soc Nephrol 2010;21:1440—3.

[76] Mahan J, Warady B, Committee C. Assessment and treatment of short stature in pediatric patients with chronic kidney disease: a consensus statement. Ped Nephrol 2006;21:917—30.

[77] Carbajo E, Lopez JM, Santos F, et al. Histologic and dynamic changes induced by chronic metabolic acidosis in the rat growth plate. J Am Soc Nephrol 2001;12:1228—34.

[78] Lefebvre A, de Vernejoul MC, Gueris J, et al. Optimal correction of acidosis changes progression of dialysis osteodystrophy. Kidney Int 1989;36:1112—8.

[79] May RC, Hara Y, Kelly RA, et al. Branched-chain amino acid metabolism in rat muscle: Abnormal regulation in acidosis. Am J Physiol 1987;252:E712—8.

[80] Hara Y, May RC, Kelly RA, et al. Acidosis not azotemia stimulates branched-chain amino acid catabolism in uremic rats. Kidney Int 1987;32:808—14.

[81] Reaich D, Channon SM, Scrimgeour CM, et al. Ammonium chloride-induced acidosis increases protein breakdown and amino acid oxidation in humans. Am J Physiol 1992;263: E735—9.

[82] Bailey JL, Wang X, England BK, et al. The acidosis of chronic renal failure activates muscle proteolysis in rats by augmenting transcription of genes encoding proteins of the ATP-dependent, ubiquitin-proteasome pathway. J Clin Invest 1996;97:1447—53.

[83] Price SR, Mitch WE. Metabolic acidosis and uremic toxicity: Protein and amino acid metabolism. Semin Nephrol 1994;14: 232—7.

[84] Williams B, Hattersley J, Layward E, et al. Metabolic acidosis and skeletal muscle adaptation to low protein diets in chronic uremia. Kidney Int 1991;40:779—86.

[85] Scialla JJ, Appel LJ, Astor BC, et al. Estimated net endogenous acid production and serum bicarbonate in African Americans with chronic kidney disease. Clin J Am Soc Nephrol 2011;6: 1526—32.

[86] Ballmer PE, McNurlan MA, Hulter HN, et al. Chronic metabolic acidosis decreases albumin synthesis and induces negative nitrogen balance in humans. J Clin Invest 1995;95:39—45.

[87] Verove C, Maisonneuve N, El Azouzi A, Boldron A, Azar R. Effect of the correction of metabolic acidosis on nutritional status in elderly patients with chronic renal failure. J Renal Nutr 2002;12:223—4.

[88] Movilli E, Zani R, Carli O, et al. Correction of metabolic acidosis increases albumin concentrations and decreases kinetically evaluated protein intake in haemodialysis patients. Nephrol Dial Transplant 1998;13:1719—22.

[89] Brady JP, Hasbargen JA. Correction of metabolic acidosis and its effect on albumin in chronic hemodialysis patients. Am J Kidney Dis 1998;31:35—40.

[90] Movilli E, Viola BF, Camerini C, et al. Malnutrition and wasting in renal disease. J Renal Nutr 2009;19:172—7.

[91] England BK, Chastain J, Mitch WE. Extracellular acidification changes protein synthesis and degradation in BC3H-1 myocytes. Am J Physiol 1991;260:C277—82.

[92] Isozaki Y, Mitch WE, England BK, et al. Interaction between glucocorticoids and acidification results in stimulation of proteolysis and mRNAs of proteins encoding the ubiquitin-proteasome pathway in BC3H-1 myocytes. Proc Natl Acad Sci USA 1996;93:1967—71.

[93] Bailey JL, England BK, Long RC, et al. Experimental acidemia and muscle cell pH in chronic acidosis and renal failure. Am J Physiol 1995;269:C706—12.

[94] May RC, Bailey JL, Mitch WE, et al. Glucocorticoids and acidosis stimulate protein and amino acid catabolism in vivo. Kidney Int 1996;49:679—83.

[95] Mitch WE, Medina R, Greiber S, et al. Metabolic acidosis stimulates muscle protein degradation by activating the ATP-dependent pathway involving ubiquitin and proteasomes. J Clin Invest 1994;93:2127—33.

[96] Mitch WE, Goldberg AL. Mechanisms of muscle wasting: The role of the ubiquitin-proteasome system. N Engl J Med 1996; 335:1897—905.

[97] Price SR, England BK, Bailey JL, et al. Acidosis and glucocorticoids concomitantly increase ubiquitin and proteasome subunit mRNAs in rat muscle. Am J Physiol 1994;267: C955—60.

[98] Bailey JL, Price SR, Zheng B, et al. Chronic kidney disease causes defects in signaling through the insulin receptor

substrate/phosphatidylinositol-3-kinase/Akt pathway: Implications for muscle atrophy. J Am Soc Nephrol 2006;17:1388–94.

[99] Workeneh BT, Mitch WE. Review of muscle wasting associated with chronic kidney disease. Am J Nutr 2010;91: 11285–325.

[100] Franch HA, Raissi S, Wang X, et al. Acidosis impairs insulin receptor substrate-1-associated phosphoinositide-3-kinase signaling in muscle cells: consequences on proteolysis. Am J Physiol 2004;287:F700–6.

[101] Zheng B, Ohkawa S, Li H, Roberts-Wilson TK, Price SR. FOXO3a mediates signaling crosstalk that coordinates ubiquitin and atrogin-1/MAFbx expression during glucocorticoid-induced skeletal muscle atrophy. FASEB J 2010;24:2660–9.

[102] Hu Z, Wang H, Lee IH, Du J, Mitch WE. Endogenous glucocorticoids and impaired insulin signaling are both required to stimulate muscle wasting under pathophysiological conditions in mice. J Clin Invest 2009;119:3059–69.

[103] Du J, Wang X, Miereles C, et al. Activation of caspase-3 is an initial step triggering accelerated muscle proteolysis in catabolic conditions. J Clin Invest 2004;113:115–23.

[104] DeFronzo RA, Beckles AD. Glucose intolerance following chronic metabolic acidosis in man. Am J Physiol 1979;236: E328–34.

[105] Price SR, Bailey JL, Wang X, et al. Muscle wasting in insulinopenic rats results from activation of the ATP-dependent, ubiquitin-proteasome pathway by a mechanism including gene transcription. J Clin Invest 1996;98:1703–8.

[106] Wang X, Du J, Klein JD, et al. Exercise ameliorates chronic kidney disease-induced defects in muscle protein metabolism and progenitor cell function. Kidney Int 2009;76: 751–9.

[107] Clapp EL, Bevington A. Exercise-induced biochemical modifications in muscle in chronic kidney disease: Occult acidosis as a potential factor limiting the anabolic effect of exercise. J Renal Nutr 2011;21:57–60.

[108] Wahl P, Zinner C, Achtzehn S, et al. Effect of high- and low-intensity exercise and metabolic acidosis on levels of GH, IGF-1, IGFBP-3 and cortisol. Growth Hormone and IgF Research 2010;20:380–5.

[109] Abramowitz MK, Hostetter TH, Melamed ML. Association of serum bicarbonate levels with gait speed and quadriceps strength in older adults. Am J Kidney Dis 2011;58:29–38.

[110] Schechter P, Shi JD, Rabkin R. Renal tubular cell protein breakdown in uninephrectomized and ammonium chloride-loaded rats. J Am Soc Nephrol 1994;5:1201–7.

[111] Franch HA, Curtis PV, Mitch WE. Mechanisms of renal tubular cell hypertrophy: mitogen-induced suppression of proteolysis. Am J Physiol 1997;273:C843–51.

[112] Cuervo AM, Dice JF. Lysosomes, a meeting point of proteins, chaperones and proteases. J Mol Med 1998;76:6–12.

[113] Franch HA, Sooparb S, Du J, et al. A mechanism regulating proteolysis of specific proteins during renal tubular cell growth. J Biol Chem 2001;276:19126–31.

[114] Preisig PA, Franch HA. Renal epithelial cell hyperplasia and hypertrophy. Sem Nephrol 1995;15:327–40.

[115] Meireles CL, Price SR, Pereira AML, et al. Nutrition and chronic renal failure in rats. What is an optimal dietary protein? J Am Soc Nephrol 1999;10:2367–73.

[116] Kalhoff H, Manz F, Diekmann L, et al. Decreased growth rate of low-birth-weight infants with prolonged maximum renal acid stimulation Acta Ped 1993;82:522–7.

[117] Graham KA, Reaich D, Channon SM, et al. Correction of acidosis in hemodialysis decreases whole-body protein degradation. J Amer Soc Nephrol 1997;8:632–7.

[118] Graham KA, Reaich D, Channon SM, et al. Correction of acidosis in CAPD decreases whole body protein degradation. Kidney Int 1996;49:1396–400.

[119] Bergstrom J, Alvestrand A, Furst P. Plasma and muscle free amino acids in maintenance hemodialysis patients without protein malnutrition. Kidney Int 1990;38:108–14.

[120] Lofberg E, Wernerman J, Anderstam B, et al. Correction of metabolic acidosis in dialysis patients increases branched-chain and total essential amino acid levels in muscle. Clin Nephrol 1997;48:230–7.

[121] Mochizuki T. The effect of metabolic acidosis on amino and keto acid metabolism in chronic renal failure. Nippon Jinzo Gakkai Shi 1991;33:213–24.

[122] Kirschbaum B. Spurious metabolic acidosis in hemodialysis patients. Am J Kidney Dis 2000;35:1068–71.

[123] Uribarri J, Levin NW, Delmez J, et al. Association of acidosis and nutritional parameters in hemodialysis patients. Am J Kidney Dis 1999;34:493–9.

[124] Frassetto LA, Todd KM, Morris Jr RC, et al. Estimation of net endogenous noncarbonic acid production in humans from diet potassium and protein contents. Am J Clin Nutri 1998;68:576–83.

[125] Berkemeyer S, Remer T. Anthropometrics provide a better estimate of urinary organic acid anion excretion than a dietary mineral intake-based estimate in children, adolescents, and young adults. J Nutri 2006;136:1203–8.

[126] Remer T, Dimitriou T, Manz F. Dietary potential renal acid load and renal net acid excretion in healthy, free-living children and adolescents. Am J Clin Nutri 2003;77:1255–60.

[127] Chiu YW, Mehrotra R. What should define optimal correction of metabolic acidosis in chronic kidney disease? Semin Dial 2010; 23:411–4.

[128] Adeva MM, Souto G. Diet-induced metabolic acidosis. Clin Nutr 2011;30:416–21.

[129] Stein A, Moorhouse J, Iles-Smith H, et al. Role of an improvement in acid-base status and nutrition in CAPD patients. Kidney Int 1997;52:1089–95.

Prevention and Management of Cardiovascular Disease in Kidney Disease and Kidney Failure

Pranav S. Garimella, Daniel E. Weiner, Mark J. Sarnak

Tufts University School of Medicine, Tufts Medical Center, Boston, MA, USA

INTRODUCTION

Cardiovascular disease (CVD) is the leading cause of morbidity and mortality in persons with chronic kidney disease (CKD) and accounts for over 50% of deaths in patients with end stage renal disease (ESRD) [1]. CKD is a powerful risk state for the development of coronary artery disease (CAD), leading the National Kidney Foundation (NKF) and the American College of Cardiology/American Heart Association (ACC/AHA) to recommend that CKD be considered a CAD risk equivalent [2,3]. While traditional cardiovascular risk factors, such as smoking, hypertension, diabetes, dyslipidemia and older age, are more prevalent in patients with CKD than the general population, a number of non-traditional risk factors, including oxidative stress and inflammation, protein-energy wasting (PEW), anemia, fluid overload and arterial calcification, may also contribute to the increase in morbidity and mortality in this population (Table 9.1) [3].

In this chapter, we discuss the major traditional cardiovascular risk factors (hypertension, dyslipidemia, diabetes, and left ventricular hypertrophy (LVH)), as well as less traditional risk factors like PEW, and then review strategies to prevent and manage heart failure and coronary disease in dialysis patients as well as patients with stages 3–4 CKD. Care of kidney transplant recipients, diagnostic cardiovascular testing, the use of specific biomarkers, and other CVD outcomes, such as stroke, peripheral artery disease, pericardial and valvular diseases, are beyond the scope of this chapter (see Chapter 34 for information about nutritional management of kidney transplant recipients). Details on the mechanisms of PEW, inflammation, uremia, oxidative and carbonyl stress are covered in Chapters 4, 5, 7, 11 and 12.

CARDIOVASCULAR RISK FACTORS

Hypertension

EPIDEMIOLOGY Hypertension is both a cause and result of CKD and is found in 75–85% of patients with CKD with its prevalence increasing as glomerular filtration rate (GFR) declines [4].

Dialysis

EPIDEMIOLOGY Most studies have shown that there is a 'U' shaped relationship between pre-dialysis blood pressure and both CVD outcomes and all-cause mortality [5–8]. Possible explanations for the association of low blood pressure with adverse outcomes include that low blood pressure may reflect the severity of cardiovascular disease and PEW [9]. Ambulatory blood pressure monitoring (ABPM) may be an option to guide clinical decision making in dialysis patients since pre and post dialysis blood pressure measures may vary significantly and have been shown to be imprecise measures of ABP [10].

TRIALS AND RECOMMENDATIONS No randomized controlled trials (RCTs) have evaluated target blood pressure and hard clinical outcomes in dialysis patients and current clinical practice guidelines are extrapolations of studies from the general population. The Kidney Disease Outcomes Quality Initiative (KDOQI) guidelines recommend pre and post-dialysis blood pressure goals of <140/90 mmHg and <130/80 mmHg, respectively (level C recommendation) [11]. Although meta-analyses and some trials have suggested a benefit with use of antihypertensive agents in dialysis patients [12,13], both because of heterogeneity and small sample sizes, data supporting specific target blood pressure values and preferred antihypertensive agents remain

TABLE 9.1 Traditional and Unique Cardiovascular Disease (CVD) Risk Factors in Persons with Kidney Disease

Traditional CVD Risk Factors	CVD Risk Factors Unique to Persons with Kidney Disease
• Male sex	• Anemia
• Hypertension	• Abnormal bone mineral metabolism
• Higher LDL cholesterol	
• Lower HDL cholesterol	• Uremia and oxidative inflammation
• Diabetes	
• Smoking	• Malnutrition and PEW
• Physical inactivity	• RAAS over-activity
• Menopause	• Volume overload
• Family history of coronary disease	• Electrolyte imbalances
	• Albuminuria
• Left ventricular hypertrophy	• "Under treatment"

HDL, high-density lipoprotein; LDL, low-density lipoprotein; PEW, protein-energy wasting; RAAS, renin angiotensin aldosterone system.
Modified from: Am J Kidney Dis. 2010;56(2): 399–417.

weak. Accordingly a recent Kidney Disease: Improving Global Outcomes (KDIGO) consensus committee concluded that there was insufficient data to develop a new guideline on blood pressure management in dialysis patients [14].

CKD Stages 1–4

EPIDEMIOLOGY The pathogenesis of hypertension in CKD is multifactorial with the major mechanisms thought to be salt and water retention as well as activation of the renin-angiotensin-aldosterone system (RAAS). Hypertension is an independent risk factor for progression of CKD as well as development of CVD, and blood pressure management targets both these complications.

TRIALS AND RECOMMENDATIONS Post hoc analyses of RCTs indicate that more intensive blood pressure control (e.g. ~MAP <92 versus 102 mmHg) may reduce kidney outcomes in individuals with proteinuria [15–17] (Figure 9.1). There are no RCTs in CKD populations however which demonstrate that tight blood pressure control reduces CVD outcomes or all cause mortality.

Individual RCTs as well as meta-analyses of RCTs have demonstrated that the use of RAAS inhibitors reduces the progression of kidney disease in diabetics and non-diabetics [16–20], particularly in those with proteinuria [19,21,22]. The combined use of angiotensin converting enzyme inhibitors (ACE-I) and angiotensin receptor blockers (ARB) decreases proteinuria to a greater extent than either drug alone [23,24] however, in studies of individuals with mild proteinuria, dual blockade was associated with an increased risk of worsening of kidney function including

progression to ESRD without improvement in CVD outcomes or mortality [23,24]. Hence dual blockade with both an ACE-I and ARB is not routinely recommended, although trials are ongoing to evaluate dual blockade in individuals with diabetes and proteinuric kidney disease.

Prior guidelines recommended target blood pressure in diabetic and non-diabetic kidney disease of <130/80 mmHg with either ACE-I or ARB being preferred agents in those with either diabetes or a urine protein to creatinine ratio (PCR) >200 mg/mg [11,25]. Preliminary data collated during the development of the new KDIGO blood pressure guideline suggests a blood pressure target of <130/80 mmHg in both diabetes and non-diabetes in individuals with >30 mg/day of albuminuria (or equivalent) and 140/90 mmHg in those with <30 mg/day. The greater the levels of proteinuria, the stronger the grade of the recommendation [26]. Finally, RAAS inhibitors are recommended in both diabetes and non-diabetes in those with >30 mg/day of albuminuria (or equivalent), again with a stronger grade of recommendation in those with higher levels of proteinuria.

Dyslipidemia

Abnormalities in lipoprotein metabolism are common in patients with kidney disease and may vary depending on the stage of kidney disease [27]. Total cholesterol levels may be normal or low in patients with advanced kidney disease, the latter possibly perhaps reflecting PEW [28].

Dialysis

EPIDEMIOLOGY Hemodialysis (HD) and peritoneal dialysis (PD) patients have increased levels of triglycerides and lipoprotein-a (Lp-a) compared to patients with milder forms of kidney dysfunction, with PD patients, potentially reflecting constant dextrose absorption, having particularly atherogenic lipid profiles. The linear association between increasing levels of cholesterol and CAD related mortality seen in the general population is less evident in patients with kidney disease. Observational studies have demonstrated a "reverse epidemiology" between total cholesterol levels and mortality in dialysis patients; i.e. increased risk at low cholesterol levels (Figure 9.2) [29–32], with evidence that malnutrition and chronic inflammation may affect modifiers on this association [31].

TRIALS AND RECOMMENDATIONS Two trials, 4D (Die Deutsche Diabetes Dialyse) study, in which HD patients with diabetes and high serum low density

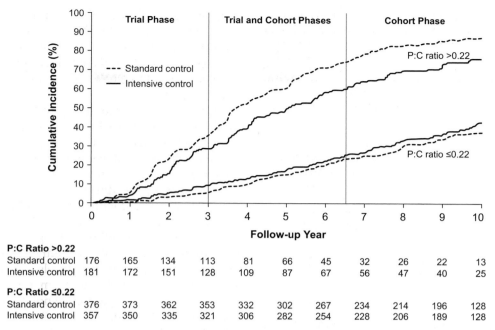

P:C Ratio >0.22										
Standard control	176	165	134	113	81	66	45	32	26	22	13
Intensive control	181	172	151	128	109	87	67	56	47	40	25

P:C Ratio ≤0.22										
Standard control	376	373	362	353	332	302	267	234	214	196	128
Intensive control	357	350	335	321	306	282	254	228	206	189	128

FIGURE 9.1 Cumulative incidence of the composite primary outcome, according to baseline proteinuria status. Among patients with baseline proteinuria, which was defined as a urinary protein-to-creatinine ratio (P:C) of more than 0.22, those who received intensive blood-pressure control had a significantly lower cumulative incidence of the composite primary outcome (a doubling of the serum creatinine level, end-stage renal disease, or death) than those who received standard blood-pressure control (hazard ratio in the intensive-control group, 0.73; 95% confidence interval [CI], 0.58 to 0.93; P = 0.01). However, the between-group difference was not significant among patients with a P:C of 0.22 or less (hazard ratio, 1.18; 95% CI, 0.93 to 1.50; P = 0.16). The values at the bottom of the graph are numbers of patients. *Reproduced with permission from N Engl J Med. 2010;363(10):918–29.*

lipoprotein (LDL) were treated with atorvastatin or placebo, and AURORA (Use of Rosuvastatin in subjects On Regular haemodialysis: an Assessment of survival and cardiovascular events) in which HD patients were treated with rosuvastatin or placebo, failed to demonstrate a significant reduction in mortality or other CVD outcomes despite reduction in LDL levels [33,34]. The

SHARP (Study of Heart and Renal Protection) trial evaluated the efficacy of simvastatin and ezetimibe compared with placebo in lowering cardiovascular outcomes in patients with CKD and dialysis [35]. Results for the dialysis subgroup in SHARP do not appear dissimilar from those seen in 4D or AURORA, showing no significant benefit, although given the absence of

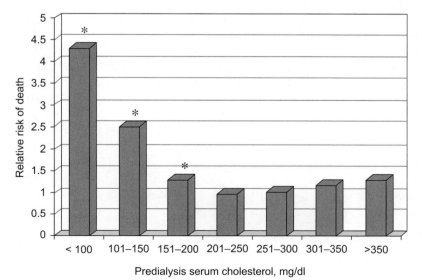

FIGURE 9.2 Relative risk (RR) of death in hemodialysis patients according to serum cholesterol concentration compared to the reference group. *Reproduced with permission from Am J Kidney Dis. 1990;15(5):458–82.*

a statistical difference between dialysis and nondialysis participant in SHARP (where there was a statistically significant benefit for prevention of major atherosclerotic events), the overall interpretation remains open to debate (Figure 9.3). Based on the results of the SHARP trial the U.S. Food and Drug Administration (FDA) has approved the use of simvastatin/ezetimibe combination for lipid lowering and cardiovascular disease risk reduction in persons with CKD not on dialysis [36]. Current KDOQI guidelines from 2005, predating these trials, recommend lowering LDL to <100 mg/dL and triglycerides to <500 mg/dL in adult dialysis patients [11]. There are no clinical trials focusing on PD, although results from SHARP in the subgroup of PD individuals suggest a possible benefit [35].

CKD Stages 1–4

EPIDEMIOLOGY Dyslipidemia is very common in CKD, occurring in over 50% of patients with nephrotic range proteinuria [37]. Like the dialysis population, the presence of malnutrition and inflammation may alter the association between total cholesterol levels and mortality [38].

TRIALS AND RECOMMENDATIONS Data supporting use of statins in secondary prevention of CVD comes from post hoc analysis of trials of the general population. A meta-analysis of 26 such trials which included 25,017 participants with stage 3 or 4 CKD reported a significant reduction in proteinuria, all cause and cardiovascular mortality and nonfatal CVD outcomes compared to placebo, without an effect on progression of CKD [39]. In 970 diabetic participants with eGFR between 30–60 mL/min/1.73 m^2 in the Collaborative Atorvastatin Diabetes Study (CARDS) trial, there was a 42% reduction in major CVD events among patients taking atorvastatin compared to placebo [40]; however, atorvastatin did not reduce mortality. In the JUPITER trial (Rosuvastatin to Prevent Vascular Events in Men and Women with Elevated C-Reactive Protein), a secondary analysis of patients with CKD (eGFR <60 mL/min/1.73 m^2) demonstrated a 45% reduction in first cardiovascular events and all-cause mortality among men and women with LDL-C <130 mg/dL and elevated C-reactive protein with rosuvastatin compared to placebo [41]. Among 6247 participants with CKD not on dialysis included in SHARP, there was a reduced incidence of CVD mortality, nonfatal myocardial infarction and stroke (9.5 versus 11.9 percent) among patients treated with simvastatin and ezetimibe compared to placebo; similar to CARDS, there was no difference in all-cause mortality by treatment group [42].

Current KDOQI guidelines published before the above mentioned studies were completed recommend lowering LDL cholesterol to <100 mg/dL in patients with CKD stage 5 (or non-HDL cholesterol to <130 mg/dL if they have LDL <100 mg/dL and triglycerides >200 mg/dL) [43]. Further data are needed to determine populations that will derive the greatest benefit and cost-effectiveness of lipid-lowering interventions.

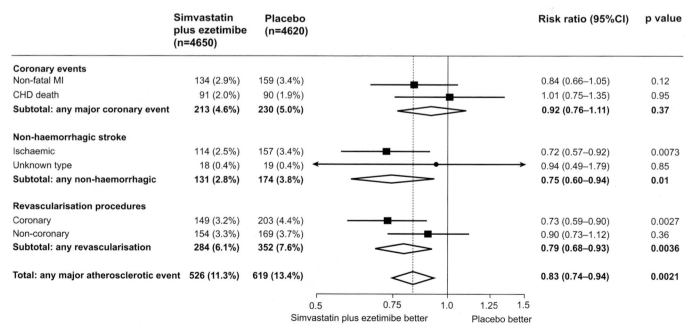

	Simvastatin plus ezetimibe (n=4650)	Placebo (n=4620)		Risk ratio (95%CI)	p value
Coronary events					
Non-fatal MI	134 (2.9%)	159 (3.4%)		0.84 (0.66–1.05)	0.12
CHD death	91 (2.0%)	90 (1.9%)		1.01 (0.75–1.35)	0.95
Subtotal: any major coronary event	**213 (4.6%)**	**230 (5.0%)**		**0.92 (0.76–1.11)**	**0.37**
Non-haemorrhagic stroke					
Ischaemic	114 (2.5%)	157 (3.4%)		0.72 (0.57–0.92)	0.0073
Unknown type	18 (0.4%)	19 (0.4%)		0.94 (0.49–1.79)	0.85
Subtotal: any non-haemorrhagic	**131 (2.8%)**	**174 (3.8%)**		**0.75 (0.60–0.94)**	**0.01**
Revascularisation procedures					
Coronary	149 (3.2%)	203 (4.4%)		0.73 (0.59–0.90)	0.0027
Non-coronary	154 (3.3%)	169 (3.7%)		0.90 (0.73–1.12)	0.36
Subtotal: any revascularisation	**284 (6.1%)**	**352 (7.6%)**		**0.79 (0.68–0.93)**	**0.0036**
Total: any major atherosclerotic event	**526 (11.3%)**	**619 (13.4%)**		**0.83 (0.74–0.94)**	**0.0021**

0.5   0.75   1.0   1.25   1.5
Simvastatin plus ezetimibe better   Placebo better

FIGURE 9.3 Major atherosclerotic events subdivided by type. MI, myocardial infarction; CHD, coronary heart disease. *Reproduced with permission from Lancet. 2011;377(9784):2181–92.*

Diabetes Mellitus

Diabetes is the most common cause of kidney failure in the United States and is present in approximately 40–50% of incident dialysis patients [44]. The risk of developing kidney failure among diabetics has declined over the last 20 years, possibly reflecting better glycemic control and use of kidney-protective medications that block the RAAS [44].

Dialysis

EPIDEMIOLOGY Diabetes is an independent risk factor for all-cause mortality, cardiovascular mortality and nonfatal CVD events in dialysis patients [45,46].

TRIALS AND RECOMMENDATIONS Post hoc analysis from 4D found that HbA1C values > 8% were associated with a 2-fold increase in sudden cardiac death compared to HbA1C values <6% [47]. However, data from other large observational studies of dialysis patients are conflicting, with some not revealing an association between HbA1C levels and survival in dialysis patients [47–49] (Figure 9.4), while others report a monotonic increase in mortality with higher HbA1C levels, especially in nonanemic patents [50,51]. It is important to recognize that uncontrolled diabetes can worsen retinopathy and diabetic neuropathy and increase the risk of vascular complications, thus necessitating a fine balance to avoid both hyperglycemia and hypoglycemia

in this high risk population. Current KDOQI guidelines for therapy reflect American Diabetes Association (ADA) recommendations with a target Hb1A of <7% [11]. However there are no RCT's to support tight control in this population, and individual decision making is required [52]. Extrapolating from studies in populations with high co-morbid disease burden, we feel that, in many patients, higher targets are reasonable because of increased risks versus benefit.

CKD Stages 1–4

EPIDEMIOLOGY In patients with CKD, diabetes significantly increases the risk of mortality and adverse CVD outcomes [53]. While the first sign of impaired kidney function in most diabetics typically is the development of low levels of urinary albumin (microalbuminuria), with subsequent increased urinary albumin excretion (macroalbuminuria) and reduction in eGFR, a smaller proportion may develop a sustained decline in eGFR without ever developing albuminuria [54].

TRIALS AND RECOMMENDATIONS A number of observational studies have shown that sustained hyperglycemia is a risk factor for development of microalbuminuria [55–57], and that a reduction of HbA1C level is associated with significant decrease in microalbuminuria and microvascular complications [58,59].

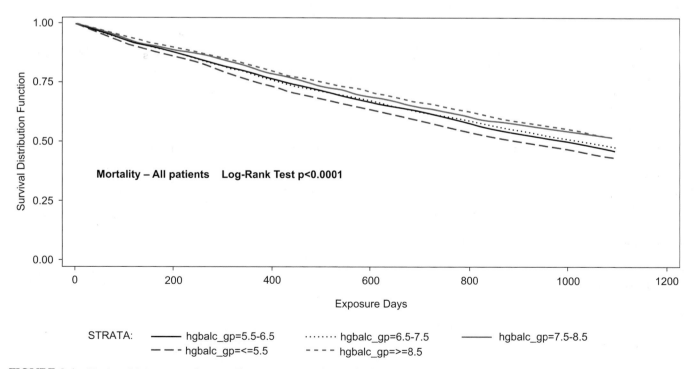

FIGURE 9.4 Kaplan–Meier survival curve. Shown are survival rates for baseline HgbA1c groups. *Reproduced with permission from Clin J Am Soc Nephrol. 2010;5(9):1595–601.* This figure is reproduced in color in the color plate section.

The benefit of strict glycemic control on macrovascular and CVD outcomes is less clear [60]. While some evidence suggests a reduction in cardiovascular mortality among patients with type 1 DM who maintain near normoglycemia (HbA1C ~7%) [61], other trials have shown that intense glucose control is instead associated with increased mortality and significantly more episodes of hypoglycemia [62,63]. Data from the recently published ACCORD (Action to Control Cardiovascular Risk in Diabetes) study which randomized over 10,000 patients who had type 2 diabetes for at least 10 years to an intensive glucose control regimen (target HbA1C <6%) vs. regular control (target HbA1C <7%) found an increased risk of all-cause mortality and cardiovascular mortality in the intensive control group [64]. Although life threatening hypoglycemia was not the cause for increased mortality, these results question whether tight control is indicated in patients with long standing diabetes (such as CKD patients). Of note however, ACCORD excluded participants with frequent or recent serious hypoglycemic events and those with a serum creatinine level of more than 1.5 mg/dL [63]. The ADA currently recommends maintaining the HbA1C level below 7%, but suggests less stringent control in some patients with type 2 diabetes, specifically those with comorbidities and a reduced life expectancy [65].

Left Ventricular Hypertrophy

LVH is a common complication in all stages of CKD including dialysis. It represents an adaptation on the part of the myocardium to pressure and fluid overload and is also considered a traditional risk factor for adverse CVD outcomes.

Dialysis

EPIDEMIOLOGY The prevalence of LVH as detected by echocardiography among incident dialysis patients is reported to be as high as 75% [66–68]. Dialysis patients are host to a number of modifiable risk factors that potentiate the development of LVH including hypertension, volume overload states, arteriovenous fistulas (AVF) and anemia. LVH is an independent risk factor for mortality and adverse CVD outcomes like heart failure [69–71].

TRIALS AND RECOMMENDATIONS Evidence based management guidelines for LVH in ESRD and CKD are lacking due to the absence of RCTs. Due to the effect of LVH on mortality and CV outcomes, current KDOQI guidelines recommend that an echocardiogram be performed in all patients at the initiation of dialysis once patients have achieved dry weight [11]; however, there

is no statement of clinical interventions in response to the results of the echocardiogram. Targeting achievement of dry weight and controlling blood pressure are also recommended with indirect evidence in support of these recommendations [72]. For example, frequent nocturnal hemodialysis has shown to improve blood pressure control, reduce the need for anti-hypertensive medications and decrease the prevalence of LVH [73,74]. However, correction of anemia with epoetin has not been shown to prevent or cause regression on LVH in randomized trials [75,76].

CKD Stages 1–4

EPIDEMIOLOGY The prevalence of LVH increases as kidney function declines [67]. LVH is independently associated with worsening kidney function, progression to dialysis and development of cardiovascular outcomes [77,78].

TRIALS AND RECOMMENDATIONS Despite a number of potentially modifiable risk factors for development of LVH, success in prevention and regression of established LVH has been limited. Similar to dialysis, correction of anemia in CKD stages 3–4 has not been shown to prevent progression of LVH or worsening of kidney function [79,80] and in some studies has been associated with worsening of cardiac outcomes [81]. Maintaining blood pressure targets and utilization of blood pressure agents as outlined above is recommended.

Malnutrition, Protein Energy Wasting and Inflammation

EPIDEMIOLOGY The complex syndrome of nutritional deficiency, muscle wasting and chronic inflammation that occur in persons on dialysis has been given a number of names including uremic cachexia, malnutrition-inflammation atherosclerosis syndrome, or malnutrition-inflammation complex. The term protein energy wasting (PEW) has now been recommended by the International Society of Renal Nutrition and Metabolism (ISRNM) [82], indicating that these abnormalities in protein energy metabolism go beyond just nutritional intake and cannot be corrected solely by dietary modification. The prevalence of malnutrition is high, especially among dialysis patients, where prevalence ranges from 15–50% [83,84]. Hypoalbuminemia, a surrogate marker for malnutrition has been associated with increased cardiovascular mortality in dialysis patients [85–87]; however, mortality associated with hypoalbuminemia may reflect chronic inflammation rather than exclusively malnutrition [88,89]. Markers of chronic inflammation, such as elevated C-reactive protein (CRP) and interleukin-6 (IL-6), have been associated with increased morbidity and mortality [90–92]. In addition, sarcopenia and lower fat mass, commonly seen in dialysis patients is associated with increased mortality and morbidity [93,94].

TRIALS AND RECOMMENDATIONS Scoring systems such as Malnutrition-Inflammation Score (MIS) [95] and the Objective Score of Nutrition on Dialysis (OSND) [96] have been devised to identify and predict dialysis patients at risk of increased mortality and morbidity, but further studies are needed to see if any interventions to improve these scores will affect clinical outcomes. Several studies have evaluated different methods of improving nutrition and lean body mass in malnourished and sarcopenic dialysis patients. For example, in short-term studies, interventions like recombinant human growth hormone and anabolic steroids with or without exercise training have increased lean body mass, improved quality of life and improved surrogate markers of cardiovascular disease [97–99]. Critically, longer and more rigorous studies are needed to fully assess safety and evaluate whether there is a beneficial impact on mortality and other important outcomes. Similarly, while oral protein supplements are associated with lower mortality in observational studies [100] and intradialytic parenteral nutrition with a rise in serum albumin levels [101], there are no large clinical trials which have evaluated the effects of these interventions on hard clinical outcomes. The current guidelines from KDOQI recommend a daily protein intake of 1.2 g/kg body weight and 30–35 kcal/kg body weight among maintenance dialysis patients [102]. While aerobic exercise programs among dialysis patients have shown to increase peak oxygen consumption and self reported physical functioning [103], the utility of exercise for preventing CVD in this population is still unknown.

Other Risk Factors

Smoking, obesity and lack of exercise are other traditional risk factors for CVD in CKD patients. Smoking is associated with adverse cardiovascular outcomes in all stages of CKD [104] and also may promote progression of CKD [105,106]. Smoking cessation is associated with a decrease in the risk of CVD outcomes in dialysis patients [107], and all patients, regardless of CKD status, should be encouraged to quit smoking. Obesity, independent of diabetes is a risk factor for development and progression of CKD and development of CVD in the earlier stages of CKD [108,109]. Overweight and obese patients in the early stages of CKD should be encouraged to lose weight (details of nutrition and weight loss in CKD are discussed in Chapters 29, 30 and 46) and all patients with CKD should be encouraged

to exercise at a moderate intensity for 30 minutes most, if not all, days per week [11]. Patients who are not currently physically active should start at very low levels and durations, and gradually progress to this recommended level.

MANAGEMENT OF CVD

Coronary Artery Disease

Epidemiology

CAD is a common cause of CVD morbidity and mortality among patients with kidney disease [1]. The prevalence of CAD among incident dialysis patients may be as high as 40% [110]. The incidence of acute coronary syndromes (ACS) among dialysis patients in the United States Renal Data System (USRDS) Dialysis Morbidity and Mortality study was 29 per 1000 patient years, with risk factors for ACS being similar to the general population — older age, male sex, diabetes, and known CAD [111]. In the same study, outcomes for dialysis patients with myocardial infarction (MI) were extremely poor with 50% and 80%, 1-year and 3-year mortality rates respectively. Even after revascularization with coronary artery by-pass grafting (CABG), mortality rates are exceedingly high with arrhythmias being the cause of death in approximately 25% of these patients [112].

Therapy of Ischemic Heart Disease

MEDICAL THERAPY Most trials evaluating prevention and treatment of CAD excluded patients with advanced CKD/ESRD; therefore recommendations are based either on observational studies in CKD, subgroups analyses of patients with earlier stages of CKD from general population studies, or extrapolation from trials in the general population [113]. Despite the adverse prognosis associated with MI in the setting of CKD, standard therapeutic strategies are less rigorously applied to these patients [114]. It remains to be determined whether this is due to therapeutic nihilism or appropriate avoidance of specific interventions. No trials have exclusively addressed anti-platelet therapy for secondary prevention of CAD in CKD/ESRD patients, but post-hoc analysis of the Hypertension Optimal Treatment (HOT) study demonstrated that the addition of aspirin resulted in fewer adverse CV events; however this was not statistically significant, possibly due to small sample size [115]. In the absence of active gastrointestinal bleeding, aspirin therapy should be considered for all CKD patients with ACS. The increased bleeding risk with aspirin in dialysis patients necessitates an individualized approach when prescribing it for primary or secondary prevention. In patients with stable angina, ACE-I and ARBs have similar benefit in CKD subgroups compared to those without CKD [116,117]. However, use of ACE/ARB should be used with additional caution in patients with advanced CKD given the increased risk of hyperkalemia. Beta blockers have only been studied to a limited extent in CAD populations with CKD, but there is evidence to suggest that they confer a mortality benefit among CKD patients with CAD [118]. Recent data also suggests that beta blockers may reduce all cause and sudden cardiac death in dialysis patients with ischemic heart disease [119]. Statin therapy is discussed above.

REVASCULARIZATION Clinical outcomes for CKD patients with ACS are better after revascularization compared to medical management alone [120–122] and the American College of Cardiology Foundation/American Heart Association recommend that an early invasive strategy (i.e., diagnostic angiography with intent to perform revascularization) is reasonable in patients with mild and moderate CKD [123]. Observational data from USRDS suggests that dialysis patients also have a better long-term survival after CABG compared to angioplasty or stenting [124], however it is important to note that these data predate the use of drug eluting stents and furthermore that they are limited by selection bias. In a recent retrospective propensity matched analysis of patients with advanced CKD and ACS, therapy with drug eluting stents (DES) did not significantly improve death, MI or target vessel revascularization compared with bare metal stents (BMS) at 2 years of follow-up [125] (Table 9.2).

Heart Failure

Epidemiology

Both the prevalence and incidence of heart failure are high in patients with kidney disease especially those with ESRD. Over 40% of patients receiving dialysis have prevalent heart failure [1,46], with data from USRDS also demonstrating incident heart failure rates of 329 per 1000 patient years in CKD patients, compared to just 97 for those without kidney failure. Rates of hospitalization and death due to heart failure are also significantly higher in patients with ESRD than those without kidney disease [1]. In a large meta-analysis of patients with heart failure, those with moderate–severe kidney disease or any kidney disease had 2.3 and 1.5 times risk of death compared to those without kidney disease respectively [126].

Treatment of Heart Failure

Volume control, by ultrafiltration is an extremely important component of heart failure therapy in dialysis patients [127]. The maintenance of euvolemia can be challenging, with factors like intra-dialytic hypotension precluding adequate fluid removal. In such patients, limited evidence suggests that switching to daily nocturnal dialysis may improve fluid balance and cardiac function [128]. PD may also represent an under-utilized option. In patients with earlier stages of CKD, diuretics form the mainstay of therapy for volume control, although no data exist comparing different diuretic therapies for treating heart failure across the spectrum of CKD.

Carvedilol is the only beta-blocker to have been studied in a randomized trial in dialysis patients with heart failure and dilated cardiomyopathy and demonstrated a significant reduction in mortality compared with placebo [129] (Figure 9.5). No trials of ACE-I or ARBs focusing on patients with heart failure and CKD have been performed. In a single center retrospective analysis of ESRD patients admitted with cardiac events (ACS and heart failure), the use of an ACE-I was found to confer a long-term mortality benefit of nearly 37% compared with its non use [130]. Aldosterone blockers have not been studied in large trials in CKD and safety with regard to hyperkalemia has not as yet been demonstrated, particularly in those patients using concomitant ACE-I and/or ARB. Trials of ARBs while demonstrating a reduction in the development of heart failure in patients with CKD stage 3–5 and proteinuria have not shown a mortality benefit [18,20]. Digoxin should be used with extreme caution in dialysis patients given the potential for more side effects. Furthermore, observational data have suggested increased mortality with

TABLE 9.2 Two-Year Clinical Outcomes

Outcome	DES (n = 431)	BMS (n = 31)	Rate Difference (95% CI)	P
Death	39.4% (170/431)	37.4% (161/431)	2.1% (−4.3–8.5)	0.5
MI	16.0% (69/431)	19.0%b982/431)	−3.0% (−8.2–2.1)	05
TVR	13.0% (56/431)	17.6% (76/431)	−4.6% (−9.5–0.3)	0.06

BMS, bare-metal stent; CI, confidence interval; DES, drug-eluting stent;; MI, myocardial infarction; TVR, target-vessel revascularization.
Reproduced with permission from Am J Kidney Dis. 2011;57(2):202–11.

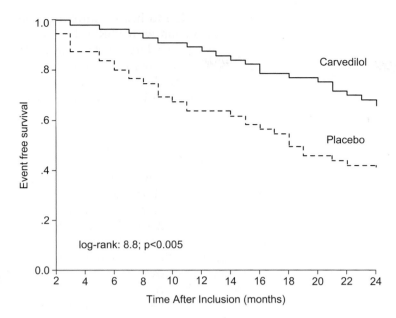

FIGURE 9.5 Kaplan–Meyer curves for all-cause mortality during 24-month follow-up cumulative survival rate according to use of carvedilol. *Reproduced with permission from J Am Coll Cardiol. 2003;41(9):1438–44.*

use of digoxin in this population, although admittedly these studies may be limited by indication bias [131].

CONCLUSION

Persons with CKD and ESRD have a significant burden of CVD. Aggressive risk factor modification and treatment of CVD should be considered in the care of this population, keeping in mind these individuals are also at a higher than normal risk of adverse outcomes from the interventions themselves, stressing the role of individualized care. Further clinical studies of CVD should focus on and include patients with kidney disease.

References

[1] US Renal Data System. USRDS 2010 Annual Data Report: Atlas of Chronic Kidney Disease and End-Stage Renal Disease in the United States. National Institutes of Health, National Institute of Diabetes and Digestive and Kidney Diseases: Bethesda, MD; 2010.

[2] K/DOQI clinical practice guidelines for chronic kidney disease: evaluation, classification, and stratification. Am J Kidney Dis 2002;39:S1–266.

[3] Sarnak MJ, Levey AS, Schoolwerth AC, et al. Kidney disease as a risk factor for development of cardiovascular disease: a statement from the American Heart Association Councils on Kidney in Cardiovascular Disease, High Blood Pressure Research, Clinical Cardiology, and Epidemiology and Prevention. Circulation 2003;108:2154–69.

[4] Buckalew Jr VM, Berg RL, Wang SR, Porush JG, Rauch S, Schulman G. Prevalence of hypertension in 1,795 subjects with chronic renal disease: the modification of diet in renal disease study baseline cohort. Modification of Diet in Renal Disease Study Group. Am J Kidney Dis 1996;28:811–21.

[5] Li Z, Lacson Jr E, Lowrie EG, et al. The epidemiology of systolic blood pressure and death risk in hemodialysis patients. Am J Kidney Dis 2006;48:606–15.

[6] Zager PG, Nikolic J, Brown RH, et al. "U" curve association of blood pressure and mortality in hemodialysis patients. Medical Directors of Dialysis Clinic, Inc. Kidney Int 1998;54:561–9.

[7] Port FK, Hulbert-Shearon TE, Wolfe RA, et al. Predialysis blood pressure and mortality risk in a national sample of maintenance hemodialysis patients. Am J Kidney Dis 1999;33:507–17.

[8] Foley RN, Herzog CA, Collins AJ. Blood pressure and long-term mortality in United States hemodialysis patients: USRDS Waves 3 and 4 Study. Kidney Int 2002;62:1784–90.

[9] Udayaraj UP, Steenkamp R, Caskey FJ, et al. Blood pressure and mortality risk on peritoneal dialysis. Am J Kidney Dis 2009;53:70–8.

[10] Agarwal R, Peixoto AJ, Santos SF, Zoccali C. Pre- and post-dialysis blood pressures are imprecise estimates of interdialytic ambulatory blood pressure. Clin J Am Soc Nephrol 2006;1:389–98.

[11] K/DOQI clinical practice guidelines for cardiovascular disease in dialysis patients. Am J Kidney Dis 2005;45:S1–153.

[12] Agarwal R, Sinha AD. Cardiovascular protection with antihypertensive drugs in dialysis patients: systematic review and meta-analysis. Hypertension 2009;53:860–6.

[13] Heerspink HJ, Ninomiya T, Zoungas S, et al. Effect of lowering blood pressure on cardiovascular events and mortality in patients on dialysis: a systematic review and meta-analysis of randomised controlled trials. Lancet 2009;373:1009–15.

[14] Levin NW, Kotanko P, Eckardt KU, et al. Blood pressure in chronic kidney disease stage 5D-report from a Kidney Disease: Improving Global Outcomes controversies conference. Kidney Int 2009;77:273–84.

[15] Sarnak MJ, Greene T, Wang X, et al. The effect of a lower target blood pressure on the progression of kidney disease: long-term follow-up of the modification of diet in renal disease study. Ann Intern Med 2005;142:342–51.

[16] Appel LJ, Wright Jr JT, Greene T, et al. Intensive blood-pressure control in hypertensive chronic kidney disease. N Engl J Med 2010;363:918–29.

[17] Upadhyay A, Earley A, Haynes SM, Uhlig K. Systematic review: blood pressure target in chronic kidney disease and

proteinuria as an effect modifier. Ann Intern Med 2011;154:541—8.

[18] Brenner BM, Cooper ME, de Zeeuw D, et al. Effects of losartan on renal and cardiovascular outcomes in patients with type 2 diabetes and nephropathy. N Engl J Med 2001;345:861—9.

[19] Jafar TH, Schmid CH, Landa M, et al. Angiotensin-converting enzyme inhibitors and progression of nondiabetic renal disease. A meta-analysis of patient-level data. Ann Intern Med 2001;135:73—87.

[20] Lewis EJ, Hunsicker LG, Clarke WR, et al. Renoprotective effect of the angiotensin-receptor antagonist irbesartan in patients with nephropathy due to type 2 diabetes. N Engl J Med 2001;345:851—60.

[21] Agodoa LY, Appel L, Bakris GL, et al. Effect of ramipril vs. amlodipine on renal outcomes in hypertensive nephrosclerosis: a randomized controlled trial. JAMA 2001;285:2719—28.

[22] Jafar TH, Stark PC, Schmid CH, et al. Progression of chronic kidney disease: the role of blood pressure control, proteinuria, and angiotensin-converting enzyme inhibition: a patient-level meta-analysis. Ann Intern Med 2003;139:244—52.

[23] Kunz R, Friedrich C, Wolbers M, Mann JF. Meta-analysis: effect of monotherapy and combination therapy with inhibitors of the renin angiotensin system on proteinuria in renal disease. Ann Intern Med 2008;148:30—48.

[24] MacKinnon M, Shurraw S, Akbari A, Knoll GA, Jaffey J, Clark HD. Combination therapy with an angiotensin receptor blocker and an ACE inhibitor in proteinuric renal disease: a systematic review of the efficacy and safety data. Am J Kidney Dis 2006;48:8—20.

[25] Chobanian AV, Bakris GL, Black HR, et al. Seventh report of the Joint National Committee on Prevention, Detection, Evaluation, and Treatment of High Blood Pressure. Hypertension 2003;42:1206—52.

[26] NKF Annual Meeting. Las Vegas, 2011.

[27] Kwan BC, Kronenberg F, Beddhu S, Cheung AK. Lipoprotein metabolism and lipid management in chronic kidney disease. J Am Soc Nephrol 2007;18:1246—61.

[28] Attman PO, Samuelsson O, Alaupovic P. Lipoprotein metabolism and renal failure. Am J Kidney Dis 1993;21:573—92.

[29] Iseki K, Yamazato M, Tozawa M, Takishita S. Hypocholester-olemia is a significant predictor of death in a cohort of chronic hemodialysis patients. Kidney Int 2002;61:1887—93.

[30] Kalantar-Zadeh K, Block G, Humphreys MH, Kopple JD. Reverse epidemiology of cardiovascular risk factors in maintenance dialysis patients. Kidney Int 2003;63:793—808.

[31] Liu Y, Coresh J, Eustace JA, et al. Association between cholesterol level and mortality in dialysis patients: role of inflammation and malnutrition. JAMA 2004;291:451—9.

[32] Lowrie EG, Lew NL. Death risk in hemodialysis patients: the predictive value of commonly measured variables and an evaluation of death rate differences between facilities. Am J Kidney Dis 1990;15:458—82.

[33] Fellstrom BC, Jardine AG, Schmieder RE, et al. Rosuvastatin and cardiovascular events in patients undergoing hemodialysis. N Engl J Med 2009;360:1395—407.

[34] Wanner C, Krane V, Marz W, et al. Atorvastatin in patients with type 2 diabetes mellitus undergoing hemodialysis. N Engl J Med 2005;353:238—48.

[35] Baigent C, Landray MJ, Reith C, et al. The effects of lowering LDL cholesterol with simvastatin plus ezetimibe in patients with chronic kidney disease (Study of Heart and Renal Protection): a randomised placebo-controlled trial. Lancet 2011;377:2181—92.

[36] Food and Drug Administration. New Drug Application 21-687/S-039: Vytorin (ezetimibe/simvastatin) and New Drug Application

21-445/S-033: Zetia (ezetimibe). Endocrinologic and Metabolic Drugs Advisory Committee Meeting November 2, 2011.

[37] Weiner DE, Sarnak MJ. Managing dyslipidemia in chronic kidney disease. J Gen Intern Med 2004;19:1045—52.

[38] Kovesdy CP, Anderson JE, Kalantar-Zadeh K. Inverse association between lipid levels and mortality in men with chronic kidney disease who are not yet on dialysis: effects of case mix and the malnutrition-inflammation-cachexia syndrome. J Am Soc Nephrol 2007;18:304—11.

[39] Navaneethan SD, Pansini F, Perkovic V, et al. HMG CoA reductase inhibitors (statins) for people with chronic kidney disease not requiring dialysis. Cochrane Database Syst Rev 2009:CD007784.

[40] Colhoun HM, Betteridge DJ, Durrington PN, et al. Effects of Atorvastatin on Kidney Outcomes and Cardiovascular Disease in Patients with Diabetes: An Analysis From the Collaborative Atorvastatin Diabetes Study (CARDS). Am J Kidney Dis 2009;54:810—9.

[41] Ridker PM, MacFadyen J, Cressman M, Glynn RJ. Efficacy of rosuvastatin among men and women with moderate chronic kidney disease and elevated high-sensitivity C-reactive protein: a secondary analysis from the JUPITER (Justification for the Use of Statins in Prevention-an Intervention Trial Evaluating Rosu-vastatin) trial. J Am Coll Cardiol 2009;55:1266—73.

[42] Sharp Collaborative G. Study of Heart and Renal Protection (SHARP): randomized trial to assess the effects of lowering low-density lipoprotein cholesterol among 9,438 patients with chronic kidney disease. Am Heart J 2010;160:785—94. e710.

[43] K/DOQI clinical practice guidelines for bone metabolism and disease in chronic kidney disease. Am J Kidney Dis 2003;42:S1—201.

[44] Incidence of end-stage renal disease attributed to diabetes among persons with diagnosed diabetes — United States and Puerto Rico. MMWR Morb Mortal Wkly Rep 1996-2007;59:1361—6.

[45] Cheung AK, Sarnak MJ, Yan G, et al. Atherosclerotic cardiovascular disease risks in chronic hemodialysis patients. Kidney Int 2000;58:353—62.

[46] Harnett JD, Foley RN, Kent GM, Barre PE, Murray D, Parfrey PS. Congestive heart failure in dialysis patients: prevalence, incidence, prognosis and risk factors. Kidney Int 1995;47:884—90.

[47] Drechsler C, Krane V, Ritz E, Marz W, Wanner C. Glycemic control and cardiovascular events in diabetic hemodialysis patients. Circulation 2009;120:2421—8.

[48] Williams ME, Lacson Jr E, Wang W, Lazarus JM, Hakim R. Glycemic control and extended hemodialysis survival in patients with diabetes mellitus: comparative results of traditional and time-dependent Cox model analyses. Clin J Am Soc Nephrol 2010;5:1595—601.

[49] Shurraw S, Majumdar SR, Thadhani R, Wiebe N, Tonelli M. Glycemic control and the risk of death in 1,484 patients receiving maintenance hemodialysis. Am J Kidney Dis 2010;55:875—84.

[50] Kalantar-Zadeh K, Kopple JD, Regidor DL, et al. A1C and survival in maintenance hemodialysis patients. Diabetes care 2007;30:1049—55.

[51] Ricks J, Molnar MZ, Kovesdy CP, et al. Glycemic control and cardiovascular mortality in hemodialysis patients with diabetes: a 6-year cohort study. Diabetes 2012;61:708—15.

[52] Halevy D, Vemireddy M. Is a target hemoglobin A1c below 7% safe in dialysis patients? Am J Kidney Dis 2007;50:166. author reply 166—167.

[53] Weiner DE, Tighiouart H, Elsayed EF, et al. The framingham predictive instrument in chronic kidney disease. J Am Coll Cardiol 2007;50:217—24.

[54] Molitch ME, Steffes M, Sun W, et al. Development and progression of renal insufficiency with and without albuminuria in adults with type 1 diabetes in the diabetes control and complications trial and the epidemiology of diabetes interventions and complications study. Diabetes Care 2010;33:1536—43.

[55] Chase HP, Jackson WE, Hoops SL, Cockerham RS, Archer PG, O'Brien D. Glucose control and the renal and retinal complications of insulin-dependent diabetes. JAMA 1989;261:1155—60.

[56] Coonrod BA, Ellis D, Becker DJ, et al. Predictors of microalbuminuria in individuals with IDDM. Pittsburgh Epidemiology of Diabetes Complications Study. Diabetes Care 1993;16:1376—83.

[57] Krolewski AS, Laffel LM, Krolewski M, Quinn M, Warram JH. Glycosylated hemoglobin and the risk of microalbuminuria in patients with insulin-dependent diabetes mellitus. N Engl J Med 1995;332:1251—5.

[58] Effect of intensive blood-glucose control with metformin on complications in overweight patients with type 2 diabetes (UKPDS 34). UK Prospective Diabetes Study (UKPDS) Group. Lancet 1998;352:854—65.

[59] Reichard P, Nilsson BY, Rosenqvist U. The effect of long-term intensified insulin treatment on the development of microvascular complications of diabetes mellitus. N Engl J Med 1993;329:304—9.

[60] Shurraw S, Hemmelgarn B, Lin M, et al. Association between glycemic control and adverse outcomes in people with diabetes mellitus and chronic kidney disease: a population-based cohort study. Arch Intern Med 2011;171:1920—7.

[61] Nathan DM, Cleary PA, Backlund JY, et al. Intensive diabetes treatment and cardiovascular disease in patients with type 1 diabetes. N Engl J Med 2005;353:2643—53.

[62] Zoungas S, Patel A, Chalmers J, et al. Severe hypoglycemia and risks of vascular events and death. N Engl J Med 2010;363:1410—8.

[63] Gerstein HC, Miller ME, Byington RP, et al. Effects of intensive glucose lowering in type 2 diabetes. N Engl J Med 2008;358:2545—59.

[64] Gerstein HC, Miller ME, Genuth S, et al. Long-term effects of intensive glucose lowering on cardiovascular outcomes. N Engl J Med 2011;364:818—28.

[65] Standards of medical care in diabetes — 2011. Diabetes care 2011;34(Suppl. 1):S11—61.

[66] Foley RN, Parfrey PS, Harnett JD, et al. Clinical and echocardiographic disease in patients starting end-stage renal disease therapy. Kidney Int 1995;47:186—92.

[67] Levin A, Singer J, Thompson CR, Ross H, Lewis M. Prevalent left ventricular hypertrophy in the predialysis population: identifying opportunities for intervention. Am J Kidney Dis 1996;27:347—54.

[68] Stack AG, Saran R. Clinical correlates and mortality impact of left ventricular hypertrophy among new ESRD patients in the United States. Am J Kidney Dis 2002;40:1202—10.

[69] Parfrey PS, Foley RN, Harnett JD, Kent GM, Murray DC, Barre PE. Outcome and risk factors for left ventricular disorders in chronic uraemia. Nephrol Dial Transplant 1996;11:1277—85.

[70] Shlipak MG, Fried LF, Cushman M, et al. Cardiovascular mortality risk in chronic kidney disease: comparison of traditional and novel risk factors. JAMA 2005;293:1737—45.

[71] Zoccali C, Benedetto FA, Mallamaci F, et al. Prognostic impact of the indexation of left ventricular mass in patients undergoing dialysis. J Am Soc Nephrol 2001;12:2768—74.

[72] Ozkahya M, Toz H, Qzerkan F, et al. Impact of volume control on left ventricular hypertrophy in dialysis patients. J Nephrol 2002;15:655—60.

[73] Chertow GM, Levin NW, Beck GJ, et al. In-center hemodialysis six times per week versus three times per week. N Engl J Med 2010;363:2287—300.

[74] Culleton BF, Walsh M, Klarenbach SW, et al. Effect of frequent nocturnal hemodialysis vs conventional hemodialysis on left ventricular mass and quality of life: a randomized controlled trial. JAMA 2007;298:1291—9.

[75] Levin A, Djurdjev O, Thompson C, et al. Canadian randomized trial of hemoglobin maintenance to prevent or delay left ventricular mass growth in patients with CKD. Am J Kidney Dis 2005;46:799—811.

[76] Parfrey PS, Foley RN, Wittreich BH, Sullivan DJ, Zagari MJ, Frei D. Double-blind comparison of full and partial anemia correction in incident hemodialysis patients without symptomatic heart disease. J Am Soc Nephrol 2005;16:2180—9.

[77] Paoletti E, Bellino D, Gallina AM, Amidone M, Cassottana P, Cannella G. Is left ventricular hypertrophy a powerful predictor of progression to dialysis in chronic kidney disease? Nephrol Dial Transplant 2010;26:670—7.

[78] Weiner DE, Tighiouart H, Vlagopoulos PT, et al. Effects of anemia and left ventricular hypertrophy on cardiovascular disease in patients with chronic kidney disease. J Am Soc Nephrol 2005;16:1803—10.

[79] Roger SD, McMahon LP, Clarkson A, et al. Effects of early and late intervention with epoetin alpha on left ventricular mass among patients with chronic kidney disease (stage 3 or 4): results of a randomized clinical trial. J Am Soc Nephrol 2004;15:148—56.

[80] Drueke TB, Locatelli F, Clyne N, et al. Normalization of hemoglobin level in patients with chronic kidney disease and anemia. N Engl J Med 2006;355:2071—84.

[81] Singh AK, Szczech L, Tang KL, et al. Correction of anemia with epoetin alfa in chronic kidney disease. N Engl J Med 2006;355:2085—98.

[82] Fouque D, Kalantar-Zadeh K, Kopple J, et al. A proposed nomenclature and diagnostic criteria for protein-energy wasting in acute and chronic kidney disease. Kidney Int 2008;73:391—8.

[83] Cianciaruso B, Brunori G, Kopple JD, et al. Cross-sectional comparison of malnutrition in continuous ambulatory peritoneal dialysis and hemodialysis patients. Am J Kidney Dis 1995;26:475—86.

[84] Young GA, Kopple JD, Lindholm B, et al. Nutritional assessment of continuous ambulatory peritoneal dialysis patients: an international study. Am J Kidney Dis 1991;17:462—71.

[85] Cooper BA, Penne EL, Bartlett LH, Pollock CA. Protein malnutrition and hypoalbuminemia as predictors of vascular events and mortality in ESRD. Am J Kidney Dis 2004;43:61—6.

[86] Foley RN, Parfrey PS, Harnett JD, Kent GM, Murray DC, Barre PE. Hypoalbuminemia, cardiac morbidity, and mortality in end-stage renal disease. J Am Soc Nephrol 1996;7:728—36.

[87] Kalantar-Zadeh K, Kilpatrick RD, Kuwae N, et al. Revisiting mortality predictability of serum albumin in the dialysis population: time dependency, longitudinal changes and population-attributable fraction. Nephrol Dial Transplant 2005;20:1880—8.

[88] de Mutsert R, Grootendorst DC, Indemans F, Boeschoten EW, Krediet RT, Dekker FW. Association between serum albumin and mortality in dialysis patients is partly explained by inflammation, and not by malnutrition. J Ren Nutr 2009;19:127—35.

[89] Eustace JA, Astor B, Muntner PM, Ikizler TA, Coresh J. Prevalence of acidosis and inflammation and their association with low serum albumin in chronic kidney disease. Kidney Int 2004;65:1031—40.

[90] Honda H, Qureshi AR, Heimburger O, et al. Serum albumin, C-reactive protein, interleukin 6, and fetuin a as predictors of malnutrition, cardiovascular disease, and mortality in patients with ESRD. Am J Kidney Dis 2006;47:139—48.

[91] Muntner P, Hamm LL, Kusek JW, Chen J, Whelton PK, He J. The prevalence of nontraditional risk factors for coronary heart disease in patients with chronic kidney disease. Ann Intern Med 2004;140:9—17.

[92] Tripepi G, Mallamaci F, Zoccali C. Inflammation markers, adhesion molecules, and all-cause and cardiovascular mortality in patients with ESRD: searching for the best risk marker by multivariate modeling. J Am Soc Nephrol 2005;16(Suppl. 1):S83—88.

[93] Huang CX, Tighiouart H, Beddhu S, et al. Both low muscle mass and low fat are associated with higher all-cause mortality in hemodialysis patients. Kidney Int 2010;77:624—9.

[94] Noori N, Kopple JD, Kovesdy CP, et al. Mid-arm muscle circumference and quality of life and survival in maintenance hemodialysis patients. Clin J Am Soc Nephrol 2010;5:2258—68.

[95] Rambod M, Bross R, Zitterkoph J, et al. Association of Malnutrition-Inflammation Score with quality of life and mortality in hemodialysis patients: a 5-year prospective cohort study. Am J Kidney Dis 2009;53:298—309.

[96] Beberashvili I, Azar A, Sinuani I, et al. Objective Score of Nutrition on Dialysis (OSND) as an alternative for the malnutrition-inflammation score in assessment of nutritional risk of haemodialysis patients. Nephrol Dial Transplant 2010;25:2662—71.

[97] Feldt-Rasmussen B, Lange M, Sulowicz W, et al. Growth hormone treatment during hemodialysis in a randomized trial improves nutrition, quality of life, and cardiovascular risk. J Am Soc Nephrol 2007;18:2161—71.

[98] Kopple JD, Cheung AK, Christiansen JS, et al. Opportunity & Trade: a large-scale randomized clinical trial of growth hormone in hemodialysis patients. Nephrol Dial Transplant 2011;26:4095—103.

[99] Johansen KL, Painter PL, Sakkas GK, Gordon P, Doyle J, Shubert T. Effects of resistance exercise training and nandrolone decanoate on body composition and muscle function among patients who receive hemodialysis: A randomized, controlled trial. J Am Soc Nephrol 2006;17:2307—14.

[100] Lacson E, Wong W, Zebrowski B, Wingard R, Hakim RM. Outcomes associated with intradialytic oral nutritional supplements in patients undergoing maintenance hemodialysis. Am J Kidney Dis In Press 2012.

[101] Czekalski S, Hozejowski R. Intradialytic amino acids supplementation in hemodialysis patients with malnutrition: results of a multicenter cohort study. J Ren Nutr 2004;14:82—8.

[102] Clinical practice guidelines for nutrition in chronic renal failure. K/DOQI, National Kidney Foundation. Am J Kidney Dis 2000;35:S1—140.

[103] Johansen KL. Exercise and chronic kidney disease: current recommendations. Sports Med 2005;35:485—99.

[104] Orth SR, Hallan SI. Smoking: a risk factor for progression of chronic kidney disease and for cardiovascular morbidity and mortality in renal patients — absence of evidence or evidence of absence? Clin J Am Soc Nephrol 2008;3:226—36.

[105] Shankar A, Klein R, Klein BE. The association among smoking, heavy drinking, and chronic kidney disease. Am J Epidemiol 2006;164:263—71.

[106] Yacoub R, Habib H, Lahdo A, et al. Association between smoking and chronic kidney disease: a case control study. BMC Public Health 2010;10:731.

[107] Foley RN, Herzog CA, Collins AJ. Smoking and cardiovascular outcomes in dialysis patients: The United States Renal Data System Wave 2 Study. Kidney Int 2003;63:1462—7.

[108] Hsu CY, McCulloch CE, Iribarren C, Darbinian J, Go AS. Body mass index and risk for end-stage renal disease. Ann Intern Med 2006;144:21—8.

[109] Elsayed EF, Sarnak MJ, Tighiouart H, et al. Waist-to-hip ratio, body mass index, and subsequent kidney disease and death. Am J Kidney Dis 2008;52:29—38.

[110] Cheung AK, Sarnak MJ, Yan G, et al. Cardiac diseases in maintenance hemodialysis patients: results of the HEMO Study. Kidney Int 2004;65:2380—9.

[111] Trespalacios FC, Taylor AJ, Agodoa LY, Abbott KC. Incident acute coronary syndromes in chronic dialysis patients in the United States. Kidney Int 2002;62:1799—805.

[112] Herzog CA, Strief JW, Collins AJ, Gilbertson DT. Cause-specific mortality of dialysis patients after coronary revascularization: why don't dialysis patients have better survival after coronary intervention? Nephrol Dial Transplant 2008;23:2629—33.

[113] Charytan D, Kuntz RE. The exclusion of patients with chronic kidney disease from clinical trials in coronary artery disease. Kidney Int 2006;70:2021—30.

[114] Fox CS, Muntner P, Chen AY, et al. Use of evidence-based therapies in short-term outcomes of ST-segment elevation myocardial infarction and non-ST-segment elevation myocardial infarction in patients with chronic kidney disease: a report from the National Cardiovascular Data Acute Coronary Treatment and Intervention Outcomes Network registry. Circulation 2010;121:357—65.

[115] Ruilope LM, Salvetti A, Jamerson K, et al. Renal function and intensive lowering of blood pressure in hypertensive participants of the hypertension optimal treatment (HOT) study. J Am Soc Nephrol 2001;12:218—25.

[116] Brugts JJ, Boersma E, Chonchol M, et al. The cardioprotective effects of the angiotensin-converting enzyme inhibitor perindopril in patients with stable coronary artery disease are not modified by mild to moderate renal insufficiency: insights from the EUROPA trial. J Am Coll Cardiol 2007;50:2148—55.

[117] Solomon SD, Rice MM, K AJ, et al. Renal function and effectiveness of angiotensin-converting enzyme inhibitor therapy in patients with chronic stable coronary disease in the Prevention of Events with ACE inhibition (PEACE) trial. Circulation 2006;114:26—31.

[118] Ezekowitz J, McAlister FA, Humphries KH, et al. The association among renal insufficiency, pharmacotherapy, and outcomes in 6,427 patients with heart failure and coronary artery disease. J Am Coll Cardiol 2004;44:1587—92.

[119] Tangri N, Shastri S, Tighiouart H, et al. beta-blockers for prevention of sudden cardiac death in patients on hemodialysis: A propensity score analysis of the HEMO Study. Am J Kidney Dis 2011.

[120] Keeley EC, Kadakia R, Soman S, Borzak S, McCullough PA. Analysis of long-term survival after revascularization in patients with chronic kidney disease presenting with acute coronary syndromes. The American journal of cardiology 2003;92:509—14.

[121] Medi C, Montalescot G, Budaj A, et al. Reperfusion in patients with renal dysfunction after presentation with ST-segment elevation or left bundle branch block: GRACE (Global Registry of Acute Coronary Events). JACC Cardiovasc Interv 2009;2:26—33.

[122] Szummer K, Lundman P, Jacobson SH, et al. Influence of renal function on the effects of early revascularization in non-ST-elevation myocardial infarction: data from the Swedish Web-System for Enhancement and Development of Evidence-Based Care in Heart Disease Evaluated According to Recommended Therapies (SWEDEHEART). Circulation 2009;120:851—8.

[123] Wright RS, Anderson JL, Adams CD, et al. 2011 ACCF/AHA focused update incorporated into the ACC/AHA 2007 Guidelines for the Management of Patients with Unstable Angina/Non-ST-Elevation Myocardial Infarction: a report of the American College of Cardiology Foundation/American Heart Association Task Force on Practice Guidelines developed in collaboration with the American Academy of Family Physicians, Society for Cardiovascular Angiography and Interventions, and the Society of Thoracic Surgeons. J Am Coll Cardiol 2011;57:e215–367.

[124] Herzog CA, Ma JZ, Collins AJ. Comparative survival of dialysis patients in the United States after coronary angioplasty, coronary artery stenting, and coronary artery bypass surgery and impact of diabetes. Circulation 2002;106:2207–11.

[125] Charytan DM, Varma MR, Silbaugh TS, Lovett AF, Normand SL, Mauri L. Long-term clinical outcomes following drug-eluting or bare-metal stent placement in patients with severely reduced GFR: Results of the Massachusetts Data Analysis Center (Mass-DAC) State Registry. Am J Kidney Dis 2011;57:202–11.

[126] Smith GL, Lichtman JH, Bracken MB, et al. Renal impairment and outcomes in heart failure: systematic review and meta-analysis. J Am Coll Cardiol 2006;47:1987–96.

[127] Kalantar-Zadeh K, Regidor DL, Kovesdy CP, et al. Fluid retention is associated with cardiovascular mortality in patients undergoing long-term hemodialysis. Circulation 2009;119:671–9.

[128] Chan CT, Floras JS, Miller JA, Richardson RM, Pierratos A. Regression of left ventricular hypertrophy after conversion to nocturnal hemodialysis. Kidney Int 2002;61:2235–9.

[129] Cice G, Ferrara L, D'Andrea A, et al. Carvedilol increases two-year survivalin dialysis patients with dilated cardiomyopathy: a prospective, placebo-controlled trial. J Am Coll Cardiol 2003;41:1438–44.

[130] McCullough PA, Sandberg KR, Yee J, Hudson MP. Mortality benefit of angiotensin-converting enzyme inhibitors after cardiac events in patients with end-stage renal disease. J Renin Angiotensin Aldosterone Syst 2002;3:188–91.

[131] Chan KE, Lazarus JM, Hakim RM. Digoxin associates with mortality in ESRD. J Am Soc Nephrol 2010;21:1550–9.

10

Assessment of Protein and Energy Nutritional Status

Lara B. Pupim, Cathi J. Martin, T. Alp Ikizler

Department of Medicine, Division of Nephrology, Vanderbilt University, Medical Center, Nashville, TN, USA

INTRODUCTION

Assessment and monitoring of protein and energy nutritional status are crucial to prevent, diagnose and treat protein and energy wasting (PEW), a condition highly prevalent and strongly correlated with increased morbidity and mortality in multiple patient populations, including patients with kidney disease [1—14] (see Chapters 11 and 12). Protein and energy nutritional status refers to the quantitative and qualitative status of protein in non-muscle (visceral) and muscle (somatic) components of body protein mass, in addition to the status of energy balance and stores [2,15,16]. Assessment of protein and energy nutritional status is a broad and complex topic, which involves indirect measures of visceral protein concentrations, somatic protein stores, energy expenditure and requirements, as well as precise measurements of protein and energy homeostasis.

DEFINITION OF PROTEIN AND ENERGY WASTING

Currently, there is inconsistency regarding the terms and definitions used to characterize the abnormalities observed in nutritional status in the setting of other comorbidities, especially in chronic kidney disease (CKD). This is due to the fact that a number of other diseases that may influence nutritional status commonly coexist in CKD. Accordingly, the International Society of Renal Nutrition and Metabolism has suggested the use of a uniform definition in the setting of CKD (protein-energy wasting — PEW) to allow a more systematic and rational approach to both research and clinical management of patients with CKD [17]. According to this definition, PEW is the state of decreased body stores of protein and energy fuels (that is, body protein and fat masses). In PEW, net nutrient intake (i.e. intake corrected for losses) is often lower than nutrient requirements, at least during its genesis, ultimately leading to various metabolic abnormalities, decreased tissue function, and loss of lean body mass [15,18]. Further, PEW is a condition that is often associated and interrelated with other, sometimes many, diseases, so that it can be secondary to or causative of an underlying disease. PEW is also often associated with diminished functional capacity related to metabolic stresses. Therefore, a clinically meaningful assessment of protein and energy nutritional status should be not only able to assess the risk of morbidity and mortality resulting from PEW, but also to simultaneously distinguish the causes and consequences of both PEW and any underlying diseases. A meaningful method should also determine whether there is a possibility of benefit from nutritional interventions to treat PEW [18].

Assessment of protein and energy nutritional status usually requires multiple different measurements [19]. There is no definitive single method to assess nutritional status and responses to nutritional intervention that can be considered as a "gold standard", and a number of the proposed methods are currently being used concomitantly (Figure 10.1). In this chapter, we will describe these various types of methods to assess protein and energy nutritional status. Our aim is to expand, update and evaluate data on the readily available indirect methods to assess protein stores and energy balance and to discuss more precise techniques to estimate protein and energy homeostasis. Considerations concerning methods of assessment for PEW that must be modified for people who have kidney disease or kidney

Nutritional Management of Renal Disease
http://dx.doi.org/10.1016/B978-0-12-391934-2.00010-2

FIGURE 10.1 Methods to assess protein and energy nutritional status. SRBP; serum retinol-binding protein, SIGF-I, serum insulin-like growth factor-1, SCRP: serum C-reactive protein, BIA; bioelectrical impedance analysis, DEXA; dual energy X-ray absorptiometry, ADP; air-displacement plethysmography, SGA; Subjective Global Assessment, MIS: Malnutrition Inflammation Score.

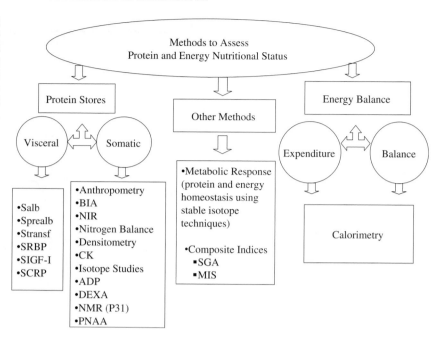

failure or which are specific to these latter conditions will be addressed as appropriate.

ASSESSMENT OF PROTEIN MASS

In order to have a healthy life, an adult must be able to maintain neutral nitrogen balance. Nitrogen balance can be defined as the difference between the intake and loss of nitrogen. A positive or negative protein balance is used to determine the adequacy of protein intake of the patient. Nitrogen balance is dependent on two components: protein anabolism and protein catabolism. Protein anabolism usually is highly dependent on dietary nutrient intake. Neutral nitrogen balance can be achieved with a dietary protein intake (DPI) of 0.6 g/kg/day or even lower in most normal adults, when energy intake is adequate and sufficient high biological value protein is ingested [20–23]. However, if protein and energy requirements are not met from the diet, compensatory mechanisms are activated to maintain neutral nitrogen balance [24,25]. These mechanisms include a reduction in protein breakdown and amino acid oxidation, ultimately leading to more efficient utilization of nutrients [25]. Still, it should be noted that these compensatory responses are limited to some extent, and there is a minimum requirement for DPI. If the protein requirements are not met, a state of net protein loss ensues and is reflected as a worsening in protein nutritional status. In most cases, direct and precise measures of nitrogen balance are not readily available, and indirect measures of protein balance

(e.g., a comparison of the difference between protein intake and nPNA) or an assessment of body protein mass are necessary. The most commonly used measures for assessing body protein mass are serum (visceral) protein concentrations and somatic protein mass.

Visceral Protein Concentrations

Visceral protein concentrations refer to biochemical markers present in serum that are used to identify protein deficiency. These markers are circulating proteins that estimate the size of the visceral protein pool in the body [15]. Almost all circulating visceral proteins have certain physiologic roles such as serving as carriers or binders or having an active involvement in vital functions, such as the immune system. The most readily available and commonly used laboratory tests for visceral protein concentrations are depicted in Table 10.1. These include serum albumin, serum prealbumin (transthyretin), and serum transferrin, although this latter protein has more limitations as a marker of nutritional or PEW status. Other less available markers are serum retinol-binding protein, insulin-like growth factor-1 (IGF-I), pseudocholinesterase, and ribonuclease. Finally, certain positive acute-phase reactants (APRs) have been proposed as "nutritionally-related" markers, since an increase in their concentrations is usually associated with a decrease in most of the visceral protein concentrations. These APRs include C-reactive protein (CRP), ceruloplasmin, complement components, fibrinogen, plasminogen-activator inhibitor-1, antiproteases, serum amyloid A, and fibronectin.

TABLE 10.1 Methods to Assess Serum Protein Concentrations in Kidney Disease Patients

Methods	Advantages	Disadvantages	Clinical Application
Serum albumin	Readily available Inexpensive Excellent outcome predictor	Long half-life (late marker) Influenced by extra-cellular volume Reduced by inflammatory response	Diagnosis and/or screening Longitudinal evaluation[#] Clinical and research
Serum prealbumin (transthyretin)	Relatively readily available Inexpensive Excellent outcome predictor Short half-life (subtle changes) Low influence of extra-cellular volume	Increases as kidney function diminishes Reduced by inflammatory response	Diagnosis and/or screening Longitudinal evaluation[#] Clinical and research
Serum transferrin	Readily available Inexpensive Short half-life Low influence of extra-cellular volume	Influenced by iron stores Reduced by inflammatory response Not validated in large scale studies	Diagnosis and/or screening Longitudinal evaluation[#] Clinical and research
Retinol-binding Protein	Short half-life (can detect early changes)	Limited availability Expensive Increases as kidney function diminishes Reduced by inflammatory response Decreased in hyperthyroidism Decreased in vitamin A deficiency	Diagnosis and/or screening Longitudinal evaluation[#] Research
Serum IGF-I	Good association with other proteins Short half-life (subtle changes)	Limited availability Expensive to measure Acutely affected by dietary intake Not validated in large scale studies	Diagnosis and/or screening Longitudinal evaluation[#] Research

[#]*Repeated measurements in the same patient allow detection of more subtle changes in order to guide nutritional interventions.*
IGF-I; Insulin-like growth factor-I.

Serum Albumin

Serum albumin is a convenient, rather inexpensive and readily available laboratory test and, by far, the most extensively studied serum protein. Several studies have shown a strong correlation between low levels of serum albumin and increased risk of morbidity and mortality in many patient populations [26–29]. It has been suggested that serum albumin is a marker of overall health status rather than simply a nutritional marker, an appropriate distinction when one understands its complex physiology. The concentration of serum albumin is the net result of its synthesis, breakdown, body pool size, volume of distribution, and exchange between intra- and extra-vascular spaces, as well as losses from the body [30,31]. Albumin is a highly water-soluble protein, located mainly in the extra-cellular space, with a total body pool of approximately 300 g (3.5 to 5.3 g/kg) in a normal average-weighted (70 kg) man. Approximately two-thirds of this pool is in the extravascular space and the ratio of intra- to extravascular albumin concentration varies in different tissues. Albumin is synthesized in the liver and secreted into the bloodstream, where it rapidly equilibrates within the intra- and extravascular compartments. Albumin has a half-life of approximately 20 days. Equilibration between intra- and extra-vascular albumin compartments is slower than within the intra-vascular space, varying from 7 to 10 days, depending on the tissue.

Inadequate DPI is characterized by a decrease in the rate of albumin synthesis [32], which, in the short-term, may have little impact on serum albumin levels, since albumin has a relatively low turnover rate and a large pool size. Serum albumin concentrations may actually increase during short-term fasting because of contraction of the intravascular space. Similarly, in the long-term, low protein intake and decreased protein synthesis may be compensated by decreased albumin breakdown and also a shift from the extravascular to the intravascular space, thereby maintaining serum albumin concentrations. Indeed, studies have shown that long-term protein and energy restriction in healthy subjects and patients with anorexia nervosa leads to significant decreases in body weight and somatic protein mass but with no or only small reductions in serum albumin concentrations [18]. Because the exchange between intravascular and extravascular albumin pools can be large, small variations in the rate of this exchange can preserve serum albumin levels over time, even when a low DPI is maintained.

In addition to decreased DPI, hypoalbuminemia can be caused by underlying pathological conditions and diseases, such as hepatic and inflammatory disorders, which engender a decrease in albumin synthesis and/or increase in albumin degradation [33–37]. Serum albumin levels below 3.0 g/dL are usually due to some cause other than solely low nutrient intake. Inflammatory processes may increase also trans-capillary losses of albumin into the extravascular space and lead to a decrease in serum concentrations despite an increase in its fractional synthesis rate [38–39]. Interestingly, in two studies, serum albumin levels failed to increase in patients with cancer after 21 days of intensive nutritional therapy [40] and in nursing home patients after enteral feeding [29]. This suggests that the underlying inflammatory stress present in some disease conditions may perpetuate hypoalbuminemia in spite of adequate protein and energy intakes [41]. Decreased albumin synthesis from liver failure and from albumin losses by the gastrointestinal tract, from the kidney in certain kidney diseases, or from tissue injuries such as wounds, burns, and peritonitis can also lead to hypoalbuminemia.

Serum albumin is an important prognostic marker in kidney disease patients. Many studies have shown the predictive power of serum albumin for clinical outcomes, especially in the end-stage renal disease (ESRD) population. Serum albumin levels below 2.5 g/dL (normal range, about 3.9–5.5 g/dL) have been associated with a risk of death 20 times greater as compared to a reference level of 4.0–4.5 g/dL in maintenance hemodialysis (MHD) patients, and levels of 3.5–4.0 g/dL were associated with a doubling of the risk of death [42,43]. Serum albumin levels may also decrease in kidney disease due to an inflammatory response or hypervolemia, both of which are highly prevalent in this patient population

[44–46]. While longitudinal studies evaluating the validity of serum albumin as a nutritional marker in the presence of inflammation and volume status are limited, available data suggest that serum albumin levels are indeed directly related to nutritional intake, and that serum albumin is a useful nutritional marker even in the presence of inflammation in ESRD patients [46,47].

Serum Prealbumin (Transthyretin)

Serum prealbumin is the carrier protein for retinol-binding protein and thyroxin. It has certain advantages for nutritional assessment as compared to serum albumin, as it is less abundant than serum albumin in the body and its half life is 2–3 days, making serum prealbumin a more sensitive test to detect subtle changes in visceral protein pools [48–50]. Other advantages of serum prealbumin are that it can be easily measured; it is less affected by liver disease than many other serum proteins, and it has a high ratio of essential to nonessential amino acids, making it a distinct marker for protein synthesis [51,52]. In addition, the serum prealbumin concentration is not affected by hydration status [53]. Low nutrient intake decreases serum prealbumin levels, which can be restored by re-feeding [54,55] which is a characteristic of a useful tool to monitor nutritional supplementation [48]. Similar to serum albumin, serum prealbumin has been reported to be a reliable outcome predictor in many patient populations, including patients with kidney disease [50, 56–60]. Limitations of its use as a marker to monitor nutritional status and intervention include the possible increase of serum prealbumin in acute alcohol intoxication [61], during prednisone therapy and while using progestational agents [62]. Serum prealbumin levels may decrease during zinc deficiency [63] and infections [64,65] as well as in response to cytokine and hormone infusions [66,67], suggesting a similar profile as serum albumin with regard to inflammatory response.

Moreover, because the protein components of prealbumin are degraded by the kidney, serum prealbumin levels tend to rise as glomerular filtration rate (GFR) falls, and it may not be a reliable tool to assess protein stores in patients with progressive kidney disease. However, in ESRD patients, in whom GFR is relatively stable and has essentially disappeared, serum prealbumin may be a useful tool. A serum level below 29 mg/dL has been recommended to indicate PEW [2,68]. Of note, this value is within the normal range (i.e. 10–40 mg/dL) for populations with normal GFR.

Serum Transferrin

The primary function of serum transferrin is to transport iron in the plasma. It has a half-life of 8–10 days and a small body pool, making it sensitive to nutritional changes [49,69,70]. It can be directly measured or estimated by measurements of the serum total iron-binding capacity (TIBC) as follows: serum transferring = (0.8 * TIBC) − 43. The normal range for serum transferrin is between 250–300 mg/dL. Low levels of serum transferrin (<200 mg/dL) have been associated with poor clinical outcome in malnourished children and other hospitalized patient populations [71–72]. Increases in serum transferrin levels have also been observed with nutritional supplementation [73]. In patients with CKD, assessment of serum transferrin as a marker of protein stores is problematic [74]. Specifically, iron metabolism is altered in advanced CKD, which can significantly affect serum transferrin concentrations. In addition, routine iron loading in ESRD patients, losses due to the nephrotic syndrome and gastrointestinal diseases, and, as with all the visceral proteins, any condition associated with inflammatory response or liver failure will affect serum transferrin concentrations [75,76]. Therefore, serum transferrin is not a recommended tool for monitoring nutritional status in patients with ESRD [77].

Retinol-Binding Protein

Retinol-binding protein transports retinol and is linked with serum prealbumin in a constant molar ratio. The half-life of retinol-binding protein is about 10 hours and, as with serum prealbumin, it has a small body pool and is a more specific marker of subtle changes in protein stores. Similar to serum albumin and serum prealbumin, retinol-binding protein levels decrease during inflammatory states. In addition, serum retinol-binding protein levels decrease with hyperthyroidism and vitamin A deficiency. In patients with CKD, the use of retinol-binding protein as a nutritional marker is more complicated than serum prealbumin, since it is metabolized in the proximal tubular cells, making the serum levels and the half-life of RBP dependent on the level of kidney function [78].

Insulin-Like Growth Factor-I

Insulin-like growth factor-I (IGF-I) is a growth factor structurally related to insulin. It is produced and released primarily by the liver, mainly in response to growth hormone. It has the benefit of a short half-life (2–6 hours). Since it is 95% bound to its specific binding proteins, its daily serum concentrations normally vary minimally [79]. IGF-I levels fall rapidly during fasting and increase with re-feeding. Therefore, IGF-I concentrations have been used to assess nutritional status in different patient populations [80–83]. Serum IGF-I concentrations may be affected by liver disease and growth hormone levels, which modulates its release from its binding proteins [79].

Limited studies in ESRD patients suggest that serum IGF-I correlates more closely with markers of somatic protein mass, compared to serum albumin and serum transferrin [83]. Changes over time in serum IGF-I concentrations in MHD patients are associated with changes in other nutritional parameters and can predict these changes, especially serum albumin [84,85]. On the other hand, since serum IGF-I concentrations may vary rapidly, over several days, in response to major changes in nutrient intake, the mechanisms by which serum IGF-I indicates the body somatic protein mass are unclear.

C-Reactive Protein

CRP is a positive APR that correlates negatively with serum visceral protein concentrations. During inflammatory processes there is release of cytokines, which mediate an increase in hepatic synthesis of such APRs as CRP and suppression of the synthesis of negative-phase reactants, such as serum albumin [86]. Serum CRP is not a nutritional marker per se, but it is important to understand its role in the overall assessment of nutritional status. For example, in the face of low serum albumin or prealbumin levels (which can be considered negative APRs because serum levels may fall quickly during inflammation), it is important to evaluate for potential non-nutritional sources of protein depletion. If serum CRP levels are simultaneously high, sources of infection and/or other causes of inflammation should be investigated and if possible, resolved, along with nutritional supplementation, as appropriate.

In CKD, levels of serum C-reactive protein have been strongly and negatively correlated with concentrations of serum albumin, and hypoalbuminemic patients have significantly higher serum values of CRP as compared to MHD patients with normal serum albumin [45,87,88]. C-reactive protein has been shown to be a strong predictor of death in patients undergoing MHD [87,89,90].

Somatic Protein Mass

Assessment of somatic protein mass is an essential component of the evaluation of nutritional status in CKD patients [91,92]. Evaluation of somatic protein mass involves determining body composition by measuring the individual compartments of water, fat, bone, muscle and visceral organs [2]. The techniques described in the subsequent sections of this chapter will discuss the various compartment models in detail and compare the benefits and drawbacks with a special emphasis on patients with CKD. When evaluating these techniques, the effects of aging, level of physical fitness, disease processes and feasibility of the tests should also be considered [93].

Muscle mass comprises the majority of somatic protein and will be the focus of this discussion.

Generally, somatic protein mass is relatively preserved at the expense of other body fuels, i.e., glycogen and fat, until severe catabolic illnesses occur, ultimately leading to PEW. There are many techniques available to determine body composition. These include anthropometry, bioelectrical impedance (BIA), dual energy X-ray absorptiometry (DEXA), prompt neutron activation analysis (PNAA) and hydro-densitometry. Table 10.2 illustrates several techniques and describes their advantages, disadvantages, and clinical applications.

Anthropometry

Anthropometric measurements have been used for decades and include height and weight, calculated body mass index (BMI), skinfold thickness, usually overlying the biceps, triceps and subscapular areas, mid-arm circumference (MAC) and calculated mid-arm muscle circumference (MAMC), diameter or area [94]. A detailed description of these techniques can be found elsewhere [95]. This technique is a two-compartment model that involves measuring skinfolds and circumferences at standardized sites, usually on the

TABLE 10.2 Different Methods for Assessing Somatic Protein Stores and Body Composition According to Compartment Models

Methods	Advantages	Disadvantages	Clinical Application
TWO-COMPARTMENT			
Anthropometry BIA* NIR*	Easy, fast, and safe Can be done at bedside Non-invasive Inexpensive Low inter- and intra-observer variability*	High inter-observer variability (anthropometry) Dependent on operator skills Influenced by extra-cellular volume Regression equations derived from healthy subjects*	Diagnosis and/or screening Longitudinal evaluation# Clinical and research
THREE-COMPARTMENT			
Creatinine kinetics (CK) Isotope dilution* TBK* DEXA**	Easy and safe (CK) Inexpensive (CK) Not influenced heavily by extra-cellular volume Accurate	Relatively invasive Time-consuming (CK) Moderately expensive	Diagnosis and/or screening Longitudinal evaluation# Clinical and research
FOUR-COMPARTMENT			
ADP PNAA**	Easy, fast, and safe Non-invasive Small influence of extra-cellular volume Accommodates most body types Accurate	Expensive Not readily available Requires time-consuming analysis	Diagnosis and/or screening Longitudinal evaluation# Research
FIVE-COMPARTMENT			
NMR	Very accurate Ability to delineate organ size and body fat distribution	Very expensive Not readily available Requires specialized personnel Validity in abnormal water balance is not well established	Diagnose and/or screening Research

#*Repeated measurements in the same patient allow detection of subtle changes in order to guide nutritional interventions.*
* *Research only.*
** *Minimal radiation exposure.*
BIA, bioelectrical impedance analysis; NIR: near infrared interactance, TBK: total body potassium; DEXA, dual energy X-ray absorptiometry; ADP: air displacement plethysmography; PNAA, prompt neutron activation analysis, NMR: nuclear magnetic resonance spectroscopy.

right side of the body or, for stage 5 CKD patients, the side which does not have a vascular access. Generally, measurements are repeated three times, averaged and compared to percentiles of the normal population. The most commonly used standards are those reported by Jelliffe [96,97] based upon European male military personnel and low-income American women, and those reported by Frisancho, which are based upon white males and females who participated in the United States Health and Nutrition and Evaluation Survey (NHANES) [98,99]. There is a rather poor correlation between these two standards for classifying patients, and most clinicians prefer the Frisancho calculations as being the most accurate for the US population. In fact, 20 to 30% of healthy control subjects would be considered malnourished based upon these standards. These measurements can indirectly quantify the major compositional determinants of body weight and are well suited for identifying levels of lean (fat-free) body mass and total body fat in healthy individuals [100,101]. Since almost half of the body's fat mass is found in the subcutaneous layer, these measurements can provide a reasonably accurate assessment of total body fat. Anthropometry has the advantages of being inexpensive and easy to perform at the bedside, and there are well-established norms for comparison of healthy populations based on the NHANES III survey data. However, it has been suggested that they may have limitations for specific patient populations, such as ESRD, because of the severely limited database and lack of correction for hydration status, which can vary greatly in ESRD patients, and the effects of chronic illness [18].

Among various anthropometric measurements, the BMI tends to overestimate body fat and is not sensitive for detecting small changes in body composition [102−104]. In addition, the calculation used to determine BMI [BM (kg) / height^2 (m^2)], as an estimate of body fat mass, may not apply to people outside the normal ranges of body weight, muscle mass, total body water or height. However, BMI is a convenient, labor saving and inexpensive measurement, and it does correlate strongly with mortality in patients undergoing MHD (please see Chapter 12).

The techniques for measuring MAMC, MAC and TSF are subjective and dependent on the technique of the measurer [94]. There has been a reported difference of as much as 10% in these measurements performed on the same individual, even when the measurements were repeated by the same observer, and this is likely to be greater when more than one observer is involved in the measurements on the same subject [105]. In addition, this technique is not valid in patients who have had recent large shifts in body water, as is frequently seen in patients with ESRD or advanced liver disease. Another shortcoming of anthropometry is the poor correlation

reported between visceral protein stores and upper arm measurements. In general, anthropometry is insensitive for detecting subtle changes in body composition as compared to other methods. However, anthropometric measurements can be useful when an individual patient is being monitored serially and when the measurements are used in conjunction with other nutritional indices [106].

With regard to patients with CKD, there are several important implications. Specifically, the patient undergoing MHD should be assessed on the side opposite the vascular access. In addition, caution should be used when comparing these measurements to the established norms, since the measurements may vary in accordance with alterations in fluid status. Among CKD patients, anthropometric measurements in patients with advanced CKD are perhaps among the least accurate. Attempts have been made to establish anthropometric standards for the dialysis population [107,108]; the validity of these standards needs to be confirmed with larger studies.

Bioelectrical Impedance Analysis

Bioelectrical impedance analysis (BIA) is a technique that has proven to be safe, generally acceptable to patients, and easy to use [109,110]. BIA is used for determining fluid management and increasingly for evaluating protein-energy status. BIA is based on a two-compartment model that determines total body water (TBW) and soft tissue (i.e. fat mass [FM] and fat-free mass [FFM]) [111]. It is based upon the principle that the impedance of a cylindrical conductor is related to its length, cross-sectional area and applied signal frequency. Impedance is the vector sum of resistance and reactance. Figure 10.2 illustrates the detailed configuration for determining bioelectrical impedance. Mammalian tissues conduct an electrical current in proportion to their water and electrolyte content. Lean body tissues, which contain body fluids and electrolytes, have highly conductive, low resistance electrical pathways. Skin, bone and fat, on the other hand, are very poor conductors and offer high resistance [112]. Reactance is defined as the opposition to the flow of electrical current due to the electrical capacitance such as is found in the cell membrane wall. Because of this property of the cell, cell membranes are the only component that offers reactance to electrical currents. The resistance and reactance components are aligned in both parallel and series orientations in the human body [113]. Resistance is defined as the extra-cellular and intra-cellular fluid content, while the reactance is based on the cell membrane content. In FFM, these fluid compartments are parallel components separated by cell membranes; therefore, parallel models are more accurate for determining their impedance.

FIGURE 10.2 Schematic diagram of technical considerations for BIA. Reprinted with permission from Biodynamics Corporation, Seattle, WA, USA.

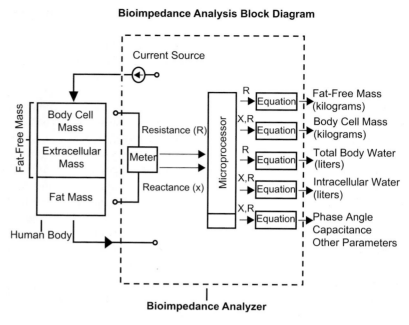

BIA is usually measured by attaching two electrodes on the arm at the mid-wrist and the middle finger, and two electrodes on the leg of the same side at the mid-ankle and foot just proximal to the second and third toe. The electrodes are connected to a small machine that emits a tiny imperceptible current and that measures the resistance and reactance. The entire process can be performed at the bedside and takes less than five minutes. BIA can be assessed through single frequency or multi-frequency electrical currents. The single frequency BIA is performed at 50 KHz and assumes a penetration of 50 to 60% intracellular space, whereas multi-frequency BIA measures extra-cellular water with the lower frequency and TBW at a higher frequency of 500 KHz to 1 to 2 KHz [114]. There is disparity regarding the accuracy between the two methods. Although arms and legs account for only 35% of total body volume, 85% of total body resistance is represented in these limbs [115–117]. Reactance, thought by some to represent cell integrity and nutritional health since cell walls and membranes possess electrical capacitance, has not been as widely investigated as resistance.

Phase angle is a calculation that is derived from BIA and that was originally used as a tool to diagnose metabolic disorders. Phase angle is defined as the arc tangent of the reactance to resistance ratio multiplied by 180 degrees and reflects the relative contribution of reactance to overall impedance. It has been found to positively correlate with total body protein and muscle mass as well as muscle strength [112]. The two compartments that are defined by BIA are extra-cellular mass (ECM), which is primarily fluid and fat mass, and body cell mass (BCM), which is by far the most metabolically active portion of the body [118]. The ratio of ECM to BCM is a known sensitive marker of PEW, and this ratio commonly increases when PEW is present; the phase angle appears to reflect the prognostic significance of PEW. Consequently, a change in the ECM: BCM ratio is probably associated with a change in the phase angle. A phase angle of less than 4 degrees is associated with a significant increase in the risk of death in patients undergoing MHD, while a phase angle of less than 3 degrees is related to a threefold increase in mortality [119]. Conversely, high phase angle readings appear to be consistent with large quantities of intact cell membranes of skeletal muscle and body cell mass. Although the phase angle may not be reliable in certain populations for detecting depletion of edema-free lean body mass, it may be superior in its ability to identify patients who have clinically important PEW and a poor prognosis [110,120].

There are some important limitations to accuracy of BIA in the body composition analysis of CKD patients, especially in patients who have nephrotic syndrome or advanced CKD. Since patients with advanced CKD usually exhibit abnormal water balance, this can result in inaccurate estimations of fat-free, edema-free body mass and fat mass [121]. Therefore, for accurate results, BIA should be conducted when the MHD patient is in an edema-free or near edema-free state; for example, at the end of a hemodialysis session. BIA should be assessed on the non-vascular access side in MHD patients. In peritoneal dialysis patients, BIA should be performed with the peritoneal cavity drained of dialysate [122]. In addition, the software packages that provide the calculations compare results to normal healthy individuals rather than to specific disease populations. However, there are recently published standards based on the MHD population that are now available for comparison [123].

Near Infrared Interactance

Near infrared interactance (NIR) is based on light absorption and reflection using a near infrared light emission. It is a non-invasive, simple and rapid method for assessing the percentage of body fat. The device is commercially available and portable. The main body of the instrument is connected via a light cable to a tiny light-emitting sensor. The NIR sensor window is attached to a light shield prior to placing it on the mid upper arm to ensure that no external light interferes with the estimation of percent body fat [124]. NIR measurements are obtained in a matter of seconds while the device is on the patient's arm. This device is moderately expensive and has been used more extensively in Europe. Drawbacks of NIR include possible errors from measuring only one site (the upper arm), the possibility of other light source contamination in measurement, and unproven validity of the predictive equations used to determine body fat when applied to advanced CKD and chronic dialysis patients. Nonetheless, its diagnostic and prognostic value has been shown in several studies involving MHD patients [106, 124–126]. For patients undergoing MHD, it is recommended that NIR be performed 10 to 20 minutes after the termination of dialysis on the non-access arm.

Densitometry

Densitometry provides a two-compartment model, measuring FM and FFM. It is based on the assumption that fat has a density constant of 0.9 kg/L, and the fat-free component has a density of 1.1 kg/L. Densitometry measures body mass and volume and calculates body density by using Siri's equation for Caucasian populations [% fat = $4.95/(D - 4.5) \times 100$] and Shuttle's equation for African Americans [% fat = $4.374/(D - 3.928) \times 100$]. The "gold standard" of densitometry is underwater weighing [127]. However, the process requires a special facility and can take anywhere from 30 to 45 minutes. In addition, the method may be uncomfortable for the subject, since it requires them to remain underwater for several seconds, and may be associated with technical difficulty for obese, elderly, or debilitated subjects when they attempt to get into or out of the water tank.

Creatinine Kinetics

Creatinine kinetics is based upon the principle that creatinine production is proportional to FFM and that in the steady state creatinine production is equal to the sum of creatinine excretion and metabolic degradation [128]. This technique has correlated well with other methods for assessing lean body mass (i.e., fat-free, edema-free mass) [129]. However, the procedure requires the subject to collect his urine for a 24-hour period and, preferably, to keep the collection on ice, which may make this method less acceptable to the patient. There are only a few studies using creatinine kinetics to estimate lean body mass. Also, intake of meat (skeletal muscle, myocardium) may contribute 30% or more of urine creatinine excretion in normal adults, and this must be taken into consideration when calculating creatinine kinetics. Therefore, the reliability of this technique is not well established.

Diluted Isotope Studies

Isotope dilution is generally considered a more accurate method than multi-frequency BIA for determining body FM from TBW. It can be used in three and four compartment models to evaluate body composition [127]. This procedure involves using isotopically labeled elements that are either ingested orally or administered intravenously and measuring their concentration in saliva, plasma and urine. The most commonly used isotopic compound for measuring TBW is deuterium oxide (D_2O). The next most common isotopic compound for assessing TBW is doubly-labeled water ($H_2^{18}O$), which has a smaller isotopic exchange rate with non-aqueous compounds making it the preferred isotope. However, its cost is prohibitive for widespread use [103,130]. Tritium labeled water has been used previously, but it is used less commonly now because it is radioactive. The advantages of isotope dilution techniques include the greater accuracy of TBW measurements as compared to densitometry and its moderate cost. Further, the measurements are less likely to be compromised by errors of technique [131]. However, these studies are somewhat invasive, requiring blood collection and also the consumption of the tracers, and the analysis is time-consuming [103]. They are used only for research purposes.

Air-Displacement Plethysmography

Air-displacement plethysmography (ADP) requires placing the subject in an egg-shaped, airtight fiberglass chamber, and uses pressure-volume relationships and body weight to derive TBW [132,133]. ADP is similar to densitometry using water displacement (see above), except body volume is measured by the displacement of air rather than water. In ADP, TBW is measured by determining the volume of air displaced by the subject's body when the subject sits inside the chamber. The subject's body volume is calculated indirectly by subtracting the volume of air remaining inside the chamber when the subject is inside, from the volume of air in the chamber when it is empty.

ADP offers several advantages over other more established methods including the fact that it can accommodate a variety of body sizes, the study procedure is rapid (6–10 minutes), the measurement process is safe and comfortable, and it is completely automated and non-invasive [134–135]. However, the instrument is expensive, requires frequent calibration and establishment of isothermal conditions for each test, and is dependent upon a highly trained technician. There are significant gender differences with ADP. ADP underestimates FM in males and slightly overestimates FM in females [134,136]. In addition, the validity, reliability and practicality of ADP in various populations, including ESRD patients has not yet been well defined.

Dual Energy X-Ray Absorptiometry

Dual energy X-ray absorptiometry (DEXA) was initially used for the detection of osteoporosis by measuring bone density. Today, DEXA is also a leading "high tech" method for measuring body composition [112]. Unlike BIA, DEXA gives a direct measure of body composition based on a three-compartment model: FM, FFM, and bone density [137]. DEXA is arguably one of the most accurate determinations of body composition that is available and has a precision error of 0.5 to 3.0% and an accuracy error of 3.0 to 9.0% [131,138]. With this technique, body composition is calculated by ascertaining the amount of radiation attenuated by the bone or soft tissue while low and high-energy radiograph beams (70 kVp and 140 kVp, respectively) are transmitted to the subject [112,139]. This technique requires the subject to lie on the examination surface as a scanning arm performs a series of transverse movements at 1 cm intervals while emitting photons at the two energy levels indicated above. The soft tissue mass reduces photon flux much less than bone mineral density, and differential absorption of the photons is measured and processed by the DEXA software to estimate bone mineral density, FM, and FFM [139]. Each study can be performed in 6 to 15 minutes with minimal radiation exposure (<5 mrem) and minor discomfort to the patient. Because of the minimal radiation exposure, serial measurements can be safely obtained [94].

DEXA offers many advantages, including the fact that it is suitable for virtually all ages and body sizes. It is easy to obtain, has excellent precision, and can also provide regional body composition. In addition, it has been shown to be quite sensitive for the detection of small changes in body composition, which makes it a very useful tool. However, it also has several limitations including cost, which is a major factor. The DEXA instrument itself can cost more than US $100,000, and there is also the expense of trained

personnel to operate it. It is not a portable device; patients must come to a center for evaluation. Hence, there is a much bigger time commitment for the patient. Thus, patient acceptance of this examination may be less than other methods. As with most other methods, hydration status of the patient must be considered for each evaluation, an important consideration for patients with kidney disease [113,134]. Although the DEXA technology continues to improve, the accuracy of this technique for individuals who do not have stable fluid balance, such as the ESRD population, is not yet well defined [131,132].

Prompt Neutron Activation Analysis

This four-compartment method has been available for twenty years and is considered to be the most accurate available technique for determining body composition. Prompt neutron activation analysis (PNAA) involves irradiating the subject with neutrons and measuring the gamma rays that are emitted by the individual during the procedure [140]. This method offers quantitative assessment of nutritionally relevant components of body composition including total body nitrogen, which remains the most direct measure of total body protein, and total body potassium [141,142]. Although this technique is considered to give the most accurate assessment of total body protein, the prohibitive cost and limited availability of the instrument and facility make this method highly impractical for the general population. The radiation exposure to the subjects, approximately 0.2 mSv, is equivalent to the average chest X-ray [143], which can be a significant detriment and limits the feasibility of making serial measurements on patients. There are few studies using PNAA to assess nutritional status in patients with CKD. However, it has been demonstrated that this method is much more sensitive for detecting nitrogen depletion in these patients. Total body nitrogen correlated significantly with DPI, calculated from the urea nitrogen appearance, as well as total energy intake and is inversely associated with increased mortality [143].

Nuclear Magnetic Resonance Spectroscopy

Nuclear magnetic resonance spectroscopy, particularly using P-31, can provide unique and quantitative data that are not available from routine laboratory tests and is the method of choice for examining muscle wasting [144]. This technique employs a five-compartment model that offers the ability to delineate organ size and structure, body fat distribution, total body water and muscle size without exposing the patient to radiation. In addition, it is very sensitive for detecting inflammatory processes in the muscle. The major drawback with this technique is cost, which is prohibitive for general clinical use [130].

Composite Indices

These indices, which are derived from the combination of a variety of nutritional, clinical and/or inflammatory measurements, include subjective global assessment (SGA), the composite nutritional index (CNI) and the malnutrition-inflammation score (MIS). Overall, they are clinically useful tools for evaluating nutritional status in a broader perspective, including medical history, symptoms, and physical parameters.

Subjective Global Assessment

Subjective global assessment is a simple assessment method that draws on the experience of a clinician to make an overall assessment of nutritional status in a standardized way. SGA is the most commonly used composite index in CKD patients. It is based on a 7-point scale and is comprised of a medical history and a physical examination (Table 10.3). The medical history includes an anthropometric component involving present weight and height and comparing them to weight and height from the past two weeks as well as the previous six months. A score is assigned on a scale from 1 to 7 based on the amount of weight lost or gained compared to previous measurements. Disease states and comorbidities are also considered in order to take into account metabolic stress and nutritional requirements. In addition, gastrointestinal symptoms are evaluated based upon the frequency, duration, and severity of symptoms such as diarrhea, anorexia, nausea and vomiting. Finally, the patient is evaluated on functional capacity, which involves assessing how much difficulty the patient has carrying out normal activities of daily living. The physical assessment involves a hands-on examination of the patient by the practitioner. Loss of subcutaneous fat stores and muscle wasting are evaluated by observation and palpation. In addition, edema is evaluated in patients with a serum albumin of <2.8 g/dL, and ascites may be assessed in patients undergoing MHD [145]. When this examination has been completed, an overall SGA rating is assigned to the patient and ranges from a rating of 1 or 2 for severe malnutrition (severe PEW) indicating significant physical signs in most categories, 3−5 for mild-moderate malnutrition (mild-moderate PEW) indicating no clear indication of normal status or severe malnutrition, and a 6 or 7 for very mild malnutrition (very mild PEW) to well-nourished (normal protein-energy status) [124,146].

The use of SGA has been mainly limited to patients with cancer, gastrointestinal surgical disorders and CKD rather than healthy populations. The direct

TABLE 10.3 Different Components of Subjective Global Assessment

Medical History		Physical Examination		
Component	Outcomes	Component	Sites	Outcomes
Weight history	Changes in dry weight − rate and pattern of loss >5−10%	Subcutaneous fat stores	Biceps, triceps, fat pads under eyes	Declining circumference Hollow under eyes
Diet intake review	Comparison to usual intake − degree and duration	Muscle wasting	Temple, quadriceps, deltoid, clavicle and shoulder, ribs, knee, calf, inter-osseous muscle, ribs, scapula	Prominent bone structure, flat or hollow areas
Gastrointestinal symptoms	Frequency and severity of symptoms that last more than 2 weeks	Edema	Extremities and facial features	Swelling when at dry weight
Functional status	Assess changes from baseline related to nutrition	Ascites (HD only)	Abdomen	Swelling in abdominal area after treatment
Acute stresses	Increased metabolic demands			

CLASSIFICATION OF RATINGS	
1 or 2	Severe malnutrition
3, 4 or 5	Moderate malnutrition
6 or 7	Mild to normal nutrition

HD, hemodialysis.

relationship of SGA to various components of nutritional status has not been determined [147], and the reliability and validity remain somewhat controversial. Indeed, the very nature of this assessment is a subjective evaluation, and scores can vary from practitioner to practitioner, although reliability between trained observers is good [145]. The accuracy, reproducibility, and consistency of the SGA should be improved by using initial standard training, specific procedures, and an ongoing review of the procedures and results. It is important to point out that SGA does not replace formal nutrition assessment methods, but can be used as a screening tool in conjunction with other measurements of PEW in order to determine the aggressiveness with which nutritional intervention should be conducted and to prioritize the intensity with which protein-energy status should be monitored in an individual patient. Research has shown that SGA is not a sensitive test or reliable predictor of the degree of PEW although it can differentiate severely wasted patients from those with normal protein-energy status [147,148]. Overall SGA scores have been shown to correlate fairly strongly with clinical outcomes in many studies, including those conducted in MHD patients [148]. There are data to indicate that SGA responds to nutritional therapy in MHD patients [149].

Composite Nutritional Index

Composite Nutritional Index takes into account SGA, anthropometric indices, and serum albumin to draw nutritional scores; a score of zero indicates normal nutrition and increasing scores indicates worsening nutritional status [150]. Jones et al. compared SGA and CNI scores in 72 patients undergoing MHD and found that SGA scores discriminated between best- versus worst-nourished patients as judged by the composite score [151]. However, a number of patients with evidence of significant PEW on the CNI presented with normal SGA scores.

Malnutrition Inflammation Score

The Malnutrition Inflammation Score utilizes a revised form of the SGA scoring system and adds BMI, serum albumin, and total iron-binding capacity (TIBC) to create a more quantitative score [152]. The MIS has been identified as a strong outcome predictor in MHD patients [153]. Its exclusive feature, as compared to other indices, is the inclusion of indicators of inflammation, which rely on measures of TIBC, normally affected by iron metabolism, which is altered in CKD [74]. The inclusion of serum albumin, which is also influenced by inflammation, also affects the reliability of all composite indices including MIS and CNI. Therefore,

as with any method for assessing nutritional status, SGA, CNI, and MIS should be used in conjunction with other clinical, nutritional and metabolic techniques for evaluating the patient. Prospective controlled studies, including a large and representative sample of CKD patients of all stages, are needed to establish these tools for clinical and research applicability.

ASSESSMENT OF PROTEIN AND ENERGY HOMEOSTASIS

As previously mentioned, whenever possible, one should assess biomarkers that directly measure nutritional status and PEW and that predict clinically important outcomes (Table 10.4). When not possible, many surrogate markers are acceptable for each disease or condition to be evaluated. Further, a meaningful biomarker should not only diagnose PEW and predict important clinical outcomes but also measure the metabolic response to nutritional interventions. The nutritional markers discussed so far can accomplish these goals to some extent. However, they are limited in terms of preciseness and may not detect subtle changes in protein and energy stores, either quantitatively or qualitatively. In addition, the concentrations of visceral proteins and the somatic protein stores are not measures of metabolic abnormalities. The assessment of metabolic abnormalities, such as the balance between protein synthesis and breakdown as well as energy intake and expenditure, can be a precise way to detect metabolic changes and/or metabolic responses to interventions. This type of assessment has low variability, high sensitivity and specificity, and is able to detect subtle and narrow changes. Further, the metabolic responses can be assessed in very short periods of time (hours), allowing each patient to be studied as his own control, and therefore decreasing inter-patient and intra-patient variability. In this respect, measurements of nitrogen balance and/or protein homeostasis using stable isotope tracer techniques are potential

TABLE 10.4 Proposed Characteristics of an Ideal Marker of Protein-Energy Status

- Readily available
- Inexpensive
- Short half-life (for measurement of serum proteins not body composition)
- Good outcome predictor
- Good association with other nutritional markers
- Distinguishes nutritional disorders from inflammatory, acidemic or other causes of PEW
- Measures metabolic responses to nutritional interventions
- Low influence of extra-cellular volume

approaches to accomplish these goals. These techniques satisfy all of these foregoing criteria and provide minimal risk to the patient. Further, metabolic studies of protein, carbohydrate, and lipids using stable isotopes, in addition to assessment of energy expenditure, are complex techniques that provide information on the link between nutrition, substrate metabolism, and substrate oxidation, which should be especially useful in the research setting.

Nitrogen Balance

Nitrogen balance can be described as a measure of the net change in total body protein. This is based on the assumption that, except in azotemic individuals, almost all nitrogen in the body is found in protein. Protein contains approximately 16% nitrogen by weight, so 1 gram of nitrogen represents 6.25 grams of protein [154]. Accordingly, classical nitrogen balance techniques are a powerful, sensitive and usually accurate tool for assessing the nutritional and metabolic response to changes in nutritional status. A major factor responsible for the precision and sensitivity of this technique is the precise control of the activities, diet and environment of an individual during the studies [155].

Normal, healthy adults are in neutral balance with a nitrogen balance that is equal to about + 0.5 g/d (to account for unmeasured nitrogen losses from sweat, skin desquamation, hair and nail growth, respiration, flatus and, if present, sputum and salivary losses and menstruation). During neutral nitrogen balance, whole body protein synthesis is equal to whole body protein degradation [156]. If nitrogen balance is positive, the subject is in a net anabolic state, whereas if the nitrogen balance is negative, the subject is in a net catabolic state such as from starvation or inadequate protein intake. This is an excellent tool for determining the amount of protein that is required for a subject to maintain a neutral or positive nitrogen balance depending on the individual's nutritional goals. However, it is not a tool that can be used in routine clinical practice, and specially equipped centers are required to conduct nitrogen balance studies. Measurement of nitrogen balance requires meticulous detail, and a period of equilibration of 10 to 14 days is usually necessary before the effects of nutritional intervention can be assessed. After nitrogen equilibration is attained, it is generally necessary to measure nitrogen balance over a period of no less than five to ten days [157–159].

Despite the apparent advantages, there are important limitations inherent to the classical nitrogen balance

technique. Most of the measurement errors, such as losses of food on cooking, losses of feces and urine on toilet paper or in collection containers lead to falsely positive balances. Further, the facilities necessary to carry out these studies are not widely available for general clinical use, are very expensive and the studies are time consuming. These facilities not only require special laboratory facilities, but also trained metabolic unit personnel and a metabolic kitchen with special facilities and skilled personnel to prepare carefully quantified diets.

A less expensive but less precise estimate of nitrogen balance can be made by measuring urinary urea nitrogen and dietary nitrogen intake during the same 24-hour period. The following equations can be used to measure nitrogen appearance [160]. Nevertheless, the calculated results can be considered to provide only crude estimates of nitrogen balance [155].

$$\text{Total nitrogen appearance (TNA; g/day)}$$
$$= \text{urine N (g/day)} + \text{dialysate N (g/day)}$$
$$+ \text{fecal N (g/day)}$$
$$+ \text{change in body urea N (g/day)}^1$$

$$\text{Urea nitrogen appearance (UNA; g/day)}$$
$$= \text{urine urea N (g/day)} + \text{dialysate urea N (g/day)}$$
$$+ \text{change in body urea N (g/day)}$$

$$\text{Non-urea nitrogen appearance (NUNA; g/day)}$$
$$= \text{urine N (g/day)} + \text{dialysate N (g/day)}$$
$$+ \text{fecal N (g/day)} - \text{urine urea N (g/day)}$$
$$- \text{dialysate urea nitrogen (g/day)}$$

$$\text{TNA g/day} = 1.19 \text{ UNA g/day} + 1.27 \text{ g/day}$$

For patients with CKD, nitrogen balance must be adjusted for changes in the body urea nitrogen pool (i.e. the urea volume of distribution) by measuring the serum urea nitrogen serially. Using linear regression, the change in the urea pool can then be estimated and used to calculate nitrogen balance. An alternative approach for measuring nitrogen output has been designed for ESRD patients using the calculation of the normalized protein nitrogen appearance (nPNA or nPCR) or urea nitrogen appearance (UNA) to estimate nitrogen output as long as the patient is edema-free and in a metabolically steady state. nPNA and UNA are less precise measures of total nitrogen output as compared to the direct measurement

---

[1]For nondialyzed patients with chronic kidney disease, the dialysate total N and urea N = 0; for anuric CAPD patients, the urine total N and urea N = 0.

of nitrogen in dialysate, urine and feces. Total nitrogen output, estimated from the UNA or nPNA then can be compared to estimated DPI to provide a rough estimate of nitrogen balance.

Assessment of Protein Homeostasis

Even though nitrogen balance is an excellent tool for determining protein requirements, it does not take into account the turnover of protein in the body, a process much greater than the DPI or net protein degradation as estimated by nPNA or total nitrogen output [161]. The balance between protein breakdown and synthesis is the determinant of the net nitrogen balance. Protein balance is then a condition where protein synthesis and protein breakdown are equal or not significantly different, a condition in which edema-free lean body mass is supposed to be stable. Protein homeostasis can be measured most readily at the whole-body level and at the skeletal muscle level. An effective method for assessing protein homeostasis and also total protein synthesis and breakdown is the use of the primed continuous infusion of isotopic tracers, such as leucine, valine and lysine for the whole-body component, and phenylalanine for the skeletal muscle component.

^{13}C-leucine is a common, stable (i.e., nonradioactive) isotopic tracer used for metabolic studies at the whole-body level. The rate of appearance of endogenous leucine is an estimate of whole-body protein breakdown and can be calculated by dividing the labeled leucine [^{13}C-leucine] infusion rate by the plasma ^{13}C-ketoisocaproate (KIC) enrichment [162]. It is normally expressed as mg/kg/min or, ideally, as mg/kg of fat-free, edema-free mass/min and should be corrected for any infused or lost amino acids during the study hours. The method also requires determination of breath ^{13}CO$_2$ production, which can be calculated by multiplying the rate of total carbon dioxide production or pulmonary expiration (VCO$_2$) by the breath ^{13}CO$_2$ enrichment. The rate of whole-body leucine oxidation during steady state infusion of the ^{13}C-labeled leucine isotope can be calculated by dividing the breath ^{13}CO$_2$ production rate by 0.8 (correction factor for the retention of ^{13}CO$_2$ in the bicarbonate pool) and by the plasma KIC enrichment [162]. The non-oxidative leucine disappearance rate is an estimate of whole-body protein synthesis, and it can be determined indirectly by subtracting leucine oxidation from the corrected total leucine rate of disappearance. Therefore, determination of the rates of whole-body protein breakdown and protein synthesis, using labeled leucine as a tracer, are rather complex but yet precise methods derived from the endogenous rate of leucine appearance, leucine oxidation rate, and the non-oxidative leucine rate of disappearance, respectively,

assuming that 7.8% of whole-body protein is comprised of leucine [163].

Similar calculations are used to assess protein turnover in skeletal muscle using the arterio-venous differences within a muscle bed, usually the forearm or the leg. However, the plasma enrichment of labeled phenylalanine [(ring-^{2}H$_5$)-phenylalanine] is measured instead of leucine, valine or lysine. This is due to the fact that phenylalanine is neither synthesized de novo nor metabolized by skeletal muscle. Therefore, the rate of appearance of unlabelled phenylalanine reflects muscle protein breakdown and the rate of disappearance of labeled phenylalanine estimates muscle protein synthesis [164]. The measurements are adjusted for blood or plasma flow through the muscle, and data are generally expressed as μg/100 mL of blood or plasma flow/min [165].

In addition to measuring whole body and skeletal muscle turnover, stable isotopes can be used to measure the fractional synthetic rate of individual proteins, such as albumin and transferrin [162,165]. Finally, skeletal muscle biopsies can be used in both in vitro [166] and in vivo studies in animals and human subjects to investigate protein synthesis and breakdown or amino acid kinetics [167–169]. Although technically complex, it provides a means of measuring the transport rates of natural amino acids directly rather than inferring from the kinetics of its analogues, which may be different from one another. These techniques enable analysis of trans-membrane transport of amino acids, the intracellular concentrations of many amino acids and their metabolites, the rates of protein breakdown and synthesis, the intra-muscular de novo synthesis of amino acids, and concentrations of many other intracellular compounds in muscle [168,169].

Studies in CKD patients have shown the utility and validity of stable isotope techniques as precise tools for evaluating metabolic responses to nutritional interventions, as well as the metabolic responses to the hemodialysis procedure. Several investigators have studied the metabolic effects of hemodialysis on whole body and skeletal muscle turnover and energy metabolism [170–173]. These techniques have been recently applied to measure the metabolic response to intradialytic parenteral nutrition in MHD patients [174]. The technique has been shown to be feasible and reliable for these research purposes. In addition, it has been successfully applied to estimate fractional synthetic rates of body proteins in MHD patients [175].

Despite the many advantages related to the use of stable isotope kinetic studies, these techniques also have certain inherent errors and limitations. There is considerable variability of protein synthesis and degradation throughout the day as well as problems associated with isotope reentry into cells and isotope recycling in and out of proteins and peptides throughout the studies. In general, it is difficult to perform long-term continuous isotope studies, and a minimum of 3–4 weeks is required between studies in a given individual. There is also a significant cost associated with these studies. Therefore, the superiority of these techniques over classical nitrogen balance studies for measuring protein balance is not conclusively justified, although stable isotope studies have other unique strengths. In many circumstances, the two techniques may be considered complementary.

Assessment of Energy Homeostasis

Energy balance is a major requirement for human cell function and is determined by energy intake and energy expenditure. Energy intake is derived almost exclusively from dietary carbohydrates, lipids and proteins. These substrates are metabolized and converted into chemical energy (in the form of ATP and other energy metabolites) and used for growth and maintenance of body tissues [16]. If nutrient intake is inadequate to meet energy requirements, the result will be loss of body weight, and a gradual decrease in carbohydrate and lipid stores [176]. Body protein stores may also be metabolized under these circumstances to generate the required energy, causing major metabolic alterations, such as acidemia, ketosis, loss of nitrogen, and dehydration.

Common terminology in energy balance includes total energy expenditure and its components: basal metabolic rate, resting energy expenditure (REE), physical activity, energy requirement and the thermic effect of food. The REE, also known as resting metabolic rate, is the metabolism of the body at rest, reflected as the heat production of the body when in a state of complete mental and physical rest and in the post-absorptive state (i.e., after a 12-hour of fast) [177]. The REE reflects the energy requirements to maintain and conduct normal metabolic activity of muscle, brain, liver, kidney, and other cells at rest [16]. On the other hand, nutrient intake, exercise performance, sleep, changes in the external temperature and disease states or external manipulations (e.g., hemodialysis) may change heat production and therefore, the REE. The thermic effect of food refers to the increase in energy expenditure above the REE that occurs after a meal. It is a consequence of the extra energy consumed due to digestion, absorption and metabolism of nutrients. Energy expenditure of physical activity is the energy required to perform body motion. In sedentary individuals, REE is the largest component of energy expenditure, encompassing about 65–80% of total daily energy expenditure. To prevent body wasting (fat and/or lean masses), the energy intake must be equal to the total expenditure

during the same period [16,177]. The World Health Organization has defined energy requirement as "the level of energy intake from food that will balance energy expenditure when the individual has a body size and composition, and level of physical activity, consistent with long term good health; and that will allow for the maintenance of economically necessary and sociably desirable physical activity. In children, pregnant or lactating women the energy requirement includes the energy needs associated with the deposition of tissues or the secretion of milk at rates consistent with good health" [178].

Energy balance is neutral when the number of calories absorbed equals the amount of energy expended for body processes and activities, with no weight change. When available energy exceeds the capacity of the body to expend it, a positive energy balance exists, causing weight gain with excess energy stored in the body primarily as adipose tissue. Adipose tissue will be maintained, increase or become depleted, depending on the energy balance over time. When energy intake is not adequate for the requirement, a negative energy balance will occur, utilizing adipose stores and other potential fuels (carbohydrates and proteins), usually causing weight loss.

As with protein assessment, it is important to define the alterations in energy metabolism in specific populations prior to assessing the energy needs. With regard to patients with CKD, earlier studies concluded that energy requirement was similar between Stage 2–5 CKD patients and healthy subjects, both before and after initiation of renal replacement therapy [179–181]. However, recent studies suggest that the REE is higher in diabetic CKD patients [182] and MHD patients, especially after adjusting for fat-free mass [183,184]. Further, several studies have shown that REE increases during the hemodialysis procedure in the postabsorptive state [171,183,185]. Overall, an energy intake of approximately 25–30 kcal/kg/day usually maintains visceral and somatic protein stores and nitrogen balance in patients with earlier stages of CKD, including patients ingesting a low protein diet and in patients undergoing MHD [77]. It is important to keep in mind that since energy intake is prescribed based on weight, and in virtue of all the fluid/body weight variability found in patients with CKD, desirable rather than actual body weight should be used. Another important point is that even though their energy requirements are the same as for healthy population, CKD patients often ingest less than 35 kcal/kg/day, especially as glomerular filtration rate decreases below 15 mL/min, mainly due to anorexia [186]. This is an important consideration, because appropriate energy intake is necessary for adequate utilization of protein, which is particularly important when low protein diets are prescribed. Also, the level of energy requirement is increased during concurrent illnesses, particularly those requiring hospitalization.

Resting energy expenditure may be assessed by using standard equations and by indirect and direct measurements. The simplest method to estimate REE (kcal/day) is the calculation by the Harris–Benedict equation:

$$\text{Men: REE} = 66 + (13.7 \times \text{weight}) + (5 \times \text{height}) - (6.8 \times \text{age})$$

$$\text{Women: REE} = 655.1 + (9.6 \times \text{weight}) + (1.8 \times \text{height}) - (4.7 \times \text{age})$$

where weight is expressed in kg, height in cm, and age in years. Currently, there are limited data on the best predictive REE equation suitable for patients undergoing maintenance dialysis.

Although there is a general consensus that direct measures are always more precise than indirect ones, this may not be the case for energy assessment, where the term "indirect" refers to the assessment of energy expenditure generally performed by measuring oxygen consumption (VO_2) and carbon dioxide production (VCO_2), and "direct" in this context means measuring the direct heat transfer [187]. Measurements of REE by indirect calorimetry, in general, are well correlated with direct calorimetry values, and in addition, provide an appreciation of the substrates that are oxidized in the course of expending energy. Direct calorimetry measures the heat production directly, but it is much more difficult and costly to perform and gives no information concerning the substrates utilized to generate the heat. Nonetheless, direct calorimetry is traditionally considered the gold standard for measurements of energy expenditure. However, indirect calorimetry is not only more convenient, but it is particularly suitable if nutritional assessment is desirable [177,188]. Since energy balance grossly equals energy intake minus energy expenditure, and indirect calorimetry is usually measured for short periods of time with the subjects in the postabsorptive state, measurement of energy balance by indirect calorimetry is mainly the measurement of energy output. Energy expenditure in clinical studies is almost invariably performed by indirect calorimetry [189]. Estimates are available so that short periods of assessment may be used to estimate 24-hour REE [189].

The most precise technique to indirectly measure calorimetry (by CO_2 and O_2 exchange) is the whole-room indirect calorimetry (metabolic chamber) [189]. These are small rooms usually furnished with a bed and/or chair, toilet facilities and telephone to allow the patient to be able to stay inside it comfortably enough for an adequate period of measurement. The metabolic chamber is designed to monitor patients for several days at a time. The metabolic rate is calculated based on the measurement of VO_2 and VCO_2, using standard estimation equations to calculate values of REE [189].

Another method of indirect calorimetry is to use the metabolic cart, which involves placing a plastic mask or ventilated hood to the patient's face to prevent the escape of expired air from the system. The air is drawn through the system and integrated into an O_2 and CO_2 analyzer attached to a computer for data analysis and storage, including all the parameters measured by the chamber (VO_2, VCO_2, metabolic rate, and RQ) [189]. The metabolic carts are widely used in clinical practice and for research purposes. The accuracy of such carts is inferior to whole-room indirect calorimetric chamber [190] because of some inherent technical limitations. For example, patients sometimes react adversely to a mask, mouthpiece, or ventilated hood and become agitated, with involuntarily hyperventilation, generating inappropriate high rates of VO_2 and VCO_2. A small percentage of subjects also experience a training effect, with REE decreasing significantly with repeated studies [190]. Finally, some masks do not fit securely around the mouths and noses of patients, particularly those with PEW, resulting in a leak of respiratory gases, and these systems are not comfortable or practical to use for long periods of time [190]. These limitations should be taken into account in clinical practice and in most of the research protocols, because a metabolic cart is the most commonly used indirect calorimetry technique and a metabolic chamber is only available in a very limited number of centers.

As previously discussed, total energy expenditure is composed of REE, the thermal effect of food, and physical activity, assuming an ideal situation of a postabsorptive state for measuring the REE. Total energy expenditure also can be precisely and directly measured by the doubly labeled water technique, a safe and non-invasive technique, yet not of widespread use. It is done by oral ingestion or intravenous injection of two stable isotopes of water, i.e. $H_2^{18}O$ and ^2H_2O, as a bolus. The disappearance of the ^2H in the ^2H_2O is similar to the water flux alone, but the disappearance of the ^{18}O in the $H_2^{18}O$ is also lost in carbon dioxide (as $C^{18}O_2$). The difference in the flux rates of these two tracers is a direct function of VCO_2 and can be used to calculate oxidation of carbohydrates, lipids and proteins (amino acids).

SUMMARY AND RECOMMENDATIONS

There are many different methods available for assessing protein and energy status. Some are easy to perform, readily available and inexpensive, while others are sophisticated, not available in many centers, and either expensive or with an unfavorable cost-benefit ratio. In the research setting, complex and precise methods to assess protein and energy metabolism, i.e. stable isotope tracer techniques, although not of widespread availability, are the methods of choice to measure acute changes or responses to metabolic interventions, minimizing variability and errors.

In Stage 1–3 CKD patients, measurement of serum albumin every 6 months along with body weight is sufficient to screen for any nutritional abnormalities. The frequency should be increased to every 3–4 months in later stages of CKD. Renal transplant recipients should be considered at similar risk as Stage 3–5 CKD patients due to underlying kidney disease and use of immunosuppressive medications that may influence metabolic milieu. In ESRD patients undergoing maintenance hemo- or peritoneal dialysis, nutritional screening should include monthly assessments of serum albumin, dry weight, and SGA every 3–6 months. In addition to interpreting absolute values for certain thresholds, trends over time should be considered. A consistent decrease greater than 0.3 g/dL in serum albumin levels should initiate a more comprehensive assessment such as dietary interviews, anthropometry, dual-energy X-ray absorptiometry, and even more sophisticated methods, if available. Direct measures of inflammatory status, such as serum CRP, is of significant use in this setting and can be employed to monitor targeted therapies. For all indirect methods, repeated measures and technical standardization are extremely important to reduce variability of results. Patients with acute kidney injury, especially individuals in the intensive care unit, represent a challenge for appropriate assessment of nutritional status. Acute illness influences almost all components of body composition and significantly alters visceral protein concentrations. Use of biochemical indices with shorter half-lives that are more responsive to nutritional therapy such as serum prealbumin should be considered in these patients. Similarly, changes in fluid status must be taken into account when assessing body composition. Regardless of the method, it is important to keep in mind that none is perfect and definitive, and the results should always be analyzed in the clinical context of each individual patient.

References

[1] Allison SP. Malnutrition, disease, and outcome. Nutrition 2000;16:590–3.

[2] Ikizler TA, Hakim RM. Nutrition in end-stage renal disease. Kidney Int 1996;50:343–57.

[3] Ikizler TA, Himmelfarb J. Nutrition in Acute Renal Failure. Adv Ren Replace Ther 1997;4:54–63.

[4] Feroze U, Noori N, Kovesdy CP, Molnar MZ, Martin DJ, Reina-Patton A, et al. Quality-of-life and mortality in hemodialysis patients: roles of race and nutritional status. Clin J Am Soc Nephrol 2011;6:1100–11.

[5] Bistrian BR, Blackburn GL, Vitale J, Cochran D, Naylor J. Prevalence of malnutrition in general medical patients. Jama 1976;235:1567–70.

[6] Hill GL, Blackett RL, Pickford I, Burkinshaw L, Young GA, Warren JV, et al. Malnutrition in surgical patients. An unrecognised problem. Lancet 1977;1:689–92.

[7] Sharma R, Florea VG, Bolger AP, Doehner W, Florea ND, Coats AJ, et al. Wasting as an independent predictor of mortality in patients with cystic fibrosis. Thorax 2001;56:746–50.

[8] Campos AC, Matias JE, Coelho JC. Nutritional aspects of liver transplantation. Curr Opin Clin Nutr Metab Care 2002;5:297–307.

[9] Angus DC, Linde-Zwirble WT, Lidicker J, Clermont G, Carcillo J, Pinsky MR. Epidemiology of severe sepsis in the United States: analysis of incidence, outcome, and associated costs of care. Crit Care Med 2001;29:1303–10.

[10] Guarnieri G, Faccini L, Lipartiti T, Ranieri F, Spangaro F, Giuntini D, et al. Simple methods for nutritional assessment in hemodialyzed patients. Am J Clin Nutr 1980;33:1598–607.

[11] Young GA, Swanepoel CR, Croft MR, Hobson SM, Parsons FM. Anthropometry and plasma valine, amino acids, and proteins in the nutritional assessment of hemodialysis patients. Kidney Int 1982;21:492–9.

[12] Schoenfeld PY, Henry RR, Laird NM, Roxe DM. Assessment of nutritional status of the national cooperative dialysis study population. Kidney Int 1983;23:80–8.

[13] Wolfson M, Strong CJ, Minturn RD, Gray DK, Kopple JD. Nutritional status and lymphocyte function in maintenance hemodialysis patients. Am J Clin Nutr 1984;37:547–55.

[14] Cianciaruso B, Brunori G, Kopple JD, Traverso G, Panarello G, Enia G, et al. Cross-sectional comparison of malnutrition in continuous ambulatory peritoneal dialysis and hemodialysis patients. Am J Kidney Dis 1995;26:475–86.

[15] Sardesai VM. Fundamentals of nutrition. In: Dekker M, editor. Introduction to clinical nutrition. New York: Sardesai, V.M; 1998. p. 1–13.

[16] Sardesai VM. Requirements for energy, carbohydrates, fat, and proteins. In: Dekker M, editor. Introduction to clinical nutrition. New York: Sardesai, V.M; 1998. p. 1–13.

[17] Fouque D, Kalantar-Zadeh K, Kopple J, et al. A proposed nomenclature and diagnostic criteria for protein-energy wasting in acute and chronic kidney disease. Kidney Int 2008;73:391–8.

[18] Jeejeebhoy KN. Nutritional assessment. Nutrition 2000;16: 585–90.

[19] Association AD. Identifying patients at risk: ADA's definitions for nutrition screening and nutrition assessment. Council on Practice (COP) Quality Management Committee. J Am Diet Assoc 1994;94:838–9.

[20] Requirements EaP. Report of a Joint FAO/WHO Ad Hoc Expert Committee. Technical Report Series 1973;522.

[21] Borah MF, Schoenfeld PY, Gotch FA, Sargent JA, Wolfson M, Humphreys MH. Nitrogen balance during intermittent dialysis therapy of uremia. Kidney Int 1978;14:491–500.

[22] Ginn HE, Frost A, Lacy WW. Nitrogen balance in hemodialysis patients. Am J Clin Nutr 1968;21:385–93.

[23] Kopple JD, Shinaberger JH, Coburn JW, Sorensen MK, Rubini ME. Optimal dietary protein treatment during chronic hemodialysis. Trans Am Soc Artif Int Organs 1969;15:302–8.

[24] Motil KJ, Matthews DE, Bier DM, Burke JF, Munro HN, Young VR. Whole-body leucine and lysine metabolism: response to dietary protein intake in young men. Am J Physiol 1981;240:E712–721.

[25] Price SR, Mitch WE. Metabolic acidosis and uremic toxicity: protein and amino acid metabolism. Semin Nephrol 1994;14:232–7.

[26] Anderson CF, Wochos DN. The utility of serum albumin values in the nutritional assessment of hospitalized patients. Mayo Clin Proc 1982;57:181–4.

[27] Reinhardt GF, Myscofski JW, Wilkens DB, Dobrin PB, Mangan Jr JE, Stannard RT. Incidence and mortality of hypoalbuminemic patients in hospitalized veterans. JPEN J Parenter Enteral Nutr 1980;4:357–9.

[28] Apelgren KN, Rombeau JL, Twomey PL, Miller RA. Comparison of nutritional indices and outcome in critically ill patients. Crit Care Med 1982;10:305–7.

[29] Kaw M, Sekas G. Long-term follow-up of consequences of percutaneous endoscopic gastrostomy (PEG) tubes in nursing home patients. Dig Dis Sci 1994;39:738–43.

[30] Jeejeebhoy KN. Nutritional assessment. Gastroenterol Clin North Am 1998;27:347–69.

[31] Klein S. The myth of serum albumin as a measure of nutritional status. Gastroenterology 1990;99:1845–6.

[32] Kirsch R, Frith L, Black E, Hoffenberg R. Regulation of albumin synthesis and catabolism by alteration of dietary protein. Nature 1968;217:578–9.

[33] Kashihara T, Fujimori E, Oki A, et al. Protein-losing enteropathy and pancreatic involvement in a case of connective tissue disease. Gastroenterol Jpn 1992;27:246–51.

[34] Chiu NT, Lee BF, Hwang SJ, Chang JM, Liu GC, Yu HS. Protein-losing enteropathy: diagnosis with (99m)Tc-labeled human serum albumin scintigraphy. Radiology 2001;219:86–90.

[35] Kaysen GA, Rathore V, Shearer GC, Depner TA. Mechanisms of hypoalbuminemia in hemodialysis patients. Kidney Int 1995;48:510–6.

[36] Cueto Manzano AM. Hypoalbuminemia in dialysis. Is it a marker for malnutrition or inflammation? Rev Invest Clin 2001;53:152–8.

[37] Moshage HJ, Janssen JA, Franssen JH, Hafkenscheid JC, Yap SH. Study of the molecular mechanism of decreased liver synthesis of albumin in inflammation. J Clin Invest 1987;79:1635–41.

[38] Fleck A, Raines G, Hawker F, Trotter J, Wallace PI, Ledingham IM, et al. Increased vascular permeability: a major cause of hypoalbuminaemia in disease and injury. Lancet 1985;1:781–4.

[39] Caglar K, Peng Y, Pupim LB, Flakoll PJ, Levenhagen D, Hakim RM, et al. Inflammatory signals associated with hemodialysis. Kidney Int 2002;62:1408–16.

[40] Gray GE, Meguid MM. Can total parenteral nutrition reverse hypoalbuminemia in oncology patients? Nutrition 1990;6:225–8.

[41] Friedman AN, Fadem SZ. Reassessment of albumin as a nutritional marker in kidney disease. J Am Soc Nephrol 2010;21:223–30.

[42] Lowrie EG, Lew NL. Death risk in hemodialysis patients: The predictive value of commonly measured variables and an evaluation of death rate differences between facilities. Am J Kidney Dis 1990;15:458–82.

[43] Mehrotra R, Duong U, Jiwakanon S, Kovesdy CP, Moran J, Kopple JD, et al. Serum albumin as a predictor of mortality in peritoneal dialysis: comparisons with hemodialysis. Am J Kidney Dis 2011;58:418–28.

[44] Kaysen GA, Dubin JA, Muller HG, Mitch WE, Rosales LM, Levin NW. Relationships among inflammation nutrition and physiologic mechanisms establishing albumin levels in hemodialysis patients. Kidney Int 2002;61:2240–9.

[45] Kaysen GA. The microinflammatory state in uremia: causes and potential consequences. J Am Soc Nephrol 2001;12:1549–57.

[46] Kaysen GA, Chertow GM, Adhikarla R, Young B, Ronco C, Levin NW. Inflammation and dietary protein intake exert competing effects on serum albumin and creatinine in hemodialysis patients. Kidney Int 2001;60:333–40.

[47] Ikizler TA, Wingard RL, Harvell J, Shyr Y, Hakim RM. Association of morbidity with markers of nutrition and inflammation in chronic hemodialysis patients: a prospective study. Kidney Int 1999;55:1945–51.

[48] Beck FK, Rosenthal TC. Prealbumin: a marker for nutritional evaluation. Am Fam Physician 2002;65:1575–8.

[49] Neyra NR, Hakim RM, Shyr Y, Ikizler TA. Serum transferrin and serum prealbumin are early predictors of serum albumin in chronic hemodialysis patients. J Ren Nutr 2000;10:184–90.

[50] Chertow GM, Ackert K, Lew NL, Lazarus JM, Lowrie EG. Prealbumin is as important as albumin in the nutritional assessment of hemodialysis patients. Kidney Int 2000;58:2512–7.

[51] Spiekerman AM. Nutritional assessment (protein nutriture). Anal Chem 1995;67:429R–36R.

[52] Spiekerman AM. Proteins used in nutritional assessment. Clin Lab Med 1993;13:353–69.

[53] Mears E. Outcomes of continuous process improvement of a nutritional care program incorporating serum prealbumin measurements. Nutrition 1996;12:479–84.

[54] Group PiNCC. Measurement of visceral protein status in assessing protein and energy malnutrition: standard of care. Prealbumin in Nutritional Care Consensus Group. Nutrition 1995;11:169–71.

[55] Cano NJ, Fouque D, Roth H, Aparicio M, Azar R, Canaud B, et al. Intradialytic parenteral nutrition does not improve survival in malnourished hemodialysis patients: A 2-year multicenter, prospective, randomized study. J Am Soc Nephrol 2007;18:2583–91.

[56] Ingenbleek Y, DeVisscher M, DeNayer P. Measurement of prealbumin as index of protein-calorie malnutrition. Lancet 1972;2:106–8.

[57] Ingenbleek Y, Van Den Schrieck HG, De Nayer P, De Visscher M. Albumin, transferrin and the thyroxine-binding prealbumin/retinol-binding protein (TBPA-RBP) complex in assessment of malnutrition. Clin Chim Acta 1975;63:61–7.

[58] Mittman N, Avram MM, Oo KK, Chattopadhyay J. Serum prealbumin predicts survival in hemodialysis and peritoneal dialysis: 10 years of prospective observation. Am J Kidney Dis 2001;38:1358–64.

[59] Duggan A, Huffman FG. Validation of serum transthyretin (prealbumin) as a nutritional parameter in hemodialysis patients. J Ren Nutr 1998;8:142–9.

[60] Rambod M, Kovesdy CP, Bross R, Kopple JD, Kalantar-Zadeh K. Association of serum prealbumin and its changes over time with clinical outcomes and survival in patients receiving hemodialysis. Am J Clin Nutr 2008;88:1485–94.

[61] Staley MJ. Fructosamine and protein concentrations in serum. Clin Chem 1987;33:2326–7.

[62] Oppenheimer JH, Werner SC. Effect of prednisone on thyroxine-binding proteins. J Clin Endocrinol Metab 1966;26:715–21.

[63] Le Moullac B, Gouache P, Bleiberg-Daniel F. Regulation of hepatic transthyretin messenger RNA levels during moderate protein and food restriction in rats. J Nutr 1992;122:864–70.

[64] Winkler MF, Gerrior SA, Pomp A, Albina JE. Use of retinol-binding protein and prealbumin as indicators of the response to nutrition therapy. J Am Diet Assoc 1989;89:684–7.

[65] Hedlund JU, Hansson LO, Ortqvist AB. Hypoalbuminemia in hospitalized patients with community-acquired pneumonia. Arch Intern Med 1995;155:1438–42.

[66] Nieken J, Mulder NH, Buter J, Vellenga E, Limburg PC, Piers DA, et al. Recombinant human interleukin-6 induces a rapid and reversible anemia in cancer patients. Blood 1995;86:900–5.

[67] O'Riordain MG, Ross JA, Fearon KC, Maingay J, Farouk M, Garden OJ, et al. Insulin and counterregulatory hormones influence acute-phase protein production in human hepatocytes. Am J Physiol 1995;269:E323–330.

[68] Hakim RM, Levin N. Malnutrition in hemodialysis patients. Am J Kidney Dis 1993;21:125–37.

[69] Huebers HA, Finch CA. The physiology of transferrin and transferrin receptors. Physiol Rev 1987;67:520–82.

[70] Fletcher JP, Little JM, Guest PK. A comparison of serum transferrin and serum albumin as nutritional parameters. J Parenter Enteral Nutr 1987;11:144.

[71] Briassoulis G, Zavras N, Hatzis T. Malnutrition, nutritional indices, and early enteral feeding in critically ill children. Nutrition 2001;17:548–57.

[72] Han PD, Burke A, Baldassano RN, Rombeau JL, Lichtenstein GR. Nutrition and inflammatory bowel disease. Gastroenterol Clin North Am 1999;28:423–43. ix.

[73] Taylor SJ, Fettes SB, Jewkes C, Nelson RJ. Prospective, randomized, controlled trial to determine the effect of early enhanced enteral nutrition on clinical outcome in mechanically ventilated patients suffering head injury. Crit Care Med 1999;27:2525–31.

[74] Qureshi AR, Alvestrand A, Danielsson A, Divino-Filho JC, Gutierrez A, Lindholm B, et al. Factors predicting malnutrition in hemodialysis patients: a cross-sectional study. Kidney Int 1998;53:773–82.

[75] Barany P, Peterson E, Ahlberg M, Hultman E, Bergstrom J. Nutritional assessment in anemic hemodialysis patients treated with recombinant human erythropoietin. Clin Nephrol 1991;35:270–9.

[76] Roza AM, Tuitt D, Shizgal HM. Transferrin: A poor measure of nutritional status. J Parenter Enteral Nutr 1984;8:523.

[77] NKF-DOQI. Clinical practice guidelines for nutrition in chronic renal failure. K/DOQI, National Kidney Foundation. Am J Kidney Dis 2000;35:S1–140.

[78] Cano N, Di Costanzo-Dufetel J, Calaf R, Durbec JP, Lacombe P, Pascal S, et al. Labastie-Coeyrehourcq, J: Prealbumin-retinol-binding-protein-retinol complex in hemodialysis patients. Am J Clin Nutr 1988;47:664–7.

[79] Kiess W, Kessler U, Schmitt S, Funk B. Growth hormone and insulin-like growth factor 1: Basic aspects. In: Flyvbjerg A, Orskov H, Alberti KG, editors. Growth hormone and insulin-like growth factor 1. New York: Wiley; 1993. p. 1–21.

[80] Raynaud-Simon A, Perin L, Meaume S, Lesourd B, Moulias R, Postel-Vinay MC, et al. IGF-I, IGF-I-binding proteins and GH-binding protein in malnourished elderly patients with inflammation receiving refeeding therapy. Eur J Endocrinol 2002;146:657–65.

[81] Thissen JP, Ketelslegers JM, Underwood LE. Nutritional regulation of the insulin-like growth factors. Endocr Rev 1994;15:80–101.

[82] Van den Berghe GH. Acute and prolonged critical illness are two distinct neuroendocrine paradigms. Verh K Acad Geneeskd Belg 1998;60:487–518. discussion 518-420.

[83] Jacob V, Carpentier JEL, Salzano S, Naylor V, Wild G, Brown CB, et al. IGF-1, a marker of undernutrition in hemodialysis patients. Am J Clin Nutr 1990;52:39–44.

[84] Kagan A, Altman Y, Zadik Z, Bar-Khayim Y. Insulin-like growth factor-I in patients on CAPD and hemodialysis: relationship to body weight and albumin level. Adv Perit Dial 1995;11:234–8.

[85] Parker III TF, Wingard RL, Husni L, Ikizler TA, Parker RA, Hakim RM. Effect of the membrane biocompatibility on nutritional parameters in chronic hemodialysis patients. Kidney Int 1996;49:551–6.

[86] Gabay C, Kushner I. Acute-phase proteins and other systemic responses to inflammation. N Engl J Med 1999;340:448–54.

[87] Owen WF, Lowrie EG. C-reactive protein as an outcome predictor for maintenance hemodialysis patients. Kidney Int 1998;54:627–36.

[88] Harrison NA, Masterton RG, Bateman JM, Rainford DJ. C-reactive protein in acute renal failure. Nephrol Dial Transplant 1989;4:864–9.

[89] Pecoits-Filho R, Barany P, Lindholm B, Heimburger O, Stenvinkel P. Interleukin-6 is an independent predictor of mortality in patients starting dialysis treatment. Nephrol Dial Transplant 2002;17:1684–8.

[90] Panichi V, Migliori M, De Pietro S, Taccola D, Bianchi AM, Norpoth M, et al. C reactive protein in patients with chronic renal diseases. Ren Fail 2001;23:551–62.

[91] Locatelli F, Fouque D, Heimburger O, Drueke TB, Cannata-Andia JB, Horl WH, et al. Nutritional status in dialysis patients: a European consensus. Nephrol Dial Transplant 2002;17:563–72.

[92] Cano NJ, Aparicio M, Brunori G, Carrero JJ, Cianciaruso B, Fiaccadori E, et al. ESPEN Guidelines on Parenteral Nutrition: adult renal failure. Clin Nutr 2009;28:401–14.

[93] Stenvinkel P, Barany P, Chung SH, Lindholm B, Heimburger O. A comparative analysis of nutritional parameters as predictors of outcome in male and female ESRD patients. Nephrol Dial Transplant 2002;17:1266–74.

[94] Wang J, Thornton JC, Kolesnik S, Pierson Jr RN. Anthropometry in body composition. An overview. Ann N Y Acad Sci 2000;904:317–26.

[95] Chumlea WC, Guo SS, Vellas B. Assessment of protein-calorie nutrition. In: Kopple JD, Massry SG, editors. Nutritional management of renal disease. Baltimore, MD: Williams & Wilkins; 1997. p. 203–28.

[96] Jelliffe DB, Jelliffe EF. An evaluation of upper arm measurements used in nutritional assessment. Am J Clin Nutr 1980;33:2058–9.

[97] Gurney JM, Jelliffe DB. Arm anthropometry in nutritional assessment: nomogram for rapid calculation of muscle circumference and cross-sectional muscle and fat areas. Am J Clin Nutr 1973;26:912–5.

[98] Harries AD, Jones LA, Heatley RV, Rhodes J. Assessment of nutritional status by anthropometry: a comparison of different standards of reference. Hum Nutr Clin Nutr 1983;37:227–31.

[99] Frisancho AR. Nutritional anthropometry. J Am Diet Assoc 1988;88:553–5.

[100] de Onis M, Habicht JP. Anthropometric reference data for international use: recommendations from a World Health Organization Expert Committee. Am J Clin Nutr 1996;64:650–8.

[101] Vansant G, Van Gaal L, De Leeuw I. Assessment of body composition by skinfold anthropometry and bioelectrical impedance technique: a comparative study. JPEN J Parenter Enteral Nutr 1994;18:427–9.

[102] Ravasco P, Camilo ME, Gouveia-Oliveira A, Adam S, Brum G. A critical approach to nutritional assessment in critically ill patients. Clin Nutr 2002;21:73–7.

[103] Yao M, Roberts SB, Ma G, Pan H, McCrory MA. Field methods for body composition assessment are valid in healthy chinese adults. Am Soc Nutr Sci 2002:310–7.

[104] Mei Z, Grummer-Strawn LM, Pietrobelli A, Goulding A, Goran MI, Dietz WH. Validity of body mass index compared with other body-composition screening indexes for the assessment of body fatness in children and adolescents. Am J Clin Nutr 2002;75:978–85.

[105] Pollock ML, Jackson AS. Research progress in validation of clinical methods of assessing body composition. Med Sci Sports Exerc 1984;16:606–15.

[106] Noori N, Kopple JD, Kovesdy CP, Feroze U, Sim JJ, Murali SB, et al. Mid-arm muscle circumference and quality of life and survival in maintenance hemodialysis patients. Clin J Am Soc Nephrol 2010;5:2258–68.

[107] Nelson EE, Hong CD, Pesce AL, Peterson DW, Singh S, Pollak VE. Anthropometric norms for the dialysis population. Am J Kidney Dis 1990;16:32–7.

[108] Noori N, Kovesdy CP, Bross R, Lee M, Oreopoulos A, Benner D, et al. Novel equations to estimate lean body mass in maintenance hemodialysis patients. Am J Kidney Dis 2011;57:130–9.

[109] Pupim LB, Kent P, Ikizler TA. Bioelectrical impedance analysis in dialysis patients. Miner Electrolyte Metab 1999;25:400–6.

[110] Dumler F, Kilates C. Use of bioelectrical impedance techniques for monitoring nutritional status in patients on maintenance dialysis. J Ren Nutr 2000;10:116–24.

[111] Evans EM, Arngrimsson SA, Cureton KJ. Body composition estimates from multicomponent models using BIA to determine body water. Med Sci Sports Exerc 2001;33:839–42.

[112] Chertow GM. Estimates of body composition as intermediate outcome variables: are DEXA and BIA ready for prime time? J Ren Nutr 1999;9:138–41.

[113] Dumler F. Use of bioelectric impedance analysis and dual-energy X-ray absorptiometry for monitoring the nutritional status of dialysis patients. Asaio J 1997;43:256–60.

[114] Khaled MA, Kabir I, Goran MI, Mahalanabis D. Bioelectrical impedance measurements at various frequencies to estimate human body compositions. Indian J Exp Biol 1997;35:159–61.

[115] Biggs J, Cha K, Horch K. Electrical resistivity of the upper arm and leg yields good estimates of whole body fat. Physiol Meas 2001;22:365–76.

[116] Di Iorio BR, Terracciano V, Bellizzi. V: Bioelectrical impedance measurement: errors and artifacts. J Ren Nutr 1999;9:192–7.

[117] Wotton MJ, Thomas BJ, Cornish BH, Ward LC. Comparison of whole body and segmental bioimpedance methodologies for estimating total body water. Ann N Y Acad Sci 2000;904:181–6.

[118] Kotler DP, Rosenbaum K, Allison DB, Wang J, Pierson Jr RN. Validation of bioimpedance analysis as a measure of change in body cell mass as estimated by whole-body counting of potassium in adults. JPEN J Parenter Enteral Nutr 1999;23:345–9.

[119] Chertow GM, Jacobs DO, Lazarus JM, Lew NL, Lowrie EG. Phase angle predicts survival in hemodialysis patients. J Renal Nutr 1997;7:204–7.

[120] Piccoli A, Fanos V, Peruzzi L, Schena S, Pizzini C, Borgione S, et al. Reference values of the bioelectrical impedance vector in neonates in the first week after birth. Nutrition 2002;18:383–7.

[121] Woodrow G, Oldroyd B, Turney JH, Davies PS, Day JM, Smith MA. Measurement of total body water by bioelectrical impedance in chronic renal failure. Eur J Clin Nutr 1996;50:676–81.

[122] Nescolarde L, Donate T, Piccoli A, Rosell J. Comparison of segmental with whole-body impedance measurements in peritoneal dialysis patients. Med Eng Phys 2008;30:817–24.

[123] Chertow GM, Lazarus JM, Lew NL, Ma L, Lowrie EG. Bioimpedance norms for the hemodialysis population. Kidney Int 1997;52:1617–21.

[124] Elia M, Rombeau JL, Rolandelli RH. Assessment of nutritional status and body composition. In: Clinical nutrition: Enteral and tube feeding. 3rd ed. Philadelphia, PA: W. H. Saunders; 1997. p. 155–73.

[125] Kalantar-Zadeh K, Dunne E, Nixon K, Kahn K, Lee GH, Kleiner M, et al. Near infra-red interactance for nutritional

assessment of dialysis patients. Nephrol Dial Transplant 1999;14:169–75.

[126] Bross R, Chandramohan G, Kovesdy CP, Oreopoulos A, Noori N, Golden S, et al. Comparing body composition assessment tests in long-term hemodialysis patients. Am J Kidney Dis 2010;55:885–96.

[127] Fuller NJ, Jebb SA, Laskey MA, Coward WA, Elia M. Four-component model for the assessment of body composition in humans: comparison with alternative methods, and evaluation of the density and hydration of fat-free mass. Clin Sci (Lond) 1992;82:687–93.

[128] Keshaviah PR, Nolph KD, Moore HL, Prowant B, Emerson PF, Meyer M, et al. Lean body mass estimation by creatinine kinetics. J Am Soc Nephrol 1994;4:1475–85.

[129] Bhatla B, Moore H, Emerson P, Keshaviah P, Prowant B, Nolph KD, et al. Lean body mass estimation by creatinine kinetics, bioimpedance, and dual energy X-ray absorptiometry in patients on continuous ambulatory peritoneal dialysis. Asaio J 1995;41:M442–446.

[130] Forbes GB. Body composition. In: Ziegler EE, Filer JR LJ, editors. Present knowledge in nutrition. 7th ed. Washington, DC: International Life Sciences Institutes Press; 1996. p. 7–12.

[131] Fogelholm M, van Marken Lichtenbelt W. Comparison of body composition methods: a literature analysis. Eur J Clin Nutr 1997;51:495–503.

[132] Kyle UG, Genton L, Pichard C. Body composition: what's new? Curr Opin Clin Nutr Metab Care 2002;5:427–33.

[133] Dempster P, Aitkens S. A new air displacement method for the determination of human body composition. Med Sci Sports Exerc 1995;27:1692–7.

[134] Levenhagen DK, Borel MJ, Welch DC, Piasecki JH, Piasecki DP, Chen KY, et al. A comparison of air displacement plethysmography with three other techniques to determine body fat in healthy adults. JPEN J Parenter Enteral Nutr 1999;23:293–9.

[135] Fields DA, Goran MI, McCrory MA. Body-composition assessment via air-displacement plethysmography in adults and children: a review. Am J Clin Nutr 2002;75:453–67.

[136] Biaggi RR, Vollman MW, Nies MA, Brener CE, Flakoll PJ, Levenhagen DK, et al. Comparison of air-displacement plethysmography with hydrostatic weighing and bioelectrical impedance analysis for the assessment of body composition in healthy adults. Am J Clin Nutr 1999;69:898–903.

[137] Curtin F, Morabia A, Pichard C, Slosman DO. Body mass index compared to dual-energy X-ray absorptiometry: evidence for a spectrum bias. J Clin Epidemiol 1997;50:837–43.

[138] Abrahamsen B, Hansen TB, Hogsberg IM, Pedersen FB. Beck-Nielsen, H: Impact of hemodialysis on dual X-ray absorptiometry, bioelectrical impedance measurements, and anthropometry. Am J Clin Nutr 1996;63:80–6.

[139] Panotopoulos G, Ruiz JC, Guy-Grand B, Basdevant A. Dual X-ray absorptiometry, bioelectrical impedance, and near infrared interactance in obese women. Med Sci Sports Exerc 2001;33:665–70.

[140] Cohn SH, Brennan BL, Yasumura S, Vartsky D, Vaswani AN, Ellis KJ. Evaluation of body composition and nitrogen content of renal patients on chronic dialysis as determined by total body neutron activation. Am J Clin Nutr 1983;38:52–8.

[141] Stall S, DeVita MV, Ginsberg NS, Frumkin D, Lynn RI, Michelis MF. Body composition assessed by neutron activation analysis in dialysis patients. Ann N Y Acad Sci 2000;904:558–63.

[142] Morgan WD. Of mermaids and mountains. Three decades of prompt activation in vivo. Ann N Y Acad Sci 2000;904:128–33.

[143] Pollock CA, Ibels LS, Allen BJ, Ayass W, Caterson RJ, Waugh DA, et al. Total body nitrogen as a prognostic marker in maintenance dialysis. J Am Soc Nephrol 1995;6:82–8.

[144] Park JH, Olsen NJ. Utility of magnetic resonance imaging in the evaluation of patients with inflammatory myopathies. Curr Rheumatol Rep 2001;3:334–45.

[145] Detsky AS, Baker JP, Mendelson RA, Wolman SL, Wesson DE, Jeejeebhoy KN. Evaluating the accuracy of nutritional assessment techniques applied to hospitalized patients: methodology and comparisons. JPEN J Parenter Enteral Nutr 1984;8:153–9.

[146] McCann L. Using subjective global assessment to identify malnutrition in the ESRD patient. Nephrol News Issues 1999;13:18–9.

[147] Cooper BA, Bartlett LH, Aslani A, Allen BJ, Ibels LS, Pollock CA. Validity of subjective global assessment as a nutritional marker in end-stage renal disease. Am J Kidney Dis 2002;40:126–32.

[148] Duerksen DR, Yeo TA, Siemens JL, O'Connor MP. The validity and reproducibility of clinical assessment of nutritional status in the elderly. Nutrition 2000;16:740–4.

[149] Caglar K, Fedje L, Dimmitt R, Hakim RM, Shyr Y, Ikizler TA. Therapeutic effects of oral nutritional supplementation during hemodialysis. Kidney Int 2002;62:1054–9.

[150] Harty JC, Boulton H, Curwell J, Heelis N, Uttley L, Venning MC, et al. The normalized protein catabolic rate is a flawed marker of nutrition in CAPD patients. Kidney Int 1994;45:103–9.

[151] Jones CH, Wolfenden RC, Wells LM. Is subjective global assessment a reliable measure of nutritional status in hemodialysis? J Ren Nutr 2004;14:26–30.

[152] Kalantar-Zadeh K, Kopple JD, Block G, Humphreys MH. A malnutrition-inflammation score is correlated with morbidity and mortality in maintenance hemodialysis patients. Am J Kidney Dis 2001;38:1251–63.

[153] Kalantar-Zadeh K, Kopple JD, Humphreys MH, Block G. Comparing outcome predictability of markers of malnutrition-inflammation complex syndrome in haemodialysis patients. Nephrol Dial Transplant 2004;19:1507–19.

[154] Goldstein DJ. Assessment of nutritional status in renal diseases. In: Mitch WE, Klahr S, editors. Handbook of nutrition and the kidney. 3rd ed. Philadelphia, PA: Lippincott-Raven; 1998. p. 46–86.

[155] Kopple JD. Uses and limitations of the balance technique. JPEN J Parenter Enteral Nutr 1987;11:79S–85S.

[156] Rao M, Sharma M, Juneja R, Jacob S, Jacob CK. Calculated nitrogen balance in hemodialysis patients: influence of protein intake. Kidney Int 2000;58:336–45.

[157] Reifenstein EC, Albright F, Wells SL. The accumulation, interpretation, and presentation of data pertaining to metabolic balances, notably those of calcium, phosphorus, and nitrogen. J Clin Endoccrinol Metab 1945;5:367–95.

[158] Kopple JD, Coburn JW. Metabolic studies of low protein diets in uremia. I. Nitrogen and potassium. Medicine (Baltimore) 1973;52:583–95.

[159] Calloway DH. Nitrogen balance of men with marginal intakes of protein and energy. J Nutr 1975;105:914–23.

[160] Kopple JD, Gao XL, Qing DP. Dietary protein, urea nitrogen appearance and total nitrogen appearance in chronic renal failure and CAPD patients. Kidney Int 1997;52:486–94.

[161] Garlick PJ, Clugston GA, Swick RW, Meinertzhagen IH, Waterlow JC. Diurnal variations in protein metabolism in man. Proc Nutr Soc 1978;37:33A.

[162] Wolfe RR. Radioactive and stable isotope tracers in biomedicine. In: Principles and practice of kinetic analysis. New York: Wiley-Liss; 1992. p. 283–316.

[163] Garlick PJ, McNurlan MA, McHardy KC, Calder AG, Milne E, Fearns LM, et al. Rates of nutrient utilization in man measured by combined respiratory gas analysis and stable isotopic

[164] Barrett EJ, Revkin JH, Young LH, Zaret BL, Jacob R, Gelfand RA. An isotopic method for measurement of muscle protein synthesis and degradation in vivo. Biochem J 1987; 245:223–8.

[165] Gelfand RA, Barrett EJ. Effect of physiologic hyperinsulinemia on skeletal muscle protein synthesis and breakdown in man. J Clin Invest 1987;80:1–6.

[166] Christensen HN. Role of amino acid transport and countertransport in nutrition and metabolism. Physiol Rev 1990; 70:43–77.

[167] Shotwell MA, Kilberg MS, Oxender DL. The regulation of neutral amino acid transport in mammalian cells. Biochim Biophys Acta 1983;737:267–84.

[168] Biolo G, Zhang XJ, Wolfe RR. Role of membrane transport in interorgan amino acid flow between muscle and small intestine. Metabolism 1995;44:719–24.

[169] Biolo G, Fleming RY, Maggi SP, Wolfe RR. Transmembrane transport and intracellular kinetics of amino acids in human skeletal muscle. Am J Physiol 1995;268:E75–84.

[170] Lim VS, Bier DM, Flanigan MJ, Sum-Ping ST. The effect of hemodialysis on protein metabolism: a leucine kinetic study. J Clin Invest 1993;91:2429–36.

[171] Ikizler TA, Pupim LB, Brouillette JR, Levenhagen DK, Farmer K, Hakim RM, et al. Hemodialysis stimulates muscle and whole body protein loss and alters substrate oxidation. Am J Physiol – Endocrinol Metab 2002;282:E107–116.

[172] Goodship TH, Mitch WE, Hoerr RA, Wagner DA, Steinman TI, Young VR. Adaptation to low-protein diets in renal failure: leucine turnover and nitrogen balance. J Am Soc Nephrol 1990;1:66–75.

[173] Goodship TH, Lloyd S, Clague MB, Bartlett K, Ward MK, Wilkinson R. Whole body leucine turnover and nutritional status in continuous ambulatory peritoneal dialysis. Clin Sci (Lond) 1987;73:463–9.

[174] Pupim LB, Flakoll PJ, Brouillette JR, Levenhagen DK, Hakim RM, Ikizler TA. Intradialytic parenteral nutrition improves protein and energy homeostasis in chronic hemodialysis patients. J Clin Invest 2002;110:483–92.

[175] Caglar K, Peng Y, Pupim LB, Flakoll PJ, Levenhagen D, Hakim RM, et al. Inflammatory signals associated with hemodialysis. Kidney Int 2002;62:1408–16.

[176] Woo R, Daniels-Kush R, Horton ES. Regulation of energy balance. Annu Rev Nutr 1985;5:411–33.

[177] Bursztein S, Elwyn DH, Asakanazi J, Kinney JM. Energy metabolism, indirect calorimetry, and nutrition, Baltimore. Williams & Wilkins; 1989.

[178] Consultation, FWUE: Energy and protein requirements. Geneva: World Health Organization; 1985.

[179] Monteon FJ, Laidlaw SA, Shaib JK, Kopple JD. Energy expenditure in patients with chronic renal failure. Kidney Int 1986;30:741–7.

[180] Schneeweiss B, Graninger W, Stokenhuber F, Druml W, Ferenci P, Eichinger S, et al. Energy metabolism in acute and chronic renal failure. Am J Clin Nutr 1990;52:596–601.

[181] Olevitch LR, Bowers BM, DeOreo PB. Measurement of resting energy expenditure via indirect calorimetry among adult hemodialysis patients. J Renal Nutrit 1994;4:192–7.

[182] Avesani CM, Cuppari L, Silva AC, Sigulem DM, Cendoroglo M, Sesso R, et al. Resting energy expenditure in pre-dialysis diabetic patients. Nephrol Dial Transplant 2001;16:556–65.

[183] Ikizler TA, Wingard RL, Sun M, Harvell J, Parker RA, Hakim RM. Increased energy expenditure in hemodialysis patients. J Am Soc Nephrol 1996;7:2646–53.

[184] Neyra RN, Chen KY, Sun M, Shyr Y, Hakim RM, Ikizler TA. Increased resting energy expenditure in patients with end-stage renal disease. J Parenter Enteral Nutr 2003;27:36—42.

[185] Pupim LB, Flakoll PJ, Brouillette JR, Levenhagen DK, Hakim RM, Ikizler TA. Intradialytic Parenteral Nutrition Improves Protein and Energy Homeostasis in Chronic Hemodialysis Patients. J Clin Invest 2002;110:483—92.

[186] Levey AS, Greene T, Beck GJ, Caggiula AW, Kusek JW, Hunsicker LG, et al. Dietary protein restriction and the progression of chronic renal disease: what have all of the results of the MDRD study shown? Modification of Diet in Renal Disease Study group. J Am Soc Nephrol 1999;10: 2426—39.

[187] Simonson DC, DeFronzo RA. Indirect calorimetry: methodological and interpretative problems. Am J Physiol 1990;258: E399—412.

[188] Ferrannini E, Elia M, Ravussin E, Rising R, Durnin JVGA, Kinney JM. Indirect calorimetry: theory and practice. In: Kinney JM, Tucker HN, editors. Energy metabolism. New York: Raven Press; 1992. p. 1—113.

[189] Jequier E, Acheson K, Schutz Y. Assessment of energy expenditure and fuel utilization in man. Annu Rev Nutr 1987;7: 187—208.

[190] Leff ML, Hill JO, Yates AA, Cotsonis GA, Heymsfield SB. Resting metabolic rate: measurement reliability. JPEN J Parenter Enteral Nutr 1987;11:354—9.

Causes of Protein-Energy Wasting in Chronic Kidney Disease

Manuel Velasquez[1], Rajnish Mehrotra[2,3], Maria Wing[1], Dominic Raj[1]

[1]Division of Renal Diseases and Hypertension, The George Washington University, Washington DC, USA
[2]Division of Nephrology and Hypertension, Harbor-UCLA Medical Center, Torrance, CA, USA
[3]David Geffen School of Medicine at UCLA, Los Angeles, CA, USA

INTRODUCTION

Protein energy wasting (PEW) represents one of the most serious complications of chronic kidney disease (CKD) [1] and poses a formidable therapeutic challenge because (a) it is common and is frequently encountered not only in individuals with endstage renal disease (ESRD) who are receiving maintenance hemodialysis (HD) or chronic peritoneal dialysis (PD) therapy but also in non-dialyzed patients with CKD; (b) it is caused by a wide range of disorders or factors that may or may not be related directly to the underlying kidney disease [2]; and (c) it can cause severe and prolonged debilitation leading to poor quality of life. In addition, PEW assumes an even greater significance because it often coexists with other co-morbid risk factors, such as diabetes, inflammation, and atherosclerosis, and is powerfully associated with all-cause mortality, adding further to the excess morbidity and mortality in the ESRD population [3,4].

In recent years, it has become increasingly apparent that the wasting syndromes attributed to PEW are not merely the result of undernutrition with reduced intake of protein and energy but may also involve other factors or conditions that reduce muscle mass or increase fat loss and/or energy expenditure. Based on new findings concerning syndromes of muscle wasting, malnutrition, and inflammation in individuals with acute kidney injury (AKI), or CKD, the International Society of Renal Nutrition and Metabolism (ISRNM) expert panel proposed in a 2008 report new terminologies and definitions related to wasting, cachexia, malnutrition, and inflammation [5]. The new term "protein-energy wasting", previously referred to as "protein-energy-malnutrition" is now defined as the state of decreased body stores of protein and energy fuels (that is, body protein and fat masses). "Kidney disease wasting" is used by some nephrologists to refer to the occurrence of PEW in CKD or AKI, regardless of the cause. Since many causes of PEW in CKD or AKI are similar to the causes of PEW in other chronic or acute diseases, many nephrologists prefer to use the term PEW for protein and/or energy wasting that occurs in kidney disease. This emphasizes the similarity for most causes of PEW in these various disease states. Cachexia refers to a severe form of PEW that occurs infrequently in kidney disease. Diagnostic criteria for PEW are shown in Table 11.1. While markers of chronic inflammation or other novel biomarkers can be useful clues for the existence of PEW, such measures do not define the condition.

This chapter focuses on the causes of PEW in CKD and examines the evidence for the role of molecular, biochemical, nutritional, as well as environmental factors involved in the pathogenesis of PEW. It is anticipated that knowledge gained from this large body of scientific evidence may prove useful for developing strategies for the prevention and treatment of this common and debilitating disorder.

CAUSES OF PEW IN CKD

PEW may be viewed as a complex heterogeneous disorder that results from an interplay of multiple factors that directly or indirectly alter protein metabolism and energy balance. There are many causes of PEW in CKD, and these encompass a wide variety of

TABLE 11.1 Protein-Energy-Wasting Diagnostic Criteria Suggested by the PEW Consensus Conferences [5]

PRIMARY CRITERIA

1. Biochemical markers
Albumin <3.8 g/dL (BCG)[†]
Prealbumin (transthyretin) <30 mg/dL (dialysis pts)[†]
Total cholesterol <100 mg/dL[†]

2. Body composition indices
Body Mass Index <22 kg/m^2 (<65 years) or <23 kg/m^2 (>65 years)
Unintentional weight loss >5% over 3 mo or 10% over 6 mo
Total body fat percentage <10%

3. Muscle mass
Muscle wasting 5% over 3 mo or 10% over 6 mo
Reduced mid-arm muscle circumference area
Creatinine appearance

4. Dietary intake
Unintentional ↓dietary protein intake (DPI) <0.80 g/kg/day[‡]
(Evidence indicates that ≤1.0 g protein/kg/day may engender protein wasting in some patients.)
Unintentional ↓dietary energy intake (DEI) <25 Kcal/kg/day
(Data indicate that some patients may need ≥30 kg/kg/day.)

SUPPORTIVE CRITERIA

1. Appetite, food intake, and energy expenditure
Appetite assessment
Food frequency questionnaires

2. Body mass and composition
Total body nitrogen or potassium
Energy-beam based methods:
Dual-emission X-ray absorptiometry
Bioelectric Impedance Analysis
Near Infrared Reactance

3. Other laboratory biomarkers
Serum biochemistry: transferrin, urea, triglyceride, bicarbonate
Hormones: leptin, ghrelin, growth hormones
Inflammatory markers: CRP, IL-6, TNF-α, IL-1β, SAA
Peripheral blood cell count: lymphocyte count or percentage

4. Nutritional scoring systems
Subjective Global Assessment
Malnutrition-Inflammation Score (MIS) [87]

5. Other novel markers
14kD Actin fragment [82,97]
Gelsolin [98]

[†]Levels may vary according to GFR level
[‡]for at least 2 months.

TABLE 11.2 Causes of Protein-Energy Wasting in CKD/ESRD

1. Anorexia
2. Decreased nutrient intake
3. Endocrine disorders:
   insulin resistance
   decreased insulin-like growth factor-I
   hyperglucagonemia
   testosterone deficiency
   vitamin D deficiency
   hyperparathyroidism
4. Inflammation
5. Oxidative and carbonyl stress
6. Metabolic acidosis
7. Volume overload
8. Co-morbid conditions including diabetes and cardiac failure
9. Nutrient loss during dialysis treatment
10. Increased energy utilization
11. Abnormal protein kinetics

the mechanisms of wasting in CKD, a few general considerations merit special attention. First, the factors involved in the regulation of nutrient intake, protein metabolism, and energy balance are diverse, and their relative contribution to wasting in PEW may vary in importance depending upon the nature of the inciting stimulus or event that occurs during the evolution of the disease. Second, given the chronicity and varying co-morbid conditions associated with CKD, mechanisms that initiated PEW may not be operative at the later stages of the disease, and as kidney disease progresses to end stage, other potential mechanisms may come into play. Third, there are inherent redundancies in molecular, cellular, and biochemical events that regulate protein and energy metabolism in a given individual, as there are in the biologic activities of various peptides, cytokines, and hormones. Thus, there are independent, overlapping, and complementary or antagonistic mechanisms of action, which make it difficult to disentangle their effects on protein metabolism and/or energy balance. Nonetheless, the accumulated scientific data may provide the framework for formulating targeted interventions to prevent or reverse PEW in patients with CKD.

Anorexia

Anorexia is a cardinal manifestation of CKD. Several factors have been proposed to account for the anorexia associated with kidney disease. Evidence that uremic toxins can suppress appetite and food intake is derived from the studies of Anderstam and co-workers [6] in experimental animals showing that intraperitoneal injection of uremic plasma ultrafiltrate into normal rats inhibits ingestion of nutrients. A dose dependent effect was noticed only with the subfractions with molecular weight ranges of 1 to 5 kD and 5 to 10 kD, respectively, whereas fractions with molecular weights below 1 kD had no effect. In a subsequent study, the

conditions or disorders that ultimately leads to decreased protein and energy intake, increased protein loss or energy expenditure, or a combination of both factors as shown in Table 11.2.

PATHOPHYSIOLOGY OF PEW IN CKD

The pathophysiologic basis of PEW in CKD is multifactorial as depicted in Figure 11.1. Before discussing

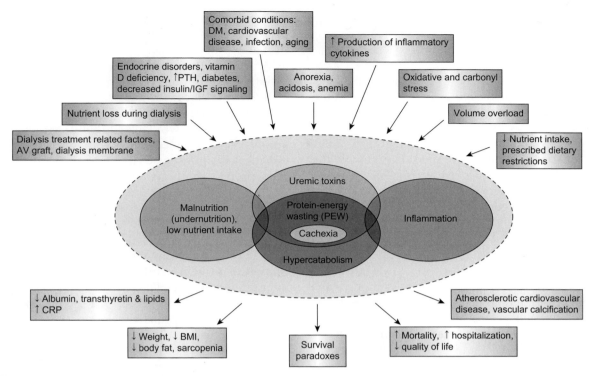

FIGURE 11.1 Schematic representation of the causes and manifestations of the protein–energy wasting syndrome in kidney disease. Reprinted from reference [5]. This figure is reproduced in color in the color plate section.

same group of investigators showed that intraperitoneal injection of a urine fraction or uremic plasma ultrafiltrate fraction inhibited carbohydrate intake by 76.3% and 45.9%, respectively [7]. An intracerebroventricular injection of 5 or 10 μl of urine middle molecule fraction (i.e., compounds with a molecular weight range of 300 to 2000 daltons) significantly inhibited carbohydrate intake. These data suggest that middle molecule compounds that accumulate in the plasma of uremic patients suppress food intake.

Decreased Nutrient Intake

Inadequate nutrient intake is considered the most important single cause of PEW in CKD and has been well documented in both adults and children with varying degrees of renal failure. The decline in dietary intake occurs early in CKD and accelerates as renal failure worsens. In children with CKD, low protein or energy intake due to anorexia is the primary reason for growth failure in this group [8]. In a prospective study Ikizler [9] showed that spontaneous dietary protein intake (calculated from 24-h urine urea excretion) of patients with CKD significantly decreases as renal function declines. This decrease is most noticeable at creatinine clearance levels below 25 mL/min. In a large cohort of adult patients with moderate to advanced CKD, Kopple et al. [10] showed that dietary protein intake and nutritional status correlated directly with the GFR. Especially, patients with a GFR of 21 mL/min/1.73 m² or lower

showed greater decline in nutritional status. Thus, dietary protein and calorie intake declines with decrease in GFR. The other factors that could contribute to decreased nutrient intake include depression, dementia and even economic barriers [11].

Impaired Gastric Motility

Several studies have documented an impairment of gastric motility in ESRD patients [12,13]. In one study more than 50% of nondiabetic ESRD patients who are receiving maintenance dialysis had abnormal gastric myoelectrical activity [14]. Furthermore, administration of prokinetic agents to hypoalbuminemic nondiabetic maintenance HD patients with occult gastroparesis was shown to improve gastric emptying, an effect that was accompanied by an increase in serum albumin [15]. The mechanism for the gastroparesis in ESRD patients is unclear, but it has been postulated that derangements in neuroendocrine signaling and imbalance in gut derived hormones may play a pathogenic role.

ENDOCRINE AND HORMONAL DISORDERS

CKD is characterized by a plethora of endocrine disorders resulting from either an increased or decreased level of hormones or impaired action at the target tissue level. We will review the association between endocrine/hormonal dysfunction and its role in the pathogenesis of PEW.

Gut-Derived Hormones

Apart from its well recognized digestive functions, the gut also produces peptides that have autocrine and paracrine as well as endocrine functions. These gut-derived peptides maintain mucosal integrity, facilitate secretion of digestive enzymes, modulate gut motility and signal to the brain regarding the presence and absorptive status of nutrients; thus, they could play an important role in the genesis of PEW.

Ghrelin is a unique hormone, principally secreted from the stomach. It acts to stimulate appetite and food intake via stimulation of the type 1a growth hormone secretagogue receptor [16]. Since ghrelin is a potent appetite-enhancer, it was initially thought that reduced levels of circulating ghrelin might be a potential mechanism for the reduced appetite seen in CKD. Surprisingly, plasma ghrelin was found to be elevated in patients with ESRD [17], and circulating ghrelin levels were found to be significantly higher in uremic patients with poor appetite when compared with uremic patients with good appetite [18]. Recent studies have shown that exogenous administration of ghrelin improves appetite and/or increases food intake in animals and humans with CKD [19,20]. Thus, exogenous administration of ghrelin appears to be a promising strategy to improve food intake in malnourished ESRD patients.

Peptide YY (PYY) is another gut-derived hormone that plays an important role in the short-term regulation of appetite [21]. This peptide is released by intestinal L cells in response to meals, suppresses appetite, and acts as a "break" to oral intake by complex mechanisms, which include vagal stimulation through interaction with the receptor Y2 (Y2R) of the hypothalamic arcuate nucleus. Increased plasma levels of PYY have been reported in patients with ESRD treated with dialysis, which could contribute to the anorexia and PEW of CKD [22].

Cholecystokinin (CCK) is an intestinal hormone known to cause early satiety and suppress appetite [23]. It is released in response to eating and induces a state of satiety via peripheral and central receptors. Because circulating levels of CCK are increased in ESRD patients, it has been suggested CCK may contribute to the premature satiety and anorexia in CKD. Experimentally, CCK administration has been shown to induce premature satiety with shortening of the eating period, and reduced nutrient intake [24].

Insulin and Insulin-Like Growth Factors (IGF)

The most common and important endocrine disorder in CKD is the development of insulin resistance [25]. Insulin is a potent anabolic hormone; even a small increase in plasma insulin stimulates protein synthesis and exerts a powerful inhibitory effect on protein catabolism [26]. Resistance to the actions of insulin has been shown to be strongly associated with increased muscle breakdown in non-diabetic chronic HD patients [27].

Insulin-like growth factor-I (IGF-I), which has a 48% amino acid sequence identity with proinsulin, enhances insulin sensitivity and independently stimulates protein synthesis and suppresses protein degradation in both experimental animals and human subjects. Kopple and associates showed that mRNA levels of IGF-IEa, IGF-II, and the IGF-I receptor are decreased in the skeletal muscle of ESRD patients [29]. There is an attenuation in the IGF-I-induced stimulation of protein synthesis and inhibition of protein degradation in skeletal muscle in CKD [28]. Among the known mechanisms for IGF-I resistance in CKD are defects in the phosphorylation and activity of the intrinsic tyrosine kinase of the IGF-I receptor and plasma inhibitors of IGF-I and elevated basal cytosolic $[Ca^{2+}]$ [29]. Bailey et al. [30] have shown that CKD causes defects in IGF-I signaling in skeletal muscle, an effect that is associated with a decrease in phosphorylation of Akt and an increase in proteolysis and muscle wasting. Another mechanism closely linked to impaired IGF-I signaling in CKD is dysfunction of skeletal muscle precursors or satellite cells, which are responsible for maintaining muscle growth and repair [31].

Interestingly, administration of thiazolidinedione (TZD) in a rodent model of insulin resistance improved insulin resistance and decreased protein degradation in muscle [32]. Furthermore, in a recent clinical study of a large cohort of incident HD patients with diabetes, non-insulin requiring type-2 diabetic subjects receiving TZDs had significantly higher body mass indices, and serum albumin levels, than those not receiving TZDs [33]. Prospective studies are needed to confirm these findings and to explore the potential beneficial role of insulin sensitizers in the treatment of ESRD patients with or at risk for PEW.

Resistance to Growth Hormone

Growth hormone (GH) regulates muscle and fat metabolism, which impacts on body composition and insulin sensitivity. Decreased or impaired action of growth hormone is another endocrine disturbance associated with CKD that may retard muscle growth and promote muscle protein catabolism [34]. Insensitivity to GH is the consequence of multiple defects in the GH/IGF-I signaling. GH activation of the Janus kinase

2-signal transducer (JAK2) and activator of transcription (STAT) signal transduction pathway is depressed in advanced CKD, and this leads to reduced IGF-I expression and resistance to IGF-I [35]. However, administration of GH has been shown to increase linear growth in children with CKD and improve net protein balance in malnourished adult ESRD patients on maintenance HD [36]. Pupim et al. [37] showed that short-term rhGH therapy (for three consecutive days) in chronic HD patients resulted in a significant accrual of whole-body protein mass, primarily through an 18% increase in whole-body protein synthesis associated with a reduction essential amino acid muscle loss. Finally, GH treatment in ESRD patients resulted in increased lean body mass and improved quality of life as well as decreased cardiovascular risk [38]. Taken together these studies indicate that rhGH improves whole-body protein synthesis in children and adults with CKD in the short-term.

Testosterone Deficiency

Testosterone regulates many physiological processes, including sexual function, muscle protein metabolism, cognitive functions, erythropoiesis, plasma lipids, and bone mineral metabolism. More than 60% of men with advanced CKD have low plasma concentrations of testosterone, and this is associated with increased mortality [39]. Treatment with nandrolone decanoate for 24 weeks, produced a two-fold increase in appendicular lean mass in patients with CKD [40]. Potential mechanisms by which testosterone deficiency might cause muscle catabolism include altered IGF-I signaling and an increase in myostatin, a protein that suppresses muscle growth.

Altered Adipokine Physiology

Adipose tissue has traditionally been viewed as a passive reservoir for storage of energy. However, in recent years it has emerged as a highly active endocrine organ that secretes a variety of bioactive peptides, known as adipokines, which mediate numerous biological and pathological processes including energy metabolism, neuroendocrine function, sex steroid metabolism, and immune function. The underlying mechanisms whereby endocrine hormones and adipokines cause anorexia and decreased nutrient intake in CKD are complex and may involve the participation of neuroendocrine pathways that control food intake and energy homeostasis (Figure 11.2).

Leptin, the protein product of the *ob*-gene, is secreted by adipocytes and acts as a lipostat mechanism to regulate food intake and energy expenditure via modulation of satiety signals in the hypothalamus [41]. An increase in the level of leptin decreases neuropeptide Y, reduces food intake, increases energy expenditure, induces weight loss, lowers plasma insulin, alters glucose homeostasis and induces muscle protein breakdown. Serum leptin concentrations are elevated in CKD patients who do not have ESRD [42], as well as in patients undergoing renal replacement therapy [43] and have been shown to be inversely correlated with dietary protein intake [44]. Longitudinal studies have also shown that increased serum leptin levels are associated with weight loss in dialysis patients [45]. Moreover, experimental studies in

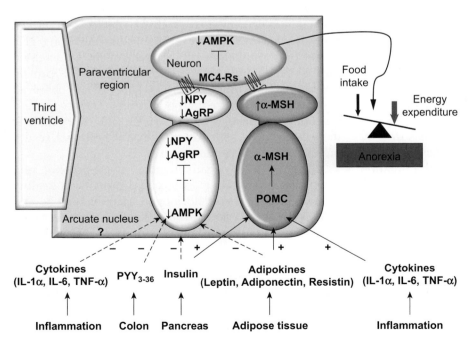

FIGURE 11.2 Orexigenic and anorexigenic mechanisms controlling energy homeostasis in CKD. Circulating hormones produced by the colon (PYY), pancreas (insulin) adipose tissue and cytokines all cause anorexia. Responses to these factors result in the modulation of the hypothalamic melanocortin signaling pathways with an increase in MC4-Rs which suppresses AMP activated protein kinase (AMPK) activity, leading to decreased food intake, increased energy expenditure, and weight loss. Reprinted with permission from Mak et al. [99]. This figure is reproduced in color in the color plate section.

leptin receptor-deficient mice made cachetic by nephrectomy have shown that uremia-associated cachexia is caused by leptin signaling through the hypothalamic melanocortin receptor 4 (MC4-R) [46]. These results suggest that increased circulating leptin may be an important mediator of uremia-associated cachexia via signaling through the central melanocortin system. However, other anorexigenic and catabolic pathways besides leptin cascade may be important.

Adiponectin is another adipocyte-derived hormone that has been shown to modulate food intake and energy homeostasis [47]. In addition, adiponectin has insulin-sensitizing, anti-atherogenic, and anti-inflammatory properties. Data regarding the role of adiponectin in PEW in CKD are limited. Despite the high prevalence of insulin resistance in CKD, circulating levels of adiponectin are increased among patients with CKD [48]. Surprisingly, in ESRD patients undergoing maintenance dialysis serum adiponectin levels were positively correlated with worse malnutrition-inflammatory scores [49]. Investigators have speculated that the apparent unfavorable effect of high adiponectin might not necessarily be related to a direct effect of adiponectin, but rather it could be a consequence of a concurrent process of wasting with a secondary increase in adiponectin levels [50].

EFFECT OF VOLUME OVERLOAD

Chronic volume overload and concomitant heart failure are frequent complications of CKD. There is increasing evidence that fluid volume overload may contribute to malnutrition in CKD patients that may contribute to PEW. For instance, volume overload is associated with inadequate dietary protein and energy intake [51] and nutritional status in maintenance PD patients [52]. In a large cohort of ESRD patients undergoing renal replacement therapy, plasma levels of the N-terminal fragment of B-type natriuretic peptide (NT-proBNP) and the extracellular fluid volume/total body water (ECFv/TBW) ratio were correlated with several markers of inflammation and poor nutrition [53,54] Furthermore, chronic fluid overload, as measured by multi-frequency bioimpedance analysis, is significantly correlated with markers of malnutrition, inflammation and atherosclerosis among PD patients [55]. These data suggest that there may be a link between the malnutrition-inflammatory state and hypervolemia in patients with CKD.

CONTRIBUTION OF CO-MORBIDITIES

A number of co-morbid diseases or conditions that are prevalent in ESRD patients may also contribute to PEW in such patients [4,56]. These include diabetes, hypertension, atherosclerosis, chronic heart failure, intercurrent catabolic illnesses such as infections, and advanced age. In addition to the hyperglycemia and insulin-resistant state in diabetes, other co-morbid disorders related to diabetes, including gastrointestinal dysfunction, hypertension ischemic vascular disease, and neuropathy may reduce food intake and add to protein wasting in CKD patients. Patients with CKD frequently sustain acute intercurrent illnesses that may also reduce food intake and induce a negative nitrogen balance. In addition, many patients with ESRD have evidence of atherosclerotic cardiovascular disease that is associated with malnutrition or PEW and increased levels of proinflammatory cytokines [4]. Because of the strong associations between malnutrition, inflammation and atherosclerosis in CKD, it has been proposed that these features constitute a specific syndrome termed "malnutrition-inflammation-atherosclerosis" (MIA), which carries a high mortality rate.

ALTERED PROTEIN KINETICS IN CKD

An increase in net proteolysis due to imbalance between protein synthesis and degradation has been reported in uremic animals [57]. The results from the human studies, however are more controversial than those from animal studies. Muscle and whole body protein turnover studies in stable advanced CKD/ESRD patients have consistently shown that there is a balanced reduction in protein synthesis and degradation, such that there is no net protein loss [58–60]. On the other hand, investigators unanimously agree that HD induces protein catabolism. Lim et al. [61] reported normal basal leucine flux, a transient decrease in protein synthesis and a negative protein balance during HD. Ikizler [62] found that protein catabolism is increased during HD, with no significant change in protein synthesis. Using multiple tracers, Raj et al. [60] observed a significant increase in both protein synthesis and breakdown during HD. However, the intra-dialytic increase in catabolism exceeded that of synthesis, resulting in net muscle protein loss.

Albumin is a negative acute phase-protein, and fibrinogen is a positive acute-phase protein. In healthy humans, albumin and fibrinogen account for ~50 and ~10% of the total liver protein synthesis, respectively. The change in albumin, fibrinogen and muscle protein synthesis rates vary according to the pathophysiological state. For instance albumin and fibrinogen synthesis rates increase in nephrotic syndrome [63]. However, in inflammatory states the synthesis rates for albumin, fibrinogen and muscle protein may show a concomitant increase or they may be discordant depending on the cause, intensity and duration of inflammation [64,65]. Giordano et al. [66] reported that synthesis rates of albumin and fibrinogen are increased in ESRD patients with normal nutritional status. Kaysen et al. found that albumin synthesis is lower in hypoalbuminemic ESRD patients, and that albumin synthesis and catabolism in ESRD are modulated by inflammation [67,68]. Cagler et al. [69] observed that the intra-dialytic increase in albumin synthesis rate (64%) was higher than that of fibrinogen (34%), but Raj et al. [70] noted that the fractional synthesis rate of fibrinogen (53.5%) tended to be larger than that of albumin (38.6%) during HD. Thus, protein catabolism appears not to be increased, even in advanced CKD, in the absence of other superimposed illness.

Peritoneal dialysis treatment provides 300 to 600 kcal/day^{-1} primarily from absorption of glucose from the use of dextrose-based dialysis solutions resulting in hyperinsulinemia in these patients. Goodship et al. [71] performed leucine turnover studies in CKD patients before and after three months of continuous ambulatory PD (CAPD) treatment. They observed that protein turnover is decreased at baseline, but the balance between synthesis and breakdown is higher and remained unchanged after three months on CAPD. Long term use of amino acid based PD fluid has been shown to induce a positive protein balance [72]. About 80% of leucine contained in the dialysate solution is absorbed through peritoneum and about 43% of the leucine absorbed is used for protein synthesis [73].

NUTRIENT LOSS DURING DIALYSIS

Chronic blood loss and losses of several nutrients, including glucose, amino acids, peptides and proteins as well as water soluble vitamins during the dialysis may contribute to the pathogenesis of PEW in ESRD patients. Raj et al. [74] studied the alanine and glutamine kinetics in ESRD patients using a three compartmental model (artery, vein and muscle) and showed that the intracellular amino acid concentration is maintained during HD by muscle protein catabolism. However, they noted that amino acid infusion during dialysis increased muscle protein turnover, with a balanced increase in both protein synthesis and breakdown [75]. On the other hand, Pupim et al. [76] demonstrated that intra-dialytic parental nutrition increases whole body protein synthesis and decreases proteolysis. Forearm muscle protein kinetics, however, showed that while protein synthesis is increased, protein breakdown is unchanged. Thus, it appears that amino acid repletion increases protein synthesis without a significant impact on muscle protein catabolism.

INFLAMMATION: AGENT PROVOCATEUR OF PEW

A large body of evidence indicates that inflammation plays a central role in the pathogenesis of PEW in CKD beyond its role in protein catabolism. For example, cytokines, such as tumor necrosis factor (TNF)-α, interleukin (IL)-1, and IL-6, can cause anorexia by acting on the central nervous system via modulation of the melanocortin signaling system to alter the release and function of several key neurotransmitters that regulate appetite and metabolic rate (Figure 11.3). IL-1 has been shown to inhibit gastric emptying, an effect mediated in part by cholecystokinin release.

It is becoming increasingly clear that intra-dialytic loss of amino acids, and the resultant deficiency of amino acids is only a part of the paradigm, the other being cytokine activation facilitating augmented protein catabolism [77]. Besides peripheral blood mononuclear cells, human skeletal muscle cells appear to have the inherent ability to express a variety of cytokines [78,79]. Muscle derived IL-6 functions as an exocrine hormone, exerting its effects on the liver and adipose tissue. Raj et al. [78] demonstrated that cytokines are released from the muscle into the vein during HD. Furthermore, they showed IL-6 leads to activation of genes promoting protein catabolism [80], efflux of amino acids from the muscle [75] and increased synthesis of hepatic acute phase proteins during HD [81] (Figure 11.4). The same group of investigators observed that caspase-3 activity in the skeletal muscle, accumulation of 14 kDa actin fragment (a measure of muscle protein breakdown) and apoptosis are increased during HD [82]. Muscle protein catabolism was positively associated with caspase-3 activity and skeletal muscle IL-6 content. These findings suggest that muscle atrophy in ESRD may also be caused by IL-6 induced activation of caspase-3 resulting in apoptosis as well as muscle proteolysis during HD (Figure 11.5).

ROLE OF METABOLIC ACIDEMIA

The National Kidney Foundation Kidney Disease and Dialysis Outcome Quality Initiative guidelines to maintain a serum bicarbonate level in ESRD patients of at least 22 mEq/L. Accordingly, Kalantar-Zadeh and associates observed that a serum bicarbonate level of >22 mEq/L had lower death risk among ESRD patients [83]. Catabolic effects of metabolic acidemia may result from an increased activity of the adenosine triphosphate (ATP)-dependent ubiquitin-proteasome and branched-chain amino acid oxidation [84]. A recent clinical trial showed that bicarbonate supplementation

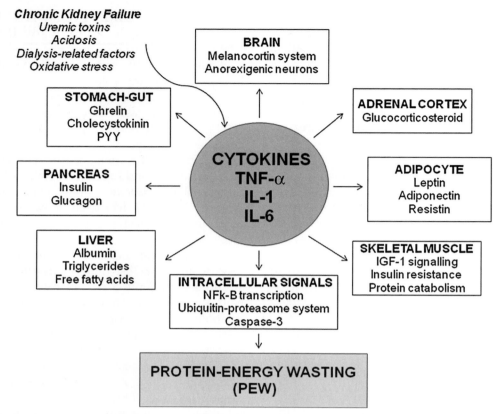

FIGURE 11.3   Central role of cytokines in the pathophysiology of protein energy wasting in CKD. This figure is reproduced in color in the color plate section.

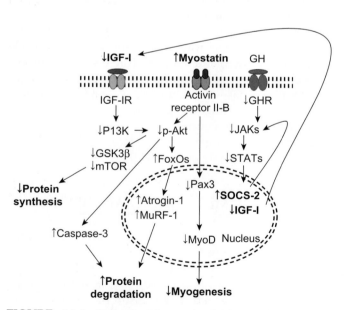

FIGURE 11.4 Pathophysiology of muscle wasting in CKD. Insulin-like growth factor (IGF)-I increases muscle mass while myostatin inhibits its development. Muscle wasting could be due to imbalance of this regulation. Phosphatidylinositol 3 kinase activity (PI3K) is key to activation of muscle proteolysis through regulation of caspase-3, and expression of atrogin-1/MAFbx. Reprinted from Mak et al. [100]. This figure is reproduced in color in the color plate section.

in patient with CKD not only improved their nutritional status but also slowed progression of the renal disease [85]. There may be advantages to increase the arterial pH beyond simply reaching the lower limit of the reference range. In a randomized, cross-over metabolic balance study of eight endstage renal disease patients treated with peritoneal dialysis, increasing the arterial pH from 7.38 to 7.44 resulted in significantly higher net positive nitrogen balances in all but one patient [86].

OXIDATIVE STRESS: OTHER KEY PATHWAYS

CKD is characterized by activation of renin-angiotensin system. Interestingly, angiotensin II infusion has been shown to induce skeletal muscle atrophy, which was associated with oxidative stress, increased expression of the E3 ligases atrogin-1/MuRF-1 and augmented ubiquitin-proteasome mediated proteolysis [87,88]. Several lines of evidence link reactive oxygen species (ROS) to muscle atrophy via redox control of proteolysis [89]. Arterio-venous balance studies have shown net release of malonaldehyde and carbonyl protein from skeletal muscle during hemodialysis

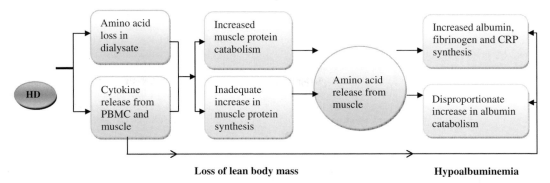

FIGURE 11.5 Integrating cytokine, amino acid kinetics and protein turnover in ESRD. Activation of cytokines during HD increases synthesis of acute phase protein, which is probably facilitated by constant delivery of amino acids derived from the muscle catabolism and intra-dialytic increase in IL-6 [101]. This figure is reproduced in color in the color plate section.

indicating increased generation of reactive oxygen species. Thus, increased oxidative stress could contribute to muscle wasting in CKD.

Nuclear factor-κB (NF-κB) is at the interface between oxidative stress and inflammation and is activated during hemodialysis [79]. NF-κB inhibits myogenesis by promoting myoblast growth and inducing loss of MyoD, which stimulates skeletal muscle differentiation and repair [90] (Figure 11.4). Another molecule, myostatin, a member of the transforming growth factor-β superfamily of signal transduction proteins is an important regulator of skeletal muscle mass and repair [91]. Systemic overexpression of myostatin in adult mice was found to induce profound muscle and fat loss analogous to that seen in human cachexia syndromes [92]. Verzola et al. [93] observed that myostatin gene expression is increased in the skeletal muscle of patients with CKD. Thus, it appears that activation of multiple pathways distinct and yet inter-related signals mediate muscle atrophy in patients with CKD.

SUMMARY AND CONCLUSION

There is an increasing incidence and prevalence of CKD in the US with poor outcomes and profound economic implications. Cardiovascular disease (CVD) is the most common cause of death in patients with CKD. Conventional risk factors of CVD and mortality (obesity, serum cholesterol, and homocysteine) may paradoxically have a protective effect in ESRD patients suggesting that nutritional status has an overriding effect on survival [94,95]. Surveys using classic measures of nutritional status indicate that approximately 20 to 75% of CKD patients show evidence for malnutrition or wasting. Results from the National Health and Nutrition Examination Survey (NHANES) III confirm that renal function is independently associated with PEW [96]. CKD patients have clinical and biochemical evidence of PEW such as anorexia, loss of

lean body mass, decreased serum albumin, pre-albumin and IGF-I, impaired response to anabolic hormones, ineffective amino acid utilization for protein synthesis and increased energy expenditure, especially in the setting of coexistent inflammation. The pathogenesis of PEW in CKD is multifactorial and involves a complex interplay of several factors or mediators that directly or indirectly affect nutrient intake, protein metabolism, and energy balance, which may vary in importance depending upon the nature of the inciting stimulus or event that occurs during the evolution of the disease. It is clear that factors, such as anorexia with inadequate food intake, acidemia due to advanced renal failure, and nutrient losses into dialysate in dialysis patients play a contributory role. More recently identified mediators of PEW include proinflammatory cytokines, insulin resistance, abnormal neuroendocrine signaling, altered physiology of adipokines and abnormal skeletal muscle protein kinetics. Clear understanding of the pathogenic mechanism and cellular signaling pathways is important to institute targeted intervention.

References

[1] Kopple JD. McCollum Award Lecture, 1996: protein-energy malnutrition in maintenance dialysis patients. [Review] [134 refs]. Am J Clin Nutr 1997;65:1544–57.

[2] Lindholm B, Heimburger O, Stenvinkel P. What are the causes of protein-energy malnutrition in chronic renal insufficiency? Am J Kidney Dis 2002;39:422–5.

[3] Rambod M, Bross R, Zitterkoph J, et al. Association of Malnutrition-Inflammation Score With Quality of Life and Mortality in Hemodialysis Patients: A 5-Year Prospective Cohort Study. Am J Kidney Dis 2008.

[4] Stenvinkel P, Heimburger O, Paultre F, et al. Strong association between malnutrition, inflammation, and atherosclerosis in chronic renal failure. Kidney Int 1999;55:1899–911.

[5] Fouque D, Kalantar-Zadeh K, Kopple J, et al. A proposed nomenclature and diagnostic criteria for protein-energy wasting in acute and chronic kidney disease. Kidney Int 2007;73:391–8.

[6] Anderstam B, Mamoun AH, Sodersten P, Bergstrom J. Middle-sized molecule fractions isolated from uremic ultrafiltrate and normal urine inhibit ingestive behavior in the rat. J Am Soc Nephrol 1996;7:2453−60.

[7] Mamoun AH, Sodersten P, Anderstam B, Bergstrom J. Evidence of splanchnic-brain signaling in inhibition of ingestive behavior by middle molecules. J Am Soc Nephrol 1999; 10:309−14.

[8] Betts PR, Magrath G. Growth pattern and dietary intake of children with chronic renal insufficiency. Br Med J 1974; 2:189−93.

[9] Ikizler TA, Greene JH, Wingard RL, et al. Spontaneous dietary protein intake during progression of chronic renal failure. J Am Soc Nephrol 1995;6:1386−91.

[10] Kopple JD, Berg R, Houser H, et al. Nutritional status of patients with different levels of chronic renal insufficiency. Modification of Diet in Renal Disease (MDRD) Study Group. Kidney Int- Suppl 1989;27:S184−94.

[11] Cohen SD, Kimmel PL. Nutritional status, psychological issues and survival in hemodialysis patients. Contrib Nephrol 2007; 155:1−17.

[12] Brown-Cartwright D, Smith HJ, Feldman M. Gastric emptying of an indigestible solid in patients with endstage renal disease on continuous ambulatory peritoneal dialysis. Gastroenterology 1988;95:49−51.

[13] Van VB, Schoonjans R, Vanholder R, et al. Dyspepsia and gastric emptying in chronic renal failure patients. Clin Nephrol 2001; 56:302−7.

[14] Lee SW, Song JH, Kim GA, et al. Effect of dialysis modalities on gastric myoelectrical activity in endstage renal disease patients. Am J Kidney Dis 2000;36:566−73.

[15] Silang R, Regalado M, Cheng TH, Wesson DE. Prokinetic agents increase plasma albumin in hypoalbuminemic chronic dialysis patients with delayed gastric emptying. Am J Kidney Dis 2001;37:287−93.

[16] Wren AM, Seal LJ, Cohen MA, et al. Ghrelin enhances appetite and increases food intake in humans. J Clin Endocrinol Metab 2001;86:5992.

[17] Yoshimoto A, Mori K, Sugawara A, et al. Plasma ghrelin and desacyl ghrelin concentrations in renal failure. J Am Soc Nephrol 2002;13:2748−52.

[18] Bossola M, Scribano D, Colacicco L, et al. Anorexia and plasma levels of free tryptophan, branched chain amino acids, and ghrelin in hemodialysis patients. J Ren Nutr 2009;19:248−55.

[19] Wynne K, Giannitsopoulou K, Small CJ, et al. Subcutaneous ghrelin enhances acute food intake in malnourished patients who receive maintenance peritoneal dialysis: a randomized, placebo-controlled trial. J Am Soc Nephrol 2005;16:2111−8.

[20] Ashby DR, Ford HE, Wynne KJ, et al. Sustained appetite improvement in malnourished dialysis patients by daily ghrelin treatment. Kidney Int 2009;76:199−206.

[21] Batterham RL, Cowley MA, Small CJ, et al. Gut hormone PYY(3-36) physiologically inhibits food intake. Nature 2002;418: 650−4.

[22] Perez-Fontan M, Cordido F, Rodriguez-Carmona A, et al. Short-term regulation of peptide YY secretion by a mixed meal or peritoneal glucose-based dialysate in patients with chronic renal failure. Nephrol Dial Transplant 2008;23:3696−703.

[23] Smith GP, Gibbs J. The satiety effect of cholecystokinin. Recent progress and current problems. Ann N Y Acad Sci 1985;448: 417−23.

[24] Wright M, Woodrow G, O'Brien S, et al. Cholecystokinin and leptin: their influence upon the eating behaviour and nutrient intake of dialysis patients. Nephrol Dial Transplant 2004;19: 133−40.

[25] DeFronzo RA, Alvestrand A, Smith D, et al. Insulin resistance in uremia. Journal of Clinical Investigation 1981;67:563−8.

[26] May RC, Kelly RA, Mitch WE. Mechanisms for defects in muscle protein metabolism in rats with chronic uremia. Influence of metabolic acidosis. J Clin Invest 1987;79: 1099−103.

[27] Siew ED, Pupim LB, Majchrzak KM, et al. Insulin resistance is associated with skeletal muscle protein breakdown in non-diabetic chronic hemodialysis patients. Kidney Int 2007;71: 146−52.

[28] Ding H, Gao XL, Hirschberg R, et al. Impaired actions of insulin-like growth factor 1 on protein synthesis and degradation in skeletal muscle of rats with chronic renal failure. Evidence for a postreceptor defect. J Clin Invest 1996;97: 1064−75.

[29] Ding H, Qing DP, Kopple JD. IGF-1 resistance in chronic renal failure: current evidence and possible mechanisms. [Review] [39 refs]. Kidney Int Suppl 1997;62:S45−7.

[30] Bailey JL, Zheng B, Hu Z, et al. Chronic kidney disease causes defects in signaling through the insulin receptor substrate/phosphatidylinositol 3-kinase/Akt pathway: implications for muscle atrophy. J Am Soc Nephrol 2006;17: 1388−94.

[31] Zhang L, Wang XH, Wang H, et al. Satellite cell dysfunction and impaired IGF-1 signaling cause CKD-induced muscle atrophy. J Am Soc Nephrol 2010;21:419−27.

[32] Wang X, Hu Z, Hu J, et al. Insulin resistance accelerates muscle protein degradation: Activation of the ubiquitin-proteasome pathway by defects in muscle cell signaling. Endocrinology 2006;147:4160−8.

[33] Brunelli SM, Thadhani R, Ikizler TA, Feldman HI. Thiazolidinedione use is associated with better survival in hemodialysis patients with non-insulin dependent diabetes. Kidney Int 2009;75:961−8.

[34] Mak RH, Cheung WW, Roberts Jr CT. The growth hormone-insulin-like factor-I axis in chronic kidney disease. Growth Horm IGF Res 2008;18:17−25.

[35] Rabkin R, Sun DF, Chen Y, et al. Growth hormone resistance in uremia, a role for impaired JAK/STAT signaling. Pediatr Nephrol 2005;20:313−8.

[36] Garibotto G, Barreca A, Russo R, et al. Effects of recombinant human growth hormone on muscle protein turnover in malnourished hemodialysis patients. J Clin Invest 1997;99: 97−105.

[37] Pupim LB, Flakoll PJ, Yu C, Ikizler TA. Recombinant human growth hormone improves muscle amino acid uptake and whole-body protein metabolism in chronic hemodialysis patients. Am J Clin Nutr 2005;82:1235−43.

[38] Feldt-Rasmussen B, Lange M, Sulowicz W, et al. Growth hormone treatment during hemodialysis in a randomized trial improves nutrition, quality of life, and cardiovascular risk. J Am Soc Nephrol 2007;18:2161−71.

[39] Carrero JJ, Qureshi AR, Parini P, et al. Low serum testosterone increases mortality risk among male dialysis patients. J Am Soc Nephrol 2009;20:613−20.

[40] Macdonald JH, Marcora SM, Jibani MM, et al. Nandrolone decanoate as anabolic therapy in chronic kidney disease: a randomized phase II dose-finding study. Nephron Clin Pract 2007;106:c125−35.

[41] Zhang Y, Proenca R, Maffei M, et al. Positional cloning of the mouse obese gene and its human homologue. Nature 1994;372:425−32.

[42] Menon V, Wang X, Greene T, et al. Factors associated with serum leptin in patients with chronic kidney disease. Clin Nephrol 2004;61:163−9.

[43] Nishizawa Y, Shoji T, Tanaka S, et al. Plasma leptin level and its relationship with body composition in hemodialysis patients. Am J Kidney Dis 1998;31:655—61.

[44] Johansen KL, Mulligan K, Tai V, Schambelan M. Leptin, body composition, and indices of malnutrition in patients on dialysis. J Am Soc Nephrol 1998;9:1080—4.

[45] Stenvinkel P, Lindholm B, Lonnqvist F, et al. Increases in serum leptin levels during peritoneal dialysis are associated with inflammation and a decrease in lean body mass. J Am Soc Nephrol 2000;11:1303—9.

[46] Cheung W, Yu PX, Little BM, et al. Role of leptin and melanocortin signaling in uremia-associated cachexia. J Clin Invest 2005;115:1659—65.

[47] Kadowaki T, Yamauchi T. Adiponectin and adiponectin receptors. Endocr Rev 2005;26:439—51.

[48] Zoccali C, Mallamaci F, Tripepi G, et al. Adiponectin, metabolic risk factors, and cardiovascular events among patients with endstage renal disease. J Am Soc Nephrol 2002;13:134—41.

[49] Dervisoglu E, Eraldemir C, Kalender B, et al. Adipocytokines leptin and adiponectin, and measures of malnutrition-inflammation in chronic renal failure: is there a relationship? J Ren Nutr 2008;18:332—7.

[50] Stenvinkel P. Adiponectin in chronic kidney disease: a complex and context sensitive clinical situation. J Ren Nutr 2011;21:82—6.

[51] Wang AY, Sanderson J, Sea MM, et al. Important factors other than dialysis adequacy associated with inadequate dietary protein and energy intakes in patients receiving maintenance peritoneal dialysis. Am J Clin Nutr 2003;77:834—41.

[52] Cheng LT, Tang W, Wang T. Strong association between volume status and nutritional status in peritoneal dialysis patients. Am J Kidney Dis 2005;45:891—902.

[53] Al-Hweish A, Sultan SS, Mogazi K, Elsammak MY. Plasma myeloperoxidase, NT-proBNP, and troponin-I in patients on CAPD compared with those on regular hemodialysis. Hemodial Int 2010;14:308—15.

[54] Paniagua R, Ventura MD, Avila-Diaz M, et al. NT-proBNP, fluid volume overload and dialysis modality are independent predictors of mortality in ESRD patients. Nephrol Dial Transplant 2010;25:551—7.

[55] Demirci MS, Demirci C, Ozdogan O, et al. Relations between malnutrition-inflammation-atherosclerosis and volume status. The usefulness of bioimpedance analysis in peritoneal dialysis patients. Nephrol Dial Transplant 2011;26:1708—16.

[56] Qureshi AR, Alvestrand A, Danielsson A, et al. Factors predicting malnutrition in hemodialysis patients: a cross-sectional study [see comments]. Kidney International 1998;53:773—82.

[57] Mitch WE. Robert H Herman Memorial Award in Clinical Nutrition Lecture, 1997. Mechanisms causing loss of lean body mass in kidney disease. Am J Clin Nutr 1998;67:359—66.

[58] Goodship TH, Mitch W, Hoer RA, et al. Adaptation to low protein diets in renal failure: Leucine turivoer and nitrogen balance. J Am Soc Nephrol 1990;1:66—75.

[59] Maroni BJ, Tom K, Masud T, et al. How is lean body mass conserved with the very-low protein diet regimen? Mineral & Electrolyte Metabolism 1996;22:54—7.

[60] Raj DS, Zager P, Shah VO, et al. Protein turnover and amino acid transport kinetics in endstage renal disease. Am J Physiol Endocrinol Metab 2004;286:E136—43.

[61] Lim VS, Bier DM, Flanigan MJ, Sum-Ping ST. The effect of hemodialysis on protein metabolism. A leucine kinetic study. J Clin Invest 1993;91:2429—36.

[62] Ikizler TA, Pupim LB, Brouillette JR, et al. Hemodialysis stimulates muscle and whole body protein loss and alters substrate oxidation. American Journal of Physiology — Endocrinology & Metabolism 2002;282:E107—16.

[63] de Sain-van der Velden MG, Kaysen GA, de MK, et al. Proportionate increase of fibrinogen and albumin synthesis in nephrotic patients: measurements with stable isotopes. Kidney Int 1998;53:181—8.

[64] Biolo G, Toigo G, Ciocchi B, et al. Metabolic response to injury and sepsis: changes in protein metabolism. Nutrition 1997;13:52S—7S.

[65] Vary TC, Kimball SR. Regulation of hepatic protein synthesis in chronic inflammation and sepsis. Am J Physiol 1992;262:C445—52.

[66] Giordano M, De FP, Lucidi P, et al. Increased albumin and fibrinogen synthesis in hemodialysis patients with normal nutritional status. J Am Soc Nephrol 2001;12:349—54.

[67] Kaysen GA, Schoenfeld PY. Albumin homeostasis in patients undergoing continuous ambulatory peritoneal dialysis. Kidney Int 1984;25:107—14.

[68] Kaysen GA, Dubin JA, Muller HG, et al. Relationships among inflammation nutrition and physiologic mechanisms establishing albumin levels in hemodialysis patients. Kidney Int 2002;61:2240—9.

[69] Caglar K, Peng Y, Pupim LB, et al. Inflammatory signals associated with hemodialysis. Kidney Int 2002;62:1408—16.

[70] Raj DS, Dominic EA, Wolfe R, et al. Coordinated increase in albumin, fibrinogen, and muscle protein synthesis during hemodialysis: role of cytokines. Am J Physiol Endocrinol Metab 2004;286:E658—64.

[71] Goodship TH, Lloyd S, Clague MB, et al. Whole body leucine turnover and nutritional status in continuous ambulatory peritoneal dialysis. Clin Sci 1987;73:463—9.

[72] Kopple JD, Bernard D, Messana J, et al. Treatment of malnourished CAPD patients with an amino acid based dialysate. Kidney Int 1995;47:1148—57.

[73] Delarue J, Maingourd C, Objois M, et al. Effects of an amino acid dialysate on leucine metabolism in continuous ambulatory peritoneal dialysis patients. Kidney Int 1999;56:1934—43.

[74] Raj DS, Welbourne T, Dominic EA, et al. Glutamine kinetics and protein turnover in endstage renal disease. Am J Physiol Endocrinol Metab 2004;288:E37—46.

[75] Raj DS, Adeniyi O, Dominic EA, et al. Amino acid repletion does not decrease muscle protein catabolism during hemodialysis. Am J Physiol Endocrinol Metab 2007;292:E1534—42.

[76] Pupim LB, Flakoll PJ, Brouillette JR, et al. Intradialytic parenteral nutrition improves protein and energy homeostasis in chronic hemodialysis patients.[comment]. Journal of Clinical Investigation 2002;110:483—92.

[77] Raj DS, Sun Y, Tzamaloukas AH. Hypercatabolism in dialysis patients. Curr Opin Nephrol Hypertens 2008;17:589—94.

[78] Raj DSC, Dominic EA, Pai A, et al. Skeletal muscle, cytokines and oxidative stress in Endstage renal disease. Kidney Int 2005;68:2338—44.

[79] Raj DS, Boivin MA, Dominic EA, et al. Haemodialysis induces mitochondrial dysfunction and apoptosis. Eur J Clin Invest 2007;37:971—7.

[80] Raj DSC, Shah H, Shah V, et al. Markers of inflammation, proteolysis and apoptosis in ESRD. Am J Kidney Dis 2003;42:1212—20.

[81] Raj DS, Moseley P, Dominic EA, et al. Interleukin-6 modulates hepatic and muscle protein synthesis during hemodialysis. Kidney Int 2008;73:1061.

[82] Boivin MA, Battah SI, Dominic EA, et al. Activation of caspase-3 in the skeletal muscle during haemodialysis. Eur J Clin Invest 2010;40:903—10.

[83] Wu DY, Shinaberger CS, Regidor DL, et al. Association between serum bicarbonate and death in hemodialysis patients: is it better to be acidotic or alkalotic? Clin J Am Soc Nephrol 2006;1:70—8.

[84] Mitch WE, Medina R, Grieber S, et al. Metabolic acidosis stimulates muscle protein degradation by activating the

adenosine triphosphate-dependent pathway involving ubiquitin and proteasomes. J Clin Invest 1994;93:2127—33.

[85] de Brito-Ashurst I, Varagunam M, Raftery MJ, Yaqoob MM. Bicarbonate supplementation slows progression of CKD and improves nutritional status. J Am Soc Nephrol 2009;20:2075—84.

[86] Mehrotra R, Bross R, Wang H, et al. Effect of high-normal compared with low-normal arterial pH on protein balances in automated peritoneal dialysis patients. Am J Clin Nutr 2009; 90:1532—40.

[87] Brink M, Price SR, Chrast J, et al. Angiotensin II induces skeletal muscle wasting through enhanced protein degradation and down-regulates autocrine insulin-like growth factor I. Endocrinology 2001;142:1489—96.

[88] Song YH, Li Y, Du J, et al. Muscle-specific expression of IGF-1 blocks angiotensin II-induced skeletal muscle wasting. J Clin Invest 2005;115:451—8.

[89] Grune T, Merker K, Sandig G, Davies KJ. Selective degradation of oxidatively modified protein substrates by the proteasome. Biochem Biophys Res Commun 2003;305:709—18.

[90] Guttridge DC, Mayo MW, Madrid LV, et al. NF-kappaB-induced loss of MyoD messenger RNA: possible role in muscle decay and cachexia. Science 2000;289:2363—6.

[91] McFarlane C, Plummer E, Thomas M, et al. Myostatin induces cachexia by activating the ubiquitin proteolytic system through an NF-kappaB-independent, FoxO1-dependent mechanism. J Cell Physiol 2006;209:501—14.

[92] Zimmers TA, Davies MV, Koniaris LG, et al. Induction of cachexia in mice by systemically administered myostatin. Science 2002;296:1486—8.

[93] Verzola D, Procopio V, Sofia A, et al. Apoptosis and myostatin mRNA are upregulated in the skeletal muscle of patients with chronic kidney disease. Kidney Int 2011;79:773—82.

[94] Beddhu S. The body mass index paradox and an obesity, inflammation, and atherosclerosis syndrome in chronic kidney disease. Semin Dial 2004;17:229—32.

[95] Kalantar-Zadeh K, Block G, Humphreys MH, Kopple JD. Reverse epidemiology of cardiovascular risk factors in maintenance dialysis patients. Kidney Int 2003;63:793—808.

[96] Garg AX, Blake PG, Clark WF, et al. Association between renal insufficiency and malnutrition in older adults: results from the NHANES III. Kidney Int 2001;60:1867—74.

[97] Workeneh BT, Rondon-Berrios H, Zhang L, et al. Development of a diagnostic method for detecting increased muscle protein degradation in patients with catabolic conditions. J Am Soc Nephrol 2006;17:3233—9.

[98] Lee PS, Sampath K, Karumanchi SA, et al. Plasma gelsolin and circulating actin correlate with hemodialysis mortality. J Am Soc Nephrol 2009;20:1140—8.

[99] Mak RH, Cheung W, Cone RD, Marks DL. Orexigenic and anorexigenic mechanisms in the control of nutrition in chronic kidney disease. Pediatr Nephrol 2005;20:427—31.

[100] Cheung WW, Rosengren S, Boyle DL, Mak RH. Modulation of melanocortin signaling ameliorates uremic cachexia. Kidney Int 2008;74:180—6.

[101] Raj DSC, Dominic EA, Wolfe RA, et al. Co-ordinated increase in albumin, fibrinogen and muscle protein synthesis during hemodialysis: Role of cytokines. Am J Physiol 2004;286: E658—64.

Protein-Energy Wasting as a Risk Factor of Morbidity and Mortality in Chronic Kidney Disease

Csaba Kovesdy[1], Kamyar Kalantar-Zadeh[2]

[1]University of Tennessee Health Science Center, Memphis TN, USA [2]Division of Nephrology and Hypertension, University of California Irvine (UCI) School of Medicine, Orange, CA, USA

INTRODUCTION

In the United States, there are currently over 450,000 individuals with End-Stage Renal Disease (ESRD) who are dependant on maintenance hemodialysis (MHD) or chronic peritoneal dialysis (CPD) treatment for their survival [1], and as many as 26 million US adults suffering from various stages of nondialysis dependent chronic kidney disease (NDD-CKD) [2]. These patients experience lower quality of life, greater morbidity, higher hospitalization rates and increased mortality as compared to the general population [1,3–5]. The annual mortality rate among MD patients in the United States continues to remain extremely high at approximately 20%, despite many recent improvements in dialytic therapies [1]. NDD-CKD patients have high mortality as well, which increases incrementally across worsening stages of CKD [3,6].

Many reports indicate that in CKD patients there is a high prevalence of protein-energy wasting (PEW), up to 40% or more, and a strong association between PEW and greater morbidity and mortality as well as lower quality of life in patients with all stages of CKD and irrespective of the dialytic techniques employed (HD vs. PD) [7–26]. Evidence indicates that nutritional decline and frailty begins before ESRD develops, often even when the reduction in glomerular filtration rate is modest, and it is likely that a decrease in dietary protein and energy intake plays an important role [11,27]. (Kim, JC et al. J Am Soc Nephrol 2012 [in press]).

In highly industrialized, affluent countries, PEW is an uncommon cause of poor outcome in the general population, whereas *over*-nutrition is associated with a greater risk of cardiovascular disease and has an immense epidemiological impact on the burden of this disease and on shortened survival [28–31]. In contrast, in CKD patients *under*-nutrition is one of the most common risk factors for adverse cardiovascular events (Figure 12.1) [32,33]. The terms "reverse epidemiology" [32–34] or "risk factor paradox (or reversal)" [35] underscore this paradoxical observation. These terms indicate that certain markers which predict a low likelihood of cardiovascular events and an improved survival in the general population, such as decreased body mass index and lower serum cholesterol, become risk factors for increased cardiovascular morbidity and death in CKD patients. Moreover, some indicators of overnutrition actually predict improved outcome in MD patients (Figure 12.2) [10,36–54].

This discrepancy has resulted in uncertainties regarding how to best manage nutrition in CKD. The strong association of PEW with adverse outcomes lead to a focus on nutritional therapies to prevent the development and to treat established PEW, but it remains unclear how to approach patients with CKD and features of over-nutrition in order to conform to widely accepted general population standards on the management of obesity and/or hypercholesterolemia, but without facilitating the development of PEW. Due to such uncertainties an in-depth understanding of the pathophysiology underlying the development of

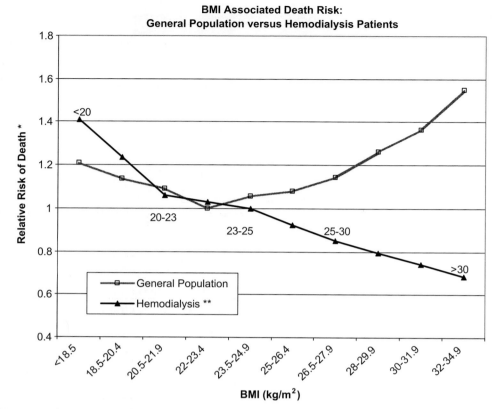

FIGURE 12.1 Reverse epidemiology of mortality risk factors in maintenance dialysis patients. Comparison between the impacts of body mass index (BMI) on all cause mortality in the general population (■) versus in maintenance hemodialysis population (▲). *Reprinted with permission from Kalantar-Zadeh et al.; used with permission from Kidney International, 2003 32. *Note that each population has a different follow-up period: 14 years for the general population versus 4 years for hemodialysis patients. **BMI stratifications are different in two populations: X-axis is based on the original graph of the general population, and the original hemodialysis BMI subgroup ranges are printed additionally along the hemodialysis curve.*

PEW in CKD, its impact on adverse outcomes and the existing interventions towards its prevention or treatment become very important. The pathophysiology of PEW and its impact on outcomes is considered to be complex, and in spite of the strong associations with mortality it remains unclear if some or all aspects of it are a direct cause of the poor outcomes, or if they are merely surrogate markers of other clinical conditions portending a poor survival [55]. Because of this complexity the various aspects of PEW have to be carefully studied in order to determine which, if any of them could be considered as truly causally related to adverse outcomes, and to thus determine which of them should be considered as targets of interventional clinical trials.

Although CKD patients are at increased risk for deficiencies of protein, energy, certain vitamins, macrominerals and trace elements, this discussion will focus on PEW, because this condition is most clearly associated with poor outcomes. This chapter reviews pertinent outcomes, the association of nutritional status with various outcomes, and the current thinking concerning the pathophysiology underlying the poor

outcomes that are associated with PEW in CKD patients.

PERTINENT OUTCOMES IN PATIENTS WITH CKD

In recent years, there has been much growth in *outcomes research* in CKD patients. The aim of much of this research has been to identify and define the scope and impact of modifiable and nonmodifiable risk factors in CKD patients. These issues are of particular importance because of the high burden on the healthcare resources that these patients represent, and their poor outcomes in spite of the available resources. Advances in statistical and epidemiological methods, the availability of robust epidemiologic techniques that account for confounding and case-mix factors, and databases from large CKD patient populations, including the United States Renal Data System (USRDS), the Kaiser-Permanente and the Veterans Healthcare Administration (VHA) databases have contributed to the advances in this field. The data generated by utilizing these

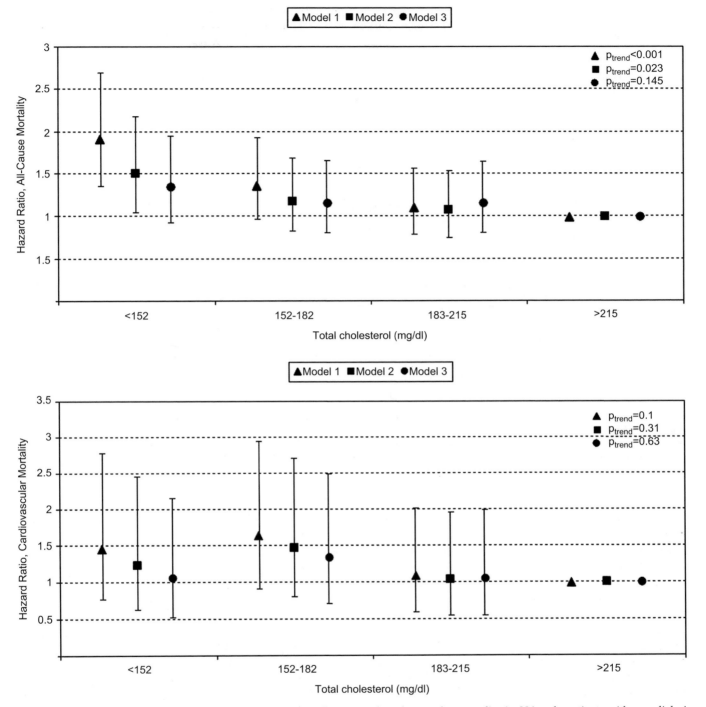

FIGURE 12.2 Association of blood cholesterol levels with all-cause and cardiovascular mortality in 986 male patients with non-dialysis dependent CKD. *Reprinted from Kovesdy et al., J Am Soc Nephrol 2007 [39].*

techniques and patient populations suggest that both PEW and inflammation play important roles in the poor outcomes of CKD patients of all disease stages.

Mortality

Mortality is the most definitive and objective outcome. The occurrence of death regardless of its etiology and type of surrounding circumstances, i.e. *all-cause mortality*, is usually used to evaluate death rate among CKD patients. This, nevertheless, includes occasional rare deaths that may not be directly related to kidney disease, such as homicides or motor-vehicle accidents. Despite such potential limitations, mortality remains the most objective and meaningful outcome in studies pertaining to CKD patients of all stages.

There is a high burden of cardiac disease and cardiovascular mortality in CKD patients suffering from PEW, accounting for more than 50% of deaths in these individuals [56,57]. Hence, mortality of CKD patients, currently about 10–20% per year in the United States (depending on CKD stage), is not only much higher than that of the general population, but the proportion of deaths from cardiovascular diseases may also be much higher in this group [1,3–5].

Because of the heterogeneity of clinical and demographic characteristics of MD patients, *standardized mortality rates* (SMR) are used in order to remove the case-mix effects of gender, age, race and the underlying causes of kidney disease such as diabetes mellitus [1,58].

Cause-specific mortality is an important constituent of overall mortality. In CKD patients, cardiovascular death is of major importance given high cardiovascular disease burden, comprising 40–50% of the total death, similar to non-CKD population. Another important cause-specific mortality is related to infectious disease, in particular among dialysis patients, and its proportion is much higher than in non-CKD populations. However, there may be substantial assessment bias in cause-specific mortality, as the source of data is usually death certificates that are not adjudicated.

Progression of CKD

Loss of kidney function is the cardinal feature of patients with NDD-CKD that determines their progression towards end-stage kidney failure and ultimately their initiation of dialysis or their demise. Furthermore, ongoing loss of residual kidney function even after the initiation of dialytic therapies retains an important role in determining survival [59,60]. Progression of CKD can be studied both as a fixed outcome measure by examining the incidence of dialysis initiation using techniques similar to the ones detailed above for mortality, or by exploring the trajectories (slopes) of the patients' kidney function measured or estimated longitudinally at various time points [61]. Both of these methods have their pertinent advantages and disadvantages. The incidence of end-stage kidney failure can be regarded as a fairly certain event with a known date of inception, but its exploration as an end point is complicated by the fact that mortality prior to its development "competes" with it; hence patients with otherwise rapid loss of kidney function could be deemed at no risk for this end point in case they expire prior to dialysis initiation. The trajectories of kidney function measured in time (slopes) may be a better way to explore progressive CKD, but their analysis is complicated by difficulties surrounding proper evaluation of kidney function (measurement vs. estimation of glomerular filtration rate), the uneven frequency of kidney function

evaluation in different patients (which could also be due to mortality intervening as a "competing" event, and hence leading to informative censoring), and the interpretation of acute kidney injury events that lead to abrupt changes in individual slopes. Nevertheless, both of these outcome measures are accepted as proper ways to study progressive CKD if applied in conjunction with proper methodologies.

Hospitalization

The length and frequency of hospitalizations are closely linked to morbidity, and CKD patients have a much higher rate of hospitalization compared to the general population, on average 10 to 15 days per year for each dialysis patient in the United States [1]. Hospitalization rates are commonly used outcome measures [1,62]. Hospitalization, however, is a less objective outcome measure when compared to mortality, since the decision to admit, retain, or discharge a patient in the hospital can be affected by subjective and nonstandardized factors, such as regional insurance or health care policies. Moreover, many hospital admissions in dialysis patients are dialysis access-related which may or may not be a direct consequence of PEW or chronic inflammation. It has, however, been argued that MD patients with PEW are more prone to develop access failure events [63].

In most outcome studies, the *hospitalization frequency* (e.g. total number of hospital admissions) and/or the total number of *hospitalization days* are calculated for a given period of time, e.g. within a 12-month period [1]. Simple or multivariate regression analyses can be used to evaluate the effect of measures of PEW on hospitalization rates and to estimate correlation coefficients [63,64]. Alternatively, Poisson regression models can be utilized to estimate the hospitalization *rate ratios* and their 95% confidence intervals (CI) to study the effect of changes in nutritional measures on hospitalization [64]. Moreover, for study subgroups or sample sizes with infrequent hospitalization, *time to first hospitalization* within a pre-determined interval can be analyzed using survival-like models [65]. The USRDS reports national end-stage kidney disease hospitalization rates in this manner as *standardized hospitalization ratios* (SHR) similar to mortality rates (SMR) [1]. In calculating the SHR, the first hospitalization event for each individual per year is considered and the subsequent hospitalizations during this interval are ignored, which may be a limitation of SHR.

Quality of Life

Monitoring patients' functional status and the subjective sense of well-being, together known as quality of life (QoL), is of particular importance in CKD patients, since the physical and emotional debility experienced especially by MD patients with PEW can be severe [66–68]. QoL measurements have become an important outcome measure and are heavily relied upon not only by physicians and scientists but also by the U.S. Food and Drug Administration and other health policy authorities as a key outcome. Although QoL measures are subjective, studies have repeatedly shown that these measures are both reproducible and reliable predictors of prospective mortality and hospitalizations in MD patients [62].

A number of instruments have been used to assess sense of well-being and functional and health status in rather broad categories, while some others have a more limited focus. Some of these tools have been validated and even modified for dialysis patients [62,68]. The Karnofsky score is based on a simple questionnaire and assesses the functional status [69]. The Short Form Health Survey with 36 questions (SF36) is one of the most commonly used instruments for QoL evaluation in dialysis patients [62,68]. It is used both as a stand-alone measure of QoL and as a core component of several major assessment tools including the Kidney Disease Quality of Life (KDQOL™) survey instrument, which has been validated for dialysis patients [70]. The Beck Depression Inventory (BDI) is another frequently used self-administered QoL questionnaire which focuses on the presence or degree of depression among dialysis patients [71].

Other Pertinent Outcome Measures

Cardiovascular events of emergency room visits may be examined given high cardiovascular burden of CKD patients. Not infrequently, composite rates are created, e.g. the composite of death and cardiovascular events [72–74]. The nature (infection, occlusion, stenosis) and frequency of dialysis access complications and the survival of different dialysis access modalities (fistula, graft, and tunneled catheter) may have some association with the nutritional and inflammatory processes in dialysis patients and, hence, can be analyzed as an outcome [75,76]. The degree of refractoriness of anemia in dialysis patients is another suggested outcome [63,75,77]. ESRD-associated anemia is a multi-factorial disorder that can be managed relatively successfully by recombinant erythropoietin (EPO) and iron therapy. The EPO and iron requirement to maintain the recommended hemoglobin concentration may rise when inflammation and/or malnutrition is present [77–80]. The ratio of the EPO dose to the hematocrit for each patient is referred to as the "EPO resistance index" [76]. Changes over time in this index can be used as

both a risk factor and an outcome measure. The EPO index is higher in dialysis patients with PEW [80], HCV infection and high serum C-reactive protein (CRP) values [76,81].

ASSOCIATION OF MEASURES OF NUTRITION WITH OUTCOMES

Many studies describe significant correlations between measures of PEW and such clinical outcomes as worsened QoL and increased rates of hospitalization and mortality in CKD patients (Table 12.1). Some indicators of PEW may also reflect the presence or the severity of inflammation [57,63,82–84]. PEW in CKD patients has recently been defined by a panel of international experts using a set of criteria that highlight the complexity of this state [82]. Based on this definition a diagnosis of PEW can be made by using the following primary criteria: (1) biochemical measures (serum albumin, prealbumin, transferrin and cholesterol); (2) measures of body mass (body mass index [BMI], unintentional weight loss and total body fat), (3) measures of muscle mass (total muscle mass, mid-arm muscle circumference and creatinine appearance); (4) measures of dietary intake (dietary protein and energy intake) and (5) integrative nutritional scoring systems (subjective global assessment of nutrition and malnutrition-inflammation score). Each of these diagnostic criteria has both practical values and limitations. For example, serum albumin, transferrin, and prealbumin are negative acute phase reactants and may reflect inflammation [84]. The nutritional scoring systems may also reflect the severity of illness in MD patients [80]. During acute catabolic states, the urea nitrogen appearance may increase transiently independent of food intake [85]. Diet records are subject to wide within-person variability, and caliper anthropometrics are subject to errors due to inter- and intra-observer variability [86]. Finally, despite the abundance of nutritional methods and the many studies of nutritional status in CKD patients, there is still no consensus as to what are the best measures of the nutritional status in these individuals. This problem is compounded because many of these measures have little or no association with each other [87]. For example an obese dialysis patient may have hypoalbuminemia, and a decreased body fat may be seen in a patient who has normal serum albumin and transferrin.

NUTRIENT INTAKE AND OUTCOMES

Anorexia, a major reason for the low nutrient intake in ESRD has been associated with 4-time higher risk of death and with increased morbidity in a study of 344

TABLE 12.1 Assessment Tools that have been Used to Evaluate Protein-Energy Wasting (PEW) in Maintenance Dialysis Patients as they Relate to Outcome

A. NUTRITIONAL INTAKE	Mortality[†]	Hospitalization[†]
A.1. Direct assessment: diet recalls, diaries with interview, and food frequency questionnaires	[335]	[159]
A.2. Indirect assessment: based on urea nitrogen appearance: nPNA (nPCR)	[102,336,337]	[102,106,338–340]
B. BODY COMPOSITION	**Mortality**	**Hospitalization**
B.1. Weight based measures: BMI, weight-for-height, and edema-free fat free weight	[51,125,127,132,341]	[132,341]
B.2. Other anthropometrics: skin fold (triceps, biceps, etc) and arm muscle circumference	[99,229]	No relevant publication detected.
B.3. Total body elements: total body nitrogen and potassium	[342,343]	No relevant publication detected.
B.4. Energy-beam methods: DEXA, BIA, NIR	[153]	[21,63]
C. LABORATORY VALUES (serum levels)	**Mortality**	**Hospitalization**
C.1. Visceral proteins/negative acute phase reactants:		
ALBUMIN	[125,154,156,157,174, 175,182,228,344–349]	[21,63,106,157–159,345, 348,349]
PREALBUMIN (Transthyretin)	[155,166–170,344]	[21]
TRANSFERRIN	[157]	[21,157]
C.2. Lipids: cholesterol, other lipids and lipoproteins	[37,38,127,174–178]	[63]
C.3. Somatic proteins and nitrogen surrogates:		
CREATININE	[155,174,185–187]	[21]
SUN	[102,127,174]	[102,106]
C.4. Positive acute phase reactants and cytokines:		
CRP, IL, TNF-α, SAA, ferritin	[20,20–25,190–192,196,197]	[21]
C.5. Blood cell counts: total lymphocyte count	[158,182,228]	No relevant publication detected.
D. NUTRITIONAL SCORING SYSTEMS	**Mortality**	**Hospitalization**
D.1. Conventional SGA and its derivatives (MIS, DMS, CANUSA, etc)	[63,126,230]	[126,230]
D.2. Non-SGA composite scores: HD-PNI, others (Wolfson, Merkus, Merckman)	[99,229,236,350]	[236,350]

[†]Numbers in Mortality and Hospitalization columns are reference numbers.
Abbreviations: nPNA: normalized protein nitrogen appearance, nPCR: normalized protein catabolic rate, BMI: body mass index, DEXA: dual energy X ray absorptiometry, BIA: bioelectrical impedance analysis, NIR: near infra-red interactance, SGA: subjective global assessment of nutritional status, DMS: dialysis malnutrition score, MIS: malnutrition inflammation score, CANUSA: Canada-USA study based modification of the SGA, HD-PNI: hemodialysis prognostic nutritional index, SUN: serum urea nitrogen, IGF-1: insulin-like growth factor 1, CRP: C-reactive protein, IL: interleukin (e.g. IL1 and IL6), TNF-α: tumor necrosis factor alpha, SAA: serum amyloid A.

hemodialysis patients in the US [88], and these findings were recently replicated by a similar study in 233 European dialysis patients [89]. However, reduced appetite can only be considered an indirect measure of dietary nutrient intake. Diet records (diaries) with or without interviews, and food recalls examine the food intake over relatively short intervals of time; i.e. usually from one or two days to one a week. They are historically among the first and most commonly utilized tools to assess directly the intake of protein and energy and other nutrients. However, they are subject to wide within-person variability due to their restricted time frame and patient unreliability [90,91]. The National Cooperative Dialysis Study (NCDS) was one of the first large scale studies that examined the diet intake in dialysis patients; 165 individuals were monitored with repeated 5-day food records [92,93]. Somewhat earlier, Thunberg et al [94]. used 3-day dietary recalls to assess food intake in 58 hemodialysis patients. Food frequency questionnaires (FFQ) comprise a set of questions about an individual's food intake history and often give multiple-choice options for the answers. Compared to diet records and recalls, the FFQ questions provide data for much more extended intervals; i.e. several weeks, months or even years, but the data generated may be less accurate [95]. The FFQ has been used extensively in epidemiological studies to evaluate the food intake among diverse populations and is a valuable tool for large cohorts and case-control studies [96]. The pattern and type of foods and nutrients can be assessed rather accurately; data concerning total food and nutrient intake tend to be less reliable. The use of FFQ in dialysis patients has been restricted to a few cross-sectional studies with small samples. Kalantar-Zadeh et al. used Block's FFQ in 30 MHD patients and 30 nondialytic controls and found that the MHD patients consumed abnormally low amounts of vitamin C, potassium and fiber [95]. Studies examining risks associated with dietary protein and/or calorie intake obtained from diet diaries have been few in number, small in size and failed to provide conclusive evidence on the risks associated with these parameters [97—100]. Evidence from these studies needs to be interpreted with caution as their small size makes these studies susceptible to type II statistical errors. Larger studies examined indirect measures of protein intake, including urine urea appearance [101] and normalized protein nitrogen appearance (nPNA, also known as normalized protein catabolic rate or nPCR) [65,100—108], indicating significant associations between these surrogates of higher protein intake and lower mortality. Some of these studies suggested that the association between nPNA and mortality may be more complex, with an increase in mortality seen in those whose nPNA was very high (>1.4 g/kg/day) [107]. Possible explanations for the higher mortality seen in those with the highest nPNA levels were outcome-associated confounding effects of body weight in smaller patients, toxic effects of a high-protein diet, a highly catabolic state caused by inflammation, or residual confounding by a behavior pattern of poor compliance in those with the highest levels of protein intake.

A significant drawback of the evidence derived from observational studies assessing associations between nPNA and outcomes is the imperfect nature of this variable as a marker of protein intake. Measured nPNA incorporates the estimated permeability of the dialyzer and is also affected by the accuracy of measured blood and dialysate flow rates [65]. Furthermore, as protein intake fluctuates from day to day due to changes in intake and catabolism [109], the monthly assessment of nPNA may not be an accurate reflection of true average protein intake, especially if the patient's protein metabolism is not in equilibrium. Further inaccuracies are incurred because of difficulties with assessment of the volume of distribution of urea in obese, malnourished, or edematous patients [110], and because of overestimation of nPNA caused by delayed equilibrium with subsequent urea rebound after dialysis, which can vary according to patient and dialysis procedure characteristics [111].

Abnormalities affecting the ingested amounts of various micronutrients (vitamins and trace elements) and imbalances of macronutrients stemming from incorrect dietary habits or prescriptions could also impact clinical outcomes, through mechanisms involving altered immune function or increased atherogenic potential [55]. The lack of arginine, glutamine, zinc, vitamin B_6 (pyridoxine), vitamin C, folic acid and levocarnitine may all adversely affect various aspects of immune function and could be instrumental in the high infectious mortality seen in ESRD [112—119]. Cardiovascular outcomes may also be affected by diet characteristics, as an atherogenic diet is imposed upon most individuals with CKD [120,121]. Recent results based on data obtained from food frequency questionnaires in MHD patients enrolled in the Nutritional and Inflammatory Evaluation (NIED) study have indicated that a higher amount of both potassium [122] and phosphorus intake [123] are associated with increased all-cause mortality especially after adjustments for protein intake.

The complex interplay between the quality and quantity of food intake could have discordant effects; for example, dietary restrictions meant to alleviate increases in serum phosphorus and potassium may result in diminished dietary protein intake and could consequently cause or worsen PEW; meanwhile prescriptions targeting increased dietary protein intake in patients with existing PEW could lead to higher phosphorus and potassium intake and worsening hyperphosphatemia and hyperkalemia. The potential effects of such dietary measures were examined in a recent epidemiologic study of 30,075 prevalent MHD patients [124], which described the risk of death associated with concomitant changes over 6 months in serum phosphorus and nPNA. While individually both lower protein intake and higher serum phosphorus were associated with higher mortality, combining these two measures indicated that the best outcomes were seen in patients whose decrease in serum phosphorus was accompanied by a concomitant increased protein intake, and those whose phosphorus and nPNA both decreased experienced the highest mortality rate [124].

BODY SIZE, BODY COMPOSITION AND OUTCOMES

The post-dialysis (dry) weight, which is usually obtained after each hemodialysis treatment among MHD patients or after emptying the abdominal dwell in CPD patients, is an easy and reliable measure of nutritional status in dialysis patients and a predictor of outcomes [51,125—127]. However, weight must be standardized by height or other confounding factors such as gender or race. Kopple et al. reported a significant correlation between standardized body weight (i.e. weight-for-height) and survival in 12,965 hemodialysis patients [128]. In another study on 3607 MHD patients [125], was shown to be a strong, independent predictor of mortality. An inverse association between the body mass index (BMI), i.e. weight (kg) divided by height (meters) squared, and risk of death has been well documented in patients on maintenance hemodialysis [42—53], with the benefit of the higher body size extending linearly even into the range of morbid obesity (BMI>35 kg/m^2). Some [129—133], but not all [134—136] studies in patients receiving peritoneal dialysis have described similar associations. Similar associations of lower BMI with higher mortality have been described in a number of studies examining patients with NDD-CKD [54,137—139].

A common criticism of the studies examining BMI is that it is not an ideal marker of obesity, as it cannot differentiate between higher weights due to increased adiposity vs. muscularity, and it cannot identify visceral adiposity, which has enhanced negative metabolic effects [140]. The concomitant application of BMI with waist circumference has emerged as a simple way to independently assess visceral adiposity and muscle mass/nonvisceral adiposity, indicating opposite associations for the two (higher mortality associated with higher waist circumference and lower mortality associated with higher BMI especially after adjustment for waist circumference) [141,142]. A further difficult issue is the reconciliation of opposite outcomes associated with higher BMI; namely the fact that while high BMI is consistently associated with lower mortality in CKD, it has also been associated with a higher risk for the development of decreased GFR and incidence of ESRD [29]. Such negative effects of obesity on kidney function could be the result of the combined effects of metabolic syndrome/insulin resistance, diabetes mellitus, hypertension and hemodynamic changes that are induced or worsened by obesity or by high protein intake, and which ultimately lead to a state of glomerular hyperfiltration [143].

The effect of weight on QoL may also be "J" or "U" shaped. Although many studies have shown that malnourished dialysis patients with decreased weight have a worse QoL, we recently showed that MHD patients with a higher BMI and body fat percentage also had less favorable QoL scores [62]. This suggests that despite the survival advantages of obese MD patients their obesity may interfere with their sense of well-being or daily activities.

The criticism concerning the crude nature of BMI as a measure of obesity is best addressed by examining body composition using more sensitive methods. Caliper anthropometry is a simple method based on measuring skin folds and extremity muscle circumference. However, compared to weight and height based measures skin fold and muscle mass measurements are less precise and have wider coefficients of variation, even if the anthropometrist is meticulous and well trained [144]. Nevertheless, they remain among classic nutritional measures for large-scale epidemiological studies of nutritional status. Chazot et al. showed that in patients undergoing hemodialysis for over 20 years, the arm-muscle circumference and triceps skin fold thickness were lower as compared to age and gender matched dialysis patients with less than 5 years of vintage [145]. Mid-arm muscle circumference has also been associated with lower mortality and with improved quality of life in another study of 792 hemodialysis patients [146].

Energy beam methods measure body composition by X-ray, electric current or light emission, and are the foundation of dual-energy X-ray absorptiometry (DEXA), bio-electrical impedance analysis, (BIA), and near infra-red interactance (NIR), respectively. DEXA has been shown to have a high degree of precision and accuracy in most validation studies [147]. Dumler et al. reported that multiple compartment measurement by DEXA provided the best current "gold standard" for body composition analysis in dialysis patients [148]. A limitation of DEXA in hemodialysis patients is its inability to differentiate between muscle mass with normal water content and excess water [147,148]. DEXA should be performed as soon as feasible following the completion of a dialysis session to avoid the effects of excess water loss or gain during or between the dialysis treatments. The same limitation pertains to BIA, a measurement which may vary widely due to fluctuations in total body water in MD patients [147—149]. NIR measurements, although less precise, appear to be independent of hydration status [150,151]. In a recent study comparing triceps skin fold, NIR, and BIA using the Segal, Kushner, and Lukaski equations to the gold standard of DEXA in maintenance hemodialysis patients found that NIR and BIA-Kushner method yielded more consistent estimates of total body fat percentage compared with the other index tests [152]. Among the energy beam measurements of body composition, a small number of studies in dialysis patients have shown associations with outcomes in dialysis patients. Chertow et al. conducted a cohort study, in 3009 adult MHD patients from 101 outpatient dialysis units who were followed for up to 12 months. Patients with narrow (low) BIA phase angle experienced an increased relative risk (RR) of death [153]. In a study of 535 hemodialysis patients Kalantar-Zadeh et al. described an association of higher adiposity measured by NIR and of fat loss over time with lower mortality and with lower QoL scores [47].

LABORATORY MEASURES AND OUTCOME

Among visceral proteins, serum albumin is the most studied laboratory measure in outcome studies in MD patients. Many studies using complex epidemiologic techniques have shown robust correlations between serum albumin concentration and mortality [7−14,154−156], hospitalization [21,63,157−159], and QoL [62] in both dialysis and NDD-CKD patients. Whether or not serum albumin is a pure marker or nutrition is debatable. Many studies by Kaysen and others point out the role of serum albumin as a negative acute phase reactant [160−162], and in a study by Struijk et al. [163] serum albumin was associated with survival in univariate analysis, but in a multivariate model that was controlled for age, hemoglobin, and presence of systemic diseases serum albumin was no longer a statistically significant predictor of mortality. At the least, decreased nutrient intake may independently lower serum albumin concentrations to a modest extent (approximately 3.0 g/dL), but very low serum albumin levels (e.g. 2.0 g/dL or less) appear to require the presence of inflammation, albumin losses (e.g., loss of albumin into the urine, the gastrointestinal tract or through peritoneal dialysis) or liver failure [33].

Serum prealbumin and transferrin have also been used to measure nutritional status in dialysis patients [87]. A theoretical advantage over serum albumin is their shorter half-lives of 1.8 and 8 days, respectively; hence these two proteins are regarded to be early predictors of changes in nutritional status [164,165]. In several studies of dialysis patients serum prealbumin was inversely related to mortality [155,166−170]. Prealbumin is also called transthyretin, because it binds

to (and carries) thyroid hormone and retinol binding protein. Serum prealbumin is elevated in CKD probably because renal degradation of retinol binding protein decreases when the kidneys fail [166]. Serum prealbumin concentrations associated with the lowest mortality risk in MD patients are about 30 mg/dL or greater. In individuals with NDD-CKD serum prealbumin may vary according to the degree of kidney insufficiency and hence it is probably not a good measure of nutritional status in these individuals [165]. Serum transferrin, as measured by total iron binding capacity (TIBC), may also be a survival predictor in dialysis patients [157,171]. However, serum transferrin levels are affected by iron stores [172]. It should also be noted that, as with serum albumin, both serum transferrin and prealbumin are negative acute phase reactants [173], and, hence, the same controversy involves the role of these latter proteins as indicators of nutritional status.

Lower, but not higher serum cholesterol is associated with poor outcomes in dialysis patients [37,38,127,174−176]. Such findings provide additional evidence for the "reverse epidemiology" theory described in dialysis patients, as compared to the general population in whom a lower serum cholesterol is a marker of improved survival [177]. The effect of other lipid components, however, may be similar to that seen in the general population; increased serum LDL or Lp(a), for instance, are associated with a poor outcome in dialysis patients [177,178], and especially in African-American dialysis patients [38]. Similar to serum albumin, effect modification by inflammation is also possible in the association of low cholesterol with mortality in dialysis patients, as shown in a study by Liu et al., where the association of lower cholesterol with increased mortality was only present in patients with elevated inflammatory markers [41]. Several studies examined the association between blood lipid levels and outcomes in NDD-CKD [13,14,39,179]; three of these used mortality as the outcome measure [14,39,179], one used cardiovascular events [13]. Only one of these studies examined patients with advanced NDD-CKD; lower total and LDL cholesterol was associated with higher all-cause and cardiovascular mortality in this study, but the association became nonsignificant after adjustments for case-mix characteristics; nevertheless, higher cholesterol and triglyceride levels were not associated with higher mortality, even after adjustments (Figure 12.2) [39]. Of the three studies that examined patients with less advanced NDD-CKD, one found a positive association between triglyceride level and adverse outcomes (but no association for total and HDL cholesterol) [14], the second found a positive association between total cholesterol and major cardiovascular events (but no association for triglycerides and

HDL cholesterol) [13], and the third one found no association between lipid levels and cardiovascular death [179]. That cholesterol levels, and especially hypercholesterolemia plays a different role in CKD patients compared to the general population is also supported by the results of several large randomized controlled clinical trials of cholesterol lowering, which have shown no benefits in dialysis patients [72,180], or only a benefit towards lowering cardiovascular event rates, but not mortality primarily in nondialysis dependent CKD patients [181].

Serum creatinine reflects a somatic protein and particularly muscle protein content and hence is also an indicator of the nutritional status (and muscle mass) in dialysis patients without residual kidney function [174,182–184]. There is a strong association between decreased serum creatinine concentrations and increased mortality in both MHD [155,174,185,186] and CPD patients [185,186]. Furthermore, an increase in serum creatinine over time is associated with a significant decrease in mortality [187]. Lower pre-transplant serum creatinine is also associated with unfavorable outcomes after transplantation [188] and a decrease in serum creatinine prior to transplantation is associated with higher mortality post-transplant [189]. Serum urea nitrogen (SUN), a rather imprecise indicator of protein intake and total nitrogen appearance is also an indicator of outcomes in dialysis patients [102,127,174]. The major determinant of total nitrogen appearance is the urea nitrogen appearance, urea being the major metabolite of protein and amino acid degradation; hence the net rate of urea production correlates closely with net protein degradation. This relationship may be stronger in dialysis patients, because they excrete little or no ammonia in the urine and hence a greater fraction of the nitrogen released from degraded protein and amino acids is converted to urea. Both serum creatinine and SUN can be affected by the dose of dialysis treatment and residual renal function, and epidemiology of these compounds should be adjusted for these factors.

Many other laboratory measures that are considered to be markers of inflammation or cardiovascular disease may be indirectly related to PEW. Serum CRP, interleukins (IL), and other positive acute phase reactants and proinflammatory cytokines have been studied with regard to their possible associations with PEW and poor outcome in CKD patients [20–25,190–192]. In patients with NDD-CKD CRP was also reported to be associated with increased progression of CKD in some [193], but not all studies [194]. Elevated CRP is reported to be more common in malnourished dialysis patients [195] and to be associated with erythropoietin resistance [76] and mortality [22–24,190–192]. Catabolic cytokines, including TNF-α, IL-1 beta and IL-6, are markers of inflammation in dialysis patients and are associated with lower mid-arm muscle circumference [196] and with increased risk of death [20,196,197]. Furthermore, in a study of NDD-CKD patients, a higher degree of inflammation (defined as a composite score based on the presence or absence of six different biomarkers of inflammation) was associated with progressive loss of kidney function [198]. Genetic polymorphisms that cause higher IL-6 levels are associated with increased mortality in dialysis patients, supporting a causal role of IL-6 in the higher mortality of this population [199]. Serum ferritin, another positive acute phase reactant and an indicator of iron stores, correlates with the degree of malnutrition [80] and is associated with hospitalization and mortality [106,157] as well as resistance to erythropoietin [76] in hemodialysis patients. Serum levels of insulin-like growth factor-I (IGF-I) correlate with protein intake, estimated from the nPNA in hemodialysis patients [200]. Some studies suggest a low level of correlation between hyperleptinemia and measures of PEW [201], but leptin levels showed no independent association with the slopes of CKD in a post-hoc analysis of the Modification of Diet in Renal Disease (MDRD) study [194]. Several studies found that paradoxically a lower, not a higher plasma homocysteine is associated with adverse outcomes in dialysis patients [202,203]; this association may be related to the higher prevalence of PEW and hypoalbuminemia in this group of patients [202,204–206]. The role of hyperhomocysteinemia in dialysis and in kidney transplant patients is also questioned by the lack of improvement in clinical outcomes with lowering of plasma homocysteine levels in randomized controlled trials [207,208]. Furthermore, in patients with NDD-CKD and diabetic nephropathy lowering of homocysteine by using high doses of vitamin B resulted in worse outcomes (progression of CKD and cardiovascular events) compared to patients receiving placebo [209].

Several serum electrolytes and solutes may be affected by nutritional intake. Serum potassium, phosphorus and bicarbonate may not be necessarily affected by protein-energy nutritional status, but abnormal serum levels may occur in circumstances where low nutrient intake plays a role [174]. Most of these measures may also be altered by non-nutritional factors and clinical judgment is necessary to accurately evaluate the significance of the aberration. Higher serum phosphorus has been associated with increased mortality in dialysis patients [174,210–213] and in patients with nondialysis dependent (NDD) CKD [214–216], and the use of phosphorus binder medications has been associated with lower mortality both in dialysis [217] and in NDD-CKD patients [218]. In addition to the increased mortality described in the above studies, higher serum phosphorus was also found to be associated with more significant loss of kidney function in NDD-CKD [216,219]. Serum potassium levels can also be affected by the quality and quantity of nutrient intake, with both hypo- and hyperkalemia being potential outcomes. Hypo- [174] and hyperkalemia [174,220,221] have been associated with an increase in all-cause mortality, and hypokalemia has also been associated with sudden cardiac arrest [222] in patients on dialysis. In patients with NDD-CKD higher [223] and lower [224] serum potassium levels have been associated with short-term mortality, and lower serum potassium has been associated with steeper slopes of estimated GFR [224]. High protein intake may increase the generation of acidic compounds with a consequent lowered serum bicarbonate and increased anion gap. Hence, a high protein intake increases the likelihood of acidemia and a propensity for increased protein catabolism. Both higher and lower serum bicarbonate levels have been associated in observational studies with increased mortality in dialysis patients [225,226], and also in patients with NDD-CKD [227]. In patients with NDD-CKD, increased serum bicarbonate levels were also associated with a decreased incidence of ESRD, suggesting a reduction in the rate of CKD progression [227].

Although not a serum chemistry, total lymphocyte count (TLC) has also been used as an indicator of PEW [228]. The Spanish Cooperative Study of Nutrition in Hemodialysis found that TLC and serum albumin were the only two nutritional measures that were associated with morbidity and mortality in hemodialysis patients [158]. A low percentage of lymphocytes has also been established as a robust predictor of mortality and hospitalization in dialysis [16–18] and in NDD-CKD patients [11]. Finally the white blood cell count (WBC count) itself has also been shown to be significantly associated with mortality both in dialysis [17–19] and in NDD-CKD [11] patients.

NUTRITIONAL SCORING SYSTEMS AND OUTCOMES

Because various nutritional measures may independently predict outcome and may assess different aspects of nutritional status, several researchers have tried to develop a composite nutritional score. Ideally, such a score would not only reflect a patient's overall nutritional status but would also predict outcomes. Wolfson et al. [99] introduced a composite score based on body weight, mid-arm muscle circumference and serum albumin, and found that 70% of hemodialysis patients were malnourished. Marckman [229] developed a nutritional scoring system based on serum transferrin, relative body weight, triceps skinfold, and mid-arm

muscle circumference. Among 16 PD and 32 MHD patients he reported that those with the worst initial composite score were more likely to die during a 24-month follow-up.

The subjective global assessment (SGA) of nutritional status was designed to evaluate surgical patients primarily with gastrointestinal diseases [172], but it has subsequently been employed in a number of epidemiological studies and clinical trials in dialysis patients [172]. The techniques for SGA have since been modified in order to more effectively evaluate the nutritional status of patients with CKD. The SGA is significantly correlated with morbidity and mortality among dialysis patients [126,230]. Some studies suggest that the SGA measures the degree of sickness as well as nutritional status [172], and the National Kidney Foundation (NKF) Kidney Disease and Dialysis Outcome Quality Initiative (K/DOQI) has recommended SGA as an appropriate nutritional assessment tool for both CPD and MHD patients [87].

The SGA has several major limitations. These include its subjective features, semi-quantitative grading restricted to only three nutritional levels, and lack of objective measures of nutrition such as weight or serum chemistries [87]. CANUSA (Canada-USA) [231] and other studies [77] have led to improved, more quantitative versions of the SGA, such as the Dialysis Malnutrition Score (DMS) [77]. Because there are epidemiological and causal associations between PEW and inflammation and measures of each of these conditions have outcome-predictive value, it is reasonable to consider a composite score that combines the measures of protein energy nutritional status and inflammation, since such a score may provide a more precise prediction of outcomes. The "Malnutrition-Inflammation Score" (MIS) is based on the SGA, body mass index, and serum albumin and transferrin concentrations [63]. In a study on 83 MHD patients, the MIS was strongly correlated with 12-month hospitalization rates and mortality [63]. In a more recent study of 378 MD patients the MIS was also significantly associated with higher mortality [24]. The MIS has also been validated as a measure of PEW in prevalent kidney transplant recipients [232], a population in which it has also been associated with anemia [233], depression [234] and higher all-cause mortality and allograft loss [235].

The hemodialysis prognostic nutrition index (HD-PNI) has been proposed by Beto et al., [236] and is based on serum creatinine and albumin concentrations and 6-month retrospective hospitalization data. The HD-PNI correlated with mortality and prospective hospitalization in a large group of MHD patients [236]. Its major limitations include the need for a sophisticated linear mathematical equation and its dependence on historical hospitalization data to predict prospective hospitalization rates.

NUTRITIONAL INTERVENTIONS AND OUTCOMES

PEW is a powerful predictor of death risk for CKD patients and if PEW is treatable, it is possible that nutritional interventions may improve outcomes in CKD patients. In a traditional sense nutritional interventions address the fact that the amount of protein and energy intake in patients with PEW is inadequate (supplementation strategies); in addition various other interventions are meant to address the quantitative and/or qualitative imbalance of nutrient intake in CKD by restricting the absorbed amount of certain nutrients (restriction strategies).

Supplementation type nutritional interventions include nutritional counseling, nutrient supplementation (through oral, enteral or parenteral routes) and a number of nondiet based strategies meant to improve protein-energy intake and alleviate PEW (vide infra). Evidence suggests that maintaining an adequate nutritional intake by using oral or parenteral supplementation in patients with a number of acute or chronic catabolic illnesses may improve their nutritional status [237—242]. In some studies, such improvement is associated with reduced morbidity and mortality and improved quality of life [243]. However, evidence as to whether nutritional support may improve morbidity and mortality in CKD patients is quite limited. There are no large-scale, randomized prospective interventional studies that have examined these questions. Among studies based on food intake, Kuhlmann et al. reported that prescription of 45 kcal/kg/d and 1.5 g protein/kg/d induced weight gain and improved serum albumin and other measures of nutritional status in malnourished MHD patients [244]. Leon et al. reported that tailored nutritional intervention improved serum albumin levels in 52 MHD patients, and this effect was observed even among patients with high serum CRP levels [245]. Several retrospective studies demonstrated a beneficial effect of intradialytic parenteral nutrition (IDPN) on clinical outcomes [246—248], but a number of other studies of IDPN failed to show improvement in nutritional status or clinical outcome in hemodialysis patients [249,250]. However, many of these studies used small sample sizes, failed to restrict study subjects to those with PEW, did not control for concurrent food intake, did not define or adjust appropriately for comorbid conditions, performed nutritional interventions for only short periods of time, or had only a short period of follow-up. A more recent study, the French Intradialytic Nutrition Evaluation Study (FineS)

compared the impact on mortality of oral nutritional supplementation with that of intradialytic parenteral nutrition in addition to the same oral intervention in 186 malnourished hemodialysis patients [251]. IDPN plus oral nutritional supplementation did not improve 2-year mortality compared to oral nutritional supplementation alone, but an increase in prealbumin of >30 mg/L within 3 months predicted a 54% decrease in mortality, reduced hospitalizations and improved general well-being, independent of the method of nutritional supplementation [251].

A number of other techniques have been employed for the prevention or treatment of PEW in CKD patients, such as maintenance of an adequate dose of dialysis, avoidance of acidemia, and aggressive treatment of superimposed catabolic illness [252]. More novel, nondietary interventions in addition to IDPN include appetite stimulants such as megestrol acetate [253], L-carnitine [254], and growth factors including recombinant human growth hormone (rhGH) [255—257], insulin-like growth factor-I (IGF-1) [258], anabolic steroids [259—261] and frequent (daily) dialysis [262,263]. Megestrol acetate is a synthetic derivate of progesterone used as an appetite stimulant, which, however, also inhibits the activity of IL-1, IL-6, and TNF-alfa [264—268]. The beneficial effects of megestrol acetate in ESRD patients are related to its appetite stimulant effects, and include improved appetite, increased energy and protein intake and increased dry weight and quality of life [269—271]. Limiting its usefulness are the many side effects of it, such as headaches, dizziness, confusion, diarrhea, hyperglycemia, thromboembolic phenomena, breakthrough uterine bleeding, peripheral edema, hypertension, adrenal suppression, and adrenal insufficiency [264]. Even though these treatments have improved nutritional parameters, none of them have yet been shown to improve morbidity or mortality. Furthermore, there is concern about potential negative effects of increased protein intake, especially if this is done in a nonselective fashion. As already mentioned above, protein-rich foods can be rich in undesirable components such as excess phosphorus and potassium [122—124]. Glomerular filtration pressure is increased by protein intake through effects on the afferent arteriole, and hence high protein intake can result in glomerular hyperfiltration and worsening proteinuria; an issue that is more relevant in nondialysis dependent CKD patients but also in ESRD patients with residual kidney function [272—274]. Furthermore, the accumulation of various protein breakdown products as a result of decreasing kidney function can result in metabolic effects such as oxidative stress, altered endothelial function, nitric oxide production or insulin resistance [275].

Concerns such as the above have resulted in the exploration of nutritional strategies aimed at optimizing both the quantity and the quality of absorbed nutrients; these involve mostly strategies of dietary protein restriction and the use of various binder agents to decrease the enteral absorption of protein breakdown products, phosphorus or potassium. A number of studies have examined the effects of protein restriction (usually applied in combination with essential amino acid/keto acid supplements to prevent PEW and its potential adverse consequences [276]) in patients with NDD-CKD, showing a beneficial effect on the progression of CKD in some [277–283], but not all studies [284]. Other benefits of supplemented low protein diets showed stable or improved serum albumin levels [281–283,285,286], decreased proteinuria [279,281,287], better preservation of residual renal function in patients receiving peritoneal dialysis [288], improved subjective global assessment scores in hemodialysis patients [282], and delayed start of hemodialysis in nondiabetic elderly patients with advanced (stage 5) NDD-CKD [289].

The main concern surrounding nonselective protein restriction is the development and/or worsening of PEW; a potential solution to this is to selectively prevent the absorption of only certain components that are responsible for dietary protein-related deleterious effects in patients with CKD (such as phosphorus [214,219], potassium [220], advanced glycation end products, indoles and phenols [290–294]) and thus allowing for the benefits of normal or increased protein intake in a way that is devoid of deleterious metabolic side-effects. The application of phosphorus binders in patients with nondialysis dependent CKD has been associated with lower mortality in observational studies [218]. The potential role of serum phosphorus

in engendering progression of CKD was also supported by small clinical trials in patients with CKD [295,296] and in laboratory animals [297–299] that showed an attenuation of progression after dietary restriction of phosphorus. Unfortunately, there are no clinical trials proving the benefits of strategies to normalize either serum phosphorus or potassium levels. Of the various uremic products resulting from intestinal protein absorption and/or abnormal metabolism and excretion indoxyl sulfate is one of the most frequently studied. Elevated indoxyl sulfate levels have been associated with vascular calcification and increased mortality in patients with CKD and ESRD [290]. The indoxyl sulfate-lowering medication AST-120 (Kremezin®, Mitsubishi, Japan) has been shown to slow progression of CKD in a number of small clinical trials [300–305]; larger randomized controlled trials are currently in progress.

Hypotheses Explaining the Link between PEW and Poor Outcomes

The mechanisms underlying the association of PEW with adverse outcomes appear complex (Figure 12.3), without a single, adequately inclusive pathophysiologic mechanism explaining the observed outcomes (Table 12.2). Comorbid illnesses may serve as a link between PEW and morbidity and mortality in CKD patients, especially since patients with the lowest serum albumin or BMI levels are more likely to have severe underlying diseases [128]. It appears less likely, though, that PEW is merely a surrogate marker of increased comorbidity, since many epidemiologic studies indicate that markers

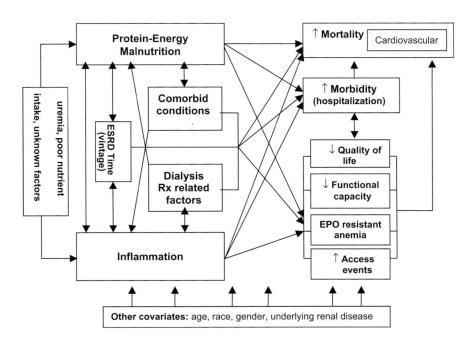

FIGURE 12.3 A hypothetical model of the complex inter-relationships between predictors (inflammation and malnutrition) and outcomes (quality of life, morbidity, and mortality).

TABLE 12.2   Hypotheses Explaining the Link Between Protein Energy Wasting and Poor Outcomes

Affected system	Effect of PEW	Mechanism of Action
Immune system	Immune deficiency	Increased susceptibility to bacterial or viral infections, poor wound healing.
Skeletal muscle	Sarcopenia Increased circulating actin	Reduced skeletal, respiratory and cardiac muscle function. Lower muscle oxidative metabolism with decreased antioxidant defense. Decrease in bioavailability of activated vitamin D and gelsolin.
Endocrine system	Loss of fat tissue Decreased adiponectin level Increased insulin resistance	Decreased sequestration of uremic toxins. Decreased production of anti-inflammatory cytokines and adiponectin. Increased levels of advanced glycation end products.
Lipoproteins	Decreased cholesterol level Proinflammatory conversion of HDL	Decreased ability to bind to circulating endotoxin, with activation of the cytokine cascade. Decreased anti-inflammatory effect of HDL.
Inflammatory cytokines	Increased CRP and IL-6 Decreased IL-10	Proinflammatory cytokines lead to endothelial dysfunction and increased atherosclerotic plaque formation.
Hematopoietic system	Increased platelet activation Increased myeloperoxidase Low hemoglobin; iron depletion	Accelerated atherogenesis; expansion of atherosclerotic plaques and/or unstable plaques.
Nutritional	Anorexia and dietary restrictions leading to decreased intake of fresh fruits and vegetables, legumes, dairy product and high-value proteins Decreased level of anti-oxidative vitamins and trace elements Reduced levels of both nutritional and activated vitamin D	Atherogenic effects of (self) imposed diet. Decreased protein intake leads to further PEW and mortality. Enhanced oxidative stress, with consequent inflammation, endothelial dysfunction, and atherosclerosis. Increased vascular calcification.
Gastrointestinal	Atrophy of gut lining Decreased intestinal secretions and altered gut flora	Decreased absorption of nutrients and increased absorption of endotoxins.

CRP: C-reactive protein.
IL-6: interleukin-6.
HDL: high density lipoprotein.
PEW: protein energy wasting.
Adapted from Kovesdy and Kalantar-Zadeh, Semin Nephrol 2009 [55].

of PEW are independently associated with increased morbidity and mortality even in patients with less severe comorbid conditions [33,306].

PEW, by virtue of its malnutrition component, may lead to impaired immune function and host resistance resulting in increased susceptibility to infections and poor wound healing [307,308]. As discussed above, deficiencies of a number of micronutrients can have a deleterious effect on the immune system [115–118]. Levocarnitine may protect against endotoxins and also suppress elaboration of tumor necrosis factor alpha (TNF-α) from monocytes [119]. Since uremia itself and associated comorbid illnesses may also compromise the immune system [309,310], it is possible that CKD patients are even more susceptible to the immune attenuating effects of the PEW. Impaired host resistance, aggravated by PEW in these individuals, may predispose to inflammatory diseases, such as hepatitis C infections, which in turn is associated with increased death in

CKD [311,312]. Indirect arguments also suggest that malnutrition might increase cardiac death as a consequence of decreased L-arginine availability and the ensuing diminished synthesis of nitric oxide [313].

The reduction in muscle mass (sarcopenia) observed in PEW may be caused by uremic toxins or by other metabolic, hormonal or neuropathic derangements. Muscle wasting may lead to reduced skeletal, respiratory and cardiac muscle function, compromising the vital functions of these organ systems; it may also restrict muscle-based oxidative metabolism and thus lead to a decreased antioxidant defense [314]. Widespread tissue damage may also lead to the emergence of circulating actin that can consume gelsolin (which is primarily produced by skeletal muscle), vitamin D binding protein and other circulating molecules with salutary and protective action [315–317]. Indeed, circulating actin and gelsolin have been associated with survival in MHD patients [318].

Several independent studies have shown a relationship between elevated serum CRP and IL-6 concentrations and risk of CV death among CKD patients [319–321]. Since inflammation may be associated with both anorexia [88] and increased net protein catabolism, inflammation may indeed be the missing link between the PEW and mortality in CKD. Inflammation may induce endothelial cell damage and endothelial dysfunction predisposing to atherosclerotic plaque formation [322]. It is important to note that inflammation may be both a cause and a consequence of PEW [206,323].

Another theory invokes the characteristics of consumed food in the mechanism of action of PEW-induced increased mortality, namely the atherogenicity of the diet resulting from imposed restrictions, as discussed above [120,121]. Furthermore, derangements of the gastrointestinal tract are characteristic of malnutrition, with atrophy of the gut lining, decreased intestinal secretions and altered gut flora leading to further reduction in gut function and the ability to absorb nutrients [324].

Gradual loss of body fat content during the progression of CKD could result in decreased sequestration of uremic toxins [325] and lower production of certain anti-inflammatory cytokines and adiponectin [326]. Furthermore, circulating lipoproteins may serve as a defense mechanism by neutralizing endotoxins intruding through the leaky GI tract [327]. This so-called "endotoxin-lipoprotein hypothesis" may explain the link between low levels of serum cholesterol and increased CV disease and death in both CKD and CHF patients; hence, higher concentration of unbound endotoxins occurring in the setting of low serum cholesterol may activate the proinflammatory cytokine cascade leading to endothelial dysfunction and atherosclerosis [327]. Increased proinflammatory conversion of HDL-cholesterol may also play a role in attenuating the pool of protective lipoproteins [328].

Other mechanisms that may be directly or indirectly related to adverse effects of malnutrition and PEW include vitamin D deficiency [329], refractory anemia and iron depletion, which may lead to increased platelet count and/or activation [330], and increased myeloperoxidase activity [331]. Not only is relative thrombocytosis associated with increased mortality [332], but in a recent study of hemodialysis patients this association was abolished by adjustment for markers of PEW [333], suggesting that the link between PEW and adverse events may be mediated at least in part by thrombocytosis.

It is very likely that the higher mortality associated with PEW be a result of a *combination* of the above mechanisms, rather than a single effect related to any of the individual components.

CONCLUSIONS

The relationship between PEW and adverse outcomes in CKD patients is so strong that it practically reverses the associations between traditional cardiovascular risk factors and outcomes seen in the general population; hence it is referred to as the "reverse epidemiology" theory. Even though no uniform approach is available for rating the overall severity of PEW in CKD patients, measures of food intake, laboratory measurements of nutritional status, body composition tools and nutritional scoring systems, are all predictors of outcome in these individuals. The pathophysiology of PEW as it relates to poor clinical outcome and the methods of treating PEW are complex, and it remains unclear which mechanism(s) of action may be primarily responsible for the association of PEW with adverse outcomes. There is strong evidence indicating that PEW contributes independently to adverse outcomes, and that nutritional therapies are beneficial for prevention and/or treatment of PEW. There is, however, a paucity of information concerning the effect of nutritional therapy on morbidity and mortality in CKD patients. Large-scale, randomized, clinical trials of the effects of nutritional interventions on clinical outcomes would greatly help to better define the causal relationships between these factors in CKD patients [334].

References

[1] U.S. Renal Data System, USRDS. 2010 Annual Data Report: Atlas of Chronic Kidney Disease and End-Stage Renal Disease in the United States. Bethesda, MD: National Institutes of Health, National Institute of Diabetes and Digestive and Kidney Diseases; 2010.

[2] Coresh J, Selvin E, Stevens LA, et al. Prevalence of chronic kidney disease in the United States. JAMA 2007;298:2038–47.

[3] Go AS, Chertow GM, Fan D, McCulloch CE, Hsu CY. Chronic kidney disease and the risks of death, cardiovascular events, and hospitalization. N Engl J Med 2004;351:1296–305.

[4] Keith DS, Nichols GA, Gullion CM, Brown JB, Smith DH. Longitudinal follow-up and outcomes among a population with chronic kidney disease in a large managed care organization. Arch Intern Med 2004;164:659–63.

[5] Kovesdy CP, Trivedi BK, Anderson JE. Association of kidney function with mortality in patients with chronic kidney disease not yet on dialysis: a historical prospective cohort study. Adv Chronic Kidney Dis 2006;13:183–8.

[6] Kovesdy CP, Trivedi BK, Anderson JE. Association of kidney function with mortality in patients with chronic kidney disease not yet on dialysis: a historical prospective cohort study. Adv Chronic Kidney Dis 2006;13:183–8.

[7] Beddhu S, Kaysen GA, Yan G, et al. Association of serum albumin and atherosclerosis in chronic hemodialysis patients. Am J Kidney Dis 2002;40:721–7.

[8] Iseki K, Kawazoe N, Fukiyama K. Serum albumin is a strong predictor of death in chronic dialysis patients. Kidney Int 1993;44:115–9.

[9] Kalantar-Zadeh K, Kilpatrick RD, Kuwae N, et al. Revisiting mortality predictability of serum albumin in the dialysis population: time dependency, longitudinal changes and population-attributable fraction. Nephrol Dial Transplant 2005;20:1880—8.

[10] Lowrie EG, Lew NL. Death risk in hemodialysis patients: the predictive value of commonly measured variables and an evaluation of death rate differences between facilities. Am J Kidney Dis 1990;15:458—82.

[11] Kovesdy CP, George SM, Anderson JE, Kalantar-Zadeh K. Outcome predictability of biomarkers of protein-energy wasting and inflammation in moderate and advanced chronic kidney disease. Am J Clin Nutr 2009;90:407—14.

[12] Menon V, Greene T, Wang X, et al. C-reactive protein and albumin as predictors of all-cause and cardiovascular mortality in chronic kidney disease. Kidney Int 2005;68:766—72.

[13] Muntner P, He J, Astor BC, Folsom AR, Coresh J. Traditional and nontraditional risk factors predict coronary heart disease in chronic kidney disease: results from the atherosclerosis risk in communities study. J Am Soc Nephrol 2005;16: 529—38.

[14] Weiner DE, Tighiouart H, Elsayed EF, et al. The relationship between nontraditional risk factors and outcomes in individuals with stage 3 to 4 CKD. Am J Kidney Dis 2008;51: 212—23.

[15] Pifer TB, McCullough KP, Port FK, et al. Mortality risk in hemodialysis patients and changes in nutritional indicators: DOPPS. Kidney Int 2002;62:2238—45.

[16] Kuwae N, Kopple JD, Kalantar-Zadeh K. A low lymphocyte percentage is a predictor of mortality and hospitalization in hemodialysis patients. Clin Nephrol 2005;63:22—34.

[17] Pifer TB, McCullough KP, Port FK, et al. Mortality risk in hemodialysis patients and changes in nutritional indicators: DOPPS. Kidney Int 2002;62:2238—45.

[18] Reddan DN, Klassen PS, Szczech LA, et al. White blood cells as a novel mortality predictor in haemodialysis patients. Nephrol Dial Transplant 2003;18:1167—73.

[19] Johnson DW, Wiggins KJ, Armstrong KA, Campbell SB, Isbel NM, Hawley CM. Elevated white cell count at commencement of peritoneal dialysis predicts overall and cardiac mortality. Kidney Int 2005;67:738—43.

[20] Bologa RM, Levine DM, Parker TS, et al. Interleukin-6 predicts hypoalbuminemia, hypocholesterolemia, and mortality in hemodialysis patients. Am J Kidney Dis 1998;32:107—14.

[21] Ikizler TA, Wingard RL, Harvell J, Shyr Y, Hakim RM. Association of morbidity with markers of nutrition and inflammation in chronic hemodialysis patients: a prospective study. Kidney Int 1999;55:1945—51.

[22] Racki S, Zaputovic L, Mavric Z, Vujicic B, Dvornik S. C-reactive protein is a strong predictor of mortality in hemodialysis patients. Ren Fail 2006;28:427—33.

[23] Zimmermann J, Herrlinger S, Pruy A, Metzger T, Wanner C. Inflammation enhances cardiovascular risk and mortality in hemodialysis patients. Kidney Int 1999;55:648—58.

[24] Kalantar-Zadeh K, Kopple JD, Humphreys MH, Block G. Comparing outcome predictability of markers of malnutrition-inflammation complex syndrome in haemodialysis patients. Nephrol Dial Transplant 2004;19:1507—19.

[25] Descamps-Latscha B, Witko-Sarsat V, Nguyen-Khoa T, et al. Advanced oxidation protein products as risk factors for atherosclerotic cardiovascular events in nondiabetic predialysis patients. Am J Kidney Dis 2005;45:39—47.

[26] Feroze U, Noori N, Kovesdy CP, et al. Quality-of-life and mortality in hemodialysis patients: roles of race and nutritional status. Clin J Am Soc Nephrol 2011;6:1100—11.

[27] Kopple JD, Greene T, Chumlea WC, et al. Relationship between nutritional status and the glomerular filtration rate: results from the MDRD study. Kidney Int 2000;57:1688—703.

[28] Byers T. Body weight and mortality. N Engl J Med 1995;333: 723—4.

[29] Hsu C, McCulloch C, Iribarren C, Darbinian J, Go A. Body mass index and risk for end-stage renal disease. Ann Intern Med 2006;144:21—8.

[30] Lew EA, Garfinkel L. Variations in mortality by weight among 750,000 men and women. J Chronic Dis 1979;32:563—76.

[31] Manson JE, Willett WC, Stampfer MJ, et al. Body weight and mortality among women. N Engl J Med 1995;333:677—85.

[32] Kalantar-Zadeh K, Block G, Humphreys MH, Kopple JD. Reverse epidemiology of cardiovascular risk factors in maintenance dialysis patients. Kidney Int 2003;63:793—808.

[33] Kalantar-Zadeh K, Kopple JD. Relative contributions of nutrition and inflammation to clinical outcome in dialysis patients. Am J Kidney Dis 2001;38:1343—50.

[34] Coresh J, Longenecker JC, Miller III ER, Young HJ, Klag MJ. Epidemiology of cardiovascular risk factors in chronic renal disease. J Am Soc Nephrol 1998;9:S24—30.

[35] Fleischmann EH, Bower JD, Salahudeen AK. Risk factor paradox in hemodialysis: better nutrition as a partial explanation. ASAIO J 2001;47:74—81.

[36] Degoulet P, Legrain M, Reach I, et al. Mortality risk factors in patients treated by chronic hemodialysis. Report of the Diaphane collaborative study. Nephron 1982;31:103—10.

[37] Iseki K, Yamazato M, Tozawa M, Takishita S. Hypocholesterolemia is a significant predictor of death in a cohort of chronic hemodialysis patients. Kidney Int 2002;61:1887—93.

[38] Kilpatrick RD, McAllister CJ, Kovesdy CP, Derose SF, Kopple JD, Kalantar-Zadeh K. Association between serum lipids and survival in hemodialysis patients and impact of race. J Am Soc Nephrol 2007;18:293—303.

[39] Kovesdy CP, Anderson JE, Kalantar-Zadeh K. Inverse association between lipid levels and mortality in men with chronic kidney disease who are not yet on dialysis: effects of case mix and the malnutrition-inflammation-cachexia syndrome. J Am Soc Nephrol 2007;18:304—11.

[40] Kovesdy CP, Kalantar-Zadeh K. Lipids in aging and chronic illness: impact on survival. Arch Med Sci 2007;3:S74—80.

[41] Liu Y, Coresh J, Eustace JA, et al. Association between cholesterol level and mortality in dialysis patients: role of inflammation and malnutrition. JAMA 2004;291:451—9.

[42] Leavey SF, Strawderman RL, Jones CA, Port FK, Held PJ. Simple nutritional indicators as independent predictors of mortality in hemodialysis patients. Am J Kidney Dis 1998;31: 997—1006.

[43] Degoulet P, Legrain M, Reach I, et al. Mortality risk factors in patients treated by chronic hemodialysis. Report of the Diaphane collaborative study. Nephron 1982;31: 103—10.

[44] Fleischmann E, Teal N, Dudley J, May W, Bower JD, Salahudeen AK. Influence of excess weight on mortality and hospital stay in 1346 hemodialysis patients. Kidney Int 1999;55:1560—7.

[45] Glanton CW, Hypolite IO, Hshieh PB, Agodoa LY, Yuan CM, Abbott KC. Factors associated with improved short term survival in obese end-stage renal disease patients. Ann Epidemiol 2003;13:136—43.

[46] Johansen KL, Kutner NG, Young B, Chertow GM. Association of body size with health status in patients beginning dialysis. Am J Clin Nutr 2006;83:543—9.

[47] Kalantar-Zadeh K, Kuwae N, Wu DY, et al. Associations of body fat and its changes over time with quality of life and

prospective mortality in hemodialysis patients. Am J Clin Nutr 2006;83:202–10.

[48] Leavey SF, McCullough K, Hecking E, Goodkin D, Port FK, Young EW. Body mass index and mortality in "healthier" as compared with "sicker" haemodialysis patients: results from the Dialysis Outcomes and Practice Patterns Study (DOPPS). Nephrol Dial Transplant 2001;16:2386–94.

[49] Lowrie EG, Li Z, Ofsthun N, Lazarus JM. Body size, dialysis dose and death risk relationships among hemodialysis patients. Kidney Int 2002;62:1891–7.

[50] Port FK, Ashby VB, Dhingra RK, Roys EC, Wolfe RA. Dialysis dose and body mass index are strongly associated with survival in hemodialysis patients. J Am Soc Nephrol 2002;13:1061–6.

[51] Wolfe RA, Ashby VB, Daugirdas JT, Agodoa LY, Jones CA, Port FK. Body size, dose of hemodialysis, and mortality. Am J Kidney Dis 2000;35:80–8.

[52] Beddhu S, Pappas LM, Ramkumar N, Samore M. Effects of body size and body composition on survival in hemodialysis patients. J Am Soc Nephrol 2003;14:2366–72.

[53] Kalantar-Zadeh K, Kopple JD, Kilpatrick RD, et al. Association of morbid obesity and weight change over time with cardiovascular survival in hemodialysis population. Am J Kidney Dis 2005;46:489–500.

[54] Kovesdy CP, Anderson JE, Kalantar-Zadeh K. Paradoxical association between body mass index and mortality in men with CKD not yet on dialysis. Am J Kidney Dis 2007;49:581–91.

[55] Kovesdy CP, Kalantar-Zadeh K. Why is protein-energy wasting associated with mortality in chronic kidney disease? Semin Nephrol 2009;29:3–14.

[56] Bergstrom J. Nutrition and mortality in hemodialysis. J Am Soc Nephrol 1995;6:1329–41.

[57] Stenvinkel P, Heimburger O, Lindholm B, Kaysen GA, Bergstrom J. Are there two types of malnutrition in chronic renal failure? Evidence for relationships between malnutrition, inflammation and atherosclerosis (MIA syndrome). Nephrol Dial Transplant 2000;15:953–60.

[58] Wolfe RA, Gaylin DS, Port FK, Held PJ, Wood CL. Using USRDS generated mortality tables to compare local ESRD mortality rates to national rates. Kidney Int 1992;42:991–6.

[59] Adequacy of dialysis and nutrition in continuous peritoneal dialysis. association with clinical outcomes. Canada-USA CANUSA. Peritoneal Dialysis Study Group. J Am Soc Nephrol 1996;7:198–207.

[60] Bargman JM, Thorpe KE, Churchill DN. Relative contribution of residual renal function and peritoneal clearance to adequacy of dialysis: a reanalysis of the CANUSA study. J Am Soc Nephrol 2001;12:2158–62.

[61] Hsu CY, Chertow GM, Curhan GC. Methodological issues in studying the epidemiology of mild to moderate chronic renal insufficiency. Kidney Int 2002;61:1567–76.

[62] Kalantar-Zadeh K, Kopple JD, Block G, Humphreys MH. Association among SF36 quality of life measures and nutrition, hospitalization, and mortality in hemodialysis. J Am Soc Nephrol 2001;12:2797–806.

[63] Kalantar-Zadeh K, Kopple JD, Block G, Humphreys MH. A malnutrition-inflammation score is correlated with morbidity and mortality in maintenance hemodialysis patients. Am J Kidney Dis 2001;38:1251–63.

[64] Sehgal AR, Dor A, Tsai AC. Morbidity and cost implications of inadequate hemodialysis. Am J Kidney Dis 2001;37:1223–31.

[65] Kalantar-Zadeh K, Supasyndh O, Lehn RS, McAllister CJ, Kopple JD. Normalized protein nitrogen appearance is correlated with hospitalization and mortality in hemodialysis patients with Kt/V greater than 1.20. J Ren Nutr 2003;13:15–25.

[66] Blake C, Codd MB, Cassidy A, O'Meara YM. Physical function, employment and quality of life in end-stage renal disease. J Nephrol 2000;13:142–9.

[67] Chen YC, Hung KY, Kao TW, Tsai TJ, Chen WY. Relationship between dialysis adequacy and quality of life in long-term peritoneal dialysis patients. Perit Dial Int 2000;20:534–40.

[68] Diaz-Buxo JA, Lowrie EG, Lew NL, Zhang H, Lazarus JM. Quality-of-life evaluation using Short Form 36: comparison in hemodialysis and peritoneal dialysis patients. Am J Kidney Dis 2000;35:293–300.

[69] Jofre R, Lopez-Gomez JM, Moreno F, Sanz-Guajardo D, Valderrabano F. Changes in quality of life after renal transplantation. Am J Kidney Dis 1998;32:93–100.

[70] Kutner NG, Zhang R, McClellan WM. Patient-reported quality of life early in dialysis treatment: effects associated with usual exercise activity. Nephrol Nurs J 2000;27:357–67.

[71] Daneker B, Kimmel PL, Ranich T, Peterson RA. Depression and marital dissatisfaction in patients with end-stage renal disease and in their spouses. Am J Kidney Dis 2001;38:839–46.

[72] Wanner C, Krane V, Marz W, et al. Atorvastatin in patients with type 2 diabetes mellitus undergoing hemodialysis. N Engl J Med 2005;353:238–48.

[73] Brenner BM, Cooper ME, de Zeeuw D, et al. Effects of losartan on renal and cardiovascular outcomes in patients with type 2 diabetes and nephropathy. N Engl J Med 2001;345:861–9.

[74] Lewis EJ, Hunsicker LG, Clarke WR, et al. Renoprotective effect of the angiotensin-receptor antagonist irbesartan in patients with nephropathy due to type 2 diabetes. N Engl J Med 2001;345:851–60.

[75] Goicoechea M, Caramelo C, Rodriguez P, et al. Role of type of vascular access in erythropoietin and intravenous iron requirements in haemodialysis. Nephrol Dial Transplant 2001;16:2188–93.

[76] Gunnell J, Yeun JY, Depner TA, Kaysen GA. Acute-phase response predicts erythropoietin resistance in hemodialysis and peritoneal dialysis patients. Am J Kidney Dis 1999;33:63–72.

[77] Kalantar-Zadeh K, Kleiner M, Dunne E, Lee GH, Luft FC. A modified quantitative subjective global assessment of nutrition for dialysis patients. Nephrol Dial Transplant 1999;14:1732–8.

[78] Kalantar-Zadeh K, Hoffken B, Wunsch H, Fink H, Kleiner M, Luft FC. Diagnosis of iron deficiency anemia in renal failure patients during the post-erythropoietin era. Am J Kidney Dis 1995;26:292–9.

[79] Madore F, Lowrie EG, Brugnara C, et al. Anemia in hemodialysis patients: variables affecting this outcome predictor. J Am Soc Nephrol 1997;8:1921–9.

[80] Kalantar-Zadeh K, Kleiner M, Dunne E, et al. Total iron-binding capacity-estimated transferrin correlates with the nutritional subjective global assessment in hemodialysis patients. Am J Kidney Dis 1998;31:263–72.

[81] Barany P, Divino Filho JC, Bergstrom J. High C-reactive protein is a strong predictor of resistance to erythropoietin in hemodialysis patients. Am J Kidney Dis 1997;29:565–8.

[82] Fouque D, Kalantar-Zadeh K, Kopple J, et al. A proposed nomenclature and diagnostic criteria for protein-energy wasting in acute and chronic kidney disease. Kidney Int 2008;73:391–8.

[83] Qureshi AR, Alvestrand A, Danielsson A, et al. Factors predicting malnutrition in hemodialysis patients: a cross-sectional study. Kidney Int 1998;53:773–82.

[84] Kaysen GA. Malnutrition and the acute-phase reaction in dialysis patients-how to measure and how to distinguish. Nephrol Dial Transplant 2000;15:1521–4.

[85] Grodstein GP, Blumenkrantz MJ, Kopple JD. Nutritional and metabolic response to catabolic stress in uremia. Am J Clin Nutr 1980;33:1411—6.

[86] Dwyer JT, Cunniff PJ, Maroni BJ, et al. The hemodialysis pilot study: nutrition program and participant characteristics at baseline. The HEMO Study Group. J Ren Nutr 1998;8:11—20.

[87] National Kidney Foundation. K/DOQI Clinical Practice Guidelines for Nutrition in Chronic Renal Failure. Am J Kidney Dis 2000;35:s1—s140.

[88] Kalantar-Zadeh K, Block G, McAllister CJ, Humphreys MH, Kopple JD. Appetite and inflammation, nutrition, anemia, and clinical outcome in hemodialysis patients. Am J Clin Nutr 2004; 80:299—307.

[89] Carrero JJ, Qureshi AR, Axelsson J, et al. Comparison of nutritional and inflammatory markers in dialysis patients with reduced appetite. Am J Clin Nutr 2007;85:695—701.

[90] Kopple JD, Shinaberger JH, Coburn JW, Sorensen MK, Rubini ME. Evaluating modified protein diets for uremia. J Am Diet Assoc 1969;54:481—5.

[91] Slomowitz LA, Monteon FJ, Grosvenor M, Laidlaw SA, Kopple JD. Effect of energy intake on nutritional status in maintenance hemodialysis patients. Kidney Int 1989;35:704—11.

[92] Lowrie EG, Laird NM, Parker TF, Sargent JA. Effect of the hemodialysis prescription of patient morbidity: report from the National Cooperative Dialysis Study. N Engl J Med 1981;305: 1176—81.

[93] Schoenfeld PY, Henry RR, Laird NM, Roxe DM. Assessment of nutritional status of the National Cooperative Dialysis Study population. Kidney Int Suppl 1983:S80—8.

[94] Thunberg BJ, Swamy AP, Cestero RV. Cross-sectional and longitudinal nutritional measurements in maintenance hemodialysis patients. Am J Clin Nutr 1981;34:2005—12.

[95] Kalantar-Zadeh K, Kopple JD, Deepak S, Block D, Block G. Food intake characteristics of hemodialysis patients as obtained by food frequency questionnaire. J Ren Nutr 2002;12:17—31.

[96] Hu FB, Manson JE, Stampfer MJ, et al. Diet, lifestyle, and the risk of type 2 diabetes mellitus in women. N Engl J Med 2001;345:790—7.

[97] Araujo IC, Kamimura MA, Draibe SA, et al. Nutritional parameters and mortality in incident hemodialysis patients. J Ren Nutr 2006;16:27—35.

[98] Herselman M, Moosa MR, Kotze TJ, Kritzinger M, Wuister S, Mostert D. Protein-energy malnutrition as a risk factor for increased morbidity in long-term hemodialysis patients. J Ren Nutr 2000;10:7—15.

[99] Wolfson M, Strong CJ, Minturn D, Gray DK, Kopple JD. Nutritional status and lymphocyte function in maintenance hemodialysis patients. Am J Clin Nutr 1984;39:547—55.

[100] Davies SJ, Russell L, Bryan J, Phillips L, Russell GI. Comorbidity, urea kinetics, and appetite in continuous ambulatory peritoneal dialysis patients: their interrelationship and prediction of survival. Am J Kidney Dis 1995;26:353—61.

[101] Beddhu S, Ramkumar N, Pappas LM. Normalization of protein intake by body weight and the associations of protein intake with nutritional status and survival. J Ren Nutr 2005;15:387—97.

[102] Acchiardo SR, Moore LW, Latour PA. Malnutrition as the main factor in morbidity and mortality of hemodialysis patients. Kidney Int Suppl 1983;16:S199—203.

[103] Allen KL, Miskulin D, Yan G, et al. Association of nutritional markers with physical and mental health status in prevalent hemodialysis patients from the HEMO study. J Ren Nutr 2002;12:160—9.

[104] Blake PG, Sombolos K, Abraham G, et al. Lack of correlation between urea kinetic indices and clinical outcomes in CAPD patients. Kidney Int 1991;39:700—6.

[105] Harter HR. Review of significant findings from the National Cooperative Dialysis Study and recommendations. Kidney Int Suppl 1983:S107—12.

[106] Teehan BP, Schleifer CR, Brown JM, Sigler MH, Raimondo J. Urea kinetic analysis and clinical outcome on CAPD. A five year longitudinal study. Adv Perit Dial 1990;6:181—5.

[107] Shinaberger CS, Kilpatrick RD, Regidor DL, et al. Longitudinal associations between dietary protein intake and survival in hemodialysis patients. Am J Kidney Dis 2006;48:37—49.

[108] Raja RM, Ijelu G, Goldstein M. Influence of Kt/V and protein catabolic rate on hemodialysis morbidity. A long-term study. ASAIO J 1992;38:M179—80.

[109] Kloppenburg WD, Stegeman CA, de Jong PE, Huisman RM. Relating protein intake to nutritional status in haemodialysis patients: how to normalize the protein equivalent of total nitrogen appearance (PNA)? Nephrol Dial Transplant 1999;14: 2165—72.

[110] Canaud B, Leblanc M, Garred LJ, Bosc JY, Argiles A, Mion C. Protein catabolic rate over lean body mass ratio: a more rational approach to normalize the protein catabolic rate in dialysis patients. Am J Kidney Dis 1997;30:672—9.

[111] Stegeman CA, Huisman RM, de RB, Joostema A, de Jong PE. Determination of protein catabolic rate in patients on chronic intermittent hemodialysis: urea output measurements compared with dietary protein intake and with calculation of urea generation rate. Am J Kidney Dis 1995;25:887—95.

[112] Hulsewe KW, van Acker BA, von Meyenfeldt MF, Soeters PB. Nutritional depletion and dietary manipulation: effects on the immune response. World J Surg 1999;23:536—44.

[113] Souba WW. Nutritional support. N Engl J Med 1997;336:41—8.

[114] Alexander JW. Immunoenhancement via enteral nutrition. Arch Surg 1993;128:1242—5.

[115] Kimmel PL, Phillips TM, Lew SQ, Langman CB. Zinc modulates mononuclear cellular calcitriol metabolism in peritoneal dialysis patients. Kidney Int 1996;49:1407—12.

[116] Erten Y, Kayatas M, Sezer S, et al. Zinc deficiency: prevalence and causes in hemodialysis patients and effect on cellular immune response. Transplant Proc 1998;30:850—1.

[117] Casciato DA, McAdam LP, Kopple JD, et al. Immunologic abnormalities in hemodialysis patients: improvement after pyridoxine therapy. Nephron 1984;38:9—16.

[118] Dobbelstein H, Korner WF, Mempel W, Grosse-Wilde H, Edel HH. Vitamin B$_6$ deficiency in uremia and its implications for the depression of immune responses. Kidney Int 1974;5: 233—9.

[119] DeSimone C, Famularo G, Tzantzoglou S, Trinchieri V, Moretti S, Sorice F. Carnitine depletion in peripheral blood mononuclear cells from patients with AIDS: effect of oral L-carnitine. AIDS 1994;8:655—60.

[120] Dolson GM. Do potassium deficient diets and K$^+$ removal by dialysis contribute to the cardiovascular morbidity and mortality of patients with end-stage renal disease? Int J Artif Organs 1997;20:134—5.

[121] Kalantar-Zadeh K, Kopple JD, Deepak S, Block D, Block G. Food intake characteristics of hemodialysis patients as obtained by food frequency questionnaire. J Ren Nutr 2002;12:17—31.

[122] Noori N, Kalantar-Zadeh K, Kovesdy CP, et al. Dietary potassium intake and mortality in long-term hemodialysis patients. Am J Kidney Dis 2010;56:338—47.

[123] Noori N, Kalantar-Zadeh K, Kovesdy CP, Bross R, Benner D, Kopple JD. Association of dietary phosphorus intake and phosphorus to protein ratio with mortality in hemodialysis patients. Clin J Am Soc Nephrol 2010;5:683—92.

[124] Shinaberger CS, Greenland S, Kopple JD, et al. Is controlling phosphorus by decreasing dietary protein intake beneficial or

harmful in persons with chronic kidney disease? Am J Clin Nutr 2008;88:1511—8.

[125] Leavey SF, Strawderman RL, Jones CA, Port FK, Held PJ. Simple nutritional indicators as independent predictors of mortality in hemodialysis patients. Am J Kidney Dis 1998;31:997—1006.

[126] Chung SH, Lindholm B, Lee HB. Influence of initial nutritional status on continuous ambulatory peritoneal dialysis patient survival. Perit Dial Int 2000;20:19—26.

[127] Degoulet P, Legrain M, Reach I, et al. Mortality risk factors in patients treated by chronic hemodialysis. Report of the Diaphane collaborative study. Nephron 1982;31:103—10.

[128] Kopple JD, Zhu X, Lew NL, Lowrie EG. Body weight-for-height relationships predict mortality in maintenance hemodialysis patients. Kidney Int 1999;56:1136—48.

[129] Adequacy of dialysis and nutrition in continuous peritoneal dialysis. association with clinical outcomes. Canada-USA (CANUSA). Peritoneal Dialysis Study Group. J Am Soc Nephrol 1996;7:198—207.

[130] Chung SH, Lindholm B, Lee HB. Influence of initial nutritional status on continuous ambulatory peritoneal dialysis patient survival. Perit Dial Int 2000;20:19—26.

[131] Hakim RM, Lowrie E. Obesity and mortality in ESRD: is it good to be fat? Kidney Int 1999;55:1580—1.

[132] Johnson DW, Herzig KA, Purdie DM, et al. Is obesity a favorable prognostic factor in peritoneal dialysis patients? Perit Dial Int 2000;20:715—21.

[133] Snyder JJ, Foley RN, Gilbertson DT, Vonesh EF, Collins AJ. Body size and outcomes on peritoneal dialysis in the United States. Kidney Int 2003;64:1838—44.

[134] Abbott KC, Glanton CW, Trespalacios FC, et al. Body mass index, dialysis modality, and survival: analysis of the United States Renal Data System Dialysis Morbidity and Mortality Wave II. Study. Kidney Int 2004;65:597—605.

[135] Aslam N, Bernardini J, Fried L, Piraino B. Large body mass index does not predict short-term survival in peritoneal dialysis patients. Perit Dial Int 2002;22:191—6.

[136] McDonald SP, Collins JF, Johnson DW. Obesity is associated with worse peritoneal dialysis outcomes in the Australia and New Zealand patient populations. J Am Soc Nephrol 2003;14:2894—901.

[137] Evans M, Fryzek JP, Elinder CG, et al. The natural history of chronic renal failure: results from an unselected, population-based, inception cohort in Sweden. Am J Kidney Dis 2005;46:863—70.

[138] Kwan BCH, Ramkumar N, Murtaugh MA, Beddhu S. Associations of body size with metabolic syndrome and mortality in moderate chronic kidney disease [abstract]. Kwan B.C.H., Ramkumar N., Murtaugh M.A. Beddhu S. Journal of the American Society of Nephrology 2006;17:99A.

[139] Jurkovitz C, Li S, Bakris G, et al. Effect of obesity on mortality in patients at high risk for kidney disease: results from KEEP [abstract]. Jurkovitz C, Li S, Bakris G, et al. J Am Soc Nephrol 2006;17:11A.

[140] Haslam DW, James WP. Obesity. Lancet 2005;366:1197—209.

[141] Kovesdy CP, Czira ME, Rudas A, et al. Body mass index, waist circumference and mortality in kidney transplant recipients. Am J Transplant 2010;10:2644—51.

[142] Postorino M, Marino C, Tripepi G, Zoccali C. Abdominal obesity and all-cause and cardiovascular mortality in end-stage renal disease. J Am Coll Cardiol 2009;53:1265—72.

[143] Wahba IM, Mak RH. Obesity and obesity-initiated metabolic syndrome: mechanistic links to chronic kidney disease. Clin J Am Soc Nephrol 2007;2:550—62.

[144] Nelson EE, Hong CD, Pesce AL, Peterson DW, Singh S, Pollak VE. Anthropometric norms for the dialysis population. Am J Kidney Dis 1990;16:32—7.

[145] Chazot C, Laurent G, Charra B, et al. Malnutrition in long-term haemodialysis survivors. Nephrol Dial Transplant 2001;16:61—9.

[146] Noori N, Kopple JD, Kovesdy CP, et al. Mid-arm muscle circumference and quality of life and survival in maintenance hemodialysis patients. Clin J Am Soc Nephrol 2010;5:2258—68.

[147] Woodrow G, Oldroyd B, Smith MA, Turney JH. Measurement of body composition in chronic renal failure: comparison of skinfold anthropometry and bioelectrical impedance with dual energy X-ray absorptiometry. Eur J Clin Nutr 1996;50:295—301.

[148] Dumler F. Use of bioelectric impedance analysis and dual-energy X-ray absorptiometry for monitoring the nutritional status of dialysis patients. ASAIO J 1997;43:256—60.

[149] Chertow GM, Lowrie EG, Wilmore DW, et al. Nutritional assessment with bioelectrical impedance analysis in maintenance hemodialysis patients. J Am Soc Nephrol 1995;6:75—81.

[150] Kalantar-Zadeh K, Block G, Kelly MP, Schroepfer C, Rodriguez RA, Humphreys MH. Near infra-red interactance for longitudinal assessment of nutrition in dialysis patients. J Ren Nutr 2001;11:23—31.

[151] Kalantar-Zadeh K, Dunne E, Nixon K, et al. Near infra-red interactance for nutritional assessment of dialysis patients. Nephrol Dial Transplant 1999;14:169—75.

[152] Bross R, Chandramohan G, Kovesdy CP, et al. Comparing body composition assessment tests in long-term hemodialysis patients. Am J Kidney Dis 2010;55:885—96.

[153] Chertow GM, Jacobs DO, Lazarus JM, Lew NL, Lowrie EG. Phase angle predicts survival in hemodialysis patients [abstract] Chertow GM, Jacobs DO, Lazarus JM, Lew NL, Lowrie EG. Journal of Renal Nutrition: The Official Journal of the Council on Renal Nutrition of the National Kidney Foundation 1997;7:204—7.

[154] Owen Jr WF, Lew NL, Liu Y, Lowrie EG, Lazarus JM. The urea reduction ratio and serum albumin concentration as predictors of mortality in patients undergoing hemodialysis. N Engl J Med 1993;329:1001—6.

[155] Noori N, Kovesdy CP, Dukkipati R, et al. Racial and ethnic differences in mortality of hemodialysis patients: role of dietary and nutritional status and inflammation. Am J Nephrol 2011;33:157—67.

[156] Avram MM, Sreedhara R, Fein P, Oo KK, Chattopadhyay J, Mittman N. Survival on hemodialysis and peritoneal dialysis over 12 years with emphasis on nutritional parameters. Am J Kidney Dis 2001;37:S77—80.

[157] Kalantar-Zadeh K, Don BR, Rodriguez RA, Humphreys MH. Serum ferritin is a marker of morbidity and mortality in hemodialysis patients. Am J Kidney Dis 2001;37:564—72.

[158] Marcen R, Teruel JL, de la Cal MA, Gamez C. The impact of malnutrition in morbidity and mortality in stable haemodialysis patients. Spanish Cooperative Study of Nutrition in Hemodialysis. Nephrol Dial Transplant 1997;12:2324—31.

[159] Fung L, Pollock CA, Caterson RJ, et al. Dialysis adequacy and nutrition determine prognosis in continuous ambulatory peritoneal dialysis patients. J Am Soc Nephrol 1996;7:737—44.

[160] Kaysen GA, Stevenson FT, Depner TA. Determinants of albumin concentration in hemodialysis patients. Am J Kidney Dis 1997;29:658—68.

[161] Kaysen GA, Yeun J, Depner T. Albumin synthesis, catabolism and distribution in dialysis patients. Miner Electrolyte Metab 1997;23:218—24.

[162] Yeun JY, Kaysen GA. Acute phase proteins and peritoneal dialysate albumin loss are the main determinants of serum

albumin in peritoneal dialysis patients. Am J Kidney Dis 1997;30:923–7.

[163] Struijk DG, Krediet RT, Koomen GC, Boeschoten EW, Arisz L. The effect of serum albumin at the start of continuous ambulatory peritoneal dialysis treatment on patient survival. Perit Dial Int 1994;14:121–6.

[164] Neyra NR, Hakim RM, Shyr Y, Ikizler TA. Serum transferrin and serum prealbumin are early predictors of serum albumin in chronic hemodialysis patients. J Ren Nutr 2000; 10:184–90.

[165] Kopple JD, Mehrotra R, Suppasyndh O, Kalantar-Zadeh K. Observations with regard to the National Kidney Foundation K/DOQI clinical practice guidelines concerning serum trans-thyretin in chronic renal failure. Clin Chem Lab Med 2002;40: 1308–12.

[166] Chertow GM, Ackert K, Lew NL, Lazarus JM, Lowrie EG. Prealbumin is as important as albumin in the nutritional assessment of hemodialysis patients. Kidney Int 2000;58: 2512–7.

[167] Chertow GM, Goldstein-Fuchs DJ, Lazarus JM, Kaysen GA. Prealbumin, mortality, and cause-specific hospitalization in hemodialysis patients. Kidney Int 2005;68:2794–800.

[168] Mittman N, Avram MM, Oo KK, Chattopadhyay J. Serum prealbumin predicts survival in hemodialysis and peritoneal dialysis: 10 years of prospective observation. Am J Kidney Dis 2001;38:1358–64.

[169] Rambod M, Kovesdy CP, Bross R, Kopple JD, Kalantar-Zadeh K. Association of serum prealbumin and its changes over time with clinical outcomes and survival in patients receiving hemodialysis. Am J Clin Nutr 2008;88:1485–94.

[170] Sreedhara R, Avram MM, Blanco M, Batish R, Avram MM, Mittman N. Prealbumin is the best nutritional predictor of survival in hemodialysis and peritoneal dialysis. Am J Kidney Dis 1996;28:937–42.

[171] Bross R, Zitterkoph J, Pithia J, et al. Association of serum total iron-binding capacity and its changes over time with nutritional and clinical outcomes in hemodialysis patients. Am J Nephrol 2009;29:571–81.

[172] Kalantar-Zadeh K, Kleiner M, Dunne E, et al. Total iron-binding capacity-estimated transferrin correlates with the nutritional subjective global assessment in hemodialysis patients. Am J Kidney Dis 1998;31:263–72.

[173] Kaysen GA. The microinflammatory state in uremia: causes and potential consequences. J Am Soc Nephrol 2001;12:1549–57.

[174] Lowrie EG, Lew NL. Death risk in hemodialysis patients: the predictive value of commonly measured variables and an evaluation of death rate differences between facilities. Am J Kidney Dis 1990;15:458–82.

[175] Gamba G, Mejia JL, Saldivar S, Pena JC, Correa-Rotter R. Death risk in CAPD patients. The predictive value of the initial clinical and laboratory variables. Nephron 1993;65:23–7.

[176] Habib AN, Baird BC, Leypoldt JK, Cheung AK, Goldfarb-Rumyantzev AS. The association of lipid levels with mortality in patients on chronic peritoneal dialysis. Nephrol Dial Transplant 2006;21:2881–92.

[177] Ritz E. Why are lipids not predictive of cardiovascular death in the dialysis patient? Miner Electrolyte Metab 1996;22: 9–12.

[178] Yang WS, Kim SB, Min WK, Park S, Lee MS, Park JS. Athero-genic lipid profile and lipoproteina.in relation to serum albumin in haemodialysis patients. Nephrol Dial Transplant 1995;10:1668–71.

[179] Shlipak MG, Fried LF, Cushman M, et al. Cardiovascular mortality risk in chronic kidney disease: comparison of traditional and novel risk factors. JAMA 2005;293:1737–45.

[180] Fellstrom BC, Jardine AG, Schmieder RE, et al. Rosuvastatin and cardiovascular events in patients undergoing hemodialysis. N Engl J Med 2009;360:1395–407.

[181] Baigent C, Landry M. Study of Heart and Renal Protection (SHARP). Kidney Int Suppl 2003:S207–10.

[182] Owen WF, Lowrie EG. C-reactive protein as an outcome predictor for maintenance hemodialysis patients. Kidney Int 1998;54:627–36.

[183] Avram MM, Fein PA, Bonomini L, et al. Predictors of survival in continuous ambulatory peritoneal dialysis patients: a five-year prospective study. Perit Dial Int 1996;16(Suppl. 1): S190–4.

[184] De Lima JJ, Vieira ML, Abensur H, Krieger EM. Baseline blood pressure and other variables influencing survival on haemo-dialysis of patients without overt cardiovascular disease. Nephrol Dial Transplant 2001;16:793–7.

[185] Avram MM, Mittman N, Bonomini L, Chattopadhyay J, Fein P. Markers for survival in dialysis: a seven-year prospective study. Am J Kidney Dis 1995;26:209–19.

[186] Lowrie EG, Huang WH, Lew NL. Death risk predictors among peritoneal dialysis and hemodialysis patients: a preliminary comparison. Am J Kidney Dis 1995;26:220–8.

[187] Kalantar-Zadeh K, Streja E, Kovesdy CP, et al. The obesity paradox and mortality associated with surrogates of body size and muscle mass in patients receiving hemodialysis. Mayo Clin Proc 2010;85:991–1001.

[188] Streja E, Molnar MZ, Kovesdy CP, et al. Associations of pretransplant weight and muscle mass with mortality in renal transplant recipients. Clin J Am Soc Nephrol 2011;6: 1463–73.

[189] Molnar MZ, Streja E, Kovesdy CP, et al. Associations of body mass index and weight loss with mortality in transplant-waitlisted maintenance hemodialysis patients. Am J Transplant 2011;11:725–36.

[190] Yeun JY, Levine RA, Mantadilok V, Kaysen GA. C-Reactive protein predicts all-cause and cardiovascular mortality in hemodialysis patients. Am J Kidney Dis 2000;35:469–76.

[191] Iseki K, Tozawa M, Yoshi S, Fukiyama K. Serum C-reactive protein (CRP) and risk of death in chronic dialysis patients. Nephrol Dial Transplant 1999;14:1956–60.

[192] Noh H, Lee SW, Kang SW, et al. Serum C-reactive protein: a predictor of mortality in continuous ambulatory peritoneal dialysis patients. Perit Dial Int 1998;18:387–94.

[193] Tonelli M, Sacks F, Pfeffer M, Jhangri GS, Curhan G. Biomarkers of inflammation and progression of chronic kidney disease. Kidney Int 2005;68:237–45.

[194] Sarnak MJ, Poindexter A, Wang SR, et al. Serum C-reactive protein and leptin as predictors of kidney disease progression in the Modification of Diet in Renal Disease Study. Kidney Int 2002;62:2208–15.

[195] Kaysen GA, Chertow GM, Adhikarla R, Young B, Ronco C, Levin NW. Inflammation and dietary protein intake exert competing effects on serum albumin and creatinine in hemo-dialysis patients. Kidney Int 2001;60:333–40.

[196] Abdullah MS, Wild G, Jacob V, et al. Cytokines and the malnutrition of chronic renal failure. Miner Electrolyte Metab 1997;23:237–42.

[197] Stenvinkel P, Lindholm B, Heimburger M, Heimburger O. Elevated serum levels of soluble adhesion molecules predict death in pre-dialysis patients: association with malnutrition, inflammation, and cardiovascular disease. Nephrol Dial Transplant 2000;15:1624–30.

[198] Fried L, Solomon C, Shlipak M, et al. Inflammatory and pro-thrombotic markers and the progression of renal disease in elderly individuals. J Am Soc Nephrol 2004;15:3184–91.

[199] Liu Y, Berthier-Schaad Y, Fallin MD, et al. IL-6 haplotypes, inflammation, and risk for cardiovascular disease in a multi-ethnic dialysis cohort. J Am Soc Nephrol 2006;17:863–70.

[200] Lindgren BF, Friis K, Ericsson F. Insulin-like growth factor I correlates with protein intake estimated from the normalized protein catabolic rate in hemodialysis patients. Am J Nephrol 2000;20:255–62.

[201] Rodriguez-Carmona A, Perez FM, Cordido F, Garcia FT, Garcia-Buela J. Hyperleptinemia is not correlated with markers of protein malnutrition in chronic renal failure. A cross-sectional study in predialysis, peritoneal dialysis and hemodialysis patients. Nephron 2000;86:274–80.

[202] Suliman M, Stenvinkel P, Qureshi AR, et al. The reverse epidemiology of plasma total homocysteine as a mortality risk factor is related to the impact of wasting and inflammation. Nephrol Dial Transplant 2007;22:209–17.

[203] Kalantar-Zadeh K, Block G, Humphreys MH, McAllister CJ, Kopple JD. A low, rather than a high, total plasma homocysteine is an indicator of poor outcome in hemodialysis patients. J Am Soc Nephrol 2004;15:442–53.

[204] Wrone EM, Zehnder JL, Hornberger JM, McCann LM, Coplon NS, Fortmann SP. An MTHFR variant, homocysteine, and cardiovascular comorbidity in renal disease. Kidney Int 2001;60:1106–13.

[205] Suliman ME, Barany P, Kalantar-Zadeh K, Lindholm B, Stenvinkel P. Homocysteine in uraemia – a puzzling and conflicting story. Nephrol Dial Transplant 2005;20:16–21.

[206] Kalantar-Zadeh K, Ikizler TA, Block G, Avram MM, Kopple JD. Malnutrition-inflammation complex syndrome in dialysis patients: causes and consequences. Am J Kidney Dis 2003;42:864–81.

[207] Bostom AG, Carpenter MA, Kusek JW, et al. Homocysteine-lowering and cardiovascular disease outcomes in kidney transplant recipients: primary results from the Folic Acid for Vascular Outcome Reduction in Transplantation trial. Circulation 2011;123:1763–70.

[208] Jamison RL, Hartigan P, Kaufman JS, et al. Effect of homocysteine lowering on mortality and vascular disease in advanced chronic kidney disease and end-stage renal disease: a randomized controlled trial. JAMA 2007;298:1163–70.

[209] House AA, Eliasziw M, Cattran DC, et al. Effect of B-vitamin therapy on progression of diabetic nephropathy: a randomized controlled trial. JAMA 2010;303:1603–9.

[210] Block GA, Hulbert-Shearon TE, Levin NW, Port FK. Association of serum phosphorus and calcium x phosphate product with mortality risk in chronic hemodialysis patients: a national study. Am J Kidney Dis 1998;31:607–17.

[211] Block GA, Klassen PS, Lazarus JM, Ofsthun N, Lowrie EG, Chertow GM. Mineral metabolism, mortality, and morbidity in maintenance hemodialysis. J Am Soc Nephrol 2004;15:2208–18.

[212] Ganesh SK, Stack AG, Levin NW, Hulbert-Shearon T, Port FK. Association of elevated serum PO4), Ca x PO4.product, and parathyroid hormone with cardiac mortality risk in chronic hemodialysis patients. J Am Soc Nephrol 2001;12:2131–8.

[213] Kalantar-Zadeh K, Kuwae N, Regidor DL, et al. Survival predictability of time-varying indicators of bone disease in maintenance hemodialysis patients. Kidney Int 2006;70:771–80.

[214] Kovesdy CP, Anderson JE, Kalantar-Zadeh K. Outcomes associated with serum phosphorus level in males with non-dialysis dependent chronic kidney disease. Clin Nephrol 2010;73:268–75.

[215] Kestenbaum B, Sampson JN, Rudser KD, et al. Serum phosphate levels and mortality risk among people with chronic kidney disease. J Am Soc Nephrol 2005;16:520–8.

[216] Voormolen N, Noordzij M, Grootendorst DC, et al. High plasma phosphate as a risk factor for decline in renal function and mortality in pre-dialysis patients. Nephrol Dial Transplant 2007;22:2909–16.

[217] Isakova T, Gutierrez OM, Chang Y, et al. Phosphorus binders and survival on hemodialysis. J Am Soc Nephrol 2009;20:388–96.

[218] Kovesdy CP, Kuchmak O, Lu JL, Kalantar-Zadeh K. Outcomes associated with phosphorus binders in men with non-dialysis-dependent CKD. Am J Kidney Dis 2010;56:842–51.

[219] Schwarz S, Trivedi BK, Kalantar-Zadeh K, Kovesdy CP. Association of disorders in mineral metabolism with progression of chronic kidney disease. Clin J Am Soc Nephrol 2006;1:825–31.

[220] Kovesdy CP, Regidor DL, Mehrotra R, et al. Serum and dialysate potassium concentrations and survival in hemodialysis patients. Clin J Am Soc Nephrol 2007;2:999–1007.

[221] Iseki K, Uehara H, Nishime K, et al. Impact of the initial levels of laboratory variables on survival in chronic dialysis patients. Am J Kidney Dis 1996;28:541–8.

[222] Pun PH, Lehrich RW, Honeycutt EF, Herzog CA, Middleton JP. Modifiable risk factors associated with sudden cardiac arrest within hemodialysis clinics. Kidney Int 2011;79:218–27.

[223] Einhorn LM, Zhan M, Hsu VD, et al. The frequency of hyperkalemia and its significance in chronic kidney disease. Arch Intern Med 2009;169:1156–62.

[224] Hayes J, Kalantar-Zadeh K, Lu JL, Turban S, Anderson JE, Kovesdy CP. Association of hypo- and hyperkalemia with disease progression and mortality in males with chronic kidney disease: the role of race. Nephron Clin Pract 2012;120:c8–16.

[225] Bommer J, Locatelli F, Satayathum S, et al. Association of pre-dialysis serum bicarbonate levels with risk of mortality and hospitalization in the Dialysis Outcomes and Practice Patterns Study (DOPPS). Am J Kidney Dis 2004;44:661–71.

[226] Wu DY, McAllister CJ, Kilpatrick RD, et al. Association between serum bicarbonate and death in hemodialysis patients: Is it better to be acidotic or alkalotic? Clin J Am Soc Nephrol 2006;1:70–8.

[227] Kovesdy CP, Anderson JE, Kalantar-Zadeh K. Association of serum bicarbonate levels with mortality in patients with non-dialysis-dependent CKD. Nephrol Dial Transplant 2009;24:1232–7.

[228] Carvounis CP, Manis T, Coritsidis G, Dubinsky M, Serpente P. Total lymphocyte count: a promising prognostic index of mortality in patients on CAPD. Perit Dial Int 2000;20:33–8.

[229] Marckmann P. Nutritional status and mortality of patients in regular dialysis therapy. J Intern Med 1989;226:429–32.

[230] Lawson JA, Lazarus R, Kelly JJ. Prevalence and prognostic significance of malnutrition in chronic renal insufficiency. J Ren Nutr 2001;11:16–22.

[231] Adequacy of dialysis and nutrition in continuous peritoneal dialysis. association with clinical outcomes. Canada-USA (CANUSA). Peritoneal Dialysis Study Group. J Am Soc Nephrol 1996;7:198–207.

[232] Molnar MZ, Keszei A, Czira ME, et al. Evaluation of the malnutrition-inflammation score in kidney transplant recipients. Am J Kidney Dis 2010;56:102–11.

[233] Molnar MZ, Czira ME, Rudas A, et al. Association between the malnutrition-inflammation score and post-transplant anaemia. Nephrol Dial Transplant 2011;26:2000–6.

[234] Czira ME, Lindner AV, Szeifert L, et al. Association between the Malnutrition-Inflammation Score and depressive symptoms in kidney transplanted patients. Gen Hosp Psychiatry 2011;33:157–65.

[235] Molnar MZ, Czira ME, Rudas A, et al. Association of the malnutrition-inflammation score with clinical outcomes in kidney transplant recipients. Am J Kidney Dis 2011;58:101—8.

[236] Beto JA, Bansal VK, Hart J, McCarthy M, Roberts D. Hemodialysis prognostic nutrition index as a predictor for morbidity and mortality in hemodialysis patients and its correlation to adequacy of dialysis. Council on Renal Nutrition National Research Question Collaborative Study Group. J Ren Nutr 1999;9:2—8.

[237] Kopple JD. The nutrition management of the patient with acute renal failure. JPEN J Parenter Enteral Nutr 1996;20:3—12.

[238] Mortelmans AK, Duym P, Vandenbroucke J, et al. Intradialytic parenteral nutrition in malnourished hemodialysis patients: a prospective long-term study. JPEN J Parenter Enteral Nutr 1999;23:90—5.

[239] Pupim LB, Flakoll PJ, Ikizler TA. Nutritional supplementation acutely increases albumin fractional synthetic rate in chronic hemodialysis patients. J Am Soc Nephrol 2004;15:1920—6.

[240] Pupim LB, Majchrzak KM, Flakoll PJ, Ikizler TA. Intradialytic oral nutrition improves protein homeostasis in chronic hemodialysis patients with deranged nutritional status. J Am Soc Nephrol 2006;17:3149—57.

[241] Stratton RJ, Bircher G, Fouque D, et al. Multinutrient oral supplements and tube feeding in maintenance dialysis: a systematic review and meta-analysis. Am J Kidney Dis 2005; 46:387—405.

[242] Czekalski S, Hozejowski R. Intradialytic amino acids supplementation in hemodialysis patients with malnutrition: results of a multicenter cohort study. J Ren Nutr 2004;14:82—8.

[243] Koretz RL. Does nutritional intervention in protein-energy malnutrition improve morbidity or mortality? J Ren Nutr 1999;9:119—21.

[244] Kuhlmann MK, Schmidt F, Kohler H. High protein/energy vs. standard protein/energy nutritional regimen in the treatment of malnourished hemodialysis patients. Miner Electrolyte Metab 1999;25:306—10.

[245] Leon JB, Majerle AD, Soinski JA, Kushner I, Ohri-Vachaspati P, Sehgal AR. Can a nutrition intervention improve albumin levels among hemodialysis patients? A pilot study. J Ren Nutr 2001; 11:9—15.

[246] Chertow GM, Ling J, Lew NL, Lazarus JM, Lowrie EG. The association of intradialytic parenteral nutrition administration with survival in hemodialysis patients. Am J Kidney Dis 1994;24:912—20.

[247] Capelli JP, Kushner H, Camiscioli TC, Chen SM, Torres MA. Effect of intradialytic parenteral nutrition on mortality rates in end-stage renal disease care. Am J Kidney Dis 1994;23:808—16.

[248] Siskind MS, Lien YH. Effect of intradialytic parenteral nutrition on quality of life in hemodialysis patients. Int J Artif Organs 1993;16:599—603.

[249] Pupim LB, Kent P, Hakim R. The potential of intradialytic parenteral nutrition: A review. Miner Electrolyte Metab 1999;25: 317—23.

[250] Foulks CJ. An evidence-based evaluation of intradialytic parenteral nutrition. Am J Kidney Dis 1999;33:186—92.

[251] Cano NJ, Fouque D, Roth H, et al. Intradialytic parenteral nutrition does not improve survival in malnourished hemodialysis patients: a 2-year multicenter, prospective, randomized study. J Am Soc Nephrol 2007;18:2583—91.

[252] Kopple JD. Nutritional status as a predictor of morbidity and mortality in maintenance dialysis patients. ASAIO J 1997;43: 246—50.

[253] Boccanfuso JA, Hutton M, McAllister B. The effects of megestrol acetate on nutritional parameters in a dialysis population. J Ren Nutr 2000;10:36—43.

[254] Semeniuk J, Shalansky KF, Taylor N, Jastrzebski J, Cameron EC. Evaluation of the effect of intravenous l-carnitine on quality of life in chronic hemodialysis patients. Clin Nephrol 2000;54: 470—7.

[255] Feldt-Rasmussen B, Lange M, Sulowicz W, et al. Growth hormone treatment during hemodialysis in a randomized trial improves nutrition, quality of life, and cardiovascular risk. J Am Soc Nephrol 2007;18:2161—71.

[256] Iglesias P, Diez JJ, Fernandez-Reyes MJ, et al. Recombinant human growth hormone therapy in malnourished dialysis patients: a randomized controlled study. Am J Kidney Dis 1998;32:454—63.

[257] Johannsson G, Bengtsson BA, Ahlmen J. Double-blind, placebo-controlled study of growth hormone treatment in elderly patients undergoing chronic hemodialysis: anabolic effect and functional improvement. Am J Kidney Dis 1999;33:709—17.

[258] Fouque D, Peng SC, Shamir E, Kopple JD. Recombinant human insulin-like growth factor-1 induces an anabolic response in malnourished CAPD patients. Kidney Int 2000;57:646—54.

[259] Johansen KL, Mulligan K, Schambelan M. Anabolic effects of nandrolone decanoate in patients receiving dialysis: a randomized controlled trial. JAMA 1999;281:1275—81.

[260] Barton PA, Chretien C, Lau AH. The effects of nandrolone decanoate on nutritional parameters in hemodialysis patients. Clin Nephrol 2002;58:38—46.

[261] Navarro JF, Mora C, Macia M, Garcia J. Randomized prospective comparison between erythropoietin and androgens in CAPD patients. Kidney Int 2002;61:1537—44.

[262] Galland R, Traeger J, Arkouche W, Cleaud C, Delawari E, Fouque D. Short daily hemodialysis rapidly improves nutritional status in hemodialysis patients. Kidney Int 2001;60: 1555—60.

[263] Galland R, Traeger J, Arkouche W, Delawari E, Fouque D. Short daily hemodialysis and nutritional status. Am J Kidney Dis 2001;37:S95—8.

[264] Bossola M, Muscaritoli M, Tazza L, et al. Malnutrition in hemodialysis patients: what therapy? Am J Kidney Dis 2005;46: 371—86.

[265] Lambert CP, Sullivan DH, Evans WJ. Effects of testosterone replacement and/or resistance training on interleukin-6, tumor necrosis factor alpha, and leptin in elderly men ingesting megestrol acetate: a randomized controlled trial. J Gerontol A Biol Sci Med Sci 2003;58:165—70.

[266] Mantovani G, Maccio A, Lai P, Massa E, Ghiani M, Santona MC. Cytokine involvement in cancer anorexia/cachexia: role of megestrol acetate and medroxyprogesterone acetate on cytokine downregulation and improvement of clinical symptoms. Crit Rev Oncog 1998;9:99—106.

[267] Mantovani G. Does megestrol acetate down-regulate interleukin-6 in patients? Support Care Cancer 2002;10:566—7.

[268] Yeh SS, Wu SY, Levine DM, et al. The correlation of cytokine levels with body weight after megestrol acetate treatment in geriatric patients. J Gerontol A Biol Sci Med Sci 2001;56: M48—54.

[269] Boccanfuso JA, Hutton M, McAllister B. The effects of megestrol acetate on nutritional parameters in a dialysis population. J Ren Nutr 2000;10:36—43.

[270] Burrowes JD, Bluestone PA, Wang J, Pierson Jr RN. The effects of moderate doses of megestrol acetate on nutritional status and body composition in a hemodialysis patient. J Ren Nutr 1999;9:89—94.

[271] Rammohan M, Kalantar-Zadeh K, Liang A, Ghossein C. Megestrol acetate in a moderate dose for the treatment of malnutrition-inflammation complex in maintenance dialysis patients. J Ren Nutr 2005;15:345—55.

[272] King AJ, Levey AS. Dietary protein and renal function. J Am Soc Nephrol 1993;3:1723—37.

[273] Wasserstein AG. Changing patterns of medical practice: protein restriction for chronic renal failure. Ann Intern Med 1993;119:79—85.

[274] de Jong PE, Anderson S, de ZD. Glomerular preload and afterload reduction as a tool to lower urinary protein leakage: will such treatments also help to improve renal function outcome? J Am Soc Nephrol 1993;3:1333—41.

[275] D'Apolito M, Du X, Zong H, et al. Urea-induced ROS generation causes insulin resistance in mice with chronic renal failure. J Clin Invest 2010;120:203—13.

[276] Menon V, Kopple JD, Wang X, et al. Effect of a very low-protein diet on outcomes: long-term follow-up of the Modification of Diet in Renal Disease (MDRD) Study. Am J Kidney Dis 2009;53:208—17.

[277] Kasiske BL, Lakatua JD, Ma JZ, Louis TA. A meta-analysis of the effects of dietary protein restriction on the rate of decline in renal function. Am J Kidney Dis 1998;31:954—61.

[278] Fouque D, Laville M. Low protein diets for chronic kidney disease in non diabetic adults. Cochrane Database Syst Rev 2009; CD001892.

[279] Chauveau P, Combe C, Rigalleau V, Vendrely B, Aparicio M. Restricted protein diet is associated with decrease in proteinuria: consequences on the progression of renal failure. J Ren Nutr 2007;17:250—7.

[280] Chang JH, Kim DK, Park JT, et al. Influence of ketoanalogs supplementation on the progression in chronic kidney disease patients who had training on low-protein diet. Nephrology Carlton 2009;14:750—7.

[281] Teplan V, Schuck O, Knotek A, et al. Effects of low-protein diet supplemented with ketoacids and erythropoietin in chronic renal failure: a long-term metabolic study. Ann Transplant 2001;6:47—53.

[282] Zakar G. The effect of a keto acid supplement on the course of chronic renal failure and nutritional parameters in predialysis patients and patients on regular hemodialysis therapy: the Hungarian Ketosteril Cohort Study. Wien Klin Wochenschr 2001;113:688—94.

[283] Prakash S, Pande DP, Sharma S, Sharma D, Bal CS, Kulkarni H. Randomized, double-blind, placebo-controlled trial to evaluate efficacy of ketodiet in predialytic chronic renal failure. J Ren Nutr 2004;14:89—96.

[284] Klahr S, Levey AS, Beck GJ, et al. The effects of dietary protein restriction and blood-pressure control on the progression of chronic renal disease. Modification of Diet in Renal Disease Study Group. N Engl J Med 1994;330:877—84.

[285] Chauveau P, Barthe N, Rigalleau V, et al. Outcome of nutritional status and body composition of uremic patients on a very low protein diet. Am J Kidney Dis 1999;34:500—7.

[286] Aparicio M, Chauveau P, De PV, Bouchet JL, Lasseur C, et al. Nutrition and outcome on renal replacement therapy of patients with chronic renal failure treated by a supplemented very low protein diet. J Am Soc Nephrol 2000;11:708—16.

[287] Di Iorio BR, Cucciniello E, Martino R, Frallicciardi A, Tortoriello R, Struzziero G. [Acute and persistent antiproteinuric effect of a low-protein diet in chronic kidney disease]. G Ital Nefrol 2009;26:608—15.

[288] Jiang N, Qian J, Sun W, et al. Better preservation of residual renal function in peritoneal dialysis patients treated with a low-protein diet supplemented with keto acids: a prospective, randomized trial. Nephrol Dial Transplant 2009;24:2551—8.

[289] Brunori G, Viola BF, Parrinello G, et al. Efficacy and safety of a very-low-protein diet when postponing dialysis in the elderly: a prospective randomized multicenter controlled study. Am J Kidney Dis 2007;49:569—80.

[290] Barreto FC, Barreto DV, Liabeuf S, et al. Serum indoxyl sulfate is associated with vascular disease and mortality in chronic kidney disease patients. Clin J Am Soc Nephrol 2009;4:1551—8.

[291] Schwedler SB, Metzger T, Schinzel R, Wanner C. Advanced glycation end products and mortality in hemodialysis patients. Kidney Int 2002;62:301—10.

[292] Roberts MA, Thomas MC, Fernando D, Macmillan N, Power DA, Ierino FL. Low molecular weight advanced glycation end products predict mortality in asymptomatic patients receiving chronic haemodialysis. Nephrol Dial Transplant 2006;21:1611—7.

[293] Liabeuf S, Barreto DV, Barreto FC, et al. Free p-cresylsulphate is a predictor of mortality in patients at different stages of chronic kidney disease. Nephrol Dial Transplant 2010;25:1183—91.

[294] Bammens B, Evenepoel P, Keuleers H, Verbeke K, Vanrenterghem Y. Free serum concentrations of the protein-bound retention solute p-cresol predict mortality in hemodialysis patients. Kidney Int 2006;69:1081—7.

[295] Barsotti G, Morelli E, Giannoni A, Guiducci A, Lupetti S, Giovannetti S. Restricted phosphorus and nitrogen intake to slow the progression of chronic renal failure: a controlled trial. Kidney Int Suppl 1983;16:S278—84.

[296] Maschio G, Oldrizzi L, Tessitore N, et al. Effects of dietary protein and phosphorus restriction on the progression of early renal failure. Kidney Int 1982;22:371—6.

[297] Ibels LS, Alfrey AC, Haut L, Huffer WE. Preservation of function in experimental renal disease by dietary restriction of phosphate. N Engl J Med 1978;298:122—6.

[298] Karlinsky ML, Haut L, Buddington B, Schrier NA, Alfrey AC. Preservation of renal function in experimental glomerulonephritis. Kidney Int 1980;17:293—302.

[299] Lumlertgul D, Burke TJ, Gillum DM, et al. Phosphate depletion arrests progression of chronic renal failure independent of protein intake. Kidney Int 1986;29:658—66.

[300] Konishi K, Nakano S, Tsuda S, Nakagawa A, Kigoshi T, Koya D. AST-120 Kremezi-initiated in early stage chronic kidney disease stunts the progression of renal dysfunction in type 2 diabetic subjects. Diabetes Res Clin Pract 2008;81:310—5.

[301] Nakamura T, Kawagoe Y, Matsuda T, et al. Oral ADSORBENT AST-120 decreases carotid intima-media thickness and arterial stiffness in patients with chronic renal failure. Kidney Blood Press Res 2004;27:121—6.

[302] Niwa T, Nomura T, Sugiyama S, Miyazaki T, Tsukushi S, Tsutsui S. The protein metabolite hypothesis, a model for the progression of renal failure: an oral adsorbent lowers indoxyl sulfate levels in undialyzed uremic patients. Kidney Int Suppl 1997;62:S23—8.

[303] Owada A, Shiigai T. Effects of oral adsorbent AST-120 concurrent with a low-protein diet on the progression of chronic renal failure. Am J Nephrol 1996;16:124—7.

[304] Shoji T, Wada A, Inoue K, et al. Prospective randomized study evaluating the efficacy of the spherical adsorptive carbon AST-120 in chronic kidney disease patients with moderate decrease in renal function. Nephron Clin Pract 2007;105:c99—107.

[305] Yorioka N, Ito T, Masaki T, et al. Dose-dependent effect of an oral adsorbent, AST-120, in patients with early chronic renal failure. J Int Med Res 2002;30:467—75.

[306] Kopple JD. McCollum Award Lecture, 1996: protein-energy malnutrition in maintenance dialysis patients. Am J Clin Nutr 1997;65:1544—57.

[307] Chinen J, Shearer WT. Secondary immunodeficiencies, including HIV infection. J Allergy Clin Immunol 2008;121:S388—92.

[308] Kalantar-Zadeh K, Kopple J. Malnutrition as a cause of morbidity and mortality in dialysis patients. In: Kopple J, Massry S, editors. Nutritional management of renal disease. 2nd ed. Philadelphia: Lipincott: Williams & Wilkins; 2004.

[309] Vanholder R, Dell'Aquila R, Jacobs V, et al. Depressed phagocytosis in hemodialyzed patients: in vivo and in vitro mechanisms. Nephron 1993;63:409—15.

[310] Vanholder R, Van LA, Dhondt AM, De SR, Ringoir S. Influence of uraemia and haemodialysis on host defence and infection. Nephrol Dial Transplant 1996;11:593—8.

[311] Kalantar-Zadeh K, Daar ES, Eysselein VE, Miller LG. Hepatitis C infection in dialysis patients: a link to poor clinical outcome? Int Urol Nephrol 2007;39:247—59.

[312] Kalantar-Zadeh K, Kilpatrick RD, McAllister CJ, et al. Hepatitis C virus and death risk in hemodialysis patients. J Am Soc Nephrol 2007;18:1584—93.

[313] Ritz E. Why are lipids not predictive of cardiovascular death in the dialysis patient? Miner Electrolyte Metab 1996;22:9—12.

[314] Argiles JM. Cancer-associated malnutrition. Eur J Oncol Nurs 2005;9(Suppl. 2):S39—50.

[315] Lee PS, Waxman AB, Cotich KL, Chung SW, Perrella MA, Stossel TP. Plasma gelsolin is a marker and therapeutic agent in animal sepsis. Crit Care Med 2007;35:849—55.

[316] Rothenbach PA, Dahl B, Schwartz JJ, et al. Recombinant plasma gelsolin infusion attenuates burn-induced pulmonary microvascular dysfunction. J Appl Physiol 2004;96:25—31.

[317] Christofidou-Solomidou M, Scherpereel A, Solomides CC, et al. Recombinant plasma gelsolin diminishes the acute inflammatory response to hyperoxia in mice. J Investig Med 2002;50: 54—60.

[318] Lee PS, Sampath K, Karumanchi SA, et al. Plasma gelsolin and circulating actin correlate with hemodialysis mortality. J Am Soc Nephrol 2009;20:1140—8.

[319] Kaysen GA. Inflammation nutritional state and outcome in end-stage renal disease. Miner Electrolyte Metab 1999;25:242—50.

[320] Bergstrom J, Lindholm B, Lacson Jr E, et al. What are the causes and consequences of the chronic inflammatory state in chronic dialysis patients? Semin Dial 2000;13:163—75.

[321] Menon V, Wang X, Greene T, et al. Relationship between C-reactive protein, albumin, and cardiovascular disease in patients with chronic kidney disease. Am J Kidney Dis 2003;42:44—52.

[322] Ross R. Atherosclerosis — an inflammatory disease. N Engl J Med 1999;340:115—26.

[323] Ling PR, Smith RJ, Kie S, Boyce P, Bistrian BR. Effects of protein malnutrition on IL-6-mediated signaling in the liver and the systemic acute-phase response in rats. Am J Physiol Regul Integr Comp Physiol 2004;287:R801—8.

[324] Ziegler TR, Evans ME, Fernandez-Estivariz C, Jones DP. Trophic and cytoprotective nutrition for intestinal adaptation, mucosal repair, and barrier function. Annu Rev Nutr 2003;23:229—61.

[325] Jandacek RJ, Anderson N, Liu M, Zheng S, Yang Q, Tso P. Effects of yo-yo diet, caloric restriction, and olestra on tissue distribution of hexachlorobenzene. Am J Physiol Gastrointest Liver Physiol 2005;288:G292—9.

[326] Mohamed-Ali V, Goodrick S, Bulmer K, Holly JM, Yudkin JS, Coppack SW. Production of soluble tumor necrosis factor receptors by human subcutaneous adipose tissue in vivo. Am J Physiol 1999;277:E971—5.

[327] Rauchhaus M, Coats AJ, Anker SD. The endotoxin-lipoprotein hypothesis. Lancet 2000;356:930—3.

[328] Kalantar-Zadeh K, Kopple JD, Kamranpour N, Fogelman AM, Navab M. HDL-inflammatory index correlates with poor outcome in hemodialysis patients. Kidney Int 2007;72:1149—56.

[329] Kovesdy CP, Kalantar-Zadeh K. Vitamin D receptor activation and survival in chronic kidney disease. Kidney Int 2008;73:1355—63.

[330] Hampl H, Kovesdy CP, Kalantar-Zadeh K. Darbepoetin alfa and chronic kidney disease. N Engl J Med 2010;362:654.

[331] Kalantar-Zadeh K, Brennan ML, Hazen SL. Serum myeloperoxidase and mortality in maintenance hemodialysis patients. Am J Kidney Dis 2006;48:59—68.

[332] Streja E, Kovesdy CP, Greenland S, et al. Erythropoietin, iron depletion, and relative thrombocytosis: a possible explanation for hemoglobin-survival paradox in hemodialysis. Am J Kidney Dis 2008;52:727—36.

[333] Molnar MZ, Streja E, Kovesdy CP, et al. High platelet count as a link between renal cachexia and cardiovascular mortality in end-stage renal disease patients. Am J Clin Nutr 2011;94: 945—54.

[334] Hakim RM. Proposed clinical trials in the evaluation of intradialytic parenteral nutrition. Am J Kidney Dis 1999;33: 217—20.

[335] Maiorca R, Cancarini GC, Brunori G, et al. Comparison of long-term survival between hemodialysis and peritoneal dialysis. Adv Perit Dial 1996;12:79—88.

[336] Genestier S, Hedelin G, Schaffer P, Faller B. Prognostic factors in CAPD patients: a retrospective study of a 10-year period. Nephrol Dial Transplant 1995;10:1905—11.

[337] Germain M, Harlow P, Mulhern J, Lipkowitz G, Braden G. Low protein catabolic rate and serum albumin correlate with increased mortality and abdominal complications in peritoneal dialysis patients. Adv Perit Dial 1992;8:113—5.

[338] Harter HR, Laird NM, Teehan BP. Effects of dialysis prescription on bone and mineral metabolism: the National Cooperative Dialysis Study. Kidney Int Suppl 1983:S73—9.

[339] Lowrie EG, Laird NM, Parker TF, Sargent JA. Effect of the hemodialysis prescription of patient morbidity: report from the National Cooperative Dialysis Study. N Engl J Med 1981;305: 1176—81.

[340] Parker TF, Laird NM, Lowrie EG. Comparison of the study groups in the National Cooperative Dialysis Study and a description of morbidity, mortality, and patient withdrawal. Kidney Int Suppl 1983:S42—9.

[341] Fleischmann E, Teal N, Dudley J, May W, Bower JD, Salahudeen AK. Influence of excess weight on mortality and hospital stay in 1346 hemodialysis patients. Kidney Int 1999;55:1560—7.

[342] Arora P, Strauss BJ, Borovnicar D, Stroud D, Atkins RC, Kerr PG. Total body nitrogen predicts long-term mortality in haemodialysis patients — a single-centre experience. Nephrol Dial Transplant 1998;13:1731—6.

[343] Pollock CA, Ibels LS, Allen BJ, et al. Total body nitrogen as a prognostic marker in maintenance dialysis. J Am Soc Nephrol 1995;6:82—8.

[344] Avram MM, Goldwasser P, Erroa M, Fein PA. Predictors of survival in continuous ambulatory peritoneal dialysis patients: the importance of prealbumin and other nutritional and metabolic markers. Am J Kidney Dis 1994;23:91—8.

[345] Blake PG, Flowerdew G, Blake RM, Oreopoulos DG. Serum albumin in patients on continuous ambulatory peritoneal dialysis — predictors and correlations with outcomes. J Am Soc Nephrol 1993;3:1501—7.

[346] Collins AJ, Ma JZ, Umen A, Keshaviah P. Urea index and other predictors of hemodialysis patient survival. Am J Kidney Dis 1994;23:272—82.

[347] Maiorca R, Cancarini GC, Brunori G, et al. Comparison of long-term survival between hemodialysis and peritoneal dialysis. Adv Perit Dial 1996;12:79—88.

[348] Churchill DN, Taylor DW, Cook RJ, et al. Canadian Hemodialysis Morbidity Study. Am J Kidney Dis 1992;19:214—34.

[349] Spiegel DM, Anderson M, Campbell U, et al. Serum albumin: a marker for morbidity in peritoneal dialysis patients. Am J Kidney Dis 1993;21:26—30.

[350] Merkus MP, Jager KJ, Dekker FW, de Haan RJ, Boeschoten EW, Krediet RT. Predictors of poor outcome in chronic dialysis patients: The Netherlands Cooperative Study on the Adequacy of Dialysis. The NECOSAD Study Group. Am J Kidney Dis 2000;35:69—79.

Effect of Nutritional Status and Changes in Protein Intake on Renal Function*

Daniel Landau[1], Ralph Rabkin[2,3]

[1]Department of Pediatrics, Soroka Medical Center, Ben Gurion University, Beer Sheva, Israel
[2]Department Medicine/Nephrology, Stanford University, Stanford, CA, USA
[3]Research Service, Veterans Affairs Palo Alto Health Care System, Palo Alto, CA, USA

INTRODUCTION

Nutrition has a significant impact on renal function and especially important is the dietary intake of protein for this component has a significant modulating effect on renal hemodynamics [1–3]. Furthermore as discussed in Chapter 14, dietary protein influences the progression of kidney disease in animals and may also do so in humans. In several species a sustained change from a low to a high-protein diet causes a decrease in renal vascular resistance, an increase in renal blood flow (RBF) and glomerular filtration rate (GFR) by 30% to 60% [4–8] and may even cause an increase in kidney size [9]. Acute oral administration of a protein load also increases RBF and GFR by similar amounts for several hours [10–13]. In normal subjects the response to animal and vegetable proteins differ; animal proteins especially red meat, increase renal hemodynamics while vegetable proteins do not appear to do so [14]. Vegetarians have a lower GFR than meat eaters [22]. Changes in renal hemodynamics are not observed after ingestion of carbohydrates or fats, suggesting that this hemodynamic response is unique to protein [4]. Mixtures of amino acids (AA) or individual AA by enteral [15] or intravenous [16–19] route mimics the response to protein with respect to RBF and GFR. In animals infused with AA single-nephron plasma flow and intra-glomerular pressure rise and transcapillary hydraulic pressure difference increases, thereby raising single nephron GFR without altering the ultrafiltration coefficient [18]. Other protein components including urea, sulfate or acid do not reproduce a meat protein-induced rise in GFR [20–22] and excretion of sodium, potassium, phosphorus, and urea increase in parallel to the increase in GFR [10].

In the USA daily protein intake averages 1.2 g/kg body weight and comprises ~15% of daily caloric intake. While far exceeding the daily protein allowance of 0.8 g/Kg (10% of energy) recommended by the Institute of Medicine [23], it is within the Institute's acceptable macronutrient distribution range of 10–35%. This upper range for protein of 35% was selected to complement the ranges for fat and carbohydrates as there was insufficient data to suggest an upper range for protein in normals. Relatively high protein (28–64% of energy) low carbohydrate diets are nowadays popular amongst overweight and obese individuals and induce weight loss by increasing fat breakdown and decreasing calorie intake, in part by suppressing appetite [24,25]. The contribution of a high protein diet to glomerular hyperfiltration seen in obese individuals was recently examined [26]. It was noted that while a high protein intake did modestly affect kidney function in obese subjects, it appears to be insufficient to fully account for their elevated GFR. High protein diets are also popular amongst athletes especially weight lifters and many consume more than 2 g/kg/day [27]. Because of the profound hemodynamic changes induced by a high protein diet and as preclinical studies in rodents have shown that a continuous high protein intake worsens kidney disease, there has been concern that a high protein intake in humans may accelerate progression of established disease and might even damage normal

---

*This chapter is based on the late Saulo Klahr's review from previous edition.

kidneys [24,27,28]. While a theoretical risk of renal damage to normal subjects does exist, there is no clear evidence to support this thesis [29,30]. There are also theoretical concerns that high protein diets could lead to nephrolithiasis because of the increase in acid load demineralization of bone [31]. On the other hand there is more support for a Western-style diet as a major risk factor for developing new onset kidney damage rather than protein alone [32,33]. The Western diet comprises highly processed and refined foods high in fat, salt, carbohydrates and red meat protein. As such it favors the development of obesity, type 2 diabetes, hypertension and cardiovascular disease, and it is associated with an increase in the incidence of chronic kidney disease [34,35].

ROLE OF SPECIFIC AA

As noted above mixtures of AA increase renal hemodynamics as seen after a protein meal, but it turns out that while many individual AA exhibit this property, not all AA do so [36]. When normal conscious dogs were given individual AA including glycine, alanine, threonine, proline, glutamic acid, aspartic acid and valine by stomach tube GFR increased. However there was no increase in GFR following cysteine or serine. Glycine is also effective in dogs when given intravenously [37]. In humans an intravenous infusion of a mixture of glucogenic AA (arginine, glycine, proline, cystine, methionine and serine) increased GFR and RPF, but neither alanine nor a mixture of branched chain AA caused a consistent alteration in renal hemodynamics [38,39]. The explanation for the failure of branched chain AA to influence renal hemodynamics is unclear and several mechanisms have been proposed. These include absence of glucagon secretion, escape from splanchnic metabolism, and differences in activation of the renin-angiotensin system and differences in renal metabolic utilization. In rats arginine infusions alone increased systemic and renal vasodilatation with an increase in RBF and GFR [40] and also does so in humans [41]. This has led to arginine infusions being used to measure renal functional reserve. The hemodynamic action of arginine is thought to be mediated through the release of nitric oxide (NO) since arginine is a substrate for NO, and its production increases during arginine infusions. Insulin also plays a permissive role in arginine's action probably by promoting renal cellular uptake of arginine [40]. In humans when arginine is infused intravenously in high doses, urinary excretion of albumin, light chains, and beta2-microglobulin increases significantly [41,42]. This appears to reflect tubular dysfunction with impaired absorption of these proteins. Other cationic AA namely lysine and ornithine also cause tubular dysfunction with lysine being particularly toxic [43].

FACTORS MEDIATING THE RENAL RESPONSE TO PROTEIN AND AMINO ACIDS

Several mechanisms have been proposed to explain the increase in RBF and GFR observed after a protein meal, during chronic protein intake or following AA loads, but the true mechanisms remain to be established. A number of potential mediators, humoral and/or local, are released in response to increased plasma AA levels and subsequently stimulate renal vasodilation. Increased protein intake stimulates secretion of growth hormone (GH), insulin-like growth factor 1 (IGF-1), glucagon, dopamine, eicosanoids, NO and renin. A role for AA as metabolic substrates or as regulators of mRNA translation in causing these endocrine changes has been suggested. The renal hemodynamic response to protein intake is also mediated by intrinsic renal processes including tubuloglomerular feedback and tubular transport.

HUMORAL MEDIATORS

Growth Hormone, IGF-1 and Glucagon

Growth hormone, IGF-1 and glucagon have been implicated in the renal vasodilation that follows a protein load [44–46]. Blood levels increase after a protein load and following their parenteral administration, RBF and GFR increase [44,47–49]. However, the role of GH in this phenomenon is questionable because RBF and GFR increase after a meat meal [11] or AA infusion [50] well before GH levels rise. Also, RPF and GFR may rise in the absence of increased levels of GH [51]. Additionally, GH deficient patients exhibit renal vasodilation after an AA infusion [50,52]. Furthermore the renal action of GH is delayed many hours and first requires stimulation of IGF-1 production that in turn mediates most of the actions of GH. In rats fed a low or high protein diet for 11 days RBF and GFR were higher in the high protein fed rats. Since serum, hepatic and glomerular IGF-1 levels were increased in the latter group it was suggested that the increase in IGF-1 might be a cause of the hyperfiltration [53]. Thus it is conceivable that GH and IGF-1 are involved in the renal response to long-term high protein intake, especially as IGF-1 expression is regulated by nutrients [49].

Glucagon release may also play a role in the increase in RBF and GFR after a protein meal. Following such a meal glucagon levels rise in parallel to the increase in GFR and effective RPF [7,46,54]. In contrast, a carbohydrate meal does not cause an increase in plasma glucagon, nor renal hemodynamics [7]. Infusion of a balanced mixture of AA also increases RBF and GFR and plasma glucagon levels [46] while a complete branched-chain AA mixture does not [39,54]. Furthermore, infusion of glucagon in humans to achieve plasma levels comparable to those obtained during arginine infusion also increases GFR and RPF [55]. However, there are contradictory results that do not support a role of glucagon [44,56,57] and those studies suggest that an increase in plasma glucagon is not needed for protein or AA-stimulated renal vasodilation and hyperfiltration [6,58,59]. Thus taken together it is possible that a combination of increased AA and increased glucagon is necessary for the hemodynamic response. Glucagon also increases sodium excretion. However, this action may be indirect because infusion of glucagon into the renal artery does not produce natriuresis. Glucagon increases circulating cyclic adenosine monophosphate (cAMP), which may in turn decrease tubular sodium absorption.

Renin-Angiotensin System

The renin-angiotensin system may regulate protein or AA-induced renal vasodilation and increases in GFR. The role played by the renin-angiotensin system may be more important during long-term changes in protein intake than with the acute administration of protein. Most studies indicate that plasma renin activity and Angiotensin II concentration do not increase during acute infusion of AA or following a meat meal [51,60,61]. Several investigators have examined the effects of ACE inhibitors on the renal hemodynamic responses to protein feeding or AA infusion. Woods et al. [2] found that infusion of captopril to dogs did not modify the increase in RPF and GFR observed after a meat meal. The same was the case in humans [62]. However, with long-term increases in dietary protein, synthesis and release of renin is augmented [63]. Renal renin messenger RNA (mRNA) was higher in rats fed a high protein diet (50% protein) than in rats fed a standard rat chow (24% protein). A lower protein intake (6% protein) decreased the activity of renal renin mRNA in rats [56]. Studies in rats infused with glycine or arginine support a role for angiotensin II in modulating the renal response to AA in conjunction with the vasodilator NO [40,64]. It appears that angiotensin II has an inhibitory effect on the action of NO released in response to AA and may do so by an inhibitory effect on proximal tubular reabsorption and activation of tubuloglomerular feedback [83]. This sequence of events is modulated by insulin which promotes AA uptake [40].

Dopamine

Because dopamine increases RPF and GFR, as well as solute excretion, intrarenal dopamine was suggested as the mediator of several renal effects of protein or AA administration [65]. A protein load increased dopamine levels in plasma (when carbidopa, a dopamine decarboxylase inhibitor, was present) and caused natriuresis and increased osmolal clearance [58]. Without carbidopa, plasma dopamine did not increase, but dopamine excretion promptly increased. Studies in humans and rats utilizing receptor antagonists have implicated the dopamine D2-like receptors but not the D1-like receptors, in the renal hemodynamic response to AA [66]. Also in a study with dopamine D3 knockout mice Luippold et al. were able to attribute this effect to the dopamine D3 receptor subtype, a member of the D2 subclass [67].

Atrial Peptides

Administration of atrial natriuretic peptide (ANP) increases GFR, but it probably does not mediate the renal hemodynamic changes observed after a meat meal or AA loading because ANP in animals increases GFR to a greater extent than RPF [68], a pattern somewhat different from that after a meat meal. Secondly there is no significant relationship between post protein meal ANP levels and the increase in renal hemodynamics [69—72].

LOCAL MEDIATORS

Eicosanoids

Protein intake conditions eicosanoid synthesis in isolated rat glomeruli [73,74]. Glomeruli from rats fed a high-protein diet produced significantly greater amounts of PGE2, 6-keto PGE1α, and thromboxane A2 under basal conditions than glomeruli from rats fed a low-protein diet. To investigate the potential role of the renin-angiotensin system in the protein-induced modulation of glomerular eicosanoid production, rats ingesting either a high-or low-protein diet were randomized to receiving an ACE inhibitor (enalapril) or no therapy. Enalapril attenuated protein-induced augmentation in glomerular eicosanoid production. This effect occurred only when enalapril was administered in vivo. The active metabolite enalaprilat did not alter PGE2 production by isolated glomeruli when added in vitro. Thus, dietary protein modulates glomerular eicosanoid synthesis in the rat, and this effect seems to be mediated by the renin-angiotensin system. Yanagisawa et al. [74] also found that addition of angiotensin II to isolated glomeruli in vitro increased eicosanoid synthesis. The increment was greater in glomeruli obtained from high-protein fed rats than in glomeruli from low-protein fed rats.

To examine the potential mechanisms by which changes in protein intake may modify eicosanoid synthesis, the activities of phospholipase A2 and phospholipase C were determined [74]. There was a significant increase in phosphatidyl ethanolamine-specific phospholipase A2 activity in glomeruli from high-protein fed rats compared with glomeruli from low-protein fed rats. In contrast, phosphatidyl specific phospholipase A2 activity was decreased significantly in glomeruli from high-protein fed rats. No significant changes in phosphatidyl inositol biphosphate (PIP2) and phospholipase C activities were detected between glomeruli of the two dietary groups. The content and activity of cyclooxygenase was significantly greater in glomeruli from high-protein fed rats than in glomeruli from low-protein fed. These studies indicate that the greater synthesis of eicosanoids in glomeruli isolated from high-protein fed rats may be mediated by increases in the amount and activity of cyclooxygenase coupled with enhanced activity of phosphoethanolamine-specific phospholipase A2. The greater release of arachidonic acid, as a result of enhanced activity of phosphoethanol-amine-specific phospholipase A2 and the increased activity of cyclooxygenase, would result in increased eicosanoid synthesis. In high-protein fed rats, inhibition of angiotensin II synthesis using an ACE inhibitor prevented the increases in activities of phospholipase A2 and cyclooxygenase observed in untreated rats. This suggests that sustained increased protein intake augments renin-angiotensin production. The increased activity of angiotensin II, in turn, conditions production of eicosanoids. Vasodilatory eicosanoids (PGE2, prostacyclin) may account for the increase in RPF and GFR observed after protein administration. Finally there is evidence that eicosanoid production is selectively enhanced in medullary but not cortical tubules, isolated from high protein fed rats. This probably occurs via activation of the PLA2-COX pathway [75].

Nitric Oxide

Many dietary factors, including protein and AA modulate nitric oxide (NO) production by inducible NO synthases or constitutive NO synthases [76]. NO plays an important regulator of systemic and renal hemodynamics, tubuloglomerular feedback, pressure natriuresis, sympathetic neurotransmitter and renin secretion, and tubular solute and water transport [77,78]. Inhibitors of L-arginine metabolism and other inhibitors of NO synthesis prevent or at least blunt

AA-stimulated renal vasodilation and the increase in GFR in rats and dogs [79–82]. Furthermore arginine, the substrate for NO production, causes an increase in GFR that correlates with an increase in urinary NO metabolites [40]. However arginine is not solely responsible for the vasodilation of AA mixtures; AA mixtures without arginine produce vasodilation and as discussed earlier, several AA alone such as glycine causes an increase in RBF and GFR [83].

INTRINSIC RENAL MECHANISMS

The third potential process involved in protein or AA-stimulated renal vasodilation is the action of intrinsic renal mechanisms including tubuloglomerular feedback and tubular transport. The kidney has a large vascular bed, and the tone of the glomerular afferent and efferent arterioles is determined not only by circulating and locally produced factors but also by specific intrarenal mechanisms such as the tubuloglomerular feedback system [40]. This system couples changes in tubular reabsorption to changes in glomerular resistances, RBF, and GFR to maintain glomerulotubular balance. In animals infused with AA single-nephron plasma flow and intra-glomerular pressure rises secondary to afferent and efferent vessel dilatation and the transcapillary hydraulic pressure difference increases, thereby raising single nephron GFR without altering the ultrafiltration coefficient and filtration fraction remains constant [18]. Absolute proximal tubular absorption increases parallel to the increase in single nephron GFR and glomerular tubular balance is maintained. Tubuloglomerular balance was studied in rats fed iso-caloric diets containing 6% or 40% casein for 10 days prior to study [84]. Rats fed the 40% casein diet required a greater tubular flow rate to initiate a decrease in single nephron GFR. A 40% to 50% decreased sensitivity of the tubuloglomerular feedback mechanism was observed, which led to the conclusion that a high-protein diet causes a failure of the normal mechanisms controlling GFR. This response may be related to a complex interplay among several hormonal systems including angiotensin or changes in vascular response to hormone action or to increased reabsorption of sodium and chloride by the thick ascending limb of the loop of Henle. The increased reabsorption of sodium chloride may be the result of marked hypertrophy of the thick ascending limb of Henle observed in rats fed a high-protein diet [85].

In summary, the mechanisms underlying the variable increase in GFR in response to an acute protein load are not well characterized. The increase in GFR may be conditioned by the previous level of dietary protein intake, protein source, other dietary components, volume status, any renal disease that may be present, activity of the renin-angiotensin system, and production of renal eicosanoids and NO. In contrast to the variable and transient response of GFR to short-term protein loads, more long-term changes in protein intake apparently affect the level of GFR in a more sustained fashion. How this change in GFR relates to the progression of renal insufficiency in humans has not been truly defined.

EFFECTS OF NUTRITIONAL STATUS OR PROTEIN DEPRIVATION ON RENAL FUNCTION

A decrease in protein intake lowers GFR and RPF in normal subjects. Normal subjects fed a calorie-deficient diet, regardless of percent calories derived from fat, protein, or carbohydrates, demonstrate a reduction in creatinine clearance [86]. Also, normal subjects with decreased intake of protein compared to the same subjects during the ingestion of a "normal" protein intake demonstrated a fall GFR and effective RPF. Prolonged deprivation of calorie and protein intake may result in calorie protein malnutrition and changes in renal function [87]. Children with calorie-protein malnutrition demonstrated significant reductions in GFR, RPF and filtration fraction [88]. These changes in renal hemodynamics were not influenced by the presence or absence of edema. Following repletion and refeeding with protein, similar increases in

GFR and RPF were observed in children with or without edema. Several studies also have revealed decreases in GFR and RPF in adults with calorie-protein malnutrition. Such decreases could be reversed toward normal by protein repletion [87] (see Table 13.1). Besides affecting renal hemodynamics, energy-protein malnutrition results in changes in acid-base balance, the kidney's concentrating ability, and the kidney's ability to excrete sodium loads (Table 13.2).

LEVELS OF PLASMA CREATININE AND SERUM UREA NITROGEN IN PATIENTS WITH PROTEIN-ENERGY MALNUTRITION

A decrease in GFR usually is associated with increased plasma levels of creatinine and urea nitrogen. However when urea or creatinine production is decreased as occurs in protein calorie deprivation, even moderate to severe impairment of renal function may not result in increased plasma levels of these compounds. Indeed plasma urea nitrogen and creatinine levels may be low or normal [89]. The decrease in creatinine production is probably the result of a decrease in muscle mass and low urea levels presumably from decreased protein intake, slower tissue-protein breakdown, and/or possibly urea reutilization [90]. Conversely, during protein repletion both serum urea nitrogen and plasma creatinine increase despite an increase in GFR [89]. The increase in urea nitrogen and

TABLE 13.1 Glomerular Filtration Rate and Renal Plasma Flow in Malnourished Subjects

		Malnourished			Repleted or Normal			
Investigator	N	C_{IN} (mL/min)	C_{PAH} (mL/min)	FF	N	C_{IN} (mL/min)	C_{PAH} (mL/min)	FF
Alleyne (1967)	8 children	47.1	249.4	0.21	14 children	92.4	321.2	0.29
	7 children	42.9	184.0	0.27				
Arroyave et al. (1961)	9 children	13.7	–	–	9 children	33.9	–	–
					17 normal children	45.0		
Gordillo et al. (1957)	10 children	23.0	108.4		25 normal children	64.0	294	0.23
Klahr (1966)	10 adults	64.1	325.8	0.20	10 adults	88.3	381.1	0.24
McCance (1951)	11 adults	119.4	–			–		
	11 adults	100.9	–			–		
Mollison (1946)	2 adults[a]	53,70	230,383[b]			–		
	2 adults	124,141	340,710[b]					

[a]*Edema was present in these subjects at the time of study. Mean values are given in mL/min. The data for adults are corrected for 1.73 m^2. The data of Arroyave and Gordillo are expressed per (m^2). The data of Alleyne are corrected for height (m^3).*

[b]*Diodone clearances. From Klahr S, Alleyne GAO. Effect of chronic protein-calorie malnutrition on the kidney. Kidney Int 1973;3 :129–141, with permission.*

N: No. of subjects; CIN: clearance of inulin (mL/min); CPAH: clearance of P-aminohippurate (mL/min); FF, filtration fraction.

TABLE 13.2 Effects of Chronic Calorie-Protein Malnutrition on Renal Function

1. Decreased renal plasma flow and glomerular filtration rate
2. Impaired concentrating ability (polyuria) with normal diluting capacity
3. Impaired ability to excrete acid loads
   a. Normal ability to decrease urine pH
   b. Decreased titratable acid excretion
4. Impaired ability to excrete salt load.

creatinine levels presumably reflect an increased rate of entry of the end products of protein and creatine metabolism into body fluids exceeding their rate of excretion. Besides affecting renal hemodynamics, energy-protein malnutrition results in changes in acid-base balance, the kidney's concentrating ability, and the kidney's ability to excrete sodium loads.

CONCENTRATION AND DILUTION OF THE URINE IN PATIENTS WITH PROTEIN-ENERGY MALNUTRITION

Polyuria and nocturia are frequent complaints of malnourished patients. The capacity to concentrate the urine in these patients is diminished. However, the ability to excrete minimally dilute urine is not reduced. Klahr et al. [91] studied the ability of patients with chronic calorie-protein malnutrition to dilute and concentrate their urine. After 14 hours of fluid deprivation urine osmolality never exceeded 600 mOsm/kg water. Protein repletion resulted in a progressive increase in urine osmolality after 14 hours of fluid deprivation. Values for solute-free water reabsorption also were depressed in malnourished individuals given mannitol and vasopressin. However, the ability of malnourished individuals to produce a dilute urine was intact. During water loading, urine osmolality averaged 57 mOsm/L, a figure comparable to normal subjects. Values for free water clearance corrected per deciliter of GFR averaged 15.8 mL, a figure similar to that in normals.

The defect in urine concentration in malnourished subjects probably results from a decrease in renal medulla osmolality, most likely a consequence of low urea levels in this area of the kidney [91]. The concentrating defect resolves slowly during protein repletion, presumably because of a markedly positive nitrogen balance in the initial weeks of protein repletion. Urinary urea excretion does not rise considerably for several weeks after dietary protein intake is initiated. Thus, rapid restoration of the renal medullary gradient for urea would not be expected. However, oral administration of urea results rapidly increases the ability to

concentrate the urine after 14 hours of fluid deprivation in malnourished subjects [91]. The marked improvement in the concentrating ability during protein repletion and the dramatic change observed following urea administration suggests that a structural alteration does not account for the concentrating defect. Rather, a functional disorder seems likely. Impaired sodium reabsorption in the ascending loop of Henle may explain the concentrating defect; however, the finding of a normal capacity to dilute the urine would argue against this postulate. Most likely, a marked decrease in urea, as an osmolal particle in the renal medulla effective in promoting the reabsorption of water from the cortical and medullary collecting ducts, accounts for the concentrating defect in protein-energy malnutrition. An excellent correlation was found during protein repletion in patients with malnutrition between the values for urine osmolality and the concomitant 24-hour nitrogen excretion. These results support the suggestion that decreased renal medullary urea concentration accounts for the renal-concentrating defect of patients with chronic protein malnutrition.

The effects of urea infusion on the urine-concentrating mechanisms of protein-depleted rats has been studied [92] and showed that the enhanced urinary osmolality was attended by (a) increased papillary hypertonicity; (b) increased urea concentration in all papillary structures; and (c) increased water removal from the descending limb. In rats fed a low-protein diet and given injections of long acting vasopressin, the administration of urea further reduced urine volume and increased urine-concentrating ability [93]. From the preceding data, it is possible to ascribe the polyuria and the renal-concentrating defect observed in malnourished subjects to decreased urea concentration in the renal medulla.

ACID EXCRETION AND ACID-BASE BALANCE IN PATIENTS WITH CALORIE-PROTEIN MALNUTRITION

Adults with chronic calorie-protein malnutrition have normal blood pH and serum bicarbonate levels [94]. However, total excretion of net acid as measured by the sum of urine ammonium plus titratable acid minus urine bicarbonate is markedly decreased in calorie-protein malnutrition. The reduced acid excretion despite normal blood pH and bicarbonate levels suggests that endogenous acid production is reduced in malnutrition [94]. Generation of hydrogen ions from metabolism usually is related to proteolysis. In normal subjects consuming a diet of constant composition, the rate of metabolic hydrogen ion production will be constant and the quantity of hydrogen excreted in the urine will equal the rate of hydrogen ion production. In severe malnutrition, hydrogen ion production is decreased. When malnourished subjects are given protein, they retain nitrogen, and even in severely malnourished children there is a marked positive balance after protein administration. Thus, fewer AA are catabolized. Also, patients with malnutrition exhibit reduced protein turnover in muscle. In addition, there is a decrease in the activities of AA-activated enzymes of liver and a decrease in urea cycle enzymes; thus, AA from muscle are incorporated preferentially into protein and there is less wasteful degradation. Little is known about organic acid excretion in malnutrition. Uric acid excretion varies widely, and it would be expected that with severe potassium deficiency the renal excretion of organic acids may be altered. The net effect of all these adaptations is a reduction in the metabolic production of acid. Renal acid excretion increases during protein repletion without a change in serum bicarbonate levels or in blood pH [94]. Administration of ammonium chloride leads to a greater degree of metabolic acidosis in malnourished patients than in the same subjects after a period of protein repletion. Klahr et al. found that although basal excretion of ammonia was lower in malnourished subjects, the increment after ammonium-chloride administration was approximately the same before and after protein repletion. However, the increment in titratable acid was four times greater in the protein-repleted state than in the malnourished state [94]. This increment is related to the greater availability of urinary phosphate, a consequence of increased dietary protein, a major source of phosphorus during the period of repletion compared to the period of profound malnutrition, when phosphorus excretion was less than 200 mg/day. A similar pattern of acid excretion occurs in children. Total urinary hydrogen excretion was greater in malnourished children after protein repletion than in the same children during their malnourished state. The percentage of hydrogen-ion excretion contributed by ammonium was approximately 75% in the malnourished state and 58% in recovered children. In adults with malnutrition the urine can be acidified to a pH as low as 4.5 during ammonium-chloride loading, suggesting no defect in the kidney's ability to produce a hydrogen gradient in distal segments of the nephron. However, it has been found that infants with malnutrition and gastroenteritis can lower their urine pH to a greater extent when they are well nourished than when malnourished [95]. Therefore, impaired ability to acidify the urine may be present in children with malnutrition. In addition, tubular damage (manifested by enzymuria) has been reported in relation to malnutrition in children [96,97].

EFFECTS OF CHRONIC PROTEIN-ENERGY MALNUTRITION ON RENAL SODIUM EXCRETION

Edema is not a constant finding in patients with chronic protein-energy malnutrition. The presence or absence of edema in these individuals seems to correlate best with the dietary history of salt intake. Intake of sodium chloride in malnourished subjects is quite variable. Among children with kwashiorkor, moderate to severe edema usually is present [98] and evident in the lower extremities, hands, and face [99]. Edema-forming states are characterized by the renal salt and water retention. Thus, in edema-forming syndromes, the rate of sodium and water excretion is lower than the concurrent rate of acquisition. Common to all edema-forming states is the apparent need for expansion of effective extracellular fluid volume. Sodium-balance studies in non-edematous malnourished patients have shown that these subjects could conserve sodium adequately when fed a diet containing 10 mEq of salt daily. By contrast, when fed a diet containing 170 mEq of sodium, these patients demonstrated a mean positive sodium balance of 420 mEq and a weight gain of 2.8 kg after 5 days of such a diet. After protein repletion, the same individuals fed an identical diet demonstrated a mean positive sodium balance of only 150 mEq and a weight gain of 1.2 kg. These balance studies suggest that subjects with protein malnutrition have impaired excretion of sodium loads [100] that improves after protein repletion.

The effects of acute sodium chloride administration also have been studied in patients with chronic protein malnutrition before and after protein repletion. These malnourished subjects had a mean GFR of 41 mL/min, which increased to 45 mL/min during extracellular volume expansion. Basal excretion of sodium in the urine averaged 20.6 mEq/min and increased to 46 mEq/min after volume expansion. Fractional sodium excretion increased from 0.5% to 0.8% with expansion. When the same individuals were studied after protein repletion, basal GFR averaged 77 mL/min and increased to 87 mL/min after administration of saline. Absolute sodium excretion increased from 112 to 1170 mEq/min, and fractional sodium excretion increased from 1.1% to 11% before and after saline expansion, respectively. Thus, the rapid intravenous administration of isotonic saline results in an almost negligible increase in fractional sodium excretion in the malnourished state. When the same studies were repeated after protein repletion, a pronounced increase in fractional sodium excretion was observed. Similar observations have been made in children with malnutrition. A smaller percentage of the saline load is excreted by children who are malnourished than by children who are protein-replete. The mechanisms of sodium retention in malnutrition are not clear, but systemic as well as intrinsic renal factors seem to have a role (Table 13.2). Decreased protein intake usually together with underlying inflammation leads to hypoalbuminemia (reviewed in [101] and is discussed in detail in Chapter 11). It is controversial whether plasma volume is decreased in malnourished subjects; however, available evidence indicates that cardiac output is diminished [102]. A decrease in cardiac output, in turn, will tend to decrease arterial pressure, leading to a fall in peritubular hydrostatic pressure and increased tubular reabsorption of salt and water. In addition, RBF and GFR are diminished greatly in malnourished subjects, leading to a decrease in the filtered load of salt and water. Simultaneously, there is increased renin-angiotensin production [102] and presumably elevated levels of circulating aldosterone, which in turn will increase the tubular reabsorption of salt and water. The combination of a decreased filtered load of salt and water plus increased tubular reabsorption leads to net sodium retention and edema formation.

EFFECTS OF MATERNAL NUTRITION ON RENAL DEVELOPMENT

Numerous epidemiological and animal experiments have reported on a reverse correlation between birth weight and common chronic diseases, including insulin resistance and diabetes, hypertension and chronic kidney disease [103–105]. The pathophysiology of this process assumes the existence of nutritional deficits during critical windows of development in the fetal and early postnatal periods. One of the outcomes of such dysregulation may be a decreased nephron number, which may lead to hypertension and chronic kidney disease with age [106].

One of the nutrients that have been shown to have a profound effect on development is vitamin A. In developing countries, vitamin A deficiency is still a serious and widespread public health problem among pregnant women and children. Vitamin A and its derivatives play a vital role in the development and homeostasis of almost every organ of the body by regulating embryogenesis, including kidney development, cell differentiation, proliferation, apoptosis, immune regulation, and metabolism [107]. Animal studies have shown that mild vitamin A deficiency leads to inborn nephron deficit in the rat [108]. Vitamin A also has an effect on energy metabolism, adipocyte differentiation, and lipid

metabolism in different organs [109], including the kidney [110]. Protein restriction may also have deleterious effects on organ development. For example, maternal gestational dietary protein restriction in mice significantly elevated adult offspring systolic blood pressure [111]. This phenomenon is associated with impaired arterial vasodilatation in male offspring, elevated serum and lung ACE activity in female and male offspring, respectively, but kidney glomerular number in females and kidney gene expression in male and female offspring appear unaffected [112].

PROTEIN ENERGY WASTING IN ADVANCED RENAL DISEASE

Patients with advanced chronic renal disease often manifest signs of protein-energy wasting as do patients with other chronic disease states such as cardiac and liver failure and chronic obstructive pulmonary disease. The prevalence of protein energy wasting in advanced CKD has been estimated to range from approximately 20% to 60% and is associated with an increase in morbidity and mortality [113–115]. This serious complication is discussed in detail in Chapters 11 and 12.

References

[1] Klahr S. Effects of protein intake on the progression of renal disease. Annu Rev Nutr 1989;9:87–108.
[2] Woods LL. Mechanisms of renal hemodynamic regulation in response to protein feeding. Kidney Int 1993;44:659–75.
[3] King AJ, Levey AS. Dietary protein and renal function. J Am Soc Nephrol 1993;3:1723–37.
[4] Shannon JA, Jolliffe N, Smith HW. The excretion of urine in the dog. IV. The effect of maintenance diet, feeding, etc., upon the quantity of glomerular filtrate. Am J Physiol 1932;101:625–38.
[5] Pullman TN, Alving AS, Oem RJ, et al. The influence of dietary protein intake on specific renal functions in normal man. J Lab Clin Med 1954;44:320–32.
[6] Schoolwerrh AC, Sandler RS, Hoffman P, et al. Effects of nephron reduction and dietary protein content on renal ammoniagenesis in the rat. Kidney Int 1975;7:397–404.
[7] Ando A, Kawata T, Hara Y, et al. Effects of dietary protein intake on renal function in humans. Kidney Int 1989;27:564–7.
[8] Brandle E, Sieberth HG, Hautmann RE. Effect of chronic dietary protein intake on the renal function in healthy subjects. Eur J Clin Nutr 1996;50:734–40.
[9] Skov AR, Toubro S, Bulow J, Krabbe K, Parving HH, Astrup A. Changes in renal function during weight loss induced by high vs low-protein low-fat diets in overweight subjects. International journal of obesity and related metabolic disorders. J Int Assoc Study Obes 1999;23:1170–7.
[10] O'Connor WJ, Summerill RA. The effect of a meal of meat on glomerular filtration rate in dogs at normal urine flows. J Physiol 1976;256:81–91.
[11] Bergstrom J, Ahlberg M, Alvestrand A. Influence of protein intake on renal hemodynamics and plasma hormone concentrations in normal subjects. Acta Med Scand 1985;217:189–96.

[12] Bosch JP, Lew S, Glabman S, et al. Renal hemodynamic changes in humans. Response to protein loading in normal and diseased kidneys. Am J Med 1986;81:809—15.

[13] Rosenberg ME, Swanson JE, Thomas BL, et al. Glomerular and hormonal responses to dietary protein intake in human renal disease. Am J Physiol 1987;253:FI083—90.

[14] Kitazato H, Fujita H, Shimotomai T, Kagaya E, Narita T, Kakei M, et al. Effects of chronic intake of vegetable protein added to animal or fish protein on renal hemodynamics. Nephron 2002;90:31—6.

[15] Lee KE, Summerill RA. Glomerular filtration rate following administration of individual amino acids in conscious dogs. Q J Exp Physiol 1982;67:459—65.

[16] Woods LL, Mizelle HL, Montani JP, et al. Mechanisms controlling renal hemodynamics and electrolyte excretion during amino acids. Am J Physiol 1986;251:F303—12.

[17] Srummvoll HK, Luger A, Prager R. Effect of amino acid infusion on glomerular filtration rate. N Engl J Med 1983;308:159—60.

[18] Meyer TW, Ichikawa I, Katz R, et al. The renal hemodynamic response to amino acid infusion in the rat. Trans Assoc Am Physicians 1983;96:76—83.

[19] ter Wee PM. Renal effects of intravenous amino acid administration in humans with and without renal disease: hormonal correlates. Semin Nephrol 1995;15:426—32.

[20] O'Connor WJ, Summerill RA. Sulphate excretion by dogs following ingestion of ammonium sulphate or meat. J Physiol 1976b;260:597—607.

[21] O'Connor WJ, Summerill RA. The excretion of urea by dogs following a meat meal. J Physiol 1976a;256:93—102.

[22] Wiseman MJ, Hunt R, Goodwin A, Gross JL, Keen H, Viberti GC. Dietary composition and renal function in healthy subjects. Nephron 1987;46:37—42.

[23] Otten JJ, HJaL DM, editors. Dietary Reference Intakes: The Essential Guide to Nutrient Requirements. National Academies Press; 2006.

[24] Bernstein AM, Treyzon L, Li Z. Are high protein, vegetable-based diets safe for kidney function? A review of the literature. J Am Diet Assoc 2007;107:644—50.

[25] Weigle DS, Breen PA, Matthys CC, et al. A high-protein diet induces sustained reductions in appetite, ad libitum caloric intake, and body weight despite compensatory changes in diurnal plasma leptin and ghrelin concentrations. AmJ Clin Nutr 2005;82:41—8.

[26] Friedman AN, Yu Z, Juliar BE, et al. Independent influence of dietary protein on markers of kidney function and disease in obesity. Kidney Int 2010;78:693—7.

[27] Martin WF, Armstrong LE, Rodriguez NR. Dietary protein intake and renal function. Nutr Metab (Lond) 2005;2:25.

[28] Friedman AN. High-protein diets: potential effects on the kidney in renal health and disease. Am J Kid Dis 2004;44:950—62.

[29] Lin J, Hu FB, Curhan GC. Associations of diet with albuminuria and kidney function decline. Clin J Am Soc Nephrol 2010;5:836—43.

[30] Knight EL, Stampfer MJ, Hankinson SE, Spiegelman D, Curhan GC. The impact of protein intake on renal function decline in women with normal renal function or mild renal insufficiency. Ann Intern Med 2003;138:460—7.

[31] Friedman AN. High-protein diets: potential effects on the kidney in renal health and disease. Am J Kid Dis 2004;44:950—62.

[32] Lin J, Fung TT, Hu FB, Curhan GC. Association of dietary patterns with albuminuria and kidney function decline in older white women: a subgroup analysis from the Nurses' Health Study. AmJ Kid Dis 2011;57:245—54.

[33] Odermatt A. The Western-style diet: a major risk factor for impaired kidney function and chronic kidney disease. Am J Physiol Renal Physiol 2011;301:F919—31.

[34] Lin J, Fung TT, Hu FB, Curhan GC. Association of dietary patterns with albuminuria and kidney function decline in older white women: a subgroup analysis from the Nurses' Health Study. Am J Kid Dis 2011;57:245—54.

[35] Odermatt A. The Western-style diet: a major risk factor for impaired kidney function and chronic kidney disease. Am J Physiol Renal Physiol 2011;301:F919—31.

[36] De Santo NG, Cirillo M, Anastasio P, Spitali L, Capasso G. Renal response to an acute oral protein load in healthy humans and in patients with renal disease or liver cirrhosis. Semin Nephrol 1995;15:433—48.

[37] Pim RF. The effects of infusing glycine and of varying the dietary protein intake on renal hemodynamics of the dog. Am J Physiol 1944;142:355—65.

[38] Castellino P, Levin R, Shohat J, et al. Effect of specific amino acid groups on renal hemodynamics in humans. Am J Physiol 1990;258:F992—7.

[39] Claris-Appiani A, Assael BM, Tirelli AS, et al. Lack of glomerular hemodynamic stimulation after infusion of branched-chain amino acids. Kidney Int 1988;33:91—4.

[40] Ruiz M, Singh P, Thomson SC, Munger K, Blantz RC, Gabbai FB. L-arginine-induced glomerular hyperfiltration response: the roles of insulin and ANG II. Am J Physiol 2008;294:R1744—51.

[41] Bello E, Caramelo C, López MD, et al. Induction of micro-albuminuria by L-arginine infusion in healthy individuals: an insight into the mechanisms of proteinuria. Am J Kidney Dis 1999;33:1018—25.

[42] Mogensen CE, Vittinghus E, Solling K. Increased urinary excretion of albumin, light chains, and beta2-microglobulin after intravenous arginine administration in normal man. Lancet 1975;2:581—3.

[43] Mogensen CE. Sølling. Studies on renal tubular protein reabsorption: partial and near complete inhibition by certain amino acids. Scand J Clin Lab Invest 1977;37:477—86.

[44] Premen AJ, Hall JE, Smith Jr MJ. Postprandial regulation of renal hemodynamics: Role of pancreatic glucagon. Am J Physiol 1985;248:F656—62.

[45] Brouhard BH, Lagrone LF, Richards GE, et al. Somatostatin limits rise in glomerular filtration rate after a protein meal. Pediatrics 1987;110:729—34.

[46] Giordano M, Castellino P, McConnell EL, et al. Effect of amino acid infusion on renal hemodynamics in humans: a dose-response study. Am J Physiol 1994;267:F703—8.

[47] Haffner 0, Zacharewicz S, Mehls 0, et al. The acute effect of growth hormone on GFR is obliterated in chronic kidney disease. Clin Nephrol 1989;32:266—9.

[48] White HL, Heinbecker P, Rolf D. Enhancing effects of growth hormone on renal function. Am J Physiol 1949;157:47—51.

[49] Rabkin R, Guest s, Schaefer F. The kidney and the insulin-like growth factor system in health and disease. In: Houston M, Holly J, Feldman E, editors. IGF and nutrition in health and disease, edn. Totawa NJ: Humana Press; 2005. p. 227—50.

[50] Hirschberg R, Kopple JD. Role of growth hormone in the amino acid-induced acute rise in renal function in man. Kidney Int 1987;32:382—7.

[51] Wada L, Don BR, Schambelan M. Hormonal mediators of amino acid-induced glomerular hyperfiltration in humans. Am J Physiol 1991;260:F787—92.

[52] Ruilope L, Rodicio J, Miranda B, et al. Renal effects of amino acid infusions in patients with panhypopituitarism. Hypertension 1988;11:557—9.

[53] Hirschberg R, Kopple JD. Response of insulin-like growth factor I and renal hemodynamics to a high- and low-protein diet in the rat. J Am Soc Nephrol 1991;1:1034—40.

[54] Castellino P, De Santo NG, Capasso G, et al. Low protein alimentation normalizes renal haemodynamic response to acute protein ingestion in type I diabetic children. Eur J Clin Invest 1989;19:78—83.

[55] Hirschberg RR, Zipser RD, Slomowitz LA, et al. Glucagon and prostaglandins are mediators of amino acid-induced rise in renal hemodynamics. Kidney Int 1988;33:1147—55.

[56] Friedlander G, Blanchet-Benque F, Nitenberg A, et al. Glucagon secretion is essential for amino acid-induced hyperfiltration in man. Nephrol Dial Transplant 1990;5:110—7.

[57] Premen AJ. Importance of the liver during glucagon-mediated increases in canine renal hemodynamics. Am J Physiol 1985;249:F319—22.

[58] Smoyer WE, Brouhard BH, Rassin OK, et al. Enhanced GFR response to oral versus intravenous arginine administration in normal adults. J Lab Clin Med 1991;118:166—75.

[59] De Santo NG, Anastasio P, Loguercio C, et al. Glucagon-independent renal hyperaemia and hyperfiltration after an oral protein load in Child A liver cirrhosis. Eur J Clin Invest 1992;22:31—7.

[60] Woods LL. Mechanisms of renal vasodilation after protein feeding: role of the renin-angiotensin system. Am J Physiol 1993;264:R601—9.

[61] Ruilope LM, Rodicio J, Garcia Robles R, et al. Influence of a low sodium diet on the renal response to amino acid infusions in humans. Kidney Int 1987;31:992—9.

[62] Slomowitz LA, Hirschberg R, Kopple JD. Captopril augments the renal response to an amino acid infusion in diabetic adults. Am J Physiol 1988;255:F755—62.

[63] Rosenberg ME, Chmielewski D, Hostetter TH. Effect of dietary protein on rat renin and angiotensinogen gene expression. J Clin Invest 1990;85:1144—9.

[64] Garcia GE, Hammond TC, Wead LM, et al. Effect of angiotensin II on the renal response to amino acid in rats. AmJ Kidney Dis 1996;28:115—23.

[65] Williams M, Young JB, Rosa RM, et al. Effect of protein ingestion on urinary dopamine excretion. Evidence for the functional importance of renal decarboxylation of circulating 3,4-dihydroxyphenylalanine in man. J Clin Invest 1986;78:1687—93.

[66] Luippold G, Schneider S, Stefanescu A, Benohr P, Muhlbauer B. Dopamine D2-like receptors and amino acid-induced glomerular hyperfiltration in humans. Br J Clin Pharmacol 2001;51:415—21.

[67] Luippold G, Pech B, Schneider S, Drescher K, Muller R, Gross G, et al. Absence of amino acid-induced glomerular hyperfiltration in dopamine D3 receptor knockout mice. Naunyn Schmiedebergs Arch Pharmacol 2006;372:284—90.

[68] Maack T, Marion ON, Camargo MI, et al. Effects of auriculin (Atrial Natriuretic Factor) on blood pressure, renal function and the renin-aldosterone system in dogs. Am J Med 1984;77:1069—75.

[69] Cavatorta A, Buzio C, Pucci F, et al. Effects of antihypertensive drugs on glomerular function in normotensive and hypertensive subjects: Hormonal aspects. J Hypertens 1991;9:S218—9.

[70] Moulin B, Dhib M, Coquerel A, et al. Atrial natriuretic peptide in the renal response to an acute protein load. Int J Clin Pharmacol Res 1990;10:211—6.

[71] Tam SC, Tang LS, Lai CK, et al. Role of atrial natriuretic peptide in the increase in glomerular filtration rate induced by a protein meal. Clin Sci 1990;78:481—5.

[72] Tam SC, Tang LS, Lai CK, Nicholls MG, Swaminathan R. Role of atrial natriuretic peptide in the increase in glomerular filtration rate induced by a protein meal. Clin Sci (Lond) 1990;78:481—5.

[73] Don BR, Blake S, Hutchison FN, et al. Dietary protein intake modulates glomerular eicosanoid production in the rat. Am J Physiol 1989;256:F711—8.

[74] Yanagisawa H, Morrissey J, Yates J, et al. Protein increases glomerular eicosanoid production and activity of related enzymes. Kidney Int 1992;41:1000—7.

[75] Yanagisawa H, Wada O. Effects of dietary protein on eicosanoid production in rat renal tubules. Nephron 1998;78:179—86.

[76] Wu G, Meininger CJ. Regulation of nitric oxide synthesis by dietary factors. Annu Rev Nutr 2002;22:61—86.

[77] Kone BC. Nitric oxide synthesis in the kidney: isoforms, biosynthesis, and functions in health. Semin Nephrol 2004;24:299—315.

[78] Mount PF, Power DA. Nitric oxide in the kidney: functions and regulation of synthesis. Acta Physiol (Oxf) 2006;187:433—46.

[79] De Nicola L, Blantz RC, Gabbai FB. Nitric oxide and angiotensin II. Glomerular and tubular interaction in the rat. J Clin Invest 1992;89:1248—56.

[80] King AJ, Troy JL, Anderson S, et al. Nitric oxide: A potential mediator of amino acid-induced renal hyperemia and hyperfiltration. J Am Soc Nephrol 1991;1:1271—7.

[81] Murakami M, Suzuki H, Ichihara A, et al. Effects of L arginine on systemic and renal haemodynamics in conscious dogs. Clin Sci 1991;81:727—32.

[82] Tolins JP, Raij L. Effects of amino acid infusion on renal hemodynamics. Role of endothelium-derived relaxing factor. Hypertension 1991;17:1045—51.

[83] Gabbai FB, De Nicola L, Garcia GE, et al. Role of angiotensin in the regulation of renal response to proteins. Seminars in nephrology 1995;15:396—404.

[84] Seney FD, Wright FS. Dietary protein suppresses feedback control of glomerular filtration in rats. J Clin Invest 1985;75:558—68.

[85] Bankir L, Bouby N, Trin-Trang-Tan MJ. Vasopressin dependent kidney hypertrophy: role of urinary concentration in protein-induced hypertrophy and in progression of chronic kidney disease. Am J Kidney Dis 1991;17:661—5.

[86] Sargent FIT, Johnson RE. The effect of diet on renal function in healthy men. Am J Clin Nutr 1956;4:466—81.

[87] Klahr S, Alleyne GAO. Effects of chronic protein-calorie malnutrition on the kidney. Kidney Int 1973;3:129—41.

[88] Alleyne GAO. The effect of severe protein-calorie malnutrition on the renal function of Jamaican children. Pediatrics 1967;39:400—11.

[89] Klahr S, Tripathy K. Evaluation of renal function in malnutrition. Arch intern Med 1966;118:322—5.

[90] Tripathy K, Klahr S, Lotero H. Utilization of exogenous urea nitrogen in malnourished adults. Metabolism 1970;19:253—62.

[91] Klahr S, Tripathy K, Garcia FT, et al. On the nature of renal concentrating defect in malnutrition. Am J Med 1967;43:84—96.

[92] Pennell JP, Sanjana V, Frey NR, et al. The effect of urea infusion on the urinary concentrating mechanism in protein depleted rats. J Clin Invest 1975;55:399—409.

[93] Crawford JB, Doyle AP, Probst JH. Service of urea in renal water conservation. Am J Physiol 1959;196:545—8.

[94] Klahr S, Tripathy K, Lorero H. Renal regulation of acid-base balance in malnourished man. Am J Med 1970;48:325—31.

[95] Barbella-Szarvas S, Domínguez L, Castro-Kolster C. Distal renal tubular dysfunction in seriously undernourished pediatric patients. Invest Clin 2010;51:5—16.

[96] Yazzie D, Dasgupta A, Okolo A, et al. Lysosomal enzymuria in protein energy malnutrition. Am J Nephrol 1998;18:9—15.

[97] Garcia Nieto V, Sánchez Almeida E, García M. Renal tubular dysfunction of vitamin-D deficiency rickets. Nephron 1996;72:364.

[98] Wareriow JC, Scrimshaw NS. The concept of kwashiorkor from a public health point of view. Bull World Health Organ 1957;16:458—64.

[99] Trowell HG, Davies JNP, Dean RFA. Kwashiorkor. London: Arnold; 1954.

[100] Klahr S, Davis TA. Changes in renal function with chronic protein-calorie malnutrition. In: Mitch WE, Klahr S, editors. Nutrition and the kidney. Boston: Little, Brown; 1988. p. 59—79.

[101] Friedman AN, Fadem SZ. Reassessment of albumin as a nutritional marker in kidney disease. J Am Soc Nephrol 2010;21:223—3.

[102] Alleyne GAO. Cardiac function in severely malnourished Jamaican children. Clin Sci 1966;30:553—62.

[103] Barker DJ. The origins of the developmental origins theory. J Intern Med 2007;261:412—7.

[104] Fanos V, Puddu M, Reali A, et al. Perinatal nutrient restriction reduces nephron endowment increasing renal morbidity in adulthood: a review. Early Hum Dev 2010;86:37—42.

[105] Lackland DT, Bendall HE, Osmond C, et al. Low birth weights contribute to high rates of early-onset chronic renal failure in the Southeastern United States. Arch Intern Med 2000;160:1472—6.

[106] Barker DJ, Bagby SP, Hanson MA. Mechanisms of disease: in utero programming in the pathogenesis of hypertension. Nat Clin Pract Nephrol 2006;2:700—7.

[107] Ross SA, McCaffery PJ, Drager UC, et al. Retinoids in embryonal development. Physiol Rev 2000;80:1021—54.

[108] Lelièvre-Pégorier M, Vilar J, Ferrier ML, et al. Mild vitamin A deficiency leads to inborn nephron deficit in the rat. Kidney Int 1998;54:1455—62.

[109] Gatica LV, Vega VA, Zirulnik F, et al. Alterations in the lipid metabolism of rat aorta: effects of vitamin A deficiency. J Vasc Res 2006;43:602—10.

[110] Yang H, Chen K, Zhang X, et al. Vitamin A deficiency results in dysregulation of lipid efflux pathway in rat kidney. Pediatr Nephrol 2010;25:1435—44.

[111] Watkins AJ, Wilkins A, Cunningham C, et al. Low protein diet fed exclusively during mouse oocyte maturation leads to behavioural and cardiovascular abnormalities in offspring. J Physiol 2008;586:2231—44.

[112] Watkins AJ, Lucas ES, Torrens C, et al. Maternal low-protein diet during mouse pre-implantation development induces vascular dysfunction and altered renin-angiotensin-system homeostasis in the offspring. Br J Nutr 2010;103:1762—70.

[113] Qureshi AR, Alvestrand A, Danielsson A, et al. Factors predicting malnutrition in hemodialysis patients: a cross-sectional study. Kidney Int 1998;53:773—82.

[114] Stenvinkel P, Heimburger 0, Paulrre F, et al. Strong association between malnutrition, inflammation, and atherosclerosis in chronic kidney disease. Kidney Int 1999;55:1899—911.

[115] lkizler TA, Hakim RM. Nutrition in end-stage renal disease. Kidney Int 1996;50:343—57.

14

Low Protein, Amino Acid and Ketoacid Diets to Slow the Progression of Chronic Kidney Disease and Improve Metabolic Control of Uremia

Denis Fouque

Department of Nephrology, Hôpital E. Herriot, Université de Lyon, Lyon, France

INTRODUCTION

For many decades, it has been recommended that patients with renal disease should modify their nutrient intakes. Depending on the disease severity, this advice is generally focused on salt, protein, potassium, calcium, phosphorus, alkaline derivatives, oxalates, citrates, products that engender uric acid, and obviously water intake. In this chapter, we will focus on the experimental and clinical effects of protein intake on renal function in patients with a chronic reduction in glomerular filtration rate (GFR) who do not have endstage renal disease (i.e., individuals with chronic renal insufficiency). We will address the potential benefits and risks of limiting the patient's protein intake to an optimal level, and how to monitor the actual intake of these diets. In addition, the clinical evidence that justifies such dietary interventions in patients with chronic renal insufficiency will be discussed.

ASSESSING THE PROGRESSION OF CHRONIC RENAL INSUFFICIENCY

One of the main questions that arises when investigators want to study nephroprotection is how progression of renal disease should be monitored. Experimental studies frequently present histological data such as glomerular sclerosis, tubular atrophy, and interstitial fibrosis in response to diet interventions. However, such data are not available in humans, since ethical considerations prevent the performance of serial kidney biopsies during dietary interventions. Since renal failure is the ultimate consequence of progressive renal disease,

renal function and its impairment is usually considered a key outcome measure in experimental as well as clinical trials. However, one of the main limitations of this approach is that renal function is directly affected by nutritional intake independently of injury to renal tissue. Thus, interpretation of traditional markers of renal function could be flawed by nutritional interventions. To illustrate this point, Levey et al. have summarized the renal function decrease during the Modification of Diet in Renal Disease study using different estimates of GFR, in both groups of usual and low protein intake diets (Figure 14.1) [1]. If we accept the ^{125}I-iothalamate renal clearance as the gold standard for GFR measurement, it is apparent that other traditional renal function markers are not as accurate measures of GFR and can lead to misinterpretation. Although it is not the aim of this chapter to present detailed information on how to monitor renal function in experimental and clinical studies, some brief comments related to nutritional influences may be warranted.

Serum creatinine has been extensively used to monitor renal function and to assess renal insufficiency in clinical trials [2]. It is now well established that serum creatinine or its derivatives are not accurate indicators of renal function [3]. Serum creatinine is derived by the conversion of creatine primarily in muscle; 1.7% of the entire muscle creatine pool is converted to creatinine daily. This conversion rate does not appear to be extremely constant, since the daily variability in this conversion rate in healthy volunteers has been reported to range from 6 to 26% [4]. Serum creatinine is also affected by creatine and creatinine intake from cooked meat [5]. Indeed, investigators report that serum creatinine increased by as much as

FIGURE 14.1   The rates of decline in renal function as measured by different techniques in Study A of the Modification of Diet in Renal Disease Study.

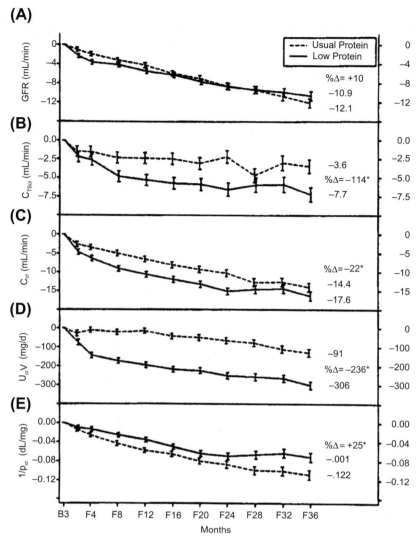

50% from normal values within two to four hours after a meal containing 225 g of boiled beef [5]. In normal adults, the half-time to achieve a new steady state in creatinine excretion following a change in creatine intake is 41 days [6]. Thus, any change in creatine intake (e.g., in intake of animal skeletal muscle) will necessitate a minimum of three half-lives to reach a new plateau, e.g., four months after the start of the new diet, and before any valid estimation of renal function from creatinine could be done. In addition, any change in the diet that leads to a variation of muscle mass will modify the creatine pool and creatinine production [7]. For instance, intensive physical exercise leading to hypertrophy of skeletal muscle will induce a rise in serum creatinine independent of renal function change.

Serum creatinine may also vary independently of renal function and food intake for additional reasons. First, there is inter-variability between measurement techniques among different clinical laboratories that can exceed 30 to 40 μmol/L for the same sample. Second, the level of serum creatinine depends on the tubular secretion of creatinine, which has a great variability, particularly when the GFR is in the range of 40 to 80 mL/min [8]. In addition, the tubular secretion of creatinine is impaired by many medicines such as trimethoprim, cimetidine, salicylate or probenecid. These drugs will generally block the tubular secretion of creatinine, thereby increasing serum creatinine without a change in GFR. Creatinine is also metabolized by extrarenal routes, mostly degraded by intestinal microorganisms, and this extrarenal clearance may vary as renal failure progresses [9].

Since it has been shown that in most renal diseases, there is a linear loss of renal function over time in more than 80% of patients, the inverse of serum creatinine (1/Screat), which also decreases linearly with time, has been used as a surrogate for estimating renal function. Unfortunately, all of the limitations that exist using the serum creatinine as an indicator of GFR also pertain to the reciprocal of the serum creatinine, thus rendering this marker poorly suitable for assessing diet impact on renal function.

Creatinine clearance, serially measured, has been proposed as an indicator of renal function loss. Creatinine clearance is not an ideal method for assessing glomerular filtration, since it exceeds the glomerular filtration rate by 10 to 15 mL/min (in healthy adults) due to active tubular secretion. As renal function deteriorates further, the tubular secretion increases disproportionately, and can overestimate renal function by 80 to 100% in cases of severe renal insufficiency [8,10]. The correlation between the creatinine clearance and true GFR is weak and improves after administering cimetidine (800 or 1200 mg), which blocks the tubule secretory part of creatinine clearance, one to two hours before commencing the urine collection [10–12]. In the pilot phase of the MDRD study, the mean correlation coefficient for the relationship between the rate of change in creatinine clearance (24-hour urine collection) and GFR (^{125}I-iothalamate clearance) was only 0.56 and 0.50 in study A and B, respectively [13]. Another important nonspecific cause of inaccurate estimation of renal function by the creatinine clearance is an incomplete urine collection. This inaccuracy tends to improve when serial, timed short-term urine collections are obtained over a 3- to 4-hour period [11,14]. Thus, to assess the effects of a given intervention on renal function in a clinical trial, creatinine clearance can be used under the following conditions: the range of renal function of patients should be wide, the treatment does not affect the tubular secretion of creatinine, and the urine collection and clearance is measured during short intervals of time [11,14]. Whether "cimetidine-treated" creatinine clearance should be performed in dietary intervention studies has not yet been validated, but perhaps should be considered when true GFR measurements cannot be employed.

Recently, a number of formulas for GFR estimation have been developed using the serum creatinine concentrations and such parameters as age, gender and body weight (Equation 1) [15–17]. These formulas appear convenient to use, can be computed directly from simple softwares or pocket organizers, and have broad applicability for the general treatment of renal disease. Levey and colleagues reanalyzed the data obtained through the MDRD study [18], and proposed a formula for true GFR based on serum creatinine, serum urea, serum albumin, age, gender and ethnicity, which is more accurate than creatinine clearance or the Cockcroft–Gault equation (Equation 2).

EQUATION 1 (COCKCROFT–GAULT EQUATION [15]):

$$CCr = [(140 - age) \times Weight]$$
$$/(Pcreat \times 72) \quad \text{for men}$$

$$CCr = [(140 - age) \times Weight]$$
$$/(Pcreat \times 85) \quad \text{for women}$$

Where CCr is creatinine clearance in mL/min, Pcreat is serum creatinine in mg/dL, age is in years and weight is in kg (from [15]).

EQUATION 2 (MDRD EQUATION [18]):

$$GFR = 170 \times [Pcreat]^{-0.999} \times [Age]^{-0.176}$$
$$\times [0.762 \text{ if patient is female}]$$
$$\times [1.180 \text{ if patient is black}]$$
$$\times [SUN]^{-0.170} \times [Alb]^{+0.318}$$

Where GFR is the glomerular filtration rate in mL/min/1.73 m^2, Pcreat is serum creatinine in mg/dL, Age in years, SUN is serum urea nitrogen in mg/dL and Alb is serum albumin in g/dL (from [18]).

More recently, Levey et al. developed a new equation for the GFR [19] called CKD-EPI, using different thresholds based on race, gender and serum creatinine:

EQUATION 3 (CKD-EPI EQUATION [19]):

Serum creatinine, μmol/L(mg/dL) Formula:

Black			
Female	≤62(≤0.7)	GFR = 166 × (Scr/0.7)$^{-0.329}$ × (0.993)^{Age}	
	>62(>0.7)	GFR = 166 × (Scr/0.7)$^{-1.209}$ × (0.993)^{Age}	
Male	≤80(≤0.9)	GFR = 163 × (Scr/0.9)$^{-0.411}$ × (0.993)^{Age}	
	>80(>0.9)	GFR = 163 × (Scr/0.9)$^{-1.209}$ × (0.993)^{Age}	
White or other			
Female	≤62(≤0.7)	GFR = 144 × (Scr/0.7)$^{-0.329}$ × (0.993)^{Age}	
	>62(>0.7)	GFR = 144 × (Scr/0.7)$^{-1.209}$ × (0.993)^{Age}	
Male	≤80(≤0.9)	GFR = 141 × (Scr/0.9)$^{-0.411}$ × (0.993)^{Age}	
	>80(>0.9)	GFR = 141 × (Scr/0.9)$^{-1.209}$ × (0.993)^{Age}	

However, although simple formulas can predict GFR with acceptable precision for routine use (Cockcroft–Gault formula overestimates GFR by only 16%, e.g.,

$7 \text{ mL/min}/1.73 \text{ m}^2$, [18]), for research purposes, more precise techniques should be used.

The GFR is considered to be the gold standard for estimating renal function and for assessing the progression of renal disease [3]. However, the GFR measurement is difficult to perform, expensive and also presents some limitations. Traditional markers such as inulin have been largely supplanted for clinical research or practice by radiotracers such as ^{125}I-iothalamate, $^{99\text{m}}\text{Tc-DTPA}$ or $^{51}\text{Cr-EDTA}$. Measurements can be done after a single injection, either subcutaneously or intravenously, and include plasma and/or urine samples collected over three to four hours. Usually, when urine samples are needed, bladder catheterization is not necessary, but may be required in cases of bladder dysfunction such as in diabetes or neurological diseases. To avoid pre-renal azotemia, it is generally recommended that a minimal urine output is ensured by ingesting a water load before the test. Anastasio and colleagues have challenged this fact while actually reporting a decrease in GFR after patients received a large oral water load (4 mL per kg body weight every 30 min) during a three-hour GFR measurement [20].

Finally, another more pragmatic approach has been recently proposed to assess the efficacy of a treatment in renal failure. "Renal death" is defined as the number of patients starting renal replacement therapy during a study [2,21]. Since it cannot formally be excluded that the death of a patient is not from renal failure origin, we have included patient deaths within the "renal death" definition, as well as the number of renal transplantations before the start of dialysis if that happens during the study.

PROTEIN INTAKE AND CHRONIC RENAL INSUFFICIENCY: EXPERIMENTAL DATA

There is ample evidence, dating from the 1920s, that elevated protein intake or amino acid infusion alter renal hemodynamics and ultimately impair renal function and tissue in normal animals or animals with experimental renal insufficiency [22–27] (for detailed reviews see [28–30]). In many of these experiments, it is somewhat difficult to clearly identify the specific role of protein per se, since sodium, energy, fluid and phosphorus intakes obviously varied and were not always controlled. In addition, in case of severe experimental nephropathy, high protein intakes may have elicited superimposed uremic toxicity and mortality not directly related to renal function or kidney damage, thus adding confounding elements [23]. We will review here the experimental data on the renal effects of a reduced protein intake.

Effects on Renal Hemodynamics

The hemodynamic effects of dietary protein have been attributed to a number of mechanisms that eventually increase GFR, induce and/or increase proteinuria, and lead to glomerulosclerosis and renal insufficiency. Candidates for these mechanisms include hormones (glucagon, insulin, insulin-like growth factor-1, angiotensin II), cytokines (prostaglandins) and kinins [31–35]. Intrarenal regulation of sodium transport may also be involved through the proximal sodium/amino acid co-transporter; activity of this transporter is enhanced in response to an increased filtered amino acid load, thus stimulating the tubuloglomerular feed-back and increasing the GFR [36]. Protein restriction in rats ablates most of the hemodynamic changes observed after renal ablation or {5/6} nephrectomy. Micropuncture studies provide direct evidence that the increase in single nephron glomerular filtration rate and increased glomerular capillary and transcapillary pressure after renal mass reduction is a cause of the accelerated glomerular injury [37]. Reducing protein intake decreases GFR in normal animals and blunts the renal hemodynamic changes induced by extensive renal ablation, i.e., increased glomerular pressure and flow. Subsequent studies in rats with less severe renal ablation showed that a low protein intake also lowers hyperfiltration and retards the onset of proteinuria and glomerular fibrosis [25,38,39]. In addition to these experimental data, low protein intakes also increase survival in these animals with reduced renal function [23].

A reduced animal protein intake (usually a diet containing 6% protein) allows a reduction in glomerular hypertension by inducing afferent arteriolar vasoconstriction, which in turn decreases the glomerular plasma flow and reduces proteinuria [37]. Protein restriction decreases the percentage of glomerular sclerosis and proteinuria. Indeed, Hostetter and colleagues reported that at four and eight months after the onset of renal insufficiency created by a {5/6}nephrectomy, glomerulosclerosis was attenuated by 50% in animals receiving a 6% protein diet, and proteinuria was lowered to 25% of that in rats receiving a 40% protein diet [25]. Of importance, these benefits were observed at different levels of renal impairment (Figure 14.2).

Micropuncture studies in {5/6}nephrectomized rats showed that a reduction in protein intake from 20% to 6% led to a reduction in single nephron GFR and intraglomerular capillary pressure to normal [27]. Of interest, proteinuria in the 6% protein diet group was reduced to one-fifth the proteinuria observed in the 20% protein

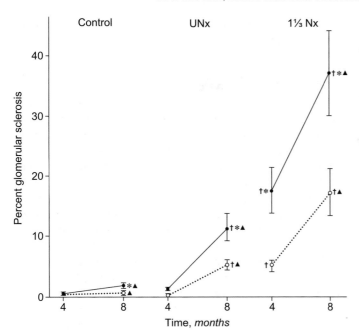

FIGURE 14.2 Percentage of sclerosed glomeruli in experimental kidney disease as compared with a control group of rats. Open circles: low protein intake; close circles: high protein intake.

diet group. Both groups of rats were hypertensive, and there was no examination of what the effects of a low protein diet would have been if the rats were normotensive [27]. Thus, whereas a low dietary protein intake that was commenced shortly after the onset of renal ablation seems to mainly blunt the increase in glomerular capillary pressure, a delayed low protein diet will reduce glomerular capillary pressure without lowering renal hyperperfusion or hyperfiltration [27,40]. These data support the deleterious impact of glomerular hypertension, and the protective role of a low protein intake on the remnant renal function in experimental renal insufficiency.

Effects on Oxidant Stress and Inflammation

Protein intake and protein trafficking through the kidney are associated with hypermetabolism [41] and oxidant stress [42]. Oxygen consumption and ammonia production decreased by about 50% when rats were fed a 12% instead of a 40% protein diet [42]. This fact is primarily explained by a decrease in net sodium reabsorption [43]. In another study, hypoxic injury of the thick ascending limb was mitigated by reducing the protein content of the diet [44]. Additional metabolic data, obtained through ^{31}P-NMR spectroscopy, also show that protein restriction reduces intracellular inorganic phosphate and pH, consistent with a decrease in oxygen consumption [45]. This decrease in oxygen demand secondary to a reduction in protein diet from 30% to 6% may be

responsible for reduced kidney production of glutathione and malondialdehyde [43,45].

Other studies have addressed the potential renal antifibrotic effect of a low protein diet. Nakayama and colleagues reported that in adriamycin-treated rats, expression of fibronectin and TGF beta in the kidney was dramatically reduced when animals received a 6% protein diet as compared with their littermates receiving a regular 20% protein diet [46]. In addition, these investigators showed a post-transcriptional reduction in fibronectin synthesis after short-term (two weeks) treatment with a low protein diet, whereas there was no difference in fibronectin gene expression. These interesting observations bear similarities to the effects of energy and protein intakes on the transcriptional and post-transcriptional regulation of IGF-1 synthesis in liver cells [47,48].

TGF-beta, a potent profibrotic agent, is decreased by intervention with low protein diets. Peters and colleagues documented two sets of findings in this regard: First, an L-arginine supplement augmented the propensity of a low protein diet (6%) to reduce the glomerular expression of TGF-beta, fibronectin and plasmin activator inhibitor 1 (PAI-1) in a model of immune glomerulonephritis [49], independent of nitric oxide metabolism. Second, whereas maximal angiotensin II blockade by very high doses of either ACEI or angiotensin II antagonists resulted in only a 45% decrease in TGF-beta gene expression and protein production, the addition of a low protein diet to other well-established nephroprotective treatments resulted in a further 20% reduction in TGF-beta expression and production, and this was associated with a similar decrease in fibronectin and PAI-1 [50]. It should be emphasized that, in both experiments the control of profibrotic mediators was associated with a concomitant decrease in proteinuria. These findings provide good evidence that a low protein diet possesses its own therapeutic actions, independent from ACEI or AII antagonists on renal scarring.

Tovar-Palacio [51] and colleagues studied the effects on kidney tissue of different amounts and types of protein intake in obese Zucker rats. These animals which had normal renal function, ingested either casein or soy protein, in an amount of 20, 30 or 45% of the food intake for two months. Urine excretion of hydrogen peroxide, a marker of oxidative stress, increased in a parallel manner to the protein intake, and for the same amount of protein in the diet, was consistently lower in the vegetal source of protein as compared with the animal one. Proteinuria followed the same trend and was lowest in the 20% soy protein diet [51]. Furthermore, renal expression of genes involved in inflammation (IL-6 and TNF-alpha), lipid metabolism (sterol-regulatory element binding protein1, SREBP-1, and fatty acid synthase, FAS), matrix accumulation (type IV collagen) and fibrosis (TGF-beta) were lowest in the 20% soy diet and highest in the 45% casein diet. Although these rats did not have kidney failure, these results strongly support a deleterious effect of high casein intake and a nephroprotective impact on low dietary protein from vegetal sources [51].

Studies have addressed the potential role of endothelin (ET) as a cause of puromycin-induced glomerulosclerosis. In addition, ET-1 gene expression has been reported to be elevated in other experiments with renal mass reduction. Nakamura et al. reported that a 6% protein diet was able to reverse proteinuria and increase ET receptor mRNA and both ET-1 mRNA and protein in puromycin-induced glomerulosclerosis as compared with rats receiving a 22% protein diet [52]. Whether this improvement occurs through a reduction in factors that stimulate ET release, e.g., TGF-beta and TNF-alpha, has not been directly proven in this experiment but represents a possibility [53].

Kruppel-like factor-15 (KLF-15) is a transcription factor that has been shown to reduce cardiac fibrosis. Gao et al. [54] studied KLF-15 in {5/6}nephrectomized rats receiving either a controlled (22%), or low protein intakes (6% or 5% + 1% ketoacids) for six months. As expected, proteinuria, glomerular sclerosis and tubular fibrosis were reduced in both LPD and LPD+KA groups, but fell to a greater extent in the LPD+KA rats [54]. Renal expression of profibrotic factors (TGF beta, fibronectin and type IV collagen) was dramatically reduced in both LPD groups, as were proinflammatory markers (TNF alpha, MCP-1 and RANTES). As a consequence of increased TGF beta and TNF alpha production in CKD rats receiving the control protein, renal KLF-15 expression was completely abolished, whereas LPD or LPD+KA almost restored KLF-15 expression to normal. For virtually all measurements, LPD+KA did improve renal KLF-15 better than LPD alone [54]. Thus, there is an extensive data set to support the renal antioxidant, anti-inflammatory and antifibrotic effects in the kidney of a reduction in protein intake in experimental kidney disease.

Effects of the Source of Dietary Proteins

As already shown above by Tovar-Palacio [51], the effect of the type of protein deserves further consideration. Based on the observation that vegetarians have lower GFR than omnivores [55,56], Williams et al. tested two different sources of protein derived from either animal or vegetable origin, casein or soya, in stable CKD rats [57]. Both regular (24%) and moderately low (12%) protein intakes of each of those two protein sources were studied. After three months of dietary feeding, glomerulosclerosis and tubular dilation were found to be significantly greater in the casein vs. the soya fed groups. Proteinuria was greatest with the 24% (99 ± 34(SD) mg/d) and 12% (64 ± 18) casein diets, lower in the 24% soya group (30 ± 5 mg/d) and lowest in the 12% (35 ± 7 mg/d) soya groups. There was no significant difference in the severity of the proteinuria or histological lesions in the 24% vs. the 12% soya groups [57]. Although these results are convincing, it should be noted that, due to the different digestibility of protein, it is possible that vegetable proteins were less absorbed by about 10% than the animal proteins, thus reducing the true protein load with the former diet. It is interesting to note that particular amino acids may elicit specific renal hemodynamic effects. A diet enriched with L-arginine, the precursor of nitric oxide (NO), has been shown to reduce glomerular hypertension and glomerulosclerosis in {5/6} nephrectomized rats [58]. Because NO is a potent vasodilation factor, locally enhanced NO production may be involved in these hemodynamic changes. L-arginine also stimulates growth hormone secretion, which may also cause renal vasodilation through release of IGF-1, and consequently, NO.

Protein and/or Energy Intake?

Venkatachalam and colleagues developed another interesting hypothesis. Since in most studies of protein reduction, it is the whole food intake that is reduced, these authors have studied the effects of energy restriction as compared with protein restriction [59]. Five groups of {5/6}nephrectomized rats were fed either a control diet, a 40% reduction in overall food, a 40% energy reduced diet, a 40% protein reduced diet, and a 40% salt reduced diet. After 21 weeks of dietary treatment, histological findings clearly showed protected kidneys in the low energy alone group, which disclosed less glomerulosclerosis as well as less interstitial inflammation, as compared with all other groups. Of interest, proteinuria was lowest in this calorie-restricted group [59]. The discrepant finding of an absence of beneficial effects of the protein-reduced diet might be explained by a too modest reduction in protein intake as compared to the control diet. In a subsequent paper, these investigators reported that two weeks after {5/6}nephrectomy, the kidney IGF-1 content and the severity of inflammatory lesions were reduced with calorie restriction [60]. Altogether, these results suggest that IGF-1 expression could be involved in the tubulo-interstitial inflammatory response and that this effect might be regulated by a low energy intake. Of interest is the fact that proteinuria was also reduced by the low calorie diet [60].

In a strain of mice (kD/kD) that develop an autoimmune interstitial nephritis, Fernandes et al. showed that a low protein diet alone did not reduce mice mortality as compared with a combination of protein and calorie restriction which induced the largest survival in animals [61]. However, the suppression of immune disease may be a more important cause of reduced mortality than any alteration in kidney metabolism or physiology in this experiment. Since in patients with CKD, reducing energy intake to a level that may induce malnutrition is not considered appropriate or justifiable, the relevance of these energy intake-reducing studies to clinical medical care may be quite limited.

It should be emphasized that the proteinuria-lowering effects of a low protein diet may impact on tubular atrophy and apoptosis [62]. Indeed, there is a toxic effect of serum albumin on tubular cells in culture [63,64]. Two sets of experiments have highlighted the role of protein delivery to the tubule as a cause of interstitial fibrosis [65] and tubule cell apoptosis [66]. Indeed, the dramatic increase in proteinuria following intraperitoneal bovine serum albumin is associated with a profound tubular apoptotic reaction. Thus, since most experiments have shown that reducing protein intake is associated with a reduction in proteinuria [67], it is possible but not proven, that a low protein intake also reduces renal apoptosis.

In summary, there is a large body of evidence from experimental research that high protein loads are hazardous to the kidney, and that a large number of the physiopathological changes that occur secondary to reduced functioning renal mass or renal insufficiency are corrected or, at most, improved by diets low in protein. However, these experiments use the extreme ends of dietary protein content, in order to identify these histological and hemodynamic changes. For example, Neugarten et al. reported that the renal injury and proteinuria of puromycin treated rats improved with a diet providing 4% protein, as compared with a group of rats receiving a 50% protein diet [68]. How do these extremely different protein diets compare with clinical studies? How do humans respond to low protein diets? What is the evidence for the nutritional safety of low protein diets? Is it possible to adhere to such diets for long periods of time? How can compliance to dietary prescription be monitored? These questions will now be addressed.

DIETARY PROTEIN INTAKE: CLINICAL STUDIES

Protein Requirements in Normal Individuals

In the United States, the daily average protein intake is about 90 to 110 g in adult men and 65 to 70 g in adult women (US Department of Agriculture, 1983), and 1.3 g/kg in most European countries. Protein intake tends to diminish by 15% by the age of 70 [69]. In women, the mean protein intake is 30 to 50% lower than in men for the same age [70], and is in accord with their 40% lower muscle mass as compared with men [71]. Thus, based on the FAO recommendations, most adults in occidental countries have protein intakes far above the recommended allowance, which currently is 0.75 g/kg/day [72]. Furthermore, it should be emphasized that the 0.75 g/kg body weight value is defined as the safety level, including two standard deviations above the average requirement obtained through individual metabolic balances, thus guarantying that at least 97.5% of subjects will attain neutral or positive nitrogen balance [72]. Fortunately, due to the Gaussian distribution of protein requirements, many normal individuals will be in neutral protein balance with a lower level of protein intake. This fact may partly explain why in maintenance dialysis, patients, some individuals present with nPNA lower than recommended and show little or no signs of protein malnutrition.

In nondialyzed patients with chronic kidney disease, from the perspective of the nutritional needs to maintain healthy body composition, there is no need to increase or decrease these recommended dietary protein levels. Indeed, in stable adult patients, most nitrogen balance and protein turn-over studies have confirmed these data (see below). In addition, it should be noted that during the progression of renal insufficiency, spontaneous alterations in nutrient intake frequently occur, generally in the form of a reduction in both energy and protein intake [73–75]. Indeed, in an NHANES survey, it was reported that in patients with an estimated GFR between 30 and 60 mL/min, spontaneous energy and protein intakes were 23.3 ± 0.7 (SEM) kcal/kg/day and 0.91 ± 0.03 g protein/kg/day, and in patients with a GFR less than 30 mL/min the values were 20.9 ± 1.0 kcal/kg/day and 0.86 ± 0.03 g protein/kg/day [76]. These findings are of particular clinical importance, because when there is a deficient energy intake, the body cannot adjust as readily to a reduction in protein intake. Thus, in the absence of a dietary control and care plan, patients with chronic renal disease will do worse nutritionally than if they were enrolled in an optimal moderately low protein and adequate energy intake diet [75,76].

Metabolic Effects of Low Protein Diets in Humans

Metabolic Adaptation to a Reduction in Protein Intake

Figure 14.3 shows the metabolic adaptation that occurs when an ad libitum protein diet (1.1 g/kg/day) is changed to a more limited protein intake

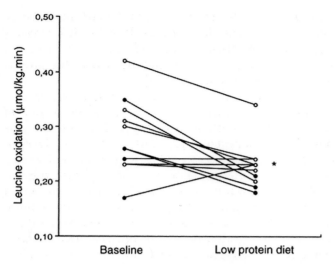

FIGURE 14.3 Total body leucine oxidation before and after a low-protein diet for three months in moderate chronic kidney disease (1.1g vs. 0.7 prot/kg/day).

(0.7 g/kg/day) in 12 patients with moderate chronic kidney disease without the nephrotic syndrome [77]. Using a whole body amino acid tracer (i.e., ^{13}C-leucine), the investigators reported a net decrease in leucine oxidation, which is considered to reflect the catabolism of excess amino acids; these findings suggest a normal adaptation in protein metabolism, similar to that reported in healthy volunteers [78]. There was no change in the patients' body weight, serum albumin, or IGF-1 after the three months of this reduced protein intake, confirming the safety of this level of protein intake (0.7 g/kg/day) in CKD [77]. Other studies have reported similar findings in CKD patients undergoing different types of diet intervention but mostly with shorter studies. Goodship et al. studied six patients with moderate CKD during short-term (one week) feeding of regular (1 g protein/kg/d) or reduced (0.6 g protein/kg/d) protein diets and with energy intakes of 32.5 kcal/kg/day [79]. Fasting leucine oxidation did not significantly change with the lower protein intake, whereas post-prandial leucine oxidation decreased by about 25% (p < 0.05). As in nephrotic patients without chronic renal failure [80], these data show that patients with mild renal insufficiency can adapt their protein metabolism during acute or chronic reductions in protein intake by reducing amino acid oxidation in both the post-prandial and the fasting state.

More restricted protein intakes have been shown to reduce amino acid oxidation by a greater magnitude. Masud et al. reported in six pre-dialysis patients that a diet providing 0.35 g protein/kg/day supplemented with either ketoacids or essential amino acids for 25 days maintained neutral nitrogen balance and body composition [81]. These diets were associated with

very low leucine oxidation rates which were not different whether patients were supplemented with ketoanalogs or essential amino acids [81]. In a long-term follow-up of these patients (16 months), the fasting leucine oxidation rate remained at the low level of 10.0 ± 2.2 μmol/kg/h [82]. With this low protein intake, these values for amino acid oxidation appear to be more reduced than was observed in studies with less restricted protein intakes [77,79], suggesting a potential "functional reserve" for protein sparing in CKD patients.

Maroni and colleagues studied patients presenting with heavy proteinuria, e.g., greater than 6 g/day, and moderate chronic renal failure (GFR, about 50 mL/min/1.73 m^2). Using leucine turnover and nitrogen balance techniques, they showed that a reduction in protein intake from 1.85 to 1.00 g protein/kg/day in these patients induced adaptive protein conserving mechanisms that were similar to these of healthy volunteers, and that these nephrotic patients were in positive nitrogen balance [83]. These results have been confirmed by Giordano et al. in seven patients with heavy proteinuria [80] who underwent a reduction in protein intake from 1.20 to 0.66 g/kg/day for one month. Endogenous leucine flux decreased by 8% (p < 0.05); hepatic albumin synthesis decreased from 18.2 to 14.9 g/1.73 m^2 (p < 0.03), and serum albumin rose from 2.88 to 3.06 g/dL (p < 0.03).

Effects of Low Protein Diets on Proteinuria

Since proteinuria has been clearly identified as an independent risk factor for progression of kidney disease, it is relevant to examine the effects of LPDs on proteinuria. As discussed above, experimental studies almost unanimously report a reduction in proteinuria when animals are placed on a low protein diet. Similar responses have been observed in humans. Rosenberg and colleagues examined the effects of a marked reduction in protein intake, from 2.0 to 0.55 g protein/kg/day, for 11 days in 12 proteinuric patients in a randomized cross-over design, [84]. There was a 35% decrease in proteinuria from 7.0 ± 3 to 4.7 ± 2 g/day, improved glomerular permselectivity, as determined by dextran clearances and from a disproportionate reduction in IgG as compared to albumin clearance; whereas there was no change in GFR and renal plasma flow [84]. A net decrease in plasma renin activity and plasma aldosterone was also noted during the low protein period, confirming experimental data.

Aparicio and coworkers confirmed this reduction in proteinuria during therapy with low protein diets (LPDs) for a longer period of time [67]. These latter investigators reported a decrease in proteinuria from 3.2 ± 1.2 to 1.8 ± 1.1 g/day (p < 0.01) in 15 patients with advanced chronic renal insufficiency after six months of very low protein intakes (0.3 g/kg/day) supplemented with ketoacids, whereas serum albumin increased concomitantly in these patients from 36.5 ± 4.0 to 40.8 ± 3.2 g/L (p < 0.01) (Figure 14.4) [67].

When Giordano et al. [80] changed seven patients with the nephrotic syndrome from a 1.2 g protein/kg/day to a 0.66 g protein/kg/day protein diet, proteinuria decreased by 38%, and there was a linear relationship between the reduction in proteinuria and the achieved reduction in protein intake, as has been previously noted by Kaysen and colleagues [85]. It was proposed that a decrease in proteinuria is a stimulus for a reduction in albumin synthesis. Furthermore, fibrinogen synthesis rate also decreased by 30% with LPDs, from 4.6 to 3.0 g/1.73 m²/day, p < 0.03; these synthesis rates, however, were still increased as compared with healthy volunteers (1.93 g/1.73 m²/day) [80]. The similar reductions in albumin and fibrinogen synthesis may be triggered by a common mechanism, presently unknown, but which is advantageously modulated by a low protein intake. Thus, not only do patients with chronic renal failure generally adapt to LPDs, but there seem to be further benefits of such LPDs diets on reduced proteinuria and its consequent metabolic disturbances in nephrotic states. In a more recent study, Bellizi et al. [86] reported in 110 CKD patients the effects of six months of treatment with three different protein intakes,

1.04, 0.78 and 0.54 g/kg BW/day, the last intake being supplemented with ketoanalogs. Proteinuria decreased significantly in the most restricted group, from 1.34 to 0.87 g/day, whereas it was not affected in the groups with higher protein intakes [86].

It is well established that ACE inhibitors and angiotensin receptor blockers (ARBs) reduce the degree of proteinuria in most renal diseases. Of interest is the additional antiproteinuric effect of a LPD given in combination with these nephroprotective medications. Ruilope et al. first described this observation in a short-term study involving 17 patients with mild CKD [87]. Enalapril, 20 mg/day, reduced proteinuria by about 20%; a 25% reduction in protein intake from 1 g/kg/day (estimated from urinary urea output) decreased proteinuria by 30%. However, the combination of both interventions induced a 55% decrease in proteinuria; this latter reduction in proteinuria was significantly greater than each separate intervention [87]. Gansevoort and colleagues [88] confirmed these findings by studying, in a crossover design, 14 patients with modest renal impairment and nephrotic range proteinuria. Enalapril, 10 mg/day, induced a reduction of proteinuria by 35%, whereas a 50% reduction in protein intake decreased proteinuria by 20%. Again, there was an additional effect of both treatments, with a 55 to 60% decrease in proteinuria by enalapril

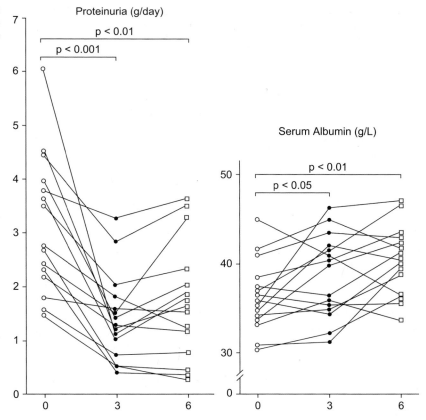

FIGURE 14.4 The decrease in proteinuria (left panel) and the increase in serum albumin (right panel) during 3 and 6 months with a very low protein diet (0.3 g/kg/day).

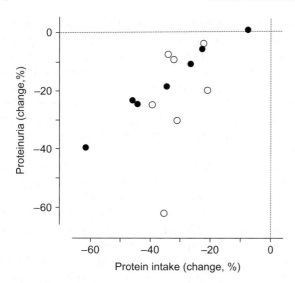

FIGURE 14.5 The relationship between the reduction in dietary protein intake and the concomitant reduction in daily proteinuria.

and low protein intake. Furthermore, as shown on Figure 14.5, there was a linear relation between the reduction in both protein intake and proteinuria [88].

Effects of the Nature of Protein Intake

As previously discussed in experimental studies, the nature of protein, e.g., from animal or vegetal sources, may impact on the renal response to the diet [51]. In humans, Kontessis et al. examined the effects of dietary protein from different sources on glomerular dynamics in seventeen healthy volunteers. Although diets were not heavily restricted (intakes averaged about 1 g/kg BW/day), a decrease in GFR (−10%), in urinary albumin excretion (−50%) and IgG clearance (−35%) was observed after three weeks of ingesting the vegetable protein diet as compared to a regular animal protein diet [89,90]. In another study of similar design, these investigators measured GFR in nine diabetic patients without severe renal involvement [89]. Both diets were isocaloric and the vegetarian diet brought 0.15 g protein/kg BW less than the animal diet. Again, there was a 15% and 40% decrease in GFR and in microalbuminuria, respectively, with the vegetable protein as compared with the animal protein diet. Interestingly, a marked decrease (−20%) in serum IGF-1, a strong GFR regulatory hormone, was also observed with the vegetarian protein diet, thus suggesting that protein intake might regulate renal hemodynamics, at least in part, through changing IGF-1 levels. The mechanisms by which vegetal protein slows progression more than animal protein are unclear. It is possible that vegetal based LPDs may slow progression of CKD more than animal based proteins because less vegetal proteins are absorbed than animal proteins.

Another study tested the effects of three different protein diets in 17 diabetic patients in a randomized crossover design [91]. Patients had macroalbuminuria and normal renal function. One diet included beef protein, 1.33 g/kg/day, the second diet was composed of 1.22 g protein/kg/day from chicken meat, and the third was a modestly LPD of 0.8 g/kg/day from vegetable sources. There was no change in GFR; macroalbuminuria decreased from 313 (beef) to 269 (chicken) and 229 μg/min (vegetarian), p < 0.05. The lipid profile improved gradually in association with the reduction in saturated fatty acid intake when patients ate the LPD as compared to the beef diet. The authors attributed the reduction in macroalbuminuria to the vascular protective effects of the polyunsaturated fatty acid enrichment mainly found in the low protein, vegetable source diet [91].

Effect of Low Protein Diets on Insulin Resistance

Abnormal insulin sensitivity and insulin resistance can be improved by a low protein diet. Gin and colleagues measured serum glucose and insulin after an oral glucose test in 10 patients with nondiabetic advanced CKD (creatinine clearance, 15 mL/min) who were given a very low protein intake (0.3 g/kg BW/day) supplemented with ketoacids [92]. Both peak serum glucose and insulin were significantly reduced after four months of diet (Figure 14.6), suggesting an improvement in insulin sensitivity [92]. In a subsequent study, these authors investigated eight patients (GFR: 13.2 ± 2.8 mL/min/1.73 m²) undergoing the same diet for three months [93]. Patients showed an improvement in fasting serum glucose from 5.0 ± 0.1 to 4.7 ± 0.1 mmol/L (p < 0.05), a decrease in fasting plasma insulin from 82.4 ± 20.7 to 48.8 ± 8.0 pmol/L (p < 0.05). More importantly, using the gold standard euglycemic insulin clamp, these workers showed a decrease in endogenous glucose production by 66% for comparable plasma insulin levels. These data clearly indicate an improved sensitivity to insulin in nondiabetic CKD patients [93].

Effect of Low Protein Diets on Dyslipidemia

As already mentioned, the sources of protein ingested can be associated with different patterns of lipid intake. Mainly, red meat intake increases dietary saturated fatty acids (in pork, lamb and beef), whereas white meat such as from chicken or turkey is associated with less saturated fatty acids. Fish and vegetable protein are mainly associated with unsaturated cardiovascular protective fatty acids. In addition, with the cooking of meat additional lipids and sodium chloride are often added to the food. Consequently, most reports show that reducing protein intake from animal source improves the patient's lipid intake and plasma lipid profile. For example, Bernard et al. reported an improvement in

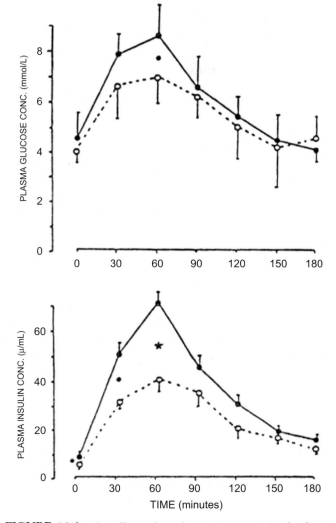

FIGURE 14.6 The effects of a reduction in protein intake during four months on plasma glucose and insulin response to an oral glucose test.

the apoA1/apoB ratio ($p < 0.03$) in 11 stage 3 CKD patients after they were switched from 1.1 g to 0.7 g protein/kg/day for three months [94]. Bellizzi and coworkers reported a 24% and 18% decrease in serum total cholesterol and triglycerides, respectively ($p < 0.001$), after six months of a very low protein intake, which is not dissimilar to the effects of treatment with a hydroxy-methylglutaryl-coenzyme A reductase inhibitor (statins) [86].

Effect of Low Protein Diets on Phosphate, Mineral and Bone Disease

Management of bone minerals and disease has emerged as one of the most important aspects of nutritional and metabolic CKD treatment, because of its impact on both bone frailty and vascular calcification. Indeed, mortality from cardiovascular disease constitutes approximately 50% of the overall mortality at

every stage of CKD, including the dialysis and transplantation. Since hyperphosphatemia and hyperparathyroidism are frequently observed even at early stages of CKD, improving serum phosphate has long been the goal of a targeted dietary counseling before dialysis. Finally, the discovery of fibroblast-growth factor-(FGF) 23, a key regulator of phosphate metabolism, has reinforced clinical and research interests in this field.

Dietary phosphate is strongly linked to protein since 1 g of food protein provides approximately 13 mg phosphorus. Not all phosphate is absorbed by the gut, only 40 to 80%, and this may be influenced by the fiber content of the diet, (i.e., phosphate from vegetarian sources will be less well absorbed than from animal sources). By contrast, calcitriol will increase the fractional rate of gut phosphate absorption. Serum phosphorus will also be influenced by renal tubular phosphorus excretion and bone metabolism. The effect of progression of CKD various alterations in phosphate metabolism have been described by Isakova and colleagues [95] who showed that serum FGF-23 increases long before the rise in serum PTH. Thus, the primary response to the oral phosphate intake is an increase in serum FGF-23 which maintains a sufficient tubular phosphate excretion; e.g., FGF-23 begins to rise when the GFR is about 80 to 60 mL/min. In addition, FGF-23 blunts the activity of the 1-α hydroxylase, blocking the synthesis of calcitriol in the proximal tubule and therefore reducing intestinal phosphate absorption. For yet unexplained reasons, during progressive CKD, FGF-23 fails to maintain normal serum phosphorus and when the GFR is about 50 mL/min, serum PTH starts to rise, which in turn compensates renal phosphorus excretion. Finally, when GFR decreases below 35 mL/min, serum phosphorus may continue to rise despite further metabolic adaptations, such as progressively increasing serum PTH. (Please also see Chapters 17, 19 and 20 for more discussion).

Why is it important to emphasize these changes in this section? First, in addition to the phosphorus-calcium abnormalities, it has been recently reported that elevated FGF-23 by itself may be independently linked to reduced survival in both healthy adults and CKD patients [96–98]. Second, the only way yet identified to reduce serum FGF-23 levels is by a reduction in phosphate intake, which usually means by reducing protein intake. Indeed, in healthy adults, it has been reported that FGF-23 expression can be directly regulated by dietary phosphorus. When adults received a daily oral load of 1 g phosphate for five days, serum FGF-23 increased by 30% whereas serum PTH did not change. In response to the increased FGF-23, there was an increase in urinary phosphate excretion and a decrease in serum calcitriol, effectively counteracting the increase in the dietary phosphorus load [99]. Restricting dietary phosphate can also reduce serum FGF-23: after five days of taking an oral phosphate binder, intestinal phosphate absorption decreased and urinary phosphorus excretion fell. Likewise, reducing the phosphate intake of 13 healthy men from 1500 to 625 mg/day induced a 30% decrease in serum FGF-23, suggesting that phosphorus intake may directly affect FGF-23 expression [99].

More recently, Moe et al. studied, in a random cross-over design in nine stage 3 CKD patients, the effects of two different diets with the same phosphorus content, e.g., 800 mg/d, one from animal sources and the other from vegetarian sources for one week each [100]. They observed during the vegetarian diet phase the known reduction in urinary phosphate excretion and serum phosphate, in response to the reduced gut absorption of phosphate bound to vegetal fibers. More interestingly, they showed for the first time a significant 28% reduction in serum FGF-23 during the vegetarian diet as compared with the mainly animal protein diet during which FGF-23 increased by 40% ($p < 0.01$) [100].

These data emphasize one reason that it is mandatory to monitor the dietary habits of CKD patients. Controlling serum phosphate below 4.4 mg/dL must include a phosphate-restricted diet. If the type and quantity of dietary protein intake is not controlled, even major increase in the hormones that control serum phosphorus (PTH and FGF-23) may not be able to compensate for the higher phosphorus intake and thereby control the development of hyperphosphatemia.

Effect of Low Protein Diets on Acidemia, Anemia and Blood Pressure

There are subsequent indirect beneficial effects of a reduction in protein intake during CKD on metabolic acidosis, hemoglobin status and blood pressure control. Indeed, Chauveau et al. showed that there is an inverse relationship between protein intake and serum bicarbonate in a cross-sectional survey of more than 7000 hemodialysis patients [101]. In ten stage 5 CKD patients receiving a supplemented very low protein diet (VLPD) for 12 months, the same investigators showed an increase in serum bicarbonate from 24.2 to 26.5 mmol/L, $p < 0.05$ [102]. From the MDRD study, Mitch and Remuzzi also estimated that a reduction of 0.20 g protein/kg/day significantly increased serum bicarbonate ($p < 0.05$) [103]. These changes mainly pertain to the acid-producing nature of animal proteins, which was identified by Claude Bernard in the late 1800s. Moving to vegetal protein will induce alkalotic urine, as observed in the majority of ruminant species. De Brito et al. demonstrated improvement in serum albumin and mid-arm muscle circumference of CKD patients and slowing of progression of their CKD after

administering oral sodium bicarbonate [104]. It should be noted that ketoacid supplements are often given as alkaline salts, and the alkali from the ketoacid supplements may play the major role in increasing serum bicarbonate in CKD patients. Thus, another benefit of reducing animal protein intake or giving the ketoacid analogs may be to increase serum bicarbonate and, by this effect, retard progression of CKD.

Anemia may be improved while reducing protein intake. Indeed, Di Iorio et al. observed an improvement in hemoglobin levels in a randomized prospective trial in 20 MHD patients receiving either a low protein intake or a VLPD supplemented with ketoacids [105]. In the VLPD group, serum hemoglobin remained stable and erythropoietin dose could be decreased by approximately 35% during the two-year duration of the trial. These investigators revealed a strong and inverse relationship between the change in patients' hemoglobin levels and serum parathyroid hormone, which is not unexpected since parathormone is responsible for a well-described resistance to the effects of erythropoietin on bone marrow. Improvement in parathyroid hormone was the consequence of the reduction of the dietary phosphate load and possibly to a higher calcium intake associated with the ketoacids. VLPDs might therefore be credited for these beneficial effects, although they could be considered as indirect.

Finally another dietary change that can be viewed positive is the fact that lowering animal protein may also reduce sodium intake, since culinary habits often add salt while cooking meat. In the ERIKA study, a six-month trial comparing three different levels of protein intake in 110 stage IV−V CKD patients, Bellizzi et al. showed a positive relationship between 24-h urinary sodium and urinary urea excretion, indicating that patients who ate less protein had the most significant reduction in sodium intake, and a greater reduction in blood pressure [86]. Thus, patients may reduce their blood pressure and lower their daily pill burden as a result of a reduced sodium intake with LPDs.

Nutritional Safety of Restricting Protein Intake

The question of whether LPDs are safe has been a subject of controversy [106] and has been examined by estimating the nutritional status and survival of patients who received LPDs for years. Chauveau et al. [102] reported regional body composition measured by DEXA and nutritional status in 10 patients receiving a very low protein diet (0.3 g protein/kg/day supplemented with amino acids and ketoanalogs) for one year. There was no change in anthropometric measures and serum albumin during the one-year follow-up [102]. DEXA analyses revealed a decrease in lean body mass during the first three months following the reduction in protein intake that was not fully corrected to baseline at one year (baseline: 46.2 kg; one year: 45.1 kg). Body fat mass increased slightly at three months and one year (baseline: 20.1 kg; one year: 21.4 kg, p < 0.01). Interestingly, there seemed to be a redistribution of lean body mass in favor of an increase in lean truncal mass, which was sustained during the one-year of follow-up [102]. It should be mentioned that during this trial, energy intake was 27.8 ± 7.6 at baseline, 31.0 ± 8.1 at three months and 29.8 ± 8.8 kcal/kg/day at one year. Thus, the alterations observed after three months of a very low protein intake spontaneously improved over time, and became of no clinical importance after one year of follow-up. These results occurred in association with the benefits observed with regard to insulin resistance, bone metabolism and reduction in uremic symptoms [102].

Long-term LPDs have been reported to be safe by other investigators [107–111]. In the MDRD study, body weight and composition were assessed every three months during the 2.2-year mean follow-up period [111]. The actual reductions in protein intake with the LPD and VLPD were less than prescribed (actual vs. prescribed: 0.71 vs. 0.58 and 1.11 vs. 1.3 g/kg BW/day, respectively, in Study A; 0.48 vs. 0.28 and 0.72 vs. 0.58 g/kg BW/day, respectively, in Study B). Furthermore, energy intake was low despite intensive counseling (range: 22.5 to 26.7 kcal/kg/day among different diet subgroups). Urinary creatinine excretion decreased during trial, most probably from a decrease in meat and thus creatinine intake from the LPD, In Study A, body weight decreased by two kg in the LPD group (from 85.4 ± 13.5 to 83.2 ± 12.8, p < 0.05), whereas there was no change in the control group, potentially underlining a reduction in nutritional status, possibly from calorie rather from protein intake since serum albumin did not change. Despite this, overall clinical and biochemical surveys, as well as end-point recording did not show evidence for nutritional impairment during a follow-up period of two to three years [111]. Figure 14.7 shows that serum albumin levels increased slightly in all groups from baseline, but this increase was greater in the low protein diet group as compared with the control group in Study A (Figure 14.7, top, solid line). The decrease in serum transferrin during the study is somewhat difficult to interpret, because iron stores and the presence of inflammation were not monitored. Finally, although statistically significant, these changes in body composition may not be of clinical importance (−2 to 0 kg for body weight and −0.5 to +0.5 % for body fat mass over 32 months). They underscore the importance for the physician to ensure that there is adequate nutritional monitoring and, where indicated, nutritional intervention in these patients (Table 14.1). Importantly, no patient was withdrawn from the MDRD study because of impaired nutritional status.

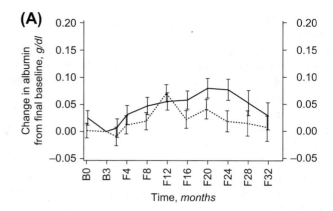

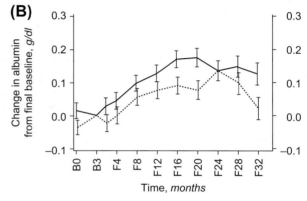

FIGURE 14.7 Mean changes in serum albumin from the end of Baseline in Study A (top) and Study B (bottom) during the Modification of Diet in Renal Disease Study.

TABLE 14.1 Estimation of Dietary Protein Intake (DPI) in a Stable Noncatabolic 70 kg Adult Patient Undertaking a 0.6 g Protein/kg/day Diet, Based on a Daily Urinary Nitrogen Appearance

UNA = 4.8 g/day

DPI = 7.25 UNA + 10.9 = 45.7 g/day

DPI/kg = 45.7/70 = 0.65 g/kg

Compliance to the diet, e.g., an upper actual protein intake no greater than 20% above prescribed intake, is considered acceptable if this patient presents a UNA no greater than 5.5 g per day.

From Kopple et al., Kidney Int 1997;52:486–94.

What is the long-term consequence of low protein diets on survival after dialysis therapy is started? Walser et al. reported that patients ingesting a very low protein diet who were carefully followed before they commenced dialysis treatments could postpone dialysis for many months, even with very low GFRs, before clinical symptoms occurred [112,113]. Aparicio and colleagues reported encouraging outcomes in 165 maintenance dialysis patients who were treated with very low protein diets before they developed endstage renal disease and commenced chronic dialysis therapy [110].

Chauveau et al. more recently re-evaluated long-term survival in 203 patients previously treated with VLPDs and amino acids/ketoacids (SVLPD) who were then treated on maintenance dialysis or received a kidney transplant [114,115]. Analyzing these patients with an unbroken follow-up for ten years after the start of renal replacement therapy, these authors clearly showed that patients who received a SVLPD before ESRD had a survival as good as patients without specific diet as reported in the French Dialysis registry, e.g., 79% at 5 years and 63% at 10 years [115]. Their results stand in contrast with those of Menon et al. who reanalyzed the late patient survival of the supplemented very low protein diet subgroup of the MDRD study [116]. Although patients who received the SVLPD had a poorer survival seven years after the termination of the MDRD study, there was no clinical or biological information on patients to document survival during those seven years, and it is difficult to incriminate 30 months of well-followed dietary intervention versus 80 months of virtually unknown follow-up [114]. However, it must be recognized that in contrast to the Menon et al. follow-up of the MDRD Trial, the studies of Walser et al. and Aparicio et al. did not have a randomized concomitant control group and used historical controls instead.

CLINICAL EVIDENCE OF THE EFFECTS OF LOW PROTEIN DIETS

It has been proposed for many years that patients with advanced kidney disease should reduce their protein intake in order to decrease uremic symptoms. A number of experimental studies in animals with CKD, usually in rats, reported beneficial effects of low protein intakes on renal function, it was proposed to test this hypothesis in humans. Before analyzing in detail these studies, some general remarks should be made. First, as discussed earlier, most animal research studies were performed using extremely high or low levels of dietary protein (e.g., unphysiological or very large differences in dietary protein content between groups), in order to identify mechanisms and explain therapeutic effects. Second, in many experiments, substantial numbers of animals died without analysis of the potential role of the diet in these deaths. Only data from the survivors were analyzed, a fact that would not apply to human research. Third, most laboratory research is short-term, in animals that do not have other chronic diseases, in contrast to the clinical status of many patients presenting with chronic kidney disease. Thus, the response to low protein diets in CKD patients may differ from experimental studies in animals. Indeed, as compared with animal research, there are specific caveats to clinical research, such as the

compliance to treatment in the effects of medications, in medicinal intakes among different patients, and in the genetic profile and phenotypes of the patients studied. These factors are among reasons why large numbers of patients are required to test a single hypothesis in a clinical trial.

Clinical Trials

More than 50 trials have assessed the effects of low protein diets in humans with renal disease. These studies have been reviewed in the Cochrane analysis [2]. In many of these trials, the methodological quality was judged to be poor, based on uncontrolled design, nonrandom allocation of diets, or the use of retrospective analyses. Furthermore, many of these reports, undertaken in the early 1970s, did not use adequate markers of renal function to assess the effect of the dietary intervention, particularly since the serum creatinine or its derivatives (creatinine clearance, 1/serum creatinine) are strongly influenced by the primary intervention, e.g., reducing protein intake (see above). Since contradictory results were often reported, we only reviewed the largest trials that were of high methodological quality, i.e., those large prospective, controlled trials with a random allocation of dietary intervention.

The study of Rosman et al. examined the effects of two different levels of protein restriction in 247 patients followed for two to four years [117,118]. Protein intake was reduced to 0.6 g/kg/day in patients who had a GFR between 60 and 30 mL/min, and 0.4 g/kg/day in those with a GFR between 30 and 10 mL/min [118]. Both of the control groups for these two low-protein diet groups were allowed an ad libitum protein intake diet. Based on the slope of the 1/serum creatinine ratio over time, it was concluded that some but not all patients benefited from the restricted diet: only males appeared to respond with significant slowing of GFR, and patients with polycystic kidney disease did not reduce their decline in GFR with a restricted diet. Measurements of urinary urea excretion indicated that protein intake with the LPD only decreased to 30 to 35% below the unrestricted protein diets, which ranged from 0.90–0.95 g/kg/day in the moderately GFR impaired group and from 0.70–0.80 g/kg/day in the more advanced CKD group. Whereas no difference in renal survival was observed between the control and LPD diet groups who had less severe CKD, in the more advanced CKD groups there was a marked improvement in renal survival in the patients treated with protein restriction as compared to the controls after four years of follow-up (percent survival off-dialysis, 60% vs. 30%, p < 0.025) [118]. The authors concluded that such dietary intervention would be more beneficial in some subgroups of patients whose CKD progresses more rapidly, such as males, and patients with glomerulonephritis. They also noted that compliance was very good after a short period of training and was sustained over time, and that protein restriction did not cause wasting [118].

The second large scale randomized study was performed by Ihle et al. in Australia and published in 1989 [108]. They studied 72 patients with advanced CKD for 18 months. Patients were randomized to receive either a control diet or a diet providing 0.4 g protein/kg/day. The actual protein intakes, estimated from urinary urea output, was approximately 0.8 and 0.6 g/kg/day, respectively, in the two diet groups. GFR was measured every six months by ^{51}Cr-EDTA clearances. The GFR decreased only in the control group (from 15 to 6 mL/min over 18 months, p < 0.01), whereas no decrease in GFR occurred in the LPD group. The number of patients who started dialysis during the trial was significantly greater in the control group (p < 0.05). Body composition varied somewhat, with a significant loss of body weight only in the LPD group, whereas there was no change in other anthropometric measures or in serum albumin in either group. There was no dietary analysis of intakes, so that an insufficient energy intake could not be ruled out to explain the loss of weight with the LPD. The authors concluded that there was a beneficial effect of this moderately reduced protein intake (p < 0.01) [108].

Two years later, Williams and colleagues published the results of three different nutritional interventions in 95 patients with advanced kidney disease [109]. After a six-month run-in period, patients were randomized to receive, for about 18 months, a 0.6 g protein/kg/day and 800 mg/day phosphorus intake, a diet providing 1000 mg phosphorus/day plus phosphate binders and without protein restriction, or a diet unrestricted in protein and phosphorus diet. Dietary compliance was estimated by urinary urea output and dietary recalls and averaged 0.7, 1.02 and 1.14 g protein/kg/day and 815, 1000 and 1400 mg phosphorus/day, respectively. Slight weight losses were observed in the low protein- and phosphorus- restricted group and the ad libitum protein- and phosphorus restricted group (−1.3 and −1.65 kg BW for these two groups, respectively). Other anthropometric measures did not change. There was no difference in the decrease in creatinine clearance over time among any of the three groups. However, the creatinine clearance is of questionable accuracy as a measure of GFR, and thus no firm conclusion on renal protection can be reliably drawn from this study [109]. Death or the commencement of dialysis therapy also did not differ among the three groups and occurred in 18 individuals prescribed the low protein and

phosphorus diet, 18 patients assigned to the low phosphorus diet, and 16 patients on the control diet.

The Northern Italian Cooperative Study Group, in 1991, reported the results of a large randomized controlled study in 456 patients with a GFR lower than 60 mL/min who were followed for two years [119]. Patients either received a control protein intake of 1 g/kg/day or a low protein intake providing 0.6 g/kg/day, both diets provided an energy intake of at least 30 kcal/kg/day. The key outcome criterion was renal survival defined as the start of dialysis therapy or the doubling of serum creatinine during the trial. Dietary protein intake was serially monitored by urinary urea output in a random sample of patients. Actual protein intakes were, however, not very different. The control group ingested, on average, 0.90 g protein/kg/day and the low protein group ate a mean of 0.78 g/kg/day, and there was a large overlap in the protein intakes between individuals from both groups (underlining the necessity for intensive dietary counseling and monitoring). There was only a borderline significant difference between the control and restricted protein groups in reaching a renal endpoint (p = 0.059) with slightly less patients in the latter group reaching the endpoint.

A smaller randomized trial from France, reported by Malvy et al., examined the effects of more severe protein restriction (0.3 g protein/kg/day) supplemented with essential amino acids and ketoacid analogs (Ketosteril®, 0.17 g/kg BW/day) vs. 0.65 g protein/kg/day in 50 patients with severe renal insufficiency (creatinine clearance lower than 20 mL/min) [107]. Patients were followed until dialysis or until the creatinine clearance decreased to less than 5 mL/min/1.73 m^2. Kaplan–Meier survival analyses did not show differences in renal survival between the two diets, but the modest sample size of the study may explain this result. There was a loss of 2.7 kg BW in the very low protein diet group over three years that was derived equally from losses of fat and lean body mass. No weight loss or body composition change was observed in the groups prescribed the 0.65 g protein/kg diet. Serum calcium was better maintained in the very low protein supplemented diet, probably due to the calcium salt content of the ketoanalogs supplement. For those patients presenting with severe renal failure at the onset of the study inclusion (GFR ≤ 15 mL/min/1.73 m^2), the "half-life" for renal death was nine months in the 0.65 g protein/kg/day as compared to 21 months in the most restricted diet (0.3 g protein/kg/day), which although not statistically significant, represents a clinically impressive difference in outcome between the patient groups.

The Modification of Diet in Renal Disease study was the largest clinical study yet performed to test the effects of low protein and low phosphorus intakes and strict blood pressure control on the progression of renal disease in more than 800 patients [1,73,120–126]. Two groups of patients were studied, one with moderate renal dysfunction (Study A, GFR: 25–55 mL/min/ 1.73 m^2) and the second with more advanced renal failure (Study B, GFR: 13–24 mL/min/1.73 m^2). The patients were randomized to receive 1 g protein/kg/ day or more vs. 0.6 g protein/kg/day and to reach a mean blood pressure of 105 or 92 mmHg in group A, and 0.6 g protein/kg/day vs. 0.3 g/kg/day plus a ketoacid supplement and comparable blood pressure goals in group B. The primary objective was the effect of both interventions, in a Latin square design and intention-to-treat analysis, on the progression of kidney disease. This was estimated by the changes in ^{125}I-iothalamate clearance measured every four months over more than two years. The mean patient follow-up was 2.2 years [122]. Actual protein intakes, estimated from urinary urea excretion, were 1.11 ± 0.19 vs. 0.73 ± 0.15 g protein/kg/day in group A (n = 585), and 0.69 ± 0.12 vs. 0.46 ± 0.15 g protein/kg/day in group B (n = 255). The overall results appeared at first glance somewhat disappointing. There was no difference between the groups with regard to the decline in GFR in Study A. In Study B, there was a borderline significantly greater rate of decline in GFR in the group prescribed the 0.6 g protein/kg/day diet vs. the ketoacid supplemented diet (p = 0.07).

These raw results require several comments. First, as shown in Figure 14.8, during the first four months of diet intervention in study A, there was a sharp initial decrease in GFR in the group with the more restricted protein intake (mean DPI, 0.73 g/kg/day). This was followed by a slower linear decrease than occurred with the larger protein intake (mean DPI, 1.11 g/kg/day). This initial four-month decrease in GFR with the lower DPI is now considered to be the consequence of the

reduction in glomerular hemodynamics that follows protein restriction [30]. Arguably, in retrospect, there should have been a run-in period that included the first several weeks of dietary protein treatment before the key GFR outcome data began to be collected. If this had been done, if the follow-up period of the study had been a bit longer, e.g., from four months after the start of the study until three years later, and if the slope of GFR decrease had remained constant, this slope would have been significantly lower in the more restricted protein group in Study A (Figure 14.8, p = 0.009) [126]. This would have indicated a beneficial effect of dietary protein restriction in reducing the rate of decrease in GFR.

Second, unexpectedly, the actual rate of progression of renal failure was lower than expected when the study was designed (i.e., in study A, the reduction in GFR was observed to be 3.8 mL/min/year rather than the projected rate of decrease of 6 mL/min/year) [120]. This had a major negative impact on the ability of this study to demonstrate statistical differences. An additional three-month period of follow-up would have been necessary to correct for this reduction in GFR decline. Thus, it is tempting to classify this large clinical trial as inconclusive rather than negative. In addition, when patients were followed in an open fashion after the end of the study and up to 44 months of diet, the difference in the cumulative incidence of ESRD or death reached borderline significance in the patients who were assigned to the lower protein diet (p = 0.056, Figure 14.9). It should be remembered that, in the large diabetes DCCT trial for strict blood glucose control and its effects on renal impairment, no effect was detected at two years, and the suppressive effect of strict glucose control on the development of microalbuminuria or proteinuria was only observed after four years of treatment [127].

Although not definitive, correlational analyses may give further insights into the efficacy of dietary

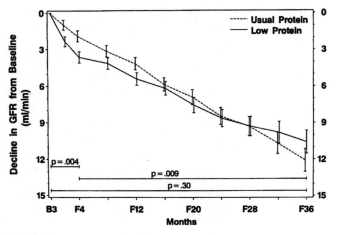

FIGURE 14.8 The glomerular filtration rate decline during the Modification of Diet in Renal Disease Study (Study A) with separate analyses including or not the first 4-month adaptation period.

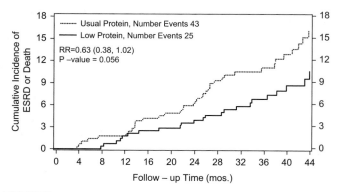

FIGURE 14.9 Occurrence of kidney failure or death in Study A of the Modification of Diet in Renal Disease Study including a 10-month additional follow-up after completion of the study (p = 0.056).

intervention. In this regard, when patients in the MDRD Study were analyzed with regard to their actual protein intake, as estimated through either diet interviews and diaries or urea nitrogen appearance, and independently of the group to which they were randomized, a strong relation was found in both Study A and Study B patients combined between the magnitude of protein intake and the GFR slope (p = 0.011) or renal death (e.g., risk of death or ESRD) (p = 0.001) [126]. Indeed, for Study B, a regression model estimated that for every reduction in 0.2 g protein/kg/day, there was a 1.15 mL/min/year reduction in GFR decline and a 49% reduction in the incidence of renal death [126]. There was no additional effect of amino acid/ketoacid supplements on retardation of progression of renal failure. This finding contradicts a previous observation made in the MDRD Feasibility Study in which a trend for a protective effect (p = 0.06) of amino acids/ketoacids was observed [125]. These latter authors suggested that the different ketoacid composition used in the MDRD Study B, and particularly the greater tryptophan content, may account for the lack of effectiveness of the ketoacids in the MDRD study [125,128].

A comparable analysis in study A showed a nonsignificant trend (p = 0.075), for a more moderate impact of protein restriction with a 0.32 mL/min/year slower GFR decline per each 0.2 g protein/kg/day reduction. Thus, these secondary analyses of the MDRD study tend to support a moderately beneficial effect of reduced protein intakes in patients with CKD. These effects were related, in a gradient fashion, to a reduction in the protein intake rather than to a well-identified degree of protein restriction that was necessary to slow progression. There was no apparent effect of either protein intake or blood pressure control in patients with polycystic kidney disease. Since these individuals constituted 25% of the total patients in the MDRD Study, this fact also contributed to the ambiguous results of the MDRD Study [129].

In 2003 Di Iorio et al. randomly evaluated in 20 patients during two years how a very low protein intake supplemented with amino acids/ketoacids will affect erythropoietin therapy [105]. Actual protein intakes were 0.49 g/kg/day plus a supplement of ketoacids vs. 0.79 g/kg/day. In the low protein diet plus ketoacids, only two patients began dialysis as compared to seven patients in the higher dietary protein group (p < 0.05). Interestingly, erythropoietin responsiveness improved in patients prescribed the very low protein-ketoacid regimen, and this improvement in erythropoietin response was inversely related to the serum parathormone level, the decrease in phosphorus intake and the decrease in serum phosphorus concentration (see above).

Mirescu et al. [130] followed 53 patients with stage IV–V CKD over a period of 60 weeks. Twenty-six patients were randomly assigned to a diet of 0.6 g protein/kg/day and 27 were assigned to a diet containing only 0.3 g protein/kg/day supplemented with ketoacids. Actual protein intakes were 0.59 ± 0.08 and 0.32 ± 0.07 g protein/kg/day respectively. There were no death and seven of the 26 patients assigned to the 0.6 g protein/kg/d diet reached endstage renal disease compared to only one of 27 who began dialysis in the very low protein/ketoacid group (p = 0.06). Serum phosphate values decreased from 1.91 ± 0.68 to 1.45 ± 0.66 mmol/L (p < 0.05) in patients with the very low protein/ketoacid diet. Otherwise, there was no change in nutritional status in the two groups and no significant difference in the GFR decrease estimated from serum creatinine. Unfortunately, the study was underpowered to examine if dietary protein restriction could slow the progression of kidney disease. The authors estimated that approximately 100 patients per group would be required to determine if there is a significant difference in the number of renal deaths associated with the very low protein/ketoacid diet.

Cianciaruso et al. [131] studied how two different levels of protein intake, 0.55 vs. 0.80 g/kg/day may influence patients with stage IV-V CKD during 18 months of observation. Two hundred and twelve patients were randomly assigned to receive the lower protein intake, and 211 patients were prescribed the higher level of dietary protein. Notably, there was a difference in the average values of protein intake between the two groups. Based on urinary urea excretion, the protein-restricted group actually ate 0.72 g protein/kg/day, while those assigned to the higher protein group ate 0.92 g protein/kg/day (p < 0.05). Serum concentrations of phosphorus, parathormone and bicarbonate did not differ between diets, and no patient was treated with a more restricted protein diet supplemented by essential amino acids/ketoacids. By contrast, values for urinary urea, sodium and phosphate excretion were all reduced in those assigned to the low-protein diet group, suggesting that exposure to toxic metabolic products was reduced by the lower protein intake. The authors found no alterations in body composition or other nutritional indices in either group. When the results were evaluated by intention-to-treat analysis, 13 patients assigned to the 0.8 g protein/kg/day diet vs. nine patients assigned to the 0.55 g protein/kg/day died or began dialysis therapy during the study.

Brunori et al. examined elderly patients with stage V CKD who were treated with a protein-restricted diet or chronic dialysis [132]. Patients were randomly assigned either to begin maintenance dialysis (n = 56 patients) or to receive a very low protein diet (0.3 g protein/kg/day) supplemented with essential amino acids/ketoacids (n = 56). After one year of observation, the survival rate was 83.7% and 87.3% in the dialysis and low protein

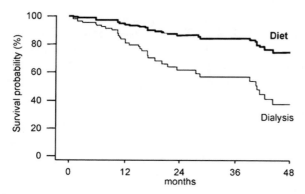

FIGURE 14.10 Survival of elderly stage V chronic kidney disease patients randomly assigned to begin dialysis treatment or to receive a very low protein diet supplemented with ketoanalogs (p = 0.01).

diet respectively (p = 0.6). Based on an intention-to-treat analysis (including analyses of those in the diet-restricted group who were switched to dialysis therapy), there was a continuous benefit of the protein-restricted diet over time (Figure 14.10). Patients assigned to chronic dialysis had a 50% higher occurrence of hospitalization. The authors concluded that there was no difference in the lifespan of elderly patients assigned to the LPD plus ketoacids vs. those treated by maintenance dialysis [132].

Meta-Analyses

Meta-analyses are considered to be second in validity for the evidence it provides, immediately behind the evidence provided by large randomized trials (considered to be level one), and equal to small randomized trials [2,132,133,133]. Three meta-analyses have been performed concerning low protein diets [2,134,135]. These reports have searched the literature by different methods to ensure the most exhaustive collection of clinical trials, including searching international databases in non-English languages. The most rigorous criteria for selecting or rejecting papers for analysis include consideration of randomized controlled trials only, since it is generally believed that nonrandomized controlled trials are more likely to give biased results than are their randomized counterparts [135].

To examine the impact of LPDS on loss of GFR, Kasiske and associates summarized a total of 24 controlled clinical trials, 13 of which were randomized [128,135]. The key outcome was the loss of GFR over time (mL/min/year) in groups receiving or not receiving a LPD. A total of 2248 patients were identified of which 1919 were enrolled in randomized studies. GFR loss was lower by 0.53 mL/min/year (95% CI, 0.08−0.98) in the lower protein intake group (p < 0.05). We have identified 10 randomized controlled trials suitable for analysis among more than 50 clinical trials

that assessed the effects of LPDs for the treatment of patients with chronic renal insufficiency [2]. Since, as seen earlier, most of these trials did not use an adequate marker of renal failure progression, we decided to define the renal death (e.g., death or the start of chronic dialysis therapy during the study) as the primary outcome. This criterion was easily obtained by analysis of published papers or by direct contact with investigators regarding both the control and the restricted dietary protein groups of patients. Gender and the nature of the renal diseases were equally distributed in control and protein restricted groups; thus, this meta-analysis avoided the likelihood that a disproportionate distribution of independent causes of more rapid progression of renal disease would influence the results. The results are depicted in Figure 14.11. Individual odds ratios are indicated at the top of Figure 14.11 and the pooled results shown on the bottom line. Overall, there were 1002 patients in the more restricted protein intake groups and 998 individuals in the higher protein intakes groups. A total of 113 renal deaths were found in the low protein diet group vs. 168 in the control group, giving an odds ratio for low protein vs. control of 0.68, with a 95% confidence interval of 0.55−0.84 (p = 0.0002, Figure 14.11). This indicates that LPDs may result in a 32% reduction for death or the need to start dialysis therapy as compared with larger or unlimited protein intakes [2]. Pedrini et al. confirmed these findings, in six trials including the MDRD study [134]. These authors reported an additional analysis for diabetic nephropathy, using different outcome measures: renal function or albuminuria. Of note is the fact that the average baseline renal function of these diabetic patients was less reduced, with a mean GFR of 77 mL/min, and the trials were of smaller size (n = 8 to 35). The overall results of this meta-analysis were also in favor of the low protein diet, with an odds ratio of 0.56 (CI:0.40−0.77, p < 0.001). However, the patients' sample size was 108, a very small number rarely seen in the meta-analytic process. Further larger scale studies in patients with diabetic nephropathy appear necessary to confirm these results.

However, it should be noted that in the meta-analyses in which renal death was used as the primary outcome, the lower protein intake might have delayed the onset of dialysis therapy by rendering the patients less uremic, by reducing the rate of generation of uremic toxins, rather than by slowing the rate of loss of GFR.

The number needed to treat (NNT) is a methodological tool used to compare the efficacy of a given treatment in different studies [136]. It theoretically represents the number of patients that must be treated by a given intervention in order to avoid one extra death or other adverse event per year. From the present meta-analysis data, NNT conferred by a low protein

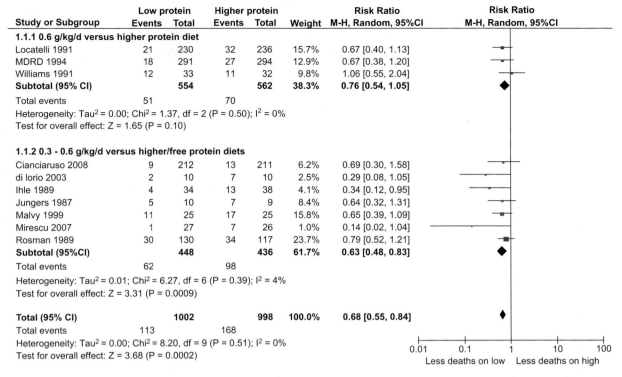

Study or Subgroup	Low protein Events	Total	Higher protein Events	Total	Weight	Risk Ratio M-H, Random, 95%CI
1.1.1 0.6 g/kg/d versus higher protein diet						
Locatelli 1991	21	230	32	236	15.7%	0.67 [0.40, 1.13]
MDRD 1994	18	291	27	294	12.9%	0.67 [0.38, 1.20]
Williams 1991	12	33	11	32	9.8%	1.06 [0.55, 2.04]
Subtotal (95% CI)		**554**		**562**	**38.3%**	**0.76 [0.54, 1.05]**
Total events	51		70			
Heterogeneity: Tau^2 = 0.00; Chi^2 = 1.37, df = 2 (P = 0.50); I^2 = 0%						
Test for overall effect: Z = 1.65 (P = 0.10)						
1.1.2 0.3 - 0.6 g/kg/d versus higher/free protein diets						
Cianciaruso 2008	9	212	13	211	6.2%	0.69 [0.30, 1.58]
di Iorio 2003	2	10	7	10	2.5%	0.29 [0.08, 1.05]
Ihle 1989	4	34	13	38	4.1%	0.34 [0.12, 0.95]
Jungers 1987	5	10	7	9	8.4%	0.64 [0.32, 1.31]
Malvy 1999	11	25	17	25	15.8%	0.65 [0.39, 1.09]
Mirescu 2007	1	27	7	26	1.0%	0.14 [0.02, 1.04]
Rosman 1989	30	130	34	117	23.7%	0.79 [0.52, 1.21]
Subtotal (95%CI)		**448**		**436**	**61.7%**	**0.63 [0.48, 0.83]**
Total events	62		98			
Heterogeneity: Tau^2 = 0.01; Chi^2 = 6.27, df = 6 (P = 0.39); I^2 = 4%						
Test for overall effect: Z = 3.31 (P = 0.0009)						
Total (95% CI)		**1002**		**998**	**100.0%**	**0.68 [0.55, 0.84]**
Total events	113		168			
Heterogeneity: Tau^2 = 0.00; Chi^2 = 8.20, df = 9 (P = 0.51); I^2 = 0%						
Test for overall effect: Z = 3.68 (P = 0.0002)						

FIGURE 14.11 A meta-analysis of randomized controlled studies of the influence of low-protein diets in reducing renal death. A square denotes the odds ratio for each trial, and the diamond the combined results of all trials; 95% confidence intervals are represented by horizontal lines.

intervention stands between 2 to 56, depending on the study. This is quite a narrow range, and favorably compares with the well-accepted mortality reduction obtained by statins in the 4S trial (NNT = 30) and WOSCOPS study (NNT = 111) [137]. This analysis gives further support to the thesis that dietary protein restriction is an effective therapeutic intervention.

CONCLUSION

Many experimental studies provide evidence for the beneficial effects of low protein intakes. These benefits include reduction in uremic toxicity, healthier nutritional status, particularly if energy intake is well maintained, reduced proteinuria and slowing of the loss of renal function and finally delay in the need for renal replacement therapy. These results have been observed with a fairly good level of evidence in large clinical trials and meta-analyses. Such low protein diets, of course, do not prevent the loss of renal function in patients with rapidly progressive renal disease. Thus, in most other patients with chronic kidney disease, perhaps excluding those with polycystic kidney disease, it may be worth prescribing a reduction in dietary protein intake, including patients receiving nephroprotective ACEIs, ARBs, or renin antagonist medications.

References

[1] Effects of diet and antihypertensive therapy on creatinine clearance and serum creatinine concentration in the Modification of Diet in Renal Disease Study. J Am Soc Nephrol Apr 1996;7(4):556−66.

[2] Fouque D, Laville M. Low protein diets for chronic kidney disease in non diabetic adults. Cochrane Database Syst Rev 2009;(3):CD001892.

[3] Levey AS. Measurement of renal function in chronic renal disease. Kidney Int Jul 1990;38(1):167−84.

[4] Edwards OM, Bayliss RI, Millen S. Urinary creatinine excretion as an index of the copleteness of 24-hour urine collections. Lancet Nov 29 1969;2(7631):1165−6.

[5] Mayersohn M, Conrad KA, Achari R. The influence of a cooked meat meal on creatinine plasma concentration and creatinine clearance. British Journal of Clinical Pharmacology Feb 1983;15(2):227−30.

[6] Mitch WE, Walser M. A proposed mechanism for reduced creatinine excretion in severe chronic renal failure. Nephron 1978;21(5):248−54.

[7] Crim MC, Calloway DH, Margen S. Creatine metabolism in men: urinary creatine and creatinine excretions with creatine feeding. The Journal of Nutrition Apr 1975;105(4):428−38.

[8] Shemesh O, Golbetz H, Kriss JP, Myers BD. Limitations of creatinine as a filtration marker in glomerulopathic patients. Kidney Int Nov 1985;28(5):830−8.

[9] Mitch WE, Collier VU, Walser M. Creatinine metabolism in chronic renal failure. Clin Sci (Lond) Apr 1980;58(4):327−35.

[10] Walser M. Assessing renal function from creatinine measurements in adults with chronic renal failure. Am J Kidney Dis Jul 1998;32(1):23−31.

[11] Zaltzman JS, Whiteside C, Cattran DC, Lopez FM, Logan AG. Accurate measurement of impaired glomerular filtration using single-dose oral cimetidine. Am J Kidney Dis Apr 1996;27(4): 504—11.

[12] Kemperman FA, Silberbusch J, Slaats EH, et al. Estimation of the glomerular filtration rate in NIDDM patients from plasma creatinine concentration after cimetidine administration. Diabetes Care Feb 1998;21(2):216—20.

[13] The Modification of Diet in Renal Disease Study: design, methods, and results from the feasibility study. Am J Kidney Dis Jul 1992;20(1):18—33.

[14] Levey AS. Assessing the effectiveness of therapy to prevent the progression of renal disease. Am J Kidney Dis Jul 1993;22(1): 207—14.

[15] Cockcroft DW, Gault MH. Prediction of creatinine clearance from serum creatinine. Nephron 1976;16(1):31—41.

[16] Walser M, Drew HH, Guldan JL. Prediction of glomerular filtration rate from serum creatinine concentration in advanced chronic renal failure. Kidney Int Nov 1993;44(5): 1145—8.

[17] Schold JD, Navaneethan SD, Jolly SE, et al. Implications of the CKD-EPI GFR estimation equation in clinical practice. Clin J Am Soc Nephrol Mar 2011;6(3):497—504.

[18] Levey AS, Bosch JP, Lewis JB, Greene T, Rogers N, Roth D. A more accurate method to estimate glomerular filtration rate from serum creatinine: a new prediction equation. Modification of Diet in Renal Disease Study Group. Ann Intern Med Mar 16 1999;130(6):461—70.

[19] Levey AS, Stevens LA, Schmid CH, et al. A new equation to estimate glomerular filtration rate. Ann Intern Med May 5 2009;150(9):604—12.

[20] Anastasio P, Cirillo M, Spitali L, Frangiosa A, Pollastro RM, De Santo NG. Level of hydration and renal function in healthy humans. Kidney Int Aug 2001;60(2):748—56.

[21] Fouque D, Laville M, Boissel JP, Chifflet R, Labeeuw M, Zech PY. Controlled low protein diets in chronic renal insufficiency: meta-analysis. BMJ Jan 25 1992;304(6821):216—20.

[22] Farr LE, Smadel JE. The effect of dietary protein on the course of nephrotoxic nephritis in rats. The Journal of Experimental Medicine Nov 30 1939;70(6):615—27.

[23] Kleinknecht C, Salusky I, Broyer M, Gubler MC. Effect of various protein diets on growth, renal function, and survival of uremic rats. Kidney Int May 1979;15(5):534—41.

[24] Brenner BM. Nephron adaptation to renal injury or ablation. Am J Physiol Sep 1985;249(3 Pt 2):F324—37.

[25] Hostetter TH, Meyer TW, Rennke HG, Brenner BM. Chronic effects of dietary protein in the rat with intact and reduced renal mass. Kidney Int Oct 1986;30(4):509—17.

[26] Mauer SM, Steffes MW, Azar S, Brown DM. Effects of dietary protein content in streptozotocin-diabetic rats. Kidney Int Jan 1989;35(1):48—59.

[27] Nath KA, Kren SM, Hostetter TH. Dietary protein restriction in established renal injury in the rat. Selective role of glomerular capillary pressure in progressive glomerular dysfunction. J Clin Invest Nov 1986;78(5):1199—205.

[28] Premen AJ. Potential mechanisms mediating postprandial renal hyperemia and hyperfiltration. Faseb J Feb 1988;2(2): 131—7.

[29] Diamond JR. Effects of dietary interventions on glomerular pathophysiology. Am J Physiol Jan 1990;258(1 Pt 2):F1—8.

[30] King AJ, Levey AS. Dietary protein and renal function. J Am Soc Nephrol May 1993;3(11):1723—37.

[31] Hirschberg R, Kopple JD. Response of insulin-like growth factor I and renal hemodynamics to a high- and low-protein diet in the rat. J Am Soc Nephrol Feb 1991;1(8):1034—40.

[32] Don BR, Blake S, Hutchison FN, Kaysen GA, Schambelan M. Dietary protein intake modulates glomerular eicosanoid production in the rat. Am J Physiol Apr 1989;256(4 Pt 2): F711—8.

[33] Jaffa AA, Vio CP, Silva RH, et al. Evidence for renal kinins as mediators of amino acid-induced hyperperfusion and hyperfiltration in the rat. J Clin Invest May 1992;89(5):1460—8.

[34] Martinez-Maldonado M, Benabe JE, Wilcox JN, Wang S, Luo C. Renal renin, angiotensinogen, and ANG I-converting-enzyme gene expression: influence of dietary protein. Am J Physiol Jun 1993;264(6 Pt 2):F981—8.

[35] Rosenberg ME, Kren SM, Hostetter TH. Effect of dietary protein on the renin-angiotensin system in subtotally nephrectomized rats. Kidney Int Aug 1990;38(2):240—8.

[36] Woods LL. Mechanisms of renal hemodynamic regulation in response to protein feeding. Kidney Int Oct 1993;44(4):659—75.

[37] Hostetter TH, Olson JL, Rennke HG, Venkatachalam MA, Brenner BM. Hyperfiltration in remnant nephrons: a potentially adverse response to renal ablation. Am J Physiol Jul 1981; 241(1):F85—93.

[38] El-Nahas AM, Paraskevakou H, Zoob S, Rees AJ, Evans DJ. Effect of dietary protein restriction on the development of renal failure after subtotal nephrectomy in rats. Clin Sci (Lond) Oct 1983;65(4):399—406.

[39] Kenner CH, Evan AP, Blomgren P, Aronoff GR, Luft FC. Effect of protein intake on renal function and structure in partially nephrectomized rats. Kidney Int May 1985;27(5):739—50.

[40] Meyer TW, Anderson S, Rennke HG, Brenner BM. Reversing glomerular hypertension stabilizes established glomerular injury. Kidney Int Mar 1987;31(3):752—9.

[41] Bankir L, Kriz W. Adaptation of the kidney to protein intake and to urine concentrating activity: similar consequences in health and CRF. Kidney Int Jan 1995;47(1):7—24.

[42] Harris DC, Tay C. Altered metabolism in the ex vivo remnant kidney. II. Effects of metabolic inhibitors and dietary protein. Nephron 1993;64(3):417—23.

[43] Nath KA, Croatt AJ, Hostetter TH. Oxygen consumption and oxidant stress in surviving nephrons. Am J Physiol May 1990; 258(5 Pt 2):F1354—62.

[44] Brezis M, Rosen SN, Epstein FH. The pathophysiological implications of medullary hypoxia. Am J Kidney Dis Mar 1989; 13(3):253—8.

[45] Jarusiripipat C, Shapiro JI, Chan L, Schrier RW. Reduction of remnant nephron hypermetabolism by protein restriction. Am J Kidney Dis Sep 1991;18(3):367—74.

[46] Nakayama M, Okuda S, Tamaki K, Fujishima M. Short- or long-term effects of a low-protein diet on fibronectin and transforming growth factor-beta synthesis in Adriamycin-induced nephropathy. J Lab Clin Med Jan 1996;127(1):29—39.

[47] Straus DS. Nutritional regulation of hormones and growth factors that control mammalian growth. Faseb J Jan 1994;8(1): 6—12.

[48] Hayden JM, Marten NW, Burke EJ, Straus DS. The effect of fasting on insulin-like growth factor-I nuclear transcript abundance in rat liver. Endocrinology Feb 1994;134(2):760—8.

[49] Peters H, Border WA, Noble NA. Tandem antifibrotic actions of L-arginine supplementation and low protein diet during the repair phase of experimental glomerulonephritis. Kidney Int Mar 2000;57(3):992—1001.

[50] Peters H, Border WA, Noble NA. Angiotensin II blockade and low-protein diet produce additive therapeutic effects in experimental glomerulonephritis. Kidney Int Apr 2000;57(4): 1493—501.

[51] Tovar-Palacio C, Tovar AR, Torres N, et al. Proinflammatory gene expression and renal lipogenesis are modulated by dietary

protein content in obese Zucker fa/fa rats. Am J Physiol Renal Physiol Jan 2011;300(1):F263−71.

[52] Nakamura T, Fukui M, Ebihara I, et al. Effects of a low-protein diet on glomerular endothelin family gene expression in experimental focal glomerular sclerosis. Clin Sci (Lond) Jan 1995;88(1):29−37.

[53] Nakamura T, Ebihara I, Fukui M, Takahashi T, Tomino Y, Koide H. Altered glomerular steady-state levels of tumour necrosis factor-alpha mRNA during nephrotic and sclerotic phases of puromycin aminonucleoside nephrosis in rats. Clin Sci (Lond) Mar 1993;84(3):349−56.

[54] Gao X, Huang L, Grosjean F, et al. Low-protein diet supplemented with ketoacids reduces the severity of renal disease in 5/6 nephrectomized rats: a role for KLF15. Kidney Int May 2011;79(9):987−96.

[55] Margetts BM, Beilin LJ, Vandongen R, Armstrong BK. Vegetarian diet in mild hypertension: a randomised controlled trial. Br Med J (Clin Res Ed) Dec 6 1986;293(6560):1468−71.

[56] Wiseman MJ, Hunt R, Goodwin A, Gross JL, Keen H, Viberti GC. Dietary composition and renal function in healthy subjects. Nephron 1987;46(1):37−42.

[57] Williams AJ, Baker F, Walls J. Effect of varying quantity and quality of dietary protein intake in experimental renal disease in rats. Nephron 1987;46(1):83−90.

[58] Katoh T, Takahashi K, Klahr S, Reyes AA, Badr KF. Dietary supplementation with L-arginine ameliorates glomerular hypertension in rats with subtotal nephrectomy. J Am Soc Nephrol Mar 1994;4(9):1690−4.

[59] Tapp DC, Wortham WG, Addison JF, Hammonds DN, Barnes JL, Venkatachalam MA. Food restriction retards body growth and prevents endstage renal pathology in remnant kidneys of rats regardless of protein intake. Lab Invest Feb 1989;60(2):184−95.

[60] Kobayashi S, Venkatachalam MA. Differential effects of calorie restriction on glomeruli and tubules of the remnant kidney. Kidney Int Sep 1992;42(3):710−7.

[61] Fernandes G, Yunis EJ, Miranda M, Smith J, Good RA. Nutritional inhibition of genetically determined renal disease and autoimmunity with prolongation of life in KDKD mice. Proc Natl Acad Sci U S A Jun 1978;75(6):2888−92.

[62] Walls J. Relationship between proteinuria and progressive renal disease. Am J Kidney Dis Jan 2001;37(1 Suppl. 2): S13−6.

[63] Dixon R, Brunskill NJ. Activation of mitogenic pathways by albumin in kidney proximal tubule epithelial cells: implications for the pathophysiology of proteinuric states. J Am Soc Nephrol Jul 1999;10(7):1487−97.

[64] Erkan E, De Leon M, Devarajan P. Albumin overload induces apoptosis in LLC-PK(1) cells. Am J Physiol Renal Physiol Jun 2001;280(6):F1107−14.

[65] Wang SN, LaPage J, Hirschberg R. Role of glomerular ultrafiltration of growth factors in progressive interstitial fibrosis in diabetic nephropathy. Kidney Int Mar 2000;57(3):1002−14.

[66] Thomas ME, Brunskill NJ, Harris KP, et al. Proteinuria induces tubular cell turnover: A potential mechanism for tubular atrophy. Kidney Int Mar 1999;55(3):890−8.

[67] Aparicio M, Bouchet JL, Gin H, et al. Effect of a low-protein diet on urinary albumin excretion in uremic patients. Nephron 1988;50(4):288−91.

[68] Neugarten J, Feiner HD, Schacht RG, Baldwin DS. Amelioration of experimental glomerulonephritis by dietary protein restriction. Kidney Int Nov 1983;24(5):595−601.

[69] Monsen ER. The 10th edition of the Recommended Dietary Allowances: what's new in the 1989 RDAs? J Am Diet Assoc Dec 1989;89(12):1748−52.

[70] Munro HN, McGandy RB, Hartz SC, Russell RM, Jacob RA, Otradovec CL. Protein nutriture of a group of free-living elderly. Am J Clin Nutr Oct 1987;46(4):586−92.

[71] Cohn SH, Vartsky D, Yasumura S, et al. Compartmental body composition based on total-body nitrogen, potassium, and calcium. Am J Physiol Dec 1980;239(6):E524−30.

[72] Energy and protein requirements. Report of a joint FAO/WHO/UNU Expert Consultation. World Health Organization Technical Report Series 1985;724:1−206.

[73] Kopple JD, Greene T, Chumlea WC, et al. Relationship between nutritional status and the glomerular filtration rate: results from the MDRD study. Kidney Int Apr 2000;57(4): 1688−703.

[74] Ikizler TA, Greene JH, Wingard RL, Parker RA, Hakim RM. Spontaneous dietary protein intake during progression of chronic renal failure. J Am Soc Nephrol Nov 1995;6(5):1386−91.

[75] Pollock CA, Ibels LS, Zhu FY, et al. Protein intake in renal disease. J Am Soc Nephrol May 1997;8(5):777−83.

[76] Garg AX, Blake PG, Clark WF, Clase CM, Haynes RB, Moist LM. Association between renal insufficiency and malnutrition in older adults: results from the NHANES III. Kidney Int Nov 2001;60(5):1867−74.

[77] Bernhard J, Beaufrere B, Laville M, Fouque D. Adaptive response to a low-protein diet in predialysis chronic renal failure patients. J Am Soc Nephrol Jun 2001;12(6):1249−54.

[78] Quevedo MR, Price GM, Halliday D, Pacy PJ, Millward DJ. Nitrogen homoeostasis in man: diurnal changes in nitrogen excretion, leucine oxidation and whole body leucine kinetics during a reduction from a high to a moderate protein intake. Clin Sci (Lond) Feb 1994;86(2):185−93.

[79] Goodship TH, Mitch WE, Hoerr RA, Wagner DA, Steinman TI, Young VR. Adaptation to low-protein diets in renal failure: leucine turnover and nitrogen balance. J Am Soc Nephrol Jul 1990;1(1):66−75.

[80] Giordano M, De Feo P, Lucidi P, et al. Effects of dietary protein restriction on fibrinogen and albumin metabolism in nephrotic patients. Kidney Int Jul 2001;60(1):235−42.

[81] Masud T, Young VR, Chapman T, Maroni BJ. Adaptive responses to very low protein diets: the first comparison of ketoacids to essential amino acids. Kidney Int Apr 1994; 45(4):1182−92.

[82] Tom K, Young VR, Chapman T, Masud T, Akpele L, Maroni BJ. Long-term adaptive responses to dietary protein restriction in chronic renal failure. Am J Physiol Apr 1995;268(4 Pt 1):E668−77.

[83] Maroni BJ, Staffeld C, Young VR, Manatunga A, Tom K. Mechanisms permitting nephrotic patients to achieve nitrogen equilibrium with a protein-restricted diet. J Clin Invest May 15 1997;99(10):2479−87.

[84] Rosenberg ME, Swanson JE, Thomas BL, Hostetter TH. Glomerular and hormonal responses to dietary protein intake in human renal disease. Am J Physiol Dec 1987;253(6 Pt 2): F1083−90.

[85] Kaysen GA, Gambertoglio J, Jimenez I, Jones H, Hutchison FN. Effect of dietary protein intake on albumin homeostasis in nephrotic patients. Kidney Int Feb 1986;29(2):572−7.

[86] Bellizzi V, Di Iorio BR, De Nicola L, et al. Very low protein diet supplemented with ketoanalogs improves blood pressure control in chronic kidney disease. Kidney Int Feb 2007;71(3): 245−51.

[87] Ruilope LM, Casal MC, Praga M, et al. Additive antiproteinuric effect of converting enzyme inhibition and a low protein intake. J Am Soc Nephrol Dec 1992;3(6):1307−11.

[88] Gansevoort RT, de Zeeuw D, de Jong PE. Additive antiproteinuric effect of ACE inhibition and a low-protein diet in human renal disease. Nephrol Dial Transplant 1995;10(4):497−504.

[89] Kontessis PA, Bossinakou I, Sarika L, et al. Renal, metabolic, and hormonal responses to proteins of different origin in normotensive, nonproteinuric type I diabetic patients. Diabetes Care Sep 1995;18(9):1233.

[90] Kontessis P, Jones S, Dodds R, et al. Renal, metabolic and hormonal responses to ingestion of animal and vegetable proteins. Kidney Int Jul 1990;38(1):136−44.

[91] de Mello VD, Zelmanovitz T, Perassolo MS, Azevedo MJ, Gross JL. Withdrawal of red meat from the usual diet reduces albuminuria and improves serum fatty acid profile in type 2 diabetes patients with macroalbuminuria. Am J Clin Nutr May 2006;83(5):1032−8.

[92] Gin H, Aparicio M, Potaux L, de Precigout V, Bouchet JL, Aubertin J. Low protein and low phosphorus diet in patients with chronic renal failure: influence on glucose tolerance and tissue insulin sensitivity. Metabolism Nov 1987;36(11):1080−5.

[93] Rigalleau V, Blanchetier V, Combe C, et al. A low-protein diet improves insulin sensitivity of endogenous glucose production in predialytic uremic patients. Am J Clin Nutr May 1997;65(5):1512−6.

[94] Bernard S, Fouque D, Laville M, Zech P. Effects of low-protein diet supplemented with ketoacids on plasma lipids in adult chronic renal failure. Miner Electrolyte Metab 1996;22(1-3):143−6.

[95] Isakova T, Wahl P, Vargas GS, et al. Fibroblast growth factor 23 is elevated before parathyroid hormone and phosphate in chronic kidney disease. Kidney Int Jun 2011;79(12):1370−8.

[96] Gutierrez OM, Mannstadt M, Isakova T, et al. Fibroblast growth factor 23 and mortality among patients undergoing hemodialysis. N Engl J Med Aug 7 2008;359(6):584−92.

[97] Gutierrez OM, Wolf M, Taylor EN. Fibroblast Growth Factor 23, Cardiovascular Disease Risk Factors, and Phosphorus Intake in the Health Professionals Follow-up Study. Clin J Am Soc Nephrol Dec 2011;6(12):2871−8.

[98] Kendrick J, Cheung AK, Kaufman JS, et al. FGF-23 associates with death, cardiovascular events, and initiation of chronic dialysis. J Am Soc Nephrol Oct 2011;22(10):1913−22.

[99] Ferrari SL, Bonjour JP, Rizzoli R. Fibroblast growth factor-23 relationship to dietary phosphate and renal phosphate handling in healthy young men. J Clin Endocrinol Metab Mar 2005;90(3):1519−24.

[100] Moe SM, Zidehsarai MP, Chambers MA, et al. Vegetarian compared with meat dietary protein source and phosphorus homeostasis in chronic kidney disease. Clin J Am Soc Nephrol Feb 2011;6(2):257−64.

[101] Chauveau P, Fouque D, Combe C, et al. Acidosis and nutritional status in hemodialyzed patients. French Study Group for Nutrition in Dialysis. Semin Dial Jul-Aug 2000;13(4):241−6.

[102] Chauveau P, Barthe N, Rigalleau V, et al. Outcome of nutritional status and body composition of uremic patients on a very low protein diet. Am J Kidney Dis Sep 1999;34(3):500−7.

[103] Mitch WE, Remuzzi G. Diets for patients with chronic kidney disease, still worth prescribing. J Am Soc Nephrol Jan 2004;15(1):234−7.

[104] de Brito-Ashurst I, Varagunam M, Raftery MJ, Yaqoob MM. Bicarbonate supplementation slows progression of CKD and improves nutritional status. J Am Soc Nephrol Sep 2009;20(9):2075−84.

[105] Di Iorio BR, Minutolo R, De Nicola L, et al. Supplemented very low protein diet ameliorates responsiveness to erythropoietin in chronic renal failure. Kidney Int Nov 2003;64(5):1822−8.

[106] Aparicio M, Chauveau P, Combe C. Are supplemented low-protein diets nutritionally safe? Am J Kidney Dis Jan 2001;37(1 Suppl. 2):S71−6.

[107] Malvy D, Maingourd C, Pengloan J, Bagros P, Nivet H. Effects of severe protein restriction with ketoanalogs in advanced renal failure. J Am Coll Nutr Oct 1999;18(5):481−6.

[108] Ihle BU, Becker GJ, Whitworth JA, Charlwood RA, Kincaid-Smith PS. The effect of protein restriction on the progression of renal insufficiency. N Engl J Med Dec 28 1989;321(26):1773−7.

[109] Williams PS, Stevens ME, Fass G, Irons L, Bone JM. Failure of dietary protein and phosphate restriction to retard the rate of progression of chronic renal failure: a prospective, randomized, controlled trial. Q J Med Oct 1991;81(294):837−55.

[110] Aparicio M, Chauveau P, De Precigout V, Bouchet JL, Lasseur C, Combe C. Nutrition and outcome on renal replacement therapy of patients with chronic renal failure treated by a supplemented very low protein diet. J Am Soc Nephrol Apr 2000;11(4):708−16.

[111] Kopple JD, Levey AS, Greene T, et al. Effect of dietary protein restriction on nutritional status in the Modification of Diet in Renal Disease Study. Kidney Int Sep 1997;52(3):778−91.

[112] Coresh J, Walser M, Hill S. Survival on dialysis among chronic renal failure patients treated with a supplemented low-protein diet before dialysis. J Am Soc Nephrol Nov 1995;6(5):1379−85.

[113] Walser M, Hill S. Can renal replacement be deferred by a supplemented very low protein diet? J Am Soc Nephrol Jan 1999;10(1):110−6.

[114] Aparicio M, Fouque D, Chauveau P. Effect of a very low-protein diet on long-term outcomes. Am J Kidney Dis Jul 2009;54(1):183.

[115] Chauveau P, Couzi L, Vendrely B, et al. Long-term outcome on renal replacement therapy in patients who previously received a keto acid-supplemented very-low-protein diet. Am J Clin Nutr Aug 5 2009.

[116] Menon V, Kopple JD, Wang X, et al. Effect of a very low-protein diet on outcomes: long-term follow-up of the Modification of Diet in Renal Disease (MDRD) Study. Am J Kidney Dis Feb 2009;53(2):208−17.

[117] Rosman JB, ter Wee PM, Meijer S, Piers-Becht TP, Sluiter WJ, Donker AJ. Prospective randomised trial of early dietary protein restriction in chronic renal failure. Lancet Dec 8 1984;2(8415):1291−6.

[118] Rosman JB, Langer K, Brandl M, et al. Protein-restricted diets in chronic renal failure: a four year follow-up shows limited indications. Kidney Int Suppl Nov 1989;27:S96−102.

[119] Locatelli F, Alberti D, Graziani G, Buccianti G, Redaelli B, Giangrande A. Prospective, randomised, multicentre trial of effect of protein restriction on progression of chronic renal insufficiency. Northern Italian Cooperative Study Group. Lancet Jun 1 1991;337(8753):1299−304.

[120] Beck GJ, Berg RL, Coggins CH, et al. Design and statistical issues of the Modification of Diet in Renal Disease Trial. The Modification of Diet in Renal Disease Study Group. Controlled Clinical Trials Oct 1991;12(5):566−86.

[121] Greene T, Bourgoignie JJ, Habwe V, et al. Baseline characteristics in the Modification of Diet in Renal Disease Study. J Am Soc Nephrol Nov 1993;4(5):1221−36.

[122] Klahr S, Levey AS, Beck GJ, et al. The effects of dietary protein restriction and blood-pressure control on the progression of chronic renal disease. Modification of Diet in Renal Disease Study Group. N Engl J Med Mar 31 1994;330(13):877−84.

[123] Short-term effects of protein intake, blood pressure, and antihypertensive therapy on glomerular filtration rate in the Modification of Diet in Renal Disease Study. J Am Soc Nephrol Oct 1996;7(10):2097−109.

[124] Levey AS, Adler S, Caggiula AW, et al. Effects of dietary protein restriction on the progression of advanced renal disease in the Modification of Diet in Renal Disease Study. Am J Kidney Dis May 1996;27(5):652−63.

[125] Teschan PE, Beck GJ, Dwyer JT, et al. Effect of a ketoacid-aminoacid-supplemented very low protein diet on the progression of advanced renal disease: a reanalysis of the MDRD feasibility study. Clin Nephrol Nov 1998;50(5):273—83.

[126] Levey AS, Greene T, Beck GJ, et al. Dietary protein restriction and the progression of chronic renal disease: what have all of the results of the MDRD study shown? Modification of Diet in Renal Disease Study group. J Am Soc Nephrol Nov 1999;10(11): 2426—39.

[127] The effect of intensive treatment of diabetes on the development and progression of long-term complications in insulin-dependent diabetes mellitus. The Diabetes Control and Complications Trial Research Group. N Engl J Med Sep 30 1993;329(14):977—86.

[128] Mitch WE, Walser M, Steinman TI, Hill S, Zeger S, Tungsanga K. The effect of a keto acid-amino acid supplement to a restricted diet on the progression of chronic renal failure. N Engl J Med Sep 6 1984;311(10):623—9.

[129] Klahr S, Breyer JA, Beck GJ, et al. Dietary protein restriction, blood pressure control, and the progression of polycystic kidney disease. Modification of Diet in Renal Disease Study Group. J Am Soc Nephrol Jun 1995;5(12):2037—47.

[130] Mircescu G, Garneata L, Stancu SH, Capusa C. Effects of a supplemented hypoproteic diet in chronic kidney disease. J Ren Nutr May 2007;17(3):179—88.

[131] Cianciaruso B, Pota A, Pisani A, et al. Metabolic effects of two low protein diets in chronic kidney disease stage 4-5 — a randomized controlled trial. Nephrol Dial Transplant Feb 2008;23(2):636—44.

[132] Brunori G, Viola BF, Parrinello G, et al. Efficacy and safety of a very-low-protein diet when postponing dialysis in the elderly: a prospective randomized multicenter controlled study. Am J Kidney Dis May 2007;49(5):569—80.

[133] Sackett DL. Rules of evidence and clinical recommendations on the use of antithrombotic agents. Chest Feb 1989;95(Suppl. 2): 2S—4S.

[134] Pedrini MT, Levey AS, Lau J, Chalmers TC, Wang PH. The effect of dietary protein restriction on the progression of diabetic and nondiabetic renal diseases: a meta-analysis. Ann Intern Med Apr 1 1996;124(7):627—32.

[135] Kasiske BL, Lakatua JD, Ma JZ, Louis TA. A meta-analysis of the effects of dietary protein restriction on the rate of decline in renal function. Am J Kidney Dis Jun 1998;31(6): 954—61.

[136] Altman DG, Andersen PK. Calculating the number needed to treat for trials where the outcome is time to an event. BMJ Dec 4 1999;319(7223):1492—5.

[137] Skolbekken JA. Communicating the risk reduction achieved by cholesterol reducing drugs. BMJ Jun 27 1998;316(7149): 1956—8.

Reducing Tryptophan Metabolites to Reduce Progression in Chronic Kidney Failure

Toshimitsu Niwa

Department of Advanced Medicine for Uremia, Nagoya University School of Medicine, Showa-ku, Nagoya, Japan

SEARCH FOR UREMIC TOXINS

The uremic syndrome is considered to be caused by an accumulation of uremic toxins due to kidney dysfunction. Ninety compounds have been identified as potential uremic toxins [1]. Sixty-eight have a molecular weight of less than 500 Da, 12 exceed 12,000 Da, and 10 have a molecular weight between 500 and 12,000 Da, 25 solutes are protein-bound. These uremic toxins are considered to be involved in a variety of symptoms which may appear in patients with stage 5 chronic kidney disease (CKD).

We applied the metabolomic analysis of comprehensive small-molecular metabolites using liquid chromatography/electrospray ionization-tandem mass spectrometry (LC/ESI-MS/MS) and principal component analysis (PCA) to identify uremic toxins accumulated in the serum of CKD rats [2]. A software created arrays of mass intensity and retention time pairs consisting of 7241 positive ions and 7475 negative ions. There were 461 positive ions and 423 negative ions, of which peak intensity was significantly higher in CKD serum than in normal serum. Indoxyl sulfate was demonstrated to be the first principal serum metabolite which differentiates CKD from normal, followed by phenyl sulfate, hippuric acid and p-cresyl sulfate.

Further, we applied the metabolomic approach to search for uremic toxins as possible indicators of the effect of AST-120 [3]. An oral sorbent AST-120 composed of spherical porous carbon particles has superior adsorption ability for certain small-molecular-weight organic compounds known to accumulate in CKD patients. Serum metabolites in normal and CKD rats before and after administration of AST-120 for 3 days were analyzed by LC/ESI-MS/MS and PCA. Indoxyl sulfate was found to be the first principal serum metabolite, which could differentiate CKD from both normal and AST-120-administered CKD rats, followed by hippuric acid, phenyl sulfate and 4-ethylphenyl sulfate. Taken together, indoxyl sulfate is the first principle serum metabolite specific for CKD as well as the best indicator of the effect of AST-120 in CKD rats.

METABOLISM OF INDOXYL SULFATE, A TRYPTOPHAN METABOLITE

We have demonstrated that indoxyl sulfate is a uremic toxin accelerating the progression of CKD [4–7]. Figure 15.1 shows the metabolism of indoxyl sulfate and the effect of an oral sorbent (AST-120: Kremezin). Indoxyl sulfate is derived from dietary protein. A part of the protein-derived tryptophan is metabolized into indole by tryptophanase in intestinal bacteria such as *Escherichia coli*. Indole is then absorbed into the blood from the intestine, and is metabolized to indoxyl sulfate in the liver, while indoxyl sulfate is normally excreted into urine. In uremia, however, the inadequate renal clearance of indoxyl sulfate leads to its elevation in serum. In fact, the serum levels of indoxyl sulfate were found to be markedly increased in both CKD rats and patients [5,8,9]. In serum, approximately 95% of indoxyl sulfate is bound to serum albumin. AST-120 reduces the serum and urine levels of indoxyl sulfate in uremic rats and patients by adsorbing indole in the intestines, consequently stimulating its excretion into feces [5,8–14]. The administration of indoxyl sulfate to {5/6}-nephrectomized rats promoted the progression of CKD accompanied by enhanced gene expression of transforming growth factor (TGF)- β1, tissue inhibitor of metalloproteinase (TIMP)-1 and proβ1(I) collagen [7,15]. These findings support the notion that indoxyl sulfate is a uremic toxin stimulating the progression of CKD by increasing renal expression of these fibrogenic genes.

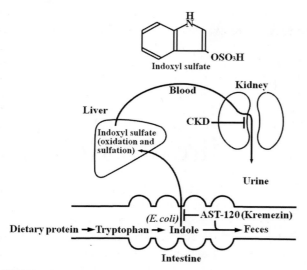

FIGURE 15.1 Metabolism of indoxyl sulfate (molecular weight: 213) and effect of AST-120 (Kremezin). (Revised from the reference [13].) Indoxyl sulfate is derived from dietary protein. A part of protein-derived tryptophan is metabolized into indole by tryptophanase in intestinal bacteria such as *Escherichia coli*. Indole is absorbed into the blood from the intestine, and is metabolized to indoxyl sulfate in the liver, it is normally excreted in urine. In chronic kidney disease (CKD), however, reduced renal clearance of indoxyl sulfate leads to its elevated serum level. AST-120 reduces the serum and urine levels of indoxyl sulfate in CKD patients by adsorbing indole in the intestines, and consequently stimulating its excretion into feces.

pathophysiological process. A progressive decline in the glomerular filtration rate (GFR) leads to increased circulating levels of endogenous protein metabolites such as indoxyl sulfate, and to the adverse effects of their overload on the remnant nephrons, especially proximal tubular cells. Indoxyl sulfate, for example, stimulates progressive tubulointerstitial fibrosis, glomerular sclerosis, and consequent progression of CKD by increasing the gene expressions of TGF-β1, TIMP-1, and proα1(I)collagen, leading to a further loss of nephrons [7,15], completing the vicious circle of progressive renal injury.

A low-protein diet delays the progression of CKD by suppressing renal TGF-β1 expression in uremic animals in which it also reduces the serum levels of indoxyl sulfate [5,12]. The administration of AST-120 decreases the serum and urine levels of indoxyl sulfate, and delays the progression of CKD by reducing the gene expression of TGF-β1, TIMP-1, and proα1(I)collagen [14,18–25]. AST-120 is widely used in Japan for the treatment of CKD patients to delay the progression of CKD. If the overload of indoxyl sulfate is alleviated by a low-protein diet or by the administration of AST-120, the chain of events leading to progressive renal injury might be interrupted.

PROTEIN METABOLITE THEORY AS A MECHANISM OF CKD PROGRESSION

We proposed the protein metabolite theory by which endogenous protein metabolites such as indoxyl sulfate play a significant role in the progression of CKD (Figure 15.2) [13,16,17]. The initial insult leads to a loss of functioning nephrons via a disease-specific

INDOXYL SULFATE INDUCES REACTIVE OXYGEN SPECIES (ROS) IN THE KIDNEY

Indoxyl sulfate induces ROS production not only in renal tubular cells but also in glomerular mesangial cells [26,27]. Indoxyl sulfate-induced ROS in renal tubular cells activate nuclear factor (NF)-κB which upregulates the expression of plasminogen activator inhibitor

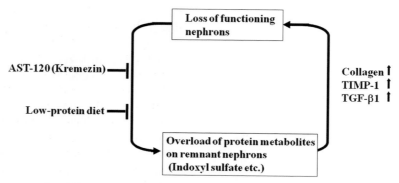

FIGURE 15.2 The protein metabolite theory, a mechanism for the progression of chronic kidney disease (CKD). (Revised from the reference [13].) Endogenous protein metabolites such as indoxyl sulfate play a significant role in the progression of CKD. The initial insult leads to a loss of functioning nephrons via a disease-specific pathophysiological process. A progressive decline in the glomerular filtration rate leads to increased circulating levels of endogenous protein metabolites such as indoxyl sulfate, and to the adverse effects of their overload on the remnant nephrons, especially proximal tubular cells. Indoxyl sulfate stimulates progressive tubulointerstitial fibrosis, glomerular sclerosis, and the progression of CKD by increasing the gene expression of transforming growth factor (TGF)-β1, tissue inhibitor of metalloproteinase (TIMP)-1 and proα1(I)collagen, leading to a further loss of nephrons and completing the vicious circle of progressive renal injury. If the overload of indoxyl sulfate is alleviated by a low-protein diet or by the administration of AST-120, the chain of events leading to further progressive renal injury might be interrupted.

(PAI)-1 [26]. Indoxyl sulfate-induced ROS in mesangial cells activate mitogen-activated protein kinases (MAPK) and cell proliferation [27]. Thus, indoxyl sulfate induces the generation of ROS in the kidneys. Administration of indoxyl sulfate reduces the superoxide scavenging activity in the kidneys of uremic rats. Therefore, indoxyl sulfate impairs the kidney's anti-oxidative system [28].

AST-120 alleviates ROS in the kidneys of uremic rats by reducing serum levels of indoxyl sulfate, and reduces the urine level of acrolein, a lipid peroxidation end product [29]. Furthermore, AST-120 increases NO synthesis in the kidneys of CKD rats by increasing the renal expressions of endothelial nitric oxide synthase and neuronal nitric oxide synthase through alleviation of indoxyl sulfate overload on the kidney [30].

ROLE OF ORGANIC ANION TRANSPORTERS IN NEPHROTOXICITY OF INDOXYL SULFATE

Figure 15.3 shows the mechanism underlying the nephrotoxicity of indoxyl sulfate. Approximately 95% of indoxyl sulfate accumulated in the blood of uremic

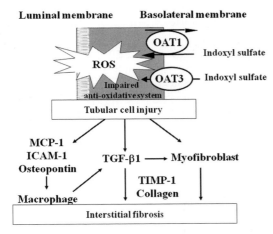

FIGURE 15.3 Nephrotoxicity of indoxyl sulfate. (Revised from the reference [48].) Indoxyl sulfate in the blood is taken up by organic anion transporters (OAT1 and OAT3) at the basolateral membrane of renal tubular cells in which it is accumulated. Indoxyl sulfate generates reactive oxygen species (ROS), reduces superoxide scavenging activity, and consequently causes tubular cell injury by impairing the kidney's anti-oxidative systems. The damaged tubular cells produce transforming growth factor (TGF)-β1 as well as chemokines such as monocyte chemotactic protein-1 (MCP-1), intercellular adhesion molecule-1 (ICAM-1), and osteopontin. These chemokines promote the infiltration of macrophages which produce TGF-β1. The secreted TGF-β1 stimulates production of tissue inhibitor of metalloproteinase (TIMP)-1 and collagen. The injured tubular cells are transformed into myofibroblasts through an epithelial-to-mesenchymal transition induced by TGF-β1. These changes facilitate interstitial fibrosis. Thus, indoxyl sulfate accelerates tubular cell injury and subsequent interstitial fibrosis.

patients is bound to serum albumin. Therefore, indoxyl sulfate is normally excreted into urine mainly via active secretion by the proximal tubular cells. Organic anion transporters (OAT1 and OAT3) play an important role in the transcellular transport of indoxyl sulfate in the tubular cells and in the induction of its nephrotoxicity [31,32]. Indoxyl sulfate in the blood is taken up by OAT1 and OAT3 at the basolateral membrane of tubular cells (OAT1: proximal, OAT3: proximal and distal), and is accumulated in the tubular cells at high concentration in CKD patients [33]. The accumulation of indoxyl sulfate generates ROS, reduces superoxide scavenging activity, and consequently causes tubular cell injury by impairing the kidney's anti-oxidative systems [28].

The damaged tubular cells produce TGF-β1 as well as chemokines such as monocyte chemotactic protein-1 (MCP-1), intercellular adhesion molecule-1 (ICAM-1), and osteopontin. These chemokines promote the infiltration of macrophages which produce TGF-β1. The secreted TGF-β1 stimulates the production of TIMP-1 and collagen. The damaged tubular cells are transformed into myofibroblasts through an epithelial-to-mesenchymal transition [34], these changes facilitate interstitial fibrosis. Thus, indoxyl sulfate accumulated in uremic serum accelerates tubular cell injury, and induces subsequent interstitial fibrosis, thus acting as a nephrotoxin.

INDOXYL SULFATE REDUCES KLOTHO AND INDUCES SENESCENCE IN THE KIDNEY

Klotho is an anti-aging gene, and mutation of the mouse Klotho gene leads to premature aging syndrome [35]. Klotho protein is expressed predominantly in the kidneys. The expression of Klotho is decreased in the kidneys of not only rat models such as hypertensive rats, {5/6}-nephrectomized rats, and diabetic rats, but also in patients with CKD [36].

We studied to clarify if indoxyl sulfate could reduce Klotho expression, and contribute to cell senescence in the kidneys of hypertensive rats [37]. Indoxyl sulfate-administered hypertensive rats showed decreased expression of Klotho, increased expression of senescence-associated β-galactosidase (SA-β-gal), p16, p21, p53 and retinoblastoma protein (Rb) in renal tubular cells, and increased tubulointerstitial fibrosis and mesangial expansion compared with hypertensive rats. Thus, administration of indoxyl sulfate to hypertensive rats reduced renal expression of Klotho, and promoted cell senescence accompanied by renal fibrosis [37].

We demonstrated that AST-120-treated CKD rats showed increased renal expression of Klotho compared with CKD rats [38]. Then, we examined whether the

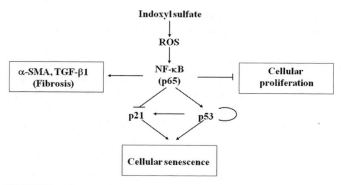

FIGURE 15.4 Schematic effects of indoxyl sulfate on proximal tubular cells. (Revised from the reference [41].) Indoxyl sulfate promotes activation (phosphorylation) of nuclear factor (NF)-κB p65 through reactive oxygen species (ROS), followed by p53 expression. Indoxyl sulfate-induced p53 expression triggers p53 accumulation. Activation and induction of NF-κB by indoxyl sulfate suppress cellular proliferation, and induce cellular senescence and expression of transforming growth factor (TGF)-β1 and α-smooth muscle actin (α-SMA), accompanied by renal fibrosis. Thus, NF-κB plays an important role in indoxyl sulfate-induced cellular senescence, fibrotic gene expression and inhibition of proliferation in proximal tubular cells.

expression of Klotho in proximal tubular cells is regulated by indoxyl sulfate using the proximal tubular cell line (HK-2) [39], because main target of indoxyl sulfate is proximal tubular cells, and Klotho is expressed in the cells as well as inner medullary collecting duct cells and distal tubular cells. Indoxyl sulfate downregulates Klotho expression in proximal tubular cells by activating NF-κB through production of ROS [40].

We investigated how indoxyl sulfate promotes CKD using cultured HK-2 cells and CKD rats [40]. Indoxyl sulfate inhibited serum-induced cell proliferation, and promoted the activation of SA-β-gal, a marker of cellular senescence, and the expression of α-smooth muscle actin (α-SMA), a marker of fibrosis, through inducing p53 expression and phosphorylation. Further, we have demonstrated that NF-κB plays an important role in indoxyl sulfate-induced cellular senescence, fibrotic gene expression and inhibition of proliferation in proximal tubular cells [41]. More notably, indoxyl sulfate accelerates proximal tubular cell senescence with progression of CKD through ROS-NF-κB-p53 pathway (Figure 15.4) [41]. AST-120, which reduces serum indoxyl sulfate level, suppressed the expression of phosphorylated NF-κB p65, p53, p21, SA-β-gal, TGF-β1 and α-SMA in the kidneys of CKD rats.

VASCULAR TOXICITY OF INDOXYL SULFATE

Indoxyl sulfate has been shown to inhibit endothelial proliferation and wound repair [42], and to stimulate the

proliferation of rat vascular smooth muscle cells [43] and human aortic smooth muscle cells [44]. The serum level of indoxyl sulfate has been associated with pentosidine and HDL-cholesterol, the risk factors of atherosclerosis in hemodialysis patients [45].

We demonstrated that indoxyl sulfate promotes aortic calcification and aortic wall thickening in hypertensive rats [46]. Osteoblast-specific proteins such as osteopontin, core binding factor 1 (Cbfa1), alkaline phosphatase (ALP), and osteocalcin are expressed in the cells embedded in the aortic calcification area. More notably, indoxyl sulfate promotes cell senescence with increased expression of SA-β-gal, p53, p21, p16, and Rb in the cells embedded in the calcification area in hypertensive rats [47]. Thus, indoxyl sulfate is a nephro-vascular toxin that may be responsible for progression of not only CKD but also cardiovascular disease (CVD) [48].

Indoxyl sulfate stimulates the generation of ROS such as superoxide by up-regulating NADPH oxidase Nox4, and induces the expressions of osteoblast-specific proteins such as Cbfa1, ALP, and osteopontin in human aortic smooth muscle cells [49]. ROS derived from NADPH oxidase Nox4 are important in inducing the transdifferentiation of human aortic smooth muscle cells into cells with a more osteoblastic phenotype. These effects of indoxyl sulfate have been observed even at a concentration of indoxyl sulfate found in hemodialysis patients [5].

Indoxyl sulfate inhibits NO production and cell viability by inducing ROS such as superoxide through the induction of NADPH oxidase Nox4 in human vascular endothelial cells [50]. Indoxyl sulfate has been shown to induce the expression of Nox4 mRNA and the production of superoxide and peroxynitrite in human vascular endothelial cells. Further, indoxyl sulfate upregulates expression of ICAM-1 and MCP-1 by oxidative stress-induced NF-κB activation [51].

Indoxyl sulfate may play a significant role in vascular disease and its higher rate of mortality observed in CKD patients [52]. Indoxyl sulfate levels exhibited an inverse relationship to renal function and a direct relationship to aortic calcification and pulse-wave velocity. The highest indoxyl sulfate tertile has proved to be a powerful predictor of overall and cardiovascular mortality in CKD patients.

Indoxyl sulfate shows pro-fibrotic, pro-hypertrophic, and pro-inflammatory effects on cardiac fibroblasts and myocytes, indicating that indoxyl sulfate might play an important role in adverse cardiac remodeling mediated via activation of the p38 MAPK, p42/44 MAPK, and NF-κB pathways [53].

AST-120 lessens the extent of atherosclerosis induced by kidney injury and alters lesion characteristics in apolipoprotein E-deficient mice, resulting in plaques with a more stable phenotype with less necrosis and reduced inflammation [54].

Oxidative stress plays a key role in the development of cardiac hypertrophy and fibrosis in CKD. AST-120 suppresses oxidative stress and reduces cardiac damage in CKD [55].

CLINICAL EFFECTS OF AST-120

We determined whether AST-120 could reduce the serum and urine levels of indoxyl sulfate and suppress the progression of CKD in undialyzed CKD patients [13]. Administration of AST-120 (6 g/day) significantly decreased the serum and urine levels of indoxyl sulfate. Those patients who showed a greater decrease in urinary indoxyl sulfate exhibited a more marked suppression in the progression of CKD.

A multicenter, randomized, double-blind, placebo-controlled, dose-ranging study of a US population was designed to examine the nephroprotective effects of 3 doses of AST-120 versus a placebo in patients with moderate to severe CKD and elevated serum indoxyl sulfate levels who were also following an adequate protein-intake diet [56]. AST-120 significantly decreased serum indoxyl sulfate levels in a dose-dependent fashion. Furthermore, significant improvement in malaise was observed in a dose-dependent fashion.

Administration of AST-120 (6 g/day) significantly reduced the plasma levels of indoxyl sulfate and TGF-β1, and improved the slope of the reciprocal of serum creatinine [57]. These results support the notion that indoxyl sulfate and TGF-β1 are involved in the progression of CKD, and that AST-120 impedes that progression, at least in part, by reducing the overproduction of TGF-β1.

AST-120 (6 g/day) was administered to CKD patients. When comparing the δGFR in the observation and intervention periods for each group, the rate of decline in GFR was found to be significantly retarded in the AST-120 group while no significant difference was observed in the control group [58]. Thus, AST-120 treatment slowed the decline in renal function in CKD patients with moderately decreased renal function.

Adding AST-120 (6 g/day) to a low-protein diet together with renin angiotensin system (RAS) blocker therapy delayed the deterioration of CKD, especially in patients with early or rapid progression [59].

The effects of AST-120 on early stage overt diabetic nephropathy have been determined in a prospective, randomized, controlled study for patients with type 2 diabetes [60]. A reduction in urinary indoxyl sulfate was observed at month 12 in the AST-120 group but not in the control group. A significant difference was observed in changes in the mean levels of serum creatinine versus time between the two groups. Thus, the administration of AST-120 initiated at an early stage of overt diabetic nephropathy stunts the progression of renal dysfunction.

The CAP-KD study (Carbonaceous oral adsorbent's effectiveness on progression of chronic kidney disease) demonstrated that AST-120 treatment (6 g/day) for 1 year significantly slowed the decline of estimated GFR (eGFR) in Japanese CKD patients compared with conventional therapy, although there was no significant improvement in the composite primary endpoint [61].

AST-120 treatment (6 g/day) for 12 months significantly reduced IL-6, proteinuria, and urinary levels of L-fatty acid binding protein (L-FABP) and 8-hydroxy-deoxyguanosine (8-OHdG), and inhibited the increase in serum creatinine in CKD patients. AST-120 may exert beneficial effects in CKD patients by protecting tubular damage partly via reduction of proteinuria and oxidative stress generation [62].

The effect of AST-120 in CKD patients has been evaluated retrospectively by the 24-month dialysis-free rate and 50% dialysis-free period [63]. The latter was significantly prolonged in the AST-120 group compared to the non-AST-120 group. When AST-120 treatment was started at a serum creatinine level below 3 mg/dL, the dialysis-free period lasted more than 24 months in the AST-120 group, compared with only 16.2 months in the non-AST-120 group. The risk of dialysis initiation was increased 3.48-fold in patients who were not administered AST-120. Thus, AST-120 was found to delay the initiation of dialysis in CKD patients.

AST-120 treatment (6 g/day) for 2 years significantly reduced arterial stiffness (pulse wave velocity) and carotid intima media thickness (IMT) in nondiabetic CKD patients before dialysis [64]. In addition, the slope of the reciprocal serum creatinine concentration over time became significantly less steep in the AST-120 group than in the non-AST-120 group. Thus, AST-120 slowed the progression not only of CKD but also of CVD.

A retrospective study examined whether AST-120 given to CKD patients in the pre-dialysis period influences their prognosis after the initiation of dialysis. AST-120 given prior to the initiation of dialysis improved the prognosis of CKD patients under dialysis [65].

AST-120 treatment (6 g/day) for 24 weeks resulted in an increase in flow-mediated endothelium-dependent vasodilatation (FMD) with a decrease in serum indoxyl sulfate and oxidized/reduced glutathione ratio in CKD patients [66].

AST-120 treatment (6 g/day) of CKD patients with congestive heart failure showed improvement in renal function tests, atrial natriuretic peptide, edema, cardio-thoracic ratio and hospital stay [67]. Thus, AST-120 contributes to the improvement of cardiac and renal

FIGURE 15.5 Uremic toxicity of indoxyl sulfate. (Revised from the reference [48].) Indoxyl sulfate induces the cellular production of reactive oxygen species (ROS) such as superoxide by activating NADPH oxidase, especially Nox4, and/or by its uptake through organic anion transporters (OAT1 and OAT3), consequently impairing cellular anti-oxidative system. It also induces ROS in renal tubular cells and glomerular mesangial cells, and stimulates the progression of chronic kidney disease (CKD), as well as inducing ROS in vascular smooth muscle cells (VSMCs), vascular endothelial cells, and cardiomyocytes, and aggravating cardiovascular disease (CVD). Moreover, indoxyl sulfate induces ROS in osteoblasts, causing osteodystrophy.

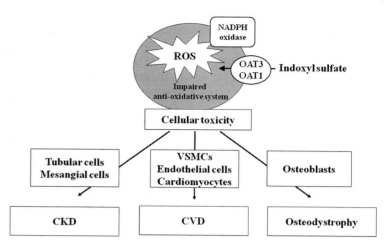

functions, and consequently improves the quality of life of patients.

A cross-sectional study examined whether AST-120 administration affects cardiac abnormalities in CKD patients. AST-120 treatment for more than 6 months prevented the development of left ventricular concentric change in predialysis CKD patients [68].

CONCLUSION

Figure 15.5 shows the overall uremic toxicity of indoxyl sulfate. It induces the cellular production of ROS such as superoxide by activating NADPH oxidase, especially Nox4, by its uptake through OAT1 and OAT3, consequently impairing the cellular anti-oxidative system. It induces ROS in renal tubular cells and glomerular mesangial cells, and stimulates the progression of CKD. It also induces ROS in vascular smooth muscle cells, vascular endothelial cells and cardiomyocytes, and aggravates CVD, as well as inducing ROS in osteoblasts, causing osteodystrophy [69,70]. Thus, the removal of indoxyl sulfate by AST-120 ameliorates the progression of not only CKD, but also CVD and osteodystrophy.

References

[1] Vanholder R, De Smet R, Glorieux G, et al. Review on uremic toxins: classification, concentration, and interindividual variability. Kidney Int 2003;63:1934—43.

[2] Kikuchi K, Itoh Y, Tateoka R, et al. Metabolomic analysis of uremic toxins by liquid chromatography/electrospray ionization-tandem mass spectrometry. J Chromatogr B 2010;878:1662—8.

[3] Kikuchi K, Itoh Y, Tateoka R, et al. Metabolomic search for uremic toxins as indicators of the effect of an oral sorbent AST-120 by liquid chromatography/tandem mass spectrometry. J Chromatogr B 2010;878:2997—3002.

[4] Niwa T. Uremic Toxicity. Indoxyl sulfate. In: Massry SG, Glassock RJ, editors. Textbook of Nephrology. Philadelphia: Lippincott Williams & Wilkins; 2001. p. 1269—72.

[5] Niwa T, Ise M. Indoxyl sulfate, a circulating uremic toxin, stimulates the progression of glomerular sclerosis. J Lab Clin Med 1994;124:96—104.

[6] Niwa T, Ise M, Miyazaki T. Progression of glomerular sclerosis in experimental uremic rats by administration of indole, a precursor of indoxyl sulfate. Am J Nephrol 1994;14:207—12.

[7] Miyazaki T, Ise M, Seo H, et al. Indoxyl sulfate increases the gene expressions of TGF-β1, TIMP-1 and proα1(I) collagen in kidneys of uremic rats. Kidney Int 1997;52(Suppl. 62): S15—22.

[8] Niwa T, Yazawa T, Ise M, et al. Inhibitory effect of oral sorbent on accumulation of albumin-bound indoxyl sulfate in serum of experimental uremic rats. Nephron 1991;57:84—8.

[9] Niwa T, Emoto Y, Maeda K, et al. Oral sorbent suppresses accumulation of albumin-bound indoxyl sulphate in serum of haemodialysis patients. Nephrol Dial Transplant 1991;6:105—9.

[10] Niwa T, Miyazaki T, Hashimoto N, et al. Suppressed serum and urine levels of indoxyl sulfate by oral sorbent in experimental uremic rats. Am J Nephrol 1992;12:201—6.

[11] Niwa T, Miyazaki T, Tsukushi S, et al. Accumulation of indoxyl-beta-D-glucuronide in uremic serum: suppression of its production by oral sorbent and efficient removal by hemodialysis. Nephron 1996;74:72—8.

[12] Niwa T, Tsukushi S, Ise M, et al. Indoxyl sulfate and progression of renal failure: effects of low-protein diet and oral sorbent on indoxyl sulfate production in uremic rats and undialyzed uremic patients. Miner Electrol Metab 1997;23:179—84.

[13] Niwa T, Nomura T, Sugiyama S, et al. The protein metabolite hypothesis, a model for the progression of renal failure: an oral sorbent lowers indoxyl sulfate levels in undialyzed uremic patients. Kidney Int 1997;52(Suppl. 62):S23—8.

[14] Miyazaki T, Aoyama I, Ise M, et al. An oral sorbent reduces overload of indoxyl sulfate and gene expression of TGF-β1 in uremic rat kidneys. Nephrol Dial Transplant 2000;15: 1773—81.

[15] Miyazaki T, Ise M, Hirata M, et al. Indoxyl sulfate stimulates renal synthesis of transforming growth factor-β1 and progression of renal failure. Kidney Int 1997;52(Suppl. 63):S211—4.

[16] Niwa T. Organic acids and the uremic syndrome: protein metabolite hypothesis in the progression of chronic renal failure. Semin Nephrol 1996;16:167—82.

[17] Niwa T, Aoyama I, Takayama F, et al. Urinary indoxyl sulfate is a clinical factor that affects the progression of renal failure. Miner Electrol Metab 1999;25:118—22.

[18] Aoyama I, Miyazaki T, Takayama F, et al. Oral adsorbent ameliorates renal TGF-β_1 expression in hypercholesterolemic rats. Kidney Int 1999;56(Suppl. 71):S193—7.

[19] Aoyama I, Miyazaki T, Niwa T. Preventive effects of an oral sorbent on nephropathy in rats. Miner Electrol Metab 1999;25:365—72.

[20] Aoyama I, Shimokata K, Niwa T. Oral adsorbent AST-120 ameliorates interstitial fibrosis and transforming growth factor-$\beta1$ expression in spontaneously diabetic (OLETF) rats. Am J Nephrol 2000;20:232—41.

[21] Aoyama I, Niwa T. Molecular insights into preventive effect of AST-120 on the progression of renal failure. Clin Exp Nephrol 2001;5:209—16.

[22] Aoyama I, Niwa T. An oral adsorbent ameliorates renal overload of indoxyl sulfate and progression of renal failure in diabetic rats. Am J Kidney Dis 2001;37(Suppl. 2):S7—12.

[23] Aoyama I, Shimokata K, Niwa T. Combination therapy with benazepril and oral adsorbent ameliorates progressive renal fibrosis in uremic rats. Nephron 2002;90:297—312.

[24] Aoyama I, Shimokata K, Niwa T. An oral adsorbent down-regulates renal expression of genes that promote interstitial inflammation and fibrosis in diabetic rats. Nephron 2002;92: 635—51.

[25] Aoyama I, Enomoto A, Niwa T. Effects of oral adsorbent on gene expression profile in uremic rat kidney: cDNA array analysis. Am J Kidney Dis 2003;41(Suppl. 1):S8—14.

[26] Motojima M, Hosokawa A, Yamato H, et al. Uremic toxins of organic anions up-regulate PAI-1 expression by induction of NF-κB and free radical in proximal tubular cells. Kidney Int 2003;63:1671—80.

[27] Gelasco AK, Raymond JR. Indoxyl sulfate induces complex redox alterations in mesangial cells. Am J Physiol Renal Physiol 2006;290:F1551—8.

[28] Owada S, Goto S, Bannai K, et al. Indoxyl sulfate reduces superoxide scavenging activity in the kidneys of normal and uremic rats. Am J Nephrol 2008;28:446—54.

[29] Taki K, Niwa T. Indoxyl sulfate-lowering capacity of oral sorbents affects prognosis of kidney function and oxidative stress in chronic kidney disease. J Ren Nutr 2007;17:48—52.

[30] Tumur Z, Niwa T. An oral sorbent AST-120 increases renal NO synthesis in uremic rats. J Ren Nutr 2008;18:60—4.

[31] Enomoto A, Takeda M, Tojo A, et al. Role of organic anion transporters in the tubular transport of indoxyl sulfate and the induction of its nephrotoxicity. J Am Soc Nephrol 2002;13:1711—20.

[32] Enomoto A, Takeda M, Taki K, T., et al. Interactions of human organic anion as well as cation transporters with indoxyl sulfate. Eur J Pharmacol 2003;466:13—20.

[33] Taki K, Nakamura S, Miglinas M, et al. Accumulation of indoxyl sulfate in OAT1/3-positive tubular cells in kidneys of patients with chronic renal failure. J Ren Nutr 2006;16:199—203.

[34] Bolati D, Shimizu H, Higashiyama Y, et al. Indoxyl sulfate induces epithelial-to-mesenchymal transition in rat kidneys and human proximal tubular cells. Am J Nephrol 2011;34:318—23.

[35] Kuro-o M, Matsumura Y, Aizawa H, et al. Mutation of the mouse klotho gene leads to a syndrome resembling aging. Nature 1997;390:45—51.

[36] Koh N, Fujimori T, Nishiguchi S, et al. Severely reduced production of Klotho in human chronic renal failure kidney. Biochem Biophys Res Commun 2001;280:1015—20.

[37] Adijiang A, Shimizu H, Higuchi Y, et al. Indoxyl sulfate reduces Klotho expression and promotes senescence in the kidneys of hypertensive rats. J Ren Nutr 2011;21:105—9.

[38] Adijiang A, Niwa T. An oral sorbent AST-120 increases Klotho expression and inhibits cell senescence in the kidney of uremic rats. Am J Nephrol 2010;31:160—4.

[39] Shimizu H, Bolati D, Adijiang A, et al. Indoxyl sulfate down-regulates renal expression of Klotho through production of ROS and activation of NF-κB. Am J Nephrol 2011;33:319—24.

[40] Shimizu H, Bolati D, Adijiang A, et al. Senescence and dysfunction of proximal tubular cells are associated with activated p53 expression by indoxyl sulfate. Am J Physiol Cell Physiol 2010;299:C1110—7.

[41] Shimizu H, Bolati D, Adijiang A, et al. NF-κB plays an important role in indoxyl sulfate-induced cellular senescence, fibrotic gene expression and inhibition of proliferation in proximal tubular cells. Am J Physiol Cell Physiol 2011;301: C1201—12.

[42] Dou L, Bertrand E, Cerini C, et al. The uremic solutes p-cresol and indoxyl sulfate inhibit endothelial proliferation and wound repair. Kidney Int 2004;65:442—51.

[43] Yamamoto H, Tsuruoka S, Ioka T, et al. Indoxyl sulfate stimulates proliferation of rat vascular smooth muscle cells. Kidney Int 2006;69:1780—5.

[44] Muteliefu G, Enomoto A, Niwa T. Indoxyl sulfate promotes proliferation of human aortic smooth muscle cells by inducing oxidative stress. J Ren Nutr 2009;19:29—32.

[45] Taki K, Tsuruta Y, Niwa T. Indoxyl sulfate and atherosclerotic risk factors in hemodialysis patients. Am J Nephrol 2007;27:30—5.

[46] Adijiang A, Goto S, Uramoto S, et al. Indoxyl sulphate promotes aortic calcification with expression of osteoblast-specific proteins in hypertensive rats. Nephrol Dial Transplant 2008;23:1892—901.

[47] Adijiang A, Higuchi Y, Nishijima F, et al. Indoxyl sulfate, a uremic toxin, promotes cell senescence in aorta of hypertensive rats. Biochem Biophys Res Commun 2010;399:637—41.

[48] Niwa T. Indoxyl sulfate is a nephro-vascular toxin. J Ren Nutr 2010;20(Suppl. 1):S2—6.

[49] Muteliefu G, Enomoto A, Jiang P, et al. Indoxyl sulphate induces oxidative stress and the expression of osteoblast-specific proteins in vascular smooth muscle cells. Nephrol Dial Transplant 2009;24:2051—8.

[50] Tumur Z, Niwa T. Indoxyl sulfate inhibits NO production and cell viability by inducing oxidative stress in vascular endothelial cells. Am J Nephrol 2009;29:551—7.

[51] Tumur Z, Shimizu H, Enomoto A, et al. Indoxyl sulfate upregulates expression of ICAM-1 and MCP-1 by oxidative stress-induced NF-κB activation. Am J Nephrol 2010;31:435—41.

[52] Barreto FC, Barreto DV, Liabeuf S, et al. Serum indoxyl sulfate is associated with vascular disease and mortality in chronic kidney disease patients. Clin J Am Soc Nephrol 2009;4:1551—8.

[53] Lekawanvijit S, Adrahtas A, Kelly DJ, et al. Does indoxyl sulfate, a uraemic toxin, have direct effects on cardiac fibroblasts and myocytes? Eur Heart J 2010;31:1771—9.

[54] Yamamoto S, Zuo Y, Ma J, et al. Oral activated charcoal adsorbent (AST-120) ameliorates extent and instability of atherosclerosis accelerated by kidney disease in apolipoprotein E-deficient mice. Nephrol Dial Transplant 2011;26:2491—7.

[55] Fujii H, Nishijima F, Goto S, et al. Oral charcoal adsorbent (AST-120) prevents progression of cardiac damage in chronic kidney disease through suppression of oxidative stress. Nephrol Dial Transplant 2009;24:2089—95.

[56] Schulman G, Agarwal R, Acharya M, et al. A multicenter, randomized, double-blind, placebo-controlled, dose-ranging

study of AST-120 (Kremezin) in patients with moderate to severe CKD. Am J Kidney Dis 2006;47:565—77.

[57] Iida S, Kohno K, Yoshimura J, et al. Carbonic-adsorbent AST-120 reduces overload of indoxyl sulfate and the plasma level of TGF-beta1 in patients with chronic renal failure. Clin Exp Nephrol 2006;10:262—7.

[58] Shoji T, Wada A, Inoue K, et al. Prospective randomized study evaluating the efficacy of the spherical adsorptive carbon AST-120 in chronic kidney disease patients with moderate decrease in renal function. Nephron Clin Pract 2007;105: c99—107.

[59] Yorioka N, Kiribayashi K, Naito T, et al. An oral adsorbent, AST-120, combined with a low-protein diet and RAS blocker, for chronic kidney disease. J Nephrol 2008;21:213—20.

[60] Konishi K, Nakano S, Tsuda S, et al. AST-120 (Kremezin) initiated in early stage chronic kidney disease stunts the progression of renal dysfunction in type 2 diabetic subjects. Diabetes Res Clin Pract 2008;81:310—5.

[61] Akizawa T, Asano Y, Morita S, et al. A multicenter, randomized, controlled trial of a carbonaceous oral adsorbent's effectiveness against the progression of chronic kidney disease: the CAP-KD study. Am J Kidney Dis 2009;54:459—67.

[62] Nakamura T, Sato E, Fujiwara N, et al. Oral adsorbent AST-120 ameliorates tubular injury in chronic renal failure patients by reducing proteinuria and oxidative stress generation. Metabolism 2011;60:260—4.

[63] Ueda H, Shibahara N, Takagi S, et al. AST-120, an oral adsorbent, delays the initiation of dialysis in patients with chronic kidney diseases. Ther Apher Dial 2007;11:189—95.

[64] Nakamura T, Kawagoe Y, Matsuda T, et al. Oral ADSORBENT AST-120 decreases carotid intima-media thickness and arterial stiffness in patients with chronic renal failure. Kidney Blood Press Res 2004;27:121—6.

[65] Ueda H, Shibahara N, Takagi S, et al. AST-120 treatment in predialysis period affects the prognosis in patients on hemodialysis. Ren Fail 2008;30:856—60.

[66] Yu M, Kim YJ, Kang DH. Indoxyl sulfate-induced endothelial dysfunction in patients with chronic kidney disease via an induction of oxidative stress. Clin J Am Soc Nephrol 2011;6:30—9.

[67] Shibahara H, Shibahara N. Cardiorenal protective effect of the oral uremic toxin absorbent AST-120 in chronic heart disease patients with moderate CKD. J Nephrol 2010;23:535—40.

[68] Nakai K, Fujii H, Kono K, et al. Effects of AST-120 on left ventricular mass in predialysis patients. Am J Nephrol 2011;33: 218—23.

[69] Nii-Kono T, Iwasaki Y, Uchida M, et al. Indoxyl sulfate induces skeletal resistance to parathyroid hormone in cultured osteoblastic cells. Kidney Int 2007;71:738—43.

[70] Iwasaki Y, Yamato H, Nii-Kono T, et al. Administration of oral charcoal adsorbent (AST-120) suppresses low-turnover bone progression in uraemic rats. Nephrol Dial Transplant 2006;21: 2768—74.

16

Altering Serum Lipids to Reduce Progression of Chronic Kidney Disease

Vito M. Campese, Samia Raju

Division of Nephrology, Keck School of Medicine, University of Southern California, Los Angeles, California

KIDNEY DISEASE AND DYSLIPIDEMIA

Dyslipidemia in patients with chronic kidney disease (CKD) is very common and it is typified by high levels of very-low-density lipoproteins, triglycerides, lipoprotein(a), small low-density lipoprotein (LDL) particles, and by impaired maturation of high-density lipoprotein cholesterol (HDL-C) [1]. Dyslipidemia may contribute to atherosclerosis and to the increased incidence of cardiovascular morbidity and mortality in this population. Evidence has also accumulated supporting the notion that lipid abnormalities may contribute to progression of CKD via the direct toxic effects of lipids and the inflammatory mechanisms common to both CKD and associated dyslipidemia [2,3].

It has been posited that dyslipidemia may affect the renal microvasculature in the same way that it affects the coronary microvasculature and it may account, at least in part, for the linkage between renal and cardiovascular diseases [4].

As with the general circulation, in the renal microcirculation macrophages may phagocytose oxidized LDL and undergo a transition to form foam cells. These foam cells release cytokines that recruit more macrophages which leads to more lipid accumulation, endothelial dysfunction and smooth muscle cells proliferation.

In addition to the effects of dyslipidemia on the renal microvasculature, accumulation of lipids in renal cells may up-regulate intracellular signaling pathways involved in inflammatory and fibrogenic responses, both of which are implicated in progressive renal injury [5].

Mesangial cells express LDL-receptors as well as scavenger receptors (SRA1 and CD36) that take-up oxidized LDL in an unregulated fashion. Activation of CD36 induces expression of the chemokines and IL-6 which is a potent stimulus for mesangial sclerosis [6]. Accumulation of ox-LDL in mesangial cells is believed to activate various growth factors and cytokines, which in turn cause mesangial cell proliferation and mesangial matrix expansion. LDL and ox-LDL stimulate the expression of monocyte chemoattractant protein-1 (MCP-1) mRNA, which increases monocyte chemotactic activity in mesangial cells [7]. LDL and ox-LDL also stimulate the expression of fibronectin mRNA and increase fibronectin protein concentrations, which induce proliferation of mesangial cells. Inflammatory cytokines cause dysregulation of LDL receptor in mesangial cells contributing to the accumulation of cholesterol and triglycerides. The cytotoxic effects of ox-LDL are evidenced by the induction of podocyte apoptosis and its ability to decrease Akt activity, deplete nephrin (an adhesion molecule specific to the glomerular slit membrane), and induce the retraction of cultured podocytes. This leads to alteration in the glomerular size-selective barrier to proteins and increased albumin diffusion into the renal parenchyma [8]. Both hypercholesterolemia and hypertriglyceremia are associated with podocyte injury, proteinuria and interstitial injury [9].

LDL and ox-LDL induce the expression of nuclear factor (NF)-κB, an essential mediator of inflammation and mesangial cell proliferation in glomerulonephritis [10]. NF-κB induces the expression of genes that encode other cytokines, chemokines, interferons, growth factors, cell adhesion molecules, and major histocompatibility complex proteins that are involved in inflammation and proliferation [11].

Lipoproteins accumulate in both glomerular and mesangial cells and within the mesangial matrix of patients with glomerular disease [12], and oxidized LDL (ox-LDL) particles are often found in renal biopsy specimens from patients with renal disease [13]. Some investigators have observed a strong correlation between triglyceride and apolipoprotein-B-containing lipoproteins and the rate of CKD progression [14]. In patients with focal and segmental glomerular sclerosis, podocytes undergo hypertrophy, foot process effacement, pseudocyst formation and detachment. This is followed by occlusion and collapse of capillaries with inclusion of foam cells and hyaline deposits that seem to contribute to the progression of the disease [15].

LIPID LOWERING AND PLEIOTROPIC EFFECTS OF STATINS

The principal action of statins is to inhibit cholesterol synthesis by inhibiting 3-hydroxy-3-methylglutaryl coenzyme A (HMG-CoA) reductase, an enzyme that controls the rate of cholesterol synthesis in the liver via the mevalonate pathway. Statins thereby effectively reduce serum levels of LDL-C. To the extent that high levels of LDL-cholesterol contribute to the progression of CKD, statins may slow this process. However, it has been postulated that the beneficial effects of statins on the kidney may be linked, at least in part, to pleiotropic effects on inflammatory cell-signaling pathways that control vascular cell migration, proliferation, and differentiation.

Besides serving as precursor of cholesterol, mevalonate also serves as a precursor for isoprenoids, such as farnesylpyrophosphate (F-PP) and geranylpyrophosphate (G-PP), a group of proteins that normally attach posttranslationally to intracellular signaling proteins, including the GTPases — Rho, Rac and Ras — and the G-proteins [16]. These signaling proteins, in turn, facilitate the interaction between growth-factor receptors and the cellular cytoskeleton [17]. By inhibiting HMG-CoA reductase, statins specifically block the synthesis of these isoprenoids and prevent the anchoring of growth factors to the cell membrane and cytoskeleton, thus hindering signal transduction to the nucleus, activation of transcription factors, and cell proliferation in the vascular endothelium.

Inhibition of the production of mevalonate and isoprenoids results in profound immunomodulatory and anti-inflammatory effects (Table 16.1 and Figure 16.1) [18−20]. Statins reduce levels of MCP-1, IL-1β, tumor necrosis factor-α, transforming growth factor-β, IL-6, PDGF, NF-κB, vascular cell adhesion molecule-1, intercellular adhesion molecule-1, fibronectin mRNA, and mesangial proteins [21−25].

Using cultured vascular smooth muscle cells and endothelial cells, Dichtl and colleagues [26] found that statins downregulate the activation of NF-κB, activator protein-1, and hypoxia-inducible factor-1α. Inhibition of NF-κB activation may decrease the release of MCP-1 and stimulate apoptosis of vascular smooth muscle cells [27]. In vitro studies indicate that statins reduce the proliferation of renal tubular epithelium by impairment of activator protein-1 binding [28,30]. as well as by preventing monocytes from maturing into macrophages, while inducing apoptosis of these cells [31]. Statins

TABLE 16.1 Anti-Inflammatory and Immunologic Effects of Statins

Anti-Inflammatory Effects	Immunologic Effects
Decrease ET-1	Decrease interferon gamma-induced MHC class II Expression
Decrease IL-6	Decrease T-cell activation
Decrease VCAM-1 and ICAM-1	Decrease monocyte activation
Decrease PDGF	Increase transplant survival?
Decrease NF-κB activation	Increase resistance to complement
Decrease endothelial cell activation	Increase inhibition of leukocyte function antigen-1
Decrease leukocyte-endothelial cell adhesion	
Decrease pro-inflammatory cytokines (particularly MCP-1)	
Decrease CRP	
Increase NO	
Increase PPAR-α	
Induce apo A-I expression	
Inhibit LDL oxidation	
Inhibit histamine release by basophils	

Apo A-I = apolipoprotein A-I; CRP = C-reactive protein; ET-1 = endothelin-1; ICAM-1 = intercellular adhesion molecule-1; IL-6 = interleukin-6; LDL = low-density lipoprotein; MCP-1 = monocyte chemoattractant protein-1; MHC = major histocompatibility complex; NF-κB = nuclear factor kappaB; NO = nitric oxide; PDGF = platelet-derived growth factor; PPAR-α = peroxisome proliferator-activated receptor-α; VCAM-1 = vascular cell adhesion molecule-1. *Reproduced with permission from Ref # [20].*

downregulate surface integrin adhesion molecules and inactivate Rho GTPases, thus preventing monocytes adhesion to endothelial cells, and blunting the earliest manifestations of atherosclerosis [29]. Statins also protect against the oxidation of LDL and thereby reduce oxidative stress [30,31].

Finally, statins have been shown to up-regulate and stabilize endothelial NO synthase (eNOS), while increasing the bioavailability of NO, a potent vasodilator with apparent anti-inflammatory actions and beneficial effects on platelet aggregation, neutrophil adhesion, and cell proliferation [32,33].

STATINS IN EXPERIMENTAL KIDNEY DISEASE

Substantial evidence supports the notion that statins may reduce the progression of kidney disease through

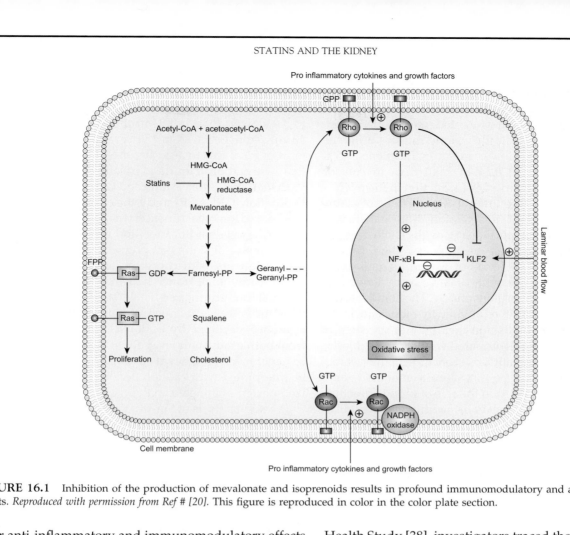

FIGURE 16.1 Inhibition of the production of mevalonate and isoprenoids results in profound immunomodulatory and anti-inflammatory effects. *Reproduced with permission from Ref # [20].* This figure is reproduced in color in the color plate section.

their anti-inflammatory and immunomodulatory effects in several experimental models.

Atorvastatin has been shown to increase eNOS activity and NO availability in aging rats, and to reduce tubular injury after acute renal ischemia [34]. Statins reduce left ventricular hypertrophy and proteinuria in Dahl salt-sensitive rats [35] and the rate of glomerulosclerosis in the renal ablation model of CKD in rats [1].

In a rat model of glomerulonephritis, Yoshimura and coworkers [36] showed that simvastatin suppressed mesangial cell proliferation, mesangial matrix expansion, and macrophage infiltration into the glomeruli. Lovastatin also attenuated glomerular macrophage infiltration and albuminuria in a rat model of puromycin aminonucleoside nephrosis [37].

EFFECTS OF DYSLIPIDEMIA AND STATINS ON THE PROGRESSION OF KIDNEY DISEASE IN HUMAN SUBJECTS

CKD Patients

Epidemiological and clinical evidence support the notion that dyslipidemia is a risk factor for CKD progression in human subjects and that lipid lowering agents may slow disease progression. In the Physician's Health Study [38], investigators traced the probability of ensuing renal dysfunction over a period of 14 years in 4483 apparently healthy males (baseline plasma creatinine level <1.5 mg/dL. After 14 years, 134 subjects (3%) had an elevated creatinine ≥1.5 mg/dL and 244 (5.4%) had reduced CrCl ≤55 mL/min. The odds of renal disease progression were directly related to baseline blood lipid levels.

The Helsinki Heart Study documented an association between dyslipidemia and progressive kidney disease in 2702 middle-aged dyslipidemic men. Renal function deteriorated by a mean 3% over 5 years, and although hypertension contributed to this change, the decline was faster in men with an LDL:HDL ratio >4.4 than in those with a ratio <3.2. Multiple regression analyses indicated that the only measures having a significant effect on the observed phenomenon were an increased LDL-HDL ratio (more rapid progression) and an increased HDL-C level (slower progression) [39].

Equally substantial, albeit inconclusive, is the evidence that lipid-lowering agents may help preserve renal function in patients with CKD.

A meta-analysis of 15 studies involving a total of 1384 patients and averaging 24 weeks in duration showed that statins reduced albuminuria (in 11 studies) and proteinuria (in 4 studies) in 13 of 15 studies. The reduction in albumin or protein excretion was greater among studies with greater baseline albuminuria or proteinuria [40].

In a meta-analysis of 27 studies with 39,704 participants, the change in the weighted mean differences for eGFR was statistically significantly different (1.22 mL/min per yr slower in statin recipients; 95% confidence interval [CI] 0.44 to 2.00) than in control subjects, corresponding to a 76% reduction in the overall rate of loss. In subgroup analysis, the benefit of statin therapy for slowing of progression was statistically significant in studies of participants with cardiovascular disease (0.93 mL/min per year slower than control subjects; 95% CI 0.10 to 1.76) but was not significantly different for participants with diabetic or hypertensive kidney disease or glomerulonephritis. The standardized mean difference for the reduction in albuminuria or proteinuria as a result of statin therapy was statistically significant (-0.58 g/24 h compared with control subjects; CI, -0.99–0.17). The authors concluded that statin therapy seems to reduce proteinuria modestly and results in a small reduction in the rate of kidney function loss, especially in populations with cardiovascular disease [41].

A prospective, controlled, open-label study by Bianchi et al. [42] showed that atorvastatin 10–40 mg/d reduced proteinuria and the rate of progression of kidney disease in 56 patients with CKD. Patients had proteinuria more than 1 g/24 h, hypercholesterolemia, and were already receiving treatment with angiotensin-converting enzyme inhibitors, angiotensin II type 1 receptor blockers, or a combination of the two. After one year, the atorvastatin-treated patients displayed a significant drop in urine protein excretion (from 2.2 ± 0.1 to 1.2 ± 1.0 g/24 h; $P < 0.01$) and only a nonsignificant fall in creatinine clearance (from 51 ± 1.8 to 49.8 ± 1.7 mL/min). By contrast, patients treated with placebo manifested no change in proteinuria and a marked decrease in creatinine clearance (from 50 ± 1.9 to 44.2 ± 1.6 mL/min; $P < 0.01$).

Secondary and post hoc analyses of renal function in landmark statin trials have also underscored the renoprotective effects of statins. A post hoc analysis of nearly 690 out of 3384 participants in the Cholesterol and Recurrent Events (CARE) study with GFR estimated from the MDRD (Modification of Diet in Renal Disease) equation < 60 mL/min per 1.73 m^2), demonstrated that the MDRD-GFR decline in the pravastatin group was not significantly different from that in the placebo group (0.1 mL/min per 1.73 m^2/yr slower; 95% CI, -0.2 to 0.4; $P = 0.49$). However, there was a significant stepwise inverse relation between MDRD-GFR before treatment and slowing of renal function loss with pravastatin use, with more benefit in those with lower MDRD-GFR at baseline ($P = 0.04$). The rate of change in MDRD-GFR in the pravastatin group was 0.6 mL/min per 1.73 m^2/yr slower than placebo (95% CI, -0.1 to 1.2; $P = 0.07$) in those with MDRD-GFR < 50 mL/min, and 2.5 mL/min per 1.73 m^2/yr slower (95% CI, 1.4 to 3.6 slower; $P = 0.0001$) in those with MDRD-GFR < 40 mL/min per 1.73 m^2/yr. Pravastatin also reduced rates of renal loss to a greater extent in participants with than without proteinuria at baseline ($P = 0.006$) [43].

In the Greek Atorvastatin and Coronary Heart Disease Evaluation (GREACE) study, the effect of atorvastatin, 10 to 80 mg/d, on renal function was compared with "usual care" (lifestyle modification and standard drug therapy not exclusive of statins) in previously untreated dyslipidemic patients with coronary heart disease. At study end, creatinine clearance had increased by 12% in the atorvastatin group versus 4.9% in the "usual care" patients who were given statins, whereas creatinine clearance declined by 5.2% ($P < 0.0001$) in patients from both groups who had either stopped taking statins or never received them at all [44]. These findings should be interpreted with caution because of the nonrandomized design of the data analysis.

In a sub-analysis of the Treating to New Targets (TNT) study, Shepherd et al. [45] investigated the effect of intensive lipid lowering on renal function using 10 mg vs. 80 mg of atorvastatin in patients with coronary heart disease. 10,001 patients with LDL cholesterol levels <130 mg/dL were randomized to double-blind therapy with atorvastatin, 10 mg/day or 80 mg/day. Estimated glomerular filtration rate (eGFR), using the MDRD equation, was compared at baseline and at the end of follow-up in 9656 participants with complete renal data. Mean eGFR at baseline was 65.6 ± 11.4 mL/min/1.73 m^2 in the atorvastatin 10 mg group and 65.0 ± 11.2 mL/min/1.73 m^2 in the atorvastatin 80 mg group.

At the end of the five-year study period, mean change in eGFR showed an increase of 3.5 ± 0.14 mL/min/1.73m^2 with atorvastatin 10 mg and 5.2 ± 0.14 mL/min/1.73m^2 with atorvastatin 80 mg ($P < 0.0001$ for treatment difference). The expected five-year decline in renal function was not observed in this study. Estimated GFR improved in both TNT treatment groups, but the significantly greater increase with 80 mg versus 10 mg of atorvastatin suggests a dose-related benefit. A weakness of this study was the absence of an untreated control group. The reasons for the increase in GFR in the atorvastatin treated group are unclear. This could be due to improved availability of nitric oxide, and/or to decreased inflammation. Whether this increase in eGFR translates into histological benefits to the kidney is uncertain at the time.

The Study of Heart and Renal Protection (SHARP) was a double-blind trial that included 9270 patients with CKD who were randomly assigned to simvastatin, 20 mg, plus exetimibe, 10 mg, daily versus matching placebo. Allocation to simvastatin plus ezetimibe yielded an average serum LDL cholesterol difference of 0.85 mmol/L during a median follow-up of 4.9 years and produced a 17% reduction in major atherosclerotic events. In the 6247 patients not on dialysis at randomization, allocation to simvastatin plus ezitimibe produced a significant reduction in the urinary albumin:creatinine ratio in patients with microalbuminuria or proteinuria. But it did not produce significant reductions in the incidence of end-stage renal disease or doubling of serum creatinine [46].

In all, these studies indicate that several questions remain unanswered regarding the postulated renoprotective effect of statins. Do statins reduce proteinuria? Are statins different than other lipid-lowering agents with regard to CKD progression? Are there differences in the antiproteinuric and kidney protective effects of various statins?

Kidney Transplant Patients

Dyslipidemia is very common among kidney transplant patients, and it affects up to 74% of recipients [47]. Dyslipidemia has been implicated in the development of chronic allograft nephropathy [48]. Consequently, lipid-lowering agents are commonly used in this population not only to reduce the risk for atherosclerotic vascular disease, but also to extend graft preservation. However, to date the clinical evidence to support the therapeutic benefit of statins in transplantation is inconclusive.

Administration of pravastatin and losartan reduced inflammation and fibrosis in a rat model of chronic cyclosporine-induced nephropathy independently of any hypolipidemic or hypotensive properties [49]. In a prospective study of cardiac transplantation, patients given pravastatin soon after surgery experienced less frequent cardiac rejection and better survival after 1 year than untreated individuals [50]. A retrospective analysis of 77 renal transplant recipients showed that at 12 months post-surgery, patients given statins manifested higher creatinine clearance and reduced fractional interstitial area and collagen III deposition than patients who were not treated [51]. In another study, renal transplant recipients randomly assigned to pravastatin for 4 months had one-half the rate of acute rejection as did placebo recipients (25% vs. 58%, $P < 0.01$) [52].

By contrast, use of simvastatin starting 2 weeks after renal transplantation did not reduce acute rejection compared to a control group treated with fibrate or placebo despite a significant reduction in total and LDL-cholesterol in the simvastatin compared with the placebo-treated group [53].

In the Assessment of Lescol in Renal Transplant (ALERT) trial, a double-blind, placebo-controlled study of 2102 renal transplant patients with total cholesterol levels of 155 to 348 mg/dL, participants were randomly assigned to fluvastatin, 40 mg or 80 mg, versus placebo and followed up for 5 to 6 years. Patients given fluvastatin experienced a 32% decrease in LDL-cholesterol levels and a not statistically significant reduction in the risk of major adverse cardiac events, the primary endpoint for this trial. In this study there was no improvement in the incidence of acute rejection, renal graft loss or doubling of serum creatinine levels, nor was active therapy associated with less deterioration in the GFR over time than was placebo [54]. Patients taking fluvastatin did not experience an increase in adverse effects reflecting its lower risk of interaction with calcineurin inhibitors compared with some other statins. Fluvastatin, pravastatin and rosuvastatin may be reasonable choices in renal transplant recipients given their low degree of interaction with calcineurin inhibitors.

In summary, although statins reduce cardiovascular risk in hyperlipidemic patients who have undergone renal transplantation, their routine use to prevent acute or chronic rejection is not supported by the evidence. Additional studies are needed to determine what role statins might play in the prevention of chronic allograft nephropathy.

Are All Statins Equally Effective in Reducing Proteinuria and CKD Progression?

All statins reduce LDL-cholesterol, albeit to different extents. The common belief is that to the extent that statins reduce LDL-cholesterol they should be commensurately effective in reducing cardiovascular disease and CKD progression. However, concerns that this might not be the case, at least with regard to CKD progression, arose with the introduction of rosuvastatin into the market.

Clinical trial data suggested that rosuvastatin use was associated with a dose-dependent increase in urine protein excretion and micro-hematuria, whereas this effect was not apparent with other statins [55]. The explanation provided was that this proteinuria was of tubular origin and characterized mainly by increased levels of low-molecular-weight proteins (e.g., alpha-1 microglobulin). The cause of tubular proteinuria was attributed to inhibition of HMG CoA reductase in the renal tubular cells. However, this explanation could not justify the increase in micro-hematuria [56].

A pooled analysis of renal function data from the rosuvastatin clinical development program, in which a diverse group of >10,000 persons received recommended doses for up to 3.8 years with a median duration of 8 weeks, showed that treated subjects had lower serum creatinine levels, as well as increased eGFR compared with baseline, both early and later in the course of treatment [57]. Beneficial effects were consistent across all demographic subgroups, including in patients with eGFR <60 mL/min/1.73 m^2, patients with baseline proteinuria, and patients with hypertension and/or diabetes, and were independent of the extent of lipid lowering. In contrast, placebo recipients showed no change in either serum creatinine levels or eGFR. Comparative analysis of rosuvastatin's renal effects in its recommended dose range (5–40 mg) with atorvastatin (10–80 mg), simvastatin (10–80 mg), pravastatin (10–40 mg), or placebo showed no difference in urine dipstick protein excretion among patients who received rosuvastatin, versus other statins or placebo. The investigators concluded that rosuvastatin, like other statins, may arrest the progression of renal disease.

These studies were reassuring. However, the majority of participants in these studies had normal to mildly impaired kidney function and had no significant proteinuria at the time of randomization.

Similarly reassuring was a small prospective, open-label, randomized trial of 20 weeks duration involving only 44 patients by Verma et al. [58] who showed that rosuvastatin 10 mg/day therapy increased eGFR by 11%.

In contrast to the above studies, in the JUPITER (Justification for the Use of Statins in Prevention: an Intervention Trial Evaluating Rosuvastatin), a randomized, double-blind, placebo-controlled, multicenter trial in apparently healthy men (≥50 yrs) and women (≥60 yrs), Ridker et al. [59] randomized (1:1 ratio) 17,802 participants to receive rosuvastatin, 20 mg daily, or placebo. The study showed that healthy persons without hyperlipidemia but with elevated high-sensitivity C-reactive protein levels treated with rosuvastatin manifested a reduced incidence of cardiovascular events compared with participants treated with placebo. In this study, after 12 months of treatment, eGFR was reduced equally in the rosuvastatin and in the placebo group. This study did not show any beneficial or adverse effects of rosuvastatin on eGFR irrespective of whether participants had a baseline eGFR greater or lower than 60 mL/min/1.73 m^2 [60].

The ECLIPSE Study was designed to compare the efficacy and safety of force-titrated treatment with rosuvastatin (10–40 mg) with that of atorvastatin (10–80 mg) in 1036 high-risk patients with hypercholesterolemia. The study showed that increasing doses of rosuvastatin produced a dose-related increase in the incidence of proteinuria (from 0.2 to 1.8%) and hematuria (from 2.9 to 4.0%), whereas this effect was not apparent with atorvastatin. Despite these differences, the authors concluded that rosuvastatin and atorvastatin were similarly well tolerated [61].

PLANET 1 was a prospective randomized study of the effects of rosuvastatin, 10 mg/day, rosuvastatin, 40 mg/day, or atorvastatin, 80 mg/day, on proteinuria and eGFR in 353 patients with diabetes mellitus and CKD. The primary end-point was the change in urinary protein/creatinine ratio from baseline to week 52. Secondary end-points included changes in eGFR from baseline to weeks 26 and 52. The study showed that patients treated with atorvastatin by 52 weeks manifested an average decrease in urine protein/creatinine excretion of 12.6% and no significant change in eGFR. By contrast, patients treated with rosuvastatin manifested no significant change in urine protein/creatinine excretion and a significant and dose-related decrease in eGFR [62].

PLANET 2 was a prospective evaluation of proteinuria and renal function in 237 patients with non-diabetes-induced CKD who were randomized to rosuvastatin, 10 mg/day, rosuvastatin, 40 mg/day, or atorvastatin, 80 mg/day. The primary end-point was the change in urinary protein/creatinine ratio from baseline to week 52. Secondary end-points included changes in eGFR from baseline to weeks 26 and 52. The study showed that patients treated with atorvastatin manifested a 24.6% decrease in the urinary protein/creatinine excretion ratio. By contrast, patients treated with rosuvastatin manifested no significant change in urine protein/creatinine excretion and a significant and dose-related decrease in eGFR. The differential effects on proteinuria and eGFR in the treatment groups were not a result of lipid lowering.

In summary, the current evidence indicates that the renoprotection of statins is not a class effect and particular caution has to be used with high doses of rosuvastatin in patients with proteinuria and pre-existing CKD.

References

[1] Vaziri ND. Dyslipidemia of chronic renal failure: the nature, mechanisms, and potential consequences. AJP – Renal Physiol 290:F262–F272.

[2] Kasiske BL, O'Donnell MP, Cowardin W, Keane WF. Lipids and the kidney. Hypertension 1990;15:443–50.

[3] Schaeffner ES, Kurth T, Curhan GC, et al. Cholesterol and the risk of renal dysfunction in apparently healthy men. J Am Soc Nephrol 2003;14:2084–91.

[4] Chade AR, Brosh D, Higano ST, et al. Mild renal insufficiency is associated with reduced coronary flow in patients with non-obstructive coronary artery disease. Kidney Int 2006;69:266–71.

[5] Oda H, Keane WG. Recent advances in statins and the kidney. Kidney Int Suppl 1999;71:S2–5.

[6] Massy ZA, Kim Y, Guijarro C, Kasiske B, Keane WF, O'Donnell MP. Low-density lipoprotein-induced expression of interleukin-6, a marker of human mesangial cell inflammation: Effects of oxidation and modulation by lovastatin. Biochem Biophys Res Commun 2000;267:536–40.

[7] Rovin BH, Tan LC. LDL stimulates mesangial fibronectin production and chemoattractant expression. Kidney Int 1993;43:218–25.

[8] Bussolati B, Deregibus MC, Fonsato V, et al. Statins prevent oxidized LDL-induced injury of glomerular podocytes by

activating the phosphatidylinositol 3-kinase/AKT-signaling pathway. J Am Soc Nephrol 2005;16:1936—47.

[9] Joles JA, Kunter U, Janssen U, Kriz W, Rabelink TJ, Koomans HA, et al. Early mechanisms of renal injury in hypercholesterolemic or hypertriglyceridemic rats. J Am Soc Nephrol 2000;11:669—83.

[10] Guijarro C, Egido J. Transcription factor-κB (NF-κB) and renal disease. Kidney Int 2001;59:415—24.

[11] Kuldo JM, Ogawara KI, Werner N, et al. Molecular pathways of endothelial cell activation for (targeted) pharmacological intervention of chronic inflammatory diseases. Curr Vasc Pharmacol 2005;3:11—39.

[12] Yoshimura A, Nemoto T, Sugenoya Y, et al. Effect of simvastatin on proliferative nephritis and cell-cycle protein expression. Kidney Int Suppl 1999;71:S84—7.

[13] Magil AB. Interstitial foam cells and oxidized lipoprotein in human glomerular disease. Mod Pathol 1999 Jan;12(1):33—40.

[14] Samuelsson O, Mulec H, Knight-Gibson C, Attman PO, Kron B, Larsson R, et al. Lipoprotein abnormalities are associated with increased rate of progression of human chronic renal insufficiency. Nephrol Dial Transplant 1997;12:1908—15.

[15] Noel LH. Morphological features of primary focal and segmental glomerulosclerosis. Nephrol Dial Transplant 1999; 14(Suppl. 3):53—7.

[16] Pierre-Paul D, Gahtan V. Noncholesterol-lowering effects of statins. Vasc Endovascular Surg 2003;37:301—13.

[17] Mason JC. Statins and their role in vascular protection. Clin Sci (Lond) 2003;105:251—66.

[18] Mason JC. Statins and their role in vascular protection. Clin Sci (Lond) 2003;105:251—66.

[19] Crisby M. Modulation of the inflammatory process by statins. Drugs Today (Barc) 2003;39:137—43.

[20] Campese V, Park J. HMG Co-A Reductase Inhibitors and the Kidney. Kidney Int 2007;71:1215—22.

[21] Pierre-Paul D, Gahtan V. Noncholesterol-lowering effects of statins. Vasc Endovascular Surg 2003;37:301—13.

[22] Massy ZA, Kim Y, Guijarro C, et al. Low-density lipoprotein-induced expression of interleukin-6, a marker of human mesangial cell inflammation: effects of oxidation and modulation by lovastatin. Biochem Biophys Res Commun 2000;267:536—40.

[23] Kim SY, Guijarro C, O'Donnell MP, et al. Human mesangial cell production of monocyte chemoattractant protein-1: modulation by lovastatin. Kidney Int 1995;48:363—71.

[24] Chen HC, Guh JY, Shin SJ, Lai YH. Pravastatin suppress superoxide and fibronectin production of glomerular mesangial cells induced by oxidized-LDL and high glucose. Atherosclerosis 2002;160:141—6.

[25] Guijarro C, Kim Y, Schoonover CM, et al. Lovastatin inhibits lipopolysaccharide-induced NF-kappaB activation in human mesangial cells. Nephrol Dial Transplant 1996;11:990—6.

[26] Dichtl W, Dulak J, Frick M, et al. HMG-CoA reductase inhibitors regulate inflammatory transcription factors in human endothelial and vascular smooth muscle cells. Arterioscler Thromb Vasc Biol 2003;23:58—63.

[27] Zelvyte I, Dominaitiene R, Crisby M, Janciauskiene S. Modulation of inflammatory mediators and PPARgamma and NFkappaB expression by pravastatin in response to lipoproteins in human monocytes in vitro. Pharmacol Res 2002;45:147—54.

[28] Vrtovsnik F, Couette S, Prie D, et al. Lovastatin-induced inhibition of renal epithelial tubular cell proliferation involves a p21ras activated, AP-1-dependent pathway. Kidney Int 1997;52:1016—27.

[29] Yoshida M, Sawada T, Ishii H, et al. HMG-CoA reductase inhibitor modulates monocyte-endothelial cell interaction under physiological flow conditions in vitro: involvement of

Rho GTPase-dependent mechanism. Arterioscler Thromb Vasc Biol 2001;21:1165—71.

[30] Laufs U, La Fata V, Plutzky J, Liao JK. Upregulation of endothelial nitric oxide synthase by HMG CoA reductase inhibitors. Circulation 1998;97:1129—35.

[31] Hernández-Perera O, Pérez-Sala D, Navarro-Antolín J, et al. Effects of the 3-hydroxy-3-methylglutaryl-CoA reductase inhibitors, atorvastatin and simvastatin, on the expression of endothelin-1 and endothelial nitric oxide synthase in vascular endothelial cells. J Clin Invest 1998;101:2711—9.

[32] Wolfrum S, Jensen KS, Liao JK. Endothelium-dependent effects of statins. Arterioscler Thromb Vasc Biol 2003;23:729—36.

[33] Blantz RC, Munger K. Role of nitric oxide in inflammatory conditions. Nephron 2002;90:373—8.

[34] Sabbatini M, Pisani A, Uccello F, et al. Atorvastatin improves the course of ischemic acute renal failure in aging rats. J Am Soc Nephrol 2004;15:901—9.

[35] Zhou M-S, Jaimes EA, Raij L. Atorvastatin prevents end-organ injury in salt-sensitive hypertension: role of eNOS and oxidant stress. Hypertension 2004;44:186—90.

[36] Yoshimura A, Nemoto T, Sugenoya Y, et al. Effect of simvastatin on proliferative nephritis and cell-cycle protein expression. Kidney Int Suppl 1999;71:S84—7.

[37] Park Y-S, Guijarro C, Kim Y, et al. Lovastatin reduces glomerular macrophage influx and expression of monocyte chemoattractant protein-1 mRNA in nephrotic rats. Am J Kidney Dis 1998;31:190—4.

[38] Schaeffner ES, Kurth T, Curhan GC, et al. Cholesterol and the risk of renal dysfunction in apparently healthy men. J Am Soc Nephrol 2003;14:2084—91.

[39] Mänttäri M, Tiula E, Alikoski T, Manninen V. Effects of hypertension and dyslipidemia on the decline in renal function. Hypertension 1995;26:670—5.

[40] Douglas K, O'Malley PG, Jackson JL. Meta-Analysis: The effect of statins on albuminuria. Ann Intern Med 2006;145:117—24.

[41] Sandhu S, Wiebe N, Fried LF, Tonelli M. Statins for Improving Renal Outcomes: A Meta-Analysis. J Am Soc Nephrol 2006;17: 2006—16.

[42] Bianchi S, Bigazzi R, Caiazza A, Campese VM. A controlled, prospective study of the effects of atorvastatin on proteinuria and progression of kidney disease. Am J Kidney Dis 2003;41: 565—70.

[43] Tonelli M, Moyé L, Sacks FM, et al. for the Cholesterol and Recurrent Events (CARE) Trial Investigators. Effect of pravastatin on loss of renal function in people with moderate chronic renal insufficiency and cardiovascular disease. J Am Soc Nephrol 2003;14:1605—13.

[44] Athyros VG, Mikhailidis DP, Papageorgiou AA, et al. The effect of statins versus untreated dyslipidaemia on renal function in patients with coronary heart disease: a subgroup analysis of the Greek atorvastatin and coronary heart disease evaluation (GREACE) study. J Clin Pathol 2004;57:728—34.

[45] Shepherd J, Kastelein JJ, Bittner V, Deedwania P, Breazna A, Dobson S, et al. Effect of intensive lipid lowering with atorvastatin on renal function in patients with coronary heart disease: the Treating to New Targets (TNT) study. Clin J Am Soc Nephrol 2007 Nov;2(6):1131—9.

[46] Baigent C, Landray MJ, Reith C, et al. The effects of lowering LDL cholesterol with simvastatin plus ezitimibe in patients with chronic kidney disease (Study of Heart and Renal Protection): a randomized placebo-controlled trial. Lancet 2011;377:2181—92.

[47] Katznelson S, Wilkinson AH, Kobashigawa JA, et al. The effect of pravastatin on acute rejection after kidney transplantation—a pilot study. Transplantation 1996;61:1469—74.

[48] Isoniemi H, Nurminen M, Tikkanen MJ, et al. Risk factors predicting chronic rejection of renal allografts. Transplantation 1994;57:68—72.

[49] Li C, Sun BK, Lim SW, et al. Combined effects of losartan and pravastatin on interstitial inflammation and fibrosis in chronic cyclosporine-induced nephropathy. Transplantation 2005;79:1522—9.

[50] Kobashigawa JA, Katznelson S, Laks H, et al. Effect of pravastatin on outcomes after cardiac transplantation. N Engl J Med 1995;333:621—7.

[51] Masterson R, Hewitson T, Leikis M, et al. Impact of statin treatment on 1-year functional and histologic renal allograft outcome. Transplantation 2005;80:332—8.

[52] Katznelson S, Wilkinson AH, Kobashigawa JA, et al. The effect of pravastatin on acute rejection after kidney transplantation — a pilot study. Transplantation 1996;61:1469—74.

[53] Kasiske BL, Heim-Duthoy KL, Singer GG, et al. The effects of lipid-lowering agents on acute renal allograft rejection. Transplantation 2001;72:223—7.

[54] Fellström B, Holdaas H, Jardine AG, et al. on behalf of the Assessment of Lescol in Renal Transplantation (ALERT) Study Investigators. Effect of fluvastatin on renal end points in the assessment of lescol in renal transplant (ALERT) trial. Kidney Int 2004;66:1549—55.

[55] Scott LJ, Curran MP, Figgitt DP. Rosuvastatin: a review of its use in the management of dyslipidemia. Am J Cardiovasc Drugs 2004;4(2):117—38.

[56] Kostapanos MS, Milionis HJ, Gazi I, Kostara C, Bairaktari ET, Elisaf M. Rosuvastatin increases alpha-1 microglobulin urinary excretion in patients with primary dyslipidemia. J Clin Pharmacol 2006;46:1337—43.

[57] Vidt DG, Cressman MD, Harris S, et al. Rosuvastatin-induced arrest in progression of renal disease. Cardiology 2004;102:52—60.

[58] Verma A, Ranganna KM, Reddy RS, Verma M, Gordon NF. Effect of rosuvastatin on C-reactive protein and renal function in patients with chronic kidney disease. Am J Cardiol 2005;96(9):1290—2.

[59] Ridker PM, Danielson E, Fonseca FA, Genest J, Gotto Jr AM, Kastelein JJ, et al. Rosuvastatin to prevent vascular events in men and women with elevated C-reactive protein. N Engl J Med 2008;359:2195—207.

[60] Ridker PM, MacFadyen J, Cressman M, Glynn RJ. Efficacy of rosuvastatin among men and women with moderate chronic kidney disease and elevated high-sensitivity C-reactive protein: a secondary analysis from the JUPITER (Justification for the Use of Statins in Prevention-an Intervention Trial Evaluating Rosuvastatin) trial. J Am Coll Cardiol 2010;55:1266—73.

[61] Faergeman O, Hill L, Windler E, Wiklund O, Asmar R, Duffield E, et al. Efficacy and tolerability of rosuvastatin and atorvastatin when force-titrated in patients with primary hypercholesterolemia: results from the ECLIPSE study. Cardiology 2008;111:219—28.

[62] De Zeeuw D. Atorvastatin Beats Rosuvastatin in Protecting Kidneys in Diabetic and Nondiabetic Patients. XLVII European Renal Association-European Dialysis and Transplant Association (ERA-EDTA) Congress. Presented June 27, 2010.

17

Disorders of Phosphorus Homeostasis: Emerging Targets for Slowing Progression of Chronic Kidney Disease

Orlando M. Gutiérrez

Division of Nephrology, Department of Medicine, School of Medicine and Department of Epidemiology,
School of Public Health, University of Alabama at Birmingham, Birmingham, AL, USA

INTRODUCTION

Studies have shown that rates of cardiovascular disease events and death increase in a linear fashion as kidney function declines [1,2]. This has led to an increased emphasis on uncovering potentially modifiable risk factors for kidney disease progression in individuals with early stages of chronic kidney disease (CKD) in the hopes that slowing progression will improve long-term outcomes. To date, however, relatively few factors have emerged as effective targets for slowing progression of CKD, representing an important unmet need in nephrology research. High serum phosphorus concentrations are an established risk factor for cardiovascular disease events and death, particularly among individuals with CKD [3–6]. Although the mechanisms for these associations remain incompletely understood, a considerable body of evidence suggests a direct causal relationship between higher serum phosphorus concentrations and cardiovascular disease [7–12]. In addition, excess phosphorus stimulates the secretion of hormonal regulators of phosphorus metabolism such as parathyroid hormone (PTH) and fibroblast growth factor 23 (FGF23) [13–15], elevated levels of which have emerged as robust risk factors for cardiovascular disease events and mortality [3,16–18]. Phosphorus excess has been implicated in the pathogenesis of kidney injury via similar mechanisms [17–39], suggesting that disorders of phosphorus metabolism may be promising therapeutic targets for attenuating kidney function decline in CKD patients. Since dietary phosphorus intake plays a central role in the pathogenesis of disordered phosphorus homeostasis in CKD, these findings have fueled renewed interest in restricting dietary phosphorus consumption as a potential therapy for preserving residual kidney function in CKD patients. The focus of the current section will be to review the evidence both supporting and refuting this possibility, critically appraise current recommendations for restricting phosphorus intake in CKD, and consider the next steps required to establish the efficacy and feasibility of dietary phosphorus restriction for the preservation of kidney function in CKD patients.

ROLE OF DIETARY PHOSPHORUS INTAKE IN DISTURBANCES OF MINERAL METABOLISM IN CKD

Serum phosphorus concentrations represent a highly dynamic balance between dietary phosphorus absorption, urinary phosphorus excretion, and exchanges with bone, soft tissue, and intracellular stores [40]. The kidneys are the primary organs that regulate this balance by modulating urinary phosphorus excretion in response to changes in diet intake and bone/soft tissue turnover. Under normal conditions, diet intake makes up the majority of the obligate phosphorus load (1200–1500 mg/day in a typical westernized diet) that the kidneys must eliminate on a daily basis to maintain phosphorus balance [41]. As such, dietary phosphorus absorption is the primary target of therapeutic interventions aimed at mitigating the development of hyperphosphatemia in patients with CKD.

Dietary phosphorus is well absorbed across the entirety of the intestinal tract by a combination of passive paracellular diffusion and active transport across luminal sodium-phosphorus co-transporters type II (Npt2b) and type III (Pit1) [42]. Although passive diffusion in the duodenum and jejunum appears to be the primary route of diet phosphorus absorption, studies in Npt2b knock-out mice revealed that sodium-dependent active transport may account for as much as 45 to 50% of total intestinal phosphorus transport [43]. 1,25-dihydroxyvitamin D (1,25(OH)$_2$D) enhances active intestinal phosphorus absorption by stimulating Npt2b expression [44]. However, unlike calcium, 1,25(OH)$_2$D is not essential for absorption of phosphorus from the intestinal lumen since passive paracellular routes of diffusion allow for substantial dietary phosphorus absorption even in settings of profound 1,25(OH)$_2$D deficiency [40].

Most circulating inorganic phosphorus is freely filtered in renal glomeruli and enters renal proximal tubules. Under typical dietary conditions, 80−90% of the filtered load is reabsorbed across sodium-phosphorus co-transporters 2a and 2c (Npt2a and Npt2c) in proximal tubular cells (as well as other minor transporters) and the rest is excreted in the urine [45]. PTH and FGF23 are the primary hormones that regulate the fraction of filtered phosphorus that is reabsorbed in renal proximal tubules. Both hormones do so by down-regulating sodium-phosphorus co-transporters in renal proximal tubule cells, thereby decreasing tubular phosphorus reabsorption and augmenting urinary phosphorus excretion [41,46]. In addition, FGF23 limits dietary phosphorus absorption by lowering 1,25(OH)$_2$D concentrations via inhibition of 25-hydroxyvitamin D-1α-hydroxylase and stimulation of 24-hydroxylase, the major catabolic pathway for 1,25(OH)$_2$D [46].

Increased phosphorus intake strongly stimulates the secretion of PTH and FGF23 in order to mitigate hyperphosphatemia by enhancing urinary phosphorus excretion and, in the case of FGF23, limiting dietary phosphorus absorption via lower 1,25(OH)$_2$D [13−15]. This appears to be particularly critical for maintaining phosphorus homeostasis in CKD patients, in whom elevations in FGF23 and PTH play a key role in enhancing per-nephron urinary phosphorus excretion in the face of unrestricted phosphorus intake. A number of observations support this view. In a study of 404 patients with stage 3 or 4 CKD and secondary hyperparathyroidism randomized to either cinacalcet or placebo for 32 weeks, cinacalcet-treated patients had a 43% decrease in mean serum PTH concentrations but at the price of a 21% increase in mean serum phosphorus concentrations, due mainly to diminished urinary phosphorus excretion as a consequence of decreased PTH [47]. Similarly, in a study of rats with experimentally-induced kidney disease, intravenous injection of anti-FGF23 antibodies resulted in a decrease in urinary fractional excretion of

phosphorus via lowering FGF23 levels and consequently, a marked elevation in serum phosphorus [48], underscoring the critical importance of elevated FGF23 levels in the control of serum phosphorus in CKD. When these data are coupled with animal and human studies showing that restriction of dietary phosphorus absorption decreased, and in some cases normalized, FGF23 and PTH levels in CKD [49−59], these findings support the concept that dietary phosphorus intake plays a pivotal role in the pathogenesis of disordered phosphorus metabolism in CKD.

DISORDERS OF PHOSPHORUS HOMEOSTASIS AND KIDNEY DISEASE PROGRESSION

Phosphorus excess has long been implicated in the pathogenesis of kidney disease via a variety of proposed mechanisms (Table 17.1). In a series of experiments conducted in the 1930s, rats with normal kidney function fed diets containing markedly high amounts of inorganic phosphorus (ranging from 2 to 6.5%) for ~6 weeks developed renal tubular necrosis, diffuse renal parenchymal calcification, inflammation and associated interstitial fibrosis [60]. These effects appeared to be accentuated in the setting of kidney disease. In a classic study published by Ibels and colleagues in 1978, two groups of rats underwent subtotal nephrectomy to induce chronic uremia, after which they were fed a diet containing either a standard content of phosphorus (0.5%) or a low phosphorus content (0.04%) plus aluminum hydroxide for a total of six weeks [19]. Importantly, both diets contained similar amounts of protein. While mean serum creatinine concentrations increased to a similar degree in both groups of rats four weeks after induction of kidney disease, creatinine concentrations continued to increase afterwards in the rats placed on a standard phosphorus diet, whereas they remained stable in rats placed on a phosphorus-depleted diet. In addition, all 26 animals placed on the standard phosphorus diet died prior to the end of the six-week experimental period, whereas only 3 of the 12 animals placed on the phosphorus-restricted diet died. Histological examination of kidney tissue obtained *ex vivo* revealed significantly higher calcium and phosphorus content and interstitial fibrosis in kidneys from rats fed standard phosphorus as compared to phosphorus-depleted diets, consistent with a direct pathological effect of excess phosphorus load on renal parenchyma.

Subsequent studies showed very similar findings in rat models of kidney disease [20−22,26], in other species with experimentally-induced kidney disease including dogs and cats [24,25,61], and in studies using

TABLE 17.1 Proposed Mechanisms Underlying a Link between Excess Dietary Phosphorus Intake or Serum Phosphorus Concentrations and Kidney Disease Progression

Mechanisms	Comments
Precipitation of calcium-phosphorus microcrystals into renal parenchyma	Most common pattern of injury noted in animals fed high phosphorus diets; induces interstitial fibrosis, tubular atrophy, and proteinuria [19,20,22,23,26,27]
Stimulation of phosphaturic hormones, such as parathyroid hormone and fibroblast growth factor 23	Higher concentrations of parathyroid hormone have been associated with increased cytosolic-free calcium in renal tubules [28]; higher fibroblast growth factor 23 concentrations have been independently associated with faster kidney disease progression in observational studies [17,18,39,63]
Promotion of vascular calcification	High phosphorus intake and excess serum phosphorus concentrations have been linked to vascular calcification in the aorta, major branch vessels, and peritubular and capillary vessels within the kidneys [19,20,22]
Stimulation of inflammatory pathways	Inflammation has been causally implicated in the nephrotoxicity of excess phosphorus intake in animal models of immune-mediated glomerulonephritis [21]

oral phosphorus binders instead of dietary manipulation as the primary method of limiting intestinal phosphorus absorption [27]. Notably, a number of these studies showed that animals fed phosphorus-restricted diets had slower kidney disease progression than animals fed phosphorus-replete diets despite no differences in protein or other nutrient intake [19,21,22,25], indicating that phosphorus restriction may have salutary effects on kidney function preservation independent of the known beneficial effects of protein restriction [62].

Although the impact of phosphorus excess on CKD progression in humans has been examined in less detail, the balance of data suggest that phosphorus overload contributes to kidney function decline. Large observational studies showed that higher serum phosphorus concentrations were associated with faster kidney disease progression and higher risk of incident end stage renal disease (ESRD) independently of established risk factors, including lower baseline eGFR [34–38]. Increased plasma FGF23 — a marker of phosphorus overload — has also been shown to be a robust risk factor for kidney disease progression in CKD patients, as depicted in Figure 17.1 showing the association of FGF23 with CKD progression in individuals with advanced CKD [17,18,39,63]. Even among individuals with normal kidney function and serum phosphorus concentrations within the normal range, a higher serum phosphorus level at baseline was independently associated with higher risk of incident CKD [37], suggesting that excess serum phosphorus may impair renal health at all levels of kidney function.

Whether reducing phosphorus load, in turn, attenuates CKD progression has not been well studied and remains unclear. Nevertheless, a number of studies have shown that dietary protein restriction may help slow kidney disease progression in CKD patients, as reviewed elsewhere in this text. Since phosphorus is so closely linked to protein intake, it is possible that concomitant reductions in phosphorus intake may

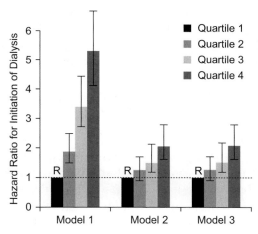

FIGURE 17.1 Hazard ratio (95% CI) for progression of kidney disease as indicated by initiation of chronic hemodialysis in patients with advanced chronic kidney disease according to quartiles of fibroblast growth factor 23 at baseline. Model 1 was adjusted for age, gender, and race. Model 2 was adjusted for variables in Model 1 plus smoking, alcohol intake, diabetes, hypertension, prevalent cardiovascular disease, Charlson score, body mass index, systolic and diastolic blood pressure, homocysteine, folate, vitamin B_{12}, treatment arm, hemoglobin, estimated glomerular filtration rate, albumin, calcium, phosphorus, 25-hydoxyvitamin D, 1,25-dihydroxyvitamin D, intact parathyroid hormone, total cholesterol, LDL-cholesterol, HDL-cholesterol, and triglycerides. Model 3 adjusted for variables in Model 2 plus medications. Quartile 1 is the referent group in all models. From reference [18].

have contributed to the beneficial effect of protein restriction. Several small human studies support this possibility. Maschio et al. showed that progression of kidney disease (as assessed by increases in the reciprocal of creatinine) was significantly slower in three groups of patients assigned to low phosphorus (600 to 750 mg per day) diets (total n = 53) than in a fourth group of patients (n = 30) consuming an unrestricted diet estimated to provide 900 mg of phosphorus per day [32,33]. Interestingly, the magnitude of the effect of phosphorus restriction on the change in the reciprocal of creatinine in this study was inversely related to baseline kidney function [33], suggesting that dietary phosphorus restriction is most beneficial when implemented in early CKD. In a study of 39 CKD patients, Barsotti et al. showed that reducing phosphorus intake (7 mg/kg/day) in CKD patients already consuming low nitrogen (protein) diets was more effective in preserving kidney function than consuming a low nitrogen diet with higher amounts of phosphorus (12 mg/kg/day) over ~1 year of follow-up [30]. In a subsequent study by the same group, 55 patients with moderate CKD (mean creatinine clearance 30 mL/min) were followed on ad libitum diets for ~12 months after which they were assigned to a low phosphorus (0.65 mg/kg/day), low nitrogen diet for an average of 21 months (n = 29), or a conventional low nitrogen diet (12 mg/kg/day of phosphorus per day) for ~17 months (n = 26) [31]. Creatinine clearance rates in both groups were noted to decline at an equal rate while consuming ad libitum diets, after which they stabilized in the group assigned to the low phosphorus, low nitrogen diet whereas they continued to decline in the conventional low nitrogen diet group. The authors interpreted these data to suggest that a low phosphorus diet confers a benefit on kidney disease progression above and beyond low protein intake in patients with moderate CKD.

While intriguing, these studies had a number of critical limitations that should merit caution when interpreting the results. First, they did not consistently isolate the effects of phosphorus restriction from the potential beneficial effects of other interventions such as protein restriction and/or more intensive medical care due to frequent study visits, making it unclear whether dietary phosphorus restriction per se was the primary beneficial intervention [28]. In addition, the number of patients studied were very small; the intervention periods were relatively short; contemporaneous, well-matched controls were not used; and changes in serum creatinine or creatinine clearance over time were not corrected for changes in muscle mass owing to decreased protein intake. Further, not all studies have reported beneficial effects of dietary phosphorus restriction, with two small studies showing

no impact of phosphorus restriction on kidney disease progression in CKD patients [64,65].

Given these limitations, at the present time there exist no quality human data to advocate dietary phosphorus restriction for the preservation of kidney function in CKD patients. Randomized controlled trials formally testing whether dietary phosphorus restriction attenuates kidney disease progression in pre-dialysis CKD patients are now needed, particularly in light of the encouraging animal and human data reviewed above.

DIETARY PHOSPHORUS RESTRICTION IN CKD: PRACTICAL CONSIDERATIONS MOVING FORWARD

Despite the lack of randomized controlled trials supporting its efficacy, restricting dietary phosphorus intake has been advocated for the management of disturbances in bone and mineral metabolism in CKD since the 1970s [58,66]. These recommendations were based upon animal and human studies showing that even modest reductions in phosphorus intake lowered PTH concentrations, attenuated parathyroid gland hyperplasia, and ameliorated high-turnover bone disease, particularly in early CKD [49—51,53,58,67]. More recently, therapy with non-calcium-based oral phosphorus binders and consumption of vegetable sources of phosphorus with low bioavailability were shown to decrease plasma FGF23 concentrations in CKD patients [52,55—57], further supporting the utility of restricting dietary phosphorus absorption in CKD. To date, however, the utilization of dietary phosphorus restriction in clinical practice has been limited by a number of practical issues, many of which will need to be addressed in the design of any future clinical trials assessing the efficacy of phosphorus restriction in slowing CKD progression.

First, the optimal timing of dietary phosphorus restriction in CKD patients needs to be more clearly defined. The only available recommendations come from the National Kidney Foundation Kidney Disease Outcome Quality Initiative (KDOQI) and the Kidney Disease Improving Global Outcomes Study Group guidelines [68,69]. Both sets of guidelines essentially advocate prescribing dietary phosphorus restriction when patients develop biochemical evidence of phosphorus overload, defined either as hyperphosphatemia or elevations of PTH above stage-specific threshold levels. However, waiting for evidence of phosphorus overload to manifest prior to instituting dietary phosphorus limitation may miss an important opportunity to ameliorate kidney injury in early CKD. Indeed, studies showed that rats with experimentally-induced kidney disease fed high phosphorus diets developed extensive renal parenchymal damage even in the absence of significant increases in serum phosphorus [20,62]. Further, CKD patients prescribed low phosphorus diets had stabilization in kidney function despite having serum phosphorus levels well within the normal range throughout the study period [31,33]. While these data suggest that implementing dietary phosphorus restriction in mild to moderate stages of CKD may help to protect residual renal function even in the absence of overt evidence of phosphorus excess, exactly how early in the course of kidney disease is optimal to maximize these potential benefits is unclear and requires further study.

Further complicating this issue is the lack of evidenced-based recommendations for the level of dietary phosphorus restriction that should be prescribed in individual patients. Although KDOQI guidelines suggest phosphorus restriction to 800–1000 mg a day in stage 3 to 5 CKD patients with hyperphosphatemia or elevated PTH levels, there exist few data to support this recommendation. Further, it seems unlikely that one target range would be suitable for such a wide spectrum of kidney disease severity. Indeed, animal studies have shown that as renal function is reduced, the nephrotoxicity of excess phosphorus is greatly enhanced [19,20], such that progressively smaller quantities of phosphorus intake are needed to induce kidney injury at lower levels of kidney function. Consistent with this, reductions in phosphorus intake that were proportional to concurrent reductions in glomerular filtration rate were shown to be necessary for maintaining normal serum phosphorus and PTH concentrations in canine models of kidney disease [58]. Whether similar stage-specific, proportional decreases in phosphorus intake are more appropriate for the treatment of disorders of mineral metabolism and preservation of kidney function than a single target range has not been well studied in humans, and remains unclear. Addressing this issue will be critical for developing rational recommendations for dietary phosphorus restriction in patients across the spectrum of kidney disease.

In addition, appropriate targets for gauging the efficacy of therapy are needed. While serum phosphorus concentrations would seem to be natural candidates, population-based data showed that even small decreases in serum phosphorus (~0.3 to 1.0 mg/dL) within the normal range were associated with decreased risks of adverse outcomes, including cardiovascular disease, progression of kidney disease, and death [4–6,36,37,70]. Targeting such small changes in serum phosphorus to gauge the efficacy of phosphorus reduction strategies in individual pre-dialysis CKD patients would be unrealistic in a clinical trial, much less in clinical practice. This is especially the case given the wide daily fluctuations in serum phosphorus concentrations

due to natural postprandial or diurnal variation [71]. FGF23 has recently been proposed as a more appropriate biomarker to gauge the efficacy of phosphorus reduction strategies given that plasma FGF23 concentrations manifest much less random variation [72]. In addition, since elevations in plasma FGF23 are among the earliest manifestations of disordered phosphorus metabolism in CKD [73], FGF23 could also potentially serve as a biomarker to help identify early-stage CKD patients with normal serum phosphorus and PTH levels who may nevertheless benefit from dietary phosphorus restriction in order to maintain phosphorus balance. Future studies will need to test this possibility and determine the most appropriate targets for assessing the efficacy of phosphorus restriction in individual patients.

Finally, given the close relationship between dietary phosphorus and protein, reasonable concerns have been raised that restricting phosphorus intake would require a reciprocal restriction in protein intake that could exacerbate protein-energy wasting in advanced CKD [74]. As such, practical strategies for safely restricting phosphorus intake in the outpatient setting need to be better defined. Importantly, numerous strategies have already been proposed, with most involving a shift in the focus of dietary phosphorus management from globally reducing phosphorus (and thus, protein) intake to optimizing the types and sources of phosphorus being consumed [75]. Such strategies include decreasing the consumption of processed foods containing high quantities of phosphorus-based food additives, consuming more vegetable-based protein sources with low phosphorus bioavailability, or increasing the consumption of foods with low phosphorus to protein ratios [75]. Before dietary phosphorus restriction can be broadly adopted in the management of patients with pre-dialysis CKD, these and the other barriers reviewed above will need to be addressed.

CONCLUSIONS

Disorders of phosphorus metabolism are strongly linked to adverse CKD outcomes, including CKD progression. Given the central role of dietary phosphorus intake in the pathogenesis of disturbances of phosphorus homeostasis in CKD, restriction of phosphorus consumption may represent an effective intervention for mitigating the decline of kidney function in CKD patients. While the balance of experimental and human data support this thesis, the lack of randomized, controlled trials examining the utility and/or feasibility of this intervention precludes the ability to recommend dietary phosphorus restriction for the attenuation of CKD progression at this time. As the phosphorus content of westernized diets will only increase in the future, initiating these trials should be a high priority, with the long-term goal of determining whether dietary phosphorus intake may be an effective and safe therapy for slowing progression of CKD.

References

[1] Weiner DE, Tighiouart H, Amin MG, et al. Chronic kidney disease as a risk factor for cardiovascular disease and all-cause mortality: a pooled analysis of community-based studies. J Am Soc Nephrol 2004;15:1307–15.

[2] Go AS, Chertow GM, Fan D, McCulloch CE, Hsu CY. Chronic kidney disease and the risks of death, cardiovascular events, and hospitalization. N Engl J Med 2004;351:1296–305.

[3] Block GA, Klassen PS, Lazarus JM, Ofsthun N, Lowrie EG, Chertow GM. Mineral metabolism, mortality, and morbidity in maintenance hemodialysis. J Am Soc Nephrol 2004;15:2208–18.

[4] Dhingra R, Sullivan LM, Fox CS, et al. Relations of serum phosphorus and calcium levels to the incidence of cardiovascular disease in the community. Arch Intern Med 2007;167: 879–85.

[5] Kestenbaum B, Sampson JN, Rudser KD, et al. Serum phosphate levels and mortality risk among people with chronic kidney disease. J Am Soc Nephrol 2005;16:520–8.

[6] Tonelli M, Sacks F, Pfeffer M, Gao Z, Curhan G. Relation between serum phosphate level and cardiovascular event rate in people with coronary disease. Circulation 2005;112:2627–33.

[7] Giachelli CM, Jono S, Shioi A, Nishizawa Y, Mori K, Morii H. Vascular calcification and inorganic phosphate. Am J Kidney Dis 2001;38:S34–7.

[8] Mathew S, Tustison KS, Sugatani T, Chaudhary LR, Rifas L, Hruska KA. The mechanism of phosphorus as a cardiovascular risk factor in CKD. J Am Soc Nephrol 2008;19:1092–105.

[9] Di Marco GS, Hausberg M, Hillebrand U, et al. Increased inorganic phosphate induces human endothelial cell apoptosis in vitro. Am J Physiol Renal Physiol 2008;294:F1381–7.

[10] Shuto E, Taketani Y, Tanaka R, et al. Dietary phosphorus acutely impairs endothelial function. J Am Soc Nephrol 2009;20: 1504–12.

[11] Lau WL, Pai A, Moe SM, Giachelli CM. Direct effects of phosphate on vascular cell function. Adv Chronic Kidney Dis 2011;18:105–12.

[12] El-Abbadi MM, Pai AS, Leaf EM, et al. Phosphate feeding induces arterial medial calcification in uremic mice: role of serum phosphorus, fibroblast growth factor-23, and osteopontin. Kidney Int 2009;75:1297–307.

[13] Antoniucci DM, Yamashita T, Portale AA. Dietary phosphorus regulates serum fibroblast growth factor-23 concentrations in healthy men. J Clin Endocrinol Metab 2006;91:3144–9.

[14] Burnett SM, Gunawardene SC, Bringhurst FR, Juppner H, Lee H, Finkelstein JS. Regulation of C-terminal and intact FGF-23 by dietary phosphate in men and women. J Bone Miner Res 2006;21:1187–96.

[15] Ferrari SL, Bonjour JP, Rizzoli R. Fibroblast growth factor-23 relationship to dietary phosphate and renal phosphate handling in healthy young men. J Clin Endocrinol Metab 2005;90: 1519–24.

[16] Gutierrez OM, Mannstadt M, Isakova T, et al. Fibroblast growth factor 23 and mortality among patients undergoing hemodialysis. N Engl J Med 2008;359:584–92.

[17] Isakova T, Xie H, Yang W, et al. Fibroblast growth factor 23 and risks of mortality and end-stage renal disease in patients with chronic kidney disease. JAMA 2011;305:2432–9.

[18] Kendrick J, Cheung AK, Kaufman JS, et al. FGF-23 Associates with death, cardiovascular events, and initiation of chronic dialysis. J Am Soc Nephrol 2011;22:1913–22.

[19] Ibels LS, Alfrey AC, Haut L, Huffer WE. Preservation of function in experimental renal disease by dietary restriction of phosphate. N Engl J Med 1978;298:122–6.

[20] Haut LL, Alfrey AC, Guggenheim S, Buddington B, Schrier N. Renal toxicity of phosphate in rats. Kidney Int 1980;17:722–31.

[21] Karlinsky ML, Haut L, Buddington B, Schrier NA, Alfrey AC. Preservation of renal function in experimental glomerulonephritis. Kidney Int 1980;17:293–302.

[22] Lumlertgul D, Burke TJ, Gillum DM, et al. Phosphate depletion arrests progression of chronic renal failure independent of protein intake. Kidney Int 1986;29:658–66.

[23] Harris DC, Falk SA, Conger JD, Hammond WS, Schrier RW. Phosphate restriction reduces proteinuria of the uninephrectomized, diabetic rat. Am J Kidney Dis 1988;11: 489–98.

[24] Brown SA, Crowell WA, Barsanti JA, White JV, Finco DR. Beneficial effects of dietary mineral restriction in dogs with marked reduction of functional renal mass. J Am Soc Nephrol 1991;1:1169–79.

[25] Finco DR, Brown SA, Crowell WA, Groves CA, Duncan JR, Barsanti JA. Effects of phosphorus/calcium-restricted and phosphorus/calcium-replete 32% protein diets in dogs with chronic renal failure. Am J Vet Res 1992;53:157–63.

[26] Koizumi T, Murakami K, Nakayama H, Kuwahara T, Yoshinari O. Role of dietary phosphorus in the progression of renal failure. Biochem Biophys Res Commun 2002;295:917–21.

[27] Nagano N, Miyata S, Obana S, et al. Sevelamer hydrochloride, a phosphate binder, protects against deterioration of renal function in rats with progressive chronic renal insufficiency. Nephrol Dial Transplant 2003;18:2014–23.

[28] Lau K. Phosphate excess and progressive renal failure: the precipitation-calcification hypothesis. Kidney Int 1989;36: 918–37.

[29] Loghman-Adham M. Role of phosphate retention in the progression of renal failure. J Lab Clin Med 1993;122:16–26.

[30] Barsotti G, Morelli E, Giannoni A, Guiducci A, Lupetti S, Giovannetti S. Restricted phosphorus and nitrogen intake to slow the progression of chronic renal failure: a controlled trial. Kidney Int Suppl 1983;16:S278–84.

[31] Barsotti G, Giannoni A, Morelli E, et al. The decline of renal function slowed by very low phosphorus intake in chronic renal patients following a low nitrogen diet. Clin Nephrol 1984;21:54–9.

[32] Maschio G, Oldrizzi L, Tessitore N, et al. Effects of dietary protein and phosphorus restriction on the progression of early renal failure. Kidney Int 1982;22:371–6.

[33] Maschio G, Oldrizzi L, Tessitore N, et al. Early dietary protein and phosphorus restriction is effective in delaying progression of chronic renal failure. Kidney Int Suppl 1983;16:S273–7.

[34] Norris KC, Greene T, Kopple J, et al. Baseline predictors of renal disease progression in the African American Study of Hypertension and Kidney Disease. J Am Soc Nephrol 2006;17(10): 2928–36. 17:2928–36.

[35] Voormolen N, Noordzij M, Grootendorst DC, et al. High plasma phosphate as a risk factor for decline in renal function and mortality in pre-dialysis patients. Nephrol Dial Transplant 2007;22:2909–16.

[36] Schwarz S, Trivedi B, Kalanter-Zadeh K, Kovesdy C. Association of disorders of mineral metabolism with progression of chronic kidney disease. Clin J Am Sco Nephrol 2006;1:825–31.

[37] O'Seaghdha CM, Hwang SJ, Muntner P, Melamed ML, Fox CS. Serum phosphorus predicts incident chronic kidney disease

and end-stage renal disease. Nephrol Dial Transplant 2011;26: 2885–90.

[38] Bellasi A, Mandreoli M, Baldrati L, et al. Chronic kidney disease progression and outcome according to serum phosphorus in mild-to-moderate kidney dysfunction. Clin J Am Soc Nephrol 2011;6:883–91.

[39] Fliser D, Kollerits B, Neyer U, et al. Fibroblast growth factor 23 (FGF23) predicts progression of chronic kidney disease: the Mild to Moderate Kidney Disease (MMKD) Study. J Am Soc Nephrol 2007;18:2600–8.

[40] Uribarri J. Phosphorus homeostasis in normal health and in chronic kidney disease patients with special emphasis on dietary phosphorus intake. Semin Dial 2007;20:295–301.

[41] Berndt T, Kumar R. Phosphatonins and the regulation of phosphate homeostasis. Annu Rev Physiol 2007;69:341–59.

[42] Sabbagh Y, Giral H, Caldas Y, Levi M, Schiavi SC. Intestinal phosphate transport. Adv Chronic Kidney Dis 2011;18:85–90.

[43] Sabbagh Y, O'Brien SP, Song W, et al. Intestinal npt2b plays a major role in phosphate absorption and homeostasis. J Am Soc Nephrol 2009;20:2348–58.

[44] Katai K, Miyamoto K, Kishida S, et al. Regulation of intestinal Na$^+$-dependent phosphate co-transporters by a low-phosphate diet and 1,25-dihydroxyvitamin D3. Biochem J 1999;343(Pt 3): 705–12.

[45] Murer H, Hernando N, Forster I, Biber J. Proximal tubular phosphate reabsorption: molecular mechanisms. Physiol Rev 2000;80:1373–409.

[46] Liu S, Quarles LD. How fibroblast growth factor 23 works. J Am Soc Nephrol 2007;18:1637–47.

[47] Chonchol M, Locatelli F, Abboud HE, et al. A randomized, double-blind, placebo-controlled study to assess the efficacy and safety of cinacalcet HCl in participants with CKD not receiving dialysis. Am J Kidney Dis 2009;53:197–207.

[48] Hasegawa H, Nagano N, Urakawa I, et al. Direct evidence for a causative role of FGF23 in the abnormal renal phosphate handling and vitamin D metabolism in rats with early-stage chronic kidney disease. Kidney Int 2010;78:975–80.

[49] Barsotti G, Cupisti A, Morelli E, et al. Secondary hyperparathyroidism in severe chronic renal failure is corrected by very-low dietary phosphate intake and calcium carbonate supplementation. Nephron 1998;79:137–41.

[50] Combe C, Aparicio M. Phosphorus and protein restriction and parathyroid function in chronic renal failure. Kidney Int 1994;46:1381–6.

[51] Combe C, Morel D, de Precigout V, et al. Long-term control of hyperparathyroidism in advanced renal failure by low-phosphorus low-protein diet supplemented with calcium (without changes in plasma calcitriol). Nephron 1995;70:287–95.

[52] Gonzalez-Parra E, Gonzalez-Casaus ML, Galan A, et al. Lanthanum carbonate reduces FGF23 in chronic kidney disease Stage 3 patients. Nephrol Dial Transplant 2011;26:2567–71.

[53] Kaye M. The effects in the rat of varying intakes of dietary calcium, phosphorus, and hydrogen ion on hyperparathyroidism due to chronic renal failure. J Clin Invest 1974;53: 256–69.

[54] Lafage MH, Combe C, Fournier A, Aparicio M. Ketodiet, physiological calcium intake and native vitamin D improve renal osteodystrophy. Kidney Int 1992;42:1217–25.

[55] Moe SM, Zidehsarai MP, Chambers MA, et al. Vegetarian compared with meat dietary protein source and phosphorus homeostasis in chronic kidney disease. Clin J Am Soc Nephrol 2011;6:257–64.

[56] Oliveira RB, Cancela AL, Graciolli FG, et al. Early control of PTH and FGF23 in normophosphatemic CKD patients: a new

target in CKD-MBD therapy? Clin J Am Soc Nephrol 2010;5: 286–91.

[57] Shigematsu T, Negi S. Combined therapy with lanthanum carbonate and calcium carbonate for hyperphosphatemia decreases serum FGF-23 level independently of calcium and PTH (COLC Study). Nephrol Dial Transplant 2012;27:1050–4.

[58] Slatopolsky E, Caglar S, Gradowska L, Canterbury J, Reiss E, Bricker NS. On the prevention of secondary hyperparathyroidism in experimental chronic renal disease using "proportional reduction" of dietary phosphorus intake. Kidney Int 1972;2:147–51.

[59] Slatopolsky E, Caglar S, Pennell JP, et al. On the pathogenesis of hyperparathyroidism in chronic experimental renal insufficiency in the dog. J Clin Invest 1971;50:492–9.

[60] Mackay EM, Oliver J. Renal damage following the ingestion of a diet containing an excess of inorganic phosphate. J Exp Med 1935;61:319–34.

[61] Ross LA, Finco DR, Crowell WA. Effect of dietary phosphorus restriction on the kidneys of cats with reduced renal mass. Am J Vet Res 1982;43:1023–6.

[62] Klahr S, Buerkert J, Purkerson ML. Role of dietary factors in the progression of chronic renal disease. Kidney Int 1983;24:579–87.

[63] Lundberg S, Qureshi AR, Olivecrona S, Gunnarsson I, Jacobson SH, Larsson TE. FGF23, albuminuria, and disease progression in patients with chronic IgA nephropathy. Clin J Am Soc Nephrol 2012.

[64] Barrientos A, Arteaga J, Rodicio JL, Alvarez Ude F, Alcazar JM, Ruilope LM. Role of the control of phosphate in the progression of chronic renal failure. Miner Electrolyte Metab 1982;7:127–33.

[65] Williams PS, Stevens ME, Fass G, Irons L, Bone JM. Failure of dietary protein and phosphate restriction to retard the rate of progression of chronic renal failure: a prospective, randomized, controlled trial. Q J Med 1991;81:837–55.

[66] Schoolwerth AC, Engle JE. Calcium and phosphorus in diet therapy of uremia. J Am Diet Assoc 1975;66:460–4.

[67] Maschio G, Tessitore N, D'Angelo A, et al. Early dietary phosphorus restriction and calcium supplementation in the prevention of renal osteodystrophy. Am J Clin Nutr 1980;33: 1546–54.

[68] National Kidney Foundation. K/DOQI Clinical Practice Guidelines for Bone Metabolism and Disease in Chronic Kidney Disease. Am J Kidney Dis 2003;42(suppl. 3):S1–202.

[69] Moe S, Drueke T, Cunningham J, et al. Definition, evaluation, and classification of renal osteodystrophy: a position statement from kidney disease: Improving Global Outcomes (KDIGO). Kidney Int 2006;69:1945–53.

[70] Foley RN, Collins AJ, Herzog CA, Ishani A, Kalra PA. Serum phosphorus levels associate with coronary atherosclerosis in young adults. J Am Soc Nephrol 2009;20:397–404.

[71] Markowitz M, Rotkin L, Rosen JF. Circadian rhythms of blood minerals in humans. Science 1981;213:672–4.

[72] Isakova T, Gutierrez OM, Wolf M. A blueprint for randomized trials targeting phosphorus metabolism in chronic kidney disease. Kidney Int 2009;76:705–16.

[73] Isakova T, Wahl P, Vargas GS, et al. Fibroblast growth factor 23 is elevated before parathyroid hormone and phosphate in chronic kidney disease. Kidney Int 2011;79:1370–8.

[74] Shinaberger CS, Greenland S, Kopple JD, et al. Is controlling phosphorus by decreasing dietary protein intake beneficial or harmful in persons with chronic kidney disease? Am J Clin Nutr 2008;88:1511–8.

[75] Gutierrez OM, Wolf M. Dietary phosphorus restriction in advanced chronic kidney disease: merits, challenges, and emerging strategies. Semin Dial 2010;23:401–6.

Alkalinization to Retard Progression of Chronic Kidney Failure

Hillel Sternlicht, Michal L. Melamed

Albert Einstein College of Medicine/Montefiore Medical Center, Bronx, NY, USA

EPIDEMIOLOGY OF METABOLIC ACIDOSIS IN KIDNEY DISEASE

Chronic kidney disease (CKD) has long been associated with metabolic acidosis [1]. As DM Lyon of Scotland noted nearly a century ago, "the processes of metabolism on an ordinary mixed diet yield daily an excess of nonvolatile acids … and these acids have to be excreted by the kidneys. When the kidneys are inadequate for this task, a retention of acid tends to occur in much the same way as urea is retained in the blood when the kidneys are gravely diseased" [2]. Since the degree of renal impairment necessary to lead to metabolic acidosis probably varies with the underlying etiology of disease and other less well understood factors, the exact prevalence of CKD induced metabolic acidosis, generally defined as a serum CO_2 <22–23 mEq/L, is unknown [3]. More recent estimates vary with the study population sampled and the bicarbonate threshold used. When serum bicarbonate <23 mEq/L is used as the cutoff, Clase and colleagues estimated 5% of CKD stage 3 patients and 33% of CKD stage 4 patients suffer from metabolic acidosis using NHANES 1988–1994 data [4]. In contrast, using identical data but a threshold of <22 mEq/L, Eustace et al. found only 3% of participants with CKD stage 3 and 20% of participants with CKD stage 4 suffer from metabolic acidosis [5].

Features associated with metabolic acidosis include age less than 65 (OR 1.7; CI 1.1–2.7). Surprisingly, traditional CKD risk factors such as hypertension, proteinuria, gender, or race were not associated with metabolic acidosis in one study [6]. The relationship between diabetes and metabolic acidosis is unclear.

Both Caravaca and Wallia documented that diabetics are less likely to develop an acidosis (OR 0.11; CI 0.03–0.3) with Moranne establishing the opposite correlation (OR 1.9; CI 1.1–3.5) [6–8]. Variations in prevalence and risk factor association are not unexpected given that most of the published literature fails to control for diuretic use, decreased protein intake or pulmonary disorders – all conditions that would affect the apparent rates of metabolic acidosis.

It is important to note that the time between collection and processing of bicarbonate samples can lead to spurious acidosis. Citing the persistence of low bicarbonate levels in dialysis patients despite using dialysate with bicarbonate concentrations of 40 mEq/L, Kirschbaum postulated that the use of central and often distant laboratories resulted in specious acidosis. Using a control group of blood samples that were centrifuged and processed locally, samples that were centrifuged and flown overnight before processing had a mean bicarbonate of 17 ± 3 mEq/L vs. 22 ± 3 mEq/L in local laboratories despite using similar enzymatic assays and no differences in other routine laboratory measurements [9]. In an editorial accompanying the article, Laski noted that "bicarbonate, like some wine, travels poorly," and postulates that the pressurized cargo hold allows CO_2 to leak out of the test tube resulting in a lower bicarbonate level [10].

MECHANISM OF ACIDOSIS IN CKD

While net acid creation varies with protein intake, a total of 1 mEq/kg body weight per day, first quantified in medical students fed a liquid soy diet, is generally

Nutritional Management of Renal Disease
http://dx.doi.org/10.1016/B978-0-12-391934-2.00018-7

cited as the standard rate of hydrogen ion production [11]. Upon establishing the mechanism of acid generation, Wrong and Davies concluded that metabolic acidosis does not develop from excess production of acids but rather from an inability to excrete a normal acid load [12]. Further experiments by Jean Oliver, Robert Platt, and J. Russell Elkinton proved that acidosis was the result of a loss in the absolute number of functioning nephrons rather than a decrease in filtration within an unchanged number of individual nephrons. Their collaborative efforts led to the "intact nephron hypothesis" which stated that, "our concept of renal failure should not be one of disordered function, but rather one of extremely efficient function by a renal remnant now too small for its task" [13]. As such, "a reduced number of hyperfunctioning intact nephrons" became the paradigm of decreased renal function in CKD [14].

ANIMAL MODELS OF KIDNEY DAMAGE WITH ACIDOSIS

Metabolic acidosis in animal models leads to further kidney damage. Using the {7/8}rat nephrectomy model to induce acidemia, Nath, Hostettor, and Hostetter noted the appearance of widespread circumferential peritubular C3 and C5b-9 deposits. Under these circumstances, ammonia facilitates the amidation of C3 which consequently stimulates the alternative pathway. This leads to the assembly of the membrane attack complex, C5b-9, which mediates tissue damage [15]. Animal models of CKD exhibit increased urinary endothelin excretion consistent with elevated endogenous renal endothelin production [15]. Using a {5/6}nephrectomy with sham control, renal cortex endothelin levels were evaluated four weeks postoperatively via cortical microdialysis. Urinary endothelin excretion in the nephrectomized rats was 346 fmol/d vs. 125 fmol/d in sham operated animals (P < 0.02). Parallel values were observed in cortical endothelin levels [16]. Both these mechanisms, complement activation and elevated endothelin levels, can increase kidney damage (see below).

ANIMAL MODELS OF TREATMENT

Bicarbonate therapy for the treatment of metabolic acidemia is nearly as old as the disease itself. Richard Bright proposed its empiric use nearly two hundred years ago [17]. In 1931, Lyon conducted a therapeutic trial by administered varying amounts of alkali to 17 uremic patients [2]. The results were published in a paper entitled, "The Alkaline Treatment of Chronic Nephritis." With little fanfare, he noted, "on alkaline treatment clinical improvement was usual," subsequently concluding, "it is possible that the lightening of the load on the kidney [via alkali administration] may have arrested the progress of the disease, and may even have allowed some regeneration of the tissue to take place" [2]. Since that time, extensive studies in animals and humans have added to the foundation laid by Bright, Lyon, and others.

Animal studies of alkali therapy have shown mixed results. Early work in the 1990s by Throssell failed to prove that bicarbonate supplementation retarded CKD progression. In {5/6}nephrectomized rats allocated to HCO_3 or NaCl supplementation, arterial pH was 7.39 in the bicarbonate supplemented rats and 6.87 in the sodium chloride fed rats after 12 weeks of therapy. All animals developed similar degrees of proteinuria (~100 mg/24 h) and blood pressure elevation. Moreover, GFR was similar between NaCl and HCO_3 groups at one month (0.77 mL/min vs. 0.64 mL/min, respectively; P > 0.05) and two months (0.62 mL/min vs. 0.66 mL/min, respectively; P > 0.05) with histological assessment revealing similar degrees of tubulointerstitial injury [18].

After demonstrating that the metabolic acidemia of CKD resulted in complement-mediated tubulointerstitial damage, Nath, Hostetter, and Hostetter investigated whether alkali therapy could mitigate this effect. After feeding {7/8}nephrectomized rats either $NaHCO_3$ or NaCl for 4—6 weeks, remnant kidney tissue was examined. Interstitial infiltration and tubular dilatation and atrophy were less pronounced in alkali supplemented rats. Immunofluorescent studies showed widespread circumferential C3 fluorescence and diffuse, granular peritubular C5b-9 complement accumulation in NaCl supplemented rats; C3 and C5b-9 accumulation was markedly diminished in the bicarbonate fed rats. In concert, these findings suggest that elevated levels of ammonia and depressed bicarbonate associated with metabolic acidemia result in both conventional and complement mediated damage to the tubulointerstitium with improvement upon correction of acidemia [15].

Gadola et al. studied the effects of administering calcium citrate on retarding GFR decline and ameliorating acid-induced morphological damage using {5/6} renal ablation to induce acidemia. After ten weeks of therapy, arterial bicarbonate concentrations were significantly higher in the calcium citrate treated (25.0 mEq/L) rats and sham operated (25.5 mEq/L) rats than the ablation-only group (17.3 mEq/L). GFR was significantly higher in the bicarbonate treated rats (92.0 μL/min·100 g) than in renal abated, acidemic animals (22 μL/min·100 g). Blinded morphologic assessment revealed fewer hypertrophied and proliferative glomeruli in the citrate-treated group at week 10 as compared to the nephrectomy-only group. Morphologic evaluation of glomerulosclerosis using such criteria as mesangial expansion and tubulointerstitial disease, characterized by tubular casts, inflammation and fibrosis, revealed 50% less damage in the citrate-treated rats vs. the acidemic CKD controls [19].

More recently, Donald Wesson and colleagues have performed several experiments revealing improvement with treatment of acidemia. Phisitkul et al., also using the {5/6}nephrectomy model, studied the effect of bicarbonate therapy on diet (protein source: casein) induced metabolic acidemia over a 12-week period using GFR and urine albumin excretion as markers of CKD progression [20]. They found that GFR was better preserved and that urinary albumin excretion was lower in the rats fed casein and sodium bicarbonate compared to casein alone or casein and sodium chloride, as long as blood pressure was controlled.

Employing a {2/3}rat nephrectomy model with dietary acid loading, Wesson and Simoni showed that tissue acid levels were important in the development of reduced GFR, and that treatment with bicarbonate led to no decline in GFR compared to a marked decline that occurred without bicarbonate treatment [21]. In a later study, Wesson and Simoni again used the {2/3} nephrectomy model and showed that the decline in eGFR in the model was mediated by endothelin and aldosterone production which were ameliorated by dietary alkali therapy. Additionally, dietary alkali worked better to preserve renal function than endothelin and aldosterone receptor antagonism [22].

OBSERVATIONAL STUDIES IN HUMANS

Several recent observational studies have suggested that metabolic acidemia (or low serum bicarbonate levels) may play a role in kidney disease progression in humans as the animal data suggest. In a study of 5422 outpatients in the Bronx, NY, Shah et al. showed that low serum bicarbonate levels (<22 mEq/L) were common in CKD stage 4 [23]. The lowest quartile of serum bicarbonate (<22 mEq/L) was associated with a faster progression of kidney disease after multivariable adjustment over 3.4 years of follow-up. This remained true with several different definitions of progression of kidney disease, including doubling of serum creatinine, reaching an eGFR of <15 mL/min/1.73m^2, a 30% decrease in eGFR and a 50% decrease in eGFR [23].

A similar study utilized data from the Modification of Diet in Renal Disease clinical trial to evaluate associations between low serum bicarbonate levels and progression of kidney disease. This study by Menon et al. included GFR measured by iothalamate clearances for the parent clinical trial [24]. Interestingly, these authors found that when using serum creatinine to estimate eGFR, results were similar to the study by Shah

et al. but when adjusting for iothalamate-measured GFR, the association between low bicarbonate levels and progression of kidney disease disappeared [24]. This suggested that possible residual confounding by the inaccuracies of estimating GFR explained the previously reported relationship between acidemia and progression of renal failure.

Raphael et al. evaluated serum bicarbonate levels and the progression of kidney disease in the African American Study of Kidney Disease [25]. This study evaluated the association between serum bicarbonate levels and a composite outcome of death, onset of dialysis and/or a GFR event. The investigators found that even using iothalamate measured GFR values, there was an association between higher bicarbonate levels and a lower risk of the composite outcome [25]. This is in contrast to the Menon et al. study which showed no association when accounting for measured GFR [22]. The Raphael study examined a different study population (all African Americans) which may account for these different results.

Human Trials

Lyon's findings were eventually confirmed in the 1970s and 1980s when papers by Blom van Assendelft, Papadoyannakis, and Jenkins demonstrated that bicarbonate supplementation did indeed decrease urea production by correcting acidemia and not simply by the dilutional effects of sodium on extracellular volume expansion [26–28]. In 1998, Rustom et al. evaluated eleven patients with a mean GFR of 46 mL/min per 1.73 m^2, a mean bicarbonate 21.2 mEq/L, and mean proteinuria of 3.2 g/d; most kidney disease was due to glomerulonephritis. After six weeks of NaHCO$_3$ therapy, serum bicarbonate, GFR, serum urea nitrogen (SUN), and proteinuria levels remained unchanged. However, median N-acetyl-β-D-glucose-aminidase (NAG) levels (no mean values were reported), a marker of tubular injury, fell by 50% (P < 0.01). Of note, no elevation in blood pressure was observed with the sodium-salt based treatment [29].

Building on Rustom's study design, Mathur et al., in 2006, conducted the first prospective randomized single blind trial among 40 patients with CKD of unspecified etiology who had an average serum creatinine of 3.10 mg/dL (GFR not noted) (Table 18.1). Participants received either bicarbonate or placebo daily and were encouraged to maintain the same dietary intake of protein and calories throughout the study. After three months of therapy, mean serum bicarbonate levels remained stable in the placebo arm at approximately 19.4 mEq/L but increased to 22.9 mEq/L in the intervention arm (P < 0.05). While there was no significant change in serum creatinine levels, mean blood urea levels were 90.3 mg/dL in the placebo group but 67.3 mg/dL in the alkali arm (P < 0.05). Moreover, "a sense of well-being was felt in half of the cases" after bicarbonate treatment [30].

A Cochrane meta-analysis of work published through 2006 — including the Rustom study but not the Mathur study — concluded that, "the evidence for the benefits and risks of correcting metabolic acidosis is very limited with no RCTs in pre-ESRD patients" [31]. Three other trials, of varying quality, have been published since the Cochrane review.

De Brito-Ashurst and colleagues conducted a partially-blinded, prospective randomized control trial of alkalinization supplementation over two years among CKD stage 4 patients from an English CKD clinic. Subjects with overt heart failure, refractory hypertension, or plasma HCO_3 <16 mEq/L or >20 mEq/L were excluded. Dietary habits were monitored closely. Finally, sevelamer hydrochloride and calcium carbonate were discontinued to avoid unintended manipulation of acid-base status. Patients were then randomized to usual care or thrice-daily $NaHCO_3$ with dose titration to achieve serum bicarbonate of $\geq$23 mEq/L. Primary endpoints included rate of GFR decline, rapidity of renal function decline (defined as a fall in CrCl of >3 mL/min·yr), and progression to dialysis (a multilateral decision initiated once CrCl <10 mL/min). An average of 1.8 g/d of bicarbonate supplement was given. After two years of therapy and 100% follow-up of the 134 patients, mean plasma bicarbonate was unchanged in the control arm and 24 mEq/L in the treatment arm. Using intention-to-treat analysis, mean blood pressure and proteinuria were similar in both groups, but the observed decline in CrCl during the two year study was 5.93 mL/min in the control group compared with 1.88 mL/min in the treatment group (P < 0.0001). Furthermore, patients receiving supplementation were 85% less likely to experience a rapid progression of CKD and 87% less likely to initiate dialysis over the interval, as compared to controls (P < 0.0001 and P < 0.001, respectively). Adverse effects including worsening hypertension and worsening edema were no more common in the treatment group; however, 6.5% of patients treated with bicarbonate reported poor palatability requiring a change in the bicarbonate formulation [32].

Phisitkul et al. recruited patients with hypertensive nephropathy who had a mean GFR between 20–60 mL/min/1.73 m^2 and a plasma bicarbonate <22 mEq/L but who had no history of diabetes, fluid overload, or cardiovascular disease. All patients underwent six months of blood pressure control at which point 1 mEq/kg·body weight sodium citrate was administered daily for two years. Patients unwilling to undergo treatment were followed as controls. The primary outcome was urinary endothelin levels, a mediator of

tubulointerstitial injury, with GFR decline as a secondary outcome. Despite lack of randomization, study characteristics were similar among the two groups of about 30 patients each, with a mean baseline GFR of 33.4 mL/min per 1.73m^2 and mean baseline bicarbonate of 20.8 mEq/L. After six months of antihypertensive therapy during which systolic pressure decreased from 161 mmHg to 132 mmHg, alkali supplementation was initiated. After two years of therapy, mean serum bicarbonate was 23.8 mEq/L in participants treated with sodium citrate and 19.6 mEq/L in untreated patients (P < 0.0001). Urinary endothelin levels were significantly lower in the sodium citrate treated group than in the untreated patients (4.83 ng/g·Cr vs. 6.92 ng/g·Cr respectively, P < 0.0001). Comparisons using linear mixed models showed that the yearly rate of eGFR decline (as measured by serum creatinine and cystatin C) was significantly slower in the sodium citrate patients than in the control group (−1.60 mL/min per 1.73 m^2 vs. −3.79 mL/min per 1.73 m^2 respectively, P < 0.001) [33].

Mahajan et al. sought to prevent advanced CKD and its attendant metabolic acidemia by performing a randomized, single-blinded prospective placebo-controlled trial of the effects of alkali therapy on the progression of early CKD in patients with hypertensive nephropathy. Patients with CKD stage 2 who had between 200 and 2000 mg of proteinuria/g·Cr/d were recruited for the trial. Patients were excluded from study who had nonhypertensive CKD, a history of cardiovascular disease, or diabetes, metabolic acidosis (serum bicarbonate <24.5 mEq/L) or evidence of fluid overload. Subjects were randomized to receive placebo, $NaHCO_3$ 0.5 mEq/kg·body weight, or NaCl daily for 5 years. Rate of GFR decline (measured by serum creatinine and cystatin C) was the primary outcome. 491 patients were drawn from a general clinic population, 349 of these fulfilled all study criteria and 120 patients were randomly assigned among the three treatment arms. Patient characteristics were similar among the three groups; the mean GFR in the three groups was 73 mL/min, and the mean venous bicarbonate was 26.2 mEq/L. Upon completion of the study, the eGFR, calculated by plasma cystatin, declined by −1.34 mL/min·yr in the alkali therapy arm vs. −2.19 mL/min·yr in the NaCl treated arm (P = 0.003 vs. HCO_3 treatment) vs. −2.37 mL/min·yr in the placebo arm (P = 0.0003 vs. HCO_3 therapy). The secondary outcome of urinary endothelin levels — a proven mediator of nephropathy progression in animals — was statistically significantly lower, by 19% and 16%, in the HCO_3 arm as compared to the placebo and NaCl arms, respectively. The adverse effect, bloating, occurred exclusively in the $NaHCO_3$ treated group [34].

Although there are no rigorously collected data published concerning the adverse effects of oral bicarbonate

TABLE 18.1 Randomized Clinical Trials of Alkali Therapy and Progression of Kidney Disease

Study	Number of Participants	Study Design	Intervention	Results
Mathur et al. [30]	40 (mean Creatinine 3.10 mg/dL)	Prospective randomized single-blind controlled trial	Sodium bicarbonate 1.2 mEq/Kg body weight for 3 months	No difference in serum creatinine levels
De Brito-Ashurst et al. [32]	134 (stage 4 CKD)	Prospective randomized, partially blinded trial	Sodium bicarbonate 1.82 g/day vs. standard treatment for 2 years	CrCl decline slower in bicarbonate treated group (1.88 vs. 5.93 mL/min/1.73 m^2) (P > 0.001)
Phisitkul et al. [33]	59 (eGFR 20−60 mL/min/1.73 m^2)	Prospective study (not randomized, no placebo, unblinded)	Sodium citrate 1meq/kg for 2 years	eGFR decline measured by creatinine slower in citrate group (−1.60 ± 0.13 vs. −3.79 ± 0.30 mL/min/yr P < 0.001)
Mahajan et al. [34]	120 (mean eGFR 73 mL/min/1.73 m^2)	Prospective randomized, placebo-controlled, blinded trial	Placebo vs. sodium bicarbonate vs. sodium chloride (0.5 mEq/kg lean body weight/day for both sodium salts)	Cystatin C eGFR higher in bicarbonate group (66.4 ± 4.9 vs. 62.7 ± 5.4 saline vs. 60.8 ± 6.3 placebo)

therapy, it appears to be well tolerated. Only a fraction of patients experienced bloating or poor palatability [28,32−34]. Furthermore, such effects may be minimized by modifying the frequency of dosing or by changing the formulation used [32,34] The principle concern among physicians has been the propensity of the sodium in the alkali formulation to increase blood pressure and worsen fluid overload. Consequently, trial populations have explicitly excluded individuals with a history of heart failure or other conditions that promote fluid overload. However, studies in humans have not suggested significant changes in blood pressure or volume status, and only one trial has documented worsening blood pressure [27,28,30,32−35]. Husted, Nolph, and Maher directly examined the propensity of sodium containing compounds to cause fluid overload by evaluating volume status in subjects receiving either chloride or bicarbonate-based salt loads. Ten patients with CKD of various etiologies with creatinine clearances between 3−16 mL/min were sequentially administered 200 mEq/d of either NaCl and NaHCO$_3$ for four days followed by washout diets. Despite equimolar doses of sodium, mean sodium excretion in the cohort receiving NaHCO$_3$ was nearly equal to intake so that mean sodium balance in the NaHCO$_3$ group was similar to pre-supplementation levels. Conversely, while bicarbonate secretion was elevated in these latter subjects, net retention occurred so that mean serum bicarbonate levels increased from 18.9 mEq/L to 30.4 mEq/L. In subjects receiving NaCl, net sodium balance was positive during supplementation. Clinical evaluation demonstrated statistically significant increases in weight and systolic blood pressure in those receiving NaCl but not NaHCO$_3$ [35].

RECOMMENDATIONS

As previously noted, a Cochrane review through 2006 stated insufficient evidence to make any recommendation. The National Kidney Foundation's 2000 KDOQI guidelines on nutrition in CKD and 2003 KDOQI guidelines for metabolic acidosis in CKD patients cite evidence that serum bicarbonate levels should be maintained at ≥22 mEq/L. It was recognized that the desirable serum bicarbonate was probably greater than 22 mEq/L, but higher values could not be recommended at those times because of the lack of available data. While newer data are available from some small clinical trials that suggest that alkali supplements can slow progression of CKD, large double-blind, placebo-controlled clinical trials are warranted to evaluate the effects of alkali supplements on meaningful kidney disease outcomes. At least one such trial is underway [36].

References

[1] Widmer B, Gerhardt RE, Harrington JT, Cohen JJ. Serum electrolyte and acid base composition. The influence of graded degrees of chronic renal failure. Archives of Internal Medicine 1979;139:1099−102.

[2] Lyon DM, Dunlop DM, Stewart CP. The alkaline treatment of chronic nephritis. The Lancet 1931;218:1009−13.

[3] Kraut JA, Kurtz I. Metabolic acidosis of CKD: diagnosis, clinical characteristics, and treatment. Am J Kid Dis 2005;45:978−93.

[4] Clase CM, Kiberd BA, Garg AX. Relationship between glomerular filtration rate and the prevalence of metabolic abnormalities: results from the Third National Health and Nutrition Examination Survey (NHANES III). Nephron Clin Pract 2007;105:c178−84.

[5] Eustace JA, Astor B, Muntner PM, Ikizler TA, Coresh J. Prevalence of acidosis and inflammation and their association with low serum albumin in chronic kidney disease. Kid Internat 2004;65:1031–40.

[6] Moranne O, Froissart M, Rossert J, et al. Timing of onset of CKD-related metabolic complications. J Am Soc Nephrol 2009;20:164–71.

[7] Caravaca F, Arrobas M, Pizarro JL, Esparrago JF. Metabolic acidosis in advanced renal failure: differences between diabetic and nondiabetic patients. Am J Kid Dis 1999;33:892–8.

[8] Wallia R, Greenberg A, Piraino B, Mitro R, Puschett JB. Serum electrolyte patterns in end-stage renal disease. American Journal of Kidney Diseases 1986;8:98–104.

[9] Kirschbaum B. Spurious metabolic acidosis in hemodialysis patients. Am J Kid Dis 2000;35:1068–71.

[10] Laski ME. Penny wise and bicarbonate foolish. Am J Kid Dis 2000;35:1224–5.

[11] Goodman AD, Lemann Jr J, Lennon EJ, Relman AS. Production, excretion, and net balance of fixed acid in patients with renal acidosis. J Clin Invest 1965;44:495–506.

[12] Davies HE, Wrong O. Acidity of urine and excretion of ammonium in renal disease. Lancet 1957;273:625.

[13] Platt R. Structural and functional adaptation in renal failure. Br Med J. (Clin Res Ed) 1952;1372–7.

[14] Elkinton JR. Hydrogen ion turnover in health and in renal disease. Ann Intern Med 1962;57:660–85.

[15] Nath KA, Hostetter MK, Hostetter TH. Pathophysiology of chronic tubulo-interstitial disease in rats. Interactions of dietary acid load, ammonia, and complement component C3. J Clin Invest 1985;76:667–75.

[16] Wesson DE. Endogenous endothelins mediate increased acidification in remnant kidneys. J Am Soc Nephrol 2001;12:1826–35.

[17] Osman AA. Guy's Hospital Reports 1927;lxxvii:386.

[18] Throssell D, Brown J, Harris KP, Walls J. Metabolic acidosis does not contribute to chronic renal injury in the rat. Clin Sci (Lond) 1995;89:643–50.

[19] Gadola L, Noboa O, Marquez MN, et al. Calcium citrate ameliorates the progression of chronic renal injury. Kidney Int 2004;65:1224–30.

[20] Phisitkul S, Hacker C, Simoni J, Tran RM, Wesson DE. Dietary protein causes a decline in the glomerular filtration rate of the remnant kidney mediated by metabolic acidosis and endothelin receptors. Kidney Internat 2008;73:192–9.

[21] Wesson DE, Simoni J. Increased tissue acid mediates a progressive decline in the glomerular filtration rate of animals with reduced nephron mass. Kidney Internat 2009;75:929–35.

[22] Wesson DE, Simoni J. Acid retention during kidney failure induces endothelin and aldosterone production which lead to progressive GFR decline, a situation ameliorated by alkali diet. Kidney Int 2010;78:1128–35.

[23] Shah SN, Abramowitz M, Hostetter TH, Melamed ML. Serum bicarbonate levels and the progression of kidney disease: a cohort study. Am J Kidney Dis 2009;54:270–7.

[24] Menon V, Tighiouart H, Vaughn NS, et al. Serum bicarbonate and long-term outcomes in CKD. Am J Kidney Dis 2010;56:907–14.

[25] Raphael KL, Wei G, Baird BC, Greene T, Beddhu S. Higher serum bicarbonate levels within the normal range are associated with better survival and renal outcomes in African Americans. Kidney Int 2011;79:356–62.

[26] Blom van Assendelft PM, Mees EJ. Urea metabolism in patients with chronic renal failure: influence of sodium bicarbonate or sodium chloride administration. Metabolism 1970;19:1053–63.

[27] Papadoyannakis NJ, Stefanidis CJ, McGeown M. The effect of the correction of metabolic acidosis on nitrogen and potassium balance of patients with chronic renal failure. Am J Clin Nutr 1984;40:623–7.

[28] Jenkins D, Burton PR, Bennett SE, Baker F, Walls J. The metabolic consequences of the correction of acidosis in uraemia. Nephrology, Dialysis, Transplantation: official publication of the European Dialysis and Transplant Association – European Renal Association 1989;4:92–5.

[29] Rustom R, Grime JS, Costigan M, et al. Oral sodium bicarbonate reduces proximal renal tubular peptide catabolism, ammoniogenesis, and tubular damage in renal patients. Ren Fail 1998;20:371–82.

[30] Mathur RP, Dash SC, Gupta N, Prakash S, Saxena S, Bhowmik D. Effects of correction of metabolic acidosis on blood urea and bone metabolism in patients with mild to moderate chronic kidney disease: a prospective randomized single blind controlled trial. Ren Fail 2006;28:1–5.

[31] Roderick P, Willis NS, Blakeley S, Jones C, Tomson C. Correction of chronic metabolic acidosis for chronic kidney disease patients. Cochrane Database Syst Rev 2007:CD001890.

[32] de Brito-Ashurst I, Varagunam M, Raftery MJ, Yaqoob MM. Bicarbonate supplementation slows progression of CKD and improves nutritional status. J Am Soc Nephrol 2009;20:2075–84.

[33] Phisitkul S, Khanna A, Simoni J, et al. Amelioration of metabolic acidosis in patients with low GFR reduced kidney endothelin production and kidney injury, and better preserved GFR. Kidney Int 2010;77:617–23.

[34] Mahajan A, Simoni J, Sheather SJ, Broglio KR, Rajab MH, Wesson DE. Daily oral sodium bicarbonate preserves glomerular filtration rate by slowing its decline in early hypertensive nephropathy. Kidney Int 2010;78:303–9.

[35] Husted FC, Nolph KD, Maher JF. NaHCO$_3$ and NaCl tolerance in chronic renal failure. J Clin Invest 1975;56:414–9.

[36] Di Iorio B, Aucella F, Conte G, Cupisti A, Santoro D. A prospective, multicenter, randomized, controlled study: the Correction of Metabolic Acidosis with Use of Bicarbonate in Chronic Renal Insufficiency (UBI) Study. J Nephrol 2012;25(3):437–40.

19

Calcium, Phosphate, PTH, Vitamin D and FGF-23 in Chronic Kidney Disease

Alexandra Voinescu, Kevin J. Martin

Division of Nephrology, Saint Louis University, St. Louis, Missouri, USA

INTRODUCTION

In healthy individuals, kidneys play an important role in regulating calcium and phosphorus homeostasis through different mechanisms. Chronic kidney disease (CKD) is associated with the inability to control normal mineral homeostasis, resulting in changes in serum levels of calcium, phosphorus, parathyroid hormone (PTH), vitamin D and fibroblastic growth factor FGF-23. Secondary hyperparathyroidism is present in early stages of CKD. Leading to the development of high bone turnover, pathological fractures, vascular calcifications and other systemic manifestations. Traditionally, mineral and bone abnormalities seen in chronic kidney disease were included in the term "renal osteodystrophy". Recently, the term CKD-mineral and bone disorder (CKD-MBD) was introduced to define the biochemical abnormalities of calcium, phosphorus, PTH, or vitamin D metabolism, abnormalities in bone turnover, volume and bone mineralization, and vascular or other soft tissue calcifications. This chapter will review the calcium, phosphorus, PTH, vitamin D and FGF-23 axis, with the main focus on phosphorus and its central role in the pathophysiology and progression of CKD-MBD.

CALCIUM METABOLISM

Calcium plays an important role in bone mineralization, as well as a wide range of biological processes. Total adult calcium content is approximately 1000 g. 99% of total body calcium is in the skeleton in the form of hydroxyapatite. The remainder is contained in the extracellular fluid and soft tissues. Serum and extracellular calcium concentration in humans is tightly controlled within a narrow physiologic range that is optimal for proper cellular functions of many tissues

affected by calcium. Approximately 50% of the total serum calcium is ionized, and the remainder is bound primarily to albumin (about 40%), or complexed with anions such as phosphates and citrate (about 10%). Serum calcium levels range between 8.5 to 10.5 mg/dL (2.1 to 2.6 mM) in healthy individuals. The ionized fraction of calcium is physiologically important and is regulated by the calcium regulating hormones, parathyroid hormone (PTH) and 1,25 dihydroxy vitamin D.

The average calcium dietary intake is around 1000 mg/day, but there are wide variations. On average, 400 mg of calcium undergoes net absorption from the diet, and the unabsorbed and secreted components appear in the stool. Yet from the extracellular pool of calcium, which contains about 900 mg, 10,000 mg/day is filtered at the glomerulus, most being reabsorbed by the renal tubules, and only a few hundred milligrams appearing in urine each day. This pool is in dynamic equilibrium with calcium entering and exiting via the intestine, bone and renal tubules. The skeleton turns over about 200 mg/day of calcium, but there is wide variation (Figure 19.1).

Intestinal calcium absorption occurs through two pathways: an active, transcellular, vitamin D dependent pathway, and a passive, paracellular diffusional process. The duodenum is the major site of calcium absorption, although absorption occurs throughout the other segments of the small intestine and the colon. The active calcium uptake from the lumen across the brush border membrane occurs through TRPV5 and TRPV6 transporters located on the apical membrane. The transport of calcium through the cytosol requires a vitamin D-inducible protein, calbindin D_{9K}. At the basolateral membrane, calcium is removed from the cell by the Ca^{2+}-ATPase (PMCA1b) and a Na^+/Ca^{2+} exchanger (NCX1) [1]. Each of these steps is regulated by 1,25 $(OH)_2$ D.

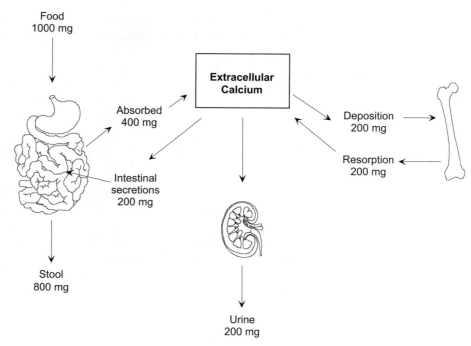

FIGURE 19.1 Diagram of calcium homeostasis showing dietary intake, the absorption and secretion of calcium by the intestine, skeletal deposition and resorption and excretion of calcium by the kidney.

In the kidney, 60% of the filtered calcium is reabsorbed in the proximal tubule mainly passively, through paracellular pathways via convection (solvent drag) and electrochemical gradients. Approximately 20% of calcium is reabsorbed in the thick ascending limb of the loop of Henle, of which about two-thirds is paracellular and the remaining is transcellular. In addition, 15% of the filtered calcium is reabsorbed in the distal convoluted tubule, the connecting tubule, and the initial part of the cortical collecting tubule. In this distal part of the nephron, calcium reabsorption actively opposes the natural electrochemical gradients. Luminal calcium enters the cells via the epithelial calcium channels, TRPV5 and TRPV6. Inside the cells, calcium binds with calbindin D28K and is transported through the basolateral membrane via Ca^{2+}-ATPase (PMCA1b) and Ca^{2+}-Na^+ exchangers (NCX1). This active transcellular transport is regulated by PTH, $1,25(OH)_2 D_3$, calcium intake and estrogens. PTH stimulates renal calcium reabsorption by upregulating the expression of the TRPV5, calbindin D28K, NCX1 and PMCA1b [2]. Vitamin D receptor (VDR) null mice and 1-alpha hydroxylase-deficient animals show down-regulation of TRPV5 and calbindin D28K demonstrating an important role of vitamin D in regulating renal calcium absorption [3]. Similarly, studies performed in VDR and 1-alpha hydroxylase knockout mice fed a high calcium rescue diet showed up-regulation of all four proteins [4]. It has also been demonstrated that estrogen upregulates the expression of TRPV5 in kidney in a $1,25-(OH)_2D_3$-independent manner [5].

VITAMIN D

Vitamin D is a multifunctional hormone that affects many essential biological functions, ranging from immune regulation to mineral ion metabolism. Vitamin D_2 (ergocalciferol) is absorbed mainly from food, and vitamin D_3 (cholecalciferol) is produced in the skin from 7-dehydrocholesterol by ultraviolet radiation. Both forms of vitamin D require further metabolism to become activated, and their respective metabolism is indistinguishable. Vitamin D is transported in the blood by the vitamin D binding protein (DBP) to the liver, where it gets converted to 25(OH)D, the major circulating metabolite of vitamin D. The final activation step, 1-hydroxylation, occurs primarily in the kidney, where 25(OH)D is 1α-hydroxylated to produce $1,25(OH)_2D$, the most active form of the hormone, responsible for most of the biological actions of vitamin D. This hydroxylation step is up-regulated by several factors, including PTH, low ambient concentrations of calcium, phosphorus, and $1,25(OH)_2D$ itself and is inhibited by FGF-23 and high levels of calcium and phosphorus. The kidney can also produce 24,25 dihydroxyvitamin D3 ($24,25(OH)_2D_3$), a relatively inactive metabolite when compared to $1,25(OH)_2D_3$. 24 hydroxylase can hydroxylate both $25(OH)D_3$ and $1,25(OH)_2D_3$. As a result, 24 hydroxylase can limit the amount of $1,25(OH)_2D_3$ in target tissues by accelerating the catabolism of $1,25(OH)_2D_3$ to $1,24,25(OH)_3D_3$ and by producing $24,25(OH)_2D_3$, thus decreasing the pool of $25(OH)D_3$ available for 1 hydroxylation [6].

1,25(OH)₂D mediates its biological effects through its own member of the nuclear hormone receptor superfamily, the vitamin D receptor (VDR), that acts as a ligand-inducible transcription factor. Ligand-bound VDR functions as a heterodimeric complex with the 9-cis retinoic acid nuclear receptor retinoid-X-receptor (RXR). The complex binds to target DNA sequences and regulates the transcription of several genes important in mediating the effects of vitamin D on calcium and skeletal metabolism and its diverse biological effects [7,8].

PHOSPHATE METABOLISM

Phosphate is an essential mineral in the body, critical for many biological processes, including bone development, cell membrane phospholipid content and function, cell signaling and energy transfer mechanism. Total adult phosphorus content is approximately 700 g. In the body, 85% of phosphate is found in bone where it is linked with calcium to form hydroxyapatite crystals. The remainder of the phosphorus is largely distributed in soft tissues (14%) and only 1% in the extracellular space [9,10]. Plasma contains both organic and inorganic forms of phosphorus. The organic phosphorus fraction, found mainly in phospholipids, accounts for approximately two-thirds of the total plasma phosphorus. Inorganic phosphorus primarily exists as phosphate (PO_4) and is the commonly measured fraction, present in concentration between 2.5 and 4.5 mg/dL. 15% of the inorganic phosphorus is bound to plasma proteins. The rest is complexed with sodium, magnesium, calcium or circulates as the free monohydrogen (HPO_4^{2-}) or dihydrogen forms ($H_2PO_4^-$). Phosphorus has a pKa of 6.8 and at normal physiologic body pH of 7.4 it primarily exists as a divalent ion in a ratio of about 4:1 HPO_4^{2-} to $H_2PO_4^-$. The term "plasma phosphorus" is used when referring to plasma inorganic phosphorus concentration, and because plasma inorganic phosphorus is nearly all in the form of the PO_4 ion, the term phosphate and phosphorus are often interchangeably used in clinical chemistry laboratory [11].

The concentration of phosphorus in the extracellular space is the result of the interactions among intestinal uptake, renal excretion, and exchanges with bone and the intracellular compartment (Figure 19.2).

The phosphate intake in the United States is on average 1000 to 1500 mg/day. Approximately 60% to 80% of dietary phosphorus is absorbed along the entire length of the intestine but is maximal in the small intestine [12,13]. Intestinal phosphate absorption occurs via two routes: a paracellular pathway involving tight junctions and driven by a passive diffusional flux and an active transcellular transport involving the type II sodium-dependent phosphate cotransporter Npt2b. The energy for this transport process is provided by the sodium gradient induced by the sodium—potassium ATPase cotransporter at the basolateral membrane [14]. In addition to Npt2b, two additional type III sodium-dependent phosphate cotransporters PiT1 and PiT2

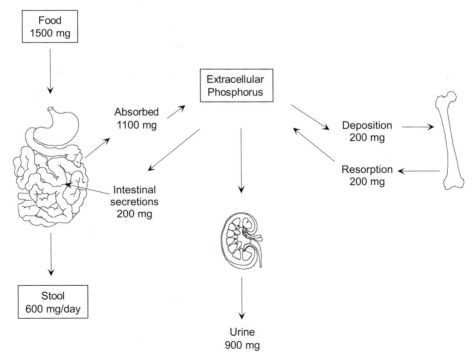

FIGURE 19.2 Diagram of phosphorus homeostasis showing dietary intake, the absorption and secretion of phosphorus by the intestine, skeletal deposition and resorption and excretion of phosphorus by the kidney.

have been found to be expressed in the intestine. The precise role of Pit transporters remains to be determined. In NaPi-IIb-$^{-/-}$ mice there is no residual sodium-dependent phosphate transport activity, suggesting that Pit mediated transporters are of limited significance in the intestine [15, 16]. The two major factors known to regulate Npt2b expression are dietary phosphate and $1,25(OH)_2D_3$. Studies in both the vitamin D receptor knockout mouse and the 1alpha-hydroxylase knockout mouse have shown that Npt2b regulation by modulating dietary phosphate occurs through a vitamin-D-independent pathway [16−18]. Other factors have been shown to modulate Npt2b expression, such as estrogens, glucocorticoids, epidermal growth factor, metabolic acidosis, matrix extracellular phosphoglycoprotein, and fibroblast growth factor 23 (FGF-23) [19−24].

The kidneys play a major role in maintaining phosphorus balance by excreting the net amount of the absorbed phosphorus. As phosphorus is not significantly bound to albumin, most of the phosphorus is filtered freely at the glomerulus. At steady state, 80−90% of the filtered phosphorus is reabsorbed by the kidneys. The proximal tubule reabsorbs 70% to 80% of filtered phosphorus through type II sodium-phosphate co-transporters Npt2a and Npt2c, expressed at the apical membrane of renal proximal tubule cells. Recently, type III phosphate transporter PiT-2 has been shown to contribute to phosphate absorption in the proximal tubules. Knockout studies in mice have shown that 70% of the renal phosphate absorption is mediated by Npt2a and approximately 30% by Npt2c. Double-knockout Npt2a/Npt2c mice still exhibit some renal phosphate reabsorption, indicating a role for PiT-2 in this process [25−28]. Phosphate transport across the basolateral membrane remains a poorly understood process. Several phosphate transport pathways have been postulated, including a phosphate-anion exchanger, passive diffusion, or phosphate transport via type II sodium-phosphate co-transporters.

Several factors have been shown to modulate renal phosphate transport. Phosphate depletion, insulin-like growth factor-1, growth hormone, thyroid hormone, $1,25(OH)_2$ vitamin D_2 stimulate phosphate reabsorption [28−31]. Factors that inhibit phosphate reabsorption include parathyroid hormone (PTH), fibroblast growth factor (FGF)-23, phosphate loading, volume expansion, metabolic acidosis, glucocorticoids, and calcitonin [32−34]. The main hormones that regulate renal phosphate handling are PTH and FGF-23.

PARATHYROID HORMONE

Parathyroid hormone is an 84 amino acid protein which is synthesized in the parathyroid gland and stored in secretary granules for release in response to a reduction in the levels of ionized calcium. Following release, it has a relatively short half-life in plasma of just minutes and is cleaved into a variety of fragments of the hormone in the liver and kidney. The principal regulator of PTH secretion is the levels of ionized calcium. PTH secretion can also be regulated by phosphate and by 1,25-dihydroxy vitamin D. The regulation of PTH secretion in response to changes in ionized calcium is mediated by the calcium-sensing receptor, a G-protein-7 membrane spanning receptor, which can also be utilized as a therapeutic target for the control of PTH secretion (see below). The regulation of PTH by 1,25-dihydroxy vitamin D is a direct effect of PTH gene transcription. The precise mechanism of the regulation of PTH secretion by phosphate is not entirely understood, but may involve effects on the EGF receptor.

Parathyroid hormone binds to type I PTH receptor in proximal tubular cells to activate cAMP-protein kinase A (PKA) and the phospholipase C-protein kinase C (PKC) signal transduction pathways. Activation of both signaling pathways leads to internalization of the sodium-phosphate cotransporters Npt2a and Npt2c. The removal of Npt2a from the apical brush border membrane in response to PTH requires the presence of the sodium-proton exchanger regulatory factor 1 (NHERF1). After removal of the exchanger from the brush border in response to PTH, Npt2a is sent to early endosomes and then to lysosomes, where subsequent proteolytic degradation of the transporter occurs [33,35,36].

Measurement of PTH is essential for the assessment of abnormalities in PTH secretion, and particularly in the assessment of the disturbances in bone and mineral metabolism in the setting of chronic kidney disease. The measurement of PTH has been complicated by the existence of circulating PTH fragments and although assay technology has evolved to two-site immunometric assays, circulating PTH fragments continue to be problematic, especially in the setting of chronic kidney disease.

FIBROBLAST GROWTH FACTOR 23 (FGF-23)

Hypophosphatemia with inappropriate urinary phosphate excretion can occur in the absence of hyperparathyroidism, suggesting the presence of non-PTH phosphaturic factors. The term "phosphatonin" was originally described as a circulating factor that caused renal phosphate wasting in patients with tumor-induced osteomalacia (TIO) or oncogenic osteomalacia, paraneoplastic syndrome characterized by renal phosphate wasting, aberrant vitamin D metabolism, and osteomalacia. Search for phosphatonin in patients with TIO led to the identification of fibroblast growth factor-23 (FGF-23). The clinical characteristics in oncogenic osteomalacia overlap those in hereditary hypophosphatemic rickets, including hypophosphatemia as a result of renal phosphate wasting, normocalcemia, inappropriately normal $1,25(OH)_2D$ levels for the degree of hypophosphatemia, and skeletal defects caused by osteomalacia. In addition to FGF-23, other phosphatonins have been identified: secreted frizzled-related protein 4 (sFRP4), matrix extracellular phosphoglycoprotein (MEPE), fibroblast growth factor-7 (FGF-7) [37−44]. FGF-23 is the bone-derived phosphatonin that has been extensively studied, and was found to play a critical role in normal physiology and altered mineral metabolism in CKD. FGF-23 is predominately expressed in osteocytes and osteoblasts in the skeleton, but low levels of unclear significance can be found in pericyte-like cells that surround the venous sinusoids of the bone marrow, ventrolateral thalamic nuclei, heart, thymus, and small intestine [45,46].

The kidney is the main target organ for FGF-23. When recombinant FGF-23 is injected in animals, it induces a rapid decline in renal phosphate reabsorption, resulting in hypophosphatemia, low serum calcitriol levels and bone demineralization. FGF-23 activates FGF receptors on the basolateral membrane of the renal tubules resulting in decreased expression of Npt2a and Npt2c on the apical surface of the tubular cell. The reduction in the number of Npt2a by FGF-23 seems to be independent of PTH [47]. FGF-23 also suppresses the 1α-hydroxylase enzyme (CYP27B1) in the renal tubule, the enzyme which stimulates the conversion of 25-hydroxyvitamin D to $1,25(OH)_2D$. FGF-23 also enhances the expression of 24-hydroxylase (CYP24), which converts $1,25(OH)_2D$ to inactive metabolites in the proximal renal tubules [48,49]. FGF exerts its biological functions by binding and activation of its cognate FGF receptor (FGFR) in the presence of klotho, a type I membrane receptor with homology to beta-glycosidases [50,51]. The transmembrane and secreted forms of klotho proteins may collectively affect the aging process in mammals [52]. Klotho expression is restricted to a few tissues, including the distal convoluted tubules in the kidney, parathyroid glands, sinoatrial node, pituitary and choroid plexus in the brain. It is still unclear how FGF-23 exerts its physiological effects on the proximal tubule in the kidney while klotho appears to be expressed in the distal tubular epithelial cells. Klotho is expressed at the cell surface but is also present in the plasma as two secreted forms. The membrane bound form can be cleaved to generate a second circulating species, and either of these forms of klotho could possibly bind to FGF-23 and FGFRs. In klotho-deficient mice, the FGF-23 concentration is increased but is ineffective in controlling serum phosphate levels. In conclusion, klotho is a co-receptor that specifically increases the sensitivity of FGF receptors to FGF-23 [36,50,51,53].

Besides its effect on tubular phosphate handling, FGF-23 may control PTH synthesis and secretion. Injection of FGF-23 in animals rapidly decreases PTH secretion within 10 minutes through the MAPK pathway; it also inhibits PTH gene expression in parathyroid glands. In addition, FGF-23 increases 1 alpha hydroxylase expression in bovine parathyroid cells, which may contribute to reduce PTH gene transcription [36,54,55].

FGF-23 gene expression in bone is regulated by phosphate and $1,25(OH)_2D$. Phosphate loading in mice increases FGF-23 levels, but the data in humans are conflicting. Few studies have failed to demonstrate increase in serum FGF-23 levels in response to phosphate loading, whereas phosphate restriction has been associated with a small, but significant, decrease in circulating FGF-23 levels. Extracellular phosphorus did not directly stimulate FGF-23 mRNA levels or FGF-23 gene promoter activity in osteoblastic cultures [56−60]. $1,25(OH)_2D$ stimulates FGF-23 production both in vivo and in vitro. This effect seems to be mediated through the vitamin D receptor since vitamin D receptor-null mice did not show an increase in FGF-23 levels after $1,25(OH)_2D_3$ administration. FGF-23 secretion is also regulated by local bone-derived factors, such as phosphate-regulating gene with homologies to endopeptidases on the X chromosome (PHEX) and dentin matrix protein 1 (DMP1) [45,61]. $1,25(OH)_2D_3$ is also able to suppress PHEX mRNA levels in bone cells, and reductions in PHEX can result in increased FGF-23 expression in osteocytes. Therefore, it is plausible that $1,25(OH)_2D_3$ upregulates FGF-23 production in part indirectly by downregulation of PHEX expression [62−66].

ALTERATIONS IN MINERAL METABOLISM IN CKD

Phosphate retention begins at an early stage of chronic kidney disease, due to a gradual decline in filtered phosphate load. Serum phosphate is maintained within normal limits until the GFR falls to less than approximately 30 mL/min [12,67]. Hyperphosphatemia is delayed until the later stages of CKD by the rise in serum concentration of PTH and FGF-23. In the early course of kidney disease, phosphorus retention stimulates FGF-23 and PTH secretion, which in turn suppress tubular phosphate reabsorption, causing increased renal phosphate excretion. FGF-23 suppresses the production of $1,25(OH)_2D$ at the same time, which limits intestinal phosphate absorption, and causes increases in PTH levels with development of secondary hyperparathyroidism. Because $1,25(OH)_2D$ is also a potent inducer of klotho expression in the kidney, decreased levels of 1,25(OH)$_2$D reduce klotho expression. FGF-23 suppresses PTH release via stimulating the dimeric klotho-FGF receptor at the parathyroid glands, but resistance to the effect of FGF-23 appears as kidney function declines because of decreased klotho expression in the parathyroid glands and kidney. Thus, as renal function continues to decline, hyperphosphatemia develops progressively due to insufficient renal excretion despite high levels of PTH and FGF-23. Increased bone resorption can also contribute to hyperphosphatemia seen in CKD and end-stage renal disease patients that occurs in response to chronically elevated PTH levels [68–72].

Hyperphosphatemia decreases serum calcium levels through physicochemical binding and suppresses 1 alpha-hydroxylase activity, resulting in decreased levels of 1,25(OH)$_2$D. This reduction in 1,25(OH)$_2$D causes direct increase in PTH secretion. Several studies in animal models have shown a direct role of phosphorus on parathyroid gland cells, resulting in parathyroid hyperplasia and secondary hyperparathyroidism, independent of serum calcium and 1,25(OH)$_2$D [73–75]. High extracellular phosphate concentrations may affect the regulation of intracellular calcium in parathyroid cells, resulting in the inhibition of phospholipase A2 (PLA2) and the formation of arachidonic acid (AA), a potent inhibitor of PTH release [76]. Studies by Ritter et al. demonstrated that hyperphosphatemia is associated with reduced expression of the calcium-sensing receptor, thereby decreasing the ability of the parathyroid gland to respond to changes in ionized calcium [77]. In addition, high phosphate intake induces cell growth through transforming growth factor-α (TGF-α) mediated via the epidermal growth factor receptor, thus worsening the parathyroid hyperplasia and the resultant secondary hyperparathyroidism [78]. The effect of phosphate on PTH gene expression involves changes in the parathyroid gland cytosolic proteins that bind to the PTH mRNA 3′ untranslated region (3′UTR) and determine PTH mRNA stability. Further studies have shown decreased PTH mRNA degradation in animals with uremia [79,80]. In conclusion, the mechanisms by which PTH secretion is regulated by phosphorus are multifactorial.

PHOSPHATE AND CARDIOVASCULAR DISEASE (CVD)

Epidemiologic data suggest that higher serum phosphate levels are associated with increased CVD morbidity and mortality in both general population and CKD populations. The Framingham Offspring Study evaluated 3368 participants with no history of CKD or CVD and found that serum phosphate levels >3.5 mg/dL were associated with an estimated 55% increased CVD risk [81]. In a post hoc analysis of the Cholesterol and Recurrent Events (CARE) study, participants with serum phosphate >4 mg/dL had a 50% greater risk of myocardial infarction (HR, 1.50; 95% CI, 1.05 to 2.16) and a 43% greater risk of developing heart failure (HR, 1.43; 95% CI, 0.95 to 2.14) compared with those with serum phosphate of 2.5 to 3.4 mg/dL. Each 1 mg/dl higher phosphorus levels was associated with a 27% increased risk for all-cause mortality (HR, 1.27; 95% CI, 1.02 to 1.59) [82]. The relationship between phosphate excess and CV risk has also been studied in CKD patients. In a study of 3490 veterans with CKD stage III–IV, each 1 unit increase in serum phosphate was associated with a significant 35% increased risk for acute myocardial infarction (HR, 1.35; 95% CI, 10.9–1.66) and a 23% greater risk of mortality (HR, 1.23; 95% CI, 1.12–1.36) after adjustments for co-morbid conditions [83]. Another large prospective longitudinal study performed in nondialysis CKD patients was the Chronic Renal Insufficiency Standards Implementation Study (CRISIS), which involved 1203 patients. In CKD stages 3 to 4 patients, all-cause and cardiovascular mortality risk increased as serum phosphorus increased [84]. Phosphate was initially identified as a cardiovascular risk factor in dialysis patients in 1998 in a cohort of 6407 hemodialysis patients, followed by another study done in 2004 in 40,538 patients from the US Renal Data System (USRDS), where there was a linear association of higher serum phosphate concentrations with a greater risk of cardiovascular hospitalizations [85,86]. In another study done in dialysis population (14,829 hemodialysis patients), the fully adjusted risk of cardiovascular events was greater with incremental higher serum phosphate concentrations [87].

Multiple studies performed in dialysis patients confirmed the association of higher phosphate levels with mortality, although slight differences in the inflection point (the point at which phosphate level becomes significantly associated with increased all-cause mortality) varied from 5.0 to 5.5 mg/dL [86], >5.5 mg/dL [88], 6.0 to 7.0 mg/dL [89], and >6.5 mg/dL [90].

The mechanisms underlying the increase in cardiovascular morbidity and mortality associated with disturbances in phosphate metabolism are not fully understood, but may involve direct effects of increased phosphate on renal bone disease and vascular calcification, as well as modulation of circulating serum hormones, such as FGF-23, PTH, and calcitriol. Serum phosphate level has also been associated with CKD progression and left ventricular hypertrophy, which are known to contribute to cardiovascular disease and death [91,92]. FGF-23 is now thought to be a main regulator of phosphate homeostasis and high FGF-23 levels were found to be an independent predictor of mortality in both incident and prevalent dialysis patients [93,94]. In both studies, the results were independent of serum phosphate, and the correlation between high FGF-23 and mortality remained significant even in patients with normophosphatemia. It is unclear whether increased FGF-23 levels are directly toxic or are a surrogate marker of the toxicity of other factors that have been implicated in the development of vascular disease. Several recent studies demonstrated that high FGF-23 levels were associated with impaired vasoreactivity and arterial stiffness, increased left ventricular mass index and increased prevalence of left ventricular hypertrophy in CKD patients [93,95—97].

Another possible mechanism by which phosphate may influence cardiovascular risk is by stimulating PTH and inhibiting the activation of vitamin D. PTH excess and activated vitamin D deficiency have been associated with cardiovascular risk in some observational studies. Activated vitamin D (calcitriol) potentially suppresses the renin-angiotension-aldosterone system and regulates cardiomyocyte proliferation and hypertrophy [85,86,98,99]. FGF-23 inhibits 1-alpha-hydroxylase in the kidney, resulting in decreasing 1,25 dihydroxyvitamin D synthesis. Further studies are needed to identify if phosphate results in increased cardiovascular disease through a mechanism that involves vitamin D. Regardless of the underlying mechanisms, it is important to consider phosphate levels as a key factor to chronic kidney disease-mineral and bone disorder (CKD-MBD).

PHOSPHATE AND VASCULAR CALCIFICATIONS

Vascular calcification has been known to be a common complication of chronic kidney disease for many years. Calcium phosphate deposition is the hallmark of vascular calcifications and can occur in blood vessels, myocardium and cardiac valves. There are two types of arterial calcifications. Intimal calcification occurs within atherosclerotic plaques. Arterial medial calcification or Monckeberg's sclerosis occurs at the internal elastic lamina of the media layer. This type of vascular calcification is more common in patients with chronic kidney disease, diabetes mellitus, and advanced aging. Similar to intimal calcification, the presence of arterial medial calcification is a powerful and independent prognostic marker for all cause and cardiovascular mortality in end stage renal disease patients [100].

The presence of atherosclerotic vascular disease is often associated with the development of plaques and occlusive lesions. Medial wall calcification is known to be associated with increased arterial stiffness and reduced vascular compliance and increased pulse wave velocity. These hemodynamic changes lead to left ventricular hypertrophy, compromised coronary blood flow during diastole, and increased cardiovascular and all-cause mortality. Arterial medial calcification can also involve the small arterioles of the skin, causing calciphylaxis, a condition associated with extremely high mortality rates in dialysis patients [101,102].

Vascular calcification can be detected by a number of radiologic techniques. Plain radiography is the simplest technique used to detect the presence or absence of vascular calcification. Although some degree of differentiation between medial compared to intimal calcification can be detected on plain radiographs, this technique is insensitive and difficult to quantify [100]. Other techniques that have been used include vascular ultrasonography which can identify calcified plaques and calcified media, and intravascular ultrasonography, a more accurate technique that allows for measurement of absolute cross-sectional luminal areas [103,104]. For coronary artery calcifications, other non-invasive techniques such as tomography-based approaches (electron beam CT [EBCT] and multislice CT [MSCT]) permit assessment and quantification of the extent of calcifications. Braun et al. reported that EBCT has a sensitivity of 93% and a specificity of 73% when angiography was used as the reference standard. These CT-based techniques do not allow to differentiate atherosclerotic calcifications and medial calcifications [101,105].

Bellasi et al. compared different simple, non-invasive techniques to detect calcifications with those obtained using EBCT for coronary artery calcium scoring (CACS) in 140 prevalent hemodialysis patients [106]. All patients underwent EBT imaging, a lateral X-ray of the lumbar abdominal aorta, an echocardiogram, and measurement of pulse pressure (PP). Calcification of the abdominal aorta was scored as 0—24 divided into tertiles, echocardiograms were graded as 0—2 for absence or presence of calcification of the mitral and aortic valve and pulse pressure was divided in quartiles. The likelihood ratio (95% confidence interval [CI]) of coronary artery calcification score by EBCT of greater or equal to 100 was 1.79 (1.09, 2.96) for calcification of either valve and 7.50 (2.89, 19.5) for participants with a lateral abdominal radiographic-score greater or equal to 7. In contrast, no association was present between pulse pressure and EBCT calcification score [106].

The 2009 KDIGO guidelines recommended the use of plain lateral abdominal radiography or echocardiography to detect the presence or absence of coronary artery calcification in end-stage renal disease patients [107].

The prevalence of vascular calcifications varies according to age, method of detection, site of measurement, time on dialysis, and diabetic status. Goodman et al. found that coronary artery calcifications occur more frequently in young dialysis patients (between 20 and 30 years of age) compared to either normal subjects of the same age and sex or older adults with normal renal function [108]. Another study showed that coronary artery calcification by EBCT increased with advancing age in patients on dialysis and that the calcification scores were 2.5-fold to 5-fold higher in the dialysis patients than in age-matched non-dialysis patients with angiographically proven coronary artery disease [105]. An autopsy study done in 54 cases was designed to compare morphology and immunohistology of coronary arteries and coronary plaques of patients with ESRD and matched nonrenal patients who had died from a cardiac event. The magnitude of atherosclerotic plaque burden and intimal thickness in the dialysis patients was similar with non-uremic controls. Coronary plaques in patients with end-stage renal disease were characterized by increased media thickness and marked calcification [109]. The prevalence of detectable coronary and peripheral artery calcifications in dialysis patients ranges from 30% to 92%, according to age, sex, dialysis duration, and site of measurement [105,110,111]. The earliest and the most common site of calcification is the ankles, followed in frequency by the abdominal aorta, feet, pelvis, and hands and wrists in radiographs. Valvular calcifications are also common in dialysis patients. EBCT studies showed a prevalence of 45–59% in the mitral valve and 34–55% in the aortic valve [105,112].

There are limited data concerning the prevalence of coronary artery calcification using CT in CKD patients not yet on dialysis. Kramer et al. evaluated the association between CKD and coronary artery calcification among 2660 patients in the Dallas Heart Study age 30 to 65 years. No association was noted between stage 1 to 2 CKD and increased coronary artery calcifications scores. Compared with no CKD, stage 3 to 5 CKD was associated with increased risk of having increased coronary artery calcification, particularly very high calcification scores. This was largely due to the inclusion of patients with diabetes as there was no significant association between increased coronary artery calcification scores and the nondiabetic population with stage 3 to 5 CKD [113].

Several studies have demonstrated that coronary artery calcification is associated with increased mortality in dialysis patients. In a prospective study done in 110 dialysis patients, the authors correlated the amount of baseline vascular calcification (as assessed by ultrasonography at four different anatomic sites) with survival during a period of more than 4 years of follow-up. The results of this study showed that the presence and extent of vascular calcifications were strong predictors of cardiovascular and all-cause mortality [114].

One study followed 127 incident hemodialysis patients prospectively after baseline EBCT and demonstrated that the severity of coronary artery calcification at the time of initiation of hemodialysis was an important predictor of long-term survival. Even after adjustment for age, race, gender, and diabetes, a baseline CAC >400 was associated with a greater than fourfold increase in mortality [115].

Hyperphosphatemia has been linked to arterial calcifications in several human observational studies and in cell culture models. In a small study of dialysis patients, the mean serum phosphorus concentration was higher among the patients with coronary artery calcification [108]. Adeney et al. involved 439 participants from the Multi-Ethnic Study of Atherosclerosis who had moderate CKD and no clinical cardiovascular disease. After adjustment for demographics and estimated GFR, each 1 mg/dL increment in serum phosphate concentration was associated with a 21% (P = 0.002), 33% (P = 0.001), 25% (P = 0.16), and 62% (P = 0.007) greater prevalence of coronary artery, thoracic, aortic valve, and mitral valve calcification, respectively [116]. The relationship between serum phosphate levels and vascular calcification was also evaluated in the general population. In 3015 healthy young adults in the prospective Coronary Artery Risk Development in Young Adults (CARDIA) study, phosphorus levels were measured at baseline, and presence of coronary artery calcium was assessed by computed tomography 15 years later. Serum phosphate levels >3.9 mg/dL had a 52% greater risk of coronary artery calcifications as compared with those with a phosphate level <3.3 mg/dL (adjusted OR, 1.52; 95% CI, 1.04–2.22) [117]. High phosphate level was also found to be associated with vascular stiffness in general population. The association between serum phosphorus levels and arterial stiffness as estimated by an ankle brachial pressure index (ABPI) was examined in 581 participants in the Third National Health and Nutrition Examination Survey with normal renal function. There was a strong association between the highest quartile of serum phosphorus (3.7 to 5.0 mg/dL) and high ABPI compared to the reference group (3.1 to 3.4 mg/dL) after multivariate adjustment (adjusted OR, 4.78%; 95% CI, 1.73–13.2; P = 0.003) [118,119]. The findings from previous studies suggest that high phosphate level is a risk factor for development of vascular calcifications. Lowering serum phosphate level with a non-calcium based phosphate binder was found to slow the progression of vascular calcification in end-stage renal disease patients [120,121]. Several animal studies pointed to a role of elevated phosphorus in vascular calcification. Uremic rats treated for 3 months with a high phosphate diet showed aortic medial calcification and was decreased by treatment with the non-calcium phosphate binder, sevelamer [122].

Vascular calcification is a highly regulated process and occurs as a result of (1) phenotypic transformation of vascular smooth muscle cells (VSMCs) into osteochondrogenic-like cells; (2) the stimulation of these cells to actively synthesize mineralization-initiating matrix vesicles; (3) VSMC apoptosis with release of calcifying apoptotic vesicles; and (4) an imbalance of systemic and locally produced promoters and inhibitors of mineralization.

Several studies have described the ability of serum phosphorus to potently stimulate the phenotypic transformation of vascular smooth muscle cells into osteoblasts capable of producing a pro-mineralizing milieu. In a hyperphosphatemic environment (Pi > 2.4 mM), the VCMS culture systems revealed both osteochondrogenic phenotypic change and mineralization through sodium-dependent phosphate transporter, Pit-1. These in vitro and animal experiments results demonstrate that phosphate plays a key role in controlling vascular calcifications [123–125].

CONTROL OF SERUM PHOSPHATE IN CKD

In 2003, the National Kidney Foundation released the KDOQI clinical practice guidelines for bone metabolism and disease in chronic kidney disease. KDOQI recommended targeting phosphorus level of 2.7 to 4.6 mg/dL in patients with CKD stage 3 and 4 and 3.5 to 5.5 mg/dL in those with CKD stage 5D. In contrast to the KDOQI guidelines, KDIGO guidelines from 2009 reaffirmed the need for treatment to normalize phosphate level in CKD stage 3 to 5 and toward normal serum phosphate levels in CKD stage 5D patients, although these guidelines did not recommend specific target values.

The current recommendations are to initiate treatment when serum phosphate levels are above the normal range. However, waiting until frank hyperphosphatemia develops may not be the correct approach. In early experimental studies done in uremic dogs, dietary phosphorus reduction in proportion to the reduction in GFR was effective in preventing the development of hyperparathyroidism during a period of 2 years of observation, suggesting a critical role for phosphate retention in the elevation of parathyroid hormone [126]. Alternative biomarkers, such as FGF-23 or the urinary phosphate excretion may become important measures of altered phosphorus metabolism not reflected in serum levels, and may indicate the need for treatment in earlier stages of CKD, before the onset of hyperphosphatemia.

The treatment strategies routinely used to lower serum phosphate levels include dietary phosphate restriction, decreasing intestinal absorption by administration of phosphate binders and removal of phosphorus with dialysis therapy. Despite these measures, less than 50% of dialysis patients meet target levels for serum phosphorus [127]. In another study done in 1,814 CKD patients (SEEK study), only 15% of patients had a serum phosphate level <4.6 mg/dL at a GFR of 20–29 mL/min [67]. The reasons for the suboptimal phosphate control are multifactorial, including late referral to nephrology with subsequent late start of dietary phosphate restriction, and fear that tight phosphate restriction may represent a risk for protein malnutrition. Once phosphate-lowering advice is initiated, other challenges appear, including poor adherence to dietary restrictions, pill burden and cost of the medications once the phosphate binders are prescribed. Hence, solid knowledge of sources of dietary phosphorus is essential to the clinical management of patients with advanced CKD.

DIETARY PHOSPHORUS RESTRICTION

Several studies have looked at dietary phosphate restriction and its effects on abnormalities of bone and mineral metabolism, progression of renal dysfunction and mortality.

In patients with advanced CKD, where urinary phosphate excretion is severely impaired, dietary absorption becomes a critical determinant of serum phosphate concentration. Hemodialysis patients absorb approximately 60% of dietary phosphorus compared with 80% absorption in healthy volunteers consuming identical study meals. The use of activated vitamin D analogues further increases intestinal phosphorus absorption [128].

Since phosphorus exists in virtually all living organisms, it is found in most foods. Dietary sources of phosphorus include the organic phosphorus, found in foods high in protein, such as meat, dairy products, eggs, grains, legumes, nuts; and inorganic phosphorus found in food additives and preservatives. Table 19.1 shows a partial list of phosphorus content in different group of foods.

Any strategy to control dietary phosphorus intake in CKD patients has to consider the actual content of phosphorus in food, as well as the bioavailability of phosphorus from various food sources. Organic phosphorus in animal proteins is hydrolyzed in the intestinal tract and then absorbed into the circulation as inorganic phosphate [129]. Usually, 40 to 60% of organic phosphate in animal proteins is absorbed in the gastrointestinal tract. By comparison, plant-derived phosphorus from seeds, legumes, nuts is less easily absorbed because it is in the form of phytic acid or phytate. Because the human intestine does not secrete phytase, the enzyme required for absorption, the bioavailability of phosphorus from plant-derived food is usually less than 50% [130].

TABLE 19.1 Phosphorus Content of Selected Foods (USDA)

Food	Portion Size	P (mg)	Protein (g)	P/Protein
Chicken	140 g	286	43	6.65
Turkey	3 oz	208	24	8.7
Beef	3 oz	200	26.4	7.6
Pork	3 oz	224	22	7.4
Veal	3 oz	212	31	6.8
Lamb	3 oz	167	22	7.4
Fish	3 oz	230	20.23	11.36
Crab	3 oz	240	16.5	14.5
Egg (whole)	1 large	99	6.29	15.7
Egg (white)	1 large	5	3.6	1.4
Cheese	1 oz	133	6.6	20
Milk	1 cup	222	7.9	28
Bread	1 slice	25	3.4	7.3
Cereals	1 cup	259	5.2	49.8
Peanuts	1 oz	101	6.7	15.1
Almonds	1 oz	134	6	22.3
Beans	1 cup	183	12	15
Lentils	1 cup	356	17.9	19.9
Rice, white	1 cup	74	4	18.4
Rice, brown	1 cup	162	5	32

TABLE 19.2 Phosphate Content (mg) of Selected Beverages (based on 12 oz serving)

Beverage	Phosphate (mg)
Coke	69.9
Pepsi-Cola	57
Diet Cherry Coke	56
Diet Pepsi	50
Dr. Pepper	45
Hires Root Beer	22
Fruitworks	53 to 140
Gatorade	36
Tropicana Fruit Drinks	37 to 93

INORGANIC PHOSPHORUS AND FOOD ADDITIVES

Phosphorus is the main component of many food additives and preservatives. Phosphorus-containing additives, the most rapidly growing source of phosphorus over the past two decades, are increasingly being added to processed foods, such as enhanced meats, processed or spreadable cheeses, frozen meals, baked products, and beverages. These phosphate salts are used to extend shelf life, to preserve moisture or color, and to enhance flavor. The phosphate additives found in different preparations (e.g. sodium phosphate, potassium phosphate, calcium phosphate, phosphoric acid, various pyrophosphates and polyphosphates), are not protein-bound, and are more readily available for absorption, being almost 100% absorbed [131,132]. Since 1990, phosphorus-containing food additives in the general US population has doubled and will continue to increase as the American demand for convenience and fast foods escalates. Depending on individual food choices, phosphorus intake from additives could

contribute up to 1 g/day [133,134]. The contribution of inorganic phosphorus from processed foods was determined in an experiment performed with eight graduate students who participated in a randomized, crossover study where two dietary patterns were fed. For one 4-week period, volunteers were fed commercial foods free of phosphate additives; during the second 4-week period, they were fed commercially available foods very similar to those in the control diet, but containing phosphate additives (e.g. processed cheese instead of natural cheese, meats with added phosphates instead of fresh meats, colas rather than citric-acid containing soft drinks, etc.). These substitutions increased the phosphorus intake by an average of 1154 mg/day, while keeping the intake of protein and calcium unchanged [135,136].

Soft drink manufacturers add different amounts of phosphate to the beverages to enhance flavor. Many but not all clear-colored beverages or teas are low in phosphate. Table 19.2 shows the phosphorus content of some commonly used beverages [43,137].

Another source of dietary phosphorus which has become increasingly recognized in the literature and may increase the total phosphorus content is the "enhancement" of meat and dairy products. Uncooked meat and poultry products are frequently enhanced by food processors using sodium and potassium phosphate salts. Enhanced meat and poultry products may increase phosphorus and potassium content by almost two- to three-fold, respectively [138]. The federal guidelines require manufacturers to include a statement of enhancement with specifications of the additives used, but they are not quantified, and many consumers are not aware that they are purchasing an altered product. Phosphate salts are also used in ham and bacon to improve color and flavor, and to reduce oxidation and stabilize proteins. Different types of cheese contain various amounts of phosphorus, from less than 100 mg (e.g. Brie cheese) to almost 1000 mg per serving of combined organic and inorganic phosphorus in processed soft cheese [10,132,137].

Some of the multivitamin supplements contain significant amounts of phosphorus (e.g. Centrum 1 tablet contains 48 mg phosphorus/serving) and it is important to be aware of them when designing a low phosphorus diet in CKD patients [10].

Patient education regarding high phosphorus foods is an important component of the management of hyperphosphatemia. To determine the effect of limiting the intake of phosphorus-containing food additives on serum phosphorus levels among patients with end-stage renal disease, Sullivan et al. assessed 279 patients with elevated baseline serum phosphorus level >5.5 mg/dL. Intervention group (n = 145) received education on avoiding foods with phosphorus additives. After 3 months, there was a 0.6 mg/dL decline in average phosphorus level among intervention participants compared with control participants (95% confidence interval, −1.0 mg/dL to −0.1 mg/dL). The authors found that educating patients with ESRD to avoid phosphorus-containing food additives resulted in modest but clinically significant improvement in serum phosphorus levels [139].

The Food and Drug Administration requires products to include a nutrition facts label that lists the content of several important nutrients, including calories, cholesterol, sodium, protein, and calcium. However, many nutrition labels fail to list phosphorus content, making it difficult for patients to know how much phosphorus they are ingesting. In one study, Sullivan and colleagues found that phosphorus content was not listed on any of 38 representative chicken products purchased in grocery stores even though 92% of these products contained phosphorus additives [140].

Educating dialysis patients to limit their intake of additive containing food products represents important dietary recommendations. However, following such recommendations can be challenging for multiple reasons. The availability of additive-free products in grocery stores may be limited. Additive-free products are more expensive and require more effort to prepare, which may represent serious limitation for dialysis patients with physical or social challenges. In addition, ingredient lists are generally not present on fast food items, making it difficult to identify the presence of phosphorus containing additives. Knowing that a product contains a phosphorus additive does not allow an accurate estimate of its phosphorus content.

There is a need for labeling changes and hopefully in the future the policymakers will mandate that phosphorus content of foods be included on the nutrition facts label. This will encourage manufacturers to limit the use of phosphorus additives, will help patients limit their phosphorus intake, will guide providers to better instruct patients, and will help researchers to accurately assess dietary intake.

DIETARY PHOSPHORUS, PROTEIN INTAKE AND PHOSPHORUS-PROTEIN RATIO

Foods rich in protein are an important source of dietary phosphorus, thus dietary restriction of phosphorus is frequently associated with a decrease in dietary protein intake. This can lead to malnutrition and protein-energy wasting (PEW), important risk factors for death in maintenance dialysis patients [141]. A 3-year study of 30,075 prevalent maintenance hemodialysis patients showed that decrease in serum phosphorus associated with a concomitant decrease in protein intake increased the risk of death. The patients whose serum phosphorus decreased and whose normalized protein equivalent of total nitrogen appearance (nPNA) increased over 6 months had greater survival, with a case mix—adjusted death risk ratio of 0.90 (95% confidence limits: 0.86, 0.95; P < 0.001), whereas those whose phosphorus increased but whose nPNA decreased or those whose phosphorus and nPNA both decreased had worse mortality with risk ratio of 1.11 (1.05, 1.17; P < 0.001) and 1.06 (1.01, 1.12; P = 0.02), respectively. The authors concluded that the risk of controlling serum phosphorus by restricting dietary protein intake may outweigh the benefit of controlled phosphorus and may lead to greater mortality [142].

Noori et al. conducted a cohort study in 224 maintenance hemodialysis patients to examine the survival predictability of dietary phosphorus and the ratio of phosphorus (in mg) to protein intake (in g). Both higher phosphorus intake and greater dietary phosphorus to protein ratio were associated with increased death risk in dialysis patients, even after adjustments for serum phosphorus, type of phosphate binder used, and dietary protein, energy, and potassium intake [143]. The ratio of phosphorus to protein may represent a better dietary phosphorus metric for CKD patients. The metric phosphorus to protein ratio was also recommended by the Kidney Disease Outcomes Quality Initiative (KDOQI) guidelines. There is great variation in the ratio of phosphorus to protein among different protein sources. Low phosphorus to protein ratios are found in nondairy animal-derived foods, including egg whites, while whole eggs, dairy products, legumes, and fast foods have higher phosphorus to protein ratios. Egg whites are an excellent source of protein, with a low phosphorus to protein ratio and a low-cholesterol content. Taylor et al. conducted a pilot dietary intervention study in 13 hemodialysis patients who substituted pasteurized liquid egg whites for meat at one meal per day. Serum phosphorus level decreased significantly by 0.9 mg/dL over six weeks, while serum albumin level tended to increase. Pasteurized liquid egg white products were well tolerated and may become an important dietary protein source for CKD patients [144].

Sherman and his colleagues measured the phosphorus and protein content of 44 food products, including 30 refrigerated or frozen precooked meat, poultry, and fish items, using Association of Analytical Communities official method. The authors found that the ratio of phosphorus to protein content ranged from 6.1 to 21.5 mg of phosphorus per 1 g of protein. The mean ratio was 14.6 mg/g in the 19 food products with a label listing phosphorus as an additive compared with 9.0 mg/g in the 11 items without listed phosphorus [145]. For example, whey protein has a low phosphorus to protein ratio, making it an excellent source of protein supplementation, without worsening of hyperphosphatemia [146].

In addition to the phosphate content of a food, measures targeting a decrease in phosphorus levels should also depend upon an understanding of the ability to absorb phosphorus within the gastrointestinal tract. In contrast to highly bioavailable phosphorus additives, plant-derived phosphorus is poorly absorbed by humans. One of the few studies done on the absorbability and metabolic consequences of dietary phosphorus from different food sources involved 16 young Finnish females that were fed five experimental diets: a control diet that contained 500 mg of phosphorus, and four diets containing the same amounts of phosphorus (~1500 mg), but from different sources, such as meat, cheese, whole grains, or phosphate supplements. Each diet was consumed for one day, during which time serum levels of phosphate and 24-hour urinary phosphate excretion were measured. Based on serum phosphorus and urinary phosphate excretion, phosphorus contained in meat, cheese and supplements appeared to absorb better than phosphorus from whole grains, suggesting lower intestinal absorption of phosphorus with the grain-based diet. Moe et al. conducted a crossover trial in nine patients with CKD stage 3 or 4 (estimated GFR 25 to 40 mL/min) and normal serum phosphorus to directly compare a grain/soy (vegetarian)-based protein diet to a meat/dairy (meat)-based protein diet with equivalent nutrients. The study demonstrated that 7 days of the vegetarian diet resulted in lower serum phosphorus levels, decreased FGF-23 levels and a trend toward decreased 24-hour urinary phosphorus excretion [147].

In conclusion, renal patients should be educated on how to substitute protein sources with high phosphorus bioavailability, such as enhanced meats, processed cheese, or fast food, with sources that have low bioavailability, such as whole-grain and unprocessed foods [148,149].

While changing the therapeutic approach towards decreasing the amount of foods that are high in phosphorus additives and those with high phosphorus to protein ratio seems to help control the phosphorus, more human studies are needed to support the efficacy of these approaches.

PHOSPHORUS REMOVAL WITH DIALYSIS

Phosphate is unevenly distributed throughout the body, being predominantly localized in the intracellular space. Hence majority of the phosphate removed during dialysis is derived from the intracellular space. The kinetics of phosphate removal differ significantly from classic urea kinetics. During the first phase of dialysis, there is a rapid decline in phosphate level due to phosphate removal from the extracellular space, followed by a second phase, during which phosphate removal continues at a lower rate, but plasma phosphate level does not further decline, as a consequence of active phosphate mobilization from a pool other than the extracellular fluid. The rate of change in plasma phosphate levels is most likely determined by the rate of phosphate transfer from one or more intracellular compartments to plasma compartment. A large rebound of phosphate occurs within a couple of hours after termination of dialysis, reaching about 80% of predialysis values [150–152].

Phosphate removal varies among the different modalities of dialysis. With conventional, thrice-weekly hemodialysis (4 hours), phosphate removal ranges from 600 to 900 mg per treatment (1800 to 2700 mg per week). Conventional hemodiafiltration improves phosphate removal (1170 mg per treatment), but overall, conventional, intermittent hemodialysis is largely inadequate for elimination of the total amount of phosphate absorbed in one week (4000 to 5000 mg) from a standard protein intake [153,154]. In short daily hemodialysis, the amount of phosphate removal depends on session length and frequency of sessions. A study by Ayus et al. compared 51 patients treated with conventional hemodialysis (three sessions/week of 4 hours each) with 26 patients treated with short daily hemodialysis (6 sessions/week of 3 hours each). There was a significant decrease in serum phosphate levels in patients on short daily hemodialysis from baseline of 6.26 ± 2.57 to 4.58 ± 1.06 at 6 months ($P < 0.0001$) and 4.20 ± 1.16 at 12 months ($P < 0.0001$), compared with conventional hemodialysis, where baseline phosphate levels were 4.98 ± 1.49 and increased to 5.02 ± 1.14 at 12 months. 70% of patients in the short hemodialysis group were taken off phosphate binders at the end of the study period. They also found that phosphate level was independently associated with a reduction in left ventricular mass index, likely through increases in vascular compliance [155]. Phosphate is effectively removed with nocturnal hemodialysis. Mucsi et al. compared eight patients on conventional hemodialysis (three sessions/week of 4 hours each) with eight patients on nocturnal hemodialysis (six sessions/week of 8 hours each) The weekly phosphate removal was more than twice with nocturnal hemodialysis as compared to conventional hemodialysis, with significantly lower average serum phosphate level in the nocturnal hemodialysis group (4 mg/dL vs. 6.5 mg/dL) [156]. A more recent, randomized trial involved 52 patients who were assigned to receive nocturnal hemodialysis 6 times weekly or conventional hemodialysis three times weekly. In the nocturnal hemodialysis group, the average predialysis serum phosphate levels were reduced from 5.5 ± 1.5 to 4.4 ± 1.7 mg/dL, and phosphate binders were reduced or discontinued in 73% of the patients [157]. In-center three times weekly nocturnal hemodialysis has been shown to improve phosphate management. Bugeja et al. reported their results in 39 patients who were switched from three times weekly conventional hemodialysis to three times weekly in-center nocturnal hemodialysis. After conversion to in-center nocturnal hemodialysis, median phosphate levels decreased from 5.9 to 3.7 mg/dL, and the mean daily dosage of phosphate binders declined from 6.2 to 4.9 pills/day at study end [158].

Many peritoneal and intrinsic factors influence phosphate transport and clearance during peritoneal dialysis. Weekly average phosphate removal in patients on CAPD has been reported to be around 70 mmol (2170 mg) with 4×2 L exchanges per day and 105 mmol (3250 mg) with 4×3 L exchanges per day [159]. Peritoneal phosphate clearance is lower than clearance of small water-soluble substances. One study by Bammens et al. reported that phosphate clearance was about 20% lower than creatinine clearance and approximately 50% lower than urea clearance. Some studies have shown that peritoneal phosphate clearance correlates better with creatinine clearance than with urea removal [160,161]. In a retrospective study which involved 129 peritoneal dialysis patients, there was a strong correlation between peritoneal phosphate and creatinine clearance. In the multivariate regression analysis, peritoneal phosphate clearance was independently associated with peritoneal creatinine clearance and not with Kt/V urea, indicating that peritoneal creatinine clearance can be used as a surrogate marker for peritoneal phosphate clearance [160].

Peritoneal phosphate clearance is influenced by different peritoneal dialysis modalities and across different peritoneal membrane transport characteristics. For patients in the high transport category, no difference in phosphate clearance is observed between CAPD and CCPD. For patients in the high average, low average and low transport category, peritoneal phosphate clearance is higher with CAPD than with CCPD, while creatinine clearance does not differ. These results suggest that in high average, low average and low transporters, peritoneal phosphate clearance may be increased by increasing cycler dwell times, and by increasing number of exchange for high transporter patients. All patients may benefit from increased convective peritoneal phosphate clearance through higher ultrafiltration rates. However, there are no available studies on the effect of increased ultrafiltration rates on peritoneal phosphate clearance [160,162].

In conclusion, weekly phosphate removal with different dialysis modalities is inadequate in relation to the weekly dietary phosphate intake, and additional therapy may be required. Many CKD patients and majority of dialysis patients require administration of oral phosphate binders to control serum phosphate levels.

PHOSPHATE BINDERS

Aluminum Salts

Aluminum hydroxide, an effective phosphate binder, was the binder of choice for many years, but due to the gradual tissue accumulation of absorbed aluminum, long-term use of this binder was found to be associated with cognitive disturbances, osteomalacia, refractory, microcytic anemia and myopathy. There is no evidence to suggest that even low levels of exposure to aluminum is safe for chronic use [163–166].

Calcium-Based Binders

Calcium acetate and calcium carbonate are inexpensive and effective in controlling hyperphosphatemia. Calcium carbonate has poor solubility in a nonacid environment, which is required for optimal calcium-phosphate interaction, and many patients with severe renal failure have achlorhydria or are taking H_2-blockers. Calcium acetate, on the other hand, is more soluble at a higher pH. Several studies have found calcium acetate to be more effective in binding intestinal phosphate per mmol of administered elemental calcium than calcium carbonate. The clinical significance of this effect is unclear, with few studies reporting equivalent rates of hypercalcemia [167–169]. Hypercalcemia is most likely to occur when these binders are used in combination with a vitamin D analogue. Long-term use of calcium-based phosphate binders may contribute to soft tissue and vascular calcification. They can also result in oversuppression of parathyroid hormone and the development of adynamic bone disease [108,170,171].

Sevelamer

Sevelamer hydrochloride (Renagel) and sevelamer carbonate (Renvela) are nonaluminum, noncalcium phosphate-binding polymers that bind phosphate through ion exchange. Since sevelamer carbonate does not decrease serum bicarbonate levels, it may be more appropriate for patients at risk for metabolic acidosis, although it has been less studied. The two agents appear to be equivalent in their ability to control phosphate levels. This was demonstrated in a double-blind, randomized study of 79 hemodialysis patients, who were randomly assigned to either sevelamer carbonate or sevelamer hydrochloride for 8 weeks, followed by a crossover to the other regimen for an additional 8 weeks of treatment. Sevelamer carbonate and seve-lamer hydrochloride were equivalent in controlling serum phosphorus, while serum bicarbonate levels increased with sevelamer carbonate [172,173]. Many clinical studies have shown that sevelamer is effective in lowering serum phosphate level and is generally well tolerated. Furthermore, sevelamer binds bile acids and decreases fecal bile acid excretion and lowers LDL cholesterol [174−177].

Several randomized clinical trials that compared sevelamer and calcium salts demonstrated similar phos-phate-lowering abilities [120,178,179]. In the prospective Treat-to-goal (TTG) trial, 200 hemodialysis patients were assigned to receive sevelamer or a calcium-based phos-phate binder. At one year, sevelamer and calcium-based binders provided equivalent control of serum phosphate levels (5.1 ± 1.2 vs. 5.1 ± 1.4 mg/dL, respectively), but serum calcium concentration was significantly higher in the calcium-treated group (P = 0.002). The use of sev-elamer was also associated with a lower incidence of hypercalcemia (15% vs. 16%) and a decreased incidence of low PTH levels (30% vs. 57%) [179]. Other randomized clinical studies conducted to compare sevelamer to calcium-based binders showed beneficial effects of seve-lamer on biochemical parameters, including C-reactive protein (CRP), LDL cholesterol, uric acid, fetuin-A, and FGF-23. The favorable outcome of these potential treat-ment benefits with sevelamer has yet to be determined [53,180−182].

The results of the studies on progression of vascular calcification with sevelamer vs. calcium-based phos-phate binders have been contradictory. In the Treat-to-goal (TTG) trial, the median percentage change in coronary artery calcium (CAC) score from baseline was significantly greater with calcium-based binders than with sevelamer at both 26 weeks (14% vs. 0%, P = 0.002) and 52 weeks (25% vs. 6%, P = 0.04) [121].

The Renagel in New Dialysis (RIND) was a prospective, randomized study that compared the effect of sevelamer and calcium-based binders on the progression of vascular calcification in 129 incident hemodialysis patients. Subjects treated with calcium-based phosphate binders showed more rapid and more severe increases in CAC score when compared with those receiving sev-elamer hydrochloride (P = 0.056 at 12 months, P = 0.01 at 18 months) [120]. By comparison, the Calcium Acetate Renagel Evaluation 2 (CARE-2) trial was a noninferiority trial designed to compare the effects of sevelamer and calcium-based phosphate binder on progression of coro-nary artery calcification. After 12 months of therapy, no significant difference was observed in progression of the coronary artery calcification between these two groups. The study was limited by its short duration, substantial drop-out rates, and the inclusion of a higher proportion of diabetic patients. The same effects of treatment on coronary artery calcification were also found in the Phosphate Binder Impact on Bone Remodeling and Coronary Calcification (BRiC) study, who assigned 101 hemodialysis patients to sevelamer or calcium acetate. Due to the inconsistencies among these study results, larger studies will need to determine the effect of sevelamer on vascular calcification [182−184].

A few studies have evaluated the mortality with sevelamer vs. calcium-based phosphate binders. In a post-hoc analysis of the RIND study, mortality rate at a median follow-up of 44 months was higher in calcium-treated patients (10.6/100 patient years, 95% CI 6.3−14.9) than sevelamer-treated patients (5.3/100 patient years, 95% CI 2.2−8.5; P = 0.05). With multivar-iate analysis, there was a greater risk of death for patients treated with calcium-based phosphate binders (hazard ratio 3.1, CI 1.23−7.61; P = 0.016) [115]. A meta-analysis of the results of five randomized trials consisting of 2429 patients, showed a similar risk differ-ence for all cause mortality between sevelamer hydro-chloride and calcium-based agents (risk difference, −2%; 95% CI, −6 to 2) [185]. The Dialysis Clinical Outcomes Revisited (DCOR) study enrolled 2103 hemo-dialysis patients who were assigned to treatment with either sevelamer hydrochloride or calcium (70% to calcium acetate and 30% to calcium carbonate). The primary analysis showed no significant difference in mortality between the two groups (hazard ratio with sevelamer, 0.93; 95% CI, 0.79 to 1.10), although secondary analyses reported all-cause hospitalization rates and hospital days being lower in the sevelamer group. In conclusion, there are no clear data to suggest the benefits of using sevelamer to improve clinically relevant end points when compared with other calcium-based binders [186,187].

Lanthanum is a rare earth element. Lanthanum carbonate is another phosphate binder able to bind phosphate across a wide pH range. Short-term trials have assessed the efficacy of lanthanum carbonate in lowering serum phosphate levels, improvements in iPTH, and potentially decreasing FGF-23 levels [188–191]. At present, no studies have assessed the effect of lanthanum on vascular calcification or mortality. Clinical studies that compared lanthanum with other phosphate binders evaluated mainly the effect on biochemical parameters and on bone histology. Lanthanum and calcium-based phosphate binders appear to be similarly effective in reducing serum phosphate concentrations in patients with end-stage renal disease. In the largest trial, the proportion of patients who had documented episodes of hypercalcemia was significantly smaller among the patients receiving lanthanum (4.3%) than among those receiving standard care, in majority of cases, calcium-based phosphate binders (8.4%) [192,193]. Few small trials have compared the effects of lanthanum and calcium carbonate on bone histology. In general, there were no adverse effects with lanthanum. More of the patients who received calcium were found to have histologic features of a dynamic bone disease [193,194]. However, the long-term safety of lanthanum and its effects on the bone and other organs, remain uncertain.

In conclusion, given the importance of hyperphosphatemia in the high morbidity and mortality of patients with chronic kidney disease, combined therapeutic measures to restore phosphate balance include dietary phosphate restriction, modification of dialysis prescription, and administration of phosphate binders.

THERAPY WITH VITAMIN D STEROLS

Because decrease in calcitriol production plays an important role in developing and maintaining secondary hyperparathyroidism, the use of vitamin D sterols represent an important part of the treatment of hyperparathyroidism in patients with chronic kidney disease. The use of vitamin D sterols suppresses the secretion of PTH, increase the absorption of both calcium and phosphorus from the gut and appears to be associated with a survival advantage in hemodialysis and CKD patients [195–197]. There are six active vitamin D derivatives currently available: calcitriol, alfacalcidol, doxercalciferol, 22-oxacalcitriol, falecalcitriol and paricalcitol. In the United States the available agents include calcitriol, paricalcitol and doxercalciferol.

Calcitriol is the natural form of active vitamin D produced by the human body, and was the first agent used for treatment of hyperparathyroidism. Early studies with calcitriol in experimental animals as well as clinical studies suggested that intermittent intravenous form of calcitriol was more effective and better tolerated than oral calcitriol, thought to be due to greater delivery of the vitamin D metabolite to peripheral target tissues other than the intestine [198]. Subsequent studies have shown that both intermittent oral and intravenous bolus therapy were equally effective with regard to PTH suppression and side effects [199].

The vitamin D analog, paricalcitol, was introduced and developed to try to obtain a more selective action on the parathyroid gland, while minimizing the effects of vitamin D sterols to cause hypercalcemia and hyperphosphatemia. In experimental animals, paricalcitol was effective in suppressing PTH with less hypercalcemia and hyperphosphatemia found than calcitriol [200]. However, direct head to head randomized studies in patients are limited. A double-blind, randomized, multi-center study compared the safety and effectiveness of intravenous paricalcitol and calcitriol in suppressing PTH concentrations among 263 hemodialysis patients. The primary end point was the greater than 50% reduction in baseline PTH, and the secondary end points were the occurrence of hypercalcemia and elevated Ca × P product. Paricalcitol treatment reduced PTH concentrations more rapidly with fewer sustained episodes of hypercalcemia and increased Ca × P product than calcitriol therapy [201].

Doxercalciferol, a prohormone that can be hepatically activated into a VDR agonist, appeared to have the potential for lesser toxicity and has proven its efficacy by reducing PTH levels. Studies with oral and intravenous formulations of doxercalciferol showed that both preparations are well tolerated and able to lower plasma PTH, with less frequent hypercalcemia seen with intravenous treatment [202]. There have been no comparative studies of doxercalciferol with other VDR agonists.

CALCIMIMETICS

Calcimimetics, such as cinacalcet, are positive allosteric modulators of the CaSR, which bind reversibly to the membrane-spanning portion of the CaSR and lower the threshold for receptor activation by extracellular calcium, leading to a decrease in circulating PTH levels [203]. Several prospective randomized studies done in dialysis patients with uncontrolled hyperparathyroidism have found that the use of the calcimimetics produces a dose-dependent reduction in the plasma PTH concentration and a decrease in the serum calcium and phosphate levels [204–207].

One of the most common side effects seen with calcimimetics is hypocalcemia, thought to occur after decreased mobilization of calcium from bone caused by reduced PTH levels. This can be managed by adjustments in calcium-based phosphate binders, reductions in cinacalcet dose, or using a combination with low doses of vitamin D sterols in patients with moderate to severe hyperparathyroidism [208].

The ADVANCE trial was a prospective, randomized, controlled trial designed to evaluate the effects of cinacalcet plus low-dose vitamin D on vascular and cardiac valve calcification in 360 prevalent adult hemodialysis patients. The results of the study showed that coronary artery calcifications and valvular calcifications were significantly lower in the cinacalcet plus low-dose vitamin D group than the vitamin D sterol alone group [209].

If medical therapy cannot achieve sustained control of hyperparathyroidism, consideration should be given to parathyroidectomy. This is usually reserved for patients with severe hyperparathyroidism in whom medical therapy cannot be tolerated.

CONCLUSION

Disorders of bone and mineral metabolism are common in chronic kidney disease. The abnormalities begin early in the course of declining renal function and progress steadily. A knowledge of the pathophysiology has led to important therapeutic strategies which can be applied to correct the abnormalities. Studies continue to demonstrate that these therapies will result in improved patient outcomes.

References

[1] van de Graaf SF, Hoenderop JG, Bindels RJ. Regulation of TRPV5 and TRPV6 by associated proteins. Am J Physiol Renal Physiol 2006;290(6):F1295−302.

[2] van Abel M, et al. Coordinated control of renal Ca(2+) transport proteins by parathyroid hormone. Kidney Int 2005;68(4):1708−21.

[3] Hoenderop JG, et al. Renal Ca^{2+} wasting, hyperabsorption, and reduced bone thickness in mice lacking TRPV5. J Clin Invest 2003;112(12):1906−14.

[4] Hoenderop JG, et al. Modulation of renal Ca^{2+} transport protein genes by dietary Ca^{2+} and 1,25-dihydroxyvitamin D3 in 25-hydroxyvitamin D3-1alpha-hydroxylase knockout mice. FASEB J 2002;16(11):1398−406.

[5] Van Abel M, et al. 1,25-dihydroxyvitamin D(3)-independent stimulatory effect of estrogen on the expression of ECaC1 in the kidney. J Am Soc Nephrol 2002;13(8):2102−9.

[6] Omdahl JL, Morris HA, May BK. Hydroxylase enzymes of the vitamin D pathway: expression, function, and regulation. Annu Rev Nutr 2002;22:139−66.

[7] Lowe KE, Maiyar AC, Norman AW. Vitamin D-mediated gene expression. Crit Rev Eukaryot Gene Expr 1992;2(1):65−109.

[8] Ozono K, Sone T, Pike JW. The genomic mechanism of action of 1,25-dihydroxyvitamin D3. J Bone Miner Res 1991;6(10):1021−7.

[9] Moe S. Disorders of phosphate metabolism in CKD. In: Hsu C, editor. Calcium and Phosphate Management in Chronic Kidney Disease. Springer; 2010. p. 13−28.

[10] Uribarri J. Phosphorus homeostasis in normal health and in chronic kidney disease patients with special emphasis on dietary phosphorus intake. Semin Dial 2007;20(4):295−301.

[11] Moe SM, Sprague SM. Chronic Kidney Disease-Mineral Bone Disorder. In: The Kidney. Elsevier Saunders; 2011:2021−49.

[12] Craver L, et al. Mineral metabolism parameters throughout chronic kidney disease stages 1-5 − achievement of K/DOQI target ranges. Nephrol Dial Transplant 2007;22(4):1171−6.

[13] Harrison HE, Harrison HC. Intestinal transport of phosphate: action of vitamin D, calcium, and potassium. Am J Physiol 1961;201:1007−12.

[14] Hilfiker H, et al. Characterization of a murine type II sodium-phosphate cotransporter expressed in mammalian small intestine. Proc Natl Acad Sci U S A 1998;95(24):14564−9.

[15] Marks J, Debnam ES, Unwin RJ. Phosphate homeostasis and the renal-gastrointestinal axis. Am J Physiol Renal Physiol 2010;299(2):F285−96.

[16] Sabbagh Y, et al. Intestinal npt2b plays a major role in phosphate absorption and homeostasis. J Am Soc Nephrol 2009;20(11):2348−58.

[17] Capuano P, et al. Intestinal and renal adaptation to a low-Pi diet of type II NaPi cotransporters in vitamin D receptor- and 1alphaOHase-deficient mice. Am J Physiol Cell Physiol 2005;288(2):C429−34.

[18] Katai K, et al. Regulation of intestinal Na+-dependent phosphate co-transporters by a low-phosphate diet and 1,25-dihydroxyvitamin D3. Biochem J 1999;343(Pt 3):705−12.

[19] Borowitz SM, Granrud GS. Glucocorticoids inhibit intestinal phosphate absorption in developing rabbits. J Nutr 1992;122(6):1273−9.

[20] Marks J, et al. Matrix extracellular phosphoglycoprotein inhibits phosphate transport. J Am Soc Nephrol 2008;19(12):2313−20.

[21] Miyamoto K, et al. Inhibition of intestinal sodium-dependent inorganic phosphate transport by fibroblast growth factor 23. Ther Apher Dial 2005;9(4):331−5.

[22] Stauber A, et al. Regulation of intestinal phosphate transport. II. Metabolic acidosis stimulates Na(+)-dependent phosphate absorption and expression of the Na(+)-P(i) cotransporter NaPi-IIb in small intestine. Am J Physiol Gastrointest Liver Physiol 2005;288(3):G501−6.

[23] Xu H, et al. Regulation of the human sodium-phosphate cotransporter NaP(i)-IIb gene promoter by epidermal growth factor. Am J Physiol Cell Physiol 2001;280(3):C628−36.

[24] Xu H, et al. Regulation of intestinal NaPi-IIb cotransporter gene expression by estrogen. Am J Physiol Gastrointest Liver Physiol 2003;285(6):G1317−24.

[25] Beck L, et al. Targeted inactivation of Npt2 in mice leads to severe renal phosphate wasting, hypercalciuria, and skeletal abnormalities. Proc Natl Acad Sci U S A 1998;95(9):5372−7.

[26] Segawa H, et al. Npt2a and Npt2c in mice play distinct and synergistic roles in inorganic phosphate metabolism and skeletal development. Am J Physiol Renal Physiol 2009;297(3):F671−8.

[27] Tenenhouse HS, et al. Differential effects of Npt2a gene ablation and X-linked Hyp mutation on renal expression of Npt2c. Am J Physiol Renal Physiol 2003;285(6):F1271−8.

[28] Villa-Bellosta R, et al. The Na+-Pi cotransporter PiT-2 (SLC20A2) is expressed in the apical membrane of rat renal proximal tubules and regulated by dietary Pi. Am J Physiol Renal Physiol 2009;296(4):F691−9.

[29] Bianda T, et al. Effects of short-term insulin-like growth factor-I or growth hormone treatment on bone turnover, renal phosphate reabsorption and 1,25 dihydroxyvitamin D3 production in healthy man. J Intern Med 1997;241(2):143−50.

[30] Ishiguro M, et al. Thyroid hormones regulate phosphate homoeostasis through transcriptional control of the renal type IIa sodium-dependent phosphate co-transporter (Npt2a) gene. Biochem J 2010;427(1):161—9.

[31] Kurnik BR, Hruska KA. Mechanism of stimulation of renal phosphate transport by 1,25-dihydroxycholecalciferol. Biochim Biophys Acta 1985;817(1):42—50.

[32] Ambuhl PM, et al. Regulation of renal phosphate transport by acute and chronic metabolic acidosis in the rat. Kidney Int 1998;53(5):1288—98.

[33] Blaine J, Weinman EJ, Cunningham R. The regulation of renal phosphate transport. Adv Chronic Kidney Dis 2011;18(2): 77—84.

[34] Laron Z, Crawford JD, Klein R. Phosphaturic effect of cortisone in normal and parathyroidectomized rats. Proc Soc Exp Biol Med 1957;96(3):649—51.

[35] Pfister MF, et al. Parathyroid hormone leads to the lysosomal degradation of the renal type II Na/Pi cotransporter. Proc Natl Acad Sci U S A 1998;95(4):1909—14.

[36] Prie D, Urena Torres P, Friedlander G. Latest findings in phosphate homeostasis. Kidney Int 2009;75(9):882—9.

[37] Berndt T, et al. Secreted frizzled-related protein 4 is a potent tumor-derived phosphaturic agent. J Clin Invest 2003;112(5): 785—94.

[38] Cai Q, et al. Brief report: inhibition of renal phosphate transport by a tumor product in a patient with oncogenic osteomalacia. N Engl J Med 1994;330(23):1645—9.

[39] Jonsson KB, et al. Fibroblast growth factor 23 in oncogenic osteomalacia and X-linked hypophosphatemia. N Engl J Med 2003;348(17):1656—63.

[40] Kumar R. Tumor-induced osteomalacia and the regulation of phosphate homeostasis. Bone 2000;27(3):333—8.

[41] Rowe PS, et al. MEPE has the properties of an osteoblastic phosphatonin and minhibin. Bone 2004;34(2):303—19.

[42] Shimada T, et al. Cloning and characterization of FGF23 as a causative factor of tumor-induced osteomalacia. Proc Natl Acad Sci U S A 2001;98(11):6500—5.

[43] White KE, et al. Autosomal dominant hypophosphataemic rickets is associated with mutations in FGF23. Nat Genet 2000;26(3):345—8.

[44] Yamashita T, Yoshioka M, Itoh N. Identification of a novel fibroblast growth factor, FGF-23, preferentially expressed in the ventrolateral thalamic nucleus of the brain. Biochem Biophys Res Commun 2000;277(2):494—8.

[45] Liu S, et al. Regulation of fibroblastic growth factor 23 expression but not degradation by PHEX. J Biol Chem 2003;278(39): 37419—26.

[46] Liu S, et al. Pathogenic role of Fgf23 in Hyp mice. Am J Physiol Endocrinol Metab 2006;291(1):E38—49.

[47] Kuro-o M. Klotho as a regulator of fibroblast growth factor signaling and phosphate/calcium metabolism. Curr Opin Nephrol Hypertens 2006;15(4):437—41.

[48] Shimada T, et al. FGF-23 is a potent regulator of vitamin D metabolism and phosphate homeostasis. J Bone Miner Res 2004;19(3):429—35.

[49] Shimada T, et al. Targeted ablation of Fgf23 demonstrates an essential physiological role of FGF23 in phosphate and vitamin D metabolism. J Clin Invest 2004;113(4):561—8.

[50] Kurosu H, et al. Regulation of fibroblast growth factor-23 signaling by klotho. J Biol Chem 2006;281(10):6120—3.

[51] Urakawa I, et al. Klotho converts canonical FGF receptor into a specific receptor for FGF23. Nature 2006;444(7120):770—4.

[52] Kuro-o M, et al. Mutation of the mouse klotho gene leads to a syndrome resembling ageing. Nature 1997;390(6655): 45—51.

[53] Segawa H, et al. Correlation between hyperphosphatemia and type II Na-Pi cotransporter activity in klotho mice. Am J Physiol Renal Physiol 2007;292(2):F769—79.

[54] Ben-Dov IZ, et al. The parathyroid is a target organ for FGF23 in rats. J Clin Invest 2007;117(12):4003—8.

[55] Krajisnik T, et al. Fibroblast growth factor-23 regulates parathyroid hormone and 1alpha-hydroxylase expression in cultured bovine parathyroid cells. J Endocrinol 2007;195(1): 125—31.

[56] Ferrari SL, Bonjour JP, Rizzoli R. Fibroblast growth factor-23 relationship to dietary phosphate and renal phosphate handling in healthy young men. J Clin Endocrinol Metab 2005;90(3): 1519—24.

[57] Liu S, et al. Fibroblast growth factor 23 is a counter-regulatory phosphaturic hormone for vitamin D. J Am Soc Nephrol 2006;17(5):1305—15.

[58] Nakai K, Komaba H, Fukagawa M. New insights into the role of fibroblast growth factor 23 in chronic kidney disease. J Nephrol 2010;23(6):619—25.

[59] Nishida Y, et al. Acute effect of oral phosphate loading on serum fibroblast growth factor 23 levels in healthy men. Kidney Int 2006;70(12):2141—7.

[60] Perwad F, et al. Dietary and serum phosphorus regulate fibroblast growth factor 23 expression and 1,25-dihydroxyvitamin D metabolism in mice. Endocrinology 2005;146(12):5358—64.

[61] Lorenz-Depiereux B, et al. DMP1 mutations in autosomal recessive hypophosphatemia implicate a bone matrix protein in the regulation of phosphate homeostasis. Nat Genet 2006;38(11): 1248—50.

[62] Collins MT, et al. Fibroblast growth factor-23 is regulated by 1alpha,25-dihydroxyvitamin D. J Bone Miner Res 2005;20(11): 1944—50.

[63] Hines ER, et al. 1,25-dihydroxyvitamin D3 down-regulation of PHEX gene expression is mediated by apparent repression of a 110 kDa transfactor that binds to a polyadenine element in the promoter. J Biol Chem 2004;279(45):46406—14.

[64] Liu S, Quarles LD. How fibroblast growth factor 23 works. J Am Soc Nephrol 2007;18(6):1637—47.

[65] Ramon I, et al. Fibroblast growth factor 23 and its role in phosphate homeostasis. Eur J Endocrinol 2010;162(1):1—10.

[66] Saito H, et al. Circulating FGF-23 is regulated by 1alpha,25-dihydroxyvitamin D3 and phosphorus in vivo. J Biol Chem 2005;280(4):2543—9.

[67] Levin A, et al. Prevalence of abnormal serum vitamin D, PTH, calcium, and phosphorus in patients with chronic kidney disease: results of the study to evaluate early kidney disease. Kidney Int 2007;71(1):31—8.

[68] Hruska KA, et al. Hyperphosphatemia of chronic kidney disease. Kidney Int 2008;74(2):148—57.

[69] Komaba H, et al. Depressed expression of Klotho and FGF receptor 1 in hyperplastic parathyroid glands from uremic patients. Kidney Int 2010;77(3):232—8.

[70] Martin KJ, Gonzalez EA. Prevention and control of phosphate retention/hyperphosphatemia in CKD-MBD: what is normal, when to start, and how to treat? Clin J Am Soc Nephrol 2011;6(2):440—6.

[71] Silver J, Naveh-Many T. Phosphate and the parathyroid. Kidney Int 2009;75(9):898—905.

[72] Tsujikawa H, et al. Klotho, a gene related to a syndrome resembling human premature aging, functions in a negative regulatory circuit of vitamin D endocrine system. Mol Endocrinol 2003;17(12):2393—403.

[73] Almaden Y, et al. Direct effect of phosphorus on PTH secretion from whole rat parathyroid glands in vitro. J Bone Miner Res 1996;11(7):970—6.

[74] Nielsen PK, Feldt-Rasmussen U, Olgaard K. A direct effect in vitro of phosphate on PTH release from bovine parathyroid tissue slices but not from dispersed parathyroid cells. Nephrol Dial Transplant 1996;11(9):1762—8.

[75] Slatopolsky E, et al. Phosphorus restriction prevents parathyroid gland growth. High phosphorus directly stimulates PTH secretion in vitro. J Clin Invest 1996;97(11):2534—40.

[76] Almaden Y, et al. Effect of high extracellular phosphate concentration on arachidonic acid production by parathyroid tissue in vitro. J Am Soc Nephrol 2000;11(9):1712—8.

[77] Ritter CS, et al. Reversal of secondary hyperparathyroidism by phosphate restriction restores parathyroid calcium-sensing receptor expression and function. J Bone Miner Res 2002;17(12):2206—13.

[78] Cozzolino M, et al. A critical role for enhanced TGF-alpha and EGFR expression in the initiation of parathyroid hyperplasia in experimental kidney disease. Am J Physiol Renal Physiol 2005;289(5):F1096—102.

[79] Silver J, et al. Regulation of the parathyroid hormone gene by vitamin D, calcium and phosphate. Kidney Int Suppl 1999;73:S2—7.

[80] Yalcindag C, Silver J, Naveh-Many T. Mechanism of increased parathyroid hormone mRNA in experimental uremia: roles of protein RNA binding and RNA degradation. J Am Soc Nephrol 1999;10(12):2562—8.

[81] Dhingra R, et al. Relations of serum phosphorus and calcium levels to the incidence of cardiovascular disease in the community. Arch Intern Med 2007;167(9):879—85.

[82] Tonelli M, et al. Relation between serum phosphate level and cardiovascular event rate in people with coronary disease. Circulation 2005;112(17):2627—33.

[83] Kestenbaum B, et al. Serum phosphate levels and mortality risk among people with chronic kidney disease. J Am Soc Nephrol 2005;16(2):520—8.

[84] Eddington H, et al. Serum phosphate and mortality in patients with chronic kidney disease. Clin J Am Soc Nephrol 2010;5(12):2251—7.

[85] Block GA, et al. Association of serum phosphorus and calcium x phosphate product with mortality risk in chronic hemodialysis patients: a national study. Am J Kidney Dis 1998;31(4):607—17.

[86] Block GA, et al. Mineral metabolism, mortality, and morbidity in maintenance hemodialysis. J Am Soc Nephrol 2004;15(8):2208—18.

[87] Slinin Y, Foley RN, Collins AJ. Calcium, phosphorus, parathyroid hormone, and cardiovascular disease in hemodialysis patients: the USRDS waves 1, 3, and 4 study. J Am Soc Nephrol 2005;16(6):1788—93.

[88] Noordzij M, et al. The Kidney Disease Outcomes Quality Initiative (K/DOQI) Guideline for Bone Metabolism and Disease in CKD: association with mortality in dialysis patients. Am J Kidney Dis 2005;46(5):925—32.

[89] Kalantar-Zadeh K, et al. Survival predictability of time-varying indicators of bone disease in maintenance hemodialysis patients. Kidney Int 2006;70(4):771—80.

[90] Tentori F, et al. Mortality risk for dialysis patients with different levels of serum calcium, phosphorus, and PTH: the Dialysis Outcomes and Practice Patterns Study (DOPPS). Am J Kidney Dis 2008;52(3):519—30.

[91] Strozecki P, et al. Parathormon, calcium, phosphorus, and left ventricular structure and function in normotensive hemodialysis patients. Ren Fail 2001;23(1):115—26.

[92] Voormolen N, et al. High plasma phosphate as a risk factor for decline in renal function and mortality in pre-dialysis patients. Nephrol Dial Transplant 2007;22(10):2909—16.

[93] Gutierrez OM, et al. Fibroblast growth factor 23 and mortality among patients undergoing hemodialysis. N Engl J Med 2008;359(6):584—92.

[94] Jean G, et al. High levels of serum fibroblast growth factor (FGF)-23 are associated with increased mortality in long haemodialysis patients. Nephrol Dial Transplant 2009;24(9):2792—6.

[95] Kirkpantur A, et al. Serum fibroblast growth factor-23 (FGF-23) levels are independently associated with left ventricular mass and myocardial performance index in maintenance haemodialysis patients. Nephrol Dial Transplant 2011;26(4):1346—54.

[96] Mirza MA, et al. Circulating fibroblast growth factor-23 is associated with vascular dysfunction in the community. Atherosclerosis 2009;205(2):385—90.

[97] Yilmaz MI, et al. FGF-23 and vascular dysfunction in patients with stage 3 and 4 chronic kidney disease. Kidney Int 2010;78(7):679—85.

[98] Li YC, et al. 1,25-Dihydroxyvitamin D(3) is a negative endocrine regulator of the renin-angiotensin system. J Clin Invest 2002;110(2):229—38.

[99] O'Connell TD, et al. 1,25-Dihydroxyvitamin D3 regulation of cardiac myocyte proliferation and hypertrophy. Am J Physiol 1997;272(4 Pt 2):H1751—8.

[100] London GM, et al. Arterial media calcification in end-stage renal disease: impact on all-cause and cardiovascular mortality. Nephrol Dial Transplant 2003;18(9):1731—40.

[101] Goodman WG, et al. Vascular calcification in chronic kidney disease. Am J Kidney Dis 2004;43(3):572—9.

[102] Vanholder R, et al. Chronic kidney disease as cause of cardiovascular morbidity and mortality. Nephrol Dial Transplant 2005;20(6):1048—56.

[103] Nishioka T, et al. Clinical validation of intravascular ultrasound imaging for assessment of coronary stenosis severity: comparison with stress myocardial perfusion imaging. J Am Coll Cardiol 1999;33(7):1870—8.

[104] Porter TR, et al. Intravascular ultrasound study of angiographically mildly diseased coronary arteries. J Am Coll Cardiol 1993;22(7):1858—65.

[105] Braun J, et al. Electron beam computed tomography in the evaluation of cardiac calcification in chronic dialysis patients. Am J Kidney Dis 1996;27(3):394—401.

[106] Bellasi A, et al. Correlation of simple imaging tests and coronary artery calcium measured by computed tomography in hemodialysis patients. Kidney Int 2006;70(9):1623—8.

[107] Group, KDIGOKCMW, KDIGO. clinical practice guideline for the diagnosis, evaluation, prevention, and treatment of chronic kidney disease—mineral and bone disorder (CKD—MBD). Kidney Int Suppl 2009;(Suppl. 113):S1—S130.

[108] Goodman WG, et al. Coronary-artery calcification in young adults with end-stage renal disease who are undergoing dialysis. N Engl J Med 2000;342(20):1478—83.

[109] Schwarz U, et al. Morphology of coronary atherosclerotic lesions in patients with end-stage renal failure. Nephrol Dial Transplant 2000;15(2):218—23.

[110] Goldsmith DJ, et al. Vascular calcification in long-term haemodialysis patients in a single unit: a retrospective analysis. Nephron 1997;77(1):37—43.

[111] Meema HE, Oreopoulos DG, deVeber GA. Arterial calcifications in severe chronic renal disease and their relationship to dialysis treatment, renal transplant, and parathyroidectomy. Radiology 1976;121(2):315—21.

[112] Raggi P, et al. Cardiac calcification in adult hemodialysis patients. A link between end-stage renal disease and cardiovascular disease? J Am Coll Cardiol 2002;39(4):695—701.

[113] Kramer H, et al. Association between chronic kidney disease and coronary artery calcification: the Dallas Heart Study. J Am Soc Nephrol 2005;16(2):507–13.

[114] Blacher J, et al. Arterial calcifications, arterial stiffness, and cardiovascular risk in end-stage renal disease. Hypertension 2001;38(4):938–42.

[115] Block GA, et al. Mortality effect of coronary calcification and phosphate binder choice in incident hemodialysis patients. Kidney Int 2007;71(5):438–41.

[116] Adeney KL, et al. Association of serum phosphate with vascular and valvular calcification in moderate CKD. J Am Soc Nephrol 2009;20(2):381–7.

[117] Foley RN, et al. Serum phosphorus levels associate with coronary atherosclerosis in young adults. J Am Soc Nephrol 2009;20(2):397–404.

[118] Kendrick J, et al. Relation of serum phosphorus levels to ankle brachial pressure index (from the Third National Health and Nutrition Examination Survey). Am J Cardiol 2010;106(4):564–8.

[119] Kendrick J, Kestenbaum B, Chonchol M. Phosphate and cardiovascular disease. Adv Chronic Kidney Dis 2011;18(2):113–9.

[120] Block GA, et al. Effects of sevelamer and calcium on coronary artery calcification in patients new to hemodialysis. Kidney Int 2005;68(4):1815–24.

[121] Chertow GM, Burke SK, Raggi P. Sevelamer attenuates the progression of coronary and aortic calcification in hemodialysis patients. Kidney Int 2002;62(1):245–52.

[122] Cozzolino M, et al. The effects of sevelamer hydrochloride and calcium carbonate on kidney calcification in uremic rats. J Am Soc Nephrol 2002;13(9):2299–308.

[123] Giachelli CM. The emerging role of phosphate in vascular calcification. Kidney Int 2009;75(9):890–7.

[124] Li X, Yang HY, Giachelli CM. Role of the sodium-dependent phosphate cotransporter, Pit-1, in vascular smooth muscle cell calcification. Circ Res 2006;98(7):905–12.

[125] Sugita A, et al. Cellular ATP synthesis mediated by type III sodium-dependent phosphate transporter Pit-1 is critical to chondrogenesis. J Biol Chem 2011;286(4):3094–103.

[126] Rutherford WE, et al. Phosphate control and 25-hydroxycholecalciferol administration in preventing experimental renal osteodystrophy in the dog. J Clin Invest 1977;60(2):332–41.

[127] Young EW, et al. Magnitude and impact of abnormal mineral metabolism in hemodialysis patients in the Dialysis Outcomes and Practice Patterns Study (DOPPS). Am J Kidney Dis 2004;44(5 Suppl. 2):34–8.

[128] Ramirez JA, et al. The absorption of dietary phosphorus and calcium in hemodialysis patients. Kidney Int 1986;30(5):753–9.

[129] Kayne LH, et al. Analysis of segmental phosphate absorption in intact rats. A compartmental analysis approach. J Clin Invest 1993;91(3):915–22.

[130] Sandberg AS, et al. Extrusion cooking of a high-fibre cereal product. 1. Effects on digestibility and absorption of protein, fat, starch, dietary fibre and phytate in the small intestine. Br J Nutr 1986;55(2):245–54.

[131] Kalantar-Zadeh K, et al. Understanding sources of dietary phosphorus in the treatment of patients with chronic kidney disease. Clin J Am Soc Nephrol 2010;5(3):519–30.

[132] Murphy-Gutekunst L. Hidden phosphorus: where do we go from here? Journal of Renal Nutrition: the official journal of the Council on Renal Nutrition of the National Kidney Foundation 2007;17(4):e31–6.

[133] Calvo MS, Park YK. Changing phosphorus content of the U.S. diet: potential for adverse effects on bone. J Nutr 1996;126(Suppl. 4):1168S–80S.

[134] Uribarri J. Phosphorus additives in food and their effect in dialysis patients. Clin J Am Soc Nephrol 2009;4(8):1290–2.

[135] Bell RR, et al. Physiological responses of human adults to foods containing phosphate additives. J Nutr 1977;107(1):42–50.

[136] Uribarri J, Calvo MS. Hidden sources of phosphorus in the typical American diet: does it matter in nephrology? Semin Dial 2003;16(3):186–8.

[137] Murphy-Gutekunst L. Hidden phosphorus in popular beverages. Nephrol Nurs J 2005;32(4):443–5.

[138] Sherman RA, Mehta O. Phosphorus and potassium content of enhanced meat and poultry products: implications for patients who receive dialysis. Clin J Am Soc Nephrol 2009;4(8):1370–3.

[139] Sullivan C, et al. Effect of food additives on hyperphosphatemia among patients with end-stage renal disease: a randomized controlled trial. JAMA 2009;301(6):629–35.

[140] Sullivan CM, Leon JB, Sehgal AR. Phosphorus-containing food additives and the accuracy of nutrient databases: implications for renal patients. J Ren Nutr 2007;17(5):350–4.

[141] Shinaberger CS, et al. Longitudinal associations between dietary protein intake and survival in hemodialysis patients. Am J Kidney Dis 2006;48(1):37–49.

[142] Shinaberger CS, et al. Is controlling phosphorus by decreasing dietary protein intake beneficial or harmful in persons with chronic kidney disease? Am J Clin Nutr 2008;88(6):1511–8.

[143] Noori N, et al. Association of dietary phosphorus intake and phosphorus to protein ratio with mortality in hemodialysis patients. Clin J Am Soc Nephrol 2010;5(4):683–92.

[144] Taylor LM, et al. Dietary egg whites for phosphorus control in maintenance haemodialysis patients: a pilot study. J Ren Care 2011;37(1):16–24.

[145] Sherman RA, Mehta O. Dietary phosphorus restriction in dialysis patients: potential impact of processed meat, poultry, and fish products as protein sources. Am J Kidney Dis 2009;54(1):18–23.

[146] Fouque D, et al. Use of a renal-specific oral supplement by haemodialysis patients with low protein intake does not increase the need for phosphate binders and may prevent a decline in nutritional status and quality of life. Nephrol Dial Transplant 2008;23(9):2902–10.

[147] Moe SM, et al. Vegetarian compared with meat dietary protein source and phosphorus homeostasis in chronic kidney disease. Clin J Am Soc Nephrol 2011;6(2):257–64.

[148] Gutierrez OM, Wolf M. Dietary phosphorus restriction in advanced chronic kidney disease: merits, challenges, and emerging strategies. Semin Dial 2010;23(4):401–6.

[149] Karp HJ, et al. Acute effects of different phosphorus sources on calcium and bone metabolism in young women: a whole-foods approach. Calcif Tissue Int 2007;80(4):251–8.

[150] DeSoi CA, Umans JG. Phosphate kinetics during high-flux hemodialysis. J Am Soc Nephrol 1993;4(5):1214–8.

[151] Kooienga L. Phosphorus balance with daily dialysis. Semin Dial 2007;20(4):342–5.

[152] Spalding EM, Chamney PW, Farrington K. Phosphate kinetics during hemodialysis: Evidence for biphasic regulation. Kidney Int 2002;61(2):655–67.

[153] Hou SH, et al. Calcium and phosphorus fluxes during hemodialysis with low calcium dialysate. Am J Kidney Dis 1991;18(2):217–24.

[154] Minutolo R, et al. Postdialytic rebound of serum phosphorus: pathogenetic and clinical insights. J Am Soc Nephrol 2002;13(4):1046–54.

[155] Ayus JC, et al. Effects of short daily vs. conventional hemodialysis on left ventricular hypertrophy and inflammatory markers: a prospective, controlled study. J Am Soc Nephrol 2005;16(9):2778–88.

[156] Mucsi I, et al. Control of serum phosphate without any phosphate binders in patients treated with nocturnal hemodialysis. Kidney Int 1998;53(5):1399–404.

[157] Culleton BF, et al. Effect of frequent nocturnal hemodialysis vs conventional hemodialysis on left ventricular mass and quality of life: a randomized controlled trial. JAMA 2007;298(11):1291–9.

[158] Bugeja A, et al. In-center nocturnal hemodialysis: another option in the management of chronic kidney disease. Clin J Am Soc Nephrol 2009;4(4):778–83.

[159] Messa P, et al. Behaviour of phosphate removal with different dialysis schedules. Nephrol Dial Transplant 1998;13(Suppl. 6):43–8.

[160] Badve SV, et al. Peritoneal phosphate clearance is influenced by peritoneal dialysis modality, independent of peritoneal transport characteristics. Clin J Am Soc Nephrol 2008;3(6):1711–7.

[161] Sedlacek M, Dimaano F, Uribarri J. Relationship between phosphorus and creatinine clearance in peritoneal dialysis: clinical implications. Am J Kidney Dis 2000;36(5):1020–4.

[162] Kuhlmann MK. Phosphate elimination in modalities of hemodialysis and peritoneal dialysis. Blood Purif 2010;29(2):137–44.

[163] Malluche HH. Aluminium and bone disease in chronic renal failure. Nephrol Dial Transplant 2002;17(Suppl. 2):21–4.

[164] Parkinson IS, et al. Fracturing dialysis osteodystrophy and dialysis encephalopathy. An epidemiological survey. Lancet 1979;1(8113):406–9.

[165] Salusky IB, et al. Aluminum accumulation during treatment with aluminum hydroxide and dialysis in children and young adults with chronic renal disease. N Engl J Med 1991;324(8):527–31.

[166] Wills MR, Savory J. Aluminium poisoning: dialysis encephalopathy, osteomalacia, and anaemia. Lancet 1983;2(8340):29–34.

[167] Emmett M, et al. Calcium acetate control of serum phosphorus in hemodialysis patients. Am J Kidney Dis 1991;17(5):544–50.

[168] Navaneethan SD, et al. Benefits and harms of phosphate binders in CKD: a systematic review of randomized controlled trials. Am J Kidney Dis 2009;54(4):619–37.

[169] Sheikh MS, et al. Reduction of dietary phosphorus absorption by phosphorus binders. A theoretical, in vitro, and in vivo study. J Clin Invest 1989;83(1):66–73.

[170] Kurz P, et al. Evidence for abnormal calcium homeostasis in patients with adynamic bone disease. Kidney Int 1994;46(3):855–61.

[171] Schaefer K, Umlauf E, von Herrath D. Reduced risk of hypercalcemia for hemodialysis patients by administering calcitriol at night. Am J Kidney Dis 1992;19(5):460–4.

[172] Delmez J, et al. A randomized, double-blind, crossover design study of sevelamer hydrochloride and sevelamer carbonate in patients on hemodialysis. Clin Nephrol 2007;68(6):386–91.

[173] Pai AB, Shepler BM. Comparison of sevelamer hydrochloride and sevelamer carbonate: risk of metabolic acidosis and clinical implications. Pharmacotherapy 2009;29(5):554–61.

[174] Chertow GM, et al. Long-term effects of sevelamer hydrochloride on the calcium x phosphate product and lipid profile of haemodialysis patients. Nephrol Dial Transplant 1999;14(12):2907–14.

[175] Chertow GM, et al. Poly[allylamine hydrochloride] (RenaGel): a noncalcemic phosphate binder for the treatment of hyperphosphatemia in chronic renal failure. Am J Kidney Dis 1997;29(1):66–71.

[176] Goldberg DI, et al. Effect of RenaGel, a non-absorbed, calcium- and aluminium-free phosphate binder, on serum phosphorus, calcium, and intact parathyroid hormone in end-stage renal disease patients. Nephrol Dial Transplant 1998;13(9):2303–10.

[177] Slatopolsky EA, Burke SK, Dillon MA. RenaGel, a nonabsorbed calcium- and aluminum-free phosphate binder, lowers serum phosphorus and parathyroid hormone. The RenaGel Study Group. Kidney Int 1999;55(1):299–307.

[178] Ferramosca E, et al. Potential antiatherogenic and anti-inflammatory properties of sevelamer in maintenance hemodialysis patients. Am Heart J 2005;149(5):820–5.

[179] Suki WN, et al. Effects of sevelamer and calcium-based phosphate binders on mortality in hemodialysis patients. Kidney Int 2007;72(9):1130–7.

[180] Caglar K, et al. Short-term treatment with sevelamer increases serum fetuin-a concentration and improves endothelial dysfunction in chronic kidney disease stage 4 patients. Clin J Am Soc Nephrol 2008;3(1):61–8.

[181] Koiwa F, et al. Sevelamer hydrochloride and calcium bicarbonate reduce serum fibroblast growth factor 23 levels in dialysis patients. Ther Apher Dial 2005;9(4):336–9.

[182] Qunibi W, et al. A 1-year randomized trial of calcium acetate vs. sevelamer on progression of coronary artery calcification in hemodialysis patients with comparable lipid control: the Calcium Acetate Renagel Evaluation-2 (CARE-2) study. Am J Kidney Dis 2008;51(6):952–65.

[183] Barreto DV, et al. Phosphate binder impact on bone remodeling and coronary calcification—results from the BRiC study. Nephron Clin Pract 2008;110(4):c273–83.

[184] Tonelli M, Pannu N, Manns B. Oral phosphate binders in patients with kidney failure. N Engl J Med 2010;362(14):1312–24.

[185] Tonelli M, et al. Systematic review of the clinical efficacy and safety of sevelamer in dialysis patients. Nephrol Dial Transplant 2007;22(10):2856–66.

[186] Raggi P, et al. Ten-year experience with sevelamer and calcium salts as phosphate binders. Clin J Am Soc Nephrol 2010;5(Suppl. 1):S31–40.

[187] St Peter WL, et al. A comparison of sevelamer and calcium-based phosphate binders on mortality, hospitalization, and morbidity in hemodialysis: a secondary analysis of the Dialysis Clinical Outcomes Revisited (DCOR) randomized trial using claims data. Am J Kidney Dis 2008;51(3):445–54.

[188] Albaaj F, Hutchison AJ. Lanthanum carbonate (Fosrenol): a novel agent for the treatment of hyperphosphataemia in renal failure and dialysis patients. Int J Clin Pract 2005;59(9):1091–6.

[189] Chiang SS, Chen JB, Yang WC. Lanthanum carbonate (Fosrenol) efficacy and tolerability in the treatment of hyperphosphatemic patients with end-stage renal disease. Clin Nephrol 2005;63(6):461–70.

[190] Finn WF, Joy MS, Hladik G. Efficacy and safety of lanthanum carbonate for reduction of serum phosphorus in patients with chronic renal failure receiving hemodialysis. Clin Nephrol 2004;62(3):193–201.

[191] Shigematsu T, Negi S. Combined therapy with lanthanum carbonate and calcium carbonate for hyperphosphatemia decreases serum FGF-23 level independently of calcium and PTH (COLC Study). Nephrol Dial Transplant 2011.

[192] Finn WF. Lanthanum carbonate vs. standard therapy for the treatment of hyperphosphatemia: safety and efficacy in chronic maintenance hemodialysis patients. Clin Nephrol 2006;65(3):191–202.

[193] Freemont AJ, Hoyland JA, Denton J. The effects of lanthanum carbonate and calcium carbonate on bone abnormalities in patients with end-stage renal disease. Clin Nephrol 2005;64(6):428–37.

[194] Malluche HH, et al. Improvements in renal osteodystrophy in patients treated with lanthanum carbonate for two years. Clin Nephrol 2008;70(4):284–95.

[195] Shoben AB, et al. Association of oral calcitriol with improved survival in nondialyzed CKD. J Am Soc Nephrol 2008;19(8): 1613—9.

[196] Teng M, et al. Survival of patients undergoing hemodialysis with paricalcitol or calcitriol therapy. N Engl J Med 2003;349(5):446—56.

[197] Teng M, et al. Activated injectable vitamin D and hemodialysis survival: a historical cohort study. J Am Soc Nephrol 2005;16(4): 1115—25.

[198] Slatopolsky E, et al. Marked suppression of secondary hyperparathyroidism by intravenous administration of 1, 25-dihydroxy-cholecalciferol in uremic patients. J Clin Invest 1984;74(6):2136—43.

[199] Quarles LD, et al. Prospective trial of pulse oral vs. intravenous calcitriol treatment of hyperparathyroidism in ESRD. Kidney Int 1994;45(6):1710—21.

[200] Slatopolsky E, et al. A new analog of calcitriol, 19-nor-1,25-(OH)$_2$D$_2$, suppresses parathyroid hormone secretion in uremic rats in the absence of hypercalcemia. Am J Kidney Dis 1995;26(5):852—60.

[201] Sprague SM, et al. Paricalcitol vs. calcitriol in the treatment of secondary hyperparathyroidism. Kidney Int 2003;63(4): 1483—90.

[202] Maung HM, et al. Efficacy and side effects of intermittent intravenous and oral doxercalciferol (1alpha-hydroxyvitamin D(2)) in dialysis patients with secondary hyperparathyroidism: a sequential comparison. Am J Kidney Dis 2001;37(3):532—43.

[203] Nemeth EF, et al. Pharmacodynamics of the type II calcimimetic compound cinacalcet HCl. J Pharmacol Exp Ther 2004;308(2): 627—35.

[204] Block GA, et al. Cinacalcet for secondary hyperparathyroidism in patients receiving hemodialysis. N Engl J Med 2004;350(15): 1516—25.

[205] Lindberg JS, et al. The calcimimetic AMG 073 reduces parathyroid hormone and calcium x phosphorus in secondary hyperparathyroidism. Kidney Int 2003;63(1):248—54.

[206] Moe SM, et al. Achieving NKF-K/DOQI bone metabolism and disease treatment goals with cinacalcet HCl. Kidney Int 2005;67(2):760—71.

[207] Quarles LD, et al. The calcimimetic AMG 073 as a potential treatment for secondary hyperparathyroidism of end-stage renal disease. J Am Soc Nephrol 2003;14(3):575—83.

[208] Block GA, et al. Combined therapy with cinacalcet and low doses of vitamin D sterols in patients with moderate to severe secondary hyperparathyroidism. Nephrol Dial Transplant 2008;23(7):2311—8.

[209] Raggi P, et al. The ADVANCE study: a randomized study to evaluate the effects of cinacalcet plus low-dose vitamin D on vascular calcification in patients on hemodialysis. Nephrol Dial Transplant 2011;26(4):1327—39.

20

Phosphate Metabolism and Fibroblast Growth Factor 23 in Chronic Kidney Disease

Jessica Houston, Tamara Isakova, Myles Wolf

Division of Nephrology and Hypertension, University of Miami Miller School of Medicine, Miami, FL, USA

INTRODUCTION

Elemental Phosphorus in the Environment

The existence of elemental phosphorus was first recorded in the late 17th century, when alchemist Henning Brand extracted a white powder after distilling urine [1]. Due to the chemiluminescent property observed during its generation, the element was named Phosphorus, meaning "bearer of light", from the Latin word fōsforos. Elemental phosphorus, with chemical symbol P and atomic number 15, is a highly reactive, multivalent nonmetal of the nitrogen group. There are three allotropic forms of phosphorus in the inanimate environment: white, red and black. White phosphorus, the least stable allotrope, is a poisonous, soft and waxy solid that combusts spontaneously when exposed to oxygen, producing white fumes of phosphorus pentoxide (P_4O_{10}). Heat, in the absence of air, converts white phosphorus to red phosphorus. Red phosphorus is more stable, does not readily ignite and is not poisonous. Black phosphorus, the most stable allotrope, is formed by heating white phosphorus under pressure; the resulting product resembles graphite. Due to the highly reactive nature of elemental phosphorus, it is present in its maximally oxidized, anionic state, as phosphate (PO_4) and is primarily found in phosphate rocks [2].

The United States is a global leader in the production and consumption of phosphate rocks, which are used to manufacture industrial products. White phosphorus, prepared commercially from mined phosphate rocks, is burned to yield P_4O_{10} and subsequently hydrolyzed or washed with sulfuric acid to yield the desired phosphoric acid (H_3PO_4). Phosphoric acid is the basis for many compounds, mainly fertilizers, but also nerve toxins, matches, detergents, plastics, pesticides, steel products, and food additives [2].

Nomenclature

Dietary phosphorus is largely bound *in vivo* to proteins and carbon containing molecules [3]. In scientific literature, the term phosphorus is often used interchangeably with phosphate when referring to dietary intake and distribution. However, since phosphorus occurs almost exclusively in the anionic form, PO_4, we use the term *phosphate* throughout this chapter.

Understanding the dynamic physiologic process of human phosphate metabolism requires the use of additional definitions, which we list below. Simply stated, phosphate *balance* is input minus output. During *neutral phosphate balance*, the amount of phosphate absorbed in the intestine is equivalent to the amount of urinary and fecal losses. In health, neutral balance is typically found in men aged <65 and premenopausal, nonpregnant women after they achieve peak bone mass at approximately 30 years of age. *Negative phosphate balance* is induced when excretion exceeds absorption and is often coupled with significant bone loss. Negative phosphate balance can occur in postmenopausal women and with chronic glucocorticoid excess, hyperparathyroidism, increased fibroblast growth factor 23 (FGF-23), and calcitriol (1,25D) deficiency. Conversely, *positive phosphate balance* occurs when absorption exceeds fecal and urinary excretion. Typically, this occurs during childhood, adolescence, pregnancy, and lactation to accommodate proper skeletal growth.

Phosphate homeostasis is the physiological process of regulating net phosphate balance. Homeostasis and metabolism are used interchangeably in this chapter. A steady state indicates that the net flux of phosphate in and out of the cellular compartments is balanced.

When describing dietary sources of phosphate, the terms *organic* and *inorganic* will be used. Organic refers to phosphate that is naturally bound to intracellular, carbon-containing molecules and proteins. In contrast, inorganic phosphate is naturally, freely circulating in the unbound form. Additionally, we will use the term inorganic when referring to food sources that contain synthetically produced inorganic phosphate in the form of phosphate salts [4,5]. *Bioavailability* of different dietary phosphate sources refers to the relative ability of phosphate to be absorbed in the gastrointestinal tract.

PHOSPHATE METABOLISM IN HEALTH

Body Distribution of Phosphate

Phosphate plays a critical role in myriad cell structures and processes, including ATP generation, hormonal signaling, bone mineralization, cell signaling, and tissue oxygenation. Although both inorganic and organic phosphate are present in cells, the majority is organic and incorporated as a structural component of cellular phospholipid membranes and as a molecular component of phosphorylated energy compounds and long chained nucleic acids [6].

Figure 20.1 represents the distribution of total body phosphate. The total body phosphate content of an adult human is approximately 700 g, of which approximately 85% is found in the skeleton bound to calcium in the form of hydroxyapatite $[Ca_{10}(PO_4)_6(OH)_2]$. The remainder is primarily distributed in soft tissues, with less than 1% of the entire phosphate content existing in the extracellular fluid. Thirty percent of the extracellular phosphate is inorganic, whereas 70% is organic, existing in the form of phosphate esters, phosphorylated intermediate molecules involved in energy generation and storage, and as phospholipids in cell membranes. Fifteen percent of the inorganic portion of the extracellular phosphate circulates freely as the monohydrogen (HPO_4) or dihydrogen (H_2PO_4) forms, and represents the measured serum value [7]. Thus, measured serum

phosphate only represents a small amount of the total body phosphate [7,8].

Circulating phosphate is able to freely move into and out of cells due to a modest extracellular phosphate gradient across the plasma membrane. The direction of phosphate movement is dependent on physiological needs. Serum phosphate levels can decrease as a result of intracellular phosphate shifts, a process that is dependent on insulin, glucose, catecholamines, and acid—base status [9]. Thus, during metabolic processes, such as oxidative phosphorylation and glycolysis, phosphorylation of organic compounds induces a low intracellular phosphate concentration. In the presence of insulin, intracellular influx of phosphate is stimulated, thereby replenishing the intracellular phosphate concentration and leading to a decrease in serum phosphate [8]. This phenomenon explains the observation of postprandial decline in serum phosphate levels [10].

Phosphate Homeostasis

An adequate amount of phosphate is necessary to support a neutral homeostatic state. States of deficiency impair skeletal mineralization, while phosphate excess may promote soft tissue calcification. Hypophosphatemia may be caused by malnutrition, malabsorption or urinary wasting; each can lead to decreased bone mineralization. Phosphate homeostasis is maintained through concerted effects on gastrointestinal absorption, exchanges with bone, soft tissues and intracellular stores, and renal excretion (Figure 20.2). It is hormonally regulated by FGF-23, 1,25D and parathyroid hormone (PTH).

Intestinal Absorption of Phosphate

Dietary phosphate absorption in the gastrointestinal tract occurs at the duodenum, jejunum and the ileum.

FIGURE 20.1   Total phosphate distribution. Sections of the pie chart indicate proportions of phosphate distribution throughout the body. The figure is reproduced in color in the color plate section.

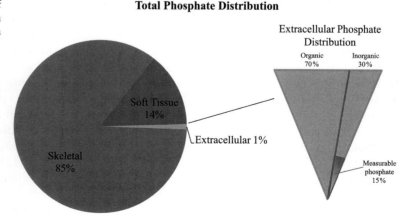

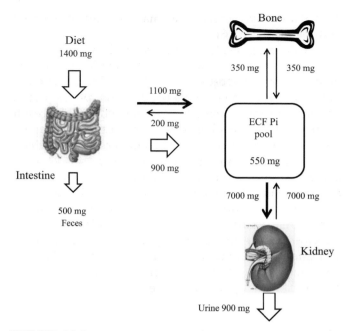

FIGURE 20.2 Phosphate metabolism in the bone, kidney and intestine. Phosphate regulation by three primary organs: kidney, bone and intestine. ECF Pi: extracellular fluid phosphorus. The figure is reproduced in color in the color plate section.

In vivo studies in rats have shown that the duodenum and jejunum are the primary sites of intestinal phosphate absorption [11,12], and recent reports have also localized phosphate absorption to the ileum in mice [12,13]. Intestinal phosphate absorption is mediated by both passive paracellular diffusion and active transport [14]. Passive paracellular diffusion through tight junction complexes across the intestinal mucosa is driven by the relative phosphate concentration gradient at the lumen. In this way, phosphate traverses the intestinal cellular membrane in the space between adjacent enterocytes of the epithelium. Active, cell mediated transport is enhanced by the presence of 1,25D and occurs via sodium-phosphate (NaPi) co-transporters located on the luminal surface of epithelial cells of the small intestine.

The maximal absorption rate of phosphate is variable and depends on the amount and type of dietary phosphate and the absorptive capacity of the body that varies according to physiological needs. In health, active transport, stimulated by 1,25D, prevails with dietary phosphate deprivation [6]. Conversely, diffusive paracellular absorption dominates with high phosphate consumption. As phosphate consumption increases, the rate at which absorption occurs may decline, but the total amount of phosphate absorbed continually increases. The bioavailability of dietary phosphate introduces additional variability in absorption rates and constitutes an important consideration. The percentage of phosphate absorption will be higher or lower depending on the type and source of phosphate consumed (see below, section on Bioavailability of phosphate: naturally bound vs. synthetic salts). Furthermore, dietary cations, such as calcium and magnesium, can complex with phosphate in the gut lumen to form nonabsorbable salts [15]. As the cationic content of these minerals in the diet changes, the amount of complexed phosphate changes, thereby changing the net amount of available phosphate for absorption. The body adapts to the frequent changes in supply and demand by inducing activation of stored sodium phosphate co-transporters and synthesis of 1,25D.

Accumulating evidence has implicated NaPi-2b as the key sodium-phosphate co-transporter involved in intestinal absorption of phosphate [16]. Animal studies have shown that maximal phosphate absorption occurs in the duodenum where expression of NaPi-2b is highest, a pattern similar to that of humans [17]. Sodium and phosphate are transported through the co-transporter with a stoichiometry of 3:1 ($Na+:HPO_4^{2}$). Given the relatively high affinity of phosphate for NaPi-2b [18,19], this complex is often utilized in the setting of dietary phosphate depletion [20]. Various hormones influence NaPi-2b expression and intestinal phosphate transport, including epidermal growth factor [21], 1,25D and FGF-23 [22]. Importantly, recent studies of knockout mice have demonstrated the NaPi-2b activity can occur independent of 1,25D [23], and that distinct pathways for regulation of this channel exist in isolated circumstances of low dietary phosphate or increased 1,25D [24,25].

Typically, 33% of the ingested phosphate is excreted in the stool. While fecal excretion is not the primary regulatory mechanism of phosphate excretion, changes in fecal excretion can occur in response to alterations in dietary intake and 1,25D levels. In the case of the latter, dietary phosphate absorption will be decreased as a result of reduced active transport leading to increased stool excretion of phosphate. In addition, diminished intestinal calcium absorption due to 1,25D deficiency will result in less calcium absorption and greater luminal availability of calcium, which complexes with phosphate and thereby further decreases phosphate absorption, leading to increased excretion in the stool [15].

Distribution into Tissues

Once phosphate is absorbed in the intestine, it is distributed to bone, blood or cellular components, as determined by physiological requirements. The bone acts as a reservoir for minerals, such as calcium, magnesium and phosphate ions. Phosphate ions exist in the bone primarily as the calcium-phosphate salt, hydroxyapatite. As a result, phosphate movement in and out of bone matrix occurs mainly as a consequence of calcium deposition and resorption. Phosphate deposition, in concert with calcium, is regulated by osteoblasts. With proper orientation and sufficient energy, the ions combine with hydroxide and bicarbonate ions to form the mature hydroxyapatite salt, and the influx of minerals into the circulation declines. This cyclic process functions in continuous balance as the bone mineral salts are broken down and distributed throughout the body.

Renal Handling of Phosphate

Phosphate and calcium are freely filtered by the glomerulus. Once in the tubule, the desired amount of minerals is reabsorbed, and excess waste is excreted in the urine. This process helps to regulate the serum mineral levels and maintains a proper homeostatic balance. The main site for reabsorption of phosphate filtered by the glomerulus is the proximal tubule, which reclaims 80% of the filtered phosphate. The rest is reabsorbed at the distal tubule (10%) and the loop of Henle and collecting duct (<1%). Typically in health, the fractional excretion in the urine represents approximately 10% of the filtrate. However, this value is variable because it depends on the amount of phosphate consumed and on renal function.

Absorbed dietary phosphate that is in excess of physiological need is excreted by the kidney. Thus, approximately 60% of the consumed organified phosphate is excreted in the urine [26] (Figure 20.2). Consequently, urinary excretion is the key mechanism involved in preservation of phosphate balance and normal serum levels. Molecular alterations in proximal tubular reabsorption accommodate extreme divergences in dietary phosphate intake. Specifically, the quantity of type II sodium phosphate co-transporters, NaPi-2a and NaPi-2c, located on the epithelial cells of the proximal tubule, allows for this flexibility. In order to maintain phosphate homeostasis, phosphate traverses the proximal tubule against the electrochemical gradient from the urine via NaPi-2a and NaPi-2c and subsequently enters the bloodstream down the electrochemical gradient. The amount of sodium phosphate co-transporters on the apical surface of the proximal tubule is hormonally regulated and dependent on physiological needs.

With high dietary phosphate consumption, expression of sodium phosphate co-transporters in the proximal tubule and phosphate reabsorption declines. Conversely, with low dietary phosphate intake, the channels are upregulated and proximal tubular reabsorption increases. For example, in the immediate postprandial setting [10] or in the event that serum phosphate rises, a series of renal compensatory events occur: the amount of phosphate filtered at the glomerulus increases, followed by a decrease in available NaPi2a and NaPi2c co-transporters on the apical surface of the proximal tubular cell and the resultant decline in proximal tubular reabsorption of phosphate. Subsequently, urinary phosphate excretion rises in excess of dietary phosphate absorption. The net loss of phosphate from the body helps to maintain phosphate balance.

Hormonal Regulation of Phosphate Homeostasis

Under normal conditions, phosphate homeostasis is tightly regulated by FGF-23, 1,25D, and PTH, which exert effects on the gastrointestinal tract, kidney, bone and parathyroid gland.

FGF-23

FGF-23 is the primary phosphate regulating hormone. It is a 251 amino acid protein, produced by osteocytes and osteoblasts in the bone in adults and by other tissues during development. There are two commercially available ELISAs to measure FGF-23: an intact assay, which detects the full length protein, and the c-terminus assay, which detects c-terminal fragments. FGF-23 was originally identified as a central cause of rare disorders of phosphate homeostasis, including X-linked hypophosphatemia, autosomal dominant hypophosphatemic rickets, autosomal recessive hypophosphatemic rickets, fibrous dysplasia, and tumor-induced osteomalacia [27]. These phosphate wasting syndromes of FGF-23 excess manifest as hypophosphatemia due to isolated renal phosphate wasting, severe rickets or osteomalacia, inappropriately low 1,25D levels for the degree of hypophosphatemia, and variable PTH. These components of FGF-23 physiology were confirmed in transgenic mice engineered to overexpress FGF-23 [28,29], and mice administered exogenous FGF-23 [30,31]. Conversely, manifestations of hyperphosphatemia with excessive 1,25D persist in states of FGF-23 depletion, such as FGF-23 knockout mice [32] and patients with tumoral calcinosis due to inactivating mutations in GALNT3, a gene that encodes for a glucosylating enzyme that stabilizes the intact FGF-23 molecule [33].

FGF-23 exerts its primary biological functions to regulate mineral metabolism by binding to FGF receptors (FGFR) in the presence of klotho, a type I transmembrane protein which is primarily expressed in the kidney and parathyroid glands and that markedly increases the binding affinity of FGF-23 for FGFR [34]. Once FGF-23 binds to the FGFR-klotho complex, it exerts specific physiological functions to maintain normal phosphate homeostasis. First, FGF-23 acts to inhibit the conversion of 25-hydroxyvitamin D to 1,25D by diminishing the activity of renal 1α-hydroxylase and stimulating the catabolic 24-hydroxylase, which catalyzes 1,25D degradation [35,36]. Second, FGF-23 production promotes increased phosphaturia, through a similar mechanism as PTH: reducing expression of type II sodium phosphate co-transporters (NaPi-2a and NaPi-2c) that regulate proximal tubular reabsorption on the apical surface of the proximal tubular cell [37]. High PTH and FGF-23 induce a rapid decline in the concentration of sodium phosphate co-transporters on the plasma membrane through internalization in endocytotic vesicles and lysosomal destruction leading to decreased phosphate reabsorption at the proximal tubule. In contrast, low PTH and FGF-23 increase the capacity of the proximal tubule to reabsorb phosphate by a rapid shift of sodium phosphate co-transporters from intracellular vesicles to the plasma membrane. Third, under normal physiologic conditions, FGF-23 binding to FGFR-klotho on the parathyroid glands inhibits PTH secretion [38].

FGF-23 levels are regulated in health through classic negative feedback loops. For example, dietary phosphate loading stimulates FGF-23 secretion [39,40], which increases phosphaturia and suppresses renal 1,25D production. In contrast, phosphate restriction leads to a decline in FGF-23 levels [39,40], which promotes renal phosphate reabsorption and intestinal phosphate absorption due to increased 1,25D production. In this way, FGF-23 helps to maintain serum phosphate within a narrow range, despite wide fluctuations in dietary phosphate intake. FGF-23 levels are also regulated by 1,25D levels [41], and there is recent evidence to suggest that PTH increases FGF-23 secretion in health [42]. How dietary phosphate loading is sensed is unknown, yet unraveling this mechanism is a critical component of understanding FGF-23 physiology. FGF-23 regulation in CKD is presented in later sections of this chapter.

Vitamin D and PTH

While emerging evidence on FGF-23 physiology points to the key role of this novel hormone in phosphate metabolism, 1,25D and PTH also have important roles in the regulation of phosphate homeostasis (discussed in further detail in Chapters 17, 19 and 21). As discussed above, the presence of 1,25D facilitates an increase in dietary phosphate absorption in the small intestine via up-regulation of NaPi-2b. Additionally, 1,25D stimulates a rise in FGF-23 and decreases levels of PTH. Though the primary effect of PTH is to regulate calcium metabolism, it has secondary effects on phosphate homeostasis. First, PTH stimulates renal 1,25D synthesis. Second, PTH decreases proximal tubular reabsorption of phosphate, via the same mechanism as FGF-23, i.e. through down-regulation of NaPi2a and

NaPi2c on the brush border of the proximal tubule. Finally, PTH stimulates FGF-23 secretion.

PHOSPHATE METABOLISM ACROSS THE SPECTRUM OF CKD

CKD is a systemic disease that affects multiple physiologic processes, including regulation of bone and mineral metabolism. Bone and mineral abnormalities begin early in the course of CKD, and with progressive loss of kidney function, the prevalence of mineral metabolism disorders becomes nearly universal. Below we review the pathophysiology of disordered phosphate metabolism and the role of FGF-23 across the spectrum of CKD.

Early CKD

Whereas elevation in serum phosphate is a late event in the course of CKD, disturbances in regulatory hormones and urinary markers of mineral metabolism already begin as early as stage 2 CKD (Figure 20.3) [43]. Indeed, the common biochemical phenotype in early and mid-stage CKD is characterized by low 1,25D, elevated PTH and FGF-23, and normal serum phosphate and calcium levels [43–45]. Fractional urinary excretion of phosphate is typically increased, while urinary calcium losses are diminished [43,44]. These observations in concert with the finding that elevated FGF-23 and PTH are consistently associated with increased fractional urinary excretion of phosphate have led to the following pathophysiologic framework. With progressive decline in kidney function the ability to excrete dietary phosphate load decreases in parallel. Elevations in FGF-23 and PTH serve to maintain normophosphatemia in early CKD through their phosphaturic actions [27]. Higher FGF-23 levels also lead to a progressive decline in 1,25D levels [46] and consequently diminished dietary phosphate absorption. In advanced CKD, these compensatory mechanisms are no longer sufficient, resulting in a decline in 24-hour urinary phosphate excretion and a progressive rise in serum phosphate levels despite persistent elevations in levels of FGF-23 and PTH.

While this framework is widely accepted several questions remain unanswered. First, unlike fractional urinary phosphate excretion, 24-hour urinary phosphate excretion does not correlate with FGF-23 levels and appears to decline in the course of CKD prior to a rise in serum phosphate levels [43]. Whether this decrease is a function of diminished urinary excretion and thus a sign of positive phosphate balance or due to ineffective dietary phosphate absorption and neutral phosphate balance remains undefined. Second, early in the course

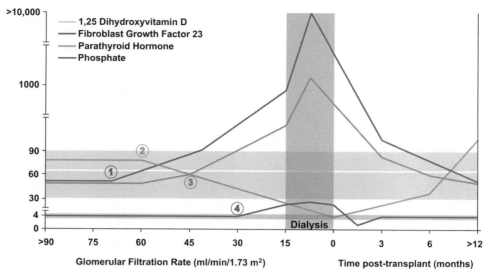

FIGURE 20.3 Temporal aspects of disordered phosphate metabolism in CKD. The x axis: represents the eGFR in the predialysis period (left); represents time after kidney transplantation in the postdialysis period (right). The y axis represents circulating concentrations of the individual analytes with the temporal changes in and normal ranges of individual analytes (C-terminal FGF-23 [RU/mL] – red; 1,25D [pg/mL] – yellow; PTH [pg/mL] – green; phosphate [mg/dL] – blue). Increased FGF-23 is the earliest abnormality in mineral metabolism in CKD and causes the subsequent decline in 1,25D levels that free PTH from feedback inhibition and lead to secondary hyperparathyroidism. All of these changes occur before serum phosphate levels increase. In early post-transplantation, FGF-23 and PTH levels rapidly decline and are variable thereafter. Tertiary FGF-23 excess contributes to post-transplantation hypophosphatemia and slow recovery of normal 1,25D production. *This figure is reproduced from Wolf [27], with permission from the American Society of Nephrology. Copyright © [2010] American Society of Nephrology. All rights reserved.* The figure is reproduced in color in the color plate section.

of CKD serum phosphate levels appear to drop modestly, at a time when FGF-23 levels are already on the rise [43]. This suggests that stimuli other than those related to phosphate handling might be important for FGF-23 secretion early in the course of CKD (see below).

Numerous human and animal studies provide support for the early and compensatory elevation of FGF-23 in CKD. Rats with experimental glomerulonephritis developed significantly elevated circulating FGF-23 within 10 days of renal injury [47]. At that time, serum creatinine was only subtly increased and serum phosphate remained unchanged. Increased PTH and reduced 1,25D achieved statistical significance at day 20. These results parallel the findings in human physiological studies of CKD and, collectively, provide evidence in favor of elevated FGF-23 levels being the first mineral metabolism abnormality in the course of CKD [48]. Further, circulating FGF-23 levels are elevated in patients with early stage CKD, perhaps as early as estimated glomerular filtration rates (eGFR) <90 mL/min per 1.73 m^2 [49]. A small study suggested that a rise in FGF-23 levels preceded PTH excess among those with early CKD [10]. The investigators found that FGF-23 levels were two times the normal limit and were significantly higher than healthy controls, while PTH remained within the normal range for both CKD and healthy participants [10]. A study examining bone biopsies of children with CKD demonstrated that FGF-23 expression in bone is increased by stage 2 [50].

Finally, in a large and racially diverse cohort of patients with stage 2-4 CKD, FGF-23 was elevated in 72% of participants, and elevated FGF-23 was more prevalent at higher eGFR than elevated PTH or serum phosphate, which was normal in most patients (Figure 20.4) [43]. Though these cross-sectional studies provide preliminary data suggesting that a rise in FGF-23 precedes an increase in PTH and serum phosphate, longitudinal studies examining changes in hormone levels over time among individuals are necessary to provide definitive evidence of the pathophysiological sequence that is currently presumed.

Though the exact mechanism of early FGF-23 secretion in CKD is unclear, several preliminary hypotheses have been put forward. First, renal injury itself may be an initial stimulus for FGF-23 secretion in early CKD by causing increased production of a factor that stimulates FGF-23 secretion or decreased expression of a tonic inhibitor [43]. Alternatively, deficiency of klotho, the obligatory co-receptor for FGF-23 receptor, has been suggested as an initiation trigger for FGF-23 excess. Klotho expression is thought to decline in parallel with rising FGF-23 levels with progressive loss of kidney function [51], suggesting progressive renal resistance to FGF-23 in CKD. Finally, kidney injury may initiate a decline in bone turnover, and consequently, an influx of phosphate into the circulation and surrounding tissues outside of bone cells. This may serve as a local stimulus for increased FGF-23 secretion from osteocytes

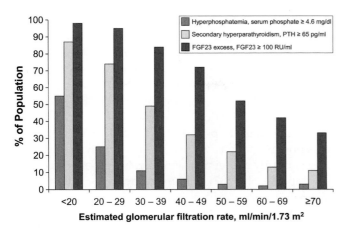

FIGURE 20.4 Prevalence of hyperphosphatemia, secondary hyperparathyroidism and elevated FGF-23 in CKD. Hyperphosphatemia was defined as serum phosphate ≥ 4.6 mg/dL, secondary hyperparathyroidism as parathyroid hormone (PTH) ≥ 65 pg/mL, and FGF-23 excess as FGF-23 ≥ 100 RU/mL. *This figure is reproduced from Isakova et al. [43], with permission from Macmillan Publishers Ltd: Kidney International. Copyright © [2011] Macmillan Publishers Ltd. All rights reserved.* The figure is reproduced in color in the color plate section.

and osteoblasts. In support of this hypothesis, Samadfam et al. demonstrated a marked increase in FGF-23 levels proportional to the degree of suppression of bone turnover in mice [52].

In addition to high FGF-23, PTH is also elevated in CKD, and often both hormones are elevated within the same individual [43]. While the observation that FGF-23 inhibits PTH secretion in health appears to conflict with the observed biochemical phenotype in CKD [38], there are at least two possible ways to reconcile these seemingly conflicting findings. First, the rise in PTH in CKD may be an indirect effect of FGF-23 via its inhibition of 1,25D production [46,47]. Second, recent evidence demonstrates resistance to FGF-23 action at the level of the parathyroid gland in advanced CKD [53,54]. Thus, high PTH in CKD patients with elevated FGF-23 levels could also be a direct effect of FGF-23 resistance resulting from down-regulation of FGFR and klotho in the parathyroid glands.

End-Stage Renal Disease

FGF-23 levels steadily rise in response to declining kidney function and can reach up to 1000-fold above the normal range by the time patients reach end stage renal disease (ESRD) [55]. While FGF-23 levels in dialysis patients directly correlate with serum phosphate levels [56,57] and with use of activated vitamin D [58], some have attributed the marked elevation of FGF-23 levels in CKD to decreased renal clearance of FGF-23 fragments [59]. A recent study of adults and children with ESRD on peritoneal dialysis used a cell-based FGF-23 bioactivity assay and Western Blots to test

whether there is accumulation of FGF-23 fragments in CKD. The investigators found that biological activity correlated strongly with FGF-23 concentrations determined by either the c-terminal or the intact FGF-23 assay, and the Western blots revealed that virtually all of the circulating FGF-23 was intact and biologically active [60]. These results underscore the importance of further studies needed to ascertain the determinants of FGF-23 levels in patients on dialysis. Two recent reports suggest that in addition to serum phosphate levels and use of active vitamin D analogs, other factors that determine FGF-23 levels in ESRD include residual renal function and dialysis vintage [57,61].

Transplant

Up to 90% of kidney transplant recipients with normal allograft function will experience hypophosphatemia due to excessive phosphaturia during the first few months after kidney transplantation [62,63], which can persist in 6–27% for months to years [64]. Until recently, the etiology of post-transplant hypophosphatemia was thought to be due to tertiary hyperparathyroidism, which is defined as chronically increased levels of PTH due to secondary hyperparathyroidism in patients during dialysis persisting into the post-transplant setting [63]. However, excessive phosphaturia can occur even with low levels of PTH, and hypophosphatemia may persist beyond normalized PTH levels [65,66]. Furthermore, 1,25D levels remain low post-transplant despite excessive PTH and hypophosphatemia, each of which should stimulate 1,25D production by the healthy allograft [67,68]. These clinical observations led to the hypothesis that mechanisms other than PTH likely contribute to post-transplant hypophosphatemia and urinary phosphate wasting [69]. This was confirmed by several reports that have shown that in the early post-transplant period, recipients exhibit a mineral metabolism phenotype reminiscent of that seen in X-linked hypophosphatemia and related hereditary hypophosphatemic disorders, namely excessive FGF-23 levels, inappropriate renal phosphate wasting and low 1,25D levels for the degree of hypophosphatemia [27].

Bhan prospectively evaluated 27 living kidney donor recipients [70]. In order to minimize potential confounding by impaired renal function, participants were chosen based on a high likelihood of immediate allograft function, and when allograft dysfunction developed, individuals' participation in the study was discontinued (prior lab results were included in the final analysis). Follow up continued for three months during which time repeated blood and urine specimens were collected. Hypophosphatemia (serum phosphate <2.6 mg/dL) occurred in 85% of patients, and 37% developed severe hypophosphatemia (serum phosphate <1.5 mg/dL), without any detection of hypercalcemia. Importantly, a strong inverse association between FGF-23 excess and decreased levels of 1,25D was found and persisted following transplantation, despite high PTH levels, a healthy allograft and hypophosphatemia. These important findings highlight the association of FGF-23 levels and the severity of hypophosphatemia in the immediate post-transplant period: FGF-23 appears to be the primary factor contributing to early post-transplant hypophosphatemia, rather than PTH. However, other studies suggest that this relationship changes in long-term post-transplant patients, among whom elevated PTH emerges as the more important contributor to urinary phosphate loss and relative hypophosphatemia by one year after transplantation and thereafter [71,72].

THE ROLE OF PHOSPHATE AND FGF-23 EXCESS IN THE PATHOPHYSIOLOGY OF CKD OUTCOMES

Progression to end-stage renal disease, cardiovascular disease morbidity and premature death are common events in CKD [73,74], and phosphate and FGF-23 dysmetabolism appear to play important roles in their pathogenesis. Below we review the experimental, observational and clinical data that implicate phosphate and FGF-23 excess as potentially causal factors and suggest possible mechanisms by which these nearly universal complications of CKD may increase the risks of adverse clinical outcomes.

The Evidence for Phosphate Excess as a Risk Factor for Adverse Outcomes

The potential connection between serum phosphate and mortality was first reported in observational cohorts of patients undergoing dialysis [75,76], but has since been extended to earlier-stage CKD and even the general population [77,78]. These epidemiologic studies have consistently reported an independent relationship between elevated serum phosphate and increased risk of death. Associations between serum phosphate and intermediate cardiovascular phenotypes, such as left ventricular hypertrophy [79] and arterial calcification [80], have also been reported. Thus, a hypothesis evolved that suggested that hyperphosphatemia may be a CKD-specific risk factor for mortality that may be directly or indirectly pathogenic.

In support of a direct causal role of phosphate excess in the pathogenesis of adverse CKD outcomes, experimental data have shown that exposure of vascular smooth muscle cells to media with high phosphate

concentrations leads to upregulation of osteoblastic factors and promotion of vascular calcification [81]. Several observational studies have reported a consistent association between serum phosphate and measures of vascular calcification [80,82–85]. Additionally, disordered phosphate metabolism, independent of its effects on vascular calcification, appears to be a risk factor for left ventricular hypertrophy [79,86]. Correction of hyperphosphatemia with daily hemodialysis has been independently associated with regression of left ventricular hypertrophy [87]. Finally, pharmacoepidemiologic studies comparing use vs. non-use of phosphate binders in incident hemodialysis patients [88] and in those with pre-dialysis CKD [89] suggested that use of binders is independently associated with improved survival. However, these studies are limited by residual confounding and selection bias, and randomized controlled trials are needed in CKD to both establish the causal relationship of phosphate excess with risk of mortality and to demonstrate the efficacy of phosphate lowering therapies on hard clinical end points [55].

Disordered phosphate metabolism may also be involved in the pathogenesis of CKD progression, as detailed in Chapter 17. Briefly, elevated serum phosphate levels are associated with rapid progression of CKD [90–92], perhaps by accelerating tubulointerstitial fibrosis [93]. In contrast, phosphate restricted diets may slow kidney function decline [94]. While residual confounding by imprecise quantification of renal function is a major limitation of these and other studies with similar findings, a recent post-hoc analysis of 331 in the randomized Ramipril Efficacy in Nephropathy (REIN) study [95] supports the hypothesis that elevated serum phosphate levels are independently associated with more rapid progression of established CKD. The investigators found that higher levels of serum phosphate were independently associated with greater adjusted risk of reaching the study's renal endpoints, and that higher baseline serum phosphate levels progressively attenuated the renoprotective effect of inhibition of the renin-angiotensin system [95]. Taken together, these findings suggest that another mechanism by which phosphate excess may contribute to increased risk of CVD morbidity and mortality may be via increased rate of progression of CKD, itself a risk factor for CVD events.

Despite these convincing observations in defense of a direct effect of phosphate, the intimate interplay between the components of mineral metabolism makes it challenging to disentangle phosphate excess from other associated factors that may also contribute to the development of adverse clinical outcomes in CKD. For example, hyperphosphatemia may enhance parathyroid hyperplasia and stimulate PTH release directly, or it may do so indirectly via inhibition of 1,25D production

[96]. Indeed, small physiologic studies have shown that interventions aimed at reducing dietary phosphate absorption can lower PTH levels and increase 1,25D levels [97,98]. Further, the link between phosphate and FGF-23 adds an additional layer of complexity (see next section for comparison of FGF-23's performance as a predictor of risk with that of serum phosphate). Moreover, the inability to reliably assess phosphate excess given diurnal and postprandial variability in serum phosphate levels [10,99] along with the subtle difference in normal serum phosphate levels that confer increased risks of adverse outcomes [77] limit the utility of serum phosphate as a prognostic tool in clinical practice.

The Evidence for FGF-23 Excess as a Risk Factor for Adverse Outcomes

The discovery and rapid characterization of FGF-23 and its role as a marker of risk for adverse outcomes could have important implications for future research and perhaps clinical care in CKD. Below we review the observations that have linked elevated FGF-23 with risks of clinical outcomes and suggest mechanisms by which FGF-23 excess may mediate these risks.

Death

As was the case with serum phosphate, the first epidemiologic study to report an association between FGF-23 and mortality was performed in the dialysis setting. A prospective, nested case-control study of 400 incident hemodialysis patients showed that higher FGF-23 levels at the initiation of dialysis were independently associated with significantly greater risk of subsequent mortality during the first year on dialysis [56]. The results were independent of serum phosphate and demonstrated a strong "dose–response"-type relationship such that ascending quartiles of FGF-23 were associated with a linear increase in risk of mortality (Figure 20.5). Furthermore, the highest FGF-23 quartile was associated with a nearly 600% increased risk of death, which was markedly greater than parallel analyses of phosphate in which mortality risk was only 20% greater in the highest vs. the lower quartiles.

This observation has been confirmed in several other studies, including studies of pre-dialysis CKD, post-kidney transplant and non-CKD patients [100–102]. For example, Isakova et al. [100] tested the hypothesis that an elevated FGF-23 was independently associated with greater risks of ESRD and mortality in the Chronic Renal Insufficiency Cohort (CRIC) study, which is a prospective, multi-center, observational study of risk factors for CKD progression and cardiovascular disease in CKD patients with baseline eGFR of 20–70 (mean 42.8 ± 13.5) mL/min/1.73 m². The investigators found that

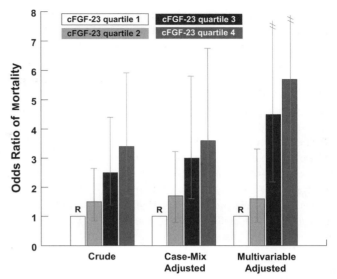

FIGURE 20.5 Odds Ratio for Death According to Quartile of FGF-23. Crude, case-mix adjusted, and multivariable adjusted odds ratios for death are shown according to quartile of cFGF-23 levels (quartile 1, <1090 reference units [RU] per milliliter; quartile 2, 1090 to 1750 RU per milliliter; quartile 3, 1751 to 4010 RU per milliliter; quartile 4, >4010 RU per milliliter). The case-mix adjusted analysis included the following variables: age, sex, race or ethnic group, blood pressure, body-mass index, facility-specific standardized mortality rate, vascular access at initiation of dialysis (fistula, graft, or catheter), cause of renal failure, urea reduction ratio, and coexisting conditions. The multivariable adjusted analysis included the case-mix variables plus phosphate, calcium, log parathyroid hormone, albumin, creatinine, and ferritin levels. Quartile 1 was the reference group in all models. I bars represent 95% confidence intervals. Asterisks indicate P < 0.05. R denotes reference. *This figure is reproduced from Gutiérrez et al. [56], with permission from the Massachusetts Medical Society. Copyright © [2008] Massachusetts Medical Society. All rights reserved.* The figure is reproduced in color in the color plate section.

elevated baseline FGF-23 was independently associated with greater risk of mortality (Figure 20.6) over a median follow-up of 3.5 years, with patients in the highest quartile of FGF-23 being at 3-fold greater adjusted risk of death compared to patients in the lowest quartile. Importantly, FGF-23 excess was the strongest predictor of mortality, stronger even than eGFR and proteinuria, which were not significantly associated with risk of death in the final adjusted models. The robust association persisted across examined eGFR cut-points (Figure 20.7), and was independent of serum phosphate or parathyroid hormone.

Kendrick et al. [103] performed a similar evaluation using stored samples from 1099 participants in the Homocysteinemia in Kidney and End-Stage Renal Disease (HOST) study, which was a multicenter, randomized, double-blind, placebo-controlled trial of folic acid and B vitamins in a population with advanced CKD. The investigators likewise found a strong independent direct association between baseline FGF-23 levels and all-cause mortality among participants with

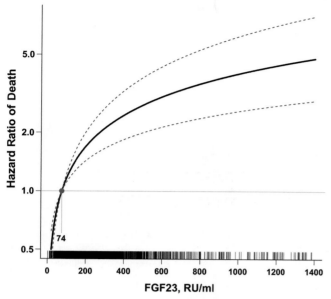

FIGURE 20.6 Multivariable-adjusted hazard function for death according to FGF-23. The median fibroblast growth factor 23 (FGF-23) level within the lowest FGF-23 quartile (74 RU/mL) served as the referent value (hazard = 1.0). The model was stratified by center and adjusted for age; sex; race; ethnicity; estimated glomerular filtration rate; natural log-transformed urine albumin-to-creatinine ratio; hemoglobin; serum albumin; systolic blood pressure; body mass index; diabetes; smoking status; low-density lipoprotein; history of coronary artery disease, congestive heart failure, stroke, and peripheral vascular disease; use of aspirin, β-blockers, statins, and angiotensin-converting enzyme inhibitors or angiotensin II receptor blockers; and serum calcium, phosphate, and natural log-transformed parathyroid hormone. Tick marks on the x-axis indicate individual observations at corresponding levels of FGF-23. The solid black line represents the multivariable-adjusted hazard of mortality as a function of the measured (nontransformed) FGF-23 level. The dashed lines indicate the 95% confidence intervals. *This figure is reproduced from Isakova et al. [43], with permission from the American Medical Association. Copyright © [2011] American Medical Association. All rights reserved. The figure is reproduced in color in the color plate section.*

stage 4–5 CKD (mean eGFR of 18 mL/min/1.73 m^2; median FGF-23 of 392 RU/mL), such that individuals in the highest quartile of FGF-23 had a 2.2-fold greater adjusted risk of death than patients in the lowest quartile during a median follow-up of 2.9 years. Notably, adjustment for other markers of mineral metabolism, including serum calcium, phosphate, parathyroid hormone and vitamin D levels, did not alter these findings.

Renal Disease Progression

Elevated FGF-23 may be an independent risk factor for more rapid loss of kidney function in CKD [104,105]. In a prospective study of 177 non-diabetic CKD patients with a median follow up of 53 months, c-terminal FGF-23 levels >104 RU/mL (or intact FGF-23 levels >35 pg/mL) were associated with more rapid progression of

CKD compared to lower levels. The results were independent of age, gender, baseline eGFR, proteinuria, and serum levels of calcium, phosphate, and PTH [104]. In a study of 55 patients with diabetic nephropathy, elevated FGF-23 was associated with the composite primary outcome of death, doubling of serum creatinine, or dialysis, although the number of events was small, which prevented the implementation of detailed MV-analysis [105]. These early findings were supported by observations in the CRIC study, in which elevated FGF-23 was an independent risk factor for ESRD in patients with relatively preserved kidney function (eGFR ≥ 30 mL/min/1.73 m^2), but not in those with eGFR <30 mL/min/1.73 m^2 [100]. Moreover, in the HOST study, elevated FGF-23 levels were independently associated with greater risk of chronic dialysis initiation [103]. Notably, several independent reports show that FGF-23 levels correlate with proteinuria [43,105]. Finally, a recent study of 701 older women suggested that elevated FGF-23 may independently predict the onset of incident CKD, though the study was limited by use of the modified Modification of Diet in Renal Disease estimating equation to define CKD in the elderly population [106].

Cardiovascular Disease

FGF-23 also appears to be a risk factor for CVD events in CKD, as demonstrated in a study of 149 CKD patients, in whom an elevated baseline FGF-23 level predicted subsequent myocardial infarction, coronary, carotid and lower limb arterial interventions, non-traumatic lower extremity amputation, or death [107]. In the secondary analysis of 1099 HOST study participants Kendrick et al also found a strong relationship between higher FGF-23 levels and greater risks of acute myocardial infarction and lower extremity limb amputations [103]. Similarly, in a cohort of 833 patients with stable coronary artery disease but low prevalence of decreased eGFR, elevated FGF-23 predicted future risk of a composite of CVD events that included myocardial infarction, stroke, transient ischemic attack, and heart failure [101]. Importantly, when the components of the composite were considered individually, the authors found significant associations between elevated FGF-23 levels and greater risks of heart failure and stroke or transient ischemic attack, but not myocardial infarction. Likewise, a recent nested case-control study in the Health Professionals Follow-up Study found no significant association between baseline FGF-23 levels and future risk of nonfatal myocardial infarction and fatal coronary heart disease [108]. Notably, congestive heart failure and stroke were not evaluated in the latter study. Whether these disparate findings are indicative of specific toxicity of FGF-23 targeting the myocardium more than the arterial vasculature requires further investigation. The association of FGF-23 with markers

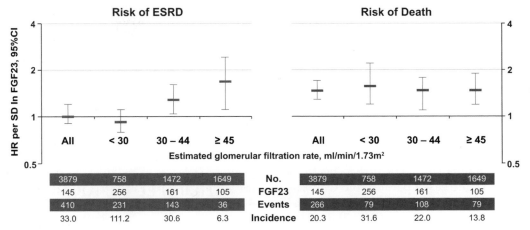

	Risk of ESRD				Risk of Death			
	3879	758	1472	1649	No.	3879	758	1472	1649
	145	256	161	105	FGF23	145	256	161	105
	410	231	143	36	Events	266	79	108	79
	33.0	111.2	30.6	6.3	Incidence	20.3	31.6	22.0	13.8

FIGURE 20.7 FGF-23 and risks of ESRD and death by baseline kidney function. Multivariable-adjusted risks of end-stage renal disease and death per unit increment in SD of natural log-transformed fibroblast growth factor 23 (FGF-23) in all participants and according to categories of baseline estimated glomerular filtration rate (GFR). See Figure 20.6 legend for adjusted variables. Error bars indicate 95% confidence intervals. HR indicates hazard ratio. *This figure is reproduced from Isakova et al. [43], with permission from the American Medical Association. Copyright © [2011] American Medical Association. All rights reserved.* The figure is reproduced in color in the color plate section.

of myocardial injury (brain natriuretic peptide [109] and troponin [110]) and with left ventricular hypertrophy (as described below) potentially supports such targeted toxicity.

Left Ventricular Hypertrophy

Several recent studies support a relationship between FGF-23 and LVH. In the first study of 124 prevalent hemodialysis patients, higher FGF-23 but not serum phosphate levels were independently associated with LVH and increased left ventricular mass index (LVMI) [111]. A second study showed that elevated FGF-23 levels were associated with increased LVMI and increased prevalence of LVH in 162 pre-dialysis CKD patients, independent of traditional risk factors and serum phosphate levels, which were not associated with LVMI or LVH [112]. Other recent studies have confirmed these initial reports [109,113—115] .

Recently, in a study of 3070 stage 2—4 CKD patients who underwent echocardiograms, Faul et al. [116] confirmed the independent association between elevated FGF-23 and LVH, and, in the first prospective study of its type, demonstrated that elevated FGF-23 predicts new-onset LVH in participants who had normal LV geometry at baseline and underwent follow-up echocardiography three years later. These prospective data suggested a possible causal role for FGF-23 in the pathogenesis of LVH, which was confirmed in a series of animal and in vitro experiments. First, the investigators showed that FGF-23 causes pathological hypertrophy of isolated cardiac myocytes in vitro via FGF receptor-dependent activation but independent of klotho, the co-receptor for FGF-23 in the kidney and parathyroid glands. Second, intra-myocardial or intravenous injection of FGF-23 in wild-type mice resulted in LVH, and

klotho deficient and klotho heterozygous mice demonstrated both elevated FGF-23 levels and LVH in a gene-dose-dependent pattern. Finally, administering an FGF receptor blocker to the {5/6}nephrectomy rat model of CKD that is known to develop LVH, severe hypertension, and elevated FGF-23, attenuated LVH without reduction in blood pressure or FGF-23. Taken together, these results provide the first evidence of a klotho-independent, causal role for FGF-23 in the pathogenesis of LVH, and suggest that chronically elevated FGF-23 levels may contribute directly to high prevalence of LVH in CKD. Given that cardiovascular disease is the primary cause of death in CKD, and LVH is an important mechanism of this relationship [117,118], these experimental findings provide support for a causal relationship between FGF-23 and mortality in this population. Furthermore, since biological activity of FGF-23 can occur in the absence of klotho, these results prompt new investigation of FGF-23 "toxicity" in other nontraditional target organs.

Vascular Calcification

The results linking FGF-23 and vascular calcification are conflicting. While several investigators were not able to find a significant relationship between FGF-23 and vascular calcification measured radiographically in individuals with healthy kidney function [119], dialysis patients [120], and patients with earlier stages of CKD [112], others did report an association with coronary calcification scores in the dialysis setting [121] and with other measures of vascular disease in the general population and in those with reduced eGFR [122,123]. For example, higher FGF-23 levels were independently associated with impaired vasoreactivity in 759 patients with normal kidney function and with arterial stiffness in 208 patients with eGFR <60 mL/min/1.73 m^2 [122]. Most recently, another report of 142 patients with CKD stages 2–5, including patients on dialysis, found that elevated FGF-23 levels were associated with higher aortic calcification scores independent of CKD stage and age [124]. Larger studies are needed to confirm or refute these findings.

Secondary Hyperparathyroidism

FGF-23 directly inhibits PTH secretion in heath [38], but in advanced CKD decreased parathyroid expression of FGFR and klotho [53,54] attenuates this effect. In contrast, in early and progressive CKD the indirect (via suppression of 1,25D synthesis [47]) stimulatory effect of elevated FGF-23 on PTH secretion appears to be more prominent and clinically important. The abundance of reports relating FGF-23 to secondary hyperparathyroidism confirms this observation. To date, several investigators have found a direct correlation between contemporaneous FGF-23 and PTH levels across the spectrum of CKD [43,46], and studies in the dialysis setting have shown that FGF-23 levels associate with severity of secondary hyperparathyroidism and PTH responsiveness to active vitamin D treatment [125,126]. Finally, in patients with severe secondary hyperparathyroidism, FGF-23 levels have been reported to decline gradually following parathyroidectomy [127], lending support to the recent animal studies that demonstrated a stimulating effect of PTH on FGF-23 secretion [42].

Bone Disease

A pathophysiologic link between FGF-23 and metabolic bone disease in CKD is biologically plausible, though few clinical studies have investigated the association. First, it has been suggested that changes in bone turnover drive FGF-23 secretion in CKD. By administering an anti-resorptive agent osteoprotegerin to several mouse models with varying degrees of coupled and uncoupled bone turnover, circulating FGF-23 concentrations markedly increased in proportion to the degree of suppression of bone turnover [52]. Second, children with CKD have been shown to have increased bone expression of FGF-23, detected as early as stage 2 [50]. Additionally, FGF-23 levels in children undergoing peritoneal dialysis were inversely correlated with indices of osteoid mineralization and bone volume [128]. Finally, it has also been proposed that phosphate released from bone under the influence of elevated PTH may perhaps induce FGF-23 secretion in CKD [129]. Importantly, it remains unclear whether FGF-23 exerts direct effects on bone cells or the signaling pathways that regulate bone formation rates.

Markers of Inflammation and Nutrition

FGF-23 may be related to inflammation in CKD, as has been suggested by the observation of a direct correlation between FGF-23 levels and C-reactive protein [130]. Additionally, limited data point to an inverse association between FGF-23 and cholesterol levels [131]. Further work is needed to delineate these relationships and their impact on adverse clinical outcomes in CKD.

THERAPEUTIC APPROACHES TO LOWERING PHOSPHATE AND FGF-23 EXCESS

Dietary phosphate restriction, dialytic phosphate removal and oral phosphate binders are interventions that are used to control hyperphosphatemia in ESRD patients. Below, we focus on the influence of dialytic, pharmocologic and other modalities on FGF-23 levels.

Dialytic Phosphate Removal

Given consistent associations between serum phosphate and FGF-23 levels in dialysis patients, it is plausible to hypothesize that the intensity of dialytic phosphate clearance would be associated with FGF-23 levels. In a recent cross-sectional analysis of adult peritoneal dialysis patients, FGF-23 levels correlated inversely with renal phosphate clearance in patients with residual renal function, but there was no significant relationship between peritoneal phosphate clearance and FGF-23 levels in patients with and without residual renal function. Intensive dialysis has been associated with improved phosphate control [132]. Prospective data on FGF-23 levels and intensive dialysis are lacking, although it can be hypothesized that given the salutary effect on hyperphosphatemia and positive phosphate balance, FGF-23 levels would be expected to decrease with frequent dialysis.

Oral Phosphate Binders

Existing phosphate binders are all moderately efficacious in lowering serum phosphate levels in hyperphosphatemic dialysis patients [133]. Few short-term physiologic studies evaluating use in earlier stages of CKD found that urinary phosphate excretion can be lowered safely by phosphate binders with infrequent development of hypophosphatemia [134,135]. Additionally, clinical data regarding impact of binders on FGF-23 levels in dialysis and in stage 3–4 CKD is beginning to accumulate [135–137]. FGF-23 levels decreased significantly from pretreatment levels in patients undergoing dialysis following four weeks of treatment with the combination of sevelamer hydrochloride and calcium carbonate [138]. Oliveira et al. showed that FGF-23 levels decreased by nearly 50% in normophosphatemic patients with CKD stages 3–4 following 6 weeks of sevelamer hydrochloride therapy [136], whereas there was no significant change in FGF-23 levels in patients treated with calcium acetate. Similarly, use of lanthanum carbonate for 4 weeks resulted in a 22% reduction in FGF-23 levels in patients with stage 3 CKD and baseline serum phosphate <4.5 mg/dL. While existing reports suggest that compared to other binder classes, calcium-based binders may be less efficacious in FGF-23 lowering [136,138], larger studies are needed to verify this early signal. Finally, 2 weeks of lanthanum carbonate therapy in a pilot study of normophosphatemic stage 3–4 CKD did not result in change in FGF-23 [135], suggesting that studies of longer duration may be needed to demonstrate efficacy.

Effect of PTH-Lowering and other Therapies on FGF-23

Active vitamin D and its analogs increased dietary phosphate absorption, and 1,25D is known to stimulate FGF-23 secretion and increase FGF-23 levels on dialysis [58,139]. In contrast, there is emerging evidence that cinacalcet lowers FGF-23 levels on dialysis [140,141], in addition to its well-described phosphate and PTH-lowering effects in ESRD [142]. Interestingly, there are a handful of reports linking intravenous iron infusion with increased FGF-23 levels in both the dialysis setting [143] as well as in individuals with healthy kidney function [144], but iron deficiency appears to increase FGF-23 levels in autosomal dominant hypophosphatemic rickets [145,146]. Further work is needed to sort out the contribution of iron metabolism to mineral metabolism in CKD and in health. Finally, additional therapeutic approaches might emerge from further investigation of the NaPi-2b-inhibitors and new calcimimetics that have shown promise in early studies [147,148].

IMPACT OF DIETARY PHOSPHATE ON PHOSPHATE/FGF-23 EXCESS

Sources of Dietary Phosphate

Every living organism contains phosphate. Therefore, phosphate is found in nearly all animal- and plant-derived foods, with dairy products, vegetables, grains, and meats being major sources of dietary phosphate. The content and bioavailability of phosphate in these foods are variable and depend on the source of dietary phosphate, which can be categorized as organic or inorganic (Table 20.1).

Organic Phosphate

Organic phosphate is defined as phosphate which is naturally bound to intracellular, carbon-containing molecules and proteins, and it is naturally present in both animal and plant life. The amount of phosphate varies across the spectrum of food categories, with most meats, cereals and dairy containing the highest organified phosphate per serving, and vegetables and grains offering the lowest organified phosphate per serving [14]. As organic phosphate is naturally bound to protein, foods that are highest in organified phosphate are generally those that also contain the highest amount of protein. Phosphate bioavailability (discussed below) in these organic sources varies by food type, digestibility of dietary components, and the relative availability of NaPi-2b co-transporters in the GI tract [4], but on average ranges from 40–60%. The organified phosphate in meat is easily hydrolyzed in the GI tract and relatively well absorbed in the small intestine, though organified phosphate in dairy products offers decreased digestibility. In plant sources, such as vegetables, legumes and grains, a majority of the phosphate is in the form of phytate. Since humans do not express the enzyme phytase, most of the organified phosphate in plants is not easily digested or absorbed [149].

Animal-Based Phosphate

Animal-based foods, such as dairy products, meat, poultry and fish, are rich in protein and typically contain an abundant supply of "natural", organic phosphate. In animal sources, phosphate exists mostly in intracellular compartments and is easily hydrolyzed in the intestinal tract and absorbed. Animal sources often contribute up to 60% of the daily intake of total phosphate [149], most of which is digested and absorbed. The bioavailability of total phosphate from animal-based foods is higher than that of plant-based foods (discussed below) [4,5]. To highlight this concept, Karp et al. [150] reported that when healthy humans consumed an equal amount of dietary phosphate from either plant or animal sources, urinary phosphate excretion was higher among those who consumed animal protein [151]. Moreover, among animal sources, the proportion of phosphate bioavailability varies greatly. While meat is generally highly digestible and offers high relative bioavailability, red meat and fish contain more phosphate than poultry [152]. Interestingly, the phosphate content in dairy products is variable, with differing phosphate bioavailability across dairy food types (milk vs. cheese) and even within the same class, for example, low-fat vs. whole milk [14]. Further, whole eggs, including the yolk, contain more phosphate than egg whites: one large

TABLE 20.1   Selection of High Phosphate Foods [4,149,158]

Low Bioavailability (10—30%)

ORGANIC	
Plant	
	Seeds
	Beans
	Legumes
	Peas
	Nuts
	Bread
	Almonds
	Peanuts
	Lentils
	Chocolate

Moderate Bioavailability (40—60%)

ORGANIC	
Animal	
	Dairy products
	Meat
	Poultry
	Fish
	Egg yolk
	Egg white

High Bioavailability (100%)

INORGANIC	
Additives	
	Chicken nuggets
	Pot pies
	Hot dogs
	Bacon
	Deli meats
	Canned meat
	Processed cheese
	Instant pudding and sauces
	Refrigerated bakery products
	Muffins
	Ready to eat cereal
	Breakfast bars
	Colas
	Fruit juices
	Nestea Cool Iced Tea
	Dry powdered beverages
	Liquid nondairy creamer
	Flavored milk

whole egg contains 6 g of protein and 86 mg of phosphate, whereas an egg white from one large egg contains 4 g of protein and only 5 mg of phosphate [152]. This is one important example of how dietary phosphate and protein can be dissociated, which has important implications for patients undergoing dialysis in whom high protein intake is desirable but must be balanced by avoiding excessive phosphate loading.

Plant-Based Phosphate: The Role of Phytate

A large portion (75%) of the "natural" phosphate in plants is in the storage form of phytic acid or phytate (myo-inositol hexakisphosphate). Humans and animals do not express the enzyme phytase, which is required to break down phytate and release the component phosphate. The bound form of phosphate found in plants is largely unavailable for absorption in humans, as humans have limited capacity to hydrolyze ingested phytate to release the component phosphate for absorption [153]. Despite the high total phosphate content in plant-derived sources, the phosphate bioavailability and actual intestinal phosphate absorption is relatively low. While current estimates suggest that humans absorb approximately 60% of total dietary phosphate intake, this percentage may be substantially lower among vegetarians. Importantly, while many fruits and vegetables contain only small amounts of phosphate, organic phosphate is abundant in some plant seeds, nuts, and legumes. Though much of the phosphate in seeds, nuts, and legumes is phytate-bound and offers a lower fractional rate of intestinal absorption, very large quantities of seeds, nuts and legumes can cause excessive phosphate burden [5].

Inorganic Phosphate

Inorganic phosphate is defined as phosphate which does not naturally occur, but is artificially added during processing in the form of biochemical compounds, such as preservatives and salts. Inorganic sources of phosphate are often added to foods to extend shelf life, improve taste and color. In baked goods, phosphate additives (ammonium phosphate) are added as leavening agents that promote growth of yeast [154]. Inorganic phosphate is commonly found in highly processed, convenience food items, such as frozen meats and dinners, processed meats, spreadable cheeses, dressings, colas, cereals, and bakery items. On food labels, inorganic phosphate is listed in many forms and typically contain the letters "phos" or the words, phosphate or polyphosphates [155] (discussed below).

Bioavailability of Phosphate: Naturally Bound vs. Synthetic Salts

As discussed above, phosphate in food is present either as natural, organic phosphate or synthetic, inorganic phosphate. Depending on the source, the total phosphate content can vary greatly. In addition to the amount of total phosphate, it is crucial to consider which sources offer greater phosphate bioavailability. Sources that offer greater bioavailability can be absorbed in the intestinal tract at a greater proportion than those that offer lower bioavailability. These variations are dependent on the molecular composition of the phosphate ion: protein-bound, phytate-bound or salt-based phosphate. In food sources, such as plants, the organic phosphate ion is mostly phytate-bound, offering lower digestibility, decreased intestinal absorption and lower relative bioavailability. In contrast, animal sources, such as meat, contain organic phosphate ions that are bound to protein or carbon containing molecules, offering greater digestibility, increased intestinal absorption and higher relative bioavailability [156]. Inorganic phosphate in food sources are mostly salt-based additives that readily dissociate as they are not protein-bound; these sources offer high digestibility, increased intestinal absorption and the highest relative bioavailability. In fact, inorganic phosphate is absorbed at nearly 100%, as compared to organic animal-based phosphate at only 40–60%. Organic plant-based food sources are even less bioavailable and are absorbed at only 10–30% [4].

Additives: Revolutions in Technology and Disease

The dramatic evolution in food technology has revolutionized the way in which people produce and consume food. The industrial revolution provided the framework for mass production of commodity-based, convenience foods by developing ultraprocessed products in place of natural foods [157]. The modernized world of ultraprocessed foods offers attractive advantages; they are accessible, palatable and require little to no preparation.

Phosphoric acid, a derivative of elemental phosphate that is converted to synthetic phosphate compounds, is commonly used in the processing of food sources to extend shelf life, improve taste and color and as leavening agents (Table 20.2). Meat producers are increasingly adding these artificial compounds to the meats for preservation, enhanced appearance and flavor. Beverages are often produced with inorganic phosphate to improve flavor. Yet, individual packages of the same product may contain divergent amounts of inorganic phosphate, depending on the specific formula used at

TABLE 20.2 Hidden Phosphate Additives on Food Labels [175]

Phosphate Additives			
Phosphate Salt	**Alternate Names**	**Function**	**Product**
Disodium phosphate	Sodium phosphate; dibasic; DSP/A; disodium monohydrogen; orthophosphate; disodium monophosphate	Texturizer	Imitation cheese, buttermilk
Monosodium phosphate	Monosodium dihydrogen orthophosphate; sodium phosphate disbasic	Emulsifier	Sports drink, whole egg
Potassium tripolyphosphate	Pentapostassium triphosphate; KTPP	Moisture retention	Poultry products
Sodium acid pyrophosphate	SAPP; disodium dihydrogen pyrophosphate; acid sodium pyrophosphate	Color	French fries, instant mashed potatoes
Sodium hexametaphosphate	HMP; sodium polyphosphate; Graham's salt	Reduce purge, emulsifier	Frozen fish fillet
Sodium tripolyphosphate	Sodium triphosphate; pentasodium triphosphate; STPP; STP	Flavor enhancer	Instant noodles, reduced sodium meats
Tetrasodium pyrophosphate	Sodium pyrophosphate; tetrasodium diphosphate; sodium diphosphate; TSPP	Moisture retention	Sausage, deli meats
Trisodium triphosphate	Sodium phosphate; tribasic; TSP; TSPA; trisodium monophosphate	Antimicrobial	Cheese

various manufacturing companies. Another challenge associated with processing is the addition of yeast, a leavening agent that contains phytase, which provides the necessary enzyme to release phosphate from plant-based foods [154]. As a result, intestinal phosphate absorption increases from foods that otherwise would have low phosphate bioavailability. Thus, individual food choices have a major impact on phosphate consumption, and a disproportionate amount of the phosphate load come from inorganic sources of phosphate. Consequently, diets that consist predominately of convenience, processed foods and fast foods may increase dietary phosphate intake by an additional 1000 mg/day [149]. Further, a diet consisting of mostly processed foods will result in higher total phosphate absorption and will provide a higher fractional phosphate excretion than a diet of similar phosphate content, but primarily fresh, unprocessed foods [149]. Therefore, consideration of inorganic phosphate is necessary when evaluating dietary intake.

Inadequacy of Food Labels and Nutritional Software

A vital tool in controlling dietary consumption is the listing of content on the nutrition facts panel of a food label. However, foods sold in the United States are not required to list the phosphate content on the label [149], and fast food and restaurant consumption make it even more difficult to determine the amount of phosphate in food [158]. Some manufacturers voluntarily quantify the phosphate content on labels. It is reflective of both organic and inorganic sources of phosphate, which do not offer the same amount of phosphate bioavailability. An accurate system to differentiate between organic and inorganic forms of phosphate in food is not currently available. The only means of identifying phosphate-containing food sources is the ingredient list on the food label. Due to the multitude of phosphate-additive names that can appear on a given food label, an average patient with CKD may find it difficult to select low phosphate food items. Many products identify phosphate-containing foods only as "enhanced" and do not list components of the "enhancement" solution, often phosphate-based, further complicating the issue [26,158]. The scope of this dilemma has been highlighted through chemical analyses of a number of common food items, with results showing that actual phosphate contents and estimates predicted by nutrient databases or product labels varied widely [159,160]. Strict regulations for product labeling of phosphate content, specifically phosphate-containing additives used in the preparation and package of food items, are needed to overcome this problem.

In addition to hindering the clinical management of CKD patients, the lack of reliable dietary assessment tools that capture both organic and inorganic dietary phosphate intake presents an obstacle in the research community. The nutrition databases generated by the United States of Department of Agriculture contain incomplete data on additive-based phosphate because the Food and Drug Administration does not mandate food manufacturers to disclose on food labels the amount of phosphate additives they use [161]. As dietary intake of phosphate in the form of additives is not accounted and phosphate additives are more readily absorbed from the gastrointestinal tract than organic forms, actual dietary phosphate exposure can differ vastly from estimated intake. This discrepancy is especially accentuated among individuals who consume large amounts of the highly processed foods that contain the most additives, most notably minorities and the poor.

Non-Western Vegetarian Diet: The Best of Both Worlds

The approach of reducing global phosphate intake should probably shift to emphasizing and optimizing the type, source and bioavailability of dietary phosphate that is consumed. Evidence has shown that restricting dietary phosphate intake in combination with phosphate binders may decrease the phosphate burden, even in the setting of normal serum phosphate [135]. However, adherence to this strategy is difficult because protein sources contain high amounts of phosphate. Thus, higher protein intake is associated with greater phosphate intake [5], and dietary phosphate restriction often necessitates reduction in protein intake. Reduction in dietary protein intake is undesirable in many clinical settings, such as ESRD, because it can contribute to protein wasting and perhaps, decreased survival in dialysis patients [162]. Therefore, there is a need to dissociate phosphate and protein content in foods. The phosphate (mg) to protein (g) ratio may be a more appropriate measure than absolute phosphate content to optimize protein intake while minimizing phosphate intake. The phosphate to protein ratio highlights foods high in phosphate but similar in protein content and foods that have low phosphate and high protein contents. Noori et al. recommend a phosphate to protein ratio of less than 10 mg/g, for example, egg whites without additives that contain a ratio of 2 mg/g [4,5].

Grain-based vegetarian diets also have a desirable phosphate to protein ratio because a large portion of the phosphate is phytate-bound and not absorbed. Animal studies showed that rats with CKD fed a grain-based vegetarian diet compared with standard meat-based, synthetic casein diets had lower serum phosphate, urinary phosphate excretion and FGF-23 levels [151]. A small human study of nine CKD participants with mean eGFR of 32.3 mL/min/1.72 m^2, mean serum phosphate of 3.5 mg/dL, and mean FGF-23 of

78 RU/mL demonstrated significant clinical differences between grain-based vegetarian and meat based diets. One week of a grain-based diet led to a 9% decline in serum phosphate and a 27% decrease in FGF-23 levels. This study demonstrated a high correlation between 24-hour fractional excretion of phosphate and 2-hour fasting urine collection among those consuming the grain-based vegetarian diet but not with those on the meat-based diet. This preliminary evidence suggests that grain-based vegetarian sources of protein may be advantageous for CKD patients [156]. In light of these findings, a strategy of selectively replacing food sources with high phosphate bioavailability, such as enhanced meats, with those of modest phytate content, like organic plant sources, may be efficacious in limiting dietary phosphate absorption while balancing protein intake. Safe and effective use of dietary phosphate interventions may theoretically reduce risks of CKD progression, adverse cardiovascular outcomes and may have an important public health role. Larger studies that follow patients over time are necessary to confirm the effectiveness of an organic plant-based diet and to evaluate the sustainability of this approach.

Potential Interactions: Phosphate and Other Nutrients

It is important to consider the interactions of phosphate with other food components, which can alter the net absorption of phosphate and other significant nutrients in the intestine. In addition to diminished phosphate bioavailability in plant-based diets, the phytic acid in these foods can also form insoluble complexes with other essential minerals, such as magnesium, zinc, and iron, reducing net intestinal absorption of these minerals and potentially exacerbating deficiency in CKD. Studies have demonstrated that the fractional absorption of these minerals are inhibited by phytic acid [163–165]. Optimally designed diets with maximal molar ratios of phytate to essential minerals are necessary to avoid side effects, and further studies are necessary to determine a dose-dependent relationship. A second crucial component to consider is the relative amount of calcium in the diet. Dietary calcium intake likely influences the intestinal absorption of dietary phosphate through molecular bonds and the formation of insoluble calcium phosphate salts, which are not well absorbed. The absorptive flux of the calcium to phosphate ratio acts in concert with available calcitriol [111]. Metabolic balance studies of normal individuals have demonstrated significant reduction in intestinal phosphate absorption when patients were administered over 1000 mg per day of calcium [166]. In CKD, high intake of calcium-based binders prevent phosphate absorption from diets of moderate phosphate intake [167]. Additionally, in states of 1,25D deficiency

diminished intestinal calcium absorption will result in greater intestinal availability of calcium, which will complex with phosphate and thereby further decrease dietary phosphate absorption, leading to increased stool excretion of phosphate [15].

QUESTIONS AND CONTROVERSIES

Despite an extensive body of basic and epidemiologic research that supports disordered phosphate metabolism and FGF-23 excess as potential targets for interventions in CKD, gaps in fundamental knowledge of pathophysiology remain, and hard clinical data are lacking to support use of existing therapies. These questions and resulting controversies are briefly summarized below.

The first area of confusion centers on the overall assessment of mineral balance in patients with CKD. Though phosphate retention and positive calcium balance are assumed to be common complications of progressive kidney disease, detailed balance studies performed before calcium-based binders and vitamin D analogs were available suggest otherwise [15,168]. Indeed, these studies show that phosphate balance was negative in patients with advanced CKD, a finding recently confirmed in three patients with stage 3–4 CKD, in whom phosphate balance was estimated to be −167 mg/24 h [169]. Comprehensive data on such assessments in the current era across the full spectrum of CKD are not available; instead, there are studies limited to evaluations of individual components of mineral handling. Findings from these studies and from experiments conducted in animal models of CKD reveal important alterations in homeostatic processes involved in regulation of mineral balance, such as dietary phosphate absorption [43,170]. These changes can affect the interpretation of results in studies of mineral metabolism in CKD. For example, if one performs a study in patients with CKD, in whom he or she believes, based on assumptions derived from study of normal physiology, that 60% of dietary phosphate should be excreted in the urine, but the findings show that only 50% of intake is excreted, then the investigator is tempted to conclude that there is phosphate retention. However, the alternate explanation for the findings could be diminished dietary phosphate absorption in CKD due to 1,25D deficiency. This scenario demonstrates that reliance on assumptions for the relationship between urinary output and estimated dietary intake that are extrapolated from balance studies performed in the steady state assessment of balance in healthy individuals can lead to inaccurate conclusions in CKD.

Lack of a definitive assessment of mineral balance across the spectrum of CKD and the potential impact of available treatments on mineral balance has compounded the debate about binder choice. In addition to paucity of data from randomized controlled trials on patient-level hard clinical outcomes with phosphate binders, to date, there is no information on what different phosphate binders accomplish with respect to overall mineral balance. Do calcium-based binders lead to positive calcium balance in CKD? Is there a threshold effect at a specific dose? Does the impact on calcium balance vary according to CKD stage? What happens to phosphate balance with use of any phosphate binder? How effective is dietary phosphate restriction in impacting phosphate balance? If effective in the short-term, is dietary phosphate restriction feasible in the long-term? These important questions remain unanswered.

Use of active vitamin D and its analogs also generates uncertainty. Though the newer analogs were designed to have less calcemic and phosphatemic actions, hypercalcemia and hyperphosphatemia still occur with use of these agents. Questions regarding effects on calcium and phosphate balance in CKD of these newer analogs alone and in combination with different phosphate binders have not been addressed.

Another important area that remains under investigation is the initial stimulus for FGF-23 secretion in CKD. While human physiologic studies have shown that increased dietary phosphate intake over several days leads to elevated FGF-23 levels, the role of diet in increased FGF-23 secretion in CKD remains poorly defined. Only a single study to date has shown that 2 weeks of increased dietary phosphate intake in CKD stage 3—4 results in FGF-23 elevation [135]. However, it remains uncertain whether stimuli other than dietary phosphate intake can induce osteocytes to increase FGF-23 production. For example, whether minute changes in serum phosphate are sensed at the level of bone is not clear. Alternatively, other messengers yet to be discovered may exist.

The role of klotho in FGF-23 secretion also remains poorly defined in CKD. Trans-membrane klotho is the co-receptor for FGF-23 in the kidney and parathyroid glands [34]. Although renal klotho expression is reduced in animal models of CKD [51], it is unknown if this induces renal resistance to FGF-23 leading to elevated FGF-23 (primacy of klotho), or if elevated FGF-23 reduces klotho expression (primacy of FGF-23). Furthermore, no studies examined klotho levels as a risk factor for CKD outcomes.

While controversial due to lack of randomization, treatment of ESRD and CKD patients with active vitamin D is associated with a survival benefit compared with no treatment [171,172]. Calcitriol stimulates FGF-23 secretion and thus, treating dialysis patients with active vitamin D would be expected to raise FGF-23 levels. This presents a possible paradox: elevated FGF-23 is associated with mortality, yet active vitamin D, which raises FGF-23, is associated with survival. Several explanations could reconcile these findings. Active vitamin D could raise FGF-23 in ESRD [139], but since levels are already >100-fold above normal, further elevation might be clinically insignificant. Second, just as the PTH response to active vitamin D varies across patients, the FGF-23 response is likely also variable. Thus, active vitamin D-treated patients who do well on dialysis may be those who exhibit a modest FGF-23 response to treatment, whereas those who die early despite therapy may exhibit a greater increase in FGF-23. Third, active vitamin D therapy conferred a survival benefit despite its tendency to also raise serum phosphate, which is associated with mortality [76,173]. Similarly, the effect of FGF-23 on mortality could be modified by treatment with active vitamin D: although a higher baseline FGF-23 is a risk factor for mortality, the incremental risk of a further modest increase due to active vitamin D therapy could be outweighed by the other benefits of therapy [174]. Research is needed to untangle these possibilities.

CONCLUSIONS

A substantial body of observational data has now established phosphate and FGF-23 excess as strong independent risk factors for adverse outcomes in CKD. Additional studies are needed to evaluate the efficacy of existing and novel pharmacological and dietary interventions to safely modify phosphate and FGF-23 excess and to determine whether these strategies will improve hard clinical end points in CKD.

Acknowledgments

TI was supported by NIH grant K23DK087858. MW was supported by NIH grants R01DK076116 and R01DK081374.

DISCLOSURES

Dr. Wolf has served as a consultant or received honoraria from Abbott Laboratories, Amgen, Ardelyx, Baxter, Cytochroma, Davita, Genzyme, Lutipold, Novartis, Mitsubishi and Shire. Dr. Isakova has served as a consultant or received honoraria from Genzyme and Shire.

References

[1] Phosphorus Krafft F. From elemental light to chemical element. Angew Chem Int Ed Engl 1969 Sep;8(9):660—71.
[2] USGS Minerals Information: Phosphate Rock. Phosphate Rock Statistics and Information 2011 [cited 19.08.11]. Available from: http://minerals.usgs.gov/minerals/pubs/commodity/phosphate_rock/

[3] Boaz M, Smetana S. Regression equation predicts dietary phosphorus intake from estimate of dietary protein intake. J Am Diet Assoc. 1996 Dec;96(12):1268−70.

[4] Noori N, Sims JJ, Kopple JD, Shah A, Colman S, Shinaberger CS, et al. Organic and inorganic dietary phosphorus and its management in chronic kidney disease. Iran J Kidney Dis 2010 Apr;4(2):89−100.

[5] Kalantar-Zadeh K, Gutekunst L, Mehrotra R, Kovesdy CP, Bross R, Shinaberger CS, et al. Understanding sources of dietary phosphorus in the treatment of patients with chronic kidney disease. Clin J Am Soc Nephrol 2010 Mar;5(3):519−30.

[6] Kutchal H. The Gastrointestinal System: Digestion and Absorption. In: Berne R, Levy MN, Koeppen BM, Stanton BA, editors. Physiology. 5th ed. Philadelphia: Elsevier; 2004. p. 595−622.

[7] Moe SM. Disorders Involving Calcium, Phosphorus, and Magnesium. In: Lerma E, editor. Kidney Disease and Hypertension, Part I. Elsevier Inc.; 2008. p. 215−38.

[8] Favus M, Bushinsky DA, Lemann J. Regulation of Calcium, Magnesium, and Phosphate Metabolism. In: Christakos S, Holick MF, editors. Primer on the Metabolic Bone Diseases and Disorders of Mineral Metabolism. 6th ed. Washington, DC: American Society for Bone and Mineral Research; 2006. p. 76−83.

[9] Kestenbaum B. Phosphate metabolism in the setting of chronic kidney disease: significance and recommendations for treatment. Seminars in dialysis 2007 Jul-Aug;20(4):286−94.

[10] Isakova T, Gutierrez O, Shah A, Castaldo L, Holmes J, Lee H, et al. Postprandial mineral metabolism and secondary hyperparathyroidism in early CKD. J Am Soc Nephrol 2008 Mar;19(3):615−23.

[11] Walling MW. Intestinal Ca and phosphate transport: differential responses to vitamin D3 metabolites. Am J Physiol 1977 Dec;233(6):E488−94.

[12] Radanovic T, Wagner CA, Murer H, Biber J. Regulation of intestinal phosphate transport. I. Segmental expression and adaptation to low-P(i) diet of the type IIb Na(+)-P(i) cotransporter in mouse small intestine. Am J Physiol Gastrointest Liver Physiol 2005 Mar;288(3):G496−500.

[13] Stauber A, Radanovic T, Stange G, Murer H, Wagner CA, Biber J. Regulation of intestinal phosphate transport. II. Metabolic acidosis stimulates Na(+)-dependent phosphate absorption and expression of the Na(+)-P(i) cotransporter NaPi-IIb in small intestine. Am J Physiol Gastrointest Liver Physiol 2005 Mar;288(3):G501−6.

[14] Uribarri J. Phosphorus homeostasis in normal health and in chronic kidney disease patients with special emphasis on dietary phosphorus intake. Seminars in dialysis 2007 Jul-Aug;20(4):295−301.

[15] Liu SH, Chu HI. Studies on calcium and phosphorus metabolism with special reference to pathogenesis and effect of dihydrotachysterol (A.T. 10) and iron. Medicine 1943;22:103−61.

[16] Amanzadeh J, Reilly Jr RF. Hypophosphatemia: an evidence-based approach to its clinical consequences and management. Nat Clin Pract Nephrol 2006 Mar;2(3):136−48.

[17] Marks J, Srai SK, Biber J, Murer H, Unwin RJ, Debnam ES. Intestinal phosphate absorption and the effect of vitamin D: a comparison of rats with mice. Exp Physiol 2006 May;91(3):531−7.

[18] Forster IC, Virkki L, Bossi E, Murer H, Biber J. Electrogenic kinetics of a mammalian intestinal type IIb Na(+)/P(i) cotransporter. J Membr Biol. 2006;212(3):177−90.

[19] Villa-Bellosta R, Sorribas V. Role of rat sodium/phosphate cotransporters in the cell membrane transport of arsenate. Toxicol Appl Pharmacol 2008 Oct 1;232(1):125−34.

[20] Sabbagh Y, Giral H, Caldas Y, Levi M, Schiavi SC. Intestinal phosphate transport. Adv Chronic Kidney Dis 2011 Mar;18(2):85−90.

[21] Xu H, Collins JF, Bai L, Kiela PR, Ghishan FK. Regulation of the human sodium-phosphate cotransporter NaP(i)-IIb gene promoter by epidermal growth factor. Am J Physiol Cell Physiol 2001 Mar;280(3):C628−36.

[22] Miyamoto K, Ito M, Kuwahata M, Kato S, Segawa H. Inhibition of intestinal sodium-dependent inorganic phosphate transport by fibroblast growth factor 23. Ther Apher Dial 2005 Aug;9(4):331−5.

[23] Segawa H, Kaneko I, Yamanaka S, Ito M, Kuwahata M, Inoue Y, et al. Intestinal Na-P(i) cotransporter adaptation to dietary P(i) content in vitamin D receptor null mice. Am J Physiol Renal Physiol 2004 Jul;287(1):F39−47.

[24] Marks J, Debnam ES, Unwin RJ. Phosphate homeostasis and the renal-gastrointestinal axis. Am J Physiol Renal Physiol 2010 Aug;299(2):F285−96.

[25] Katai K, Miyamoto K, Kishida S, Segawa H, Nii T, Tanaka H, et al. Regulation of intestinal Na+-dependent phosphate co-transporters by a low-phosphate diet and 1,25-dihydroxy-vitamin D3. Biochem J 1999 Nov 1;343(Pt 3):705−12.

[26] Gutierrez OM, Wolf M. Dietary phosphorus restriction in advanced chronic kidney disease: merits, challenges, and emerging strategies. Seminars in dialysis 2010 Jul-Aug;23(4):401−6.

[27] Wolf M. Forging forward with 10 burning questions on FGF-23 in kidney disease. J Am Soc Nephrol 2010 Sep;21(9):1427−35.

[28] Shimada T, Yoneya T, Hino R, Takeuchi Y, Fukumoto S, Yamashita T. Transgenic mice expressing FGF-23 demonstrate hypophosphatemia with low serum 1,25-dihydroxyvitamin D and rickets/osteomalacia. J Bone Miner Res. 2001;16:S151.

[29] Larsson T, Marsell R, Schipani E, Ohlsson C, Ljunggren O, Tenenhouse HS, et al. Transgenic mice expressing fibroblast growth factor 23 under the control of the alpha1(I) collagen promoter exhibit growth retardation, osteomalacia, and disturbed phosphate homeostasis. Endocrinology 2004 Jul;145(7):3087−94.

[30] Shimada T, Muto T, Urakawa I, Yoneya T, Yamazaki Y, Okawa K, et al. Mutant FGF-23 responsible for autosomal dominant hypophosphatemic rickets is resistant to proteolytic cleavage and causes hypophosphatemia in vivo. Endocrinology 2002 Aug;143(8):3179−82.

[31] Saito H, Kusano K, Kinosaki M, Ito H, Hirata M, Segawa H, et al. Human fibroblast growth factor-23 mutants suppress Na+-dependent phosphate co-transport activity and 1alpha,25-dihydroxyvitamin D3 production. J Biol Chem. 2003 Jan 24;278(4):2206−11.

[32] Sitara D, Razzaque MS, Hesse M, Yoganathan S, Taguchi T, Erben RG, et al. Homozygous ablation of fibroblast growth factor-23 results in hyperphosphatemia and impaired skeletogenesis, and reverses hypophosphatemia in Phex-deficient mice. Matrix Biol. 2004 Nov;23(7):421−32.

[33] Benet-Pages A, Orlik P, Strom TM, Lorenz-Depiereux B. An FGF-23 missense mutation causes familial tumoral calcinosis with hyperphosphatemia. Hum Mol Genet. 2005 Feb 1;14(3):385−90.

[34] Urakawa I, Yamazaki Y, Shimada T, Iijima K, Hasegawa H, Okawa K, et al. Klotho converts canonical FGF receptor into a specific receptor for FGF-23. Nature 2006 Dec 7;444(7120):770−4.

[35] Shimada T, Kakitani M, Yamazaki Y, Hasegawa H, Takeuchi Y, Fujita T, et al. Targeted ablation of Fgf23 demonstrates an essential physiological role of FGF-23 in phosphate and vitamin D metabolism. J Clin Invest 2004;113(4):561−8.

[36] Shimada T, Hasegawa H, Yamazaki Y, Muto T, Hino R, Takeuchi Y, et al. FGF-23 is a potent regulator of vitamin D metabolism and phosphate homeostasis. J Bone Miner Res. 2004;19(3):429−35.

[37] Kronenberg HM. NPT2a − the key to phosphate homeostasis. N Engl J Med 2002 Sep 26;347(13):1022−4.

[38] Ben-Dov IZ, Galitzer H, Lavi-Moshayoff V, Goetz R, Kuro-o M, Mohammadi M, et al. The parathyroid is a target organ for FGF-23 in rats. J Clin Invest 2007 Dec;117(12):4003−8.

[39] Burnett SM, Gunawardene SC, Bringhurst FR, Juppner H, Lee H, Finkelstein JS. Regulation of C-terminal and intact FGF-23 by dietary phosphate in men and women. J Bone Miner Res. 2006 Aug;21(8):1187−96.

[40] Ferrari SL, Bonjour JP, Rizzoli R. FGF-23 relationship to dietary phosphate and renal phosphate handling in healthy young men. J Clin Endocrinol Metab 2004 Dec 21.

[41] Liu S, Tang W, Zhou J, Stubbs JR, Luo Q, Pi M, et al. Fibroblast growth factor 23 is a counter-regulatory phosphaturic hormone for vitamin D. J Am Soc Nephrol 2006 May;17(5):1305−15.

[42] Lavi-Moshayoff V, Wasserman G, Meir T, Silver J, Naveh-Many T. PTH increases FGF-23 gene expression and mediates the high-FGF-23 levels of experimental kidney failure: a bone parathyroid feedback loop. Am J Physiol Renal Physiol 2010 Oct;299(4):F882−9.

[43] Isakova T, Wahl P, Vargas GS, Gutierrez OM, Scialla J, Xie H, et al. Fibroblast growth factor 23 is elevated before parathyroid hormone and phosphate in chronic kidney disease. Kidney Int 2011 Jun;79(12):1370−8.

[44] Craver L, Marco MP, Martinez I, Rue M, Borras M, Martin ML, et al. Mineral metabolism parameters throughout chronic kidney disease stages 1−5 − achievement of K/DOQI target ranges. Nephrol Dial Transplant 2007 Apr;22(4):1171−6.

[45] Levin A, Bakris GL, Molitch M, Smulders M, Tian J, Williams LA, et al. Prevalence of abnormal serum vitamin D, PTH, calcium, and phosphorus in patients with chronic kidney disease: results of the study to evaluate early kidney disease. Kidney Int 2007 Jan;71(1):31−8.

[46] Gutierrez O, Isakova T, Rhee E, Shah A, Holmes J, Collerone G, et al. Fibroblast growth factor-23 mitigates hyperphosphatemia but accentuates calcitriol deficiency in chronic kidney disease. J Am Soc Nephrol 2005 Jul;16(7):2205−15.

[47] Hasegawa H, Nagano N, Urakawa I, Yamazaki Y, Iijima K, Fujita T, et al. Direct evidence for a causative role of FGF-23 in the abnormal renal phosphate handling and vitamin D metabolism in rats with early-stage chronic kidney disease. Kidney Int 2010 Nov;78(10):975−80.

[48] Isakova T, Wolf MS. FGF-23 or PTH: which comes first in CKD? Kidney Int 2010 Nov;78(10):947−9.

[49] Pavik I, Jaeger P, Kistler AD, Poster D, Krauer F, Cavelti-Weder C, et al. Patients with autosomal dominant polycystic kidney disease have elevated fibroblast growth factor 23 levels and a renal leak of phosphate. Kidney Int 2011 Jan;79(2):234−40.

[50] Pereira RC, Juppner H, Azucena-Serrano CE, Yadin O, Salusky IB, Wesseling-Perry K. Patterns of FGF-23, DMP1, and MEPE expression in patients with chronic kidney disease. Bone 2009 Dec;45(6):1161−8.

[51] Kuro-o M. Klotho in chronic kidney disease − what's new? Nephrol Dial Transplant 2009 Jun;24(6):1705−8.

[52] Samadfam R, Richard C, Nguyen-Yamamoto L, Bolivar I, Goltzman D. Bone formation regulates circulating concentrations of fibroblast growth factor 23. Endocrinology 2009 Nov;150(11):4835−45.

[53] Galitzer H, Ben-Dov IZ, Silver J, Naveh-Many T. Parathyroid cell resistance to fibroblast growth factor 23 in secondary hyperparathyroidism of chronic kidney disease. Kidney Int 2010 Feb;77(3):211−8.

[54] Komaba H, Goto S, Fujii H, Hamada Y, Kobayashi A, Shibuya K, et al. Depressed expression of Klotho and FGF receptor 1 in hyperplastic parathyroid glands from uremic patients. Kidney Int 2010 Feb;77(3):232−8.

[55] Isakova T, Gutierrez OM, Wolf M. A blueprint for randomized trials targeting phosphorus metabolism in chronic kidney disease. Kidney Int 2009 Oct;76(7):705−16.

[56] Gutierrez OM, Mannstadt M, Isakova T, Rauh-Hain JA, Tamez H, Shah A, et al. Fibroblast growth factor 23 and mortality among patients undergoing hemodialysis. N Engl J Med 2008 Aug 7;359(6):584−92.

[57] Isakova T, Xie H, Barchi-Chung A, Vargas G, Sowden N, Houston J, et al. Fibroblast growth factor 23 in patients undergoing peritoneal dialysis. Clin J Am Soc Nephrol 2011 Nov;6(11):2688−95.

[58] Wesseling-Perry K, Pereira RC, Sahney S, Gales B, Wang HJ, Elashoff R, et al. Calcitriol and doxercalciferol are equivalent in controlling bone turnover, suppressing parathyroid hormone, and increasing fibroblast growth factor-23 in secondary hyperparathyroidism. Kidney Int 2011 Jan;79(1):112−9.

[59] Larsson T, Nisbeth U, Ljunggren O, Juppner H, Jonsson KB. Circulating concentration of FGF-23 increases as renal function declines in patients with chronic kidney disease, but does not change in response to variation in phosphate intake in healthy volunteers. Kidney Int 2003 Dec;64(6):2272−9.

[60] Shimada T, Urakawa I, Isakova T, Yamazaki Y, Epstein M, Wesseling-Perry K, et al. Circulating fibroblast growth factor 23 in patients with end-stage renal disease treated by peritoneal dialysis is intact and biologically active. J Clin Endocrinol Metab 2010 Feb;95(2):578−85.

[61] Viaene L, Bammens B, Meijers BK, Vanrenterghem Y, Vanderschueren D, Evenepoel P. Residual renal function is an independent determinant of serum FGF-23 levels in dialysis patients. Nephrol Dial Transplant 2011 Oct 24.

[62] Ambuhl PM, Meier D, Wolf B, Dydak U, Boesiger P, Binswanger U. Metabolic aspects of phosphate replacement therapy for hypophosphatemia after renal transplantation: impact on muscular phosphate content, mineral metabolism, and acid/base homeostasis. Am J Kidney Dis 1999;34(5):875−83.

[63] Levi M. Post-transplant hypophosphatemia. Kidney Internat 2001;59(6):2377−87.

[64] Felsenfeld AJ, Gutman RA, Drezner M, Llach F. Hypophosphatemia in long-term renal transplant recipients: effects on bone histology and 1,25-dihydroxycholecalciferol. Mineral & Electrolyte Metab 1986;12(5-6):333−41.

[65] Parfitt AM, Kleerekoper M, Cruz C. Reduced phosphate reabsorption unrelated to parathyroid hormone after renal transplantation: implications for the pathogenesis of hyperparathyroidism in chronic renal failure. Mineral & Electrolyte Metab 1986;12(5-6):356−62.

[66] Green J, Debby H, Lederer E, Levi M, Zajicek HK, Bick T. Evidence for a PTH-independent humoral mechanism in post-transplant hypophosphatemia and phosphaturia. Kidney Internat 2001;60(3):1182−96.

[67] Riancho JA, de Francisco AL, del Arco C, Amado JA, Cotorruelo JG, Arias M, et al. Serum levels of 1,25-dihydroxy-vitamin D after renal transplantation. Min Electrol Metab 1988;14(6):332−7.

[68] Steiner RW, Ziegler M, Halasz NA, Catherwood BD, Manolagas S, Deftos LJ. Effect of daily oral vitamin D and calcium therapy, hypophosphatemia, and endogenous 1-25 dihydroxycholecalciferol on parathyroid hormone and

phosphate wasting in renal transplant recipients. Transplantation 1993;56(4):843—6.

[69] Seeherunvong W, Wolf M. Tertiary excess of fibroblast growth factor 23 and hypophosphatemia following kidney transplantation. Pediatr Transplant 2011 Feb;15(1):37—46.

[70] Bhan I, Shah A, Holmes J, Isakova T, Gutierrez O, Burnett SM, et al. Post-transplant hypophosphatemia: Tertiary 'Hyper-Phosphatoninism'? Kidney Int 2006 Oct;70(8):1486—94.

[71] Sirilak S, Chatsrisak K, Ingsathit A, Kantachuvesiri S, Sumethkul V, Stitchantrakul W, et al. Renal phosphate loss in long-term kidney transplantation. Clin J Am Soc Nephrol 2012 Feb;7(2):323—31.

[72] Evenepoel P, Meijers BK, de Jonge H, Naesens M, Bammens B, Claes K, et al. Recovery of hyperphosphatoninism and renal phosphorus wasting one year after successful renal transplantation. Clin J Am Soc Nephrol 2008 Nov;3(6):1829—36.

[73] Go AS, Chertow GM, Fan D, McCulloch CE, Hsu CY. Chronic kidney disease and the risks of death, cardiovascular events, and hospitalization. N Engl J Med 2004 Sep 23;351(13): 1296—305.

[74] Landray MJ, Emberson JR, Blackwell L, Dasgupta T, Zakeri R, Morgan MD, et al. Prediction of ESRD and death among people with CKD: the Chronic Renal Impairment in Birmingham (CRIB) prospective cohort study. Am J Kidney Dis 2010 Dec;56(6):1082—94.

[75] Block GA, Klassen PS, Lazarus JM, Ofsthun N, Lowrie EG, Chertow GM. Mineral metabolism, mortality, and morbidity in maintenance hemodialysis. J Am Soc Nephrol 2004 Aug;15(8): 2208—18.

[76] Kalantar-Zadeh K, Kuwae N, Regidor DL, Kovesdy CP, Kilpatrick RD, Shinaberger CS, et al. Survival predictability of time-varying indicators of bone disease in maintenance hemodialysis patients. Kidney Int 2006 Aug;70(4):771—80.

[77] Kestenbaum B, Sampson JN, Rudser KD, Patterson DJ, Seliger SL, Young B, et al. Serum phosphate levels and mortality risk among people with chronic kidney disease. J Am Soc Nephrol 2005 Feb;16(2):520—8.

[78] Tonelli M, Sacks F, Pfeffer M, Gao Z, Curhan G. Relation between serum phosphate level and cardiovascular event rate in people with coronary disease. Circulation 2005 Oct 25;112(17):2627—33.

[79] Strozecki P, Adamowicz A, Nartowicz E, Odrowaz-Sypniewska G, Wlodarczyk Z, Manitius J. Parathormon, calcium, phosphorus, and left ventricular structure and function in normotensive hemodialysis patients. Ren Fail. 2001 Jan;23(1):115—26.

[80] Goodman WG, Goldin J, Kuizon BD, Yoon C, Gales B, Sider D, et al. Coronary-artery calcification in young adults with end-stage renal disease who are undergoing dialysis. N Engl J Med 2000 May 18;342(20):1478—83.

[81] Jono S, McKee MD, Murry CE, Shioi A, Nishizawa Y, Mori K, et al. Phosphate regulation of vascular smooth muscle cell calcification. Circ Res. 2000 Sep 29;87(7):E10—7.

[82] Blacher J, Guerin AP, Pannier B, Marchais SJ, London GM. Arterial calcifications, arterial stiffness, and cardiovascular risk in end-stage renal disease. Hypertension 2001 Oct;38(4):938—42.

[83] Cozzolino M, Brancaccio D, Gallieni M, Slatopolsky E. Pathogenesis of vascular calcification in chronic kidney disease. Kidney Int 2005 Aug;68(2):429—36.

[84] Moe SM, O'Neill KD, Reslerova M, Fineberg N, Persohn S, Meyer CA. Natural history of vascular calcification in dialysis and transplant patients. Nephrol Dial Transplant 2004 Sep;19(9):2387—93.

[85] Adeney KL, Siscovick DS, Ix JH, Seliger SL, Shlipak MG, Jenny NS, et al. Association of serum phosphate with vascular and valvular calcification in moderate CKD. J Am Soc Nephrol 2008 Dec 10.

[86] Galetta F, Cupisti A, Franzoni F, Femia FR, Rossi M, Barsotti G, et al. Left ventricular function and calcium phosphate plasma levels in uraemic patients. J Intern Med 2005 Oct;258(4): 378—84.

[87] Culleton BF, Walsh M, Klarenbach SW, Mortis G, Scott-Douglas N, Quinn RR, et al. Effect of frequent nocturnal hemodialysis vs conventional hemodialysis on left ventricular mass and quality of life: a randomized controlled trial. JAMA 2007 Sep 19;298(11):1291—9.

[88] Isakova T, Gutierrez OM, Chang Y, Shah A, Tamez H, Smith K, et al. Phosphorus binders and survival on hemodialysis. J Am Soc Nephrol 2009 Feb;20(2):388—96.

[89] Kovesdy CP, Kuchmak O, Lu JL, Kalantar-Zadeh K. Outcomes associated with phosphorus binders in men with non-dialysis-dependent CKD. Am J Kidney Dis 2010 Nov;56(5):842—51.

[90] Schwarz S, Trivedi BK, Kalantar-Zadeh K, Kovesdy CP. Association of disorders in mineral metabolism with progression of chronic kidney disease. Clin J Am Soc Nephrol 2006 Jul;1(4): 825—31.

[91] Voormolen N, Noordzij M, Grootendorst DC, Beetz I, Sijpkens YM, Manen JG, et al. High plasma phosphate as a risk factor for decline in renal function and mortality in pre-dialysis patients. Nephrol Dial Transplant 2007 Oct;22(10):2909—16.

[92] Norris KC, Greene T, Kopple J, Lea J, Lewis J, Lipkowitz M, et al. Baseline predictors of renal disease progression in the African American Study of Hypertension and Kidney Disease. J Am Soc Nephrol 2006 Oct;17(10):2928—36.

[93] Haut LL, Alfrey AC, Guggenheim S, Buddington B, Schrier N. Renal toxicity of phosphate in rats. Kidney Int 1980 Jun;17(6):722—31.

[94] Barsotti G, Giannoni A, Morelli E, Lazzeri M, Vlamis I, Baldi R, et al. The decline of renal function slowed by very low phosphorus intake in chronic renal patients following a low nitrogen diet. Clinical Nephrology 1984 Jan;21(1):54—9.

[95] Zoccali C, Ruggenenti P, Perna A, Leonardis D, Tripepi R, Tripepi G, et al. Phosphate may promote CKD progression and attenuate renoprotective effect of ACE inhibition. J Am Soc Nephrol 2011 Oct;22(10):1923—30.

[96] Cunningham J, Locatelli F, Rodriguez M. Secondary hyperparathyroidism: pathogenesis, disease progression, and therapeutic options. Clin J Am Soc Nephrol 2011 Apr;6(4):913—21.

[97] Mak RH, Turner C, Thompson T, Powell H, Haycock GB, Chantler C. Suppression of secondary hyperparathyroidism in children with chronic renal failure by high dose phosphate binders: calcium carbonate versus aluminium hydroxide. Br Med J (Clin Res Ed) 1985 Sep 7;291(6496):623—7.

[98] Portale AA, Booth BE, Halloran BP, Morris Jr RC. Effect of dietary phosphorus on circulating concentrations of 1,25-dihydroxyvitamin D and immunoreactive parathyroid hormone in children with moderate renal insufficiency. J Clin Invest 1984 Jun;73(6):1580—9.

[99] Markowitz M, Rotkin L, Rosen JF. Circadian rhythms of blood minerals in humans. Science (New York, NY 1981 Aug 7;213(4508):672—4.

[100] Isakova T, Xie H, Yang W, Xie D, Anderson AH, Scialla J, et al. Fibroblast growth factor 23 and risks of mortality and end-stage renal disease in patients with chronic kidney disease. JAMA 2011 Jun 15;305(23):2432—9.

[101] Parker BD, Schurgers LJ, Brandenburg VM, Christenson RH, Vermeer C, Ketteler M, et al. The associations of fibroblast growth factor 23 and uncarboxylated matrix Gla protein with mortality in coronary artery disease: the Heart and Soul Study. Ann Intern Med 2010 May 18;152(10):640—8.

[102] Wolf M, Molnar MZ, Amaral AP, Czira ME, Rudas A, Ujszaszi A, et al. Elevated fibroblast growth factor 23 is a risk factor for kidney transplant loss and mortality. J Am Soc Nephrol 2011 May;22(5):956—66.

[103] Kendrick J, Cheung AK, Kaufman JS, Greene T, Roberts WL, Smits G, et al. FGF-23 associates with death, cardiovascular events, and initiation of chronic dialysis. J Am Soc Nephrol 2011 Oct;22(10):1913—22.

[104] Fliser D, Kollerits B, Neyer U, Ankerst DP, Lhotta K, Lingenhel A, et al. Fibroblast growth factor 23 (FGF-23) predicts progression of chronic kidney disease: the Mild to Moderate Kidney Disease (MMKD) Study. J Am Soc Nephrol 2007 Sep;18(9):2600—8.

[105] Titan SM, Zatz R, Graciolli FG, Dos Reis LM, Barros RT, Jorgetti V, et al. FGF-23 as a predictor of renal outcome in diabetic nephropathy. Clin J Am Soc Nephrol 2011 Feb;6(2):241—7.

[106] Semba RD, Fink JC, Sun K, Cappola AR, Dalal M, Crasto C, et al. Serum fibroblast growth factor-23 and risk of incident chronic kidney disease in older community-dwelling women. Clin J Am Soc Nephrol 2012 Jan;7(1):85—91.

[107] Seiler S, Reichart B, Roth D, Seibert E, Fliser D, Heine GH. FGF-23 and future cardiovascular events in patients with chronic kidney disease before initiation of dialysis treatment. Nephrol Dial Transplant 2010 Dec;25(12):3983—9.

[108] Taylor EN, Rimm EB, Stampfer MJ, Curhan GC. Plasma fibroblast growth factor 23, parathyroid hormone, phosphorus, and risk of coronary heart disease. Am Heart J 2011 May;161(5):956—62.

[109] Seiler S, Cremers B, Rebling NM, Hornof F, Jeken J, Kersting S, et al. The phosphatonin fibroblast growth factor 23 links calcium-phosphate metabolism with left-ventricular dysfunction and atrial fibrillation. Eur Heart J 2011 Nov;32(21):2688—96.

[110] Ford ML, Smith ER, Tomlinson LA, Chatterjee PK, Rajkumar C, Holt SG. FGF23 and osteoprotegerin are independently associated with myocardial damage in chronic kidney disease stages 3 and 4. Another link between chronic kidney disease-mineral bone disorder and the heart. Nephrol Dial Transplant 2012 Feb;27(2):727—33.

[111] Hsu HJ, Wu MS. Fibroblast growth factor 23: a possible cause of left ventricular hypertrophy in hemodialysis patients. The American Journal of the Medical Sciences 2009 Feb;337(2):116—22.

[112] Gutierrez OM, Januzzi JL, Isakova T, Laliberte K, Smith K, Collerone G, et al. Fibroblast growth factor 23 and left ventricular hypertrophy in chronic kidney disease. Circulation 2009 May 19;119(19):2545—52.

[113] Mirza MA, Larsson A, Melhus H, Lind L, Larsson TE. Serum intact FGF-23 associate with left ventricular mass, hypertrophy and geometry in an elderly population. Atherosclerosis 2009 Dec;207(2):546—51.

[114] Canziani ME, Tomiyama C, Higa A, Draibe SA, Carvalho AB. Fibroblast growth factor 23 in chronic kidney disease: bridging the gap between bone mineral metabolism and left ventricular hypertrophy. Blood Purif 2011;31(1-3):26—32.

[115] Kirkpantur A, Balci M, Gurbuz OA, Afsar B, Canbakan B, Akdemir R, et al. Serum fibroblast growth factor-23 (FGF-23) levels are independently associated with left ventricular mass and myocardial performance index in maintenance haemodialysis patients. Nephrol Dial Transplant 2011 Apr;26(4):1346—54.

[116] Faul C, Amaral AP, Oskouei B, Hu MC, Sloan A, Isakova T, et al. FGF-23 induces left ventricular hypertrophy. J Clin Invest 2011 Nov 1;121(11):4393—408.

[117] Silberberg JS, Barre PE, Prichard SS, Sniderman AD. Impact of left ventricular hypertrophy on survival in end-stage renal disease. Kidney Int 1989 Aug;36(2):286—90.

[118] Levy D, Garrison RJ, Savage DD, Kannel WB, Castelli WP. Prognostic implications of echocardiographically determined left ventricular mass in the Framingham Heart Study. N Engl J Med 1990 May 31;322(22):1561—6.

[119] Roos M, Lutz J, Salmhofer H, Luppa P, Knauss A, Braun S, et al. Relation between plasma fibroblast growth factor-23, serum fetuin-A levels and coronary artery calcification evaluated by multislice computed tomography in patients with normal kidney function. Clinical Endocrinology 2008 Apr;68(4):660—5.

[120] Inaba M, Okuno S, Imanishi Y, Yamada S, Shioi A, Yamakawa T, et al. Role of fibroblast growth factor-23 in peripheral vascular calcification in non-diabetic and diabetic hemodialysis patients. Osteoporos Int 2006 Oct;17(10):1506—13.

[121] Srivaths PR, Goldstein SL, Silverstein DM, Krishnamurthy R, Brewer ED, Elevated FGF. 23 and phosphorus are associated with coronary calcification in hemodialysis patients. Pediatr Nephrol 2011 Jun;26(6):945—51.

[122] Mirza MA, Larsson A, Lind L, Larsson TE. Circulating fibroblast growth factor-23 is associated with vascular dysfunction in the community. Atherosclerosis 2009 Aug;205(2):385—90.

[123] Mirza MA, Hansen T, Johansson L, Ahlstrom H, Larsson A, Lind L, et al. Relationship between circulating FGF-23 and total body atherosclerosis in the community. Nephrol Dial Transplant 2009 Oct;24(10):3125—31.

[124] Desjardins L, Liabeuf S, Renard C, Lenglet A, Lemke HD, Choukroun G, et al. FGF-23 is independently associated with vascular calcification but not bone mineral density in patients at various CKD stages. Osteoporos Int 2012 Jul;23(7):2017—25.

[125] Nakanishi S, Kazama JJ, Nii-Kono T, Omori K, Yamashita T, Fukumoto S, et al. Serum fibroblast growth factor-23 levels predict the future refractory hyperparathyroidism in dialysis patients. Kidney Int 2005 Mar;67(3):1171—8.

[126] Kazama JJ, Sato F, Omori K, Hama H, Yamamoto S, Maruyama H, et al. Pretreatment serum FGF-23 levels predict the efficacy of calcitriol therapy in dialysis patients. Kidney Int 2005 Mar;67(3):1120—5.

[127] Sato T, Tominaga Y, Ueki T, Goto N, Matsuoka S, Katayama A, et al. Total parathyroidectomy reduces elevated circulating fibroblast growth factor 23 in advanced secondary hyperparathyroidism. Am J Kidney Dis 2004 Sep;44(3):481—7.

[128] Wesseling-Perry K, Pereira RC, Wang H, Elashoff RM, Sahney S, Gales B, et al. Relationship between plasma fibroblast growth factor-23 concentration and bone mineralization in children with renal failure on peritoneal dialysis. J Clin Endocrinol Metab 2009 Feb;94(2):511—7.

[129] Komaba H, Fukagawa M. FGF-23-parathyroid interaction: implications in chronic kidney disease. Kidney Int 2010 Feb;77(4):292—8.

[130] Manghat P, Fraser WD, Wierzbicki AS, Fogelman I, Goldsmith DJ, Hampson G. Fibroblast growth factor-23 is associated with C-reactive protein, serum phosphate and bone mineral density in chronic kidney disease. Osteoporos Int 2010 Nov;21(11):1853—61.

[131] Ashikaga E, Honda H, Suzuki H, Hosaka N, Hirai Y, Sanada D, et al. Impact of fibroblast growth factor 23 on lipids and atherosclerosis in hemodialysis patients. Ther Apher Dial 2010 Jun;14(3):315—22.

[132] Chertow GM, Levin NW, Beck GJ, Depner TA, Eggers PW, Gassman JJ, et al. In-center hemodialysis six times per week versus three times per week. N Engl J Med 2010 Dec 9;363(24):2287—300.

[133] Tonelli M, Pannu N, Manns B. Oral phosphate binders in patients with kidney failure. N Engl J Med 2010 Apr 8;362(14):1312—24.

[134] Sprague SM, Abboud H, Qiu P, Dauphin M, Zhang P, Finn W. Lanthanum carbonate reduces phosphorus burden in patients with CKD stages 3 and 4: a randomized trial. Clin J Am Soc Nephrol 2009 Jan;4(1):178—85.

[135] Isakova T, Gutierrez OM, Smith K, Epstein M, Keating LK, Juppner H, et al. Pilot study of dietary phosphorus restriction and phosphorus binders to target fibroblast growth factor 23 in patients with chronic kidney disease. Nephrol Dial Transplant 2011 Feb;26(2):584—91.

[136] Oliveira RB, Cancela AL, Graciolli FG, Dos Reis LM, Draibe SA, Cuppari L, et al. Early control of PTH and FGF-23 in normophosphatemic CKD patients: a new target in CKD-MBD therapy? Clin J Am Soc Nephrol 2010 Feb;5(2):286—91.

[137] Gonzalez-Parra E, Gonzalez-Casaus ML, Galan A, Martinez-Calero A, Navas V, Rodriguez M, et al. Lanthanum carbonate reduces FGF-23 in chronic kidney disease Stage 3 patients. Nephrol Dial Transplant 2011 Aug;26(8):2567—71.

[138] Koiwa F, Kazama JJ, Tokumoto A, Onoda N, Kato H, Okada T, et al. Sevelamer hydrochloride and calcium bicarbonate reduce serum fibroblast growth factor 23 levels in dialysis patients. Ther Apher Dial 2005 Aug;9(4):336—9.

[139] Nishi H, Nii-Kono T, Nakanishi S, Yamazaki Y, Yamashita T, Fukumoto S, et al. Intravenous calcitriol therapy increases serum concentrations of fibroblast growth factor-23 in dialysis patients with secondary hyperparathyroidism. Nephron 2005;101(2):c94—9.

[140] Wetmore JB, Liu S, Krebill R, Menard R, Quarles LD. Effects of cinacalcet and concurrent low-dose vitamin D on FGF-23 levels in ESRD. Clin J Am Soc Nephrol 2010 Jan;5(1):110—6.

[141] Koizumi M, Komaba H, Nakanishi S, Fujimori A, Fukagawa M. Cinacalcet treatment and serum FGF-23 levels in haemodialysis patients with secondary hyperparathyroidism. Nephrol Dial Transplant 2011 Jul 5.

[142] Block GA, Martin KJ, de Francisco AL, Turner SA, Avram MM, Suranyi MG, et al. Cinacalcet for secondary hyperparathyroidism in patients receiving hemodialysis. N Engl J Med 2004 Apr 8;350(15):1516—25.

[143] Takeda Y, Komaba H, Goto S, Fujii H, Umezu M, Hasegawa H, et al. Effect of intravenous saccharated ferric oxide on serum FGF-23 and mineral metabolism in hemodialysis patients. Am J Nephrol 2011;33(5):421—6.

[144] Schouten BJ, Hunt PJ, Livesey JH, Frampton CM, Soule SG. FGF-23 elevation and hypophosphatemia after intravenous iron polymaltose: a prospective study. J Clin Endocrinol Metab 2009 Jul;94(7):2332—7.

[145] Farrow EG, Yu X, Summers LJ, Davis SI, Fleet JC, Allen MR, et al. Iron deficiency drives an autosomal dominant hypophosphatemic rickets (ADHR) phenotype in fibroblast growth factor-23 (Fgf23) knock-in mice. Proc Natl Acad Sci USA 2011 Nov 15;108(46):E1146—55.

[146] Imel EA, Peacock M, Gray AK, Padgett LR, Hui SL, Econs MJ. Iron modifies plasma FGF-23 differently in autosomal dominant hypophosphatemic rickets and healthy humans. J Clin Endocrinol Metab 2011 Nov;96(11):3541—9.

[147] Martin KJ, Bell G, Huang S, Pickthorn K, Kaskas MO, Bernardo M, et al. The effect of KAI-4169, a novel treatment for chronic kidney disease-mineral and bone disorder, on serum phosphorus kinetics post-hemodialysis [Abstract]. J Am Soc Nephrol 2011;22:398A.

[148] Schiavi SC, Tang W, Bracken C, O'Brien SP, Song W, Boulanger J, et al. Npt2b deletion attenuates hyperphosphatemia associated with CKD. J Am Soc Nephrol 2012 Oct;23(10):1691—700.

[149] Uribarri J, Calvo MS. Hidden sources of phosphorus in the typical American diet: does it matter in nephrology? Seminars in dialysis 2003 May-Jun;16(3):186—8.

[150] Karp HJ, Vaihia KP, Karkkainen MU, Niemisto MJ, Lamberg-Allardt CJ. Acute effects of different phosphorus sources on calcium and bone metabolism in young women: a whole-foods approach. Calcif Tissue Int 2007 Apr;80(4):251—8.

[151] Moe SM, Chen NX, Seifert MF, Sinders RM, Duan D, Chen X, et al. A rat model of chronic kidney disease-mineral bone disorder. Kidney Int 2009 Jan;75(2):176—84.

[152] Taylor LM, Kalantar-Zadeh K, Markewich T, Colman S, Benner D, Sim JJ, et al. Dietary egg whites for phosphorus control in maintenance haemodialysis patients: a pilot study. J Ren Care 2011 Mar;37(1):16—24.

[153] Iqbal TH, Lewis KO, Cooper BT. Phytase activity in the human and rat small intestine. Gut 1994 Sep;35(9):1233—6.

[154] Food Ingredient and Color: International Food Information Council (IFIC) and U.S. Food and Drug Administration. Types of Food Ingredients 2010 [cited 2011 December 7]. Available from: www.fda.gov/food/foodingredientspackaging/ucm094211.htm#types

[155] Sullivan C, Sayre SS, Leon JB, Machekano R, Love TE, Porter D, et al. Effect of food additives on hyperphosphatemia among patients with end-stage renal disease: a randomized controlled trial. JAMA 2009 Feb 11;301(6):629—35.

[156] Moe SM, Zidehsarai MP, Chambers MA, Jackman LA, Radcliffe JS, Trevino LL, et al. Vegetarian compared with meat dietary protein source and phosphorus homeostasis in chronic kidney disease. Clin J Am Soc Nephrol 2011 Feb;6(2):257—64.

[157] Ludwig DS. Technology, diet, and the burden of chronic disease. JAMA 2011 Apr 6;305(13):1352—3.

[158] Sullivan CM, Leon JB, Sehgal AR. Phosphorus-containing food additives and the accuracy of nutrient databases: implications for renal patients. J Ren Nutr 2007 Sep;17(5):350—4.

[159] Sherman RA, Mehta O. Phosphorus and potassium content of enhanced meat and poultry products: implications for patients who receive dialysis. Clin J Am Soc Nephrol 2009 Aug;4(8):1370—3.

[160] Oenning LL, Vogel J, Calvo MS. Accuracy of methods estimating calcium and phosphorus intake in daily diets. J Am Diet Assoc 1988 Sep;88(9):1076—80.

[161] Karalis M, Murphy-Gutekunst L. Patient education. Enhanced foods: hidden phosphorus and sodium in foods commonly eaten. J Ren Nutr 2006 Jan;16(1):79—81.

[162] Shinaberger CS, Greenland S, Kopple JD, Van Wyck D, Mehrotra R, Kovesdy CP, et al. Is controlling phosphorus by decreasing dietary protein intake beneficial or harmful in persons with chronic kidney disease? Am J Clin Nutr 2008 Dec;88(6):1511—8.

[163] Bohn T, Davidsson L, Walczyk T, Hurrell RF. Phytic acid added to white-wheat bread inhibits fractional apparent magnesium absorption in humans. Am J Clin Nutr 2004 Mar;79(3):418—23.

[164] Hallberg L, Rossander L, Skanberg AB. Phytates and the inhibitory effect of bran on iron absorption in man. Am J Clin Nutr 1987 May;45(5):988—96.

[165] Turnlund JR, King JC, Keyes WR, Gong B, Michel MC. A stable isotope study of zinc absorption in young men: effects of phytate and alpha-cellulose. Am J Clin Nutr 1984 Nov;40(5):1071—7.

[166] Spencer H, Kramer L, Norris C, Osis D. Effect of calcium and phosphorus on zinc metabolism in man. Am J Clin Nutr 1984 Dec;40(6):1213—8.

[167] Schiller LR, Santa Ana CA, Sheikh MS, Emmett M, Fordtran JS. Effect of the time of administration of calcium acetate on phosphorus binding. N Engl J Med 1989 Apr 27;320(17):1110—3.

[168] Litzow JR, Lemann Jr J, Lennon EJ. The effect of treatment of acidosis on calcium balance in patients with chronic azotemic renal disease. J Clin Invest 1967 Feb;46(2):280—6.

[169] Hill KM, Martin B, Moe SM, McCabe GP, Weaver CM, Peacock M. Effect of calcium carbonate supplement on phosphate balance and homeostasis in patients with stage 3 and 4 chronic kidney Disease [Abstract]. J Am Soc Nephrol 2011;22:4A.

[170] Moe SM, Radcliffe JS, White KE, Gattone 2nd VH, Seifert MF, Chen X, et al. The pathophysiology of early stage chronic kidney disease-mineral bone disorder (CKD-MBD) and response to phosphate binders in the rat. J Bone Miner Res 2011 Nov;26(11):2672—81.

[171] Teng M, Wolf M, Lowrie E, Ofsthun N, Lazarus JM, Thadhani R. Survival of patients undergoing hemodialysis with paricalcitol or calcitriol therapy. N Engl J Med 2003 Jul 31;349(5):446—56.

[172] Shoben AB, Rudser KD, de Boer IH, Young B, Kestenbaum B. Association of oral calcitriol with improved survival in nondialyzed CKD. J Am Soc Nephrol 2008 Aug;19(8):1613—9.

[173] Teng M, Wolf M, Ofsthun MN, Lazarus JM, Hernan MA, Camargo Jr CA, et al. Activated injectable vitamin D and hemodialysis survival: a historical cohort study. J Am Soc Nephrol 2005 Apr;16(4):1115—25.

[174] Holick MF. Vitamin D deficiency. N Engl J Med 2007 Jul 19;357(3):266—81.

[175] Murphy-Gutekunst L, Uribarri J. Hidden Phosphorus-Enhanced Meats: Part 3. J Ren Nutr 2005;15(4):E1—4.

Vitamin D in Kidney Disease

Marta Christov, Ravi Thadhani

Division of Endocrinology, Massachusetts General Hospital and Department of Medicine,
Harvard Medical School, Boston, MA, USA

NORMAL VITAMIN D METABOLISM

Synthesis and Breakdown of Vitamin D

Vitamins are a class of organic compounds essential for the survival of an organism. In most cases they must be obtained from the diet. Vitamin D is unusual among vitamins in that it can also be synthesized in the body. In the skin, UV light converts 7-dehydrocholesterol to cholecalciferol (Vitamin D_3) (Figure 21.1). Generically, the term "Vitamin D" refers to a group of related compounds, which include cholecalciferol (Vitamin D_3), as well as ergocalciferol (Vitamin D_2), a plant- and fungal-derived calciferol. Cholecalciferol and ergocalciferol are inactive precursors that must undergo further modification and are sometimes referred to as "nutritional vitamin D". Both in vivo (D_3) and nutritionally obtained (D_2, D_3) calciferols undergo hydroxylation at the 25th carbon, primarily in the liver, to become 25-hydroxyvitamin D (25OH D), also known as calcidiol (25OH D_2 is ercalcidiol; in this chapter "calcidiol" will refer to both D_2 and D_3 25-hydroxylated compounds). Several cytochrome P450 enzymes can catabolize this hydroxylation step, including CYP2R (in testes, skin, ubiquitous), CYP27A1 (in liver, intestine), CYP2J2 (in liver, heart, brain), and CYP3A4 (in liver, intestine) [1]. Calcidiol (25OH D) is a prohormone that needs further modification via hydroxylation at the 1st carbon to yield 1,25(OH)$_2$ dihydroxyvitamin D (1,25OH$_2$ D), or calcitriol, the active hormone. This latter reaction is catalyzed by the enzyme 1-α hydroxylase (a product of the gene CYP27B1), which is most abundantly, but not exclusively found in the kidney. 1-α-hydroxylase synthesis is regulated by parathyroid hormone (PTH), calcium, phosphorus, fibroblast growth factor 23 (FGF23), estrogen, calcitonin and 1,25OH$_2$ D [2].

Both 25OH D and 1,25OH$_2$ D are inactivated by the enzyme 24-hydroxylase (product of the gene CYP24A1),

with 1,25OH$_2$ D being the preferred binding substrate. CYP24A1 is expressed not only in the kidney, but also in multiple other tissues, such as intestine, macrophages, skin, lung, bone, pancreas, ovary, brain, and thyroid [1]. CYP24A1 expression and 24-hydroxylase production are induced most strongly by 1,25OH$_2$ D, as part of a negative feedback loop. PTH and FGF23 also affect CYP24A1 expression. Many other compounds induce CYP24A1, including drugs such as rifampicin, carbamazepine and phenobarbital [1]. CYP24A1 expression is also increased in a number of malignancies, where it is associated with a poor prognosis.

In addition to the kidney, cells from the skin, gastrointestinal tract, immune system, and brain (and others) express the 1-α-hydroxylase enzyme, and are able to produce 1,25OH$_2$ D, albeit at lower concentrations [1]. For example, if the expression of the 1-α-hydroxylase enzyme (by measuring mRNA or protein levels) or activity of the enzyme in kidney tissues is rated as "strong", tissues such as pancreas, colon, brain, placenta, and endothelium have an "intermediate" expression or activity, and tissues such as breast, ovary, parathyroid, and adrenal medulla have a "weak" expression or activity [3]. Importantly, 1-α-hydroxylase expression in these "non-classical" vitamin D-responsive cells is under cell-function specific, rather than mineral-metabolic, control. In monocytes, for example, pathogen exposure triggers 1-α-hydroxylase and VDR expression via toll-like receptors [4]. Given the ubiquitous expression of the vitamin D receptor (VDR), a significant role for autocrine/paracrine actions of 1,25OH$_2$ D has emerged. To what extent local production versus systemic supply of the active hormone accounts for many or all of the effects outside the mineral metabolism axis discussed in this chapter is not yet clear.

In the circulation, both 25OH D and 1,25OH$_2$ D exist in protein-bound forms, largely to albumin or vitamin D binding protein (DBP), with a very small

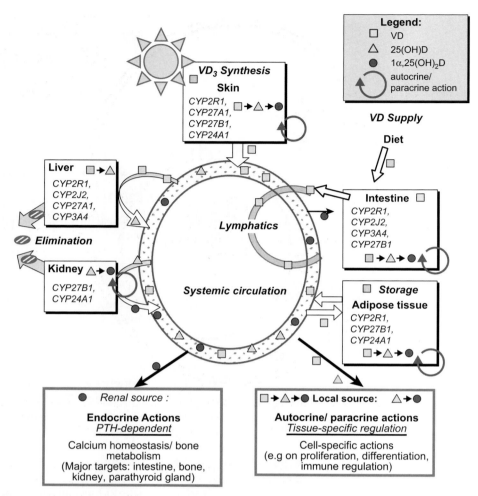

FIGURE 21.1 Vitamin D metabolites in the circulation and enzymes from the vitamin D synthetic pathway at major sites of endocrine and autocrine/paracrine functions of $1,25OH_2$ D. Note that many locations can synthesize $1,25OH_2$ D from its precursors. CYP2R1, CYP2J2, CYP27A1 and CYP3A4 can synthesize 25OH D. CYP27B1 synthesizes $1,25OH_2$ D and CYP24A1 degrades both 25OH D and $1,25OH_2$ D. Red arrows denote tissues that can respond to $1,25OH_2$ D, red circles, $1,25OH_2$ D and yellow triangles, 25OH D. *(Reprinted, with permission from Schuster, 2011.)* This figure is reproduced in color in the color plate section.

unbound (free) fraction. 25OH D bound to DBP is filtered in the urine and reuptake via the megalin/cubilin system in the proximal tubule ensures intracellular delivery of 25OH D as a substrate for 1-α-hydroxylase. Disruption of the reuptake system leads to loss of DBP in the urine and, in some animal models, vitamin D deficiency [5]. Mice with a genetic deletion of DBP, however, are normocalcemic and have normal tissue levels of $1,25OH_2$ D despite immeasurable serum levels of the hormone and prohormone, suggesting that DBP may serve as a serum "storage" form of 25OH D [6]. The total amount of DBP capable of binding 25OH D, as well as the affinity of DBP for 25OH D may be important modifiers of total 25OH D levels with respect to tissue levels effects [7,8].

Actions of $1,25OH_2$ D

$1,25OH_2$ D functions classically as a nuclear hormone. It enters the nucleus where it binds to the vitamin D receptor

(VDR). The VDR complexes with the retinoic acid X receptor (RXR) to form a heterodimer able to recognize specific DNA sequences known as vitamin D response elements (VDREs). When the $1,25OH_2$ D/VDR/RXR complex binds to VDREs, it is able to recruit transcription factors and increase or decrease transcription of genes involved in bone and calcium metabolism, and multitude of signaling pathways affecting cellular proliferation, differentiation, or function (Figure 21.2).

In addition, it has been suggested that $1,25OH_2$ D has rapid, nongenomic effects by activating apical voltage-dependent calcium channels and increasing intracellular calcium, a process that may or may not require the VDR [9]. The nongenomic effects also include triggering of downstream signaling pathways in diverse tissues that affect cell differentiation, apoptosis, and proliferation [10].

In CKD, $1,25OH_2$ D action is impaired due to several mechanisms (Table 21.1). The absolute levels of active

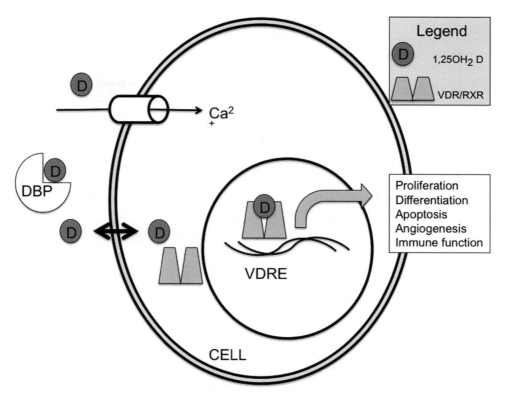

FIGURE 21.2 Cellular actions of 1,25OH$_2$ D, denoted with red circles. 1,25OH$_2$ D has classical gene-regulatory actions mediated by the VDR/RXR complex in the nucleus, which recruits transcriptional activators and remodeling factors upon 1,25OH$_2$ D binding. 1,25OH$_2$ D also acts as non-classical activator of calcium channels in a VDR-independent manner. This figure is reproduced in the color plate section.

hormone are reduced, as highlighted below. Expression of the VDR is most potently upregulated by calcitriol, and thus VDR levels are also reduced with calcitriol deficiency. In addition, VDR/RXR dimerization and target DNA binding, as well as recruitment of transcriptional co-factors are impaired in uremia leading to defects in downstream gene transcription [11].

Classically, vitamin D compounds serve as endocrine hormones to regulate calcium and phosphorus balance, and both directly and indirectly affect parathyroid hormone synthesis and bone turnover. Vitamin D deficiency thus has significant effects on bone metabolism and disease in CKD; these aspects of vitamin D physiology will be reviewed in Chapter 19. Emerging evidence, however, suggests that Vitamin D has physiological effects outside the mineral metabolism axis. Below we will review the alterations in metabolism of vitamin D in CKD, as well as the implications for vitamin D deficiency.

PREVALENCE AND ETIOLOGY OF DEFICIENCY IN THE VITAMIN D AXIS IN CKD

Definitions

We will discuss two forms of vitamin D deficiency: deficiency of the prohormone, 25OH D, and deficiency of the hormone, 1,25OH$_2$ D. As will be discussed below, several potential etiologies may lead to either 25OH D or 1,25OH$_2$ D deficiency, although the former clearly can lead to the latter. The approaches to correction of these deficiencies differ: 25OH D deficiency usually is treated with oral vitamin D precursors, or nutritional vitamin D (cholecalciferol, ergocalciferol), while 1,25OH$_2$ D deficiency can be treated with either versions of the active

TABLE 21.1 Factors and Conditions that Impair 1,25(OH)$_2$ D Synthesis and Activity in CKD

SYNTHESIS
Decreased substrate concentration
Reduced delivery of substrate to tubule cells due to low GFR
Reduced nephron mass
Inhibition of 1-α-hydroxylase by FGF23 or acidosis
Inability of 1-α-hydroxylase to respond to PTH

ACTIVITY
Decreased VDR expression
Decreased VDR/RXR dimerization and target DNA binding

For references and details, see text. FGF23 = fibroblast growth factor 23. VDR = vitamin D receptor. VDR/RXR = VDR receptor complex.

hormone itself (calcitriol, paricalcitol, maxacalcitol), or 1-α-hydroxylated versions of the hormone (doxercalciferol, alphacalcidol) which need to be 25-hydroxylated in the liver [12].

The prevalence of 25OH D deficiency is common in populations with normal renal function [13,14], although it seems to be increased in patients with CKD, potentially due to uremic effects both on production (reduced production in the skin of the precursor, reduced production in the liver of 25OH D) and on catabolism (loss in the urine, increased degradation via 24-hydroxylase enzyme which is upregulated in CKD). Importantly, as the final activation step to make the active $1,25OH_2$ D hormone occurs in the kidney, CKD patients are uniquely susceptible to development of $1,25OH_2$ deficiency.

Prevalence of 25OH D Deficiency

Controversy exists regarding the definition of vitamin 25OH D sufficiency. Generally, 25OH D levels below 30 ng/mL (75 nM) are considered insufficient, and levels below 15 or 20 ng/mL (37.5 or 50 nM) are considered deficient [15]. While the prevalence of 25OH D deficiency is variable across populations and latitudes [13,14], it is increased in CKD and end stage renal disease (ESRD) patients. For example, a cross-sectional study of 201 US patients across latitudes with CKD stage 3 and 4 reported that between 71 and 83% of patients were insufficient for 25OH D [16]. Another cross-sectional study of 160 Canadian patients from a single center reported that 98.7% of individuals were insufficient or deficient for 25OH D [17]; these results are consistent in other reports [18]. In the ESRD population, similar values are reported in PD [19] and HD patients [20,21].

Etiologies: Reduced Precursor and Calcidiol Synthesis (Table 21.2)

Decreased sun exposure likely plays a part in reducing cholecalciferol levels in CKD and ESRD patients. For example, in a CKD population of 144 patients from Brazil, who live in a subtropical area with abundant sunlight, only 39.6% had 25OH D levels <30 ng/mL, compared with >70% of patients in US, Canada or Britain [22]. In the 201 CKD stage 3 and 4 patients from across the US discussed previously, there was a correlation of calcidiol levels with geographic location within the US, with individuals in Florida having higher levels compared with individuals from other sites [16]. However, the change in calcidiol levels in CKD patients between winter and fall (after sun exposure), was modest and may reflect uremic effects on skin

TABLE 21.2   Etiologies for Vitamin D Deficiency in CKD Patients

REDUCED PRECURSOR SYNTHESIS/ABSORPTION

Decreased sun exposure
Decreased synthesis of D3 in skin with age
Decreased synthesis of D3 in skin in uremia
Decreased synthesis of D3 in skin in black people
Decreased absorption from diet high in polyunsaturated fat or fructose

REDUCED CALCITRIOL SYNTHESIS

Decreased conversion to calcidiol in liver in uremia
Decreased delivery of calcidiol to proximal tubule
Decreased uptake of calcidiol by proximal tubule

INCREASED DEGRADATION/LOSS

Increased expression of 24-hydroxylase enzyme
Increased loss in urine or peritoneal fluid (bound to DBP)

For references and details, see text. D3 = cholecalciferol. DBP = vitamin D binding protein.

cholecalciferol production (see below). One possible mechanism for decreased sun exposure aside from geography may be due to decreased overall activity and time spent outside among CKD patients.

With age, the conversion of 7-dehydrocholesterol to cholecalciferol is also impaired, with a 70-year old individual being able to generate only ~25% of the vitamin D_3 that a 20-year-old person makes for the same duration of sun exposure [23]. Since renal dysfunction affects predominantly an older population, decreased precursor synthesis likely contributes to 25OH D deficiency. In addition, the uremic state also impairs the production of cholecalciferol in the skin of dialysis patients, despite normal levels of the precursor 7-dehydrocholesterol, through an unknown mechanism [24].

Other factors identified by epidemiological studies associated with low 25OH D in the CKD and ESRD populations are diabetes, female sex, elevated iPTH levels [21,25], hypoalbuminemia, and black race [26]. Mechanistically, synthesis of cholecalciferol in darker pigmented skin (as present in the African-American population) is reduced presumably due to melanin-related absorption of UV light [23]. Adipose tissue is a potential storage compartment for both 25OH D and $1,25OH2$ D [1]. Interestingly, obesity is also a risk factor for hypovitaminosis D in CKD, although the mechanism for this is not clear [27].

In addition to decreased precursor synthesis in the skin, recent evidence from animal models suggests impaired conversion of cholecalciferol to calcidiol in the uremic state [28]. These investigators found that the ability of liver P450 enzymes to hydroxylate either vitamin D_3 or 1-α-hydroxyvitamin D_3 at the 25th carbon was impaired in the uremic animals, in a PTH-dependent manner; moreover, levels of the P450 isoforms were reduced in this model. Whether similar impairments in hepatic production of calcidiol exist in humans remains to be determined.

Etiologies: Increased Loss or Metabolism (Table 21.2)

Other potential factors leading to low 25OH D levels may be the loss of DBP (and its accompanying 25OH D bound to it) in patients with proteinuria or on peritoneal dialysis [29]. For example, in a multicenter cohort of 1847 patients with early CKD (including diabetics), albuminuria was correlated with low 25OH D and $1,25OH_2$ D levels [30]. In 115 patients with type I diabetes and microalbuminuria, increased urinary loss of DBP correlated with low $1,25OH_2$ D levels [31]. This increased loss may be due to dysfunction of the megalin/cubilin system seen in animals with early diabetic nephropathy and postulated to exist in patients, potentially accounting for increased prevalence of 25OH D deficiency [32]. On the other hand, treatment of 13 patients with CKD with antiproteinuric therapy for 4–6 weeks had no effect on serum total 25OH D, $1,25OH_2$ D or serum levels of DBP, despite a decrease in urinary DBP losses [33]. Thus, the mechanism of vitamin D deficiency in patients with albuminuria or proteinuria remains unclear.

Finally, metabolism of 25OH D may also be increased in CKD [34]. In an animal model of CKD, Helvig et al. reported increased expression of the 24-hydroxylase gene in the kidney [35]. This was also observed in several human biopsies from patients with CKD, suggesting that increased activity of the 24-hydroxylase may contribute to low 25OH D levels by inactivating them. Thus, one would expect that 24-hydroxylated vitamin D compounds would be increased in CKD. Levels of $24,25OH_2$ D (the initial product of 25OH D metabolism) however, have been previously reported low in the CKD and ESRD populations [36,37].

Etiologies: Effect of Diet

Dietary composition may affect overall 25OH D levels. In a 2-year study of 152 individuals without known renal dysfunction, all of whom were receiving 700 IU per day vitamin D_3 supplements, a diet rich in mono-unsaturated fats was associated with an increase in 25OH D levels, while a diet rich in polyunsaturated fats had the opposite effect [38]. Whether similar effects exist in CKD or ESRD patients is not known. CKD and ESRD patients may restrict their diets either due to symptoms of uremia, or on the advice of health care practitioners and thus may potentially affect nutritional vitamin D absorption. The exact mechanism by which dietary fat affects vitamin D supplement or nutritional vitamin D absorption is not clear. Potentially, an oily vehicle for vitamin D supplements leads to better absorption, although the evidence is limited [39]. In addition, in a rat model of CKD, a diet high in fructose was associated with 25OH D insufficiency compared with a diet high in glucose [40]. To what extent the fructose content of an average American diet, lower than the 60% used in the study, has similar effects in patients with CKD is also not clear.

Prevalence and Etiology of $1,25OH_2$ D Deficiency (Figure 21.3)

$1,25OH_2$ D deficiency develops with loss of renal function, with about 30% of patients with CKD stage 3 having levels <30 pg/mL and greater than 80% of patients with stage 4 and 5 CKD being similarly deficient [41]. 25OH D deficiency, as discussed earlier, is common in CKD patients. The contribution of 25OH D to $1,25OH_2$ D levels was illustrated in 5 dialysis patients, where supplementation with 25OH D_3 to achieve serum levels on average of 108 ng/mL over 4 weeks led to tripling and near normalization of $1,25OH_2$ D levels [42].

In addition to prohormone deficiency, loss of nephron mass may contribute to low $1,25OH_2$ D levels by a reduction in the absolute numbers of cells capable of generating $1,25OH_2$ D. In the kidney, $1,25OH_2$ D generation is hampered by reduced delivery of the prohormone 25OH D to the proximal tubule, as GFR decline as well as decrease in the megalin receptor expression are both observed with CKD [11]. The 1-α-hydroxylase enzyme's ability to respond to PTH activation is also impaired, and enzyme expression appears to be further inhibited by acidosis in a PTH-independent manner [11]. Research into the phosphate-regulating hormone FGF23 has added another explanation, whereby the early rise of FGF23 in renal failure acts to inhibit the 1-α-hydroxylase enzyme production [41,43]. This hypothesis is consistent with findings from animal studies, where lack of FGF23 leads to significant up-regulation of the 1-α-hydroxylase gene and elevated $1,25OH_2$ D levels [44]. Finally, loss of vitamin D binding protein in proteinuric renal disease also may contribute to the reduction of $1,25OH_2$ D in some patients.

IMPLICATIONS

Increased Mortality

Altered vitamin D metabolism in the CKD and ESRD populations affects calcium turnover and bone health.

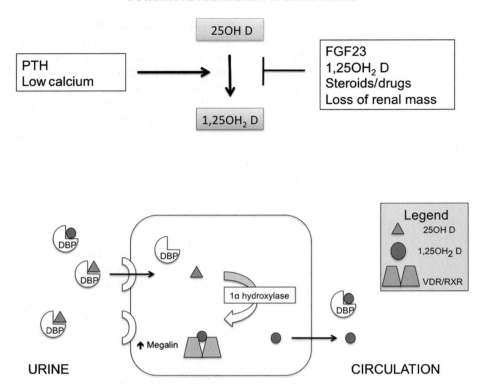

FIGURE 21.3   Factors affecting 1,25OH$_2$ D production. In CKD/ESRD, elevated FGF23 and loss of renal mass likely contribute to the decreased synthesis of 1,25OH$_2$ D. In the lower panel, reduction in 25OHD/DBP delivery to the proximal tubule cell, as well as decrease in the megalin receptor and the 1-α-hydroxylase amount contribute to reduced 1,25OH$_2$ D synthesis. This figure is reproduced in color in the color plate section.

More significantly, vitamin D deficiency (both 25OH D and 1,25OH$_2$ D) has been linked in observational studies with additional patient-level outcomes, such as increased morbidity and mortality. In addition, vitamin D deficiency has been associated with congestive heart failure, hypertension, diabetes, malignancy, and immune function [14]. Given the ubiquitous presence of the vitamin D receptor among cell types, these associations support a tissue-level function for vitamin D outside organismal control of mineral metabolism. In addition, multiple tissues have been found to have low levels of the 1-α-hydroxylase enzyme and may thus participate in local conversion of calcidiol to calcitriol for autocrine or paracrine functions.

A retrospective analysis of patients starting hemodialysis suggested that those with the lowest 25OH D levels (<10 ng/mL) at initiation had an increased risk of all cause mortality compared with those patients who were vitamin D replete [20]. This increased risk of mortality was most evident in those who had received no active vitamin D therapy. In CKD patients, a prospective study also found that low 25OH D levels were an independent predictor of mortality and progression to ESRD [25].

It should be emphasized that the above studies, as well as other studies that will be outlined below, show association between 25OH D deficiency and outcomes but do not prove causation. Thus, in the study above, a patient with a high risk of death may have low 25OH D levels as a secondary phenomenon. The question of whether association indicates causation will not be resolved until prospective interventional studies assess changes in outcomes.

Cardiovascular Effects

In patients without renal dysfunction, vitamin D deficiency is associated with cardiovascular risk factors and increased cardiovascular mortality [45–47]. Similar findings are seen in patients with renal dysfunction. For example, in 230 patients on peritoneal dialysis, 25OH D levels <47.5 nmol/L (~20 ng/mL) were associated with increased cardiovascular events in those with a preserved ejection fraction and/or absence of left ventricular hypertrophy [19]. In 1108 German diabetic dialysis patients, 25OH D deficiency (<25 nmol/L) was associated with a 3 fold increased risk of sudden cardiac death compared to patients who were sufficient; in addition, cardiovascular events and all cause mortality were also increased in this population [48]. And among children with vitamin D deficient rickets, half had echocardiographic changes consistent with LV dysfunction, which resolved after therapy (confounded by hypophosphatemia and hypocalcemia, however) [49].

In addition to being inversely linked to adverse cardiovascular events, 25OH D deficiency has been linked to vessel stiffness and coronary calcifications. For example, among 394 patients with CKD in the multi-ethnic study of atherosclerosis cohort, those with 25OH D levels <15 ng/mL had a trend towards increased incident coronary artery calcification (CAC) scores [50]. In 210 predialysis CKD patients (CKD stage 4 and 5), 25OH D levels were associated with X-ray based calcification scores [51]. In 197 prevalent kidney transplant recipients who had CAC and thoracic aorta calcification assessed on average 4.4 years apart, lower 25OH D levels were associated with CAC progression [52]. Finally, in 43 children with CKD, measurements of peripheral arterial reflective properties (as a surrogate measure of aortic stiffness), correlated negatively with vitamin D levels [53].

Several potential mechanisms may be behind the observed cardiovascular effects. 25OH D is a known regulator of the renin-angiotensin system and treatment with calcitriol leads to renin suppression in wild-type animals [54]. VDR is present on vascular smooth muscle cells (VSMC) and calcitriol can affect VSMC proliferation [55]. VDRA can increase the expression of calcification inhibitors such as matrix-gla protein and osteopontin in vascular cells and decrease the expression of proinflammatory cytokines [56]. Thus, vitamin D may simultaneously modify the VSMC phenotype and dampen the activated renin-angiotensin-aldosterone system (RAAS)'s effects on the vasculature.

Kidney Disease Progression

Low 25OH D levels are also associated with faster progression of CKD. Among 168 CKD patients, 25OH D levels predicted disease progression to ESRD [25]. In NHANES III, 25OH D levels <15 ng/mL were associated with increased risk of incident ESRD, especially in non-Hispanic black people [57]. Finally, among 207 older adults from the Cardiovascular Health Study with initial GFR > 60 mL/min and GFR loss over 4 years of follow-up, those with 25OH D levels <15 ng/mL had 68% greater adjusted risk for rapid GFR loss compared with individuals with 25OH D levels ≥30 ng/mL, independent of serum PTH, calcium or phosphorus [58]. This magnitude of risk was greater than the risk for GFR loss conferred by co-morbidities such as hypertension or diabetes.

A potential mechanism may be the suppressive role that vitamin D plays in regulating the RAAS axis [54], and interfering with the effects of RAAS activation is a proven reno-protective strategy in certain CKD populations. The effect of low 25OH D on GFR loss was strongest among individuals with diabetes [58].

Several animal studies have shown that VDRA therapy in models of diabetic nephropathy can ameliorate disease progression and synergize with angiotensin receptor blockade in reducing proteinuria and reducing glomerular sclerosis [59,60]. In addition to its effect on renin expression, VDRA therapy in animal studies is suggested to have anti-fibrotic as well as anti-proliferative effects, which may contribute to potential renoprotection.

Immune System Effects

Several molecules in the vitamin D pathway, including the 1-α-hydroxylase and the VDR are expressed in macrophages [4], and 1-α-hydroxylase expression is induced in the setting of infection. Specifically, activation of toll-like receptors leads to up-regulation of $1,25OH_2$ D and VDR production. This enables the macrophage to elaborate antimicrobial peptides, such as cathelicidin, which have been shown to have antimicrobial properties. In a retrospective study of maintenance hemodialysis patients, low cathelicidin levels were modestly associated with $1,25OH_2$ D levels and predicted increased infectious disease mortality [61].

Anemia

Anemia is a common complication of late CKD and ESRD, contributing to decreased quality of life, use of recombinant erythropoeisis-stimulating agents, and potentially leading to transfusion dependence. While loss of renal mass and erythropoietin deficiency, iron-deficiency, and increased inflammation are the drivers behind the development of anemia, low vitamin D levels have been recently associated with this as well. In a cross-sectional study of 1661 CKD patients from the SEEK (Study to Evaluate Early Kidney Disease, mean eGFR 47 mL/min) cohort, lower 25OH D levels were associated with lower Hgb [62]. These investigators also found an independent association between Hgb and $1,25OH_2$ D in this population, with an increased prevalence of anemia of 5.4-fold in those patients who had both 25OH D and $1,25OH_2$ D deficiency [62]. In a 106 male patients with diabetic CKD (mean eGFR 55 mL/min), 25OH D levels were also correlated with Hgb independent of albuminuria or eGFR [63]. And, in a retrospective analysis of 142 prevalent hemodialysis patients, Kiss et al. found significant association between 25OH D levels and Hgb [64]. Finally, in a retrospective cohort study of a CKD population of 153 patients, those whose 25OH D levels improved from insufficient into the normal range, had on average a 24% reduction in ESA dose, while those who became

25OH D insufficient had a non-significant increase in ESA dose [65].

Mechanistically, in vitro studies suggest that $1,25OH_2$ D therapy can increase the responsiveness of red cell precursors to erythropoietin by increasing the expression of the erythropoietin receptor and leading to increased proliferation of precursors [66,67]. These observations have been extended to clinical studies, where treatment with calcitriol was shown to increase hemoglobin [68,69].

Given that several studies found independent association of 25OH D deficiency and Hgb, supplementation with $1,25OH_2$vitamin D precursors has also been evaluated. Among 81 prevalent hemodialysis patients, ergocalciferol supplementation over 4 months reduced the ESA dose in 57% of patients, although it increased the ESA dose in 43% [70]. Among a different population of 158 hemodialysis patients, 1 year supplementation with cholecalciferol led to an overall reduced darbopoetin dose, although not increase in the average Hgb levels [71].

Insulin Resistance

Impaired glucose metabolism is frequently found in patients with CKD. Some short-term studies with vitamin D supplementation in dialysis patients have shown increased insulin sensitivity and secretion (reviewed in [72]). In a large cohort of adults, some of whom had impaired renal function (NHANES III), lower 25OH D levels were associated with insulin resistance independent of eGFR [73]. A cross-sectional study of 120 non-diabetic CKD patients found that insulin levels were decreased in patients treated with activated vitamin D [74]. Currently, one study on the effect of 6 month supplementation with cholecalciferol on measures of insulin resistance is ongoing [75].

Neuromuscular Function

Vitamin D deficiency is associated with impairment of muscle function, and meta-analyses have suggested that supplementation with vitamin D can reduce the risk of falls in the elderly [14]. ESRD patients are at increased risk of fractures compared with an age-matched population without impaired renal function, and muscle wasting and weakness may contribute to this increased risk [76]. Decreased calcitriol production may be one mechanism contributing to muscle weakness, as a placebo controlled trial in elderly women with age-related loss of renal function (measured 24 h CrCl < 60 mL/min/1.73 m^2) showed a reduction in falls over 3 years in those women treated with calcitriol irrespective of treatment with hormone replacement therapy [77].

INTERVENTIONS

Definitions

Active vitamin D analogs are compounds that can either activate the VDR or need a non-renal modification via a hydroxylation step at the 25th carbon to become active. The types of vitamin D preparations, both active and nutritional available for use in the US (and abroad) are listed in Table 21.3.

Active D Analogs

Effects on Survival

While epidemiological data linking vitamin D deficiency to outcomes is critical for hypothesis generation, interventional studies linked to outcomes provide further evidence of an association. Several studies have shown improved survival in the ESRD population with supplementation with calcitriol or related compounds, also known as vitamin D receptor agonists (VDRA). For example, when examining a historical cohort of over 50,000 incident dialysis patients, Teng et al. found a 20% survival advantage among those who had received VDRAs compared with those who did not [78]. In a subsequent retrospective study, which also was able to look at underlying 25OH D levels, of 1000 patients initiating hemodialysis, Wolf et al. found that all cause mortality was lower in those treated with active D analogs irrespective of underlying 25OH D level [20]. In addition, the

TABLE 21.3   Types of Vitamin D Preparations, Both Active and Nutritional, Available for Use in the US (and Abroad)

Vitamin D Preparations	Type of Analog	Notes (Route of Administration, Brand Name, Availability)
ACTIVE D ANALOGS		
Calcitriol	VDRA, D_3	IV, PO Calcijex, Rocaltrol
Paricalcitol	VDRA, D_2	IV, PO Zemplar
Doxercalciferol	Missing 25(OH), D_2	IV, PO Hectorol
Maxacalcitol	VDRA, D_3	Not available in US
PRECURSORS AND PROHORMONES		
Ergocalciferol	D_2 precursor	Drisdol, generic
Cholecalciferol	D_3 precursor	Calciol, generic
25(OH) vitamin D	D_3 prohormone	Not available in US

Modified, with permission, from Kalantar-Zadeh and Kovesdy, 2009. VDRA = vitamin D receptor agonist.

same investigators found that VDRA therapy abolished the 35% increase in mortality in black incident hemodialysis patients compared with non-hispanic whites [79]. Follow-up randomized trials to further test these hypotheses are pending.

Several VDRAs are currently available for clinical use in the US, including calcitriol, and paricalcitol (maxacalcitol, another VDRA, is not available in the US); doxercalciferol is a 1-α-hydroxylated D_2 derived compound that needs further hydroxylation in the liver and is thus technically a pro-hormone, although will be included in the VDRA group. The main indication for use of VDRAs is treatment of secondary hyperparathyroidism and all are able to suppress PTH levels, although with different frequency of side-effects [80]. However, these compounds appear non-equivalent in their effects on pathways other than the PTH axis. For example, one retrospective study looking at survival of dialysis patients treated with calcitriol vs. paricalcitol found decreased mortality in the patients treated with paricalcitol [81]. This observation was subsequently confirmed in a different dialysis population of 7731 patients followed for a median of 3 years [82]. This study also found that doxercalciferol appeared identical to paricalcitol with respect to its effect on mortality.

Effects on Cardiovascular Function

The potential mechanisms of improved mortality may involve beneficial effects of vitamin D on cardiovascular function. This is suggested because animals deficient either for the VDR or for the 1-α-hydroxylase gene develop cardiac hypertrophy, which in the latter study was rescued by exogenous $1,25OH_2$ D administration [83,84]. In addition, in hypertensive rats, paricalcitol reduced left ventricular abnormalities and improved diastolic function [85]. And in humans, in 15 patients with ESRD, calcitriol infusion leading to partial reduction of PTH led to reversal of myocardial hypertrophy [86].

However, one study in nephrectomized animals suggested that VDRA administration increases vascular calcification [87] independent of effects on the calcium-phosphate product. This has been followed by a study in children with ESRD suggesting that elevated $1,25OH_2$ D levels were associated with increased carotid intima-media thickness and calcification score [88,89]. In the PRIMO study, which randomized 227 stage 3 and 4 CKD patients to 2 μg paricalcitol or placebo, there was no reduction in left ventricular mass index by cardiac MRI or in standard measures of diastolic function by echocardiogram, however cardiac related hospitalizations were fewer in the treated group after 48 weeks [90]. Finally, in the ADVANCE study, which assessed CAC scores in 360 hemodialysis patients randomized to cinacalcet plus low dose calcitriol or paricalcitol

versus a flexible VDRA dose, there was a trend towards a smaller increase in the CAC score in the group assigned to less total VDRA exposure (the cinacalcet group), compared with the flexible VDRA group after 52 weeks [91]; however, it is not clear that VDRA doses achieved were significantly different. Thus, treatment with VDRAs may have a U-shaped effect on cardiovascular disease and outcome in patients with kidney failure, with either too little, or too much VDRAs having adverse consequences.

Effects on Proteinuria

Building on small trials that examined the effect of VDRAs on proteinuria in CKD patients [92–94], the Vitamin D Receptor Activator for Albuminuria Lowering (VITAL) study randomized 281 patients with diabetic CKD and albuminuria to two doses of daily oral paricalcitol vs. placebo [95]. After 24 weeks, only the higher paricalcitol dose significantly lowered albuminuria. This change was associated with blood pressure lowering, as well as stable GFR lowering, both of which returned towards baseline during the withdrawal phase of the trial [95]. The mechanism of GFR lowering was not clear, but the authors postulate it may be related to the effect of VDRAs on creatinine metabolism. While encouraging, these results highlight the limitations of VDRA therapy, as a higher number of adverse events and study withdrawals occurred in the high paricalcitol group.

Effects on the Immune System

Given the expression of vitamin D metabolism pathway genes in immune cells, and the correlation of low vitamin D levels with infectious susceptibility, the effect of both VDRA and vitamin D precursor supplementation on immune function in the CKD/ESRD populations is of great interest. One group of investigators showed that paricalcitol therapy increased the proportion of "inflammatory" peripheral monocytes expressing high levels of the VDR (and thus showing vitamin D responsiveness) among seven ESRD patients [96]. Recently, another group using a retrospective study of 508 Japanese prevalent hemodialysis patients assessed hospitalization rates for acute respiratory infections over an average of 5 years [97]. While only 11% of patients experienced the primary outcome over that time, the incidence of hospitalization was lower among those who had been treated with VDRAs compared to those who had not been.

25OHD

Cholecalciferol or ergocalciferol (precursor) supplementation has also been explored in the CKD and

ESRD populations, given the wide expression of the 1-α-hydroxylase enzyme, with an expectation of affecting local, tissue-level conversion to calcitriol. In addition, several studies have shown that precursor supplementation can increase serum levels of 1,25OH$_2$ D in hemodialysis patients, presumably via nonrenal 1-α-hydroxylation, since this effect was observed even in nephrectomized individuals [98,99].

Recently, Bhan and colleagues found that ergocalciferol supplementation and correction of underlying 25OH D deficiency can boost cathelicidin levels in healthy adults [100]. Cholecalciferol and paricalcitol therapy in seven ESRD patients decreased inflammatory cytokines and increased calcitriol-responsive gene expression in peripheral blood monocytes [96]. Whether these changes in immune system molecules (cytokines) and cells (monocytes) lead to patient-level benefit in the ESRD population is the subject of active investigation in the DIVINE trial, where 25OH D deficient incident hemodialysis patients are treated with ergocalciferol for 12 weeks and measures of immune fitness, such as cathelicidin levels, as well as infectious, cardiovascular, and all-cause complications and mortality assessed (www.clinicaltrials.gov NCT00892099).

Cholecalciferol supplementation also may decrease the need for VDRA and phosphate binder therapy, as was shown in a study of 158 prevalent hemodialysis patients. After one year of cholecalciferol, serum levels of phosphate decreased, and serum 25OH D and 1,25OH$_2$ D increased, leading to fewer patients on sevelamer and paricalcitol therapy [71].

Route of Administration

The formulation as well as route of administration may influence how well patients with CKD or ESRD respond to vitamin D compounds. For example, the vehicle in which vitamin D$_3$ is suspended (oily vs. not) may influence absorption of precursors from the gut [39].

With respect to calcitriol, several studies have examined the oral vs. intravenous routes of administration. For example, Levine and Song found no difference in PTH suppression between hemodialysis patients after 22 weeks of either oral or intravenous calcitriol therapy [101]. Similarly, Turk et al. found no difference of mineral metabolism parameters at 6 months of therapy, although the effects on inflammatory cytokines interleukin-1 and interleukin-6 at 3 months differed in favor of the intravenous route [102]. In addition, co-administration with certain phosphate binders may reduce the absorption of calcitriol, as assessed by Pierce et al. This study, performed by the makers of lanthanum, found that sevelamer, but not lanthanum limited the amount of calcitriol absorbed in healthy volunteers [103].

OTHER COMPOUNDS

CYP24A1 Inhibitors

Other compounds are also being explored for the treatment of vitamin D deficiency in the CKD and ESRD population. Given the increased expression of the 24-hydroxylase gene product in renal biopsies, the Canadian company Cytochroma has developed vitamin D analogs with antagonism for the 24-hydroxylase $\pm$ partial agonism for the VDR, currently in phase I/II clinical trials [104]. Their hope is that a pure 24-hydroxylase inhibitor will increase the half-life of endogenous and/or exogenous vitamin D compounds, based on observations from the CYP24A1 knockout mouse where in the absence of 24-hydroxylase activity, exogenously administered 1,25OH$_2$ D levels remained elevated [105].

Alphacalcidol (1-Alpha-Hydroxycholecalciferol)

Alphacalcidol (also called alfacalcidol), a vitamin D$_3$ derivative, can bypass the renal 1-α-hydroxylase due to its pre-existing hydroxyl group at the 1st carbon, and can then undergo hydroxylation in the liver to yield 1,25OH$_2$ D. This compound has been used in Europe and effectively suppresses PTH in dialysis patients. Interestingly, one recent crossover study in five dialysis patients found that 6 weeks of alphacalcidol therapy did not suppress iPTH levels (while equal calcitriol doses did), but were able to raise 1,25(OH)$_2$ D levels [106], also in CKD patients [107]. In the largest trial to date in ESRD patients, there was no difference in PTH suppression or incidence of hypercalcemia and hyperphosphatemia between alphacalcidol and paricalcitol over 16 weeks in 80 chronic hemodialysis patients [108]. No information regarding non-mineral metabolism outcomes in the CKD/ESRD population is available at this time, although clinical trials are in process (www.clinicaltrials.gov, NCT01364688).

THERAPEUTIC CONSIDERATIONS

Therapeutic guidelines on vitamin D supplementation for CKD and ESRD patients focus on PTH suppression as a measure of effectiveness, and hyperphosphatemia and hypercalcemia as trigger point side-effects to alter the dosing regiment [109,110]. For example, current guidelines recommend measuring 25OH D serum levels if PTH is elevated in CKD stage 3 and 4 patients, and then repletion with a goal of lowering PTH. It is likely beneficial to supplement the CKD patients with hypovitaminosis D even if PTH levels are in the normal range. Thus, we suggest maintaining 25OH D levels above

30 ng/mL in CKD patients, irrespective of PTH, provided hypercalcemia is not present.

Similarly, VDRA therapy is currently guided by PTH levels both in the late CKD and ESRD populations. A challenging situation for the clinician is the dialysis patient with low PTH levels, for whom VDRA therapy would otherwise not be prescribed. In those individuals, we consider supplementing with vitamin D pro-hormones (ergocalciferol, cholecalciferol). Addition of low-dose VDRA in these patients may have beneficial effects based on prior mortality studies, although currently no clinical trials and corresponding guidelines exist to support this use. Randomized clinical trials with patient-level outcomes will be crucial to guide future therapy.

SUMMARY

Vitamin D compounds are crucial for the optimal function of many organ systems beyond those in the calcium/phosphorus/bone axis. The pervasiveness of vitamin D deficiency in the chronic kidney disease population clearly contributes to increased adverse outcomes, including increased mortality, cardiovascular morbidity, infectious complications, and anemia. Optimal targets for supplementation for both precursor compounds (e.g. ergocalciferol), and active analogs (e.g. paricalcitol, calcitriol) with respect to non-calciotropic effects are not yet established. Clinical trials elucidating these important questions are ongoing but more are needed to definitively guide practice.

Acknowledgement

Dr. Thadhani is supported by NIH K24 DK094872, and is a consultant to Fresenius Medical Care NA.

References

[1] Schuster I. Cytochromes P450 are essential players in the vitamin D signaling system. Biochim Biophys Acta 2011 Jan;1814(1):186—99.

[2] Omdahl JL, Morris HA, May BK. Hydroxylase enzymes of the vitamin D pathway: expression, function, and regulation. Annu Rev Nutr 2002;22:139—66.

[3] Townsend K, Evans KN, Campbell MJ, Colston KW, Adams JS, Hewison M. Biological actions of extra-renal 25-hydroxy-vitamin D-1alpha-hydroxylase and implications for chemoprevention and treatment. J Steroid Biochem Mol Biol 2005 Oct;97(1—2):103—9.

[4] Hewison M. Vitamin D and the intracrinology of innate immunity. Mol Cell Endocrinol 2010 Jun 10;321(2):103—11.

[5] Nykjaer A, Fyfe JC, Kozyraki R, Leheste JR, Jacobsen C, Nielsen MS, et al. Cubilin dysfunction causes abnormal metabolism of the steroid hormone 25(OH) vitamin D(3). Proc Natl Acad Sci USA 2001 Nov 20;98(24):13895—900.

[6] Safadi FF, Thornton P, Magiera H, Hollis BW, Gentile M, Haddad JG, et al. Osteopathy and resistance to vitamin D toxicity in mice null for vitamin D binding protein. J Clin Invest 1999 Jan;103(2):239—51.

[7] Powe CE, Ricciardi C, Berg AH, Erdenesanaa D, Collerone G, Ankers E, et al. Vitamin D-binding protein modifies the vitamin D-bone mineral density relationship. J Bone Miner Res 2011 Jul;26(7):1609—16.

[8] Chun RF, Lauridsen AL, Suon L, Zella LA, Pike JW, Modlin RL, et al. Vitamin D-binding protein directs monocyte responses to 25-hydroxy- and 1,25-dihydroxyvitamin D. J Clin Endocrinol Metab 2010 Jul;95(7):3368—76.

[9] Wali RK, Kong J, Sitrin MD, Bissonnette M, Li YC. Vitamin D receptor is not required for the rapid actions of 1,25-dihydroxy-vitamin D3 to increase intracellular calcium and activate protein kinase C in mouse osteoblasts. J Cell Biochem 2003 Mar 1;88(4):794—801.

[10] Mizwicki M, Norman A. Vitamin D sterol/VDR conformational dynamics and nongenomic actions. In: Feldman D, Pike JW, Adams JS, editors. 3rd ed. Amsterdam; Boston: Academic Press; 2011.

[11] Dusso A, Slatopolsky E. Vitamin D and renal disease. In: Feldman D, Pike JW, Adams JS, editors. 3rd ed. Amsterdam; Boston: Academic Press; 2011.

[12] Kalantar-Zadeh K, Kovesdy CP. Clinical outcomes with active versus nutritional vitamin D compounds in chronic kidney disease. Clin J Am Soc Nephrol 2009 Sep;4(9):1529—39.

[13] Thomas MK, Lloyd-Jones DM, Thadhani RI, Shaw AC, Deraska DJ, Kitch BT, et al. Hypovitaminosis D in medical inpatients. N Engl J Med 1998 Mar 19;338(12):777—83.

[14] Holick MF. Vitamin D deficiency. N Engl J Med 2007 Jul 19;357(3):266—81.

[15] Holick MF, Binkley NC, Bischoff-Ferrari HA, Gordon CM, Hanley DA, Heaney RP, et al. Evaluation, treatment, and prevention of vitamin D deficiency: an Endocrine Society clinical practice guideline. J Clin Endocrinol Metab 2011 Jul;96(7):1911—30.

[16] LaClair RE, Hellman RN, Karp SL, Kraus M, Ofner S, Li Q, et al. Prevalence of calcidiol deficiency in CKD: a cross-sectional study across latitudes in the United States. Am J Kidney Dis 2005 Jun;45(6):1026—33.

[17] Bouchard J, Ouimet D, Vallee M, Lafrance JP, Leblanc M, Senecal L, et al. Comparison of the prevalence of calcidiol insufficiency in predialysis and osteoporotic populations. Int Urol Nephrol 2009 Dec;41(4):983—8.

[18] Zehnder D, Landray MJ, Wheeler DC, Fraser W, Blackwell L, Nuttall S, et al. Cross-sectional analysis of abnormalities of mineral homeostasis, vitamin D and parathyroid hormone in a cohort of pre-dialysis patients. The chronic renal impairment in Birmingham (CRIB) study. Nephron Clin Pract 2007;107(3):c109—16.

[19] Wang AY, Lam CW, Sanderson JE, Wang M, Chan IH, Lui SF, et al. Serum 25-hydroxyvitamin D status and cardiovascular outcomes in chronic peritoneal dialysis patients: a 3-y prospective cohort study. Am J Clin Nutr 2008 Jun;87(6):1631—8.

[20] Wolf M, Shah A, Gutierrez O, Ankers E, Monroy M, Tamez H, et al. Vitamin D levels and early mortality among incident hemodialysis patients. Kidney Int 2007 Oct;72(8):1004—13.

[21] Jean G, Charra B, Chazot C. Vitamin D deficiency and associated factors in hemodialysis patients. J Ren Nutr 2008 Sep;18(5):395—9.

[22] Cuppari L, Carvalho AB, Draibe SA. Vitamin D status of chronic kidney disease patients living in a sunny country. J Ren Nutr 2008 Sep;18(5):408—14.

[23] Holick MF. Sunlight and vitamin D for bone health and prevention of autoimmune diseases, cancers, and cardiovascular disease. Am J Clin Nutr 2004 Dec;80(Suppl. 6):1678S–88S.

[24] Jacob AI, Sallman A, Santiz Z, Hollis BW. Defective photoproduction of cholecalciferol in normal and uremic humans. J Nutr 1984 Jul;114(7):1313–9.

[25] Ravani P, Malberti F, Tripepi G, Pecchini P, Cutrupi S, Pizzini P, et al. Vitamin D levels and patient outcome in chronic kidney disease. Kidney Int 2009 Jan;75(1):88–95.

[26] Bhan I, Dubey A, Wolf M. Diagnosis and management of mineral metabolism in CKD. J Gen Intern Med 2010 Jul;25(7):710–6.

[27] Urena-Torres P, Metzger M, Haymann JP, Karras A, Boffa JJ, Flamant M, et al. Association of kidney function, vitamin d deficiency, and circulating markers of mineral and bone disorders in CKD. Am J Kidney Dis 2011 Oct;58(4):544–53.

[28] Michaud J, Naud J, Ouimet D, Demers C, Petit JL, Leblond FA, et al. Reduced hepatic synthesis of calcidiol in uremia. J Am Soc Nephrol 2010 Sep;21(9):1488–97.

[29] Koenig KG, Lindberg JS, Zerwekh JE, Padalino PK, Cushner HM, Copley JB. Free and total 1,25-dihydroxyvitamin D levels in subjects with renal disease. Kidney Int 1992 Jan;41(1):161–5.

[30] Isakova T, Gutierrez OM, Patel NM, Andress DL, Wolf M, Levin A. Vitamin D deficiency, inflammation, and albuminuria in chronic kidney disease: complex interactions. J Ren Nutr 2011 Jul;21(4):295–302.

[31] Thrailkill KM, Jo CH, Cockrell GE, Moreau CS, Fowlkes JL. Enhanced excretion of vitamin D binding protein in type 1 diabetes: a role in vitamin D deficiency? J Clin Endocrinol Metab 2011 Jan;96(1):142–9.

[32] Kaseda R, Hosojima M, Sato H, Saito A. Role of megalin and cubilin in the metabolism of vitamin D(3). Ther Apher Dial 2011 Jun;15(Suppl. 1):14–7.

[33] Doorenbos CR, de Cuba MM, Vogt L, Kema IP, van den Born J, Gans RO, et al. Antiproteinuric treatment reduces urinary loss of vitamin D-binding protein but does not affect vitamin D status in patients with chronic kidney disease. J Steroid Biochem Mol Biol 2011 Sep 21.

[34] Petkovich M, Jones G. CYP24A1 and kidney disease. Curr Opin Nephrol Hypertens 2011 Jul;20(4):337–44.

[35] Helvig CF, Cuerrier D, Hosfield CM, Ireland B, Kharebov AZ, Kim JW, et al. Dysregulation of renal vitamin D metabolism in the uremic rat. Kidney Int 2010 Sep;78(5):463–72.

[36] Ishimura E, Nishizawa Y, Inaba M, Matsumoto N, Emoto M, Kawagishi T, et al. Serum levels of 1,25-dihydroxyvitamin D, 24,25-dihydroxyvitamin D, and 25-hydroxyvitamin D in non-dialyzed patients with chronic renal failure. Kidney Int 1999 Mar;55(3):1019–27.

[37] Haddad Jr JG, Min C, Mendelsohn M, Slatopolsky E, Hahn TJ. Competitive protein-binding radioassay of 24,25-dihydroxyvitamin D in sera from normal and anephric subjects. Arch Biochem Biophys 1977 Aug;182(2):390–5.

[38] Niramitmahapanya S, Harris SS, Dawson-Hughes B. Type of dietary fat is associated with the 25-hydroxyvitamin d3 increment in response to vitamin d supplementation. J Clin Endocrinol Metab 2011 Oct;96(10):3170–4.

[39] Grossmann RE, Tangpricha V. Evaluation of vehicle substances on vitamin D bioavailability: a systematic review. Mol Nutr Food Res 2010 Aug;54(8):1055–61.

[40] Douard V, Asgerally A, Sabbagh Y, Sugiura S, Shapses SA, Casirola D, et al. Dietary fructose inhibits intestinal calcium absorption and induces vitamin D insufficiency in CKD. J Am Soc Nephrol 2010 Feb;21(2):261–71.

[41] Gutierrez O, Isakova T, Rhee E, Shah A, Holmes J, Collerone G, et al. Fibroblast growth factor-23 mitigates hyperphosphatemia but accentuates calcitriol deficiency in chronic kidney disease. J Am Soc Nephrol 2005 Jul;16(7):2205–15.

[42] Halloran BP, Schaefer P, Lifschitz M, Levens M, Goldsmith RS. Plasma vitamin D metabolite concentrations in chronic renal failure: effect of oral administration of 25-hydroxyvitamin D3. J Clin Endocrinol Metab 1984 Dec;59(6):1063–9.

[43] Shigematsu T, Kazama JJ, Yamashita T, Fukumoto S, Hosoya T, Gejyo F, et al. Possible involvement of circulating fibroblast growth factor 23 in the development of secondary hyperparathyroidism associated with renal insufficiency. Am J Kidney Dis 2004 Aug;44(2):250–6.

[44] Shimada T, Hasegawa H, Yamazaki Y, Muto T, Hino R, Takeuchi Y, et al. FGF-23 is a potent regulator of vitamin D metabolism and phosphate homeostasis. J Bone Miner Res 2004 Mar;19(3):429–35.

[45] Dobnig H, Pilz S, Scharnagl H, Renner W, Seelhorst U, Wellnitz B, et al. Independent association of low serum 25-hydroxyvitamin D and 1,25-dihydroxyvitamin D levels with all-cause and cardiovascular mortality. Arch Intern Med 2008 Jun 23;168(12):1340–9.

[46] Martins D, Wolf M, Pan D, Zadshir A, Tareen N, Thadhani R, et al. Prevalence of cardiovascular risk factors and the serum levels of 25-hydroxyvitamin D in the United States: data from the Third National Health and Nutrition Examination Survey. Arch Intern Med 2007 Jun 11;167(11):1159–65.

[47] Scragg R, Jackson R, Holdaway IM, Lim T, Beaglehole R. Myocardial infarction is inversely associated with plasma 25-hydroxyvitamin D3 levels: a community-based study. Int J Epidemiol 1990 Sep;19(3):559–63.

[48] Drechsler C, Pilz S, Obermayer-Pietsch B, Verduijn M, Tomaschitz A, Krane V, et al. Vitamin D deficiency is associated with sudden cardiac death, combined cardiovascular events, and mortality in haemodialysis patients. Eur Heart J 2010 Sep;31(18):2253–61.

[49] Uysal S, Kalayci AG, Baysal K. Cardiac functions in children with vitamin D deficiency rickets. Pediatr Cardiol 1999 Jul-Aug;20(4):283–6.

[50] de Boer IH, Kestenbaum B, Shoben AB, Michos ED, Sarnak MJ, Siscovick DS. 25-hydroxyvitamin D levels inversely associate with risk for developing coronary artery calcification. J Am Soc Nephrol 2009 Aug;20(8):1805–12.

[51] Garcia-Canton C, Bosch E, Ramirez A, Gonzalez Y, Auyanet I, Guerra R, et al. Vascular calcification and 25-hydroxyvitamin D levels in non-dialysis patients with chronic kidney disease stages 4 and 5. Nephrol Dial Transplant 2011 Jul;26(7):2250–6.

[52] Marechal C, Coche E, Goffin E, Dragean A, Schlieper G, Nguyen P, et al. Progression of coronary artery calcification and thoracic aorta calcification in kidney transplant recipients. Am J Kidney Dis 2012 Feb;59(2):258–69.

[53] Patange AR, Valentini RP, Du W, Pettersen MD. Vitamin D deficiency and arterial wall stiffness in children with chronic kidney disease. Pediatr Cardiol 2012 Jan;33(1):122–8.

[54] Li YC, Kong J, Wei M, Chen ZF, Liu SQ, Cao LP. 1,25-Dihydroxyvitamin D(3) is a negative endocrine regulator of the renin-angiotensin system. J Clin Invest 2002 Jul;110(2):229–38.

[55] Cardus A, Parisi E, Gallego C, Aldea M, Fernandez E, Valdivielso JM. 1,25-Dihydroxyvitamin D3 stimulates vascular smooth muscle cell proliferation through a VEGF-mediated pathway. Kidney Int 2006 Apr;69(8):1377–84.

[56] Zittermann A, Koerfer R. Protective and toxic effects of vitamin D on vascular calcification: clinical implications. Mol Aspects Med 2008 Dec;29(6):423–32.

[57] Melamed ML, Astor B, Michos ED, Hostetter TH, Powe NR, Muntner P. 25-hydroxyvitamin D levels, race, and the progression of kidney disease. J Am Soc Nephrol 2009 Dec;20(12):2631–9.

[58] de Boer IH, Katz R, Chonchol M, Ix JH, Sarnak MJ, Shlipak MG, et al. Serum 25-hydroxyvitamin d and change in estimated glomerular filtration rate. Clin J Am Soc Nephrol 2011 Sep;6(9): 2141–9.

[59] Deb DK, Sun T, Wong KE, Zhang Z, Ning G, Zhang Y, et al. Combined vitamin D analog and AT1 receptor antagonist synergistically block the development of kidney disease in a model of type 2 diabetes. Kidney Int 2010 Jun;77(11):1000–9.

[60] Zhang Z, Zhang Y, Ning G, Deb DK, Kong J, Li YC. Combination therapy with AT1 blocker and vitamin D analog markedly ameliorates diabetic nephropathy: blockade of compensatory renin increase. Proc Natl Acad Sci U S A 2008 Oct 14;105(41): 15896–901.

[61] Gombart AF, Bhan I, Borregaard N, Tamez H, Camargo Jr CA, Koeffler HP, et al. Low plasma level of cathelicidin antimicrobial peptide (hCAP18) predicts increased infectious disease mortality in patients undergoing hemodialysis. Clin Infect Dis 2009 Feb 15;48(4):418–24.

[62] Patel NM, Gutierrez OM, Andress DL, Coyne DW, Levin A, Wolf M. Vitamin D deficiency and anemia in early chronic kidney disease. Kidney Int 2010 Apr;77(8):715–20.

[63] Meguro S, Tomita M, Katsuki T, Kato K, Oh H, Ainai A, et al. Plasma 25-hydroxyvitamin D is independently associated with hemoglobin concentration in male subjects with type 2 diabetes mellitus. Int J Endocrinol 2011;2011:362981.

[64] Kiss Z, Ambrus C, Almasi C, Berta K, Deak G, Horonyi P, et al. Serum 25(OH)-cholecalciferol concentration is associated with hemoglobin level and erythropoietin resistance in patients on maintenance hemodialysis. Nephron Clin Pract 2011;117(4): c373–8.

[65] Lac PT, Choi K, Liu IA, Meguerditchian S, Rasgon SA, Sim JJ. The effects of changing vitamin D levels on anemia in chronic kidney disease patients: a retrospective cohort review. Clin Nephrol 2010 Jul;74(1):25–32.

[66] Aucella F, Scalzulli RP, Gatta G, Vigilante M, Carella AM, Stallone C. Calcitriol increases burst-forming unit-erythroid proliferation in chronic renal failure. A synergistic effect with r-HuEpo. Nephron Clin Pract 2003;95(4):c121–7.

[67] Alon DB, Chaimovitz C, Dvilansky A, Lugassy G, Douvdevani A, Shany S, et al. Novel role of 1,25(OH)(2)D(3) in induction of erythroid progenitor cell proliferation. Exp Hematol 2002 May;30(5):403–9.

[68] Goicoechea M, Vazquez MI, Ruiz MA, Gomez-Campdera F, Perez-Garcia R, Valderrabano F. Intravenous calcitriol improves anaemia and reduces the need for erythropoietin in haemodialysis patients. Nephron 1998;78(1):23–7.

[69] Neves PL, Trivino J, Casaubon F, Santos V, Mendes P, Romao P, et al. Elderly patients on chronic hemodialysis with hyperparathyroidism: increase of hemoglobin level after intravenous calcitriol. Int Urol Nephrol 2006;38(1):175–7.

[70] Kumar VA, Kujubu DA, Sim JJ, Rasgon SA, Yang PS. Vitamin D supplementation and recombinant human erythropoietin utilization in vitamin D-deficient hemodialysis patients. J Nephrol 2011 Jan-Feb;24(1):98–105.

[71] Matias PJ, Jorge C, Ferreira C, Borges M, Aires I, Amaral T, et al. Cholecalciferol supplementation in hemodialysis patients: effects on mineral metabolism, inflammation, and cardiac dimension parameters. Clin J Am Soc Nephrol 2010 May;5(5):905–11.

[72] de Boer IH. Vitamin D and glucose metabolism in chronic kidney disease. Curr Opin Nephrol Hypertens 2008 Nov;17(6): 566–72.

[73] Chonchol M, Scragg R. 25-Hydroxyvitamin D, insulin resistance, and kidney function in the Third National Health and Nutrition Examination Survey. Kidney Int 2007 Jan;71(2): 134–9.

[74] Friedman DJ, Bhatt N, Hayman NS, Nichols BJ, Herman M, Nikolaev N, et al. Impact of activated vitamin D on insulin resistance in non-diabetic chronic kidney disease patients. Clin Endocrinol (Oxf) 2012 Jul;77(1):56–61.

[75] Petchey WG, Hickman IJ, Duncan E, Prins JB, Hawley CM, Johnson DW, et al. The role of 25-hydroxyvitamin D deficiency in promoting insulin resistance and inflammation in patients with chronic kidney disease: a randomised controlled trial. BMC Nephrol 2009;10:41.

[76] Jamal SA, West SL, Miller PD. Fracture risk assessment in patients with chronic kidney disease. Osteoporos Int 2012 Apr;23(4):1191–8.

[77] Gallagher JC, Rapuri PB, Smith LM. An age-related decrease in creatinine clearance is associated with an increase in number of falls in untreated women but not in women receiving calcitriol treatment. J Clin Endocrinol Metab 2007 Jan;92(1):51–8.

[78] Teng M, Wolf M, Ofsthun MN, Lazarus JM, Hernan MA, Camargo Jr CA, et al. Activated injectable vitamin D and hemodialysis survival: a historical cohort study. J Am Soc Nephrol 2005 Apr;16(4):1115–25.

[79] Wolf M, Betancourt J, Chang Y, Shah A, Teng M, Tamez H, et al. Impact of activated vitamin D and race on survival among hemodialysis patients. J Am Soc Nephrol 2008 Jul;19(7):1379–88.

[80] Sprague SM, Llach F, Amdahl M, Taccetta C, Batlle D. Paricalcitol versus calcitriol in the treatment of secondary hyperparathyroidism. Kidney Int 2003 Apr;63(4):1483–90.

[81] Teng M, Wolf M, Lowrie E, Ofsthun N, Lazarus JM, Thadhani R. Survival of patients undergoing hemodialysis with paricalcitol or calcitriol therapy. N Engl J Med 2003 Jul 31;349(5):446–56.

[82] Tentori F, Hunt WC, Stidley CA, Rohrscheib MR, Bedrick EJ, Meyer KB, et al. Mortality risk among hemodialysis patients receiving different vitamin D analogs. Kidney Int 2006 Nov;70(10): 1858–65.

[83] Zhou C, Lu F, Cao K, Xu D, Goltzman D, Miao D. Calcium-independent and 1,25(OH)2D3-dependent regulation of the renin-angiotensin system in 1alpha-hydroxylase knockout mice. Kidney Int 2008 Jul;74(2):170–9.

[84] Xiang W, Kong J, Chen S, Cao LP, Qiao G, Zheng W, et al. Cardiac hypertrophy in vitamin D receptor knockout mice: role of the systemic and cardiac renin-angiotensin systems. Am J Physiol Endocrinol Metab 2005 Jan;288(1):E125–32.

[85] Bodyak N, Ayus JC, Achinger S, Shivalingappa V, Ke Q, Chen YS, et al. Activated vitamin D attenuates left ventricular abnormalities induced by dietary sodium in Dahl salt-sensitive animals. Proc Natl Acad Sci USA 2007 Oct 23;104(43):16810–5.

[86] Park CW, Oh YS, Shin YS, Kim CM, Kim YS, Kim SY, et al. Intravenous calcitriol regresses myocardial hypertrophy in hemodialysis patients with secondary hyperparathyroidism. Am J Kidney Dis 1999 Jan;33(1):73–81.

[87] Mizobuchi M, Finch JL, Martin DR, Slatopolsky E. Differential effects of vitamin D receptor activators on vascular calcification in uremic rats. Kidney Int 2007 Sep;72(6):709–15.

[88] Shroff R, Egerton M, Bridel M, Shah V, Donald AE, Cole TJ, et al. A bimodal association of vitamin D levels and vascular disease in children on dialysis. J Am Soc Nephrol 2008 Jun;19(6):1239–46.

[89] Shroff RC, Donald AE, Hiorns MP, Watson A, Feather S, Milford D, et al. Mineral metabolism and vascular damage in children on dialysis. J Am Soc Nephrol 2007 Nov;18(11):2996–3003.

[90] Thadhani R, Appelbaum E, Pritchett Y, Chang Y, Wenger J, Tamez H, et al. Vitamin D therapy and cardiac structure and function in patients with chronic kidney disease: the PRIMO randomized controlled trial. JAMA 2012 Feb 15;307(7):674–84.

[91] Raggi P, Chertow GM, Torres PU, Csiky B, Naso A, Nossuli K, et al. The ADVANCE study: a randomized study to evaluate the effects of cinacalcet plus low-dose vitamin D on vascular

calcification in patients on hemodialysis. Nephrol Dial Transplant 2011 Apr;26(4):1327–39.

[92] Alborzi P, Patel NA, Peterson C, Bills JE, Bekele DM, Bunaye Z, et al. Paricalcitol reduces albuminuria and inflammation in chronic kidney disease: a randomized double-blind pilot trial. Hypertension 2008 Aug;52(2):249–55.

[93] Agarwal R, Acharya M, Tian J, Hippensteel RL, Melnick JZ, Qiu P, et al. Antiproteinuric effect of oral paricalcitol in chronic kidney disease. Kidney Int 2005 Dec;68(6):2823–8.

[94] Fishbane S, Chittineni H, Packman M, Dutka P, Ali N, Durie N. Oral paricalcitol in the treatment of patients with CKD and proteinuria: a randomized trial. Am J Kidney Dis 2009 Oct;54(4):647–52.

[95] de Zeeuw D, Agarwal R, Amdahl M, Audhya P, Coyne D, Garimella T, et al. Selective vitamin D receptor activation with paricalcitol for reduction of albuminuria in patients with type 2 diabetes (VITAL study): a randomised controlled trial. Lancet 2010 Nov 6;376(9752):1543–51.

[96] Stubbs JR, Idicula A, Slusser J, Menard R, Quarles LD. Cholecalciferol supplementation alters calcitriol-responsive monocyte proteins and decreases inflammatory cytokines in ESRD. J Am Soc Nephrol 2010 Feb;21(2):353–61.

[97] Tsujimoto Y, Tahara H, Shoji T, Emoto M, Koyama H, Ishimura E, et al. Active vitamin D and acute respiratory infections in dialysis patients. Clin J Am Soc Nephrol 2011 Jun;6(6):1361–7.

[98] Jean G, Terrat JC, Vanel T, Hurot JM, Lorriaux C, Mayor B, et al. Evidence for persistent vitamin D 1-alpha-hydroxylation in hemodialysis patients: evolution of serum 1,25-dihydroxy-cholecalciferol after 6 months of 25-hydroxycholecalciferol treatment. Nephron Clin Pract 2008;110(1):c58–65.

[99] Dusso A, Lopez-Hilker S, Rapp N, Slatopolsky E. Extra-renal production of calcitriol in chronic renal failure. Kidney Int 1988 Sep;34(3):368–75.

[100] Bhan I, Camargo Jr CA, Wenger J, Ricciardi C, Ye J, Borregaard N, et al. Circulating levels of 25-hydroxyvitamin D and human cathelicidin in healthy adults. J Allergy Clin Immunol 2011 May;127(5):1302–4. e1.

[101] Levine BS, Song M. Pharmacokinetics and efficacy of pulse oral versus intravenous calcitriol in hemodialysis patients. J Am Soc Nephrol 1996 Mar;7(3):488–96.

[102] Turk S, Akbulut M, Yildiz A, Gurbilek M, Gonen S, Tombul Z, et al. Comparative effect of oral pulse and intravenous calcitriol treatment in hemodialysis patients: the effect on serum IL-1 and IL-6 levels and bone mineral density. Nephron 2002 Feb;90(2):188–94.

[103] Pierce D, Hossack S, Poole L, Robinson A, Van Heusen H, Martin P, et al. The effect of sevelamer carbonate and lanthanum carbonate on the pharmacokinetics of oral calcitriol. Nephrol Dial Transplant 2011 May;26(5):1615–21.

[104] Posner GH, Helvig C, Cuerrier D, Collop D, Kharebov A, Ryder K, et al. Vitamin D analogues targeting CYP24 in chronic kidney disease. J Steroid Biochem Mol Biol 2010 Jul;121(1–2):13–9.

[105] St-Arnaud R, Arabian A, Travers R, Barletta F, Raval-Pandya M, Chapin K, et al. Deficient mineralization of intramembranous bone in vitamin D-24-hydroxylase-ablated mice is due to elevated 1,25-dihydroxyvitamin D and not to the absence of 24,25-dihydroxyvitamin D. Endocrinology 2000 Jul;141(7):2658–66.

[106] Moe S, Wazny LD, Martin JE. Oral calcitriol versus oral alfacalcidol for the treatment of secondary hyperparathyroidism in patients receiving hemodialysis: a randomized, crossover trial. Can J Clin Pharmacol 2008 Winter;15(1):e36–43.

[107] Reichel H. Low-dose alfacalcidol controls secondary hyperparathyroidism in predialysis chronic kidney disease. Nephron Clin Pract 2010;114(4):c268–76.

[108] Hansen D, Rasmussen K, Danielsen H, Meyer-Hofmann H, Bacevicius E, Lauridsen TG, et al. No difference between alfacalcidol and paricalcitol in the treatment of secondary hyperparathyroidism in hemodialysis patients: a randomized crossover trial. Kidney Int 2011 Oct;80(8):841–50.

[109] Uhlig K, Berns JS, Kestenbaum B, Kumar R, Leonard MB, Martin KJ, et al. KDOQI US commentary on the 2009 KDIGO Clinical Practice Guideline for the Diagnosis, Evaluation, and Treatment of CKD-Mineral and Bone Disorder (CKD-MBD). Am J Kidney Dis 2010 May;55(5):773–99.

[110] KDIGO clinical practice guideline for the diagnosis, evaluation, prevention, and treatment of Chronic Kidney Disease-Mineral and Bone Disorder (CKD-MBD). Kidney Int Suppl 2009 Aug;(113):S1–130.

Nutritional Management of Water, Sodium, Potassium, Chloride, and Magnesium in Kidney Disease and Kidney Failure

Nabil Haddad, Rosemarie Shim, Lee A. Hebert

The Ohio State University Medical Center, Department of Internal Medicine, Columbus, OH, USA

SODIUM AND CHLORIDE

Sodium and the Control of Extracellular Fluid Volume

Sodium is the most abundant extracellular cation. Because sodium is actively excluded from cells and because cell membranes generally are freely permeable to water, the amount of sodium in the extracellular space critically determines extracellular fluid volume (ECFV). Figure 22.1 shows that the intravascular fluid volume is a component of the ECFV and, in health, comprises approximately one-fourth of the ECFV. In many pathologic states the intravascular and interstitial fluid volume change is parallel; however, some disease states alter the distribution of fluid within the ECFV (Figure 22.2). The highest priority in ECFV volume control is to maintain the intravascular volume at an optimum level [2]. So, the goal in dietary sodium (salt) management is to reestablish or help maintain an optimal intravascular volume.

A constellation of findings, when taken together, provides the clinician with an assessment of the intravascular volume. An overview of the diagnostic approach to assessing volume status is shown in Table 22.1. In the present context, volume depletion is defined as a condition in which the patient will be benefited by increasing intravascular volume; volume expansion is defined as a condition in which the patient will be benefited by decreasing intravascular volume.

Regulation of Sodium Balance in Health

There are several organ systems that "sense" the effective circulating volume, i.e., assess the patient's "volume status": heart [3,4], arterial baroreceptors [5], liver [6], brain [7], and kidney [8]. However, it is the kidney alone that is the effector organ in sodium homeostasis. The normal kidney is able to maintain adequate volume status over a wide range of dietary sodium intake. For example, in the United States the average sodium intake is 170 mEq/day; in areas of Japan, it can approach 300 mEq/day; among certain indigenous tribes, it is less than 20 mEq/day [9,10].

Although the kidney is remarkable in its ability to defend volume status, its defense is not perfect. This is demonstrated in Figure 22.3A. When NaCl intake is decreased abruptly from 150 mEq/day to 10 mEq/day in a normal individual, urine sodium excretion gradually decreases over the next 4 days until sodium balance is achieved (i.e., urine sodium output approximates sodium intake) [9,11]. However, before this steady state (salt balance) was reached, sodium output exceeded intake, and a net loss of about 150 mEq of sodium occurred. Because normal homeostasis requires that serum sodium concentration remain constant [12], ECFV volume decreased. This is shown in Figure 22.3A by the approximate 1-kg weight loss after the reduction in sodium intake.

On the other hand, Figure 22.3B shows that acutely increasing NaCl intake gradually increases urinary sodium excretion over the next 4 days until a new steady state is reached [9,11]. During this period, a net gain of sodium occurs and is accompanied by water retention (approximately 1 kg) sufficient to maintain ECFV isotonicity.

This traditional view of sodium balance has been challenged by the concept of sodium storage [12]. In this model, when NaCl intake is increased, the

FIGURE 22.1 The normal distribution and osmolality of body water. The short horizontal arrows indicate the presence of free diffusion of water among the body water compartments.

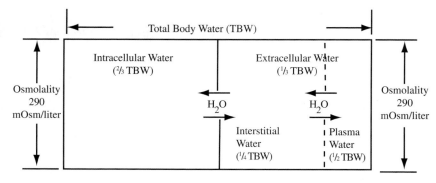

intravascular volume may increase without a concomitant increase in ECFV or body weight [12]. The clinical implications of this model have yet to be elucidated [13]. Irrespective of this debate, in patients with "salt-sensitive" hypertension, sodium retention can result in an increase in blood pressure to abnormal levels [14]. The critical determinants of "salt sensitivity" are unknown, although CKD [14], older age [15], African-ancestry [15], and adducin gene [16] are associated with salt-sensitive hypertension. The alpha-adducin gene polymorphism Gly 460Trp allele is strongly associated with impaired endothelium dependent vasodilation [17], and probably is a mechanism of sodium sensitive form of hypertension [18]. The gamma adducin gene may influence blood pressure by increasing the activity of the thiazide-sensitive sodium chloride transporter in the distal convoluted tubule [19].

Clinical Significance of Dietary Salt Intake

The 2010 U.S. Dietary Guidelines recommend that all Americans over age 50 restrict their salt intake to < 3.8 g daily (1500 mg sodium, 65 mEq sodium) in order to improve or prevent hypertension. This recommendation is also extended to those with a variety of common health conditions including hypertension. For healthy individuals under age 50, the recommended salt intake is less than 5.8 g daily (2300 mg sodium, 100 mEq sodium) [20]. There are other strong advocates of low-salt intake [21,22], including the authors of the Seventh Report of the Joint National Commission [23].

The rationale for low-salt intake is the well documented effect of low salt intake to cause reductions in blood pressure, and correlational analysis has generally shown that lower blood pressure is associated with lower cardiovascular risk. In addition, there have been a few randomized trials that suggest cardiovascular benefit from salt restriction. Nevertheless, a recent Cochrane Review meta-analysis of these randomized trials concluded that there is "still insufficient power to exclude clinically important effects of reduced dietary salt intake on mortality or cardiovascular morbidity" [24].

Adding to the uncertainty of the Cochrane meta-analysis is that the bulk of the evidence came from the Taiwan study, which contributed 58% of the patients and 85% of the cardiovascular events [25]. In that study, the patients were randomly assigned to either usual salt intake (about 230 mM/d) or diet in which half of the NaCl in the diet was substituted for by KCl. The Taiwan study showed strong benefit of the lower salt intake in the hypertensive subset (a 35% decrease in cardiovascular events). However, it is unclear whether the benefit was the result of the increased potassium intake, which has been associated with lower blood pressure and cardiovascular risk, or reduced sodium intake or both [25].

Adding further uncertainty of the cardiovascular benefits of low-salt intake are the recently reported observational studies of salt intake in patients with Type 1 diabetes [26], Type 2 diabetes [27], a prospective general population study [28], and a retrospective analysis of the ONTARGET, and TRANSCEND databases [29]. Each study demonstrated that cardiovascular events were lower in those with higher salt intake (e.g., > 200 mM sodium chloride/24 h; > 12 g of sodium chloride/24 h), but higher in those with lower salt intake < 100 mM/d (5.8 g sodium chloride). These differences persisted despite extensive risk factor adjustment.

The most recent of the observation studies [29] is noteworthy because of its large size (> 28,000 patients), long follow-up (median more than 4 years), and the large number of patients at the extremes of high salt intake (19% of the patients has estimated NaCl intakes of 260 to > 350 mM/d). This study is remarkable in three respects:

1. The cohort with the lowest mortality had generous salt intakes (130 to 260 mM/d).
2. The cohorts with highest mortality were those with either the very high salt intake (> 260 to > 350 mM/d) or the less than average salt intake (< 130 mM/d).
3. The worse outcome in those with very high salt intakes is not surprising because all of the participants in these studies were older patients with

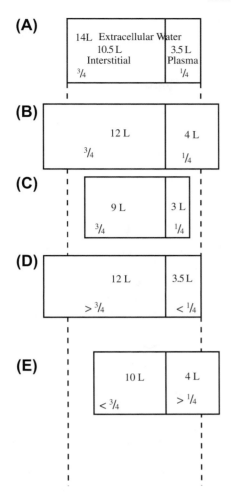

FIGURE 22.2 In a normal 70-kg person extracellular water (ECW) consists of 14 L of fluid divided between the interstitial (10.5 L) and intravascular (3.5 L) spaces (see illustration A). Illustrations B through E show how various pathologic states can alter the amount and distributions of ECW. A: Distribution of ECW. Normal interstitial volume is three-fourths of ECW. Intravascular water (mainly plasma) is one-fourth of ECW. B: Interstitial and intravascular volume increase in parallel as occurs in: congestive heart failure; high salt intake; normal salt intake in ESRD. C: Interstitial and intravascular volume decrease in parallel as occurs in: gastrointestinal losses (vomiting and diarrhea); renal losses (diuretics, salt wasting); skin losses (sweating, burns). D: Interstitial volume increases but intravascular volume decreases or remains the same: therapy with calcium channel blocker, hydralazine, minoxidil; hypoalbuminemia (liver disease, nephrotic syndrome, malnutrition). E: Intravascular volume increases but interstitial volume decreases or remains unchanged: rapid infusion of blood or colloid; head out water immersion.

cardiovascular disease or strong cardiovascular risk factors, including mild stages of CKD. However, the worse outcome in those with less than the average salt intake is surprising in light of the benefits that have been imputed to lower salt intakes because of its effect to lower blood pressure and/or prevent hypertension.

In an effort to explain how lower salt intake might increase cardiovascular risk, it has been pointed out that, although blood pressure tends to decrease with low-salt intake, there is also a brisk and chronic stimulation of the renin-angiotensin system when salt intake is less than 120 mM/d [30]. It is well established that aldosterone is vasculo-toxic and increases cardiovascular risk [31]. In addition, angiotensin II, which is upregulated by high renin levels, is pro-fibrotic [31], and causes insulin resistance [31,32]. In mice, low salt diet increases atherosclerosis probably through increased angiotensin II [33]. So, although blood pressure may be reduced by the low-salt diet, there may be countervailing metabolic changes that increase cardiovascular risk. In this respect, the effects of a low-salt diet resemble those of diuretic therapy as revealed in the ALLHAT trial. In that trial, diuretic therapy lowered blood pressure significantly better than ACE inhibitor or calcium channel blockers but did not lower overall cardiovascular risk, presumably because of the metabolic dysfunctions of diuretic therapy, which includes stimulation of the renin-angiotensin system [34,35].

An emerging viewpoint is that in most individuals a wide range of dietary salt intakes may be "safe". It is only at the extremes of salt intake, or in those who are "salt sensitive" that increased cardiovascular and renal risk is incurred [36]. It has been suggested that for an essential nutrient such as salt, evolution likely would favor survival of a species in which the margin of safety is broad, rather than narrow [36]. This hypothesis is consistent with the observed J-curve relationship between salt intake and cardiovascular risk. It has also been suggested that there may be a setpoint for salt intake that humans try to maintain. This may explain the stability of high salt intake in the US over the past 40—50 years despite the strong and persisting recommendations of public health experts to lower salt intake [37].

Of the recommended dietary approaches, the DASH diet (Dietary Approaches to Stop Hypertension) has been particularly popular. It recommends 4—5 daily servings of both fruits and vegetables, low-fat dairy products, and low saturated and total fat intake to lower blood pressure [38]. Blood pressure is reduced further if the DASH diet is combined with low salt intake (less than 100 mM daily). This blood pressure lowering effect of including a low salt intake with the DASH diet was observed in both those with or without hypertension [39].

Regulation of Sodium Balance in CKD

The ability of patients with chronic kidney disease (CKD) to maintain salt balance on a normal or nearly normal sodium intake usually remains intact until the glomerular filtration rate (GFR) falls to less than 15 mL/min (serum creatinine about 3 mg/dL) [40,41]. Below a GFR of 15 mL/min, the kidneys often are unable

TABLE 22.1 Clinical and Laboratory Assessment of Volume Status

Findings Consistent with Volume Depletion	
Finding	**Comment**
Weight loss exceeding 0.25 kg/day	Weight loss exceeding this rate is usually the result of fluid and electrolyte deficits, not caloric deficits.
Blood pressure less than usual and/or orthostatic fall in blood pressure	A fall in systolic blood pressure by greater than 20 mmHg when changing from a supine to standing position with a rise in pulse rate suggests intravascular volume depletion. Autonomic neuropathy or alpha blockers can cause orthostatic hypotension in the absence of volume depletion. If the patient has an autonomic neuropathy, the pulse will not increase upon standing.
Decreased skin turgor, cool or mottled extremities, collapsed peripheral veins	Elderly patients with arterial insufficiency can manifest these findings in the absence of volume depletion.
Elevated serum creatinine associated with a urine/plasma osmolality ratio > 1.5 mEq/L and/or urine Na concentration < 20 mEq/L	These findings also can be seen in severe congestive heart failure or hepatic failure, in the absence of volume depletion.

Findings Consistent with the Absence of Volume Depletion and/or the Presence of Volume Expansion	
Finding	**Comment**
Weight gain exceeding 0.25 kg/day	Weight gains exceeding this rate usually indicate fluid weight gains.
Onset of hypertension or worsening of previous hypertension	Those with salt-sensitive hypertension (e.g., African-Americans, elderly) are particularly susceptible to hypertension with sodium and water retention.
Left ventricular failure (orthopnea, paroxysmal nocturnal dyspnea, rales at lung bases, audible third heart sound)	Patients with left ventricular failure are volume expanded (they will benefit from measures to decrease intravascular volume) regardless of other findings related to volume status.
Peripheral edema, ascites, pleural effusions	These findings also can be the result of venous or lymphatic obstruction or severe hypoalbuminemia in the absence of volume expansion.

to increase sodium excretion sufficient to maintain satisfactory sodium balance on an average adult salt intake (120 to 170 mEq/day) [42]. So, salt intake must be reduced in such patients to avoid an increase in intravascular volume [43].

At a GFR of less than 50 mL/min but greater than 15 mL/min, mild to moderate renal sodium wasting occurs in many CKD patients, unless nephrotic syndrome or other sodium-retaining state is present [44]. At a GFR of 15–50 mL/min the CKD patient usually loses the ability to acutely reduce sodium excretion to less than 30 mEq/day [44]. So, CKD patients are particularly vulnerable to volume depletion if intake of salt is acutely reduced. However, the ability of the CKD patient to reduce urine sodium excretion may be improved if dietary sodium is lowered gradually rather than abruptly [45].

Renal sodium wasting is accentuated if sodium is ingested as $NaHCO_3$ (sodium bicarbonate) rather than NaCl. This was demonstrated when patients with various forms of CKD were fed a diet in which the source of sodium was 100 mM/d of NaCl or 100 mM/d of $NaHCO_3$. During NaCl feeding, the patients maintained

satisfactory sodium balance. However, during $NaHCO_3$ feeding, progressive negative sodium balances developed [46]. The mechanism is thought to be a decreased capacity of the kidney to reabsorb sodium, unless it is accompanied by a highly reabsorbable anion such as chloride [47].

Dietary NaCl in CKD Patients

The goal of NaCl intake in CKD is to achieve optimum intravascular volume. Assessment of volume status is discussed in Table 22.1 and Figure 22.2. Recommended levels of salt intake according to type and stage of CKD are discussed in Table 22.2.

Avoiding excess salt intake is important in CKD patients. Excessive salt intake promotes hypertension [25,48] and worsens proteinuria [49]. Both hypertension 50–52 and proteinuria [51,53], are strong risk factors for progression of CKD, likely because they are mechanisms of progression of kidney disease. Evidence that hypertension and proteinuria are mechanisms of CKD progression is provided by the following randomized

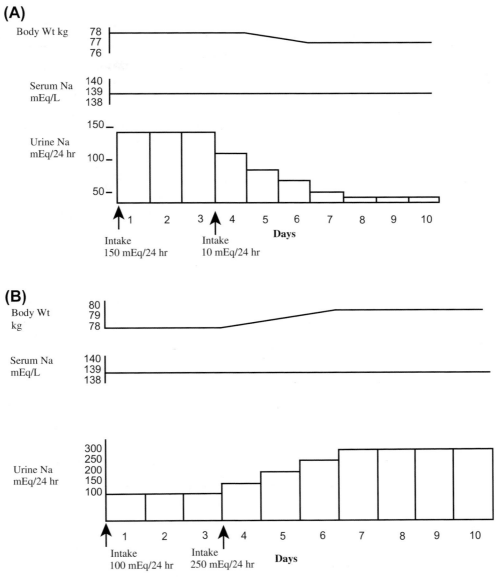

FIGURE 22.3 Change in body weight (Wt), serum sodium, and urine sodium. A: Dietary sodium intake is decreased to 10 mEq/day after a steady-state intake of 150 mEq/day. B: Dietary sodium intake increased to 250 mEq/day after steady-state intake of 100 mEq/day. (From: Simpson FO. Sodium intake, body sodium, and sodium excretion. Lancet 1988;2:25–28, with permission.)

trials: MDRD [50], AASK [51], and ESCAPE [52]. Also, experimental models of kidney disease have identified mechanisms by which proteinuria causes kidney damage [53]. Particularly relevant to the present discussion is that high-salt intake (i.e., 200 mM/d) can completely override the antiproteinuric effect of ACE inhibitors, ARBs, and CCBs [49].

Dietary prescriptions for salt usually are expressed in units that are different from the units that describe sodium (or chloride) in body fluids. This can result in confusion when the dietary prescription, which is expressed in milligrams or grams of sodium, needs to be adjusted to replace increased electrolyte losses in body fluids, which are expressed in mEq of Na or Cl. This problem is compounded if dietary NaCl intake is

supplemented with NaCl tablets (usually formulated as 1-g NaCl tablets). It is unfortunate that tradition maintains this confusing situation. It would be easier if the dietary sodium prescription were provided in mEq of sodium (or mM of NaCl) rather than in milligrams or grams of sodium. To aid the clinician, Table 22.3 is a conversion table for the dietary sodium prescription.

High-Salt Diet

High salt intakes can be consistently achieved by using foods with high salt contents (Table 22.4). NaCl tablets are also useful to increase NaCl intake. Compressed NaCl tablets, rather than enteric-coated tablets, are recommended because of more predictable

TABLE 22.2   Recommended Dietary Sodium Intake According to Type or Stage of Renal Disease

---

INCREASED NEED FOR DIETARY NACL (GENERALLY > 120 mM/DAY)

Medullary cystic disease
Fanconi's syndrome
Kidney-pancreas transplant with drainage of pancreatic secretions into the bladder
CKD of any cause associated with excessive extra renal salt losses (e.g., diarrhea, excess sweating)
Hypercalcemia-associated renal impairment (the excess dietary sodium is needed to promote renal calcium excretion)
Polyuric recovery phase from acute renal injury, such as postobstructive diuresis, or the diuretic phase of recovery from AKI

USUAL NEED FOR DIETARY NACL (GENERALLY 90 TO 120 mM/DAY)

Renal disease that is not complicated by hypertension, edema, congestive heart failure, ascites or pleural effusion

DECREASED NEED FOR DIETARY NACL (GENERALLY <100 mM/DAY)

CKD complicated by hypertension, edema, ascites, or pleural effusion. Oliguric end-stage renal disease associated with normal volume status. Congestive heart failure complicating CKD. Severe salt restriction (e.g., < 80 mM/day is not recommended because it increases mortality rate (Alderman MH: The Cochrane Review of Sodium and Health, Am J Hypertens 2011;24(8);854–856).

---

absorption of the compressed tablet. Some patients dislike NaCl tablets because in doses greater than 6 g daily a disagreeable salty aftertaste develops. The least effective means to substantially increase salt intake is to instruct the patient to add salt to the surface of food. Generally, the amount of salt actually added is small because the food becomes unpalatable if large amounts of surface salt are added. Increased dietary salt is more palatable if the salt is mixed with the food during preparation.

TABLE 22.3   Conversion Table for Dietary NACL Prescriptions (Daily Intake) for Normal Adults

	Level of Salt Intake[a]			
	Low	**Recommended**[b]	**Average**	**High**
Na				
g	2.0	2.3	3.9	4.6
mEq	88	100	170	200
NaCl				
g	5.1	5.8	9.9	11.6
mM	88	100	170	200

[a]*Molecular weights: Na 23, Cl 35.5.*
[b]*Approximately 1 to 1.3 mM/kg ideal body weight/day. This is controversial, as discussed herein.*

Low-Salt Diet

Low-salt intakes can be consistently achieved with proper dietary counseling, the use of low-salt foods (Table 22.4), salt substitutes and other flavor enhancers, and the judicious use of surface salt. Surface salt is much

TABLE 22.4   Sodium Content of Various Foods

High (Greater than 8 mEq per Serving)	Low (Less than 2 mEq per Serving)
DAIRY	
Processed American cheese	Nondairy creamer
Cottage cheese	Half and half cream
Buttermilk	
MEATS/FISH	
Processed meats	Lean beef
Bacon, sausage	Lean chicken
Canned meats	Fresh fish
Pickled herring	
Smoked salmon	
BREADS AND PASTAS	
Bread crumbs	Rice
Pita bread	Wheat germ
Bread stuffing	Cream of wheat
Cereals:	Melba toast
Corn flakes	Spaghetti
All bran	
Waffles	
English muffins	
LEGUMES, FRUITS, AND MISCELLANEOUS	
Coconut	Legumes
Refried beans	Tofu
Canned vegetables	Raw fruit
Canned soups	Raw carrots
Pickles	Lettuce
Corn chips, pretzels	Baked potato
Canned tomato products	Alcohol
Barbecue sauce	Soda
Canned gravy	Chocolate
Soy sauce	

From Mitch WE, Klahr S. Composition of common foods. In: Mitch WE, Klahr S (eds). Nutrition and the Kidney. Boston: Little Brown 1988:331, with permission.

more efficiently tasted than is salt that is mixed with food. This is the reason that a serving of potato chips, which contains about 3 to 4 mEq of NaCl, tastes much "saltier" than a serving of bread, which contains about 5 to 8 mEq/NaCl.

Low salt diets can be adhered to if processed foods are kept to a minimum and salt is avoided in food preparation. To enhance the flavor of foods cooked without salt, flavor enhancers such as pepper, paprika, curry, thyme, and oregano can be used. Salt substitutes, which consist mostly of KCl, also can be used if potassium intake does not need to be restricted. Compared to flavor enhancers, salt substitutes have the advantage of tasting "saltier". Another strategy to achieve a tasty low-salt diet is to prepare a 2 g Na diet (88 mM NaCl) and then allow {1/3} teaspoon of salt to be used as surface salt added to the meals eaten that day. The total NaCl intake would be less than 120 mM.

NaHCO₃ Therapy

Many patients with chronic kidney disease require NaHCO₃ to treat the metabolic acidosis of renal failure. An even more important reason to use NaHCO₃ is the recent evidence from randomized trials showing that sodium bicarbonate therapy in moderate dose (e.g., two 650-mg tablets twice daily) slows progression of kidney disease [54,55]. The mechanism of the kidney protection may involve suppression of pro-fibrotic cytokines such as endothelin-1. Bicarbonate therapy may also suppress activation of the alternative complement pathway in those with non-selective proteinuria [49,56]. Usually NaHCO₃ can be administered without inducing important sodium retention, as discussed earlier.

Calcium Channel Blocker Therapy and Dietary Sodium Management

Unlike other classes of antihypertensive agents, the antihypertensive effects of calcium channel blockers may not be increased by salt restriction [57], apparently because calcium channel blockers promote natriuresis [58]. Paradoxically, calcium channel blocker therapy often is associated with lower-extremity edema. Apparently, calcium channel blockers induce sufficient peripheral arteriolar vasodilatation to cause increased transmission of arterial hydrostatic pressure to tissue capillaries. As a consequence, interstitial volume increases as intravascular volume decreases. This mechanism of lower-extremity edema likely also accounts for the edema seen with other vasodilators such as minoxidil and hydralazine. Usually the edema is a benign condition, although discomfort in the joints of the swollen lower extremities is common.

Dietary salt restriction and diuretics can reduce the edema. However, vigorous salt restriction and diuretic therapy are not recommended. That can result in reducing intravascular volume to less than normal.

WATER

Water Metabolism in Health

By weight, the average human is about 70% water — two-thirds in the intracellular space and one-third in the extracellular space (Figure 22.1). Unlike sodium, in which excretion in health is adjusted to control blood volume, water excretion is adjusted to control plasma osmolality. The normal kidney has the ability to conserve water (increase urinary osmolality as high as 1200 mOsm/L) or excrete water (reduce urine osmolality to as low as 50 mOsm/L) [59].

In health, daily metabolism and intake of nutrients produces about 600 mOsm of solute that requires renal excretion. This "solute load" largely consists of urea produced from metabolism of protein and ingested Na, K, and their anions. If the urine is concentrated maximally (1200 mOsm/L) the 600 mOsm can be excreted in 0.5 liter of urine. Conversely, in states of maximum water intake, this same 600 mOsm would be excreted in about 12 liters of urine (50 mOsm/L). This 12 liters of urine can be viewed as consisting of 2 liters of isotonic urine and 10 liters of solute-free urine.

Kidney Disease and Water Intake

The urinary volume in which the daily osmolar load is excreted depends on antidiuretic hormone (ADH). In the absence of ADH the collecting duct becomes virtually impermeable to water, resulting in excretion of the dilute tubular fluid that is formed in the loop of Henle and distal tubule [60]. Plasma osmolality is the primary regulator of ADH release [61,62]. However, there are nonosmotic stimuli for ADH release as well. These include nausea [63], hypoxia [64], insulin [65], norepinephrine [66], angiotensin II [67], and severe volume depletion [68]. In health, water balance is achieved by adjusting renal excretion of water to compensate for variations in water intake and nonrenal water losses. The components of normal daily water balance in the adult are shown in Table 22.5.

Water Metabolism in CKD

Impaired ability to both concentrate and dilute the urine occurs in all forms of CKD. It occurs earlier and more severely in primary tubulointerstitial renal diseases compared to primary glomerular diseases.

TABLE 22.5 Components of Normal Daily Water Balance in the Adult

Water Intake	
Source of Water	**Water Volume (mL/day)**
Ingested as fluid	Variable[a], usually 1000−2000
Ingested as solid food	Usually 800−1000
Water production from oxidative metabolism	Usually 200−300
Total:	2000−3300

Water Output	
Routes of Water Loss	**Water Volume (mL/day)**
Urine	Variable[b], usually 1000−2200
Sweat	Negligible, except in hot environment, when several thousand ml can be lost
Stool	100
Evaporation[c]:	
Skin	450
Respiratory tract	450
Total:	2000−3300

[a]*The amount of water ingested depends on cultural influences as well as serum osmolality.*
[b]*Depends on that needed to achieve water balance.*
[c]*These are pure water losses. The losses are influenced by humidity and body temperature.*

However, in either form of CKD, when GFR falls to less than 20 mL/min in adults, the maximum urine concentration barely exceeds plasma osmolality (300 mOsm/L) and the minimum urine osmolality is approximately 200 mOsm/L [24]. So, in advanced renal insufficiency an osmolar load of 600 mOsm/day obligates a urine output of about 2 liters/day. As a consequence, urine output is usually higher than normal in advanced renal insufficiency. It is only when end-stage renal disease (ESRD) is reached that urine volume would be expected to be lower than normal regardless of fluid intake.

The impaired renal concentrating ability in CKD is related to tubular dysfunction, changes in medullary structures and tonicity, high single nephron GFR, and vasopressin resistance. These dysfunctions obligate higher urine volume in order to excrete the daily osmotic load (600−900 mOsm/day). So, patients with CKD will become dehydrated and hypernatremic if water intake is insufficient. On the other hand, CKD patients with excessive water intake will become volume overloaded and hyponatremic. Management of such patients is problematic if they become severely hyponatremic. Water restriction is not likely to efficiently reverse the hyponatremia because of impaired

ability to form a dilute urine. Also, tolvaptans likely would be ineffective because the CKD renal tubules are vasopressin resistant and vasopressin levels may already be suppressed by the hyponatremia. If severe central nervous symptoms are present, a relatively rapid rise in serum sodium, e.g., ≤ 12 mEq/L over 24 hours may be needed. If the patient is able to tolerate volume expansion, intravenous hypertonic saline infusion may be sufficient. If volume expansion is not likely to be tolerated, the patient can receive the intravenous hypertonic saline infusion along with hemofiltration to control volume status.

Table 22.6 provides recommendations for water intake in CKD patients with impaired kidney function in order to avoid the scenarios of hyponatremia or hypernatremia described above.

Possible Adverse Effects of High Fluid Intake on CKD Progression

A retrospective analysis of the MDRD Study A showed that urine volumes exceeding 2 liters/day were associated with faster GFR decline, especially in patients with polycystic kidney disease [69]. The patients with higher urine volumes showed higher blood pressure, lower serum sodium, and frankly hypotonic urine suggesting that they were intentionally taking in excess fluid ("pushing fluids"). Also, in the

TABLE 22.6 Guideline for Daily Water Intake in Adult Patients with Renal Insufficiency

PATIENTS WITH CKD BUT NOT ESRD

Measured fluid intake (not including water in solid foods) of 2000 ± 500 mL/24 h is appropriate.

Higher water intake is required if the following conditions are present:
- "Salt-wasting" renal disease
- Nephrogenic diabetes insipidus
- Fever (increase fluid intake by 50 mL/day for each 1°F of fever)
- Hyperventilation (doubling the respiratory rate increases insensible losses from respiratory tract by about 200 mL/day)
- Increased sweating (the electrolyte content of sweat is not altered by renal failure)

PATIENTS WITH OLIGURIC AKI OR ESRD

Total daily fluid intake (including solid food) should approximate:
- 600 mL[a] + urine output + extrarenal water losses[b]

The above formula should be strictly adhered to in patients vulnerable to fluid overload (hypertension, congestive heart failure, etc.) or in those with hyponatremia.

More liberal intake is appropriate in patients not vulnerable to serious adverse effects of fluid overload. In these patients it is acceptable to permit up to 3-kg weight gains between hemodialysis treatments.

[a]*600 mL/day is the difference between daily insensible water losses (900 mL) and daily water production from metabolism of carbohydrates and fat (300 mL).*
[b]*Diarrhea, nasogastric suction, etc.*
ESRD, end-stage renal disease.

African American Study of Kidney Disease (AASK) trial, greater urine volume measured at baseline was significantly and independently related to faster GFR decline [70]. Greater urine volume has also been independently associated with greater 24-h protein/creatinine (P/C) ratio [69].

The association of greater urine volume with faster GFR decline in the MDRD Study was seen at 24-h urine volumes exceeding 2 liters. On this basis, we recommend that CKD patients not "push fluids". Instead CKD patients should let their thirst dictate fluid intake. Generally, that will guard against excessive fluid intake because the thirst mechanism is intact in CKD [71].

CKD patients at increased risk of hyponatremia are those not in control of their fluid intake such as hospitalized patients, or those with diabetes in whom high serum glucose stimulates thirst [68], or patients with congestive heart failure in whom high angiotensin II levels stimulate thirst [72]. In these patients excessive water intake may exceed the impaired kidney's ability to excrete the free water load. In such patients, water intake must be controlled properly to avoid serious perturbations of water balance.

There is a common perception that high urine volumes mean greater excretion of metabolic waste products. This is incorrect. The excretion of metabolic waste products depends upon GFR, not urine volume. Also, high urine volumes lead to nocturia. Nocturia leads to disrupted sleep.

A recent population study reported that those with 24-h urine volume exceeding 3 liters had slower estimated (e) GFR decline than those with lower 24-h urine volume. This suggests that in normal individuals, above normal fluid intakes may slow the GFR decline that occurs with age [73]. The clinical significance of these findings is not clear. The observed association could represent confounding [74] including decreased meat intake because high fluid intake can suppress appetite. Decreased meat intake would lower serum creatinine and eGFR, even though the actual GFR was unchanged.

Excessive Fluid Weight Gain in Patients with ESRD

It is not uncommon for some patients with ESRD to gain 4 to 6 kg in fluid weight between hemodialysis treatments or during several days of continuous ambulatory peritoneal dialysis (CAPD) therapy. Many develop adverse effects of fluid overload such as hypertension or congestive heart failure. Often these patients are advised to "drink less fluid". However, it is unlikely that the primary mechanism of the large fluid weight gains is excess water intake. If water intake was primarily responsible, such patients would show frank hyponatremia (e.g., a 10% to 15% decrease in serum

sodium concentration). In fact, these patients are usually normonatremic. This suggests that the primary mechanism for fluid weight gain is excess salt intake, which then drives excess water intake. So, the key to managing these patients is to reduce salt intake. If their salt intake is controlled, their water intake (and fluid weight gains) will be controlled.

POTASSIUM

Normal Potassium Metabolism

Potassium is the most abundant intracellular cation. Only 2% of total body potassium is present in the extracellular space. Although the extracellular potassium concentration may not reflect total body potassium stores, measurement of serum potassium is useful because disturbances of serum potassium are clinically relevant (Table 22.7). In health the distribution of potassium between the intracellular and extracellular space is influenced primarily by insulin [75,76], catecholamines [77,78], acid—base status [79], and serum osmolality [80,81]. Approximately 80% to 95% of the daily potassium intake is excreted in the urine, and 5% to 20% is

TABLE 22.7 Major Consequences of Abnormal Plasma Potassium Concentration

---

HYPERKALEMIA

Mild (Serum Potassium 5.5 to 6.5 mEq/L)[a]

EKG: peaked T-wave, prolonged PR interval
Symptoms: often none

Moderate to Severe (Serum Potassium > 6.5 mEq/L)[a]

EKG: loss of P wave, prolonged QRS interval, intraventricular conduction abnormalities progressing to bradycardia, sine wave complexes.
Symptoms: can be asymptomatic, muscle weakness and/or stiffness, especially leg muscles, progressing to total paralysis of skeletal muscles

HYPOKALEMIA

Mild (Serum Potassium 3.0 to 3.5 mEq/L)[a]

EKG: prolonged QT interval; premature ventricular contractions, particularly in patients receiving digitalis and/or those with heart disease
Symptoms: often none, except those attributable to arrhythmia

Moderate to Severe (Serum Potassium < 3.0 mEq/L)

EKG: same as mild hypokalemia but tendency to ventricular tachycardia may be greater
Symptoms: muscle weakness that can be severe, muscle cramping

---

[a]The levels of serum potassium that provide serious signs and symptoms vary considerably among patients. Changes in serum potassium that come about gradually are usually better tolerated than those that occur acutely.
EKG, electrocardiogram.

excreted in the stool [82]. The urinary excretion of a potassium load is not abrupt; rather, it occurs over 24 to 48 hours. To prevent life-threatening hyperkalemia, much of an administered or ingested potassium load is shifted into the intracellular space. Thus, potassium homeostasis is best considered in two categories: factors regulating potassium shift into cells and factors regulating renal excretion of potassium.

Extrarenal Potassium Handling in Health and in CKD

Insulin promotes the shift of potassium into the intracellular compartment in health and in renal insufficiency [75,76,83—85]. In the absence of insulin, infusion of a hypertonic solution such as glucose can induce hyperkalemia. The increase in potassium is secondary to the increase in plasma osmolality. Hyperkalemia has also been documented in patients with renal insufficiency as a result of administration of hypertonic saline or radiocontrast agents [80,81,86].

Catecholamines such as epinephrine cause a transient increase in extracellular fluid potassium followed by a sustained reduction in extracellular fluid potassium. The transient hyperkalemic response is mediated by the α-receptors, and the hypokalemic response is mediated by the β_2 receptors [75,87—89]. Catecholamine-induced cellular potassium uptake can be impaired in renal failure and may explain the enhanced hyperkalemic response to α-adrenergic stimulation in renal failure [88,90]. Despite this, patients with hyperkalemia and ESRD experience a decrease in serum potassium levels with β-agonist therapy [78,91].

Acidemia from inorganic acids, such as the infusion of HCl or NH_4Cl, results in hyperkalemia [79]. However, metabolic acidosis that is the result of accumulation of organic acids, such as lactic acid or ketoacids, does not result in important transcellular shifts of potassium [92]. Controversy exists regarding the effect of the metabolic acidosis of renal failure on transcellular potassium shifts [89,93].

Parathyroid hormone (PTH), through its ability to increase cytosolic calcium, interferes with the cellular uptake of potassium in renal disease and may play a role in the extrarenal handling of potassium in ESRD [94—96]. Fasting in the patient with ESRD promotes hyperkalemia. This paradox is thought to result from insulinopenia and diminished response to catecholamines [87,90].

There is conflicting evidence about aldosterone's role in extrarenal potassium handling [85,87,97,98]. In healthy individuals aldosterone's role in extrarenal potassium handling is minimal [99]. In individuals who are anephric, disposal of an acute potassium load is impaired by an aldosterone receptor antagonist and is improved by an aldosterone agonist [100]. There are also reports of impaired potassium handling in patients with renal insufficiency receiving heparin and angiotensin converting enzyme (ACE) inhibitors [101].

Renal Handling of Potassium in Health and in CKD

Plasma potassium is filtered freely at the glomerulus and then is reabsorbed extensively (90% to 95%) in the proximal nephron and loop of Henle. Potassium excretion is accomplished mainly by distal tubular secretion. The renal tubular secretion of potassium is an energy-requiring process. Thus, disruption of tubular function by renal disease results in renal retention of potassium. This is in contrast to the renal handling of sodium in which damage to the kidney usually results in renal sodium wasting as a result of decreased sodium reabsorption.

In the distal collecting duct potassium can be reabsorbed or secreted. Aldosterone is the primary factor influencing renal potassium handling [102]. Increasing levels of aldosterone enhance potassium excretion by increasing the number of Na-K-ATPase pumps and sodium and potassium channels [103]. Conversely, tubular damage that blunts the response to aldosterone, i.e., renal tubular acidosis type IV, will impair renal potassium excretion. Medications that impair production or action of the renin angiotensin aldosterone system such as angiotensin converting enzyme (ACE) inhibitors, angiotensin receptor blockers (ARB), or beta blockers impair renal potassium excretion via their effect on aldosterone and may lead to hyperkalemia [104]. ACEI and ARBs are safety issues in CKD [104]. Spironolactone and eplerenone cause hyperkalemia by competitively inhibiting the action of aldosterone at its receptor. Chronic heparin therapy can inhibit aldosterone secretion [105,106]. NSAIDs may also lead to hyperkalemia by decreasing kaliuresis due to decreased glomerular filtration. Table 22.8 lists the major causes of hyperkalemia and their mechanisms.

Renal potassium excretion is linked to distal nephron sodium absorption. So, increasing delivery of sodium to the distal tubule tends to increase urinary potassium excretion. Consequently, conditions such as high-salt diet, thiazide or loop diuretic therapy, Bartter's syndrome, and other acute or chronic salt-wasting renal diseases tend to cause hypokalemia (Table 22.8). By contrast, low-salt diet or conditions that decrease distal delivery of sodium, such as congestive heart failure, tend to cause hyperkalemia. Positively charged ions such as trimethoprim and amiloride cause hyperkalemia by interfering with potassium excretion through blocking luminal sodium channels in the distal nephron [107] (Table 22.8).

Renal potassium excretion is maintained as GFR falls by increasing fractional excretion of potassium. At GFR above 15 mL/min (serum creatinine approximately 3.0

TABLE 22.8 Guidelines for Dietary Potassium Intake in Adults With CKD

CONDITION USUALLY REQUIRING REDUCED POTASSIUM INTAKE (50–60 mEQ/DAY)

Mechanism: Decreased Aldosterone Levels or Aldosterone Antagonism

Hyporenin-hypoaldosteronism
Beta blocker therapy
Chronic heparin therapy
Angiotensin-converting-enzyme inhibitor therapy
Angiotensin II receptor blockade
Trimethoprim
Spironolactone
Eplerenone
Drospirenone/ethinyl estradiol (oral contraceptive, Yaz)

Mechanism: Decreased Sodium Delivery to NaK Exchange Site in the Distal Nephron

Low NaCl intake
End-stage renal disease
Cyclosporine or tacrolimus therapy

CONDITIONS USUALLY REQUIRING AN INCREASE IN POTASSIUM INTAKE (>100 mEQ/DAY) OR CONCOMITANT USE OF POTASSIUM-SPARING DIURETICS (SPIRONOLACTONE, EPLERENONE, AMILORIDE, TRIAMETERENE)

Mechanism: Renal Potassium Wasting

Type 1 or Type 2 renal tubular acidosis
Diuretic therapy (thiazide or loop diuretics)
High-salt diet
$NaHCO_3$ therapy
Mineralocorticoid therapy (e.g., fludrocortisone, hydrocortisone)
Diuretic phase during recovery from acute tubular necrosis or obstructive uropathy
Bartter's or Gittleman's syndrome

mg/dL), hyperkalemia rarely occurs unless aldosterone secretion or function is impaired. When the GFR falls below 15 mL/min, extrarenal handling of potassium, including increased gastrointestinal excretion, becomes more important in dissipating an acute potassium load [108].

When evaluating an elevated serum potassium level in the patient with renal impairment, many factors in addition to diet play a role. As outlined earlier, fasting state, level of insulin, acid-base status, β-blocker therapy, serum PTH level, and heparin therapy can affect the plasma potassium level. Blood transfusion can be an important source of potassium because transfused blood can contain between 5 and 50 mEq/L of plasma potassium, depending on storage time of the blood [109,110].

Pseudohyperkalemia can result from lysis of erythrocytes if the venipuncture technique is flawed or if abnormally elevated levels of erythrocytes, platelets, or leukocytes are present [111–113]. These cells release intracellular potassium when the blood is allowed to clot before obtaining serum. Collecting blood in heparin to obtain plasma and using a syringe rather than a vacuum tube to collect the blood can avoid these causes of pseudohyperkalemia.

Dietary Management of Potassium in CKD

Most patients with CKD do not require aggressive dietary potassium restriction. That is, on a normal potassium intake (1 to 1.3 mEq/kg of ideal body weight/day) serum potassium will be maintained within the normal range. However, there are certain circumstances that may substantially limit renal potassium secretion in CKD, making it necessary to reduce dietary potassium intake. There also are some conditions in patients with renal disease that may increase excretion of potassium, making it necessary to increase dietary potassium intake (Table 22.8).

Each gram of dietary protein generally contains about 1 mEq of potassium. So, it is difficult to design a diet that has a low potassium intake without also having a low protein intake. Fortunately, many patients with progressive renal disease are maintained on a reduced protein intake (e.g., 0.7 to 0.8 g/kg ideal body weight/day). So, potassium intake automatically is limited.

For patients with chronic hyperkalemia, determining whether excessive potassium intake or decreased renal excretion is the cause of the hyperkalemia can best be done by obtaining a 24-h urine for creatinine and potassium while the patient is on their usual diet. The creatinine measure is done to assess the extent to which the patient has provided a complete 24-h collection [114]. If the patient presents a complete 24-h collection which shows a potassium content < 50 mEq, reducing intake of potassium further is not a feasible approach to correct the hyperkalemia. On the other hand, if the 24-h urine for potassium is much higher that 50 mEq/24 h, reducing potassium intake should be effective in controlling their hyperkalemia.

For CKD patients with chronic hypokalemia, potassium intake can be increased by increasing intake of nonprotein high-potassium food (Table 22.9).

Pharmacologic Management of Chronic Hyperkalemia in CKD

If the hyperkalemia cannot be controlled by dietary restriction of potassium and the patient is hypertensive, addition of a thiazide or loop diuretic will help control the hyperkalemia and the hypertension. Loop diuretics are preferred if the serum creatinine is > 2.0 mg/dL [70]. If the CKD patient is not hypertensive, $NaHCO_3$ therapy (e.g., one or two 650-mg tablets tid with meals) is recommended.

When there is severe impairment, i.e. GFR < 15 cc/min, a potassium binding resin (Kayexalate) may be

TABLE 22.9 Potassium Content of Food

FOODS HIGH IN POTASSIUM (GREATER THAN 6.5 mEq per serving)

Imitation sour cream
Milk
Yogurt
Ice cream
Ground beef
Liver
Steak
Ham
Turkey
Flounder
Haddock
Tuna
Wheatgerm
English muffins
Legumes[a]
Fruit[a]
Raw vegetables[a]
Potatoes[a]

FOODS LOW IN POTASSIUM (LESS THAN 2.5 mEq per serving)

Mozzarella and Swiss cheese
Parmesan cheese
Cream
Eggs
Shrimp
Breads
Rice
Spaghetti
Egg noodles
Raw grapes
Raw lemons
Alfalfa sprouts
Lettuce
Cucumber
Onion

[a]*Foods that are high in potassium but low in protein.*
From Mitch WE, Klahr S, Composition of common foods. In: Mitch WE, Klahr S, (eds). Nutrition and the Kidney, Boston: Little Brown 1988:331, with permission.

necessary to decrease dietary potassium absorption. Generally, chronic daily Kayexalate therapy is best tolerated when the resin is sprinkled on moist food (i.e., 1 tablespoon of Kayexalate (about 15 g) daily on oatmeal). Each gram of Kayexalate binds and prevents the absorption of about 1 mEq of potassium. An alternative strategy to manage chronic hyperkalemia is Kayexalate Fudge (see MicroMedix®).

Intermittent dosing of Kayexalate (i.e., 30 g) every few days is also an option. The Kayexalate should be given without sorbitol because sorbitol increases the risk of bowel necrosis, which can be fatal [115].

MAGNESIUM

Total body magnesium is distributed primarily in bone and the intracellular fluid compartment, where it is the second most abundant intracellular cation. Only 1% of total body magnesium is found in the ECFV. Magnesium is an essential co-activator for enzymatic reactions metabolizing ATP, and is a critical cellular and mitochondrial control mechanism [116]. In health, approximately 40% of dietary magnesium is absorbed by the gastrointestinal tract; the remainder is excreted in the stool [117]. Of plasma magnesium, 80% is filtered at the glomerulus. All but 3% to 5% is reabsorbed. Of the filtered load, 60% of magnesium is reabsorbed by the thick-ascending loop of Henle, 20% to 30% in the proximal tubule, and 5% in the distal tubule. In the face of low dietary magnesium intake, gastrointestinal absorption can increase to 70%, and urinary excretion can be reduced to 0.5% of the filtered load. High dietary magnesium intake has the opposite effect.

Magnesium deficiency can result from low dietary intake, or from gastrointestinal, or renal magnesium wasting that is acquired (e.g., drug related — see below) or genetic. In evaluating patients with hypomagnesemia, a 24-hour urinary magnesium content of greater than 0.5 mmol is abnormal and reflects renal magnesium wasting [58]. Several drugs have been reported to lead to renal magnesium wasting including diuretics, proton pump inhibitors, cisplatin, aminoglycosides, cyclosporine, among others (Table 22.10) [118]. The association of renal magnesium wasting with proton pump inhibitors is a newly recognized association [118,119].

Low serum magnesium can interfere with the release of PTH and result in concomitant hypocalcemia [120]. Hypomagnesemia also can result in tetany, muscle weakness, seizures, supraventricular and ventricular arrhythmias, and has been suggested to play a role in the progression of diabetic nephropathy [117,118,121]. Mutations in magnesium regulating cation channel genes cause hypomagnesemia with secondary hypocalcemia (HSH), a rare autosomal recessive disorder, and may play a mechanistic role in FSGS [116]. Hypomagnesemia can also cause renal potassium wasting

TABLE 22.10 Conditions Associated with the Renal Magnesium Wasting

Diuretics
Cisplatin-induced nephrotoxicity
Aminoglycoside-induced nephrotoxicity
Cyclosporine
Amphotericin B
Proton pump inhibitors
Foscarnet
Recovery phase of acute tubular necrosis
Acute alcohol intake
Hyperaldosteronism
Bartter's syndrome
Familial hypercalcemia
Hyperparathyroidism

TABLE 22.11 Magnesium Content of Various Foods

HIGH (GREATER THAN 20 MG PER SERVING)
Meats
Green vegetables
Legumes
Dairy products

LOW (LESS THAN 5 MG PER SERVING)
Alcohol
Processed foods
Fat

that is resistant to correction by potassium supplementation [122].

Negative magnesium balance from decreased dietary intake is rare, except in the case of alcoholism. Alcoholics usually have a diet deficient in magnesium, and alcohol may promote renal magnesium wasting [123]. Table 22.10 lists the causes of urinary magnesium wasting.

High serum magnesium levels occur almost exclusively in the face of renal insufficiency. At a GFR of less than 15 mL/min, the fractional excretion of magnesium may not increase sufficiently to prevent positive magnesium balance from occurring. This is especially true if dietary magnesium is supplemented with magnesium-containing antacids or cathartics [120]. Mild increases in plasma magnesium are well tolerated, but at levels greater than 4 mEq/L loss of deep tendon reflexes, respiratory paralysis, and heart block may occur [120].

Dialysate for both hemodialysis and peritoneal dialysis contains magnesium concentrations that are below serum concentrations to help combat positive magnesium balance [120]. Despite this, most patients undergoing dialysis have an increase in total body magnesium [124]. The positive magnesium balance in patients with ESRD may contribute to renal osteodystrophy [125]. Dietary magnesium manipulation usually is not addressed in ESRD unless the patient develops hypermagnesemia. On a diet containing the standard recommended daily allowance of magnesium (300 mg) serum magnesium levels usually will be maintained within normal limits. Table 22.11 lists the magnesium content of various food products. If dietary sources are insufficient, then supplementation with oral magnesium salts is usually sufficient. Slow release magnesium preparations are recommended. Renal magnesium wasting can be inhibited by the potassium-sparing diuretics such as amiloride.

References

[1] Whitescarver SA, Ott CE, Jackson BA, Guthrie Jr GP, Kotchen TA. Salt-sensitive hypertension: contribution of chloride. Science 1984;223(4643):1430–2.

[2] Schrier RW. Pathogenesis of sodium and water retention in high-output and low-output cardiac failure, nephrotic syndrome, cirrhosis, and pregnancy (1). N Engl J Med 1988;319(16):1065–72.

[3] Wennergren G, Henriksson BA, Weiss LG, Oberg B. Effects of stimulation of nonmedullated cardiac afferents on renal water and sodium excretion. Acta Physiol Scand 1976;97(2):261–3.

[4] de Bold AJ, Borenstein HB, Veress AT, Sonnenberg H. A rapid and potent natriuretic response to intravenous injection of atrial myocardial extract in rats. Life Sci 1981;28(1):89–94.

[5] Epstein F. Effects of arteriovenous fistula on renal hemodynamics and electrolyte excretion. J Clin Invest 1953;32:233.

[6] McCartney S, Cramb G. Effects of a high-salt diet on hepatic atrial natriuretic peptide receptor expression in Dahl salt-resistant and salt-sensitive rats. J Hypertens 1993;11(3):253–62.

[7] Sumners C, Tang W, Paulding W, Raizada MK. Peptide receptors in astroglia: focus on angiotensin II and atrial natriuretic peptide. Glia 1994;11(2):110–6.

[8] Fitzgibbons JP, Gennari FJ, Garfinkel HB, Cortell S. Dependence of saline-induced natriuresis upon exposure of the kidney to the physical effects of extracellular fluid volume expansion. J Clin Invest 1974;54(6):1428–36.

[9] Simpson FO. Sodium intake, body sodium, and sodium excretion. Lancet 1988;2(8601):25–9.

[10] Oliver WJ, Cohen EL, Neel JV. Blood pressure, sodium intake, and sodium related hormones in the Yanomamo Indians, a "no-salt" culture. Circulation 1975;52(1):146–51.

[11] Strauss MB. Surfeit and deficit of sodium. Arch Intern Med 1958;102:527–37.

[12] Heer M, Baisch F, Kropp J, Gerzer R, Drummer C. High dietary sodium chloride consumption may not induce body fluid retention in humans. Am J Physiol Renal Physiol 2000;278(4):F585–95.

[13] Humphreys MH. Salt intake and body fluid volumes: have we learned all there is to know? Am J Kidney Dis 2001;37(3):648–52.

[14] Murray RH, Luft FC, Bloch R, Weyman AE. Blood pressure responses to extremes of sodium intake in normal man. Proc Soc Exp Biol Med 1978;159(3):432–6.

[15] Campase V. Salt sensitivity in hypertension. Renal and cardiovascular implications. Hypertension 1994;23:531.

[16] Tripodi G, Valtorta F, Torielli L, Chieregatti E, Salardi S, Trusolino L, et al. Hypertension-associated point mutations in the adducin alpha and beta subunits affect actin cytoskeleton and ion transport. J Clin Invest 1996;97(12):2815–22.

[17] Perticone F, Sciacqua A, Barlassina C, Del Vecchio L, Signorello MC, Dal Fiume C, et al. Gly460Trp alpha-adducin gene polymorphism and endothelial function in untreated hypertensive patients. J Hypertens 2007;25(11):2234–9.

[18] Beeks E, Kessels AG, Kroon AA, van der Klauw MM, de Leeuw PW. Genetic predisposition to salt-sensitivity: a systematic review. J Hypertens 2004;22(7):1243–9.

[19] Dimke H, San-Cristobal P, de Graaf M, Lenders JW, Deinum J, Hoenderop JG, et al. gamma-Adducin stimulates the thiazide-sensitive NaCl cotransporter. J Am Soc Nephrol 2011;22(3):508–17.

[20] U.S.D.A, D.H.H.S. U.S. Department of Agriculture and U.S. Department of Health and Human Services: Dietary Guidelines for Americans. 7th ed. Washington, DC: U.S. Government Printing Office; 2010.

[21] He FJ, MacGregor GA. Salt reduction lowers cardiovascular risk: meta-analysis of outcome trials. Lancet 2011;378(9789):380–2.

[22] He FJ, Appel LJ, Cappuccio FP, de Wardener HE, MacGregor GA. Does reducing salt intake increase cardiovascular mortality? Kidney Int 2011;80(7):696–8.

[23] NIH. The Seventh Report of the Joint National Committee on Prevention, Detection, Evaluation, and Treatment of High Blood Pressure. In: Services, editor. USDoHaH, Washington, DC; 2004.

[24] Taylor RS, Ashton KE, Moxham T, Hooper L, Ebrahim S. Reduced dietary salt for the prevention of cardiovascular disease: a meta-analysis of randomized controlled trials (Cochrane review). Am J Hypertens 2011;24(8):843—53.

[25] Chang HY, Hu YW, Yue CS, Wen YW, Yeh WT, Hsu LS, et al. Effect of potassium-enriched salt on cardiovascular mortality and medical expenses of elderly men. Am J Clin Nutr 2006;83(6):1289—96.

[26] Thomas MC, Moran J, Forsblom C, Harjutsalo V, Thorn L, Ahola A, et al. The association between dietary sodium intake, ESRD, and all-cause mortality in patients with type 1 diabetes. Diabetes Care 2011;34(4):861—6.

[27] Ekinci EI, Clarke S, Thomas MC, Moran JL, Cheong K, MacIsaac RJ, et al. Dietary salt intake and mortality in patients with type 2 diabetes. Diabetes Care 2011;34(3):703—9.

[28] Stolarz-Skrzypek K, Kuznetsova T, Thijs L, Tikhonoff V, Seidlerova J, Richart T, et al. Fatal and nonfatal outcomes, incidence of hypertension, and blood pressure changes in relation to urinary sodium excretion. JAMA 2011;305(17):1777—85.

[29] O'Donnell MJ, Yusuf S, Mente A, Gao P, Mann JF, Teo K, et al. Urinary sodium and potassium excretion and risk of cardiovascular events. JAMA 2011;306(20):2229—38.

[30] Graudal NA, Galloe AM, Garred P. Effects of sodium restriction on blood pressure, renin, aldosterone, catecholamines, cholesterols, and triglyceride: a meta-analysis. JAMA 1998;279(17):1383—91.

[31] Haddad N, Rajan J, Nagaraja HN, Agarwal AK, Hebert LA. Usual ACE inhibitor therapy in CKD patients is associated with lower plasma aldosterone levels than usual angiotensin receptor blocker therapy. Kidney Blood Press Res. 2007;30(5):299—305.

[32] Petrie JR, Morris AD, Minamisawa K, Hilditch TE, Elliott HL, Small M, et al. Dietary sodium restriction impairs insulin sensitivity in noninsulin-dependent diabetes mellitus. J Clin Endocrinol Metab 1998;83(5):1552—7.

[33] Ivanovski O, Szumilak D, Nguyen-Khoa T, Dechaux M, Massy ZA, Phan O, et al. Dietary salt restriction accelerates atherosclerosis in apolipoprotein E-deficient mice. Atherosclerosis 2005;180(2):271—6.

[34] Hebert LA, Rovin BH, Hebert CJ. The design of ALLHAT may have biased the study's outcome in favor of the diuretic cohort. Nature Clin Pract Nephrol 2007;3(2):60—1.

[35] Rovin BH, Hebert LA. Thiazide diuretic monotherapy for hypertension: diuretic's dark side just got darker. Kidney Int 2007;72(12):1423—6.

[36] Alderman MH. The Cochrane review of sodium and health. Am J Hypertens 2011;24(8):854—6.

[37] Bernstein AM, Willett WC. Trends in 24-h urinary sodium excretion in the United States, 1957—2003: a systematic review. Am J Clin Nutr 2010;92(5):1172—80.

[38] Appel LJ, Moore TJ, Obarzanek E, Vollmer WM, Svetkey LP, Sacks FM, et al. A clinical trial of the effects of dietary patterns on blood pressure. DASH Collaborative Research Group. N Engl J Med 1997;336(16):1117—24.

[39] Sacks FM, Svetkey LP, Vollmer WM, Appel LJ, Bray GA, Harsha D, et al. Effects on blood pressure of reduced dietary sodium and the Dietary Approaches to Stop Hypertension (DASH) diet. DASH-Sodium Collaborative Research Group. N Engl J Med 2001;344(1):3—10.

[40] Bricker NS, Fine LG, Kaplan M, Epstein M, Bourgoignie JJ, Light A. Magnification phenomenon in chronic renal disease. N Engl J Med 1978;299(23):1287—93.

[41] Fine L, Kurtz I, Woolf A, Danovitch G, Emmons C, Kujubu D, et al. Pathophysiology and nephron adaptation in chronic renal failure. In: Schrier RW, Gottschalk C, editors. Diseases of the Kidney. Boston: Little, Brown; 1993. p. 1993—2703.

[42] Kahn T, Mohammad G, Stein RM. Alterations in renal tubular sodium and water reabsorption in chronic renal disease in man. Kidney Int 1972;2(3):164—74.

[43] Brod J, Bahlmann J, Cachovan M, Pretschner P. Development of hypertension in renal disease. Clin Sci (Lond) 1983;64(2):141—52.

[44] Coleman A, Arias M, Carter N, et al. The mechanism of salt wastage in chroni renal disease. Clin Invest 1966;45:1116—25.

[45] Danovitch GM, Bourgoignie J, Bricker NS. Reversibility of the "salt-losing" tendency of chronic renal failure. N Engl J Med 1977;296(1):14—9.

[46] Husted FC, Nolph KD, Maher JF. NaHCO3 and NaCl tolerance in chronic renal failure. J Clin Invest 1975;56(2):414—9.

[47] Schrier R. Tubular sodium transport. In: Gottschalk CW, editor. Diseases of the kidney. Boston: Little Brown & Co; 1993. p. 139.

[48] Pimenta E, Gaddam KK, Oparil S, Aban I, Husain S, Dell'Italia LJ, et al. Effects of dietary sodium reduction on blood pressure in subjects with resistant hypertension: results from a randomized trial. Hypertension 2009;54(3):475—81.

[49] Parikh S, Hebert LA, Rovin BH. Protecting the kidneys in lupus nephritis. Int J Clin Rheumatol 2011. p. 529.

[50] Klahr S, Levey AS, Beck GJ, Caggiula AW, Hunsicker L, Kusek JW, et al. The effects of dietary protein restriction and blood-pressure control on the progression of chronic renal disease. Modification of Diet in Renal Disease Study Group. N Engl J Med 1994;330(13):877—84.

[51] Appel LJ, Wright Jr JT. The long-term effects of a lower blood pressure goal on progression of hypertensive chronic kidney disease in African-Americans. N Engl J Med 2010;363(10):918—29.

[52] Wuhl E, Trivelli A, Picca S, Litwin M, Peco-Antic A, Zurowska A, et al. Strict blood-pressure control and progression of renal failure in children. N Engl J Med 2009;361(17):1639—50.

[53] Wilmer WA, Rovin BH, Hebert CJ, Rao SV, Kumor K, Hebert LA. Management of glomerular proteinuria: a commentary. J Am Soc Nephrol 2003;14(12):3217—32.

[54] Mahajan A, Simoni J, Sheather SJ, Broglio KR, Rajab MH, Wesson DE. Daily oral sodium bicarbonate preserves glomerular filtration rate by slowing its decline in early hypertensive nephropathy. Kidney Int 2010;78(3):303—9.

[55] Phisitkul S, Khanna A, Simoni J, Broglio K, Sheather S, Rajab MH, et al. Amelioration of metabolic acidosis in patients with low GFR reduced kidney endothelin production and kidney injury, and better preserved GFR. Kidney Int 2010;77(7):617—23.

[56] Couser WG, Nangaku M. Mechanism of bicarbonate effect in CKD. Kidney Int 2010;78(8):817; author reply 8.

[57] Nicholson JP, Resnick LM, Laragh JH. The antihypertensive effect of verapamil at extremes of dietary sodium intake. Ann Intern Med 1987;107(3):329—34.

[58] Krishna GG, Riley Jr LJ, Deuter G, Kapoor SC, Narins RG. Natriuretic effect of calcium-channel blockers in hypertensives. Am J Kidney Dis 1991;18(5):566—72.

[59] Robertson G, Berl T. Pathophysiology of water metabolism. In: Brenner B, Rector F, editors. The kidney. Philadelphia: WB Saunders; 1991. p. 677.

[60] Teitelbaum I, Berl T, Kleeman C. The physiology of renal concentrating and diluting mechanisms. In: Maxwell M, Kleeman C, Narins RG, editors. Clinical disorders of fluid and electrolyte metabolism. St Louis: McGraw-Hill; 1987. p. 79.

[61] Robertson GL. Thirst and vasopressin function in normal and disordered states of water balance. J Lab Clin Med 1983;101(3):351—71.

[62] Verney E. The antdiuretic hormone and the factors which determine its release. Proc R Soc London 1947;135:25.

[63] Robertson GL. The regulation of vasopressin function in health and disease. Recent Prog Horm Res 1976;33:333—85.

[64] Anderson RJ, Pluss RG, Berns AS, Jackson JT, Arnold PE, Schrier RW, et al. Mechanism of effect of hypoxia on renal water excretion. J Clin Invest 1978;62(4):769—77.

[65] Baylis PH, Zerbe RL, Robertson GL. Arginine vasopressin response to insulin-induced hypoglycemia in man. J Clin Endocrinol Metab 1981;53(5):935—40.

[66] Fisher DA. Norepinephrine inhibition of vasopressin anti-diuresis. J Clin Invest 1968;47(3):540—7.

[67] Keil LC, Summy-Long J, Severs WB. Release of vasopressin by angiotensin II. Endocrinology 1975;96(4):1063—5.

[68] Zerbe R, Robertson G. Osmotic and nonosmotic regulation of thirst and vasopressin secretion. In: Maxwell M, Kleeman C, Narins R, editors. Clinical disorders of fluid and electrolyte metabolism. New York: McGraw-Hill; 1987. p. 61.

[69] Hebert LA, Greene T, Levey AS, Falkenhain M, Klahr S. High urine volume and low urine osmolality are risk factors for faster progression of renal disease. Am J Kidney Dis 2003;41(5): 962—71.

[70] Brown C, Haddad N, Hebert LA. Retarding Progression of Kidney Disease. In: Feehally J, Floege J, Johnson RJ, editors. Comprehensive Clinical Nephrology. 4th ed. Philadelphia: Elsevier; 2010. p. 919—26.

[71] Argent NB, Burrell LM, Goodship TH, Wilkinson R, Baylis PH. Osmoregulation of thirst and vasopressin release in severe chronic renal failure. Kidney Int 1991;39(2):295—300.

[72] Ramsay DJ, Rolls BJ, Wood RJ. The relationship between elevated water intake and oedema associated with congestive cardiac failure in the dog. J Physiol 1975;244(2):303—12.

[73] Clark WF, Sontrop JM, Macnab JJ, Suri RS, Moist L, Salvadori M, et al. Urine Volume and Change in Estimated GFR in a Community-Based Cohort Study. Clin J Am Soc Nephrol 2011;6(11):2634—41.

[74] Chang A, Kramer H. Fluid intake for kidney disease prevention: an urban myth? Clin J Am Soc Nephrol 2011;6(11): 2558—60.

[75] DeFronzo RA, Sherwin RS, Dillingham M, Hendler R, Tamborlane WV, Felig P. Influence of basal insulin and glucagon secretion on potassium and sodium metabolism. Studies with somatostatin in normal dogs and in normal and diabetic human beings. J Clin Invest 1978;61(2):472—9.

[76] DeFronzo RA, Felig P, Ferrannini E, Wahren J. Effect of graded doses of insulin on splanchnic and peripheral potassium metabolism in man. Am J Physiol 1980;238(5):E421—7.

[77] Brown MJ, Brown DC, Murphy MB. Hypokalemia from beta2-receptor stimulation by circulating epinephrine. N Engl J Med 1983;309:1414—9.

[78] Castellino P, Bia MJ, DeFronzo RA. Adrenergic modulation of potassium metabolism in uremia. Kidney Int 1990;37(2):793—8.

[79] Adler S, Fraley DS. Potassium and intracellular pH. Kidney Int 1977;11(6):433—42.

[80] Conte G, Dal Canton A, Imperatore P, De Nicola L, Gigliotti G, Pisanti N, et al. Acute increase in plasma osmolality as a cause of hyperkalemia in patients with renal failure. Kidney Int 1990;38(2):301—7.

[81] Moreno M, Murphy C, Goldsmith C. Increase in serum potassium resulting from the administration of hypertonic mannitol and other solutions. J Lab Clin Med 1969;73(2):291—8.

[82] Rabelink TJ, Koomans HA, Hene RJ, Dorhout Mees EJ. Early and late adjustment to potassium loading in humans. Kidney Int 1990;38(5):942—7.

[83] Alvestrand A, Wahren J, Smith D, DeFronzo RA. Insulin-mediated potassium uptake is normal in uremic and healthy subjects. Am J Physiol 1984;246(2 Pt 1):E174—80.

[84] Silvia P, Brown R, Epstein F. Adaptation to potassium. Kidney Int 1977;11:466—75.

[85] Brown RS. Extrarenal potassium homeostasis. Kidney Int 1986;30(1):116—27.

[86] Goldfarb S, Cox M, Singer I, Goldberg M. Acute hyperkalemia induced by hyperglycemia: hormonal mechanisms. Ann Intern Med 1976;84(4):426—32.

[87] Allon M. Treatment and prevention of hyperkalemia in end-stage renal disease. Kidney Int 1993;43(6):1197—209.

[88] Allon M, Copkney C. Albuterol and insulin for treatment of hyperkalemia in hemodialysis patients. Kidney Int 1990;38(5): 869—72.

[89] Allon M, Shanklin N. Adrenergic modulation of extrarenal potassium disposal in men with end-stage renal disease. Kidney Int 1991;40(6):1103—9.

[90] Gifford JD, Rutsky EA, Kirk KA, McDaniel HG. Control of serum potassium during fasting in patients with end-stage renal disease. Kidney Int 1989;35(1):90—4.

[91] Montoliu J, Lens XM, Revert L. Potassium-lowering effect of albuterol for hyperkalemia in renal failure. Arch Intern Med 1987;147(4):713—7.

[92] Fulop M. Serum potassium in lactic acidosis and ketoacidosis. N Engl J Med 1979;300(19):1087—9.

[93] Blumberg A, Weidmann P, Ferrari P. Effect of prolonged bicar-bonate administration on plasma potassium in terminal renal failure. Kidney Int 1992;41(2):369—74.

[94] Massry SG. Renal failure, parathyroid hormone and extrarenal disposal of potassium. Miner Electrolyte Metab 1990;16(1):77—81.

[95] Soliman AR, Akmal M, Massry SG. Parathyroid hormone interferes with extrarenal disposition of potassium in chronic renal failure. Nephron 1989;52(3):262—7.

[96] Sugarman A, Kahn T. Parathyroid hormone impairs extrarenal potassium tolerance in the rat. Am J Physiol 1988;254(3 Pt 2):F385—90.

[97] Tuck ML, Davidson MB, Asp N, Schultze RG. Augmented aldosterone and insulin responses to potassium infusion in dogs with renal failure. Kidney Int 1986;30(6):883—90.

[98] Hiatt N, Chapman LW, Davidson MB, Sheinkopf JA. Adrenal hormones and the regulation of serum potassium in potassium-loaded adrenalectomized dogs. Endocrinology 1979;105(1):215—9.

[99] Alexander EA, Levinsky NG. An extrarenal mechanism of potassium adaptation. J Clin Invest 1968;47(4):740—8.

[100] Sugarman A, Brown RS. The role of aldosterone in potassium tolerance: studies in anephric humans. Kidney Int 1988;34(3): 397—403.

[101] Durand D, Ader JL, Rey JP, Tran-Van T, Lloveras JJ, Bernadet P, et al. Inducing hyperkalemia by converting enzyme inhibitors and heparin. Kidney Int Suppl 1988;25:S196—7.

[102] Rabinowitz L. Homeostatic regulation of potassium excretion. J Hypertens 1989;7(6):433—42.

[103] Giebish G, Malnic G, Berliner R. Renal transport and control of potassium excretion. In: Brenner B, Rector F, editors. The kidney. Philadelphia: WB Saunders; 1991. p. 283—317.

[104] Mangrum AJ, Bakris GL. Angiotensin-converting enzyme inhibitors and angiotensin receptor blockers in chronic renal disease: safety issues. Semin Nephrol 2004;24(2):168—75.

[105] Wilson I, Goetz F. Selective hypoaldosteronism after prolonged heparin administration. Am J Med 1984;36:635—9.

[106] O'Kelly R, Magee F, McKenna TJ. Routine heparin therapy inhibits adrenal aldosterone production. J Clin Endocrinol Metab 1983;56(1):108—12.

[107] Choi MJ, Fernandez PC, Patnaik A, Coupaye-Gerard B, D'Andrea D, Szerlip H, et al. Brief report: trimethoprim-induced hyperkalemia in a patient with AIDS. N Engl J Med 1993;328(10):703—6.

[108] Martin RS, Panese S, Virginillo M, Gimenez M, Litardo M, Arrizurieta E, et al. Increased secretion of potassium in the rectum of humans with chronic renal failure. Am J Kidney Dis 1986;8(2):105—10.

[109] Simon GE, Bove JR. The potassium load from blood transfusion. Postgrad Med 1971;49(6):61—4.

[110] Palmer BF. A physiologic-based approach to the evaluation of a patient with hypokalemia. Am J Kidney Dis 2010;56(6): 1184—90.

[111] Bronson WR, DeVita VT, Carbone PP, Cotlove E. Pseudo-hyperkalemia due to release of potassium from white blood cells during clotting. N Engl J Med 1966;274(7):369—75.

[112] Don BR, Sebastian A, Cheitlin M, Christiansen M, Schambelan M. Pseudohyperkalemia caused by fist clenching during phle-botomy. N Engl J Med 1990;322(18):1290—2.

[113] Hartmann R, Auditore J, Jackson D. Studies on thromboytosis. I. Hyperkalemia due to release of potassium from platelets during coagulation. J Clin Invest 1958;37:699—707.

[114] Birmingham DJ, Rovin BH, Shidham G, Nagaraja HN, Zou X, Bissell M, et al. Spot urine protein/creatinine ratios are unreliable estimates of 24 h proteinuria in most systemic lupus erythematosus nephritis flares. Kidney Int 2007;72: 865—70.

[115] Sterns RH, Rojas M, Bernstein P, Chennupati S. Ion-exchange resins for the treatment of hyperkalemia: are they safe and effective? J Am Soc Nephrol 2010;21(5):733—5.

[116] Dietrich A, Chubanov V, Gudermann T. Renal TRPathies. J Am Soc Nephrol 2010;21(5):736—44.

[117] Slatopolsky E, Hruska K, Klahr S. Disorders of phosphorus, calcium, and magnesium metabolism. In: Schrier RW, Gottschalk C, editors. Diseases of the kidney. Boston: Little, Brown; 1993. p. 2630—5.

[118] Regolisti G, Cabassi A, Parenti E, Maggiore U, Fiaccadori E. Severe hypomagnesemia during long-term treatment with a proton pump inhibitor. Am J Kidney Dis 2010;56(1):168—74.

[119] Hoorn EJ, van der Hoek J, de Man RA, Kuipers EJ, Bolwerk C, Zietse R. A case series of proton pump inhibitor-induced hypomagnesemia. Am J Kidney Dis 2010;56(1):112—6.

[120] Sutton R, Dirks J. Disturbances of calcium and magnesum metabolism. In: Brenner B, Rector F, editors. The kidney. Phil-adelphia: WB Saunders; 1991. p. 841.

[121] Pham PC, Pham PM, Pham PT, Pham SV, Pham PA. The link between lower serum magnesium and kidney function in patients with diabetes mellitus Type 2 deserves a closer look. Clin Nephrol 2009;71(4):375—9.

[122] Whang R, Flink EB, Dyckner T, Wester PO, Aikawa JK, Ryan MP. Magnesium depletion as a cause of refractory potassium repletion. Arch Intern Med 1985;145(9):1686—9.

[123] Dick M, Evans RA, Watson L. Effect of ethanol on magnesium excretion. J Clin Pathol 1969;22(2):152—3.

[124] Contiguglia SR, Alfrey AC, Miller N, Butkus D. Total-body magnesium excess in chronic renal failure. Lancet 1972;1(7764): 1300—2.

[125] Mitch W, Klahr S. Composition of common foods. In: Mitch W, Klahr S, editors. Nutrition and the kidney. Boston: Little, Brown; 1988. p. 331.

Trace Elements, Toxic Metals, and Metalloids in Kidney Disease

Sundararaman Swaminathan

Division of Nephrology, Department of Internal Medicine, University of Arkansas for Medical Sciences and
Renal Section, Medicine Service, Central Arkansas Veterans Healthcare System, Little Rock, Arkansas, USA

INTRODUCTION

Trace elements include all naturally occurring elements in the periodic table except the bulk elements. Examples of bulk elements include oxygen, hydrogen, carbon, sulfur, and nitrogen, and their requirements are in the order of grams per day. Macro-minerals include sodium, magnesium, phosphorus, chlorine, potassium and calcium, and their requirements are usually a fraction of a gram per day [1]. Trace elements are present in the body at less than 0.01% of total body mass, and their current daily recommended intake is typically less than 100 mg per day. Ultratrace elements are typically defined as those with a daily requirement of less than 1 mg per day. Trace elements may be differentiated between those with or without an established essentiality, and their source is usually from air, water, or diet. Withdrawal or absence of essential trace elements from the diet will produce functional or structural changes that are usually reversible upon replacement of the deficient element. Although all of the trace minerals important to human nutrition are elements, they are not all metals (e.g., selenium and iodine). A metalloid is a chemical element with properties in between a metal and a nonmetal. Commonly recognized metalloids include arsenic, antimony, boron, germanium, silicon and tellurium.

Trace elements serve three broad physiologic functions: (1) oxygen binding and transport — iron (Fe); (2) metabolic catalysis — manganese (Mn), molybdenum (Mo), copper (Cu), zinc (Zn), selenium (Se), and chromium (Cr); and (3) hormone effects — Se and iodine (I). In this chapter, we will review the disease processes related to alterations in trace element burden in patients with kidney disease (please see Chapters 6 and 22 for a more detailed discussion of iron). We will first focus on essential trace elements and then discuss nonessential trace elements and metals in patients with kidney disease.

ALTERATIONS IN ESSENTIAL TRACE ELEMENTS IN PATIENTS WITH KIDNEY DISEASE

We will review the current literature on alterations in individual essential trace elements in kidney disease and present them in the order of potential importance and available evidence.

Zinc

The major metabolic function of zinc is as a cofactor for many enzymes that are important for cellular activity (e.g., alcohol dehydrogenase, alkaline phosphatase, angiotensin-converting enzyme, and superoxide dismutase). Zinc is also an important component of zinc finger proteins that act as transcription factors to allow binding of proteins to deoxyribonucleic acid (DNA) and that control gene expression. Most of the zinc in the body is present in the skeletal muscle (60%) and bone (30%). The daily zinc requirement is about 8–11 mg. Most good protein sources, including oysters, poultry, meat and eggs, contain substantial zinc. Whole cereal grains are also good sources of zinc. Alcoholism, use of medications such as hydrochlorothiazide, penicillamine and ethambutol, sickle cell disease, human immunodeficiency virus (HIV) infection, liver and renal disease may result in zinc deficiency. In the general population, zinc deficiency is manifested with growth retardation, poor wound healing, decreased sexual performance, abnormal hair and nails, loss of taste (hypogeusia),

TABLE 23.1   Zinc Metabolism in Kidney Disease

- **Daily zinc requirement:** 8–11 mg
- **Dietary sources:** Oysters, poultry, meat, eggs, legumes, whole-grain cereals
- **Function:** Enzymes, zinc finger proteins
- **Specific clinical manifestations of deficiency in dialysis patients:** Erythropoietin resistance, anxiety, depression, hyperammonemia
- **Diagnostic laboratory tests:** Low serum alkaline phosphatase and decreased serum zinc levels

TABLE 23.2   Copper Metabolism in Kidney Disease

- **Daily copper requirements:** 900 μg per day
- **Dietary sources:** nuts, chocolates, meat, shellfish
- **Function:** cuproenzymes, collagen synthesis, iron metabolism
- Specific clinical manifestations of deficiency in dialysis patients: Erythropoietin resistance, anemia, neutropenia, neurodegenerative illness
- **Risk factors for deficiency:** Bariatric surgery, zinc supplementation, parenteral nutrition
- **Laboratory tests to diagnose copper deficiency:** Low serum copper and ceruloplasmin levels; serum ferritin may be high
- **Copper accumulation:** Historic, in patients dialyzed with cuprophane membrane; link to dialysis-related amyloidosis

gastrointestinal (GI) disturbances such as anorexia, abdominal pain, nausea and glossitis, and impaired folate and vitamin A absorption. Zinc excess in the body may cause rough hair, diarrhea, microcytic anemia, and hypercholesterolemia. Since zinc competes with the GI absorption of copper, manganese, and iron, excessive zinc intake may result in copper, manganese, and iron deficiency as well.

Many maintenance hemodialysis (MHD) patients suffer from zinc deficiency (Table 23.1). The mechanisms leading to zinc deficiency can include decreased dietary intake, malabsorption, and dialysate loss. In a recent study, 96% of anemic dialysis patients were found to be zinc-deficient, based on serum zinc measurements [2]. In those patients with serum zinc levels less than 80 mg/dL, the anemia responded favorably to oral zinc supplementation. In particular, many patients diagnosed with refractory anemia despite erythropoietin (EPO) therapy also had zinc deficiency anemia. Zinc replacement not only corrected the anemia but substantially lowered the EPO requirements in this population. Thus, zinc deficiency anemia should be considered in patients with erythropoietin resistance [2].

Zinc is also important for neurobehavioral function. Zinc deficiency can result in increased anxiety and depression [3–5]. A recent study reported an association between zinc deficiency and depression in MHD patients. However, there are no well-conducted studies that have examined the potential beneficial effects of zinc replacement on depressive symptoms in MHD patients. Zinc deficiency in MHD patients may also result in hyperammonemia, because ornithine transcarbomylase is a zinc-dependent enzyme; these abnormalities are well corrected with zinc replacement [6].

Copper

Copper (Table 23.2) exists in the body in two oxidative states, as cuprous (Cu^{1+}) and cupric (Cu^{2+}). Copper serves as a cofactor for many enzymes known as cuproenzymes. Copper is particularly essential for the function of several important enzymes, including superoxide dismutase (Cu/Zn SOD is an anti-oxidant), amine oxidase (monoamine oxidase), lysyl oxidase (involved in collagen synthesis), tyrosine hydroxylase, dopamine beta-hydrolase (regarding skin pigmentation), factor V (for coagulation), and cytochrome c oxidase. Cu/Zn SOD has two atoms of copper per molecule and is present at high levels in the brain and kidney, among other tissues. Copper plays an additional important function in iron metabolism which is mediated through ceruloplasmin or ferroxidase. The adult human body contains about 50 to 120 mg of copper, with the highest content in the liver (10–35 μg/g of dry weight). Copper is primarily excreted via bile (2 mg per day), and about 10 to 50 μg are lost in the urine daily. Ceruloplasmin is the major copper binding protein in the blood, and in plasma, 60 to 90% of the copper is bound to ceruloplasmin, and the remainder is loosely bound to albumin. A normal plasma copper level is about 0.9 μg per milliliter, and plasma ceruloplasmin levels are 150 to 600 μg per milliliter. In the western diet, 60% of dietary copper comes from vegetable sources (grains, nuts, chocolates), and 20% is derived from meat, fish (particularly shellfish), and poultry. In the GI tract, several minerals influence copper absorption. Dietary zinc, in particular, can decrease copper absorption through the stimulating effects of zinc on metallothionein synthesis and the subsequent binding of copper by metallothionein. Excess dietary iron can also decrease copper absorption. Previous bariatric surgery, zinc supplementation, malabsorption, proteinuria, and chronic peritoneal dialysis serve as risk factors for copper deficiency. In patients undergoing chronic peritoneal dialysis, loss of ceruloplasmin-bound copper into the dialysate may lead to copper deficiency. In patients with proteinuric kidney diseases, urinary copper losses may serve as an additional mechanism that contributes to copper deficiency.

Copper deficiency in the general population is characterized by fragile, abnormally-formed hair, depigmentation of the skin, myeloneuropathy, ataxia, edema, osteoporosis, and hematologic changes (microcytic anemia and neuropenia). In chronic dialysis patients, copper deficiency may be significantly present and remain underdiagnosed [7–11]. Symptoms of copper deficiency described in maintenance dialysis patients include immune dysfunction as evidenced by neutropenia [12], erythropoietin-resistant anemia [13], and neurodegeneration (cerebellar, spinal cord, and peripheral nerve involvement) [14]. Neurologic manifestations due to copper deficiency may be precipitated in patients who have undergone bariatric surgery [14] and in those receiving dietary zinc supplements [15]. Treatment of copper deficiency usually consists of oral copper supplementation. In patients receiving total parenteral nutrition, intravenous copper replacement may be necessary. Copper accumulation has also been described historically in patients who received hemodialysis with a cuprophane membrane which is a cellulose membrane prepared by the cuprammonium method and that contains small amounts of copper [16]. Studies have shown a potential contributory role for copper in the genesis of beta-2-microglobulin amyloidosis (also known as dialysis-induced amyloidosis) [17]. Excess copper intake (copper sulfate) can cause a syndrome of hemolysis and acute kidney injury [18].

Manganese

The total amount of manganese in the adult human body is about 12 to 20 mg. Of the organs, bone and the kidney have some of the highest concentrations of manganese. Within the cell, it is concentrated in the mitochondria and the nucleus. Manganese functions are a key component of metalloenzymes. Manganese is important in the formation of cartilage, in glucose metabolism, and in the function of enzymes such as arginase and manganese superoxide dismutase (antioxidant function). Dietary sources of manganese include wholegrain cereals, fruits, and vegetables. Blood manganese levels are often low in MHD patients [19]. Serum manganese levels correlate with the nutritional status in MHD patients [20]. A recent study showed an association between low serum manganese levels and increased carotid atherosclerosis in MHD patients [21]. In some chronic dialysis patients, serum manganese levels are increased and result in deposition of manganese in the cerebral basal ganglia (visualized as hyperintense signals on T1-weighted magnetic resonance (MR) images). These patients may present with extrapyramidal syndromes, parkinsonism, myoclonus, and vestibular-auditory syndromes [22,23].

Selenium

Selenium is an essential trace element that is important for controlling oxidative stress (via modulating glutathione peroxidase activity), immune functions, and thyroid hormone synthesis [24]. In the general population, selenium deficiency has been found in association with bone disease (endemic osteochondropathy or Kashin—Beck disease) and cancer and may increase the risk of cardiovascular diseases [25]. Keshan disease is an endemic cardiomyopathy due to selenium deficiency seen in parts of China with selenium-deficient soil [25]. Serum selenium levels are often decreased in MHD patients [8,26], and serum selenium levels correlate with nutritional status [24]. Correction of selenium deficiency results in increased glutathione peroxidase activity with a potential reduction in oxidative stress [27—29] and is also shown to reduce DNA damage [30]. In a recent population-based cohort study of 1040 MHD patients, the quartiles of serum selenium levels were inversely associated with death risk. There was especially an increase in death associated with infectious complications in the patients who had the lowest serum selenium concentrations [31]. Decreased serum selenium levels in MHD patients may be associated with increased cardiovascular risk [32]. Selenium may also have a protective effect against vascular calcification [33]. It is of interest that supplementation with Brazil nuts (the richest known food source of selenium) corrects selenium deficiency in MHD patients [34]. Selenium toxicity or selenosis is rare and is manifested by brittle hair, breath with a garlic-like odor, such gastrointestinal symptoms as nausea, vomiting and diarrhea and, rarely, acute tubular necrosis [35].

Boron

Boron, the fifth element in the periodic table, is ubiquitous in nature. Boron is mostly present in the bone and seems essential for the structure of bone [36,37]. Boron is beneficial particularly to the bone and mineral metabolism in the setting of vitamin D deficiency [38,39]. This may be particularly relevant to chronic kidney disease (CKD) and chronic dialysis patients who exhibit significant vitamin D deficiency. Exposure to boron has been implicated recently as a cause of acute kidney injury as well as a potential cause of CKD in Southeast Asia [40]. Hemodialysis treatments substantially decrease serum boron levels [41]. The consequences of boron deficiency are unknown.

Chromium

Chromium is an essential element. Its primary function is its proposed role in enhancing insulin sensitivity at the muscle cell level mediated through a binding protein known as chromomodulin. Chromium deficiency thus can result in insulin resistance. The recommended daily intake is about 30 to 35 µg per day. Rich dietary sources of chromium include egg yolks, meat, and whole grains. The effects of chromium deficiency in patients with kidney disease remain to be investigated.

Fluoride

Fluoride is an essential trace element that is important in dental and bone health. Serum and bone fluoride content are generally increased in patients with reduced kidney function [42,43]. However, there is a lack of evidence linking fluoride accumulation and bone disease in chronic dialysis patients [44]. Acute fluoride intoxication due to contamination of dialysate water has been described. These patients manifested severe pruritus, and, in some patients, fatal ventricular fibrillation [45]. The mechanisms of these fatal toxic effects include induction of profound hypocalcemia, inhibition of Na^+-K^+-ATPase and development of an explosive hyperkalemia [46].

Cobalt

Cobalt is an essential component of vitamin B_{12}. In the past, cobalt chloride was used to treat the anemia of CKD [47]. Cobalt induces erythropoiesis, acting as an inducer of hypoxia-inducible-factor (HIF) [48]. Because of its side effects, including cardiomyopathy and thyroid dysfunction, its use was discontinued [49]. There is a positive correlation between serum cobalt levels and atherosclerosis in MHD patients [21]. More rigorous studies are needed to examine the potential benefits and hazards of cobalt intake for chronic dialysis patients.

Silicon

Silicon has been thought to be an essential element involved in mineralization [50]. There is a unique affinity of silicon to aluminum, and it has been suggested that silicon deficiency could be a predisposing factor for aluminum toxicity [51]. Silicon is excreted primarily through the urine, and silicon may accumulate in chronic dialysis patients [52,53]. Silicon is detected in the liver, spleen, lungs, skin, bone, and vessels of chronic dialysis patients [54]. There is a reported association between silicon accumulation and perforating folliculitis [55] and liver and neurologic dysfunction [56,57]. Additional consequences or benefits of silicon deficiency or accumulation have not been investigated in detail in chronic dialysis patients.

ALTERATIONS IN NONESSENTIAL TRACE ELEMENTS, METALS, AND METALLOIDS IN PATIENTS WITH KIDNEY DISEASE

Aluminum

Aluminum accumulation was historically described in MHD patients as a consequence of dialysis using tap water that was contaminated with aluminum sulfate added as a purifying agent [58–60]. Aluminum is added to the water in the form of alum to remove suspended colloidal matter by a process called flocculation. Other potential sources of aluminum include dietary sources and aluminum-containing antacids [61]. Aluminum accumulates in a variety of organs in chronic dialysis patients including the lungs, skin, brain, and bone [62–64]. It is present in the mineralizing front of bone. Diabetes mellitus and citrate intake are risk factors for increased aluminum accumulation [65,66]. Dietary citrate complexes to aluminum, thereby facilitating its intestinal absorption. Aluminum accumulation has been shown to cause anemia [67,68], low-turnover bone disease [69], and dialysis dementia [70]. There are also studies that have implicated aluminum accumulation with left ventricular hypertrophy [71,72]. With improvements in water treatment and frequent monitoring of plasma aluminum levels, aluminum-related diseases have largely disappeared in the dialysis setting. Of interest, recent studies have observed tissue aluminum accumulation in patients with nephrogenic systemic fibrosis and calciphylaxis [73]. The sources and consequences of aluminum accumulation in these disease processes are unknown.

Antimony

Antimony is a nonessential metalloid. Sources of antimony exposure can include both occupational (welding and smelting) and therapeutic sources. Antimony is widely used in its pentavalent form to treat visceral leishmaniasis and as pentamidine to treat pneumocystis infection. Trivalent antimony is known to be a potent inducer of heme oxygenase [74]. Antimony therapy can induce nephrotoxicity, causing both acute kidney injury and renal tubular acidosis [75]. No data are available on blood or tissue antimony levels in patients with chronic kidney disease.

Arsenic

Arsenic is known to be nephrotoxic, particularly after acute exposure to arsine [76–78]. Patients exposed to arsine develop hemolysis, acute renal failure with cortical necrosis, chronic kidney disease, and peripheral neuropathy. Arsenic accumulates in the serum and tissues of patients with renal insufficiency [79–83]. Sources of arsenic include contaminated water and food (such as tilapia fish). Cutaneous manifestations of chronic arsenic exposure are generalized hyperpigmentation, palmoplantar hyperkeratosis, and Mee's line in the nails [84,85]. Arsenic induces oxidative stress, and chronic arsenic exposure may be a causal factor for atherosclerosis, progression of kidney disease, and increased risk of cancer [86,87].

Cadmium

Cadmium levels are increased in the blood and bone of MHD patients [8,88]. Major environmental sources of cadmium include the diet and smoking. Cadmium toxicity has been associated with increased risk of cancers, kidney disease and osteoporosis [89]. A study from Sri Lanka has suggested a link between environmental cadmium exposure and chronic kidney disease [90]. There is a significant and direct association between serum cadmium levels and endothelial dysfunction (as measured by decreased flow-mediated dilatation) in MHD patients [91]. Supporting the importance of this observation, a recent study reported an association between increased blood cadmium levels and increased 18-month all-cause mortality in diabetic MHD patients [92]. Cadmium may exert systemic toxicity through its nephrotoxic (tubular toxicity), proinflammatory and vasculotoxic/pro-atherosclerotic effects [21,93,94]. In fact, a recent study suggested an association between environmental cadmium exposure and malnutrition, inflammation, and protein-energy wasting (malnutrition-inflammation-cachexia (MIA) syndrome) in MHD patients [94]. In another recent study, elevated serum cadmium levels (>1.38 µg/L) were associated with a 10-fold increased risk of inflammation [94]. Cadmium can also induce anemia by decreasing erythropoietin production and by inducing hemolysis [95,96]. Thus, it may be important to limit cadmium accumulation in MHD patients by restricting the intake of foods with high cadmium concentrations (shellfish, particularly pacific oysters and mushrooms such as *Agaricus subrufescens* Peck) and avoiding smoking.

Gadolinium

Gadolinium contrast agents are used in magnetic resonance (MR) imaging. Chelated gadolinium is administered as a paramagnetic agent for contrast-enhanced MR imaging. Gadolinium belongs to the lanthanide series of metals, and in its free form, it is highly cytotoxic. To minimize this toxicity, gadolinium is administered in a chelated form with high kinetic stability so that under normal endogenous conditions, gadolinium dechelation would not usually occur. Most of the administered gadolinium chelate is excreted promptly through the urine, and the half-life (t1/2) of gadolinium in patients with normal kidney function is about 60 to 90 minutes. Recently, gadolinium contrast agents have been implicated in a serious fibrosing disorder known as nephrogenic systemic fibrosis (NSF) in patients with advanced renal insufficiency [97,98]. Based on this, the US Federal Drug Administration (FDA) issued a black-box warning cautioning against the use of gadolinium contrast agents in patients who have an estimated glomerular filtration

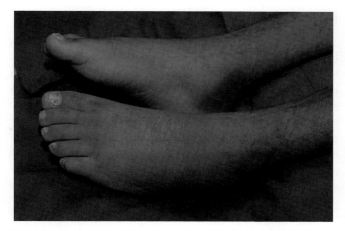

FIGURE 23.1 Gadolinium-induced nephrogenic systemic fibrosis.

rate (eGFR) less than 30 mL/min. Patients with NSF may develop fibrosis and ectopic calcification/bone formation in the dermis, subcutaneous tissues, heart, diaphragm, testes, and dura mater [99]. Clinically, this is manifested by edema, a plaque-like rash, a woody induration of the extremities, tethering of the skin, and severely restricted joint mobility (Figure 23.1). The pathology is characterized by infiltration of CD34$^+$ spindle cells and macrophages, angiogenesis, and fibrosis [100]. Patients with renal insufficiency are susceptible to gadolinium toxicity for a variety of reasons. First, administered gadolinium chelates are retained for prolonged periods of time in people with advanced CKD. The t{1/2} for gadolinium can be prolonged for up to 32 hours in MHD patients and up to 20 days in chronic peritoneal dialysis patients. Second, gadolinium contrast agents can induce iron mobilization which may, along with other endogenous metals such as zinc and calcium, induce dechelation of the gadolinium contrast (also known as transmetallation) and lead to precipitation of gadolinium phosphate. Among the gadolinium contrast agents, those with a linear structure (such as gadolinium-DTPA-BMA, Omniscan™) are less stable than the macrocyclic agents and are thus more likely to cause NSF [101]. There is a high mortality associated with NSF [99]. The use of sodium thiosulfate, rapamycin, and renal transplantation may all have a role in the treatment of NSF [98,102,103].

Germanium

Germanium is a nonessential trace element. Germanium trioxide ingestion has been linked to renal tubular toxicity in humans [104–106]. Glomeruli (foamy podocytes) and distal renal tubules (acute tubular necrosis) are specifically affected, and tissue lipofuscin accumulation and associated neuromuscular weakness are specific manifestations. Recovery of renal function from germanium toxicity is slow and incomplete [107].

Lanthanum

Lanthanum carbonate is an oral phosphate binder in use in Europe and the US. Prolonged use of lanthanum-based phosphate binders has been associated with an increase in serum lanthanum levels and accumulation of lanthanum in the bone [108]. In animal studies, orally administered lanthanum has been demonstrated to accumulate in the liver and bone [109,110]. No direct adverse effect of lanthanum accumulation has been reported in humans. Lanthanum carbonate is a commercially available intestinal phosphate binder that is prescribed for patients with advanced CKD.

Lead

Lead exposure and accumulation is a well-known cause of CKD [111,112]. Studies suggest that up to 15% of patients diagnosed with essential hypertension may have a high lead burden [113]. Blood lead levels correlate with the risk of CKD in large population studies [114]. Serum and bone lead levels are increased in chronic dialysis patients [115,116]. Overt lead nephropathy presents as a chronic tubulointerstitial disease accompanied by glucosuria, aminoaciduria, low molecular weight proteinuria, hypertension, hyperuricemia, and gout (saturnine gout) [117]. Patients with lead toxicity also have significant anemia (red blood cells may have Howell–Jolly bodies) and may present with a neuropathy. Lead that accumulates in bone can undergo recycling into the serum during states of increased bone turnover (e.g., hyperparathyroidism), and the mobilized lead might in turn cause lead toxicity [118]. Low-level chronic lead exposure has been causally linked to progression of kidney disease, and EDTA chelation has been shown to retard the rate of kidney disease progression [119].

Mercury

Mercury has been implicated in a variety of kidney diseases. Historically, mercury was used to treat syphilis and as a diuretic [120]. In addition, environmental and occupational exposure also contributed to mercury exposure and toxicity. Mercury has been implicated as a cause of acute tubular necrosis, glomerulonephritis, and CKD [121,122].

Molybdenum

Molybdenum is a constituent of molybdoenzymes that participate in oxidation-reduction reactions. It is also an important cofactor for xanthine oxidase and xanthine dehydrogenase. Molybdenum is known to be increased in the serum and hair of MHD patients [82,123]. Molybdenum may interfere with normal copper homeostasis and increase urinary copper excretion. Excessive dietary molybdenum intake may result in gout-like symptoms [124]. Other consequences of increased molybdenum levels in patients with renal insufficiency are currently unknown.

Nickel

A defined role for nickel in human physiology is lacking. Nickel levels have been reported to be both lower and higher in patients with renal insufficiency [19,20,125]. Dermatitis due to nickel has been reported in MHD patients. Nickel inhibits homocysteine synthetic pathways, and there is a negative correlation between serum nickel levels and homocysteine concentrations in MHD patients [126]. Nickel is a hypoxia-inducible-factor (HIF) mimetic and therefore has the potential to induce erythropoiesis [127–129]. Although there is an association between nickel compounds and both erythrocytosis and renal cell cancer in animals, evidence of such an association in humans link is lacking [130].

Strontium

Strontium is known to accumulate in patients with reduced kidney function. Strontium accumulates in the serum, bone, and calcified tissues of uremic patients [131–134]. Strontium can interfere with osteoblast function and mineralization [135,136]. In animal models and human studies, accumulation of strontium has been associated with osteomalacia [137,138].

Vanadium

Vanadium exists in several oxidation states with a valence of $+2$ to $+5$. Its dietary sources include cereals, mushrooms, spinach, and shellfish. There is evidence that serum vanadium levels are increased in MHD patients [8,139]. Vanadium has an effect on glucose metabolism similar to insulin and may have anabolic effects on muscle. Renal toxicity due to chronic vanadium exposure has been described in animals, but evidence of such an association is lacking in humans [140].

TRACE ELEMENT ABNORMALITIES IN RENAL-SPECIFIC SYNDROMES

In Figure 23.2, the abnormalities in trace elements and metals in various renal-specific syndromes are summarized. The implications of these associations, including proofs of causality, need additional investigation.

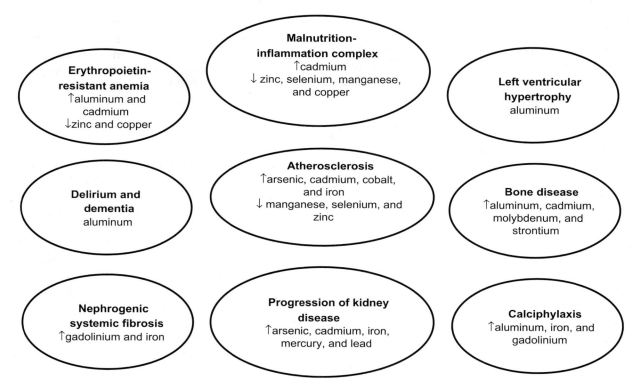

FIGURE 23.2 Trace element and metal abnormalities in renal-specific syndromes.

DIAGNOSTIC AND THERAPEUTIC APPROACHES

Trace-element disturbances have to be considered in the differential diagnosis of individual clinical presentations as well as in an epidemic setting. A high index of suspicion is critical for the diagnosis of trace-element deficiencies and toxicities. Measurement of trace elements in serum and tissue samples can be helpful in reaching the correct clinical diagnosis. Concentrations of trace elements, particularly trace metals, can be fairly precisely assessed by bulk chemical analysis methods such as atomic absorption spectroscopy (AAS) or inductively-coupled mass spectrometry (ICP-MS). There is a high level of sensitivity with these methods; the measurements give values in parts per billion with AAS and in parts per trillion with ICP-MS. However, these are tissue-destructive techniques, and there is lack of information concerning the tissue distribution of metals. To image tissue distribution of trace metals, several novel methods with high spatial resolution (i.e., the ability to image at submicron levels) in biologic samples are available [141]. These include electron microprobe (EM), laser ablation microscopy-coupled ICP-MS, and synchrotron-based X-ray fluorescence (SXRF).

Therapeutic approaches to correct trace element and metal deficiencies include dietary supplementation and use of parenteral replacement as necessary. Toxic accumulation can be treated by removing the sources of toxins. The use of appropriate chelating agents to remove the toxic element must be considered. Successful examples of chelation therapies include the use of desferroxamine to treat aluminum toxicity and the treatment of lead accumulation with EDTA chelation.

CONCLUSIONS

This review summarizes the current knowledge of what is known and not known concerning alterations in trace elements, metals, and metalloids in kidney disease and kidney failure and the syndromes that may be associated with these altered trace element burdens. Of importance to nephrology is the recognition that perturbations in trace-element metabolism may contribute to some of the major manifestations of the uremic syndrome, such as erythropoietin resistance, the malnutrition-inflammation syndrome, and atherosclerosis. For people with kidney disease and kidney failure, future studies are needed to examine the pathophysiological relevance of these associations, to develop more precise methods for assessing trace element burden, and to identify more effective therapies to treat trace element deficiency and excess.

References

[1] Mertz W. The essential trace elements. Science Sep 18 1981; 213(4514):1332−8.

[2] Fukushima T, Horike H, Fujiki S, Kitada S, Sasaki T, Kashihara N. Zinc deficiency anemia and effects of zinc therapy in maintenance hemodialysis patients. Ther Apher Dial Jun 2009;13(3):213−9.

[3] Partyka A, Jastrzebska-Wiesek M, Szewczyk B, Stachowicz K, Slawinska A, Poleszak E, et al. Anxiolytic-like activity of zinc in rodent tests. Pharmacol Rep 2011;63(4):1050−5.

[4] Cope EC, Levenson CW. Role of zinc in the development and treatment of mood disorders. Curr Opin Clin Nutr Metab Care Nov 2010;13(6):685−9.

[5] Tassabehji NM, Corniola RS, Alshingiti A, Levenson CW. Zinc deficiency induces depression-like symptoms in adult rats. Physiol Behav Oct 20 2008;95(3):365−9.

[6] Mahajan SK, Prasad AS, Rabbani P, Briggs WA, McDonald FD. Zinc deficiency: a reversible complication of uremia. Am J Clin Nutr Dec 1982;36(6):1177−83.

[7] Sahin H, Uyanik F, Inanc N, Erdem O. Serum zinc, plasma ghrelin, leptin levels, selected biochemical parameters and nutritional status in malnourished hemodialysis patients. Biol Trace Elem Res. Mar 2009;127(3):191−9.

[8] Tonelli M, Wiebe N, Hemmelgarn B, Klarenbach S, Field C, Manns B, et al. Trace elements in hemodialysis patients: a systematic review and meta-analysis. BMC Med 2009;7:25.

[9] Emenaker NJ, DiSilvestro RA, Nahman Jr NS, Percival S. Copper-related blood indexes in kidney dialysis patients. Am J Clin Nutr Nov 1996;64(5):757−60.

[10] Navarro-Alarcon M, Reyes-Perez A, Lopez-Garcia H, Palomares-Bayo M, Olalla-Herrera M, Lopez-Martinez MC. Longitudinal study of serum zinc and copper levels in hemodialysis patients and their relation to biochemical markers. Biol Trace Elem Res Dec 2006;113(3):209−22.

[11] Yilmaz MI, Saglam M, Caglar K, Cakir E, Sonmez A, Ozgurtas T, et al. The determinants of endothelial dysfunction in CKD: oxidative stress and asymmetric dimethylarginine. Am J Kidney Dis Jan 2006;47(1):42−50.

[12] Becton DL, Schultz WH, Kinney TR. Severe neutropenia caused by copper deficiency in a child receiving continuous ambulatory peritoneal dialysis. J Pediatr May 1986;108(5 Pt 1):735−7.

[13] Higuchi T, Matsukawa Y, Okada K, Oikawa O, Yamazaki T, Ohnishi Y, et al. Correction of copper deficiency improves erythropoietin unresponsiveness in hemodialysis patients with anemia. Intern Med 2006;45(5):271−3.

[14] Rounis E, Laing CM, Davenport A. Acute neurological presentation due to copper deficiency in a hemodialysis patient following gastric bypass surgery. Clin Nephrol Nov 2010;74(5):389−92.

[15] Yaldizli O, Johansson U, Gizewski ER, Maschke M. Copper deficiency myelopathy induced by repetitive parenteral zinc supplementation during chronic hemodialysis. J Neurol Nov 2006;253(11):1507−9.

[16] Kalantar-Zadeh K, Kopple JD. Trace elements and vitamins in maintenance dialysis patients. Adv Ren Replace Ther Jul 2003;10(3):170−82.

[17] Morgan CJ, Gelfand M, Atreya C, Miranker AD. Kidney dialysis-associated amyloidosis: a molecular role for copper in fiber formation. J Mol Biol Jun 1 2001;309(2):339−45.

[18] Jha V, Chugh KS. Community-acquired acute kidney injury in Asia. Semin Nephrol Jul 2008;28(4):330−47.

[19] Hsieh YY, Shen WS, Lee LY, Wu TL, Ning HC, Sun CF. Long-term changes in trace elements in patients undergoing chronic hemodialysis. Biol Trace Elem Res Feb 2006;109(2):115−21.

[20] Hosokawa S, Oyamaguchi A, Yoshida O. Trace elements and complications in patients undergoing chronic hemodialysis. Nephron 1990;55(4):375−9.

[21] Ari E, Kaya Y, Demir H, Asicioglu E, Keskin S. The correlation of serum trace elements and heavy metals with carotid artery atherosclerosis in maintenance hemodialysis patients. Biol Trace Elem Res. Dec 2011;144(1−3):351−9.

[22] da Silva CJ, da Rocha AJ, Jeronymo S, Mendes MF, Milani FT, Maia Jr AC, et al. A preliminary study revealing a new association in patients undergoing maintenance hemodialysis: manganism symptoms and T1 hyperintense changes in the basal ganglia. Am J Neuroradiol Sep 2007;28(8):1474−9.

[23] Ohtake T, Negishi K, Okamoto K, Oka M, Maesato K, Moriya H, et al. Manganese-induced Parkinsonism in a patient undergoing maintenance hemodialysis. Am J Kidney Dis Oct 2005;46(4):749−53.

[24] Liu ML, Xu G, Huang ZY, Zhong XC, Liu SH, Jiang TY. Euthyroid sick syndrome and nutritional status are correlated with hyposelenemia in hemodialysis patients. Int J Artif Organs Jul 2011;34(7):577−83.

[25] Jackson ML. Selenium: geochemical distribution and associations with human heart and cancer death rates and longevity in China and the United States. Biol Trace Elem Res Jan−Apr 1988;15:13−21.

[26] Saint-Georges MD, Bonnefont DJ, Bourely BA, Jaudon MC, Cereze P, Chaumeil P, et al. Correction of selenium deficiency in hemodialyzed patients. Kidney Int Suppl Nov 1989;27:S274−7.

[27] Richard MJ, Ducros V, Foret M, Arnaud J, Coudray C, Fusselier M, et al. Reversal of selenium and zinc deficiencies in chronic hemodialysis patients by intravenous sodium selenite and zinc gluconate supplementation. Time-course of glutathione peroxidase repletion and lipid peroxidation decrease. Biol Trace Elem Res Nov−Dec 1993;39(2−3):149−59.

[28] Loughrey CM, Young IS, Lightbody JH, McMaster D, McNamee PT, Trimble ER. Oxidative stress in haemodialysis. QJM Nov 1994;87(11):679−83.

[29] Locatelli F, Canaud B, Eckardt KU, Stenvinkel P, Wanner C, Zoccali C. Oxidative stress in end-stage renal disease: an emerging threat to patient outcome. Nephrol Dial Transplant Jul 2003;18(7):1272−80.

[30] Zachara BA, Gromadzinska J, Palus J, Zbrog Z, Swiech R, Twardowska E, et al. The effect of selenium supplementation in the prevention of DNA damage in white blood cells of hemodialyzed patients: a pilot study. Biol Trace Elem Res Sep 2011;142(3):274−83.

[31] Fujishima Y, Ohsawa M, Itai K, Kato K, Tanno K, Turin TC, et al. Serum selenium levels are inversely associated with death risk among hemodialysis patients. Nephrol Dial Transplant Oct 2011;26(10):3331−8.

[32] Marti del Moral L, Agil A, Navarro-Alarcon M, Lopez-Ga de la Serrana H, Palomares-Bayo M, Oliveras-Lopez MJ. Altered serum selenium and uric acid levels and dyslipidemia in hemodialysis patients could be associated with enhanced cardiovascular risk. Biol Trace Elem Res Dec 2011;144(1-3):496−503.

[33] Liu H, Lu Q, Huang K. Selenium suppressed hydrogen peroxide-induced vascular smooth muscle cells calcification through inhibiting oxidative stress and ERK activation. J Cell Biochem Dec 15 2010;111(6):1556−64.

[34] Stockler-Pinto MB, Lobo J, Moraes C, Leal VO, Farage NE, Rocha AV, et al. Effect of Brazil nut supplementation on plasma levels of selenium in hemodialysis patients: 12 months of follow-up. J Ren Nutr Jan 2 2012.

[35] Sutter ME, Thomas JD, Brown J, Morgan B. Selenium toxicity: a case of selenosis caused by a nutritional supplement. Ann Intern Med Jun 17 2008;148(12):970−1.

[36] Nielsen FH. Is boron nutritionally relevant? Nutr Rev Apr 2008;66(4):183—91.

[37] Devirian TA, Volpe SL. The physiological effects of dietary boron. Crit Rev Food Sci Nutr 2003;43(2):219—31.

[38] Hegsted M, Keenan MJ, Siver F, Wozniak P. Effect of boron on vitamin D deficient rats. Biol Trace Elem Res. Mar 1991;28(3): 243—55.

[39] Schaafsma A, de Vries PJ, Saris WH. Delay of natural bone loss by higher intakes of specific minerals and vitamins. Crit Rev Food Sci Nutr May 2001;41(4):225—49.

[40] Pahl MV, Culver BD, Vaziri ND. Boron and the kidney. J Ren Nutr Oct 2005;15(4):362—70.

[41] Usuda K, Kono K, Iguchi K, Nishiura K, Miyata K, Shimahara M, et al. Hemodialysis effect on serum boron level in the patients with long term hemodialysis. Sci Total Environ Nov 22 1996;191(3):283—90.

[42] Torra M, Rodamilans M, Corbella J. Serum and urine fluoride concentration: relationships to age, sex and renal function in a non-fluoridated population. Sci Total Environ Sep 4 1998; 220(1):81—5.

[43] al-Wakeel JS, Mitwalli AH, Huraib S, al-Mohaya S, Abu-Aisha H, Chaudhary AR, et al. Serum ionic fluoride levels in haemodialysis and continuous ambulatory peritoneal dialysis patients. Nephrol Dial Transplant Jul 1997;12(7):1420—4.

[44] Cohen-Solal ME, Augry F, Mauras Y, Morieux C, Allain P, de Vernejoul MC. Fluoride and strontium accumulation in bone does not correlate with osteoid tissue in dialysis patients. Nephrol Dial Transplant Mar 2002;17(3):449—54.

[45] Arnow PM, Bland LA, Garcia-Houchins S, Fridkin S, Fellner SK. An outbreak of fatal fluoride intoxication in a long-term hemodialysis unit. Ann Intern Med Sep 1 1994;121(5):339—44.

[46] McIvor ME. Acute fluoride toxicity. Pathophysiology and management. Drug Saf Mar—Apr 1990;5(2):79—85.

[47] Bowie EA, Hurley PJ. Cobalt chloride in the treatment of refractory anaemia in patients undergoing long-term haemodialysis. Aust N Z J Med Aug 1975;5(4):306—14.

[48] Maxwell PH, Wiesener MS, Chang GW, Clifford SC, Vaux EC, Cockman ME, et al. The tumour suppressor protein VHL targets hypoxia-inducible factors for oxygen-dependent proteolysis. Nature May 20 1999;399(6733):271—5.

[49] Manifold IH, Platts MM, Kennedy A. Cobalt cardiomyopathy in a patient on maintenance haemodialysis. Br Med J Dec 9 1978; 2(6152):1609.

[50] Carlisle EM. Silicon: a possible factor in bone calcification. Science Jan 16 1970;167(3916):279—80.

[51] Parry R, Plowman D, Delves HT, Roberts NB, Birchall JD, Bellia JP, et al. Silicon and aluminium interactions in haemodialysis patients. Nephrol Dial Transplant Jul 1998;13(7):1759—62.

[52] Gitelman HJ, Alderman FR, Perry SJ. Silicon accumulation in dialysis patients. Am J Kidney Dis Feb 1992;19(2):140—3.

[53] D'Haese PC, Shaheen FA, Huraib SO, Djukanovic L, Polenakovic MH, Spasovski G, et al. Increased silicon levels in dialysis patients due to high silicon content in the drinking water, inadequate water treatment procedures, and concentrate contamination: a multicentre study. Nephrol Dial Transplant Oct 1995;10(10):1838—44.

[54] van Landeghem GF, de Broe ME, D'Haese PC. Al and Si: their speciation, distribution, and toxicity. Clin Biochem Jul 1998; 31(5):385—97.

[55] Saldanha LF, Gonick HC, Rodriguez HJ, Marmelzat JA, Repique EV, Marcus CL. Silicon-related syndrome in dialysis patients. Nephron 1997;77(1):48—56.

[56] Hunt J, Farthing MJ, Baker LR, Crocker PR, Levison DA. Silicone in the liver: possible late effects. Gut Feb 1989;30(2): 239—42.

[57] Hershey CO, Ricanati ES, Hershey LA, Varnes AW, Lavin PJ, Strain WH. Silicon as a potential uremic neurotoxin: trace element analysis in patients with renal failure. Neurology Jun 1983;33(6):786—9.

[58] Savory J, Wills MR. Dialysis fluids as a source of aluminum accumulation. Contrib Nephrol 1984;38:12—23.

[59] McClure J, Fazzalari NL, Fassett RG, Pugsley DJ. Bone histoquantitative findings and histochemical staining reactions for aluminium in chronic renal failure patients treated with haemodialysis fluids containing high and low concentrations of aluminium. J Clin Pathol Nov 1983;36(11):1281—7.

[60] Ellis HA, McCarthy JH, Herrington J. Bone aluminium in haemodialysed patients and in rats injected with aluminium chloride: relationship to impaired bone mineralisation. J Clin Pathol Aug 1979;32(8):832—44.

[61] Salusky IB, Foley J, Nelson P, Goodman WG. Aluminum accumulation during treatment with aluminum hydroxide and dialysis in children and young adults with chronic renal disease. N Engl J Med Feb 21 1991;324(8):527—31.

[62] Di Paolo N, Masti A, Comparini IB, Garosi G, Di Paolo M, Centini F, et al. Uremia, dialysis and aluminium. Int J Artif Organs Oct 1997;20(10):547—52.

[63] Malluche HH, Faugere MC. Aluminum-related bone disease. Blood Purif 1988;6(1):1—15.

[64] Van de Vyver FL, De Broe ME. Aluminum in tissues. Clin Nephrol 1985;24(Suppl. 1):S37—57.

[65] Andress DL, Kopp JB, Maloney NA, Coburn JW, Sherrard DJ. Early deposition of aluminum in bone in diabetic patients on hemodialysis. N Engl J Med Feb 5 1987;316(6):292—6.

[66] Delmez JA, Slatopolsky E. Hyperphosphatemia: its consequences and treatment in patients with chronic renal disease. Am J Kidney Dis Apr 1992;19(4):303—17.

[67] Abreo K, Glass J, Sella M. Aluminum inhibits hemoglobin synthesis but enhances iron uptake in Friend erythroleukemia cells. Kidney Int Feb 1990;37(2):677—81.

[68] Muirhead N, Hodsman AB, Hollomby DJ, Cordy PE. The role of aluminium and parathyroid hormone in erythropoietin resistance in haemodialysis patients. Nephrol Dial Transplant 1991;6(5):342—5.

[69] Malluche HH, Monier-Faugere MC. Risk of adynamic bone disease in dialyzed patients. Kidney Int Suppl. Oct 1992;38:S62—7.

[70] Harrington CR, Wischik CM, McArthur FK, Taylor GA, Edwardson JA, Candy JM. Alzheimer's-disease-like changes in tau protein processing: association with aluminium accumulation in brains of renal dialysis patients. Lancet Apr 23 1994; 343(8904):993—7.

[71] Parfrey PS, Harnett JD, Barre PE. The natural history of myocardial disease in dialysis patients. J Am Soc Nephrol Jul 1991;2(1):2—12.

[72] London GM, de Vernejoul MC, Fabiani F, Marchais S, Guerin A, Metivier F, et al. Association between aluminum accumulation and cardiac hypertrophy in hemodialyzed patients. Am J Kidney Dis Jan 1989;13(1):75—83.

[73] Amuluru L, High W, Hiatt KM, Ranville J, Shah SV, Malik B, et al. Metal deposition in calcific uremic arteriolopathy. J Am Acad Dermatol Jul 2009;61(1):73—9.

[74] Drummond GS, Kappas A. Potent heme-degrading action of antimony and antimony-containing parasiticidal agents. J Exp Med 1981;153(2):245—56.

[75] Veiga JPR, Wolff ER, Sampaio RN, Marsden PD. Renal tubular dysfunction in patients with mucocutaneous leishmaniasis treated with pentavalent antimonials. Lancet 1983;322(8349):569.

[76] Phoon WH, Chan MO, Goh CH, Edmondson RP, Kwek YK, Gan SL, et al. Five cases of arsine poisoning. Ann Acad Med Singapore Apr 1984;13(Suppl. 2):394—8.

[77] Gerhardt RE, Hudson JB, Rao RN, Sobel RE. Chronic renal insufficiency from cortical necrosis induced by arsenic poisoning. Arch Intern Med Aug 1978;138(8):1267–9.

[78] Fowler BA, Weissberg JB. Arsine poisoning. N Engl J Med Nov 28 1974;291(22):1171–4.

[79] Zhang X, Cornelis R, De Kimpe J, Mees L, Lameire N. Speciation of arsenic in serum, urine, and dialysate of patients on continuous ambulatory peritoneal dialysis. Clin Chem. Feb 1997;43(2):406–8.

[80] Zhang X, Cornelis R, De Kimpe J, Mees L, Vanderbiesen V, De Cubber A, et al. Accumulation of arsenic species in serum of patients with chronic renal disease. Clin Chem Aug 1996;42(8 Pt 1):1231–7.

[81] De Kimpe J, Cornelis R, Mees L, Van Lierde S, Vanholder R. More than tenfold increase of arsenic in serum and packed cells of chronic hemodialysis patients. Am J Nephrol 1993;13(6):429–34.

[82] Ochi A, Ishimura E, Tsujimoto Y, Kakiya R, Tabata T, Mori K, et al. Trace elements in the hair of hemodialysis patients. Biol Trace Elem Res Nov 2011;143(2):825–34.

[83] Rucker D, Thadhani R, Tonelli M. Trace element status in hemodialysis patients. Semin Dial Jul-Aug 2010;23(4):389–95.

[84] Brown KG, Ross GL. Arsenic, drinking water, and health: a position paper of the American Council on Science and Health. Regul Toxicol Pharmacol Oct 2002;36(2):162–74.

[85] Rahman MM, Chowdhury UK, Mukherjee SC, Mondal BK, Paul K, Lodh D, et al. Chronic arsenic toxicity in Bangladesh and West Bengal, India — a review and commentary. J Toxicol Clin Toxicol 2001;39(7):683–700.

[86] Hsueh YM, Chung CJ, Shiue HS, Chen JB, Chiang SS, Yang MH, et al. Urinary arsenic species and CKD in a Taiwanese population: a case-control study. Am J Kidney Dis Nov 2009;54(5):859–70.

[87] Jomova K, Jenisova Z, Feszterova M, Baros S, Liska J, Hudecova D, et al. Arsenic: toxicity, oxidative stress and human disease. J Appl Toxicol Mar 2011;31(2):95–107.

[88] Vanholder R, Cornelis R, Dhondt A, Lameire N. The role of trace elements in uraemic toxicity. Nephrol Dial Transplant 2002;17(Suppl. 2):2–8.

[89] Jarup L. Cadmium overload and toxicity. Nephrol Dial Transplant 2002;17(Suppl. 2):35–9.

[90] Bandara JM, Senevirathna DM, Dasanayake DM, Herath V, Abeysekara T, Rajapaksha KH. Chronic renal failure among farm families in cascade irrigation systems in Sri Lanka associated with elevated dietary cadmium levels in rice and freshwater fish (Tilapia). Environ Geochem Health Oct 2008;30(5):465–78.

[91] Kaya Y, Ari E, Demir H, Gecit I, Beytur A, Kaspar C. Serum cadmium levels are independently associated with endothelial function in hemodialysis patients. Int Urol Nephrol 2012 Oct;44(5):1487–92.

[92] Yen TH, Lin JL, Lin-Tan DT, Hsu CW, Chen KH, Hsu HH. Blood cadmium level's association with 18-month mortality in diabetic patients with maintenance haemodialysis. Nephrol Dial Transplant Mar 2011;26(3):998–1005.

[93] Ferraro PM, Costanzi S, Naticchia A, Sturniolo A, Gambaro G. Low level exposure to cadmium increases the risk of chronic kidney disease: analysis of the NHANES 1999-2006. BMC Public Health 2010;10:304.

[94] Hsu CW, Lin JL, Lin-Tan DT, Yen TH, Huang WH, Ho TC, et al. Association of environmental cadmium exposure with inflammation and malnutrition in maintenance haemodialysis patients. Nephrol Dial Transplant Apr 2009;24(4):1282–8.

[95] Horiguchi H, Oguma E, Kayama F. Cadmium induces anemia through interdependent progress of hemolysis, body iron accumulation, and insufficient erythropoietin production in rats. Toxicol Sci. Jul 2011;122(1):198–210.

[96] Horiguchi H, Teranishi H, Niiya K, Aoshima K, Katoh T, Sakuragawa N, et al. Hypoproduction of erythropoietin contributes to anemia in chronic cadmium intoxication: clinical study on Itai-itai disease in Japan. Arch Toxicol 1994;68(10):632–6.

[97] Grobner T. Gadolinium — a specific trigger for the development of nephrogenic fibrosing dermopathy and nephrogenic systemic fibrosis? Nephrol Dialysis Transplant April 2006. 2006;21(4):1104–1108.

[98] Swaminathan S, Horn TD, Pellowski D, Abul-Ezz S, Bornhorst JA, Viswamitra S, et al. Nephrogenic systemic fibrosis, gadolinium, and iron mobilization. N Engl J Med Aug 16 2007;357(7):720–2.

[99] Swaminathan S, High WA, Ranville J, Horn TD, Hiatt K, Thomas M, et al. Cardiac and vascular metal deposition with high mortality in nephrogenic systemic fibrosis. Kidney Int Jun 2008;73(12):1413–8.

[100] Swaminathan S, Shah SV. New insights into nephrogenic systemic fibrosis. J Am Soc Nephrol 2007;18(4):2336–43.

[101] Wertman R, Altun E, Martin DR, Mitchell DG, Leyendecker JR, O'Malley RB, et al. Risk of nephrogenic systemic fibrosis: evaluation of gadolinium chelate contrast agents at four American universities. Radiology Sep 2008;248(3):799–806.

[102] Yerram P, Saab G, Karuparthi PR, Hayden MR, Khanna R. Nephrogenic systemic fibrosis: a mysterious disease in patients with renal failure — role of gadolinium-based contrast media in causation and the beneficial effect of intravenous sodium thiosulfate. Clin J Am Soc Nephrol Mar 2007;2(2):258–63.

[103] Swaminathan S, Arbiser JL, Hiatt KM, High W, Abul-Ezz S, Horn TD, et al. Rapid improvement of nephrogenic systemic fibrosis with rapamycin therapy: possible role of phospho-70-ribosomal-S6 kinase. J Am Acad Dermatol Feb 2010;62(2):343–5.

[104] Nagata N, Yoneyama T, Yanagida K, Ushio K, Yanagihara S, Matsubara O, et al. Accumulation of germanium in the tissues of a long-term user of germanium preparation died of acute renal failure. J Toxicol Sci Nov 1985;10(4):333–41.

[105] Sanai T, Okuda S, Onoyama K, Oochi N, Oh Y, Kobayashi K, et al. Germanium dioxide-induced nephropathy: a new type of renal disease. Nephron 1990;54(1):53–60.

[106] Takeuchi A, Yoshizawa N, Oshima S, Kubota T, Oshikawa Y, Akashi Y, et al. Nephrotoxicity of germanium compounds: report of a case and review of the literature. Nephron 1992;60(4):436–42.

[107] Gabardi S, Munz K, Ulbricht C. A review of dietary supplement-induced renal dysfunction. Clin J Am Soc Nephrol Jul 2007;2(4):757–65.

[108] Handley SA, Raja KB, Sharpe C, Flanagan RJ. Measurement of serum lanthanum in patients treated with lanthanum carbonate by inductively coupled plasma-mass spectrometry. Ann Clin Biochem Mar 2011;48(Pt 2):178–82.

[109] Freemont AJ, Hoyland JA, Denton J. The effects of lanthanum carbonate and calcium carbonate on bone abnormalities in patients with end-stage renal disease. Clin Nephrol Dec 2005;64(6):428–37.

[110] Behets GJ, Verberckmoes SC, Oste L, Bervoets AR, Salome M, Cox AG, et al. Localization of lanthanum in bone of chronic renal failure rats after oral dosing with lanthanum carbonate. Kidney Int May 2005;67(5):1830–6.

[111] Batuman V. Lead nephropathy, gout, and hypertension. Am J Med Sci Apr 1993;305(4):241–7.

[112] Nuyts GD, Van Vlem E, Thys J, De Leersnijder D, D'Haese PC, Elseviers MM, et al. New occupational risk factors for chronic renal failure. Lancet Jul 1 1995;346(8966):7–11.

[113] Sanchez-Fructuoso AI, Torralbo A, Arroyo M, Luque M, Ruilope LM, Santos JL, et al. Occult lead intoxication as a cause of hypertension and renal failure. Nephrol Dial Transplant Sep 1996;11(9):1775—80.

[114] Muntner P, He J, Vupputuri S, Coresh J, Batuman V. Blood lead and chronic kidney disease in the general United States population: results from NHANES III. Kidney Int Mar 2003; 63(3):1044—50.

[115] Koster J, Erhardt A, Stoeppler M, Mohl C, Ritz E. Mobilizable lead in patients with chronic renal failure. Eur J Clin Invest Apr 1989;19(2):228—33.

[116] Van de Vyver FL, D'Haese PC, Visser WJ, Elseviers MM, Knippenberg LJ, Lamberts LV, et al. Bone lead in dialysis patients. Kidney Int Feb 1988;33(2):601—7.

[117] Loghman-Adham M. Renal effects of environmental and occupational lead exposure. Environ Health Perspect Sep 1997;105(9):928—38.

[118] Kessler M, Durand PY, Huu TC, Royer-Morot MJ, Chanliau J, Netter P, et al. Mobilization of lead from bone in end-stage renal failure patients with secondary hyperparathyroidism. Nephrol Dial Transplant Nov 1999;14(11):2731—3.

[119] Lin JL, Lin-Tan DT, Hsu KH, Yu CC. Environmental lead exposure and progression of chronic renal diseases in patients without diabetes. N Engl J Med Jan 23 2003;348(4):277—86.

[120] Bomback AS, Klemmer PJ. Jack London's "mysterious malady". Am J Med May 2007;120(5):466—7.

[121] George CR. Mercury and the kidney. J Nephrol May—Jun 2011;24(Suppl. 17):S126—32.

[122] Brewster UC. Chronic kidney disease from environmental and occupational toxins. Conn Med Apr 2006;70(4):229—37.

[123] Hosokawa S, Yoshida O. Clinical studies on molybdenum in patients requiring long-term hemodialysis. ASAIO J Jul—Sep 1994;40(3):M445—9.

[124] Selden AI, Berg NP, Soderbergh A, Bergstrom BE. Occupational molybdenum exposure and a gouty electrician. Occup Med (Lond) Mar 2005;55(2):145—8.

[125] Hopfer SM, Fay WP, Sunderman Jr FW. Serum nickel concentrations in hemodialysis patients with environmental exposure. Ann Clin Lab Sci May—Jun 1989;19(3):161—7.

[126] Katko M, Kiss I, Karpati I, Kadar A, Matyus J, Csongradi E, et al. Relationship between serum nickel and homocysteine concentration in hemodialysis patients. Biol Trace Elem Res Sep 2008;124(3):195—205.

[127] Andrew AS, Klei LR, Barchowsky A. Nickel requires hypoxia-inducible factor-1 alpha, not redox signaling, to induce plasminogen activator inhibitor-1. Am J Physiol Lung Cell Mol Physiol Sep 2001;281(3):L607—15.

[128] Salnikow K, Su W, Blagosklonny MV, Costa M. Carcinogenic metals induce hypoxia-inducible factor-stimulated transcription by reactive oxygen species-independent mechanism. Cancer Res Jul 1 2000;60(13):3375—8.

[129] Huang LE, Ho V, Arany Z, Krainc D, Galson D, Tendler D, et al. Erythropoietin gene regulation depends on heme-dependent oxygen sensing and assembly of interacting transcription factors. Kidney Int Feb 1997;51(2):548—52.

[130] Sunderman Jr FW, McCully KS, Hopfer SM. Association between erythrocytosis and renal cancers in rats following intrarenal injection of nickel compounds. Carcinogenesis Nov 1984;5(11):1511—7.

[131] Canavese C, Pacitti A, Salomone M, Santoro MA, Stratta P, Mangiarotti G, et al. Strontium overload in uremic patients on regular dialytic treatment. ASAIO Trans Jul—Sep 1986;32(1): 120—2.

[132] Mauras Y, Ang KS, Simon P, Tessier B, Cartier F, Allain P. Increase in blood plasma levels of boron and strontium in hemodialyzed patients. Clin Chim Acta May 15 1986;156(3): 315—20.

[133] Smythe WR, Alfrey AC, Craswell PW, Crouch CA, Ibels LS, Kubo H, et al. Trace element abnormalities in chronic uremia. Ann Intern Med Mar 1982;96(3):302—10.

[134] Schrooten I, Elseviers MM, Lamberts LV, De Broe ME, D'Haese PC. Increased serum strontium levels in dialysis patients: an epidemiological survey. Kidney Int Nov 1999;56(5): 1886—92.

[135] Verberckmoes SC, De Broe ME, D'Haese PC. Dose-dependent effects of strontium on osteoblast function and mineralization. Kidney Int Aug 2003;64(2):534—43.

[136] Bervoets AR, Spasovski GB, Behets GJ, Dams G, Polenakovic MH, Zafirovska K, et al. Useful biochemical markers for diagnosing renal osteodystrophy in predialysis end-stage renal failure patients. Am J Kidney Dis May 2003;41(5):997—1007.

[137] Schrooten I, Cabrera W, Goodman WG, Dauwe S, Lamberts LV, Marynissen R, et al. Strontium causes osteomalacia in chronic renal failure rats. Kidney Int Aug 1998;54(2):448—56.

[138] D'Haese PC, Schrooten I, Goodman WG, Cabrera WE, Lamberts LV, Elseviers MM, et al. Increased bone strontium levels in hemodialysis patients with osteomalacia. Kidney Int Mar 2000;57(3):1107—14.

[139] Hosokawa S, Yoshida O. Vanadium in patients undergoing chronic haemodialysis. Nephrol Dial Transplant 1989;4(4): 282—4.

[140] Boscolo P, Carmignani M, Volpe AR, Felaco M, Del Rosso G, Porcelli G, et al. Renal toxicity and arterial hypertension in rats chronically exposed to vanadate. Occup Environ Med Jul 1994;51(7):500—3.

[141] Ralle M, Lutsenko S. Quantitative imaging of metals in tissues. Biometals Feb 2009;22(1):197—205.

Vitamin Metabolism and Requirements in Renal Disease and Renal Failure

Charles Chazot[1], Joel D. Kopple[2]

[1]NephroCare Tassin-Charcot, 69110 Sainte Foy Les Lyon, France
[2]Division of Nephrology and Hypertension, Torrance, CA, USA

INTRODUCTION

Kidney diseases and kidney failure commonly alter the biochemistry, metabolism and nutritional requirements for many vitamins and enhance the risk of abnormal vitamin function. Both deficiencies and abnormally high levels of vitamins occur in patients with renal failure. These abnormalities are reviewed in this chapter. Since the last edition of this book, important data have emerged such as the beneficial effect of multi-vitamins on the outcome of maintenance dialysis (MD) patients, the role of vitamin K in vascular calcification, the association of oxidant stress with cardiovascular morbidity in chronic kidney disease (CKD), and the disappointing trials on homocysteine lowering therapy. Moreover, several guidelines have been released that concern vitamin supplementation for MD patients. Vitamin D nutrition is reviewed elsewhere (Chapters 19, 21, 32, 33, 34, 35 and 36) and will not be addressed in this chapter.

STRUCTURE AND PHYSIOLOGICAL ROLE OF VITAMINS

Vitamin A

The structure and biochemistry of vitamin A in normal individuals have been reviewed [1]. Vitamin A is composed of several compounds including retinol (Table 24.1) and the biologically active retinoids which have a common structure consisting of four isoprenoid units (20 carbons) with five double bonds. Retinol, retinoic acid and retinal are the main bioactive retinoic compounds. Since the 1990s, the accepted units for vitamin A content have changed from International Units (IU) to Retinol Equivalents (RE), where 1.0 IU = 0.3 µg RE [2]. Carotenoids (40 carbon compounds) may be biologically active and are considered to be vitamin A precursors. Variable quantities of carotenoids are converted to retinol; this conversion is regulated according to the body vitamin A levels [3]. The allo-trans-β carotene is the main bioactive carotenoid. Retinoids and carotenoids are fat soluble and are predominantly found in foods derived from animals for retinyl esters and from vegetables for carotenoids [4]. During digestion, retinyl-esters are hydrolyzed in the intestinal lumen by pancreatic lipase. Retinol and carotenoids are incorporated into micelles and absorbed by enterocytes where β-carotene is converted to retinol. Retinol is esterified, combined in chylomicrons and broken down into chylomicron remnants in the lymphatic system by lipoprotein-lipase. The hepatic cells incorporate the chylomicron remnants through apo-E or B receptors. A significant part (10 to 40%) of the absorbed retinoids are oxidized or conjugated and excreted into bile and urine. At least 50% of the retinoid compounds are transferred into the perisinusoidal stellate cells of the liver where they are stored as retinyl palmitate and other retinyl-esters. In plasma, retinol is largely bound to apo-retinol binding protein (RBP 4), a 21.3 kD protein primarily synthesized in the liver and adipose tissue. This equimolar complex is bound as part of the molecule, prealbumin (also called transthyretin), and delivered to the target where it binds to RBP cell-surface receptors. Retinol is incorporated into the cell, whereas apo-RBP is released and catabolized by the kidney.

Vitamin A is necessary for normal nocturnal vision; it plays a role in the immune response, differentiation of epithelial cells and morphogenesis of solid organs

TABLE 24.1 Physicochemical and Some Clinical Characteristics of Vitamins

Vitamin	Main Compound	Solubility	MW	Protein Binding in Plasma	HD Losses	Peritoneal Losses	Body Stores	Toxicity[a]
A	Retinol	Lipid	286	Rbp+ Pre-albumin	None	Controversial[b]	Large	Yes
E	α-tocopherol	Lipid	431	Lipoproteins	None	Small	Small	Possible
K	Phylloquinone (K$_1$)	Lipid	451	Lipoproteins	Na[c]	Na[c]	Small	No
B$_1$	Thiamin	Water	337	Albumin	13–40 mL/min[d]	Low	4–10 days	No
B$_2$	Riboflavin	Water	376	Weak Albumin, IgG	27–52 mL/min[d]	High	2–3 months	No
B$_6$	Pyridoxine	Water	169	Albumin	54 mL/min[d]	= or < Urinary excretion	3–4 months	Yes
B$_{12}$	Cyanocobalamin	Water	1355	Transcobalamin Ii	Controversial[f]	None	Years	Na[c]
C	Ascorbic acid	Water	176	No	80–280 mg/session[d]	40–56 mg/day	3–4 months	Yes
Folates	Pteroylglutamic acid	Water	441	No	135 mL/min[e]	1/3 of RDA	> one year	Yes
Niacin	Nicotinic acid nicotinamide	Water	123	Weak	Very low	Na[c]	2 months	Na[c]
Biotin	Biotin	Water	244	Weak	52 mL/min[d]	Na[c]	5 weeks	None
Pantothenic acid	Pantothenic acid	Water	219	Na[c]	30 mL/min[d]	Na[c]	Several weeks	None

[a]For normal individuals.
[b]See Vitamin A section.
[c]Not available.
[d]Values obtained with low flux/low efficiency dialysis.
[e]Values obtained with high flux/high efficiency dialysis.
[f]Possible effect of convective forces.

including the kidney, and it has anti-oxidant properties [1,5]. Due to the promoting effect of 13-cis retinoic acid on cellular differentiation, it has been used to treat acute promyelocytic leukemia [6]. Large scale clinical trials failed to demonstrate a benefit of large doses of retinol and carotenoids for the prevention of cancer or cardiovascular disease [7]. An increased death rate was even reported in patients given vitamin A supplements, which may be attributed to the pro-oxidant effects of carotenoids [3]. The physiological effects of vitamin A are mediated through the retinoic acid nuclear receptor (RAR) and retinoid X receptor (RXR), which belong to the same nuclear receptor superfamily as the vitamin D receptor. Plasma vitamin A is usually measured by high pressure liquid chromatography (HPLC) which has replaced older colorimetric methods.

Vitamin E

Vitamin E is a fat soluble vitamin for which the main active compound is α-tocopherol (Table 24.1); there are other naturally occurring isomers of vitamin E as well. The main sources of vitamin E are vegetable oils, such as corn, soybean, wheat germ and sunflower oil [8]. Animal products are not rich sources of vitamin E. After intestinal absorption of vitamin E congeners, these compounds are transported with fat, mainly through the lymphatic flow, into the venous circulation [9]. In plasma, there is no specific carrier for α-tocopherol. It is carried in plasma by lipoproteins, and its plasma concentration is affected by the lipid content of blood. Assessment of the nutritional vitamin E status is difficult. HPLC is widely used to measure serum vitamin E levels [10]. The cell membrane concentration of α-tocopherol and/or its antioxidant activity might give more helpful information concerning the activity and adequacy of tissue α-tocopherol levels than plasma α-tocopherol concentrations.

Vitamin E is the main antioxidant in biological membranes, protecting phospholipid membranes from oxidative stress. Vitamin E deficiency caused by intestinal malabsorption has been reported to increase hemolysis by causing membrane fragility [10]. Vitamin E is also an antiatherogenic agent. Epidemiological studies have found a reduced risk of coronary heart disease in men and women with higher intakes of vitamin E from foods [11,12]. The mechanism of this protective effect is attributed to the decreased oxidation of LDL-cholesterol, a key step in the pathogenesis of the fatty streak, the first step in the development of the atheromatous plaque. On the other hand, vitamin E may promote synthesis and secretion of selectin, an adhesion molecule involved in the endothelial attachment of monocytes to endothelial cells, another step in atherogenesis [13]. However, as with vitamin A, large

scale clinical trials failed to demonstrate a benefit of vitamin E for the prevention of cancer or cardiovascular disease [7].

Vitamin K

Vitamin K metabolism has been well reviewed [14,15]. Two classes of compounds, phylloquinone (K_1) and menaquinones (K2), are primarily responsible for vitamin K activity. Phylloquinone (Table 24.1) is found essentially in green and leafy vegetables (e.g., spinach, kale, cabbage, and broccoli) and cow's milk. Menaquinones are of bacterial origin and are found in yogurt but are also produced by colonic bacteria. The intestinal absorption of these compounds requires biliary and pancreatic juices and occurs in the small bowel where vitamin K is incorporated into chylomicrons. The importance of intestinal bacterial synthesis of vitamin K (menaquinone) as a vitamin source is still controversial. Its importance had been emphasized because of the frequent vitamin K deficiency states associated with the use of large spectrum antibiotics. However, antibiotic therapy is not necessary for the development of vitamin K deficiency. Moreover, certain antibiotics may promote vitamin K deficiency by an independent mechanism. Antibiotics that have a N-methyl-5-thiotetrazole side chain like cefamandole and cefaperazone have a warfarin-like effect and interfere directly with the gamma-carboxylation of proteins, independently of any suppression of intestinal flora [16]. Furthermore, a vitamin K_1 deficient state is easily induced experimentally by restricting food for a few days or weeks. This leads to decreased levels of plasma descarboxyprothrombin and reduced urinary excretion of gamma-carboxyglutamic acid [17]. The uptake of vitamin K by the liver depends on β-lipoproteins and the clearance of the chylomicron remnants including its apo-E component. There is no specific carrier for vitamin K in plasma. The plasma level of phylloquinone is found to be lower in elderly individuals, as compared to young subjects [18]. Vitamin K turnover is rapid, and the body pool is small (Table 24.1). The kidney has no major role in vitamin K metabolism. The reference method for measuring plasma vitamin K levels is liquid chromatography. There is a seasonal variation in fasting plasma vitamin K concentrations, with higher levels found at the end of summer.

Vitamin K is a coenzyme for the post-translational carboxylation of glutamate residues in several proteins resulting in gamma-carboxyglutamate (Gla) residues on these latter proteins. These latter proteins are called Gla-proteins, and they may be highly functional (see below). The Gla-residue in protein binds to calcium. In the process of forming the Gla-residue, vitamin K is transformed from the hydroquinone form (KH2) to the

FIGURE 24.1 The vitamin K cycle from [235] with permission. This figure is reproduced in color in the color plate section.

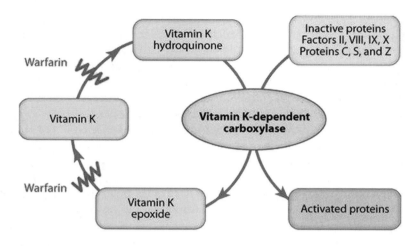

epoxide form (KO), releasing the amount of energy required to generate the carboxylation reaction (see Figure 24.1). The epoxide form of vitamin K is then recycled back to the hydroquinone form; thus, a rather small quantity of vitamin K can generate a much larger amount of the Gla proteins. Indeed, the urinary excretion of Gla residues is 200–500 times greater than the dietary intake of vitamin K. The currently known Gla-proteins are found in the coagulation cascade, in bone and dentin, in microsomes of tubular cells [19] and in atherogenic plaques. The importance of vitamin K for the normal coagulation cascade is well known. In fact, the name "vitamin K" reflects this association (K for Koagulation). The procoagulant factors which contain Gla residues, and hence require vitamin K for their post-translational carboxylation, are prothrombin (Factor II), proconvertin (Factor VII), Christmas factor (Factor IX) and Stuart factor (Factor X). The anticoagulation effect of coumarin derivatives is related to the blockade of the dithiol-dependent reductases that are necessary for the recycling of vitamin K. However, the production of several inhibitors of coagulation is also vitamin K dependent, including proteins C, S and Z. This is the explanation for the uncommon and paradoxical thrombotic complications of coumarin therapy, such as skin necrosis [20]. Two Gla-proteins are present in bone: osteocalcin and matrix Gla protein (MGP). Osteocalcin is the most abundant noncollagenous protein of bone and is a specific marker for osteoblast activity. In vitro, osteocalcin binds to hydroxyapatite and inhibits its formation. This action requires the vitamin K-dependent carboxylation of the protein. Matrix Gla-protein (MGP) regulates calcium deposition in the tissues. MGP knock-out mice present with extensive lethal vascular calcifications [21]. These carboxylated-proteins in bone play a key role in bone homeostasis. Women with hip fractures have been found to have lower plasma vitamin K levels [22]. It has been suggested

that patients receiving warfarin therapy have greater bone density loss, but this remains controversial [23].

Vitamin B₁ (Thiamin)

It has been stated that the syndrome of beriberi has been recognized for over 4000 years [24]. In 1911, an anti-beriberi principle was discovered in rice bran extracts, and in 1934 the structure of thiamin was identified. Vitamin B₁ or thiamin (Table 24.1) is a compound formed by the condensation of pyrimidine and thiazole rings. Thiamin forms esters with phosphate, functionally the most important of which are thiamin pyrophosphate (TPP), monophosphate (TMP), and triphosphate (TTP). Thiamin is rather labile and may be destroyed by heat, high pH (above 8), oxidants and ultraviolet irradiation. Thiamin is abundant in only a few food foods of animal and vegetable origin. These foods include lean pork, yeast, and legumes. Because thiamin is water soluble, foods cooked with water can be leached of significant amounts of thiamin. Thiamin is absorbed from the small intestine by active and passive processes. In plasma, thiamin is mainly bound to albumin. Most thiamin in the body is present as thiamin pyrophosphate. The availability or activity of thiamin is inhibited by alcohol, thiaminases, folate deficiency and protein-energy malnutrition. Catabolism of thiamin produces many metabolites that are excreted in the urine. In vivo, thiamin stores can be indirectly assessed by measuring the erythrocyte transketolase activity (ETKA), before (ETKA₀) and after (ETKAₛ) stimulation by thiamin pyrophosphate [25]. The ETKA stimulation index (αETKA) (i.e., the ETKA after addition of TPP X 100, divided by ETKA₀) is considered to be a more sensitive indicator of thiamin deficiency. HPLC has become the preferred method for measuring thiamin status in many laboratories [26]. HPLC can measure whole blood thiamin and RBC TPP, the active functional form of thiamin.

Thiamin pyrophosphate (TPP), in association with CoA, flavine adenine nucleotide (FAD) and nicotinamide adenine nucleotide (NAD), is a coenzyme for the oxidative decaboxylation of α-ketoacids. TPP is a coenzyme for many other enzymes, particularly those involved with carbohydrate metabolism, including pyruvate dehydrogenase. This enzyme catalyzes the conversion of pyruvate to acetyl CoA. Hence, thiamin deficiency may impair lactate utilization and lead to thiamin-responsive lactic acidosis [27]. As indicated above, thiamin is also a coenzyme for the transketolase reaction which is an integral part of the pentose phosphate pathway. Transketolase is found abundantly in myelinated structures of nervous tissues [28]. This may account for the peripheral neuropathy that occurs in beriberi. Independently of its activity as a coenzyme for transketolase, it has been suggested that thiamin may play a role in nerve impulse transmission, by interacting with sodium channels [24].

Vitamin B$_2$ or Riboflavin

Riboflavin (vitamin B$_2$) is an alloxazine derivative with a MW of 376.4 (Table 24.1). The main active riboflavin compounds are the flavin mononucleotide (FMN, an alloxazine ring combined with ribitol, a sugar moiety and phosphate) and flavin adenine dinucleotide (FAD) (FMN molecule modified by the addition of an activated adenosine monophosphate (AMP)). Riboflavin is modestly soluble in aqueous solutions, heat-stable and photosensitive. It is present in many plant and animal products, such as milk, eggs, bread, cereals, lean meats and broccoli [29]. An active sodium and glucose-dependent absorption pathway for riboflavin occurs in the proximal jejunum and is important for the transport of small quantities of this vitamin. Large amounts are absorbed from the intestine by passive diffusion. Bile salts appear to facilitate intestinal absorption of riboflavin.

After cellular uptake, riboflavin is transformed by the action of flavokinase and FAD synthetase to FMN and FAD to form functional flavoproteins. Riboflavin metabolites are excreted in urine. Flavoenzymes are involved in numerous oxidation-reduction reactions that are necessary for many metabolic pathways including energy production. The erythrocyte glutathione reductase (EGR) activity without (EGR$_o$) and with the saturation of this enzyme with FAD has been used to assess ribloflavin status [25]. The ratio of EGR with FAD $\times$ 100 divided by EGR$_o$ indicates the EGR stimulation index (α-EGR). The α-EGR is a rather reproducible and sensitive test, a high α-EGR indicating riboflavin deficiency. Riboflavin may be measured directly by a fluorometric method and by HPLC, which has been used to study CKD patients [30].

Vitamin B$_6$

Normal vitamin B$_6$ metabolism has been reviewed by Leklem [31]. Vitamin B$_6$ is composed of three derivatives of the pyridine ring: pyridoxine, pyridoxal and pyridoxamine. Some characteristics of vitamin B$_6$ are listed in Table 24.1. Phosphorylation in the 5 position is necessary for the biological activity of vitamin B$_6$. Pyridoxal-5'-phosphate (PLP) and pyridoxamine-5'-phosphate are the active coenzyme forms. Pyridoxine is mainly found in plant foods (especially wheat bran, avocado, banana, lentils, walnuts, cooked soybean and potatoes), and pyridoxal and pyridoxamine are primarily obtained from animal products (e.g., tuna, raw chicken breast, ground beef). These compounds are absorbed by a nonsaturable, passive process in the jejunum. These three vitamers are phosphorylated in the liver by pyridoxine kinase, which requires zinc and adenosine triphosphate. PLP is derived from the other vitamers by the action of a flavin mononucleotide oxidase and is transported in plasma bound to albumin and in red cells bound to hemoglobin. The major pool of PLP is in the skeletal muscle, where it is bound to glycogen phosphorylase. In liver, PLP and the other phosphorylated forms of vitamin B$_6$ are dephosphorylated by alkaline phosphatase, leading first to pyridoxal and then 4-pyridoxic acid (4-PA) by the irreversible action of a flavin adenine dinucleotide-dependent aldehyde oxidase.

Functional tests have been utilized to assess vitamin B$_6$ deficiency. Erythrocyte glutamate oxaloacetate transaminase (EGOT) or glutamic pyruvate transaminase (EGPT) activity is measured in the basal state (EGOT$_o$, EGPT$_o$) and after stimulation by adding an excess of PLP. The ratio of the stimulated to basal activity is the activation coefficient or index (α-EGOT and α-EGPT). If stores of the coenzyme (PLP) are adequate, the addition of an excess of the coenzyme will have only a small effect on the apoenzyme activity, and the ratio will be close to 1.0. If there is deficiency of PLP, the apoenzyme will be stimulated by the addition of the coenzyme, and the index value will be higher [31]. The nutritional status of vitamin B$_6$ may also be assessed by direct measurement of total pyridoxine by microbiological tests or by measurement of the urinary metabolites of tryptophan or methionine, particularly after a load of the respective amino acid is given. Currently, plasma levels of PLP and other B$_6$ compounds are usually measured using HPLC [31]. Several factors are associated with higher or lower plasma PLP levels. People over 65 years have lower plasma PLP levels than younger individuals. Females have lower levels than males. One explanation for these

TABLE 24.2   Medicines and Other Substances Interfering with Vitamin B_6 and Folic Acid Metabolism which May Contribute to Vitamin Deficiency

Vitamin B_6	Folic Acid
Isoniazide	Salicylazosulfapyridine
Hydralazine	Ethanol
Iproniazide	Diphenylhydantoin
Penicillamine	Metothrexate
Oral contraceptives	Pyrimethamine
Cycloserine	Pentamidine
Thyroxine	Trimethoprim
Theophylline	Triamterene
Caffeine	Cycloserine
Ethanol	Mysoline
	Primidone
	Barbiturates
	Yeasts, beans

findings could be differences in muscle mass. Plasma PLP levels are inversely correlated with dietary protein intake. Tobacco smoking decreases plasma B_6 levels. A large epidemiological study in normal individuals confirmed higher plasma vitamin B_6 levels in young people as compared to the elderly, and the association of increased serum acute phase proteins, alkaline phosphatase activity and impaired renal function with lower plasma B_6 levels [32]. Also, many medicines interfere with the actions or metabolism of vitamin B_6. Many of these medicines are taken by patients with CKD (Table 24.2). The intake of these medicines must be considered when evaluating studies of the dietary requirements for vitamin B_6 or when prescribing vitamin B_6 intake.

PLP is a coenzyme for almost 100 enzymatic reactions, and particularly for those enzymes involved with the metabolism of amino acids and some lipids. PLP forms a Schiff base with the ε-amino group of lysine in the enzyme. The Schiff base alters the charge of the rest of the PLP molecule and strongly increases its reactivity, particularly to other amino acids. Vitamin B_6 is essential for gluconeogenesis, by facilitating transamination and glycogen phosphorylation; for niacin formation, via the PLP dependent kinureninase which transforms tryptophan to niacin; and for normal erythrocyte metabolism, by acting as coenzyme for transaminase and influencing the O_2 affinity of hemoglobin. Vitamin B_6 facilitates the synthesis of several neurotransmitters and modulates the action of certain hormones through the binding of PLP to steroid receptors.

Vitamin C

Vitamin C (ascorbic acid, Table 24.1), whose deficiency leads to scurvy, is oxidized to dehydroascorbic acid (DHAA) which also possesses antiscorbutic activity. Ascorbic acid is mainly found in fresh fruits (e.g., blackcurrant, strawberry, lemon, orange, lime) and vegetables (e.g., broccoli, Brussels sprouts, cauliflower, cabbage). Ascorbic acid in food can be degraded by heat or extracted in cooking water. Intestinal absorption of ascorbic acid is an active, energy-requiring and saturable process. About 70 to 90% of the usual dietary vitamin C intake is absorbed, but this fraction decreases substantially when large loads of ascorbic acid are ingested. In plasma, vitamin C is nonprotein-bound and is present in a reduced form. Ascorbic acid enters the cell by active transport. The average half-life of ascorbic acid in normal adult humans is about 16 to 20 days. The body ascorbic acid pools are regulated by intestinal absorption, renal tubule reabsorption, and the catabolism of ascorbic acid [33]. Excess ascorbic acid is filtered at the glomerulus and excreted intact in the urine. The catabolic rate for ascorbic acid is directly related to the body pool size. Ascorbic acid can be oxidized to DHAA and then to a variety of compounds including L-xylose, threonic acid and oxalic acid which are excreted in urine. Oxalic acid represents 5 to 10% of the metabolites of ascorbic acid.

The methods for assessment of ascorbic acid have evolved from colorimetric methods, based on the reductive properties of ascorbic acid, to HPLC technology which is sensitive and specific [33]. The oxidized form of ascorbic acid, the ascorbyl free radical (AFR), can be detected by electron paramagnetic resonance spectroscopy. Ascorbic acid is measured in plasma, which reflects recent dietary intake, and in leukocytes, which gives a more accurate estimate of the body pool of ascorbic acid. Women usually have higher plasma ascorbic acid levels than men; smokers and elderly individuals have lower values of plasma ascorbic acid. The function of ascorbic acid is largely due to its reversible reducing power. For instance, ascorbic acid plays an important role in metal catalysed hydroxylations by reducing the metal catalyst and by allowing the metal—enzyme complex to reconstitute after it is oxidized. Perhaps the most well recognized activities of ascorbic acid are collagen synthesis via lysyl and prolyl hydroxylations, hydroxylation of peptidyl proline, enhanced secretion of procollagen that contains hydroxyproline, carnitine synthesis, hydroxylation of dopamine to form norepinephrine and of tryptophan to form serotonin, amidation of peptide hormones, intestinal iron absorption and antioxidant protection of folate and vitamin E. Potential immune activities, actions on cholesterol metabolism, and anti-cancer effects of ascorbic acid are still the subjects of investigation.

Folic Acid or Vitamin B$_9$

Folic acid (pteroylglutamic acid) is composed of three subunits: a pteridine moiety, para-aminobenzoic acid and glutamic acid (Table 24.1). Reduced forms of folic acid are present both in foods and in the human body, usually as tetrahydrofolate (THF). Folic acid is found in many foods and is present in large amounts in polyglutamate forms, usually of tetrahydrofolates or dihydrofolates, in yeast, liver, meats, green vegetables and fruits. Very sensitive to oxidation, folate is readily destroyed by extensive cooking and also by food processing such as canning or refining [34]. Intestinal absorption occurs mainly in the proximal one-third of the small bowel. Polyglutamates require the action of conjugases, present in the brush border of enterocytes, to be transformed to folate monoglutamates, such as 5-methyl-THF, formyl-THF or dihydrofolates. Another enzyme, the glutamate carboxypeptidase II anchored in the intestinal brush border, participates in polyglutamate catabolism. Devlin et al. [35] identified a H475Y DNA variant coding for this enzyme; low folate levels and hyperhomocysteinemia are associated with a 53% reduction of the enzyme activity. Cellular transport relies on specific folate membrane receptors, carriers, and cellular exit pumps. Folates are stored in the body as polyglutamates and require the action of conjugases, which are present in many tissues, to yield the biologically active monoglutamate form. However, polyglutamates may have physiological actions themselves. Actions of conjugases can be inhibited by various substances including medicines. Indeed, many medicines may inhibit the actions of folate, including ones that are commonly prescribed for CKD patients (Table 24.2). Folic acid in plasma is mainly free or loosely bound to nonspecific carriers. Delivery of folic acid to tissues requires a specific cell membrane receptor protein. Also, vitamin B$_{12}$, which like folate is involved in transmethylation reactions, is necessary for cellular transport and storage of folate. Excretion of free folate and metabolites of folic acid occurs in urine and bile. There is an enterohepatic cycle that helps to preserve the body pool of folates and that is impaired by alcohol consumption. Folate nutriture is assessed mainly by measuring serum, plasma or red cell folate levels with radioimmunological measurements which are able to detect nanogram quantities of 5-methyl THF.

The fundamental action of folate can be summarized as one carbon unit transfers [34]. Folic acid is required for DNA synthesis. The 5,10-methylene THF (requiring the vitamin B$_{12}$-dependent transmethylation of homocysteine-methionine) delivers its methyl group to deoxyuridilate, which is transformed to thymidilate and is necessary for DNA synthesis. A defect in this step in DNA synthesis leads to megaloblastosis, which occurs in all replicating cells in the body but is most striking in bone marrow cells. Folic acid plays a role in amino acid metabolism, particularly for those amino acids that are methyl donors, including the interconversion of glycine and serine, the transformation of homocysteine to methionine (Figure 24.2), and the conversion of histidine to glutamic acid. Moreover, folic acid is required for purine synthesis in the methylation of transfer RNA. Unlike vitamin B$_{12}$, folate is not involved in myelin synthesis, and therefore folate deficiency does not cause neurological disease.

Vitamin B$_{12}$

Vitamin B$_{12}$ or cobalamin (Table 24.1) has been identified as the "extrinsic factor" (i.e., present in food), which, when combined to the "intrinsic factor" (present in gastric juice), results in the absorption of the antipernicious anemia factor. The molecule of vitamin B$_{12}$ is constituted by a corrin nucleus, a nucleotide and a cobalt atom. Cobalamins are unstable in light and destroyed by strong oxidation and reduction agents. Cyanocobalamin, the pharmaceutical form of vitamin B$_{12}$, has been isolated from liver extracts. Coenzyme B$_{12}$ and methylcobalamin are the metabolically active forms. All forms of B$_{12}$ in large doses are equally potent [36]. The only source of vitamin B$_{12}$ is bacterial synthesis. Cobalamins are present in animal tissues, mostly liver, meat and seafood, but also in lesser amounts in egg yolk and milk. Very small amounts are present in fruits and vegetables. Physiological intestinal absorption follows several steps: free cobalamin is combined with a salivary peptide binder, then is released in small intestine by trypsin and is combined again with the intrinsic factor, a glycoprotein molecule of gastric origin. Absorption of the vitamin B$_{12}$-intrinsic factor complex occurs after binding to a receptor on the brush border of mucosal cells in the ileum. However, large pharmacological doses of cobalamins may be absorbed by the small intestine via passive diffusion. Three binding proteins (transcobalamins I, II and III) participate in cobalamin transport in plasma and also in the storage of vitamin B$_{12}$. Cobalamin stores can be comprised of several milligrams of vitamin B$_{12}$ and may prevent vitamin B$_{12}$ deficiency from occurring for several years after intestinal absorption ceases [37] (Table 24.1). Vitamin B$_{12}$ is not catabolized and is excreted in bile, with an efficient enterohepatic cycle. Vitamin B$_{12}$ assessment is performed using microbiologic assays and

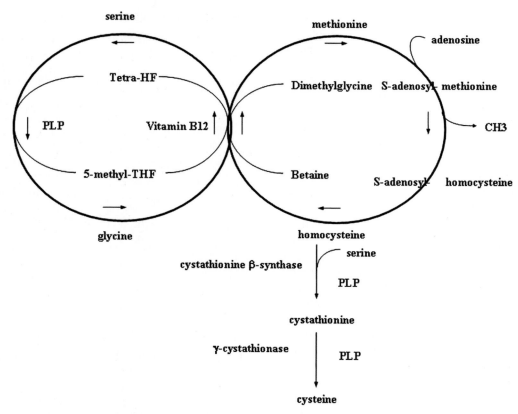

FIGURE 24.2   Role of folic acid, vitamin B_{12} and B_6 in methionine-homocysteine-cysteine metabolism.

currently by radioassays. Radioassays are not affected by antibiotic treatment.

Vitamin B_{12} has a key role in folic acid metabolism. Its essential function is the demethylation of methyltetrahydrofolate and methylation of Hcy (Figure 24.2). This step is essential for regeneration of THF, which is involved in DNA synthesis by thymidilate synthesis, and for folate delivery to tissues. In the absence of demethylation, signs of folate deficiency may occur [36]. Furthermore, vitamin B_{12} is required for myelin synthesis, as demonstrated by the severe neurological disturbances that may occur with pernicious anemia. The exact mechanism of cobalamin action on myelin is unknown.

Niacin or Vitamin B_3

Niacin has been identified as the therapeutic agent for pellagra, a condition described initially in maize-eating populations [38]. Niacin is a generic term including nicotinic acid and nicotinamide (Table 24.1). Active coenzymes are pyridine nucleotides, nicotinamide adenine dinucleotide (NAD) and NAD phosphate (NADP). High amounts of NAD and NADP (the main forms of niacin intake from foods) are present in meat, fish, legumes, coffee and tea. These compounds are hydrolyzed in the intestine to yield nicotinamide and then nicotinic acid. However, niacin bioavailability may be reduced because of its binding to carbohydrate and peptide macromolecules. Intestinal absorption by diffusion is efficient, even for large doses of niacin. Tryptophan is a precursor for niacin, and tryptophan intake alone may be sufficient to provide the RDA for nicotinic acid. Niacin is quickly removed from plasma by tissues (mainly by liver and RBC) where it is converted to coenzyme forms. Storage, mostly in the liver, is limited, and signs of pellagra may occur within 50–60 days in humans fed a corn diet deficient in niacin. Excess niacin is methylated in the liver, and the methylated metabolites are excreted in the urine. Niacin status is assessed by measuring nicotinic acid and nicotinamide in blood and red cells, using microbiological or, currently, chemical assays or HPLC. The NAD/NADP ratio in red cells, which is decreased in niacin deficiency, may be used as an indicator of niacin depletion in renal failure patients.

Pyridine nucleotides are involved in many enzymatic reactions (at least 200). These may include NAD which is mainly involved in catabolic reactions, such as oxidation of fuel molecules, and NADP, which is primarily concerned with synthesis, such as for steroids. These coenzymes are key elements for carbohydrate, fatty acid and amino acid metabolism. There is a close relationship between the metabolism of niacin and of other vitamins. Vitamin B_6 and riboflavin are necessary for niacin synthesis from tryptophan. Niacin is necessary for the synthesis of active forms of vitamin B_6, riboflavin and folic acid. Pharmacological doses of nicotinic acid reduce total cholesterol, increase the HDL-cholesterol fraction, and decrease LDL and VLDL fractions and triglycerides [39]. Another important property of nicotinamide is inhibition of the Na/Pi type IIb cotransporter (Na Pi-2b) and the type IIa cotransporter (NaPi-2a) in the intestinal brush border and in the proximal renal tubular epithelial cells of the kidneys, respectively [40]. Large doses of nicotinamide, 500 to 1500 mg/day given twice-daily, can reduce serum phosphorus concentrations in hemodialysis patients.

Biotin or Vitamin B_8

Biotin or vitamin B_8 is a bi-cyclic compound containing an ureido ring and a tetrahydrothiophene ring (Table 24.1). Although biotin is synthetized by intestinal flora, it is controversial as to whether this synthesis can satisfy the daily need for biotin in humans [41]. Main food sources of biotin are liver, egg yolk, soybean and yeast. Cereals, legumes and nuts contain moderate amounts of biotin, and fruits and vegetables are poor sources of biotin, except for cauliflower and mushrooms. Biotin absorption occurs mainly in the jejunum and requires the release of biocytin (biotinyl lysine) from ingested proteins and the action of biotinidase to free lysine and biotin, which are each absorbed by a diffusive saturable process. Long-term anticonvulsivant therapy may interfere with the binding of biotin to biotinidase. The presence of avidin, a glycoprotein which strongly binds to biotin, may impair biotin absorption. Free biotin and its metabolites are excreted in the urine. Biotin stores appear to cover biotin needs about one month. A biotin deficient diet in human volunteers leads to symptoms of deficiency in 5 weeks [42]. Biotin is assessed in plasma with microbiological assays.

Biotin mainly acts as a "CO_2 carrier" being the coenzyme for carboxylases (Acetyl CoA carboxylase, pyruvate carboxylase, propionyl CoA carboxylase, B methylcrotonyl CoA carboxylase). Biotin is covalently bound to the ε-amino group of a lysine residue of carboxylases. Thus, it plays an important role in the metabolism of carbohydrates, fatty acids and some amino acids. Experimental biotin deficiency was induced in seven healthy human volunteers who were given a biotin-free diet and an excessive intake of raw egg white (rich in avidin). In five weeks, the subjects developed mild depression, somnolence, muscle pains, hyperesthesia, anorexia and later a maculosquamous dermatitis with greyish palor and fine desquamation. All symptoms disappeared within five days of starting biotin injections [41]. Alopecia is also a common feature of biotin deficiency [42].

Pantothenic Acid or Vitamin B_5

Pantothenic acid or "chick antidermatitis factor" is formed from the combination of pantoic acid and β-alanine. Some of its characteristics are given in Table 24.1. Pantothenic acid, after passing through several biochemical steps, is incorporated into the coenzyme A (CoA) macromolecule which is comprised of pantothenic acid, adenosine monophosphate and β-mercaptoethylamine. Pantothenic acid is ubiquitous and present in large amounts in many foods, especially liver, kidney, egg yolk, fresh vegetables, royal bee jelly and ovaries of tuna and cod [43]. After CoA hydrolysis, pantothenic acid is liberated and excreted in the urine. Pantothenic acid is assessed by microbiological assays or, more currently, by radioimmunoassay.

Pantothenic acid, in its function as a cofactor for CoA, is necessary for the synthesis of many compounds including fatty acids, cholesterol, steroid hormones, molecules containing isoprenoid units (e.g., vitamins A and D), δ-aminolevulinic acid, and some neurotransmitters and amino acids. It is also necessary for energy extraction during the β-oxidation of fatty acids and oxidation of amino acids. Also, pantothenic acid and CoA play a central role in the acetylation of proteins, microtubules and histones and in the acylation of proteins with fatty acids, mainly myristic and palmitic acids. The acetylation and acylation of proteins affect both their structure and activity. In animals, pantothenic acid deficiency results in retarded growth, neuromuscular disorders, abnormalities of skin and hair and gastrointestinal symptoms. In young men fed a pantothenic-free diet for nine weeks, their main complaint was fatigue [44].

VITAMIN INTAKE IN CHRONIC RENAL DISEASE

Data regarding vitamin intake in patients with advanced CKD, except for vitamin C, are often conflicting. No data are currently available about vitamin intake for nephrotic patients. The vitamin intake with the protein-restricted diets usually prescribed to CKD patients who do not have ESRD is reported in Table 24.3 from Stein et al. [45]. Protein-restricted diets are most likely to engender low intakes of vitamin K, biotin, folic acid, B_{12}, niacin and pantothenic acid. More studies have been published regarding vitamin intakes of chronic dialysis patients. Vitamin B_6 intake is often low, according to dietary surveys of maintenance dialysis patients [46,47]. In 242 CAPD patients, Wang et al. [48] reported inadequate intakes for vitamin B_1 and B_6 and folic acid in patients with loss of residual renal function and/or low urea clearance. Martin-Del-Campo et al. [49] reported that 50% of 73 CPD patients had low intakes

TABLE 24.3 Calculated Vitamin Content of Different Diets Prescribed to Chronic Renal Failure Patients (from Stein [45])

Dietary Protein Intake	Vitamin A (μg RE[b])	Vitamin E (mg)	Vitamin K (μg)	Thiamin (mg)	Riboflavin (mg)	Biotin (μg)	Pyridoxine (mg)	Folic acid (μg)	Vitamin B_{12}(μg)	Niacin (mg)	Ascorbic Acid (mg)	Pantothenic Acid (mg)
40 g[a]	556	16.0	80	1.2	0.8	13.4	1.4	50	0.6	9.0	107	3.0
60 g[a]	570	12.0	80	1.5	1.4	17.8	1.5	80	1.2	10.5	88	4.0
80 g[a]	568	14.0	80	1.3	1.2	15.8	1.8	70	2.5	15.0	60	3.2
RDA[c]	700–900	15	80–120	1.1–1.2	1.1–1.3	30[d]	1.3–1.7[e]	400	2.4	14–16	75–90[f]	5[d]

[a]Data refer to 24 hour intake of the nutrient from the diet.
[b]RE: Retinol Equivalents.
[c]Recommended Dietary Allowance for healthy, nonpregnant, nonlactating adults.
[d]This value is not a RDA; there is inadequate scientific evidence to allow calculation of RDA. Recommended intake, termed "Adequate Intake" is used instead. It is derived from experimental data or by an approximation of observed mean intakes, as suggested by the Standing Committee on the Scientific Evaluation of Dietary Reference Intakes [234].
[e]In female and male adults below the age of 50, the RDA is 1.3 mg/d. Over the age of 50, the RDA is respectively 1.5 and 1.7 mg/d for women and men.
[f]Values of the RDA are for nonsmoking female and male adults. Add 35 mg/d for smokers [53].

of vitamin A, B_2, B_6, C, folate and niacin. Patients in the higher quartile of serum C reactive protein (CRP) levels had significantly lower intakes of riboflavin and vitamin A. Dietary habits may influence the amount of vitamins ingested by CKD or maintenance dialysis patients. For example, lower intakes of vitamin B_6 and folic acid were found when MHD patients ingested meals of processed foods rather than traditionally prepared complete dinners [50]. These data underscore the nutritional superiority of traditional foods and cooking above most processed foods. Takagi et al. [51] reported that sevelamer HCl binds a significant amount of vitamin B_6.

More extensive data have been reported for vitamin C intake. In the early days of chronic dialysis treatment, the average ascorbic acid intake of maintenance hemodialysis (MHD) patients was reported by Sullivan et al. [52] to be 34 mg/day, whereas the recommended dietary allowance (RDA) for ascorbic acid is respectively 75 mg and 90 mg/day in nonsmoking female and male adults [53]. Allman et al. [46] showed a low spontaneous intake of vitamin C in their MHD patients (69% consumed less than two-thirds of the RDA). In children undergoing MHD and CAPD, the vitamin C intake was found respectively at 51% and 77% of the RDA [54]. Prescription of a low potassium diet is likely to reduce intake of vitamin C containing foods. Both ascorbic acid and potassium are abundant in fresh fruits and leafy vegetables. Hence, restriction of foods high in potassium will reduce the intake of ascorbic acid and may predispose to vitamin C deficiency [55]. Among the prescribed restrictions in dietary intake for maintenance dialysis patients, the reduction in potassium is the one most likely to be adhered to [56], and it increases the risk of low vitamin C intake. Moreover, prolonged soaking and boiling of vegetables, which may be employed to reduce the potassium content of food, may leech out or degrade ascorbic acid. Bohm et al. [57] reported that renal transplant recipients have a vitamin C intake equal to the RDA. Hence, ingesting the RDA for vitamins will depend on many factors including the dietary prescription and the patient's adherence to the prescription, appetite, medicinal intake and superimposed illnesses (see below). The renal dietitian is the key person in the outpatient setting and in the dialysis unit to evaluate this situation and to alert the patient and the nephrologist regarding his vitamin intake and needs.

VITAMINS STATUS IN CHRONIC RENAL DISEASE

Nephrotic Syndrome

Few data have been published regarding the vitamin status in patients with nephrotic syndrome. Plasma RBP, retinol and retinyl esters levels are reported to be increased [58] even in the absence of renal failure. Data are conflicting for vitamin E in this condition. In 33 adults with the nephrotic syndrome, erythrocyte thiamin pyrophosphate and riboflavin were found to be normal by Midlyk et al. [59], whereas plasma PLP was significantly decreased. More recently, Podda et al. [60] reported a significant decrease of blood vitamin B_6 concentrations in 84 nephrotic patients as compared to controls, and there was a correlation between the blood vitamin B_6 levels and the magnitude of proteinuria. Rajbala et al. [61] found decreased serum vitamin C in 45 children presenting with the nephrotic syndrome. This was confirmed by Fydryk et al. [62] who found decreased blood vitamin C during relapse of steroid-dependent nephrotic syndrome in 18 children. Twenty-nine nephrotic patients were studied with regarding to their vitamin C and E status and compared with 25 patients with hematuria [63]. Plasma vitamin C and the ascorbate/vitamin E ratio were significantly lower in the nephrotic patients. These data suggest that for nephrotic patients, vitamin C and vitamin B_6 levels should be assessed or, alternatively, multivitamin supplements should be routinely administered.

Chronic Kidney Disease 2−5 Stages Including Dialysis Therapy

Vitamin A

In comparison to normal individuals, high plasma vitamin A levels and an increased rise in plasma vitamin A in response to a vitamin A load test was reported in CKD patients as long ago as 1945 [64]. Many authors have constantly confirmed elevated plasma concentrations of total vitamin A, RBP bound vitamin A and free vitamin A in nondialyzed CKD patients and maintenance dialysis patients, including children [45,65−70]. The increase of vitamin A in CKD is attributed to RBP metabolism. After the delivery of retinol to target tissues, the free RBP can be filtered by the glomerulus and catabolized by the tubular cells. Thus, in renal failure there is an increase in plasma RBP, and the plasma RBP/prealbumin and RBP/retinol ratios [71]. The small proportion (5%) of the RBP-retinol complex that is not bound to transthyretin normally is filtered by the glomerulus. In renal failure, this reduction in glomerular filtration may contribute to the elevated plasma levels. The complex is captured by the proximal tubular cell by a specific apical receptor, megalin, allowing for retinol recycling into the blood stream at the basolateral level of the cell. Knockout mice for megalin display a urinary loss of the RBP-retinol complex [72].

As shown many years ago, hemodialysis (HD) treatment does not change vitamin A levels [66]; indeed losses of vitamin A into dialysate would not be expected because of the relatively large size of the vitamin A-RBP-prealbumin complex. However, β-carotene, ubiquinol and lycopene have been found to be lower in MHD patients than in controls [68,73], and β-carotene and ubiquinol fall further after a single HD session. There are no published data on the dialysis kinetics of vitamin A and RBP handling in MHD patients treated with high flux membranes, convective techniques and daily dialysis. The data are conflicting as to whether vitamin A and RBP are present in the effluent peritoneal dialysate [67,74].

Whether there is an increased risk of vitamin A toxicity in individuals with CKD and in chronic dialysis patients is controversial. Intriguingly, in patients who did not have other evidence for vitamin A toxicity, a correlation between plasma vitamin A concentrations and serum calcium levels has been reported in CRF patients [75]. MHD patients who were taking modest doses of vitamin A supplements, 2500 to 15,000 IU per day, had higher serum vitamin A and calcium concentrations than those who were not. However, such correlations between plasma vitamin A and increased serum calcium or serum alkaline phosphatase have not been found consistently. The mechanism of hypercalcemia with vitamin A toxicity is related to the osteolytic action of the retinoids on bone [76]. Many chronic renal failure patients who have increased plasma vitamin A (up to 3–4 times normal levels) do not show evidence for toxicity [77,78]. Elevated plasma vitamin A in renal failure is considered by many authors to be relative, due to increased plasma RBP and to have no clinical significance as long as the vitamin A/RBP ratio is normal or low.

Vitamin A toxicity is believed to occur when plasma retinyl esters in the lipoprotein fractions increase [1,71]. Whether vitamin A accumulates in solid tissues in ordinary renal failure patients is controversial [65,78–80]. Therefore, it is not known whether the increased vitamin A levels that are commonly found in CKD and chronic dialysis patients are hazardous. In nonuremic people with vitamin A overload and toxicity, large amounts of vitamin A may accumulate in the liver. The clinical signs of vitamin A intoxication, cutaneous lesions (fissures, dryness, desquamation, yellowish appearance), headaches and CNS manifestations, joint pains, bone tenderness to palpation, anemia, hepatomegaly and muscle stiffness are not specific indicators for vitamin A toxicity.

The prognostic value of plasma vitamin A levels in MHD and renal transplant patients has been recently analyzed. In a post-hoc analysis of the 4-D study including prevalent diabetic MHD patients, Espe et al. [81] found that the lower quartiles of retinol (Figure 24.3) and RBP4 were associated with increased risk of sudden

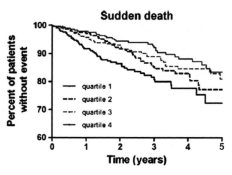

FIGURE 24.3 Influence of vitamin A plasma levels on sudden cardiac death in hemodialysis patients ([81] with permission). Quartile 1 includes patients with the lowest plasma retinol levels as assessed with HPLC.

death, infection-related and overall mortality. The lower retinol quartile remained above the normal range of plasma retinol. It confirms previous data reported in a smaller cohort of prevalent MHD patients [82]. The possible interpretation is that the lower retinol level is an indirect marker of inflammation. This is consistent with data in CPD patients by Martin-Del-Campo et al. [49] who found a significant lower vitamin A intake in the patients belonging to the higher serum CRP quartile.

Vitamin E

In nondialyzed patients with advanced CKD, plasma vitamin E levels are usually within the normal range [83]. Protein restricted diets generally provide a normal and nutritionally sufficient vitamin E intake (Table 24.3). Malnutrition may also influence vitamin E status, and lower serum α-tocopherol levels are found in malnourished CKD patients than in well-nourished individuals [84]. Peuchant et al. [85] found decreased α-tocopherol in red blood cells (RBC) from nondialyzed CKD patients who had increased erythrocyte peroxidation, as determined by elevated intraerythrocyte malonyldialdehyde (MDA) concentrations. In MHD patients, serum α-tocopherol levels have been found reported low [73], normal [83] or increased [45]. There is no difference in plasma vitamin E concentrations between pre- and postdialysis samples [73]. In CPD patients, data regarding vitamin E status are also conflictory.

Vitamin K

Few studies have systematically examined the vitamin K status of CKD and dialysis patients, and they are conflicting. Plasma vitamin K levels were found to be normal by Malyszko et al. [86] in CKD, MHD and CPD patients. Robert et al. [87] reported a high plasma level of phylloquinone in MHD patients. In contrast, a plasma low phylloquinone level was identified in some CKD (6%), MHD (29%) and PD (24%) patients [88–90]. But the plasma phylloquinone level itself is not a sensitive indicator of subclinical vitamin K deficiency. In a cohort of nondialyzed CKD 3–5 patients, the phylloquinone plasma level was found to be normal in 94% of the patients, whereas 60% and 97% had subclinical deficiency as assessed, respectively, from the proportion of uncarboxylated osteocalcin in serum and the serum level of PIVKA-2. PIVKA-2 is a protein induced by vitamin K. The absence or inhibition of PIVKA-2 leads to an increase in serum des-gamma-carboxy prothrombin; an increase in these levels is a very early manifestation of vitamin K deficiency before the prolongation of coagulation) [89].

Vitamin B_1

The EKTA stimulation index was found to be normal by Kopple et al. [91] in 15 nondialyzed advanced CKD patients who were receiving 1-mg/day thiamine HCl supplements. No relationship was observed between EKTA or the EKTA stimulation index and the level of renal function. Uremic toxins may impair thiamine function. In the early days of dialysis, Lonergan reported a dialysable compound in uremic serum that inhibited ETKA and suggested that it might be guanidosuccinic acid [92]. This inhibitory effect of uremic sera was ameliorated by dialysis treatment. Sterzel et al. [93] reported that transketolase activity of nervous tissue was inhibited by uremic plasma and by cerebrospinal fluid from uremic patients and by a low MW fraction (<500 kD) of dialysate. However, in the early years of dialysis therapy, Kopple et al. [91] did not find acute changes in ETKA observed during a single hemodialysis treatment. Kuriyama confirmed a low basal ETKA ($EKTA_o$) or stimulated ETKA ($ETKA_s$) in a group of 72 MHD, CPD and nondialysed patients with chronic renal failure, even though they had high blood thiamin levels following ingestion of supplements [94]. Other investigators reported that the blood thiamin level is usually in the normal range in MHD patients [95]. In 43 unsupplemented MHD patients, Descombes et al. found low or marginal $ETKA_o$ in 56% of patients, and the ETKA stimulation index was increased in 21% of the patients [37]. In $ETKA_o$ deficient patients, whole blood thiamin was normal. The functional deficiency was reversed with large amounts of thiamin hydrochloride (100 mg after each hemodialysis). In the same study, patients undergoing MHD with a polyacrilonitrile membrane dialyzer had lower $ETKA_o$ than those treated with cellulose acetate. Heinz et al. [96] reported that the hemodialysis procedure induces a greater decrease in plasma thiamin levels with high-flux versus low-flux membranes. Coveney et al. [97] have reported lower plasma thiamin in patients treated with extended dialysis sessions when compared to patients treated by conventional dialysis. However, no patient was found to have blood thiamin levels below the normal range.

Hence, highly permeable membranes may increase the risk of thiamin deficiency in MHD patients, presumably by increasing the thiamin losses from hemodialysis.

Blumberg et al. [47] and Boeschotten and coworkers [74] reported thiamin deficiency in 50% and 26% of CPD patients who were not receiving thiamin supplements. Losses of this vitamin into the peritoneal dialysate were substantially lower than the normal daily urine excretion of thiamin [74]. These findings suggest that even if blood thiamin levels are normal, this does not rule out a functional deficiency. Moreover, in experimental CKD rats, it has been shown that thiamine transporters are down regulated in the heart, the brain, the liver and the intestine. These observations raise questions concerning the appropriate methods for assessing thiamin status in advanced CKD and dialysis patients.

Clinical manifestations of thiamin deficiency have rarely been described in ESKD patients. Beriberi has been reported in two MHD patients [98,99]. Case reports of Wernicke's encephalopathy are increasing and have been described in MHD and CPD patients but may be frequently overlooked because the classical triad of this syndrome (confusional state, ataxia, opthalmoplegia) is present in only 20% of the cases [100–102]. In the report by Ueda et al. [102], typical pathologic lesions of Wernicke's encephalopathy were found in five patients who had been given such other diagnoses by clinicians as uremic encephalopathy, dysequilibrium syndrome, dialysis dementia, or brainstem hemorrhage. Also, chorea has been reported in two cases of thiamin deficiency in MHD patients [103]. The same authors found thiamin deficiency in 10 MHD patients presenting with mental disturbances. Nine out of 10 recovered with intravenous thiamin supplementation [104]. Infection, surgery and large glucose loads may increase the nutritional needs for thiamin, and precipitate clinical manifestations of thiamin deficiency.

Riboflavin (Vitamin B_2)

Porrini et al. [105] have reported increased αEGR activity (indicating riboflavin deficiency) in CKD patients prescribed a low protein diet. However, its clinical significance remains unknown. In dialysis patients, most studies show normal or excess riboflavin in plasma of MHD and CPD patients even when they are not prescribed vitamin supplements [37,74,106] and despite the losses of riboflavin into peritoneal dialysate [74]. However, Skoupy et al. found that 18.5% of CAPD patients had increased α-EGR [107]. More recently, riboflavin deficiency was not found in 12 pediatric CPD and MHD patients who were not receiving supplements [108]. Also in MHD patients receiving multivitamin supplements, and treated with standard or daily long HD sessions, no riboflavin deficiency was found even with the more extensive dialysis treatment [109]. No clinical syndromes associated with ribloflavin excess or deficiency have been reported in CKD or ESRD patients.

Vitamin B₆

Blunted weight gain was observed during a four week period in chronically azotemic compared to sham-operated rats and was significantly more pronounced in the rats that were fed a vitamin B₆-deficient-diet when compared to vitamin B₆-surfeit diet [110]. Most but not all surveys detect a high incidence of vitamin B₆ deficiency in both adult and pediatric advanced CKD, MHD and CPD patients. Methodologic differences in the measurements of vitamin B₆ could explain these observed differences in vitamin B₆ deficiency. The use of red cell transaminase activity ($EGOT_0$ or $EGPT_0$) as the criterion for deficiency [111] has been criticized because of the shortened life span of red cells in CKD and the higher activities of some enzymes in younger erythrocytes. Studies that assessed plasma pyridoxal-5-phosphate (PLP) concentrations also found decreased levels in most dialyzed and nondialyzed CKD patients. In a recent systematic review of vitamin B₆ status in MHD patients, Corken & Porter [112] reported a 33–56% prevalence of vitamin B₆ deficiency when low plasma PLP was used as the criterion for deficiency. Removal of vitamin B₆ by dialysis has not been confirmed. Lacour et al. [113] did not find PLP in the hemodialysis ultrafiltrate from low-flux hemodialysis. This is not surprising since PLP is bound to albumin. The effect of PLP clearance with high flux membrane is contradictory. Kasama et al. [114] observed a significant reduction of serum PLP in six MHD patients after they switched from cuprophane to cellulose triacetate, whereas Heinz et al. [96] did not find any difference in serum PLP with the same study design. No data are currently available on PLP clearance with convective techniques. Boeschotten and coworkers reported that the quantity of PLP lost into peritoneal dialysate, assessed by HPLC, is similar to the normal urinary vitamin B₆ excretion [74]. In another study of peritoneal dialysis, much lower losses of PLP were reported [115]. Moreover, additional PLP bound to proteins may be lost into peritoneal dialysate.

Vitamin B₆ deficiency in experimental animals and humans is associated with many alterations in immune function including reduced numbers of blood granulocytes and lymphocytes, decreased lymphocyte maturation, reduced blastogenic response of lymphocytes to mitogenic stimuli, delayed cutaneous hypersensitivity and decreased antibody production. B₆ deficiency may play a role in the alterations of immune function in advanced CKD. Many years ago, Dobbelstein et al.

[116] were able to reverse decreased reactivity in mixed lymphocyte culture by giving MHD patients 300 mg/day of pyridoxine HCl for two weeks. Casciato et al. [117] improved immunologic function of polymorphonuclear neutrophils and lymphocytes in eight MHD patients, most of whom had vitamin B₆ deficiency, by giving 50 mg/day of pyridoxine hydrochloride for three to five weeks.

Vitamin C

Few studies of vitamin C status are available for non-dialyzed, advanced CKD patients. Marumo [118] surprisingly found low plasma ascorbic acid levels in patients with mild to moderate CKD but not in nondialyzed individuals with advanced CKD or in MHD patients. In contrast, Clermont et al. [83] found decreased vitamin C levels, with an increased ascorbyl free radical/ascorbic acid ratio in CKD patients. Intravenous furosemide increases urinary vitamin C excretion in CKD patients [119]. In the early days of MHD treatment, Sullivan and Eisenstein described ascorbic acid deficiency in MHD patients [52]. Latter reports confirmed a high incidence of vitamin C deficiency in MHD and PD patients not given vitamin C supplements [46,47,74,83,120,121] and even in some patients receiving supplements [37]. However, Tarng et al. [122] found normal vitamin C levels in 65 nonsupplemented patients treated with MHD for a mean of 48.7 months. Ramirez et al. [95] monitored plasma ascorbic acid levels for one year after discontinuing vitamin C supplements. A dramatic decrease in plasma ascorbic acid was observed, but no patient reached a deficient level. Mydlik et al. [123] found normal plasma vitamin C levels in 32 CAPD patients not receiving ascorbic acid supplements. Recently, Zhang et al. [124] reported in that in plasma of 284 MHD and CAPD patients, 64% of the patients presented with deficiency or insufficiency for vitamin C.

Ascorbic acid is a small molecular weight (MW) and nonprotein bound molecule, which is readily dialyzable. Bohm et al. [57] measured the amount of vitamin C in dialysate and found it to range from 92 to 334 mg per treatment, with a 50% decrease in plasma ascorbic acid during an individual HD treatment and a return to pre-dialysis levels by 44 hours. Hultqvist et al. [120] found a 40% decrease in plasma ascorbic acid during a 3-hour HD treatment. In peritoneal dialysate, 56 mg of ascorbic acid were recovered in the 24-hour cycle [74]. According to Mydlik et al. [123], the peritoneal transfer of ascorbic acid was 136.4 μmoles/6 hours with 1.5% glucose in dialysate, and increased to 175.8 μmoles/6 hours with 2.5% dialysate glucose. Whereas low plasma ascorbic acid levels are not infrequently reported in MHD and CPD patients who do not receive vitamin C supplements, scurvy has been described only rarely in CKD patients. Ihle reported a MHD patient with cutaneous symptoms (pruritus, bruising and ecchymoses), impaired platelet function, a low vitamin C intake and decreased plasma and leukocyte ascorbic acid levels [125]. The defect in platelet function was similar to that reported with scurvy. Treatment with one gram of vitamin C per day for a few days rapidly corrected the ecchymoses, prolonged bleeding time and platelet dysfunction. However, fatigue and periodontal lesions are frequent in dialysis patients, and their relationship to the frequent vitamin C deficiency has never been addressed [126].

Folic Acid

Folate metabolism is altered in renal failure. CKD impairs the intestinal absorption of THF. Using in vivo perfusion of the jejunum, Said et al. [127] showed that azotemic rats had significantly lower absorption of 5-methyl THF than sham-operated controls. Using an in vitro everted jejunal sac technique, these authors found that predialysis sera obtained from MHD patients showed suppression of intestinal absorption of 5-methyl THF, whereas postdialysis sera caused significantly less suppression. In rats with chronic kidney failure, Bukhari et al. [128] demonstrated a downregulation of folic acid transporters in tissues and especially in the intestine. This could lead to decreased folate absorption. Livant et al. [129] reported that plasma conjugase activity was reduced in predialysis sera and rose to normal levels posthemodialysis. The authors suggest that there are one or more circulating heat stable compounds in uremic plasma which may inhibit plasma folate conjugase activity.

Marumo et al. [118] reported that in CKD patients who were not receiving folate supplements, serum folic acid was normal in those with mild to moderate CKD and was increased above normal in patients with advanced CKD who were not undergoing MHD. In the 1960s to 1980s, reports regarding folic acid status in MHD patients were contradictory, describing both normal and deficient status. Marked increases in plasma and red cell folate levels have been found in patients receiving folate supplements [130]. Folate pools are believed to contain sufficient quantities to satisfy folic acid requirements for at least one year [37]. Thus, at least several months, if not more than one year of follow-up, after interruption of supplementation may be necessary to assess the risk of folate depletion. Moreover, most of these studies were conducted before the advent of high flux/high efficiency HD which appears to have dramatically increased the risk of folic acid deficiency in MHD patients. Livant et al. [129] found that in 32 MHD patients treated with high flux polysulfone dialyzers, five individuals had reduced predialysis plasma folate concentrations and four had decreased red cell

folate levels. The incidence of folate deficiency might have been greater if 20 of the patients had not been prescribed folate supplements. Leblanc et al. [131] reported the folic acid clearance to be 134.7 ± 22.2 mL/min with high flux/high efficiency MHD, with a 26.3% decrease in plasma folic acid during an individual MHD treatment. But the risk of folic acid depletion with high flux membranes is not confirmed [132]. The incidence of folate deficiency in CPD patients is also controversial [47,74,133,134]. Folate losses into peritoneal dialysate averaged 107 μg/day in one study [74]. The influence of EPO therapy on folate status is reported below.

Vitamin B$_{12}$

Plasma vitamin B$_{12}$ is usually within the normal range in CKD and chronic dialysis patients even without supplementation and even with extended hemodialysis vintage [97]. Because cobalamin is a larger molecule in its own right (MW: 1355) and is also protein-bound, losses of vitamin B$_{12}$ in dialysate are low. Fehrman-Ekholm et al. [135] did not find decreased serum vitamin B$_{12}$ levels in hemodialfiltration patients. In CPD patients, no cobalamin was recovered in peritoneal fluid by Boeschoten et al. [74].

Niacin

There are few data regarding niacin status in nondialyzed and dialyzed CKD patients. Because of its rapid metabolic clearance, losses of niacin in dialysate are expected to be low. Ramirez et al. [95] did not find differences between pre- and postdialysis red cell niacin concentrations in MHD patients. No data are available on niacin losses in peritoneal dialysate. DeBari reported low concentrations of niacin in leukocytes, but normal niacin content in red cells of MHD patients [136]. Ramirez et al. [95,111] did not find evidence of low niacin levels in whole blood or erythrocytes of MHD patients who were not receiving supplements or in whom supplements had been stopped for at least one year. Pellagra (characterized by diarrhea, dementia, dermatitis) has never been reported in CKD patients, but niacin deficiency has been suggested as the cause of onycholysis in MHD patients [137].

Biotin

Uremic toxins have been shown to impair tubulin polymerization which leads to microtubule formation, and biotin counteracts the effects of uremic toxins on tubulin [138]. Biotin intake in CKD patients prescribed low protein diets has been estimated to be much lower than the RDA (Table 24.3). With the exception of an occasional deficient patient, several studies did not find biotin deficiency in chronic renal failure patients. Biotin concentrations in plasma, leukocytes and RBC were found to be high in MHD patients [139], and even higher in anuric patients and in MHD patients treated for longer periods of time [37].

Pantothenic Acid

There are few data concerning the pantothenic acid status of renal failure patients. Conflicting data have been reported regarding the pantothenic acid status in MHD patients. Debari et al. [136] found in 12 nonsupplemented MHD patients that pantothenic acid concentrations in plasma, leukocytes and red cells were significantly higher than in normal controls. Lasker et al. [140] reported normal or high concentrations of pantothenic acid in blood of six MHD and three CPD patients who were not receiving vitamin supplements. On the other hand, Mackenzie et al. [141] reported low concentrations of plasma pantothenic acid in six MHD patients who were not receiving supplemental pantothenic acid.

Kidney Transplant Patients

There are few published data regarding the vitamin status of renal transplant recipients. Plasma vitamin A levels decrease slowly toward normal after renal transplantation, Yatzidis and coworkers reported that more than 20 months may elapse in patients with a well functioning kidney transplant before plasma vitamin A levels are normal [142]. In renal transplant recipients as in MHD patients, a decreased survival has been observed in patients in the lower tertile for plasma retinol. In contrast, vitamin E and a variety of carotenoids, including β-carotene, are not associated with patient survival [143]. McGrath et al. [144] found vitamin E to be normal in 40 transplant patients, 20 of whom were receiving cyclosporine and 20 of whom were receiving azathioprine and glucocorticoids. Malyszko et al. [86] did not found vitamin K deficiency in renal transplant patients. Bohm et al. [57] reported normal plasma vitamin C levels in renal transplant recipients. The folic acid status in renal transplant patient is normal or decreased. The MTHFR genotypes, labeled 677 and 1298, have been shown to significantly influence plasma folic acid levels in a group of 733 renal transplant patients; the 677TT/1298AA group had lower plasma folic acid levels [145].

Acute Kidney Injury Patients

In patients with acute kidney injury (AKI), serum vitamin A levels were found to be normal in one study [71], decreased in another study (with normal serum RBP levels) [146] and increased in a third study of AKI patients receiving total parenteral nutrition (TPN) containing standard retinol supplementation [147]. With continuous veno-venous hemofiltration or hemodiafiltration,

plasma PLP decreased, and the calculated PLP loss was 80 nmol/day [148]; the PLP clearance was about 49% of the urea clearance and the amount of folic acid removed has been estimated to be 650 nmoles/day, with a clearance as high as 76% of urea clearance. Plasma vitamin E levels are decreased in patients with AKI, regardless of whether they are or not treated with continuous hemofiltration [149].

VITAMINS AS THERAPY FOR PEOPLE WITH KIDNEY DISEASE

Effect of Water-Soluble Vitamin Supplementation on Patient Outcomes

According to the DOPPS report, MHD patients receiving a supplementation of vitamins B_6, B_{12} and C, and folates had better nutritional status (indicated by serum albumin levels and nPNA) and a 16% decrease in mortality [150]. The reduced mortality persisted after adjustment for nutritional markers. It was not possible to distinguish the specific effects of each vitamin. Vitamin prescription varied substantially across continents, but the impact on mortality did not vary when stratified by geographic regions. The interpretation to explain this effect includes the possible plasma homocysteine (Hcy) lowering effect of these vitamins, increased appetite and protein intake with vitamin supplementation, better patient-care in chronic dialysis programs where supplements are prescribed and better socio-economical status associated with this prescription. However, the prospective trials of Hcy-lowering with vitamin supplements do not support the first hypothesis (see below).

Homocysteine Lowering Therapy

Increased plasma homocysteine (Hcy) is a recognized cardiovascular risk factor, and elevation of plasma Hcy in advanced CKD and chronic dialysis patients has been recognized for at least two decades. The possibility that reducing plasma homocysteine might improve outcomes in CKD, maintenance dialysis and renal transplant patients has been tantalizing. Homocysteine is an intermediate in the formation of cystathionine from methionine (Figure 24.2). Three vitamins, B_6, B_{12} and folates are directly involved in its synthesis and metabolism. The formation of cysteine from methionine requires vitamin B_6. PLP is a coenzyme for cystathionine synthase, which transforms methionine to cystathionine, and for cystathionase, which cleaves cystathionine to form cysteine. As suggested in Figure 24.2, PLP or folate deficiency, which occurs not infrequently in CKD and dialysis patients, could participate in the pathogenesis of increased plasma Hcy in CKD and dialysis patients. However, renal patients who have normal levels of folate, cobalamin and PLP still manifest increased plasma Hcy [151]. In advanced CKD patients and maintenance dialysis patients, plasma homocysteine levels tend to be about one and one-half to two times higher than in healthy controls and correlate inversely with the GFR [152,153]. Plasma Hcy is routinely increased (>15 µmoles/L) in dialysis patients. However, plasma Hcy levels are influenced by the nutritional status and may be low in patients with protein-energy wasting [154]. Plasma Hcy is also increased in nondialyzed children with CKD and in children undergoing MHD treatment. Arnadottir et al. [155] found that 6 months after renal transplantation, plasma Hcy had decreased by an average of 14%, but that plasma Hcy was still significantly higher in the renal transplant recipients as compared to a control group matched for renal function.

Plasma homocysteine levels are affected by the dialysis technique. Despite a greater intradialytic decrease in plasma Hcy with high vs. low flux membranes (42 vs. 32%), no difference was found in predialysis plasma Hcy levels with high- as compared to low-flux membranes during a 3-month period [156]. Recently Pedrini et al. [157] found in a randomized cross-over trial that on-line hemodiafiltration sustainly decreases predialysis Hcy level when compared to low-flux conventional HD. Vychtyl et al. [158] studied peritoneal losses of Hcy in 39 CPD patients. Daily peritoneal Hcy removal (38.9 ± 20.8 µmoles) was correlated with plasma Hcy, effluent volume, and the D/P creatinine ratio [158]. Free Hcy represented 47.5% and 75.2% of total Hcy in plasma and dialysate, respectively. It was concluded that CPD, like, MHD, is not sufficiently effective to normalize plasma Hcy levels.

More than 10 years ago, two prospective studies described the association between plasma Hcy and cardiovascular risk in chronic renal failure patients. Moustapha et al. [159] followed 167 ESRD patients for a 17.4-month period and reported an increased cardiovascular morbidity and mortality risk of 1% for each µmole rise in plasma Hcy. In CPD and MHD patients, Bostom et al. [160] found a relative risk for nonfatal and fatal cardiovascular events of 3.0 and 4.4, respectively, when comparing the highest quartile versus the lower three quartiles of plasma Hcy levels also during a follow-up period of 17.0 months. Elevated plasma Hcy is a risk factor for endothelial dysfunction and for cardiovascular disease in CKD patients [161]. However, Kalantar-Zadeh et al. [162] found an increased mortality in the lowest Hcy quartile of 367 MHD patients, even after adjustment for the nutritional and inflammatory state. These authors concluded that Hcy is an independent nutritional marker explaining the reverse association of plasma values with patient outcome. Furthermore, the role of Hcy with regard to patency of the blood access has not been confirmed. In a prospective study of 733 renal transplant recipients, Winkelmeier et al. [163] found that the risks of death and graft loss were associated with plasma Hcy levels >12 µmoles/L with hazard ratios, respectively, at 2.44 and 1.63 after adjustment. The mechanisms of homocysteine toxicity have been thoroughly reviewed [164]. Homocysteine is one of the factors in the transsulfuration-transmethylation pathways and the complex folate cycle. Its accumulation may lead to altered DNA methylation with epigenetic consequences and homocysteine binding to proteins with resulting functional deficiencies.

Many studies have examined the effects of lowering plasma Hcy levels in patients with advanced CKD, in those undergoing dialysis or in renal transplant recipients. The findings can be summarized as follows. The usual effect is a 30—50% decrease in Hcy with folic acid therapy, but with few patients attaining normal plasma Hcy levels. The magnitude of the lowering effect of folic acid is positively related to the pretreatment plasma Hcy values and negatively associated with the RBC folic acid concentration. Most clinical trials using low doses (2.5—5 mg/d) of folic acid treatment to lower plasma Hcy levels in advanced CKD and maintenance dialysis patients show about the same magnitude of reduction as in the trials that used larger folic acid doses. Bostom et al. [165] reported a more effective lowering effect of plasma Hcy with a combination of folic acid, vitamin B_6 and vitamin B_{12} in renal transplant recipients than in MHD patients. Recent prospective, large scale trials addressed the efficacy of Hcy-lowering therapy on clinical outcomes in CKD patients. The HOST trial included 2056 nondialyzed advanced CKD patients and chronic dialysis patients who were randomized in a blinded fashion to receive daily either a combination of the vitamins, folic acid, 40 mg; pyridoxine hydrochloride (vitamin B_6), 100 mg; and cyanocobalamin (vitamin B_{12}) 2 mg or placebo [153]. The average follow-up was 3.2 years. No decrease of overall mortality or CV events was observed in the treated group even though plasma Hcy fell significantly in the treated group. In a substudy of this trial, cognition was analyzed as an outcome and was not improved by the Hcy lowering therapy [166]. Heinz et al. [167] enrolled 650 MHD patients in a randomized control trial comparing a combination of folic acid, vitamins B_6 and B_{12} with placebo. Again no difference in clinical outcomes (overall and CV mortality and CV events) was found. A large prospective trial in renal transplant patients is in process (the FAVORIT trial [168]).

Vitamins and Oxalate Burden in Renal Failure

As shown in Figure 24.4, oxalate is a metabolic end product of ascorbic acid. In normal humans, urinary

FIGURE 24.4   Pathways for oxalate metabolism.

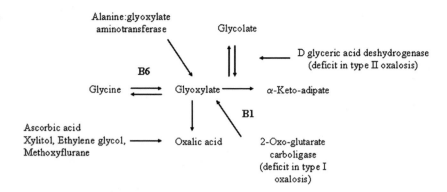

excretion of oxalate increases when these individuals are fed an ascorbic acid load. However, the relationship between ascorbic acid intake and urinary oxalate excretion is not linear, and only a fraction of the ascorbic acid ingested is normally recovered in the urine as oxalate [169]. Plasma oxalate concentrations are virtually always increased in nondialyzed advanced CKD and chronic dialysis patients [170,171]. Plasma oxalate is correlated with serum creatinine [172] and may be increased several times above normal values in renal failure patients, close to the levels found in primary hyperoxaluria. Calcium oxalate deposits are described in several tissues in advanced CKD and appear to be most pronounced in kidneys, heart, blood vessels, thyroid, and skin and to increase with the duration of MHD therapy [173]. Mydlik et al. [123] reported increased plasma oxalic acid in 32 CAPD patients (23.6 ± 7.4 µmoles/L; normal range: 2–5.5 µmoles/L) despite a large peritoneal oxalate clearance. In 15 MHD patients, plasma oxalate was increased (40.3 ± 9.8 µmoles/L) and oxalate clearance was greater with postdilutional hemofiltration (74.2% of urea clearance) then with conventional hemodialysis (58.1% of urea clearance) or postdilutional hemodiafiltration (69%) [174]. In children, there appears to be a large discrepancy between oxalate clearances in those undergoing CAPD (7.14 mL/min, n = 15) and MHD (115.6 mL/min, n = 10). Nonetheless, the weekly elimination of oxalate was similar, and blood oxalic acid levels remained high and not different between the two groups [175]. An oxalemia level >30µmoles/L has been proposed to indicate calcium-oxalate supersaturation in plasma [176].

There is strong evidence that a high vitamin C intake may contribute to hyperoxalemia and to oxalate deposition in soft tissues of CKD patients. The mechanism of oxalate accumulation with low doses of ascorbic acid is related to the decrease or absence of renal function. In such circumstances, excess ascorbic acid and the oxalate subsequently produced cannot be eliminated in the urine, unlike in normal subjects who can tolerate much higher intakes of ascorbic acid without oxalate accumulation. In MHD patients, plasma oxalate levels increased with

oral supplementation of 0.5 to 1 g/day of ascorbic acid, and cessation of ascorbic acid supplements results in a decrease in plasma oxalate [177]. The calcium oxalate saturation threshold was exceeded in 7 of 18 patients (40%) during the course of 6 months of ascorbic acid therapy, 500 mg/wk [178]. Ott et al. [179] observed bone oxalate deposits in a bone biopsy from a patient who had undergone MHD for 23 years and who had ingested 2.6 g/day of ascorbic acid for seven years. A bone biopsy in the same patient obtained before commencing ascorbic acid supplements showed no evidence for bone oxalate deposits. A case of calcium oxalate deposits in kidneys and pancreas was reported in a pediatric patient with the hemolytic uremic syndrome who received 500 mg/day of ascorbic acid by parenteral nutrition [180]. Hyperoxalemia is also associated with ascorbic acid supplementation in CPD patients [181].

Vitamin B₆ is the coenzyme for the transamination of glyoxylate to glycine (Figure 24.4). Since vitamin B₆ deficiency is not uncommon in CKD, this might contribute to increased oxalate plasma levels. Hence both decreased clearance of oxalate because of impaired renal function and impaired vitamin B₆ status may play a role. Recently Mydlik et al. [182] have reported a close relationship between the vitamin B₆ status and serum oxalate levels in MHD patients (Figure 24.5). Several attempts have been made to decrease plasma oxalate levels with pharmacological doses of pyridoxine HCl. Conflicting results were obtained. Tomson et al. [183] did not observe a significant decrease in oxalemia in 21 chronic dialysis patients treated for four months with pyridoxine HCl, 100 mg/day. In contrast, a 46% decrease of plasma oxalate was observed by Balcke et al. [184] after one month of treatment with pyridoxine HCl, 600 mg/day orally or 600 mg three times per week intravenously after hemodialysis treatment. However, the plasma oxalate level remained elevated and in the supersaturation range [171]. In a controlled study, Costello was unable to reduce plasma oxalate levels after six months of treatment with 100 mg/day of pyridoxine HCl or after four weeks of therapy with 750 mg/day of pyridoxine HCl [185]. The reason for these discrepant results is not clear.

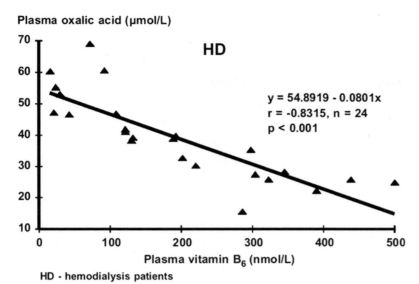

Plasma oxalic acid (µmol/L)

HD

$$y = 54.8919 - 0.0801x$$
$$r = -0.8315, n = 24$$
$$p < 0.001$$

Plasma vitamin B$_6$ (nmol/L)

HD - hemodialysis patients

FIGURE 24.5 Indirect relationship between the plasma vitamin B$_6$ and plasma oxalate concentrations in maintenance hemodialysis (HD) patients ([182] with permission).

Descombes et al. [186] reported a high plasma oxalic acid level in 33 patients receiving high flux dialysis and 50 mg of pyridoxine HCl after each dialysis treatment, indicating that current dialysis techniques and vitamin B$_6$ supplementation are not sufficient to normalize oxalic acid levels. Patients with type I or type II primary hyperoxaluria have been treated with different doses of pyridoxine (25–1000 mg/day), also with variable results [187]. Oxalate clearance differs among different filters and dialysis modalities; the most efficient ones are high-flux membranes such as polysulphone and hemodiafiltration [188]. Renal transplantation remains the most efficient therapy for hyperoxalemia [172].

Vitamins in Anemia Management

Reference is made to Chapter 25 for a comprehensive discussion of this subject. The following is a brief summary of vitamins in anemia management. Since the advent of the erythropoietin (EPO) era, concerns have been raised regarding the status of vitamins directly involved in erythropoiesis, such as vitamin B$_{12}$ and folates because of their increased consumption and the possibility that they might reduce the needed dose of EPO or iron. Mydlik et al. [189] reported a significant decrease of erythrocyte folic acid after one year of EPO therapy in 15 MHD patients. This was not confirmed by Pollock et al. [190] who did not find any difference in folates and vitamin B$_{12}$ concentrations before and after 18 months of EPO treatment in 81 MHD and 31 CPD patients. No information was given concerning folic acid or vitamin B$_{12}$ supplements in these patients.

Both the not uncommon prevalence of EPO resistance, especially of inflammatory origin, and the quest for cost reduction of EPO therapy have triggered a large number of studies to improve the iron utilization. There has been much interest concerning the potential value of ascorbic acid as an adjuvant therapy to EPO to increase hemoglobin and reduce the cost of anemia therapy, particularly in MHD and CPD patients with erythropoietin resistant anemia. Tarng et al. [122] have reported that in MHD patients hyporesponsive to EPO and with normal vitamin C levels who were treated with 300 mg of vitamin C given at the end of dialysis for 8 weeks, there was increased hematocrit and transferrin saturation and decreased EPO needs. However, only half of these patients had a positive response to vitamin C administration. Plasma oxalate levels increased slightly, but not to a statistical significant degree during the vitamin C therapy. In the last decades, numerous studies have indicated that vitamin C administration reduces anemia in renal failure. A recent meta-analysis identified 157 reports, with only six of these reports fulfilling the selection criteria [191]. The meta-analysis concludes that vitamin C (between 200 and 500 mg three times per week) increases the transferin saturation coefficient and decreases EPO needs. However, the long-term safety of such treatments is not addressed in this report, and oxalate supersaturation might have been reached in a significant number of patients with these dosages [178]. In the forthcoming KDIGO guidelines on anemia management, no adjuvants such as folates or vitamin C are recommended with EPO therapy [192].

Vitamins (Except Vitamin D) and Bone Mineral Metabolism

Besides vitamin D and its pivotal role in bone mineral metabolism (BMD), other vitamins may be involved in these complex interactions, mainly vitamins K and A and niacin. Administration of vitamin K_1 reduces urinary calcium excretion in postmenopausal women who have increased calciuria (i.e., urine Ca/creatinine ratio >0.5) [193]. Coumarin-derivatives increase urinary calcium excretion in young adults [194]. The anti-calciuric effects of vitamin K may be mediated through the carboxylation of bone proteins (i.e., osteocalcin and other Gla proteins which bind calcium). The reduced bone mineral content found in patients receiving oral anticoagulants supports the possibility that vitamin K antagonists increase urinary calcium by mobilizing bone calcium. However, a direct effect of vitamin K or its antagonists on the kidney cannot be ruled out.

The use of coumarin-derivatives in dialysis patients is associated with an increased risk of calciphyllaxis [195] and aortic valve calcification [196]. Vascular and valvular calcifications are associated with the high prevalence of cardiovascular morbidity and mortality in CKD and chronic dialysis patients. Matrix Gla-protein (MGP), a vitamin K-dependent factor, interferes with the genesis of vascular calcifications, and MGP knockout mice present with extensive lethal vascular calcifications [21]. With quantitative or functional vitamin-K deficiency, MGP is predominantly present in the uncarboxylated form (ucMGP) and can be found in the media of calcified vessels. Thus, vitamin K deficiency may play a role in the complex pathophysiology of accelerated tissue calcification in this setting. It is not known whether vitamin K therapy may prevent such calcification.

Another vitamin K-dependent protein, osteocalcin plays a role on bone mineralization. In the general population, vitamin K supplementation seems to reduce the incidence of fractures, as summarized by Fusaro et al. [197]. In MHD patients, an inverse relationship has been reported between a history of bone fractures and the plasma phylloquinone levels or the proportion of carboxylated vs. noncarboxylated osteocalcin in plasma [198]. In this latter study, serum PTH levels were found to be high (>300 ng/L) only in patients with low plasma phylloquinone concentrations. These patients also had an abnormally high incidence of the apolipoprotein E3/4 and E4/4 genotype that may indicate impaired tissue uptake of phylloquinone from chylomicrons [199]. MHD patients with adynamic bone disease who received vitamin K supplementation for one year displayed a significant increase in serum PTH, alkaline phosphatase and the cross-linked N-terminal telopeptide of type I collagen in association with a trend toward a decrease in serum osteoprotegerin, a well-recognized factor associated with vascular calcification [200].

The bone reabsorptive effects of excess vitamin A have been known for many years with a report of hypercalcemia with serum high vitamin A levels in CRF patients [201]. This condition should be considered in the differential diagnosis of hypercalcemia in renal failure patients. Elevated serum vitamin A levels and vitamin A toxicity in CKD are discussed above.

Large doses of niacin, and its amide form, niacinamide, have been proposed to treat hyperphosphatemia in CKD because of their capacity to inhibit the Na-Pi cotransporter in the GI tract [202]. The usual side-effects of the molecule, hepatotoxicity and flush, have been reduced by the change in the formulation from immediate to extended-release and are less pronounced with niacinamide than with niacin itself. A decrease in platelets may occur but is observed inconstantly. The potential advantages of niacin as a phosphate absorption inhibitor are the low cost, the absence of calcium in the medication, the potential benefits on the lipid profile, and the medicine can be taken at a time that is independent of the meal [40]. However, at present, these phosphate-lowering effects have been reported in only small cohorts of patients with no studies on long-term clinical outcomes.

Vitamins and Anti-Oxidant Therapy in Renal Disease

Oral Anti-Oxidant Therapy

It is mainly vitamin E and vitamin C that have been studied for their anti-oxidant properties in renal disease patients. There is much evidence that nondialyzed patients with CKD and individuals undergoing MHD or CPD suffer from oxidant stress and that this condition is associated with adverse cardiovascular complications [203]. This important issue is discussed in more detail in Chapters 6 and 9. Numerous studies have examined the effects of oral vitamin E supplementation on oxidant stress, and this has been extensively analyzed by Coombes and Fassett [204]. Most studies using α-tocopherol have shown that it reduces measures of oxidant stress. The most important trial is the SPACE study, a randomized controlled trial including 196 MHD patients that demonstrated the efficiency of oral vitamin E, 800 IU/day, in the secondary prevention of cardiovascular events [205]. Because many studies using statins or cardiovascular drugs in this setting have failed to demonstrate a clinical benefit, this trial remains almost unique in lowering the high burden of cardiovascular disease in CKD patients. Another study using N-acetyl-cysteine also showed reduced adverse cardiovascular events in ESRD patients [206]. Oxidant stress in CKD and dialysis patients should be a target for future studies. Other trials in small numbers of MHD and/or CAPD patients have shown that α-tocopherol therapy has a number of potentially beneficial effects including vitamin E enrichment content of LDL [207], increased erythrocyte life span or decreased EPO dose [208,209] and reduced LDL susceptibility to oxidation [210]. Studies with supplemental vitamin C have shown conflicting results with regard to the patients' oxidant status, and none of them have addressed the patients' clinical outcome.

Vitamin E-Coated Hemodialysis Membranes

These membranes have been investigated as a way to reduce oxidative stress during HD treatment. Most clinical trials with these membranes have been carried out for at least three months and have reported an increase in plasma or RBC vitamin E levels [211] and a decrease in plasma malondialdehyde (MDA) [212]. Other observed potentially beneficial effects of vitamin E coated membranes include decreased neutrophil activation, reduced decreased pro-oxidant activity of leukocytes, reduced intradialytic IL-6 production, lower serum oxidized-LDL and ADMA (asymmetrical dimethyl arginine) and reduced oxidative damage to DNA. A recent study has provided evidence that in a 6-month controlled trial the use of vitamin E-coated dialyzer membranes decreased serum CRP and oxidized-LDL levels [213]. There is currently no trial that has examined morbidity and mortality with the use of these membranes.

Oxidant Stress in Renal Transplantation

Oxidative damage is particularly likely to occur at several steps during the course of kidney transplantation. Reperfusion after cold ischemia may lead to marked oxidative bursts in the kidney. An antioxidant mixture, including 10 mg of α-tocopherol, given 30 minutes before reperfusion, was able to reduce the degree of lipid peroxidation as assessed by the plasma MDA levels [214]. Cristol et al. [215] found evidence for increased oxidative stress in 77 longstanding kidney transplant recipients, including individuals with and without chronic rejection. Evidence indicated that oxidative stress was greater in the patients with chronic rejection. However, McGrath et al. [144] did not observe differences in plasma TBARS (thiobarbituric acid reactive substances) and plasma vitamin E concentrations in patients receiving cyclosporine or azathioprine when compared to controls. Patients treated with tacrolimus were found to have increased susceptibility to oxidation when compared to cyclosporine-treated patients [216]. However, there is not enough evidence yet to recommend the routine administration of antioxidant vitamins in renal transplant recipients [217].

Potential Miscellaneous Clinical Benefits of Vitamin Therapy in CRF Patients

In a randomized, blinded, prospective clinical trial in 26 MHD patients with symptoms of peripheral neuropathy, there was dramatic improvement of symptoms in 14 patients who received pyridoxine HCl, 60 mg/day, for four weeks, but not in 12 patients who received vitamin B_{12}, 500 μg/day orally, even though the initial serum PLP was only slightly and not significantly lower than in controls [218]. However, no objective measurement of motor nerve conduction velocity was reported. Also vitamin E alone or combined with vitamin C is reported to reduce the incidence of cramps in MHD patients [219].

As indicated above, nicotinamide in large doses may inhibit the Na/Pi type IIb cotransporter (Na Pi-2b) and the type IIa cotransporter (NaPi-2a) in the intestinal brush border and in the proximal renal tubular epithelial cells of the kidneys, respectively [40]. Twice-daily doses of 500 to 1500 mg of nicotinamide can reduce serum phosphorus concentrations in maintenance hemodialysis patients by blocking intestinal absorption of phosphorus. Large, randomized, prospective clinical trials are needed to demonstrate the long-term efficacy and safety of this treatment for preventing and treating excess body burden of phosphorus in CKD and chronic dialysis patients.

RECOMMENDATIONS FOR VITAMIN SUPPLEMENTATION AND VITAMIN THERAPY IN RENAL DISEASES

Vitamin supplementation to avoid deficiency and vitamin therapy to improve complications of renal failure are important issues for renal patients, as morbidity and mortality remain high in this population. The DOPPS report [150] has stimulated new interest in water-soluble vitamin supplementation in CKD patients. Also new data or the absence of confirmation of previous ones (such as the SPACE study) has raised questions concerning the usual recommendations for fat soluble vitamins. Last but not least, vitamin supplementation, besides protein and energy intake, must not be ignored in the ongoing debate regarding the deleterious effects and prevention and treatment of malnutrition on clinical outcome in CKD and ESRD patients.

Vitamin Supplementation Across the World

The DOPPS report [150] has highlighted the wide disparity of vitamin supplementation in hemodialysis patients across the continents from 3.7% in the UK to 71.9% of MHD and CPD patients in the United States. Both the availability of specifically designed supplements for renal patients and the absence of strong clinical evidence for a positive effect of vitamin supplementation on patient outcome may explain such differences.

Existing Recommendations for Vitamin Supplementation or Therapy in Renal Patients

During the last decade, several guidelines on nutrition in renal patients have been published (see Table 24.4). A few of them have issued statements on vitamin supplementation. The DOQI guidelines on nutrition decided not to address vitamins because of lack of evidence regarding the effect of vitamin supplements on quality of life, morbidity or mortality [220]. The CARI guidelines for nondialysis CKD patients [221] propose only suggestions for vitamin supplementation because of the absence of Level I or II evidence. These guidelines suggest that CKD patients following a protein-restricted diet should receive supplementation with thiamine (>1 mg/day), B_2 (1–2 mg/day) and B_6 (1.5–2.0 mg/day of pyridoxine hydrochloride). Recently Steiber & Kopple have reviewed the vitamin status in CKD 3–5 nondialysis patients and underlined the risk of deficiency in these patients [222]. The European Best Practice Guidelines [219] recommend for MHD patients 400–800 IU/day of vitamin E based on the SPACE study for prevention of cardiovascular events and the following daily amounts for vitamin B_1 (1.1–1.2 mg), vitamin B_2 (1.1–1.3 mg), vitamin B_6 (10 mg of pyridoxine HCl), vitamin C (75–90 mg), folic acid (1 mg), vitamin B_{12} (2.4 µg), niacin (14–16 mg), biotin (30 µg) and pantothenic acid (5 mg). They do not recommend vitamin A supplementation, but transient vitamin K supplementation (10 mg/day) is suggested for patients undergoing prolonged antibiotic therapy or presenting with increased blood coagulation. Druml has summarized the needs for micronutrients in AKI receiving total parenteral nutrition [223] (see Chapter 36). The ESPEN guidelines for parenteral nutrition in adults with renal failure have emphasized the daily needs of vitamin C (up to 100 mg/day) and folates (up to 600 nmoles/day) because of losses with continuous dialysis techniques [224].

Vitamin Supplementation Reappraisal

To analyze and comment on the foregoing published recommendations, it is necessary to summarize our knowledge regarding the nutritional status of each vitamin in CKD3-5 and ESRD patients and the evidence supporting supplementation. The following recommendations for nondialyzed CKD3-5 patients also apply to nondialyzed CKD1-5 patients with the nephrotic syndrome unless stated otherwise. Not withstanding the foregoing recommendations, in locations where multivitamin preparations specifically designed for CKD and chronic dialysis patients are not available, it may be prudent to recommend that such individuals take a daily supplement of a multivitamin that provides the RDA or AI of the water soluble vitamins.

Vitamin A

Plasma vitamin A levels in CKD and maintenance dialysis patients are elevated, and vitamin A deficiency has rarely been observed, and even small supplements of vitamin A (i.e., 2500–15,000 IU, i.e. 750–4500 µg of retinol equivalents (RE)) may cause vitamin A toxicity. There is a consensus that supplemental doses of vitamin A larger then the Recommended Daily Allowance for vitamin A in normal healthy adults (i.e., 700–900 µg of RE, [53]) should not be given. However, the new findings demonstrating that low plasma retinol levels are associated with increased mortality of chronic dialysis patients [81,82] raises questions concerning this consensus. Prudence dictates that vitamin A supplements larger than the RDA should not be taken by advanced CKD or maintenance dialysis patients until more long term prospective trials demonstrate clinical benefits to greater supplements.

Since patients with the nephrotic syndrome may excrete vitamins that bind to protein, a daily intake of the RDA for vitamin A in these individuals is recommended. For renal transplant recipients, vitamin A supplements do not appear to be necessary unless patients received their renal transplant more than one or two years previously, their vitamin A intake is low and their renal function is not markedly reduced. Vitamin A supplements are probably not necessary for AKI patients unless they are given total parenteral nutrition without vitamin supplements for at least two or three weeks. Given the risks of vitamin A toxicity in advanced CKD patients, and reports of vitamin A toxicity in TPN patients with AKI receiving as little as 1500 µg of RE per day [147], it is recommended that no more then the RDA for vitamin A (800–1000 µg RE for nonpregnant, nonlactating adults) should be given for AKI patients receiving TPN as the sole nutritional source.

Vitamin E

The SPACE study [205] and the well-recognized pro-oxidant state of uremia would support the recommendation of α-tocopherol supplementation in MHD patients to prevent cardiovascular events at the dose of the SPACE study, i.e. 800 IU. However the HOPE study did not show clinical benefit of vitamin E supplements in individuals with or without chronic renal insufficiency [225,226]. Moreover, subsequent analysis of the HOPE trial and its extension (HOPE-TOO) have shown an increased risk of heart failure in patients under vitamin E supplementation [227]. In individuals without renal disease, platelet dysfunction and interference with the vitamin K-dependent

TABLE 24.4 Recommendations/Suggestions for Daily Vitamin Supplementation in Renal Patients

Origin	RDA in Healthy Subjects / Dietary reference intake [53,234,236]	Nephrotic Syndrome CKD3-5 Patients / Authors' suggestions	Non-Dialysis CKD3-5 Patients / CARI [221]	Non-Dialysis CKD3-5 Patients / Steiber & Kopple[b] [222]	MHD Patients / EBPG [219]	MHD Patients / Authors' suggestions	CPD Patients / Authors' suggestions	Acute Renal Failure Patients with TPN[a,b] / Chapter 36 [223]
Vitamin A	700–900 RE[c]	Up to RDA[d]		Up to the RDA[d]	None	None[e]	None	RDA
Vitamin E	22.5 IU	Up to RDA[d]		Up to the RDA[d]	400–800 IU	up to the RDA[d,f]	up to the RDA[d,f]	RDA
Vitamin K	80–120 µg	None		Supplements if antibiotherapy	None[g]	None[g]	None[g]	RDA
Vitamin B$_1$	1.1–1.2 mg	Unknown[h]	>1 mg	1.1–1.2 mg	1.1–1.2 mg	1.1–1.2 mg	1.1–1.2 mg	RDA×2
Riboflavin	1.1–1.3 mg	Unknown[h]	1–2 mg	??[i]	1.1–1.3 mg	1.1–1.3 mg	1.1–1.3 mg	RDA×2
Vitamin B$_6$[j]	1.3–1.7 mg	5 mg	1.5–2 mg	5 mg	10 mg	10 mg	10 mg	RDA×2
Vitamin C	75–90 mg	75–90 mg		30–60 mg	75–90 mg	75–90 mg	75–90 mg	RDA×2
Folic acid	400 µg	Unknown[h]		Up to the RDA[d]	1 mg	1 mg	1 mg	RDA×2
Vitamin B$_{12}$	2.4 µg	RDA		RDA	2.4 µg	2.4µg	2.4 µg	RDA×2
Niacin	14–16 mg	Unknown[h]		up to the RDA[d]	14–16 mg	14–16 mg	14–16 mg	RDA×2
Biotin	30 µg	Unknown[h]		Up to AI[k,l]	30 µg	30 µg	30 µg	RDA×2
Pantothenic acid	5 mg	Unknown[h]		Up to AI[k]	5 mg	5 mg	5 mg	RDA×2

[a]TPN: Total Parenteral Nutrition.
[b]Endorsed by the authors.
[c]Retinol equivalent.
[d]For patients ingesting less than the DRI.
[e]Recent data on vitamin A and survival question this usual recommendation.
[f]Caution is required after subsequent analysis and extension of the HOPE study.
[g]10 mg/d if prolonged antibiotic therapy or low food intake.
[h]Insufficient data.
[i]To supplement if restricted protein diet. Amount nonspecified.
[j]Refers to pyridoxine HCl.
[k]Refers to Adequate Intake reflecting the average intake in the normal population. There not enough data to establish RDA. Risk of deficiency in low protein diet.
[l]Absent from Steiber & Kopple review [222]. Reported by the authors of the current review.

coagulation factors have been reported with pharmacological doses of vitamin E [16]. As the SPACE trial has not been confirmed and the findings of the HOPE study follow-up and extension, it appears necessary to wait for more data before recommending a supplemental daily vitamin E intake in CKD and dialysis patients.

Vitamin K

Because of the high risk of thrombosis associated with the nephrotic condition and the frequent need of coumarin-derivatives for its prevention, vitamin K supplementation is not recommended for nephrotic patients. Since CKD and dialysis patients generally do not have evidence for vitamin K deficiency, as determined by clotting factors or clotting function, vitamin K supplements generally have not been recommended. However, it could be argued that vitamin K status should also be assessed using ucMGP and ucBGP in order to determine whether a CKD or ESRD patient should receive supplemental vitamin K. Traditionally, vitamin K supplements have been proposed for patients who are eating poorly and receiving antibiotics that may suppress intestinal bacterial flora, particularly for extended periods of time, because they are probably at increased risk for developing vitamin K deficiency. Patients receiving TPN for more than one to two weeks should receive vitamin K.

Vitamin B_1

The recommended amounts of thiamin for supplementation of MHD and CPD patients have ranged from 1 to 45 mg daily [37,46]. The thiamin intake from food is generally about 0.6 to 1.5 mg/day in patients with CKD, MHD or CPD. ETKA stimulation index and serum thiamin levels are usually normal in patients with CKD, MHD or CPD. When thiamin deficiency is present, correction is readily obtained by feeding low quantities of thiamin. Thus, we recommend a thiamin supplement of 1.1–1.2 mg/day in nondialyzed CKD3-5, MHD and CPD patients (Table 24.4). Although these patients may receive adequate thiamin from their ingested foods, their food intake is not uncommonly low, and, as indicated above, thiamin deficiency has been reported in these patients.

Riboflavin

Recommendations regarding riboflavin supplementation vary from no supplement to an amount equivalent to the RDA. Low doses of riboflavin (1 mg/day) were enough to normalize α-EGR in CAPD patients [67]. We recommend a daily riboflavin supplement equal to the RDA for CKD 3-5 and chronic dialysis patients.

Vitamin B_6

Most workers in the field agree that there is a need for routine pyridoxine supplementation in CKD, MHD, CPD patients and nephrotic patients. Recommended supplemental pyridoxine HCl doses vary from 1.2 mg/day [46] to 50 mg 3 times/week [186]. These recommended doses were not based on dose response studies, and therefore the daily vitamin need might actually be lower than was recommended. Kopple et al. [228], in a dose response study, described normalization of the EGPT index in all nondialyzed CKD patients given a supplement of 5 mg/day of pyridoxine HCl (4.1 mg/day of the pyridoxine base); in patients given a lower amount of pyridoxine HCl, the EGPT index became normal more slowly or did not normalize at all. In MHD patients, various doses of pyridoxine HCl have normalized one or more parameters of vitamin B_6 status. However, the lowest pyridoxine HCl supplement that has consistently normalized a parameter of vitamin B_6 deficiency (i.e., the EGPT index) is 10 mg per day [229]. In CAPD patients, the lowest pyridoxine HCl dose that normalized vitamin B_6 nutriture (i.e., serum PLP levels) was also 10 mg per day [115]. In eight children undergoing CPD, 10 mg daily of pyridoxine HCl increased serum PLP to twice the normal control levels [230]; lower doses of pyridoxine HCl would probably be adequate for this pediatric population. It is important to remember that the pyridoxine HCl dose that engenders a normal serum PLP level may not necessarily indicate the desirable daily dose. There may be inhibitors, altered binding or cellular transport, or discrepant intracellular concentrations, etc. for vitamin B_6 in renal failure. In the absence of evidence to the contrary, it seems sensible to accept normal plasma levels as an appropriate or criterion for determining the desirable daily vitamin B_6 dose. In MHD patients, Mydlik et al. [189] recommended 20 mg/day of pyridoxine HCl to correct or prevent a decrease in RBC vitamin B_6 levels that may occur after several months of EPO treatment. Again, this was not a dose response study. In renal transplant recipients, no dosage studies have been conducted. Based on these foregoing data, we recommended a daily of 5 mg of pyridoxine HCl for CKD3-5 patients and 10 mg for MHD and CPD patients (Table 24.4).

Pyridoxine has been given as pyridoxilate, which is a vasodilator that has been used to treat coronary artery and peripheral circulatory insufficiency. This medicine can cause oxalate nephropathy and end stage renal disease [231]. Also very high doses of pyridoxine HCl (i.e., 200 to 600 mg/day), occasionally have been associated with peripheral neuropathy in patients without renal disease [232]. CKD patients may have impaired ability to excrete metabolites of vitamin B_6. Thus, it is possible that these metabolites might accumulate and interfere with the normal, active metabolites of B_6. Indeed, 4-pyridoxic acid, the main metabolite of vitamin B_6, is excreted primarily in the urine and might be expected to accumulate in patients with renal failure, particularly in those taking vitamin B_6 supplements. Therefore, until more information is available, caution should be exercised when prescribing very large doses of pyridoxine HCl to nondialyzed CKD and maintenance dialysis patients (i.e., 100 mg/day or greater) for extended periods of time.

Vitamin C

Many studies suggest that a substantial subset of MHD and CPD patients are at risk for vitamin C deficiency if they do not receive supplements, and several authors have recommended various amounts of daily ascorbic acid. The combination of insufficient dietary intake of vitamin C and dialysate losses appears to be primarily responsible for the risk of deficiency. However, there is no clear evidence that the dietary vitamin requirement is increased in maintenance dialysis patients, at least with regard to the amount necessary to maintain normal plasma ascorbic acid levels. Indeed the lack of urinary vitamin C excretion will at least to some extent offset the dialysate losses. On the other hand, larger doses of vitamin C have been associated with increased oxalate concentrations in plasma and possibly soft tissues. It is possible that the ascorbic acid clearance with high efficiency and/or high flux hemodialyzers may increase the dietary requirement for vitamin C. However, considering the small size of ascorbic acid (molecular weight, 176), it is not likely that highly permeable dialyzers will markedly increase the dialysis losses of vitamin C. Thus, at the present time, it is recommended that nondialyzed CKD3-5, MHD and CPD patients be prescribed the nonpregnant, nonlactating adult RDA for ascorbic acid, 75−90 mg/day (Table 24.4).

Folic Acid

There is no consensus regarding the need for folate supplementation in patients with CKD patients not receiving dialysis as well as those undergoing MHD or CPD. Folic acid supplements appear to be safe for such patients, even at the range of doses prescribed to reduce plasma Hcy levels. Exceptions are the possibility that folate treatment could mask the hematological disturbances associated with vitamin B_{12} deficiency or that metabolites of folate might be toxic, possibly by inhibiting cellular transport of folate. Possible mild side effects of folate, such as nausea, headache, or vivid dreams, have been reported, usually with a dose of 5 mg/day or greater [233]. Although many of the more recent studies indicate that plasma

and red cell folate levels are usually normal in CKD and maintenance dialysis patients, some patients still have low folate concentrations. A low protein diet usually provides a folic acid daily intake below the RDA. High efficiency/high flux dialysis increases the risk of folate deficiency. Also, as indicated above, there may be endogenous as well as exogenous (i.e., from medicines) inhibitors of folic acid in renal failure, and this inhibition may not be reflected in the plasma or red cell folate levels. Hence a daily supplement of 1 mg of folic acid is recommended for CKD3-5, MHD and CPD patients (Table 24.4).

Vitamin B₁₂

Vitamin B_{12} deficiency is unusual in CKD and maintenance dialysis patients, and most authors do not think that vitamin B_{12} supplementation is necessary. On the other hand a daily supplement of about 3 μg of vitamin B_{12}, as part of a multivitamin preparation, is very safe and inexpensive and might occasionally help to prevent vitamin B_{12} deficiency.

Niacin

A low protein diet may provide only small amounts of niacin, and some studies have demonstrated niacin deficiency in dialysis patients. We therefore recommend the RDA of niacin as a supplement for CKD3-5 and chronic dialysis patients. The use of niacin as phosphate lowering therapy or as a cholesterol-lowering therapy in CKD and chronic dialysis patients requires further study.

Biotin

There is no RDA for biotin intake in healthy subjects, but there is an estimation of the biotin need referred to as the "Adequate Intake" [234]. In the absence of data to estimate the RDA, the Adequate Intake (AI) is provided. It reflects the average intake in the normal population. The need for supplemental biotin in renal failure patients is controversial. Biotin deficiency is not reported in CKD and chronic dialysis patients. However, a low protein diet provides a biotin daily intake below the AI. Again, because CKD3-5, MHD and CPD patients not uncommonly have low food intakes, it is recommended that they receive a daily biotin supplement equal to the AI for healthy adults (Table 24.4).

Pantothenic Acid

There are few data on which to base recommendations concerning the needs, if any, for supplemental pantothenic acid. Low protein diets have reduced pantothenic acid content. The reported hemodialyzer clearances of pantothenic acid in older reports are not negligible, and the clearances with high flux and/or high efficient dialysis are unknown. Low concentrations of pantothenic acid have been found in one study in unsupplemented dialysis patients [136]. As with biotin, there is no RDA for pantothenic acid in normal individuals, but only an estimation of needs; the "Adequate Intake" estimation. It is recommended that CKD3-5, MHD and CPD patients receive daily the AI for pantothenic acid.

Vitamin Supplementation in Acute Renal Failure with TPN

The micronutrient needs of acute kidney injury patients have been reviewed by Druml (see Chapter 36) [223]. Plasma or blood vitamin levels are usually found to be low in AKI, and the needs are estimated to be increased because of AKI itself and/or the marked inflammation and increased oxidant stress as well as the vitamin losses that may occur with continuous renal replacement therapy. The RDA for the fat soluble vitamins should be given daily [223]. Up to twice the RDA or the AI for the water soluble vitamins should be given daily for AKI patients (see Table 24.4).

CONCLUSIONS

It should be clear from the foregoing discussion that the nutritional requirements for many vitamins are not well defined for patients with renal disease or renal failure. Indeed, we still do not know the optimal ways to assess the nutritional status for many vitamins in CKD, ESRD and AKI patients. The blood or plasma concentrations of vitamins may be poor indicators of their functional activities. The example of vitamin K in patients with CKD 3—5 highlights the gap that remains the currently used and rather crude methods for assessing the vitamin status and our need for more precise methods. [89]. The effects of renal failure or uremic toxins on the metabolism and actions of vitamins are largely unknown. Moreover, the cohort study from DOPPS and the survival advantage associated with water-soluble vitamin prescription must be confirmed in prospective randomized trials. However, according to the ClinicalTrials.gov website, no such trials are under way. Furthermore, in the last decade, the hope that vitamin therapy targeting hyperhomocysteinemia in advanced renal failure may improve patient outcome has vanished. And the effects of niacin on intestinal phosphorus uptake, phosphorus balance and the lipid profile must be more extensively investigated. New data on vitamin needs and tolerance in CKD patients, such as with vitamins A and K, strongly challenge our traditional concepts. Many unanswered questions remain; for example, the magnitude of the hazard of increased serum oxalate concentrations in CKD and

ESRD patients and what effective methods can eradicate these increased levels. It therefore can be concluded that the field of vitamin metabolism and nutriture in renal diseases and renal failure is wide open for more basic and clinical research.

References

[1] (a) Ross AC. Vitamin A. In: Modern Nutrition in Health and Disease. 11th edition. Ross AC, Cabellero B, Cousins RJ, Tucker KL, Ziegler TR, eds. Lippincott Williams & Wilkins, Baltimore, MD, 2013; pp. 260—77. (b) Wang X-D. Carotenoids. In: Modern Nutrition in Health and Disease. 11th edition. Ross AC, Cabellero B, Cousins RJ, Tucker KL, Ziegler TR, eds. Lippincott Williams & Wilkins, Baltimore, MD, 2013; pp. 427—39

[2] Norum KR, Blomhoff R. McCollum Award Lecture, 1992: vitamin A absorption, transport, cellular uptake, and storage. Am J Clin Nutr 1992;56:735—44.

[3] Russell RM. The vitamin A spectrum: from deficiency to toxicity. Am J Clin Nutr 2000;71:878—84.

[4] Blomhoff R, Wake K. Perisinusoidal stellate cells of the liver: important roles in retinol metabolism and fibrosis. Faseb J 1991;5:271—7.

[5] Burrow CR. Retinoids and renal development. Exp Nephrol 2000;8:219—25.

[6] Randolph TR. Acute promyelocytic leukemia (AML-M3)—Part 1: Pathophysiology, clinical diagnosis, and differentiation therapy. Clin Lab Sci 2000;13:98—105.

[7] Bjelakovic G, Nikolova D, Gluud LL, Simonetti RG, Gluud C. Antioxidant supplements for prevention of mortality in healthy participants and patients with various diseases. Cochrane database of systematic reviews (Online): CD007176, 2008.

[8] Meydani M. Vitamin E. Lancet 1995;345:170—5.

[9] Pastor MC, Sierra C, Bonal J, Teixido J. Serum and erythrocyte tocopherol in uremic patients: effect of hemodialysis versus peritoneal dialysis. American journal of nephrology 1993;13:238—43.

[10] Farrell P, Roberts R. Vitamin E. In: Shills M, Olson J, Shike M, editors. Modern Nutrition in Health and Disease. Philadelphia: Lea & Febiger; 1993. p. 326—41.

[11] Rimm EB, Stampfer MJ, Ascherio A, Giovannucci E, Colditz GA, Willett WC. Vitamin E consumption and the risk of coronary heart disease in men. The New England journal of medicine 1993;328:1450—6.

[12] Stampfer MJ, Hennekens CH, Manson JE, Colditz GA, Rosner B, Willett WC. Vitamin E consumption and the risk of coronary disease in women. The New England journal of medicine 1993;328:1444—9.

[13] Faruqi R, de la Motte C, DiCorleto PE. Alpha-tocopherol inhibits agonist-induced monocytic cell adhesion to cultured human endothelial cells. J Clin Invest 1994;94:592—600.

[14] Ansell JE, Kumar R, Deykin D. The spectrum of vitamin K deficiency. Jama 1977;238:40—2.

[15] Shearer MJ. Vitamin K. Lancet 1995;345:229—34.

[16] Olson JA. Vitamin K. In: Shills M, Olson JA, Shike M, Ross AC, editors. Modern Nutrition in Health and Disease (ed 9th). Baltimore: Williams & Wilkins; 1998. p. 363—80.

[17] Suttie JW, Mummah-Schendel LL, Shah DV, Lyle BJ, Greger JL. Vitamin K deficiency from dietary vitamin K restriction in humans. Am J Clin Nutr 1988;47:475—80.

[18] Sadowski JA, Hood SJ, Dallal GE, Garry PJ. Phylloquinone in plasma from elderly and young adults: factors influencing its concentration. Am J Clin Nutr 1989;50:100—8.

[19] Friedman PA, Mitch WE, Silva P. Localization of renal vitamin K-dependent gamma-glutamyl carboxylase to tubule cells. J Biol Chem 1982;257:11037−40.

[20] Scandling J, Walker BK. Extensive tissue necrosis associated with warfarin sodium therapy. South Med J 1980;73:1470−2.

[21] Shanahan CM, Proudfoot D, Tyson KL, Cary NR, Edmonds M, Weissberg PL. Expression of mineralisation-regulating proteins in association with human vascular calcification. Z Kardiol 2000;89:63−8.

[22] Hodges SJ, Akesson K, Vergnaud P, Obrant K, Delmas PD. Circulating levels of vitamins K_1 and K_2 decreased in elderly women with hip fracture. J Bone Miner Res 1993;8:1241−5.

[23] Shea MK, Booth SL. Update on the role of vitamin K in skeletal health. Nutr Rev 2008;66:549−57.

[24] Tanphaichitr V. Thiamin. In: Shills M, Olson JA, Shike M, Ross AC, editors. Modern Nutrition in Health and Disease. Baltimore: Williams & Wilkins; 1998.

[25] Vuilleumier JP, Keller HE, Rettenmaier R, Hunziker F. Clinical chemical methods for the routine assessment of the vitamin status in human populations. Part II: The water-soluble vitamins B_1, B_2 and B_6. International journal for vitamin and nutrition research Internationale Zeitschrift fur Vitamin- und Ernahrungsforschung 1983;53:359−70.

[26] Lynch PL, Young IS. Determination of thiamine by high-performance liquid chromatography. J Chromatogr A 2000;881:267−84.

[27] Luft FC. Lactic acidosis update for critical care clinicians. J Am Soc Nephrol 12 Suppl 2001;17:S15−9.

[28] Sterzel RB, Semar M, Lonergan ET, Lange K. Effect of hemodialysis on the inhibition of nervous tissue transketolase and on uremic neuropathy. Trans Am Soc Artif Intern Organs 1971;17:77−9.

[29] McCormick D. Riboflavin. In: Shills M, Olson JA, Shike M, Ross AC, editors. Modern Nutrition in Health and Disease. Baltimore: Williams & Wilkins; 1998. p. 391−9.

[30] Mohammed HY, Veening H, Dayton DA. Liquid chromatographic determination and time − concentration studies of riboflavin in hemodialysate from uremic patients. J Chromatogr 1981;226:471−6.

[31] Leklem J. Vitamin B_6. In: Shills M, Olson JA, Shike M, Ross AC, editors. Modern Nutrition in Health and Disease. Baltimore: Williams & Wilkins; 1998.

[32] Bates CJ, Pentieva KD, Prentice A. An appraisal of vitamin B_6 status indices and associated confounders, in young people aged 4−18 years and in people aged 65 years and over, in two national British surveys. Public Health Nutr 1999;2:529−35.

[33] Jacob R. Vitamin C. In: Shills M, Olson JA, Shike M, Ross AC, editors. Modern Nutrition in Health and Disease. Baltimore: Williams & Wilkins; 1998.

[34] Herbert V. Folic acid. In: Shills M, Olson JA, Shike M, Ross AC, editors. Modern Nutrition in Health and Disease (ed 9th). Baltimore: Williams & Wilkins; 1998. p. 433−46.

[35] Devlin AM, Ling EH, Peerson JM, et al. Glutamate carboxypeptidase II: a polymorphism associated with lower levels of serum folate and hyperhomocysteinemia. Hum Mol Genet 2000;9:2837−44.

[36] Weir D, Scott J. Vitamin B_{12} "Cobalamin". In: Shills M, Olson JA, Shike M, Ross AC, editors. Modern Nutrition in Health and Disease. Baltimore: Williams & Wilkins; 1998. p. 447−58.

[37] Descombes E, Hanck AB, Fellay G. Water soluble vitamins in chronic hemodialysis patients and need for supplementation. Kidney Internat 1993;43:1319−28.

[38] Cervantes-Laurean D, McElvaney G, Moss J. Niacin. In: Shills M, Olson JA, Shike M, Ross AC, editors. Modern Nutrition in Health and Disease. Baltimore: Williams & Wilkins; 1998. p. 401−11.

[39] Kwan BC, Kronenberg F, Beddhu S, Cheung AK. Lipoprotein metabolism and lipid management in chronic kidney disease. J Am Soc Nephrol 2007;18:1246−61.

[40] Berns JS. Niacin and related compounds for treating hyperphosphatemia in dialysis patients. Seminars in Dialysis 2008;21:203−5.

[41] Tanaka K. New light on biotin deficiency. New Engl J Med 1981;304:839−40.

[42] Mock D. Biotin. In: Shills M, Olson JA, Shike M, Ross AC, editors. Modern Nutrition in Health and Disease. Baltimore: Williams & Wilkins; 1998. p. 459−66.

[43] Plesofsky-Vig N. Pantothenic acid. In: Shills M, Olson JA, Shike M, Ross AC, editors. Modern Nutrition in Health and Disease. Baltimore: Williams & Wilkins; 1998. p. 423−32.

[44] Fry PC, Fox HM, Tao HG. Metabolic response to a pantothenic acid deficient diet in humans. J Nutr Sci Vitaminol 1976;22:339−46.

[45] Stein G, Sperschneider H, Koppe S. Vitamin levels in chronic renal failure and need for supplementation. Blood Purification 1985;3:52−62.

[46] Allman MA, Truswell AS, Tiller DJ, et al. Vitamin supplementation of patients receiving haemodialysis. Med J Aust 1989;150:130−3.

[47] Blumberg A, Hanck A, Sander G. Vitamin nutrition in patients on continuous ambulatory peritoneal dialysis (CAPD). Clin Nephrol 1983;20:244−50.

[48] Wang AY, Sea MM, Ip R, et al. Independent effects of residual renal function and dialysis adequacy on dietary micronutrient intakes in patients receiving continuous ambulatory peritoneal dialysis. Am J Clin Nutr 2002;76:569−76.

[49] Martin-Del-Campo F, Batis-Ruvalcaba C, Gonzalez-Espinoza L, et al. Dietary Micronutrient Intake in Peritoneal Dialysis Patients: Relationship with Nutrition and Inflammation Status. Perit Dial Int 2012;32:183−91.

[50] Ribeiro MM, Araujo ML, Netto MP, Cunha LM. Effects of customary dinner on dietetical profile of patients undergoing hemodialysis. J Bras Nefrol 2011;33:69−77.

[51] Takagi K, Masuda K, Yamazaki M, et al. Metal ion and vitamin adsorption profiles of phosphate binder ion-exchange resins. Clin Nephrol 2010;73:30−5.

[52] Sullivan JF, Eisenstein AB. Ascorbic acid depletion in patients undergoing chronic hemodialysis. Am J Clin Nutr 1970;23:1339−46.

[53] Dietary References Intakes for vitamin C, vitamin E, Selenium and carotenoids. Washington DC: National Academy Press; 2000.

[54] Pereira AM, Hamani N, Nogueira PC, Carvalhaes JT. Oral vitamin intake in children receiving long-term dialysis. J Ren Nutr 2000;10:24−9.

[55] Kalantar-Zadeh K, Kopple JD, Deepak S, Block D, Block G. Food intake characteristics of hemodialysis patients as obtained by food frequency questionnaire. J Ren Nutr 2002;12:17−31.

[56] Durose CL, Holdsworth M, Watson V, Przygrodzka F. Knowledge of dietary restrictions and the medical consequences of noncompliance by patients on hemodialysis are not predictive of dietary compliance. J Am Dietetic Ass 2004;104:35−41.

[57] Bohm V, Tiroke K, Schneider S, Sperschneider H, Stein G, Bitsch R. Vitamin C status of patients with chronic renal failure, dialysis patients and patients after renal transplantation. International Journal for Vitamin and Nutrition Research. Internationale Zeitschrift fur Vitamin- und Ernahrungsforschung 1997;67:262−6.

[58] Mydlik M, Derzsiova K, Bratova M, Havris S. Serum vitamin A, retinyl esters and vitamin E in nephrotic syndrome. Int Urol Nephrol 1991;23:399−405.

[59] Mydlik M, Derzsiova K. Erythrocyte vitamin B_1, B_2 and B_6 in nephrotic syndrome. Miner Electrolyte Metab 1992;18:293−4.

[60] Podda GM, Lussana F, Moroni G, et al. Abnormalities of homocysteine and B vitamins in the nephrotic syndrome. Thrombosis research 2007;120:647−52.

[61] Rajbala A, Sane AS, Zope J, Mishra VV, Trivedi HL. Oxidative stress status in children with nephrotic syndrome. Panminerva Med 1997;39:165−8.

[62] Fydryk J, Jacobson E, Kurzawska O, et al. Antioxidant status of children with steroid-sensitive nephrotic syndrome. Pediatric Nephrology (Berlin, Germany) 1998;12:751−4.

[63] Warwick GL, Waller H, Ferns GA. Antioxidant vitamin concentrations and LDL oxidation in nephrotic syndrome. Ann Clin Biochem 2000;37:488−91.

[64] Popper H, Steigman F, Dyniewicz H. Plasma vitamin A level in renal diseases. Am J Clin Pathol 1945;15:272−7.

[65] Yatzidis H, Digenis P, Fountas P. Hypervitaminosis A accompanying advanced chronic renal failure. Br Med J 1975; 3:352−3.

[66] Werb R, Clark W, Lindsay R, Jones E, Linton A. Serum vitamin A levels and associated abnormalities in patients on regular dialysis treatment. Clinical Nephrology 1979;12:63−8.

[67] Mydlik M, Derzsiova K, Valek A, Szabo T, Dandar V, Takac M. Vitamins and continuous ambulatory peritoneal dialysis (CAPD). Int Urol Nephrol 1985;17:281−6.

[68] Ha TK, Sattar N, Talwar D, et al. Abnormal antioxidant vitamin and carotenoid status in chronic renal failure. QJM 1996;89: 765−9.

[69] Roehrs M, Valentini J, Bulcao R, et al. The plasma retinol levels as pro-oxidant/oxidant agents in haemodialysis patients. Nephrol Dial Transplant 2009;24:2212−8.

[70] Fassinger N, Imam A, Klurfeld DM. Serum retinol, retinol-binding protein, and transthyretin in children receiving dialysis. J Ren Nutr 2010;20:17−22.

[71] Smith FR, Goodman DS. Vitamin A transport in human vitamin A toxicity. New England J Med 1976;294:805−8.

[72] Christensen EI, Moskaug JO, Vorum H, et al. Evidence for an essential role of megalin in transepithelial transport of retinol. J Am Soc Nephrol 1999;10:685−95.

[73] de Cavanagh EM, Ferder L, Carrasquedo F, et al. Higher levels of antioxidant defenses in enalapril-treated versus non-enalapril-treated hemodialysis patients. Am J Kidney Dis 1999;34:445−55.

[74] Boeschoten EW, Schrijver J, Krediet RT, Schreurs WH, Arisz L. Deficiencies of vitamins in CAPD patients: the effect of supplementation. Nephrol Dial Transplant 1988;3:187−93.

[75] Farrington K, Miller P, Varghese Z, Baillod RA, Moorhead JF. In: Vitamin A toxicity and hypercalcaemia in chronic renal failure. Br med J (Clin Res Ed) 1981;28:1999−2002.

[76] Katz CM, Tzagournis M. Chronic adult hypervitaminosis A with hypercalcemia. Metabolism 1972;21:1171−6.

[77] Stewart WK, Fleming LW. Plasma retinol and retinol binding protein concentrations in patients on maintenance haemodialysis with and without vitamin A supplements. Nephron 1982; 30:15−21.

[78] Vahlquist A, Berne B, Berne C. Skin content and plasma transport of vitamin A and beta-carotene in chronic renal failure. Eur J Clin Invest 1982;12:63−7.

[79] Delacoux E, Evstigneeff T, Leclercq M, et al. Skin disorders and vitamin A metabolism disturbances in chronic dialysis patients: the role of zinc, retinol-binding protein, retinol and retinoic acid. Clin Chim Acta 1984;137:283−9.

[80] Stein G, Schone S, Geinitz D, et al. No tissue level abnormality of vitamin A concentration despite elevated serum vitamin A of uremic patients. Clinical Nephrology 1986;25:87−93.

[81] Espe KM, Raila J, Henze A, et al. Impact of vitamin A on clinical outcomes in haemodialysis patients. Nephrol Dial Transplant 2011;26:4054−61.

[82] Kalousova M, Kubena AA, Kostirova M, et al. Lower retinol levels as an independent predictor of mortality in long-term hemodialysis patients: a prospective observational cohort study. Am J Kidney Dis 2010;56:513−21.

[83] Clermont G, Lecour S, Lahet J, et al. Alteration in plasma antioxidant capacities in chronic renal failure and hemodialysis patients: a possible explanation for the increased cardiovascular risk in these patients. Cardiovasc Res 2000;47:618−23.

[84] Stenvinkel P, Heimburger O, Paultre F, et al. Strong association between malnutrition, inflammation, and atherosclerosis in chronic renal failure. Kidney International 1999;55:1899−911.

[85] Peuchant E, Delmas-Beauvieux MC, Dubourg L, et al. Antioxidant effects of a supplemented very low protein diet in chronic renal failure. Free Radic Biol Med 1997;22:313−20.

[86] Malyszko J, Wolczynski S, Skrzydlewska E, Malyszko JS, Mysliwiec M. Vitamin K status in relation to bone metabolism in patients with renal failure. Am J Nephrol 2002;22:504−8.

[87] Robert D, Jorgetti V, Leclercq M, et al. Does vitamin K excess induce ectopic calcifications in hemodialysis patients? Clinical Nephrology 1985;24:300−4.

[88] Holden RM, Iliescu E, Morton AR, Booth SL. Vitamin K status of Canadian peritoneal dialysis patients. Perit Dial Int 2008;28:415−8.

[89] Holden RM, Morton AR, Garland JS, Pavlov A, Day AG, Booth SL. Vitamins K and D status in stages 3−5 chronic kidney disease. Clin J Am Soc Nephrol 2010;5:590−7.

[90] Pilkey RM, Morton AR, Boffa MB, et al. Subclinical vitamin K deficiency in hemodialysis patients. Am J Kidney Dis 2007;49:432−9.

[91] Kopple JD, Dirige OV, Jacob M, Wang M, Swendseid ME. Transketolase activity in red blood cells in chronic uremia. Trans Am Soc Artif Intern Organs 1972;18:250−6.

[92] Lonergan ET, Semar M, Sterzel RB, et al. Erythrocyte transketolase activity in dialyzed patients. A reversible metabolic lesion of uremia. New Engl J Med 1971;284:1399−403.

[93] Sterzel RB, Semar M, Lonergan ET, Treser G, Lange K. Relationship of nervous tissue transketolase to the neuropathy in chronic uremia. J Clin Invest 1971;50:2295−304.

[94] Kuriyama M, Mizuma A, Yokomine R, Igata A, Otuji Y. Erythrocyte transketolase activity in uremia. Clin Chim Acta 1980;108:169−77.

[95] Ramirez G, Chen M, Boyce Jr HW, et al. Longitudinal follow-up of chronic hemodialysis patients without vitamin supplementation. Kidney Internat 1986;30:99−106.

[96] Heinz J, Domrose U, Westphal S, Luley C, Neumann KH, Dierkes J. Washout of water-soluble vitamins and of homocysteine during haemodialysis: effect of high-flux and low-flux dialyser membranes. Nephrology (Carlton, Vic) 2008;13:384−9.

[97] Coveney N, Polkinghorne KR, Linehan L, Corradini A, Kerr PG. Water-soluble vitamin levels in extended hours hemodialysis. Hemodialysis Internat 2011;15:30−8.

[98] Cage JB, Wall BM. Shoshin beriberi in an AIDS patient with end-stage renal disease. Clin Cardiol 1992;15:862−5.

[99] Gotloib L, Servadio C. A possible case of beriberi heart failure in a chronic hemodialyzed patient. Nephron 1975;14:293−8.

[100] Barbara PG, Manuel B, Elisabetta M, et al. The suddenly speechless florist on chronic dialysis: the unexpected threats of a flower shop? Diagnosis: dialysis related Wernicke encephalopathy. Nephrol Dial Transplant 2006;21:223−5.

[101] Jagadha V, Deck JH, Halliday WC, Smyth HS. Wernicke's encephalopathy in patients on peritoneal dialysis or hemodialysis. Ann Neurol 1987;21:78–84.

[102] Ueda K, Takada D, Mii A, et al. Severe thiamine deficiency resulted in Wernicke's encephalopathy in a chronic dialysis patient. Clin Exp Nephrol 2006;10:290–3.

[103] Hung SC, Hung SH, Tarng DC, Yang WC, Huang TP. Chorea induced by thiamine deficiency in hemodialysis patients. Am J Kidney Dis 2001;37:427–30.

[104] Hung SC, Hung SH, Tarng DC, Yang WC, Chen TW, Huang TP. Thiamine deficiency and unexplained encephalopathy in hemodialysis and peritoneal dialysis patients. Am J Kidney Dis 2001;38:941–7.

[105] Porrini M, Simonetti P, Ciappellano S, et al. Thiamin, riboflavin and pyridoxine status in chronic renal insufficiency. International Journal for Vitamin and Nutrition Research Internationale Zeitschrift fur Vitamin- und Ernahrungsforschung 1989;59:304–8.

[106] Ito T, Niwa T, Matsui E, Oishi N, Yagi K. Plasma flavin levels of patients receiving long-term hemodialysis. Clin Chim Acta 1972;39:125–9.

[107] Skoupy S, Fodinger M, Veitl M, et al. Riboflavin is a determinant of total homocysteine plasma concentrations in end-stage renal disease patients. J Am Soc Nephrol 2002;13:1331–7.

[108] Don T, Friedlander S, Wong W. Dietary Intakes and Biochemical Status of B Vitamins in a Group of Children Receiving Dialysis. Journal of Renal Nutrition: the official journal of the Council on Renal Nutrition of the National Kidney Foundation 2010;20:23–8.

[109] Kannampuzha J, Donnelly SM, McFarlane PA, et al. Glutathione and riboflavin status in supplemented patients undergoing home nocturnal hemodialysis versus standard hemodialysis. J Ren Nutr 2010;20:199–208.

[110] Wolfson M, Kopple JD. The effect of vitamin B_6 deficiency on food intake, growth, and renal function in chronically azotemic rats. JPEN J Parenter Enteral Nutr 1987;11:398–402.

[111] Ramirez G, Chen M, Boyce Jr HW, et al. The plasma and red cell vitamin B levels of chronic hemodialysis patients: a longitudinal study. Nephron 1986;42:41–6.

[112] Corken M, Porter J. Is vitamin B(6) deficiency an under-recognized risk in patients receiving haemodialysis? A systematic review: 2000-2010. Nephrology (Carlton, Vic) 2011;16:619–25.

[113] Lacour B, Parry C, Drueke T, et al. Pyridoxal 5'-phosphate deficiency in uremic undialyzed, hemodialyzed, and non-uremic kidney transplant patients. Clin Chim Acta 1983;127:205–15.

[114] Kasama R, Koch T, Canals-Navas C, Pitone JM. Vitamin B_6 and hemodialysis: the impact of high-flux/high-efficiency dialysis and review of the literature. Am J Kidney Dis 1996;27:680–6.

[115] Ross EA, Shah GM, Reynolds RD, Sabo A, Pichon M. Vitamin B_6 requirements of patients on chronic peritoneal dialysis. Kidney International 1989;36:702–6.

[116] Dobbelstein H, Korner WF, Mempel W, Grosse-Wilde H, Edel HH. Vitamin B_6 deficiency in uremia and its implications for the depression of immune responses. Kidney Internat 1974;5:233–9.

[117] Casciato DA, McAdam LP, Kopple JD, et al. Immunologic abnormalities in hemodialysis patients: improvement after pyridoxine therapy. Nephron 1984;38:9–16.

[118] Marumo F, Kamata K, Okubo M. Deranged concentrations of water-soluble vitamins in the blood of undialyzed and dialyzed patients with chronic renal failure. Internat J Artif Organs 1986;9:17–24.

[119] Mydlik M, Derzsiova K, Zemberova E. Influence of water and sodium diuresis and furosemide on urinary excretion of vitamin B(6), oxalic acid and vitamin C in chronic renal failure. Miner Electrolyte Metab 1999;25:352–6.

[120] Hultqvist M, Hegbrant J, Nilsson-Thorell C, et al. Plasma concentrations of vitamin C, vitamin E and/or malondialdehyde as markers of oxygen free radical production during hemodialysis. Clin Nephrol 1997;47:37–46.

[121] Wang S, Eide TC, Sogn EM, Berg KJ, Sund RB. Plasma ascorbic acid in patients undergoing chronic haemodialysis. Eur J Clin Pharmacol 1999;55:527–32.

[122] Tarng DC, Wei YH, Huang TP, Kuo BI, Yang WC. Intravenous ascorbic acid as an adjuvant therapy for recombinant erythropoietin in hemodialysis patients with hyperferritinemia. Kidney Internat 1999;55:2477–86.

[123] Mydlik M, Derzsiova K, Svac J, Dlhopolcek P, Zemberova E. Peritoneal clearance and peritoneal transfer of oxalic acid, vitamin C, and vitamin B_6 during continuous ambulatory peritoneal dialysis. Artif Organs 1998;22:784–8.

[124] Zhang K, Liu L, Cheng X, Dong J, Geng Q, Zuo L. Low levels of vitamin C in dialysis patients is associated with decreased prealbumin and increased C-reactive protein. BMC Nephrol 2011;12:18.

[125] Ihle BU, Gillies M. Scurvy and thrombocytopathy in a chronic hemodialysis patient. Aust N Z J Med 1983;13:523.

[126] Handelman GJ. Vitamin C neglect in hemodialysis: sailing between Scylla and Charybdis. Blood Purification 2007;25:58–61.

[127] Said HM, Vaziri ND, Kariger RK, Hollander D. Intestinal absorption of 5-methyltetrahydrofolate in experimental uremia. Acta Vitaminol Enzymol 1984;6:339–46.

[128] Bukhari FJ, Moradi H, Gollapudi P, Ju Kim H, Vaziri ND, Said HM. Effect of chronic kidney disease on the expression of thiamin and folic acid transporters. Nephrol Dial Transplant 2011;26:2137–44.

[129] Livant E, Tamura T, Johnston K, et al. Plasma folate conjugase activities and folate concentrations in patients receiving hemodialysis. J Nutr Biochem 1994;5:504–8.

[130] Westhuyzen J, Matherson K, Tracey R, Fleming SJ. Effect of withdrawal of folic acid supplementation in maintenance hemodialysis patients. Clinical Nephrology 1993;40:96–9.

[131] Leblanc M, Pichette V, Geadah D, Ouimet D. Folic acid and pyridoxal-5'-phosphate losses during high-efficiency hemodialysis in patients without hydrosoluble vitamin supplementation. J Ren Nutr 2000;10:196–201.

[132] Fehrman-Ekholm I, Lotsander A, Logan K, Dunge D, Odar-Cederlof I, Kallner A. Concentrations of vitamin C, vitamin B_{12} and folic acid in patients treated with hemodialysis and on-line hemodiafiltration or hemofiltration. Scandinavian Journal of Urology and Nephrology 2008;42:74–80.

[133] Henderson I, Leung A, Shenkin A. Vitamin status in continuous ambulatory peritoneal dialysis. Perit Dial Bull 1984;4:143–5.

[134] Salahudeen AK, Varma SR, Karim T, Bari MZ, Pingle A, D'Costa R. Anaemia, ferritin, and vitamins in continuous ambulatory peritoneal dialysis. Lancet 1988;1:1049.

[135] Fehrman-Ekholm I, Lotsander A, Logan K, Dunge D, Odar-Cederlöf I, Kallner A. Concentrations of vitamin C, vitamin B_{12} and folic acid in patients treated with hemodialysis and on-line hemodiafiltration or hemofiltration. Scand J Urol Nephrol 2008;42:74–80.

[136] DeBari VA, Frank O, Baker H, Needle MA. Water soluble vitamins in granulocytes, erythrocytes, and plasma obtained from chronic hemodialysis patients. Am J Clin Nutr 1984;39:410–5.

[137] Henkin Y, Oberman A, Hurst DC, Segrest JP. Niacin revisited: clinical observations on an important but underutilized drug. Am J Med 1991;91:239–46.

[138] Braguer D, Gallice P, Yatzidis H, Berland Y, Crevat A. Restoration by biotin of the in vitro microtubule formation inhibited by uremic toxins. Nephron 1991;57:192–6.

[139] Jung U, Helbich-Endermann M, Bitsch R, Schneider S, Stein G. Are patients with chronic renal failure (CRF) deficient in Biotin and is regular Biotin supplementation required? Zeitschrift fur Ernahrungswissenschaft 1998;37:363–7.

[140] Lasker N, Harvey A, Baker H. Vitamin levels in hemodialysis and intermittent peritoneal dialysis. Trans Am Soc Art Int Organs 1963;9:51–6.

[141] Mackenzie J, Ford J, Waters A, Harding N, Cattell W, Anderson B. Erythropoiesis in patients undergoing regular dialysis treatment without transfusion. Proc Eur Dial Transplant Assoc 1968;5:172–8.

[142] Yatzidis H, Digenis P, Koutsicos D. Hypervitaminosis A in chronic renal failure after transplantation. Br Med J 1976;2: 1075.

[143] Connolly GM, Cunningham R, Maxwell AP, Young IS. Decreased serum retinol is associated with increased mortality in renal transplant recipients. Clin Chem 2007;53:1841–6.

[144] McGrath LT, Treacy R, McClean E, Brown JH. Oxidative stress in cyclosporin and azathioprine treated renal transplant patients. Clin Chim Acta 1997;264:1–12.

[145] Fodinger M, Buchmayer H, Heinz G, et al. Effect of MTHFR 1298A→>C and MTHFR 677C→T genotypes on total homocysteine, folate, and vitamin B(12) plasma concentrations in kidney graft recipients. J Am Soc Nephrol 2000;11:1918–25.

[146] Druml W, Schwarzenhofer M, Apsner R, Horl WH. Fat-soluble vitamins in patients with acute renal failure. Miner Electrolyte Metab 1998;24:220–6.

[147] Gleghorn EE, Eisenberg LD, Hack S, Parton P, Merritt RJ. Observations of vitamin A toxicity in three patients with renal failure receiving parenteral alimentation. Am J Clin Nutr 1986;44:107–12.

[148] Fortin MC, Amyot SL, Geadah D, Leblanc M. Serum concentrations and clearances of folic acid and pyridoxal-5- phosphate during venovenous continuous renal replacement therapy. Intensive Care Med 1999;25:594–8.

[149] Story DA, Ronco C, Bellomo R. Trace element and vitamin concentrations and losses in critically ill patients treated with continuous venovenous hemofiltration. Crit Care Med 1999; 27:220–3.

[150] Fissell RB, Bragg-Gresham JL, Gillespie BW, et al. International variation in vitamin prescription and association with mortality in the Dialysis Outcomes and Practice Patterns Study (DOPPS). Am J Kidney Dis 2004;44:293–9.

[151] Moustapha A, Gupta A, Robinson K, et al. Prevalence and determinants of hyperhomocysteinemia in hemodialysis and peritoneal dialysis. Kidney Internat 1999;55:1470–5.

[152] Arnadottir M, Hultberg B, Nilsson-Ehle P, Thysell H. The effect of reduced glomerular filtration rate on plasma total homocysteine concentration. Scand J Clin Lab Invest 1996;56:41–6.

[153] Jamison RL, Hartigan P, Kaufman JS, et al. Effect of homocysteine lowering on mortality and vascular disease in advanced chronic kidney disease and end-stage renal disease: a randomized controlled trial. Jama 2007;298:1163–70.

[154] Suliman ME, Barany P, Divino Filho JC, et al. Influence of nutritional status on plasma and erythrocyte sulphur amino acids, sulph-hydryls, and inorganic sulphate in end-stage renal disease. Nephrol Dial Transplant 2002;17:1050–6.

[155] Arnadottir M, Hultberg B, Wahlberg J, Fellstrom B, Dimeny E. Serum total homocysteine concentration before and after renal transplantation. Kidney Internat 1998;54:1380–4.

[156] House AA, Wells GA, Donnelly JG, Nadler SP, Hebert PC. Randomized trial of high-flux vs. low-flux haemodialysis:

[157] Pedrini LA, De Cristofaro V, Comelli M, et al. Long-term effects of high-efficiency on-line haemodiafiltration on uraemic toxicity. A multicentre prospective randomized study. Nephrol Dial Transplant 2011;26:2617–24.

[158] Vychytil A, Fodinger M, Wolfl G, et al. Major determinants of hyperhomocysteinemia in peritoneal dialysis patients. Kidney Internat 1998;53:1775–82.

[159] Moustapha A, Naso A, Nahlawi M, et al. Prospective study of hyperhomocysteinemia as an adverse cardiovascular risk factor in end-stage renal disease. Circulation 1998;97:138–41.

[160] Bostom AG, Shemin D, Verhoef P, et al. Elevated fasting total plasma homocysteine levels and cardiovascular disease outcomes in maintenance dialysis patients. A prospective study. Arterioscler Thromb Vasc Biol 1997;17:2554–8.

[161] Stenvinkel P, Carrero JJ, Axelsson J, Lindholm B, Heimburger O, Massy ZA. Emerging biomarkers for evaluating cardiovascular risk in the chronic kidney disease patient: how do new pieces fit into the uremic puzzle? Clin J Am Soc Nephrol 2008;3: 505–21.

[162] Kalantar-Zadeh K, Block G, Humphreys MH, McAllister CJ, Kopple JD. A low, rather than a high, total plasma homocysteine is an indicator of poor outcome in hemodialysis patients. J Am Soc Nephrol 2004;15:442–53.

[163] Winkelmayer WC, Kramar R, Curhan GC, et al. Fasting plasma total homocysteine levels and mortality and allograft loss in kidney transplant recipients: a prospective study. J Am Soc Nephrol 2005;16:255–60.

[164] Perna AF, Ingrosso D, Violetti E, et al. Progress in uremic toxin research: hyperhomocysteinemia in uremia – a red flag in a disrupted circuit. Seminars in Dialysis 2009;22:351–6.

[165] Bostom AG, Gohh RY, Beaulieu AJ, et al. Treatment of hyperhomocysteinemia in renal transplant recipients. A randomized, placebo-controlled trial. Ann Intern Med 1997;127:1089–92.

[166] Brady CB, Gaziano JM, Cxypoliski RA, et al. Homocysteine lowering and cognition in CKD: the Veterans Affairs homocysteine study. Am J Kidney Dis 2009;54:440–9.

[167] Heinz J, Kropf S, Domrose U, et al. B vitamins and the risk of total mortality and cardiovascular disease in end-stage renal disease: results of a randomized controlled trial. Circulation 2011;121:1432–8.

[168] Bostom AG, Carpenter MA, Hunsicker L, et al. Baseline characteristics of participants in the Folic Acid for Vascular Outcome Reduction in Transplantation (FAVORIT) Trial. Am J Kidney Dis 2009;53:121–8.

[169] Tsao CS, Salimi SL. Effect of large intake of ascorbic acid on urinary and plasma oxalic acid levels. International Journal for Vitamin and Nutrition Research Internationale Zeitschrift fur Vitamin- und Ernahrungsforschung 1984;54:245–9.

[170] McConnell KN, Rolton HA, Modi KS, Macdougall AI. Plasma oxalate in patients with chronic renal failure receiving continuous ambulatory peritoneal dialysis or hemodialysis. Am J Kidney Dis 1991;18:441–5.

[171] Worcester EM, Nakagawa Y, Bushinsky DA, Coe FL. Evidence that serum calcium oxalate supersaturation is a consequence of oxalate retention in patients with chronic renal failure. J Clin Invest 1986;77:1888–96.

[172] Elgstoen KB, Johnsen LF, Woldseth B, Morkrid L, Hartmann A. Plasma oxalate following kidney transplantation in patients without primary hyperoxaluria. Nephrol Dial Transplant 2010; 25:2341–5.

[173] Fayemi AO, Ali M, Braun EV. Oxalosis in hemodialysis patients: a pathologic study of 80 cases. Arch Pathol Lab Med 1979;103: 58–62.

effects on homocysteine and lipids. Nephrol Dial Transplant 2000;15:1029–34.

[174] Mydlik M, Derzsiova K. Renal replacement therapy and secondary hyperoxalemia in chronic renal failure. Kidney Int Suppl 2001;78:S304–7.

[175] Hoppe B, Graf D, Offner G, et al. Oxalate elimination via hemodialysis or peritoneal dialysis in children with chronic renal failure. Pediatric Nephrol (Berlin, Germany) 1996;10:488–92.

[176] Ogawa Y, Machida N, Ogawa T, et al. Calcium oxalate saturation in dialysis patients with and without primary hyperoxaluria. Urol Res 2006;34:12–6.

[177] Balcke P, Schmidt P, Zazgornik J, Kopsa H, Haubenstock A. Ascorbic acid aggravates secondary hyperoxalemia in patients on chronic hemodialysis. Ann Intern Med 1984;101:344–5.

[178] Canavese C, Petrarulo M, Massarenti P, et al. Long-term, low-dose, intravenous vitamin C leads to plasma calcium oxalate supersaturation in hemodialysis patients. Am J Kidney Dis 2005;45:540–9.

[179] Ott SM, Andress DL, Sherrard DJ. Bone oxalate in a long-term hemodialysis patient who ingested high doses of vitamin C. Am J Kidney Dis 1986;8:450–4.

[180] Friedman AL, Chesney RW, Gilbert EF, Gilchrist KW, Latorraca R, Segar WE. Secondary oxalosis as a complication of parenteral alimentation in acute renal failure. Am J Nephrol 1983;3:248–52.

[181] Tomson CR, Channon SM, Parkinson IS, et al. Plasma oxalate in patients receiving continuous ambulatory peritoneal dialysis. Nephrol Dial Transplant 1988;3:295–9.

[182] Mydlik M, Derzsiova K. Vitamin B_6 and oxalic acid in clinical nephrology. J Ren Nutr 2010;20:S95–102.

[183] Tomson CR, Channon SM, Parkinson IS, Sheldon WS, Ward MK, Laker MK. Effect of pyridoxine supplementation on plasma oxalate concentrations in patients receiving dialysis. Eur J Clin Invest 1989;19:201–5.

[184] Balcke P, Schmidt P, Zazgornik J, Kopsa H, Deutsch E. Effect of vitamin B_6 administration on elevated plasma oxalic acid levels in haemodialysed patients. Eur J Clin Invest 1982;12:481–3.

[185] Costello JF, Sadovnic MC, Smith M, Stolarski C. Effect of vitamin B_6 supplementation on plasma oxalate and oxalate removal rate in hemodialysis patients. J Am Soc Nephrol 1992;3:1018–24.

[186] Descombes E, Boulat O, Perriard F, Fellay G. Water-soluble vitamin levels in patients undergoing high-flux hemodialysis and receiving long-term oral postdialysis vitamin supplementation. Artif Organs 2000;24:773–8.

[187] Will EJ, Bijvoet OL. Primary oxalosis: clinical and biochemical response to high-dose pyridoxine therapy. Metabolism 1979;28:542–8.

[188] Franssen CF. Oxalate clearance by haemodialysis—a comparison of seven dialysers. Nephrol Dial Transplant 2005;20:1916–21.

[189] Mydlik M, Derzsiova K. [Vitamin levels in the serum and erythrocytes during erythropoietin therapy in hemodialyzed patients]. Bratisl Lek Listy 1999;100:426–31.

[190] Pollock CA, Wyndham R, Collett PV, et al. Effects of erythropoietin therapy on the lipid profile in end-stage renal failure. Kidney Internat 1994;45:897–902.

[191] Deved V, Poyah P, James MT, et al. Ascorbic acid for anemia management in hemodialysis patients: a systematic review and meta-analysis. Am J Kidney Dis 2009;54:1089–97.

[192] Parfrey PS: KDIGO report on upcoming guidelines: Anemia, in Nephrology ASo (ed): 2011 Renal Week Philadelphia, 2011

[193] Knapen MH, Jie KS, Hamulyak K, Vermeer C. Vitamin K-induced changes in markers for osteoblast activity and urinary calcium loss. Calcif Tissue Int 1993;53:81–5.

[194] Jie KS, Gijsbers BL, Knapen MH, Hamulyak K, Frank HL, Vermeer C. Effects of vitamin K and oral anticoagulants on urinary calcium excretion. Br J Haematol 1993;83:100–4.

[195] Mehta RL, Scott G, Sloand JA, Francis CW. Skin necrosis associated with acquired protein C deficiency in patients with renal failure and calciphylaxis. Am J Med 1990;88:252–7.

[196] Holden RM, Sanfilippo AS, Hopman WM, Zimmerman D, Garland JS, Morton AR. Warfarin and aortic valve calcification in hemodialysis patients. J Nephrol 2007;20:417–22.

[197] Fusaro M, Crepaldi G, Maggi S, et al. Vitamin K, bone fractures, and vascular calcifications in chronic kidney disease: an important but poorly studied relationship. J Endocrinol Invest 2011;34:317–23.

[198] Kohlmeier M, Saupe J, Shearer MJ, Schaefer K, Asmus G. Bone health of adult hemodialysis patients is related to vitamin K status. Kidney Internat 1997;51:1218–21.

[199] Kohlmeier M, Saupe J, Schaefer K, Asmus G. Bone fracture history and prospective bone fracture risk of hemodialysis patients are related to apolipoprotein E genotype. Calcif Tissue Int 1998;62:278–81.

[200] Ochiai M, Nakashima A, Takasugi N, et al. Vitamin K alters bone metabolism markers in hemodialysis patients with a low serum parathyroid hormone level. Nephron 2011;117:c15–9.

[201] Wieland RG, Hendricks FH, Amat y Leon F, Gutierrez L, Jones JC. Hypervitaminosis A with hypercalcaemia. Lancet 1971;1:698.

[202] Takahashi Y, Tanaka A, Nakamura T, et al. Nicotinamide suppresses hyperphosphatemia in hemodialysis patients. Kidney Internat 2004;65:1099–104.

[203] Dursun B, Dursun E, Suleymanlar G, et al. Carotid artery intima-media thickness correlates with oxidative stress in chronic haemodialysis patients with accelerated atherosclerosis. Nephrol Dial Transplant 2008;23:1697–703.

[204] Coombes JS, Fassett RG. Antioxidant therapy in hemodialysis patients: a systematic review. Kidney Internat 2011;81:233–46.

[205] Boaz M, Smetana S, Weinstein T, et al. Secondary prevention with antioxidants of cardiovascular disease in endstage renal disease (SPACE): randomised placebo-controlled trial. Lancet 2000;356:1213–8.

[206] Tepel M, van der Giet M, Statz M, Jankowski J, Zidek W. The antioxidant acetylcysteine reduces cardiovascular events in patients with end-stage renal failure: a randomized, controlled trial. Circulation 2003;107:992–5.

[207] Mafra D, Santos FR, Lobo JC, et al. Alpha-tocopherol supplementation decreases electronegative low-density lipoprotein concentration [LDL(-)] in haemodialysis patients. Nephrol Dial Transplant 2009;24:1587–92.

[208] Cristol JP, Bosc JY, Badiou S, et al. Erythropoietin and oxidative stress in haemodialysis: beneficial effects of vitamin E supplementation. Nephrol Dial Transplant 1997;12:2312–7.

[209] Yalcin AS, Yurtkuran M, Dilek K, Kilinc A, Taga Y, Emerk K. The effect of vitamin E therapy on plasma and erythrocyte lipid peroxidation in chronic hemodialysis patients. Clin Chim Acta 1989;185:109–12.

[210] Islam KN, O'Byrne D, Devaraj S, Palmer B, Grundy SM, Jialal I. Alpha-tocopherol supplementation decreases the oxidative susceptibility of LDL in renal failure patients on dialysis therapy. Atherosclerosis 2000;150:217–24.

[211] Tarng DC, Huang TP, Liu TY, Chen HW, Sung YJ, Wei YH. Effect of vitamin E-bonded membrane on the 8-hydroxy 2'-deoxyguanosine level in leukocyte DNA of hemodialysis patients. Kidney Internat 2000;58:790–9.

[212] Omata M, Higuchi C, Demura R, Sanaka T, Nihei H. Reduction of neutrophil activation by vitamin E modified dialyzer membranes. Nephron 2000;85:221–31.

[213] Kirmizis D, Papagianni A, Belechri AM, Memmos D. Effects of vitamin E-coated membrane dialyser on markers of oxidative stress and inflammation in patients on chronic haemodialysis. Nephrol Dial Transplant 2010;26:2296—301.

[214] Varghese Z, Fernando RL, Turakhia G, et al. Calcineurin inhibitors enhance low-density lipoprotein oxidation in transplant patients. Kidney Int Suppl 1999;71:S137—40.

[215] Cristol JP, Vela C, Maggi MF, Descomps B, Mourad G. Oxidative stress and lipid abnormalities in renal transplant recipients with or without chronic rejection. Transplantation 1998;65:1322—8.

[216] Wang C, Salahudeen AK. Lipid peroxidation accompanies cyclosporine nephrotoxicity: effects of vitamin E. Kidney Internat 1995;47:927—34.

[217] Schnell-Inderst P, Kossmann B, Fischereder M, Klauss V, Wasem J. Antioxidative vitamins for prevention of cardiovascular disease for patients after renal transplantation and patients with chronic renal failure. GMS Health Technol Assess 2: Doc14, 2006.

[218] Okada H, Moriwaki K, Kanno Y, et al. Vitamin B_6 supplementation can improve peripheral polyneuropathy in patients with chronic renal failure on high-flux haemodialysis and human recombinant erythropoietin. Nephrol Dial Transplant 2000;15:1410—3.

[219] Fouque D, Vennegoor M, ter Wee P, et al. EBPG guideline on nutrition. Nephrol Dial Transplant 22 Suppl 2007;2:ii45—87.

[220] Clinical practice guidelines for nutrition in chronic renal failure. K/DOQI, National Kidney Foundation. Am J Kidney Dis 2000;35:S1—140.

[221] Voss D. Vitamins in pre-dialysis patients: The CARI Guidelines — Caring for Australians with Renal Impairment, 2005. http://www.cari.org.au/guidelines.php.

[222] Steiber AL, Kopple JD. Vitamin status and needs for people with stages 3-5 chronic kidney disease. J Ren Nutr 2011;21: 355—68.

[223] Druml W. Nutritional management of acute renal failure. J Ren Nutr 2005;15:63—70.

[224] Cano NJ, Aparicio M, Brunori G, et al. ESPEN Guidelines on Parenteral Nutrition: adult renal failure. Clinical nutrition (Edinburgh, Scotland) 2009;28:401—14.

[225] Mann JF, Lonn EM, Yi Q, et al. Effects of vitamin E on cardiovascular outcomes in people with mild-to-moderate renal insufficiency: results of the HOPE study. Kidney Internat 2004;65:1375—80.

[226] No author: Effects of ramipril on cardiovascular and microvascular outcomes in people with diabetes mellitus: results of the HOPE study and MICRO-HOPE substudy. Heart Outcomes Prevention Evaluation Study Investigators. Lancet 2000;355: 253—9.

[227] Lonn E, Bosch J, Yusuf S, et al. Effects of long-term vitamin E supplementation on cardiovascular events and cancer: a randomized controlled trial. Jama 2005;293:1338—47.

[228] Kopple JD, Mercurio K, Blumenkrantz MJ, et al. Daily requirement for pyridoxine supplements in chronic renal failure. Kidney Internat 1981;19:694—704.

[229] Kopple J. Dietary considerations in patients with advanced chronic renal failure, acute renal failure, and transplantation. In: Shills M, Olson JA, Shike M, Ross AC, editors. Diseases of the Kidney. Baltimore: Williams & Wilkins; 1998. p. 3167—210.

[230] Kriley M, Warady BA. Vitamin status of pediatric patients receiving long-term peritoneal dialysis. Am J Clin Nutr 1991;53:1476—9.

[231] Mousson C, Justrabo E, Rifle G, Sgro C, Chalopin JM, Gerard C. Piridoxilate-induced oxalate nephropathy can lead to end-stage renal failure. Nephron 1993;63:104—6.

[232] Schaumburg H, Kaplan J, Windebank A, et al. Sensory neuropathy from pyridoxine abuse. A new megavitamin syndrome. New Engl J Med 1983;309:445—8.

[233] Zazgornik J, Druml W, Balcke P, et al. Diminished serum folic acid levels in renal transplant recipients. Clinical Nephrol 1982; 18:306—10.

[234] Dietary Reference Intakes for thiamin, riboflavin, niacin, vitamin B6, Folate, pantothenic acid, biotin and cholin. Washington DC: National Academy Press; 1998.

[235] Kamali F, Wynne H. Pharmacogenetics of Warfarin. Ann Rev Med 2010;61:63—75.

[236] Dietary Reference Intakes for vitamin A, vitamin K, arsenic, boron, chromium, copper, iodin, iron, manganese, molybdenum, nickel, silicon, vanadium and zinc. Washington DC: National Academy Press; 2001.

Nutrition and Anemia in End-stage Renal Disease

Rajnish Mehrotra[1], Min Zhang[2], Yinan Li[3]

[1]Section Head, Nephrology, Harborview Medical Center, University of Washington, Seattle, WA, USA
[2]Division of Nephrology, Tianjin Union Medical Center, Tianjin, China
[3]Division of Nephrology and Hypertension, Los Angeles Biomedical Research Institute at Harbor-UCLA, Torrance, CA, USA

INTRODUCTION

Erythropoietin deficiency is a hallmark of progressive kidney disease and is the most important cause for anemia in individuals undergoing maintenance dialysis. The availability of erythropoiesis stimulating agents (ESAs) for the last two decades has revolutionized anemia management in this patient population. The concern about the potential adverse cardiovascular effects of ESAs as well as the high costs of the therapy, however, have led to re-examination of the clinical approach to the management of anemia [1–3]. In this context, the role of potentially ESA-sparing nutrients has gained renewed interest some of which may be required to replace deficits and others to be provided in surfeit. We present a review of the potential role of key nutrients and growth factors in the management of anemia in dialysis-dependent patients.

IRON

Role in Anemia of Kidney Disease

Iron is essential for hemoglobin formation in health and disease. Hence, an adequate supply of iron is essential to ensure an optimal response to ESAs.

Status in Maintenance Dialysis Patients

Iron deficiency is commonly present at the time of initiation of maintenance dialysis therapy [4,5]. Moreover, dialysis patients have a higher than normal amount of iron loss which is due to blood loss during the hemodialysis procedure, oozing of blood from the gastrointestinal tract, and frequent venipuncture. Indeed, one study has estimated that maintenance hemodialysis patients may lose three liters of blood annually from the dialysis procedure and venipuncture alone [6]. Finally, ESA therapy increases the rate of erythropoiesis and, hence, the demand for iron [7]. Thus, it is no surprise that dietary intake of iron is insufficient to maintain adequate available iron stores in most dialysis patients. Thus, clinical practice guidelines formulated both in the United States and Europe recommend routine evaluation and management of available body iron stores in dialysis patients treated with ESAs [8,9].

Evidence and Recommendations

Several studies have demonstrated that oral iron therapy is usually ineffective in either correcting the iron deficiency or in reducing the ESA dose requirements in patients undergoing maintenance dialysis [10–13]. On the other hand, several studies have consistently demonstrated the ability of intravenous iron treatment to correct the iron deficiency as well to reduce the ESA requirements [10,11,13–15]. Hence, intravenous therapy forms the cornerstone of iron supplementation in dialysis patients.

A variety of intravenous iron preparations are available in different parts of the world and include iron dextran, ferric sodium gluconate, iron sucrose, ferumoxytol, and ferric carboxymaltose [15–17]. While they have similar efficacy in the repletion or maintenance of iron stores, the safety profile of these preparations differs significantly. In a recent analysis of all the adverse events reported to the United States Food and Drug Administration, ferric sodium gluconate and iron sucrose were associated with the lowest rate of adverse events and iron dextran and ferumoxytol with the highest [18]. Compared to iron sucrose and ferric sodium gluconate, ferumoxytol was associated with significantly higher odds of any adverse event, including serious fatal and non-fatal adverse events [18]. As a result of these concerns, the use of iron dextran and ferumoxytol is substantially lower than that of the other preparations.

In clinical practice, iron repletion is performed in patients with overt iron deficiency with/without periodic administration of a small dose as maintenance therapy. Routine monitoring of iron status is needed to determine the dose and frequency of iron administration as well as to prevent iron overload. The presence of stainable iron on bone marrow is the most reliable method to diagnose iron deficiency but is not feasible for use in day-to-day clinical practice. Thus, one has to rely on serum biomarkers of which transferrin saturation and ferritin are the ones most widely used [8]. Expert groups recommend maintaining serum transferrin saturation between 20 and 50% and ferritin between 100 and 500 ng/mL [8]. However, there are significant limitations with these parameters — while transferrin (the major component of total iron binding capacity, the denominator for calculating transferrin saturation) is a negative acute phase reactant, ferritin is a positive acute phase reactant. Thus, it is not uncommon for iron deficient patients with superimposed illnesses to have serum transferrin saturation and/or ferritin levels to be within the normal range. Moreover, there is no single value of either serum transferrin saturation or ferritin that accurately identifies individuals in need of iron supplementation [11,13,15,19]. Under such circumstances, it is helpful to administer parenteral supplementation in patients with serum iron <50 μg/mL. Furthermore, serum ferritin levels higher than those recommended by expert groups do not preclude hematopoietic response to iron repletion and should be considered in patients with serum ferritin up to 1200 ng/mL but transferrin saturation <20% [20,21]. Thus, it is necessary to combine clinical judgment with a routine evaluation of laboratory parameters when making decisions regarding either the need to provide or to withhold iron supplementation.

Other noninvasive tests, like zinc protoporphyrin, reticulocyte hemoglobin, soluble transferrin receptors and percent hypochromic red cells, have been evaluated [22–25]; of these, reticulocyte hemoglobin appears to be the most promising. However, the role of these biomarkers in the day-to-day management of iron therapy in ESA-treated patients remains unclear and cannot be recommended at this time.

A little over a decade ago, the iron-regulatory peptide hepcidin was characterized [26,27]. High levels of hepcidin inhibit the availability of iron for erythropoiesis both by reducing iron absorption from the gastrointestinal tract as well as its efflux from the reticuloendothelial system and hepatocytes [27]. The serum hepcidin levels are elevated in dialysis patients and there has been interest in using it as a biomarker to guide iron administration [28–30]. The preliminary studies in this regard, however, have not been encouraging and the use of hepcidin levels to guide iron therapy cannot be recommended at this time [31].

Concern has been raised about the safety of routine use of intravenous iron in the dialysis patient population. There are two major potential risks associated with iron therapy. First, iron is known to enhance the pathogenicity of a large number of infectious microbes. Some investigators have identified a high serum ferritin level in hemodialysis patients as a risk factor for bacteremia, particularly related to catheter sepsis [32,33]. However, in a study conducted by Hoen et al. [34] anemia and not an elevated serum ferritin, emerged as a risk factor for bacteremia. As pointed out earlier, serum ferritin is also an acute phase reactant and an elevated serum ferritin may be a marker of processes that increase the susceptibility of dialysis patients to infection. Furthermore, there is no direct evidence that causally links iron therapy with an increased risk of infection in patients with kidney disease. Second, administration of large intravenous doses of iron may increase oxidative stress [35,36]. This, in turn, may accelerate atherosclerosis and increase cardiovascular morbidity or mortality. However, definitive evidence regarding the risks with iron administration in dialysis patients is lacking. Nevertheless, there is a need to strike a balance between facilitating erythropoiesis and minimizing short- and long-term risk.

To conclude, individuals with either a transferrin saturation <20% or serum ferritin <100 ng/mL can be considered to have absolute iron deficiency and require iron repletion [8]. The regimen is dependent upon whether the patient is undergoing maintenance hemodialysis or peritoneal dialysis. Individuals with apparent ESA resistance or with transferrin saturation between 20% and 50% and with serum ferritin between 100 and 800 ng/mL, may have functional iron deficiency and may also receive a trial of intravenous iron therapy [8]. Maintenance, weekly intravenous iron should be administered in hemodialysis patients to maintain TSAT between 20% and 50% and serum ferritin between 100 and 800–1200 ng/mL [8]. There is no evidence to support the use of maintenance doses of iron to patients undergoing peritoneal dialysis.

VITAMIN C

Role in Anemia of Kidney Disease

Vitamin C is a potentially useful but under-utilized adjuvant for ESA therapy in dialysis-dependent patients since it maintains iron in a reduced state. This, in turn, potentiates the intestinal absorption of iron and the enzymatic incorporation of iron into protoporphyrin, an intermediate in heme biosynthesis [37].

Status in Maintenance Dialysis Patients

Several recent clinical studies have reported that 30–50% of dialysis-dependent patients have subclinical vitamin C deficiency [38–42]; limited evidence suggests that this is more frequent in patients undergoing maintenance hemodialysis, particularly in those undergoing extended-hours treatments [42,43]. Furthermore, epidemiologic studies have demonstrated an inverse association between vitamin C levels and all-cause and cardiovascular mortality, and the occurrence of fatal and non-fatal cardiovascular events [38,41]. Whether the association is causal and/or mediated by the effect of vitamin C on ESA responsiveness or erythropoiesis has not been examined thus far.

Evidence and Recommendations

Over the last few years, at least six clinical trials have evaluated the effect of adjuvant vitamin C therapy in ESA-treated dialysis dependent patients [44–48]; the data from these studies have been summarized using at least two meta-analyses [49,50]. All except one of these studies enrolled less than 50 patients, the administered doses ranged from 500 mg once to thrice weekly, and the follow-up ranged from two to six months [49]. When administered as adjuvant therapy to ESA-treated patients with hemoglobin <11 g/dL, the weighted mean difference was 0.9 g/dL higher in patients who received vitamin C [49]. Furthermore, the weighted mean difference for the erythropoietin dose was 17 units/kg/week lower with significantly higher transferrin saturation. The latter finding, along with other suggestive evidence, indicates that administration of vitamin C may have a salutary effect on mobilization of the body iron stores [51,52].

Care needs to be exercised, since vitamin C supplements can lead to oxalate accumulation in dialysis patients [53,54]. The available data suggest that the total daily dose of ascorbic acid should not exceed 150 mg/d in individuals with chronic kidney disease; short-term studies with this dose, for up to 8 weeks, have not demonstrated any increase in serum oxalate levels [52]. There is additional concern that vitamin C may behave as an oxidant and enhance cellular toxicity in individuals with iron overload. However, the evidence to support this concern is limited.

In summary, adjuvant therapy with vitamin C may potentiate the response to ESAs in dialysis-dependent patients particularly in those with hyperferritinemia and low transferrin saturation.

VITAMIN D

Role in Anemia of Kidney Disease

The effect of vitamin D on anemia associated with chronic kidney disease and ESA requirements may be mediated by two potential mechanisms. First, secondary hyperparathyroidism associated with chronic kidney disease results in osteitis fibrosa cystica, a condition associated with bone marrow fibrosis and ESA resistance [55]. The current clinical paradigm for the treatment of secondary hyperparathyroidism consists of the use of supraphysiologic doses of 1,25 dihydroxy vitamin D or its analogs. Thus, amelioration of hyperparathyroidism may be one of the potential mechanisms for the beneficial effects of vitamin D therapy on anemia management in dialysis-dependent patients. Consistent with the importance of secondary hyperparathyroidism, uncontrolled studies have demonstrated an increase in hemoglobin levels in dialysis patients who undergo parathyroidectomy or are treated with cinacalcet, a benefit that seems to parallel the reduction in serum parathyroid hormone levels [56–59]. Second, there appears to be a direct effect of vitamin D on hematopoiesis; 1,25 dihydroxy vitamin D has a synergistic effect on the ESA-stimulated proliferation of erythroid precursors in samples obtained from dialysis-dependent patients both in vitro and in vivo [60]. Consistent with these observations, addition of calcium and 1,25 dihydroxy vitamin D to cell cultures attenuates the uremia-associated decline in the growth rate of erythroid burst- and colony-forming units [61].

Status in Maintenance Dialysis Patients

Vitamin D, synthesized either in the skin or absorbed from the diet, undergoes 25-hydroxylation in the liver and 1-α hydroxylation in the kidney to form the active 1,25 dihydroxy vitamin D [62]. There is accumulating evidence for a high prevalence of 25-hydroxy vitamin D deficiency in dialysis-dependent patients and there is an inverse association between serum 25-hydroxy vitamin D levels and death risk in this population [63,64]. In addition to low availability of substrate (25-hydroxy vitamin D), there are at least two additional mechanisms that contribute to the high prevalence of 1,25 dihydroxy vitamin D in patients with kidney diseases. First, loss of renal function is associated with a progressive increase in serum fibroblast growth factor-23 which is a potent inhibitor of 1-α hydroxlase [65]. Furthermore, reduced renal mass with progressive kidney disease is associated with reduced number of cells with 1α hydroxylase activity. Epidemiologic studies have demonstrated a lower death risk in dialysis patients treated with active vitamin D therapy [66]. However, there is no clinical trial evidence to corroborate this benefit representing a direct or indirect effect of vitamin D on erythropoiesis in mediating this benefit.

Evidence and Recommendations

There are two groups of vitamin D compounds that can potentially be used in the clinical setting — calciferols (chole- or ergocalciferol; 25-hydroxy vitamin D), or active vitamin D (1,25 dihydroxy vitamin D or its analogs). Presently, while calciferols are used to correct 25-hydroxy vitamin D deficiency, 1,25 dihydroxy vitamin D or analogs are used for the treatment of secondary hyperparathyroidism. At least one uncontrolled study has examined the effect of correction of 25-hydroxy D deficiency in hemodialysis patients with ergocalciferol on ESA requirements; the trend towards a lower dose with calciferol therapy did not reach statistical significance [67]. Similarly, small uncontrolled studies have demonstrated improvements in anemia management with aggressive treatment of secondary hyperparathyroidism with active vitamin D [68–71]. However, the quality of evidence is currently not strong enough to recommend the use of any of the vitamin D preparations for the sole purpose of facilitating anemia management.

FOLIC ACID

Role in Anemia of Kidney Disease

Like iron, folic acid is a key nutrient required for erythropoiesis. It serves as a co-factor for DNA synthesis, and its requirements are increased in the face of increased cell turnover. At least one study has demonstrated that dialysis patients with higher folic acid levels have lower mortality and fewer cardiovascular events [72]. Whether this association is mediated through salutary effect on erythropoiesis, or simply reflects better health of the patients, however, is not known.

Status in Maintenance Dialysis Patients

Folic acid, a water-soluble vitamin, is lost during dialytic therapy, particularly with high-flux hemodialysis [73,74]. Several recent reports have indicated that there is variable prevalence of folate deficiency in the dialysis population; most studies, however, report a low prevalence of folic acid deficiency in such individuals even in the absence of folate supplementation [4,73,75–80].

Evidence and Recommendations

Several published reports have suggested a role for folic acid deficiency in mediating ESA resistance in individuals undergoing maintenance dialysis [80–82]. Moreover, some reports have indicated the development of macrocytosis in individuals undergoing ESA treatment which is prevented with folate supplementation [83]. However, it appears that routine supplementation is not necessary to optimize the response to ESA therapy in most patients [84]. Hence, an expert group has recommended folate supplementation (2–3 mg/week) for dialysis patients receiving ESAs [85]; higher doses may be considered for patients with overt macrocytosis.

VITAMIN B₆ (PYRIDOXINE)

Role in Anemia of Kidney Disease

Vitamin B₆ is a co-factor in the formation of δ-amino levulinic acid, a rate-limiting step in heme biosynthesis. Vitamin B₆ also plays a potentially important role in the incorporation of iron into protoporphyrin, the final step in heme synthesis. Hence, vitamin B₆ is an important nutrient for erythropoiesis.

Status in Maintenance Dialysis Patients

There is evidence that in the absence of supplementation, there is a high prevalence of vitamin B₆ deficiency. Vitamin B₆ metabolism is impaired in individuals with ESRD. The metabolism of pyridoxal phosphate (the major active metabolite of vitamin B₆) is also impaired, and there are increased vitamin B₆ losses in the dialysate, particularly with high-flux hemodialysis [74,75,86–88]. More importantly, vitamin B₆ is consumed during treatment with ESA, and oral supplementation prevents the depletion of erythrocyte vitamin B₆ [89,90].

Evidence and Recommendations

There are at least two studies that have evaluated the role of vitamin B₆ supplementation on hemoglobin levels in dialysis patients receiving ESAs. In the first study, vitamin B_6 supplementation alone or with intravenous iron therapy, resulted in a significant increase in the hematocrit in hemodialysis patients who had microcytic and hypochromic anemia even though they had normal plasma pyridoxine levels [91]. In the second study, vitamin B_6 supplementation for hemodialysis patients with normal plasma pyridoxine levels failed to result in an increase in hematocrit [92].

It is recommended that dialysis patients receiving ESAs should be given supplemental pyridoxine hydrochloride, 100–150 mg/week.

VITAMIN B_{12}

Status in Maintenance Dialysis Patients

Vitamin B_{12} deficiency is unusual in patients undergoing maintenance dialysis because it is a large compound, is largely protein bound in serum, and hence, poorly dialyzable [4,79,93–95]. Vitamin B_{12} deficiency is uncommon even in hemodialysis patients treated with high-flux dialyzers, or with longer treatment times (>15 hours/week) [43].

Evidence and Recommendations

Although vitamin B_{12} is necessary for normal erythropoiesis, there is no direct evidence for the value of vitamin B_{12} supplementation in dialysis patients receiving ESAs. There is no demonstrable effect of vitamin B_{12} supplementation on either hemoglobin levels or darbapoietin dose in hemodialysis patients with macrocytosis [96]. Nevertheless, it may be prudent to provide low-dose vitamin B_{12} supplementation (0.25 mg/month) to dialysis patients receiving ESAs [85].

CARNITINE

Role in Anemia of Kidney Disease

Although the most important cause for the anemia associated with chronic kidney disease is erythropoietin deficiency, increased osmotic fragility leading to reduced red blood cell survival also appears to play a role [97,98]. Since L-carnitine plays a key role in lipid metabolism, it has been postulated that a deficiency of L-carnitine or alteration in carnitine metabolism may contribute to the reduction in red blood cell survival observed in uremia [99,100]. Matsumura et al. [100] demonstrated an increased red cell osmotic fragility in individuals with low carnitine levels. Furthermore, some but not all studies have demonstrated an

improvement in red blood cell fragility of dialysis patients treated with L-carnitine [101,102]. These data form the rationale for considering L-carnitine as a potentially useful adjunct for the management of anemia in dialysis patients treated with ESAs.

Status in Maintenance Dialysis Patients

L-carnitine is dialyzable, and hence, serum levels of free carnitine are sub-normal in many dialysis patients [103,104]. Moreover, uremia is associated with an increased acylcarnitine to free carnitine ratio [103,104]. Free carnitine is also reduced in skeletal muscle of some long-term hemodialysis patients [105].

Evidence and Recommendations

Several clinical trials have demonstrated an increase in hemoglobin levels in maintenance dialysis patients treated with L-carnitine without the concomitant administration of ESAs [103,105,106]. Numerous studies have also evaluated the effect of L-carnitine supplementation on ESA requirements; however, many of these are small and uncontrolled observational studies; at least six of these were randomized trials [103]. Of these six randomized controlled trials, four reported a significant reduction in the ESA dose required to maintain a similar target hematocrit level [103]. Moreover, in three of four evaluable trials, there was a significant decline in the ESA resistance index. In a summative assessment of the data in a systematic review, a common effect size of −0.75 was observed, indicating an overall significant benefit [103].

Thus, there is suggestive evidence supporting a role for L-carnitine supplementation for individuals undergoing dialysis with ESA-resistance, in the absence of other known causes of this condition. However, there is a need to validate these findings in adequately powered randomized controlled clinical trials. In the meantime, L-carnitine supplementation may be considered for patients with ESA-resistant anemia, who have not responded to other standard treatments [85].

GROWTH HORMONE AND INSULIN-LIKE GROWTH FACTOR-I (IGF-I)

Role in Anemia of Kidney Disease

In humans, IGF-I is a key mediator of the anabolic actions of growth hormone. There is in vitro and in vivo evidence that growth hormone and IGF-I directly stimulates erythropoiesis and have a synergistic effect on the response of anemia to erythropoietin therapy in mice with kidney disease [107–112]. In addition to a direct effect on erythropoiesis, administration of growth hormone and/or IGF-I has been shown to result in an increase in circulating levels of endogenous erythropoietin levels [113]. In humans, this increase in endogenous erythropoietin levels is evident with administration of recombinant growth hormone in the presence of either chronic kidney disease or growth hormone deficiency [114,115]. Furthermore, evidence suggests a causal role for IGF-I in post-kidney transplant erythrocytosis as well as in the genesis of spontaneous erythrocytosis that occasionally occurs in dialysis patients [116,117].

Evidence and Recommendations

There are no studies that have evaluated the effect of either rhGH or IGF-I administration on either the response to ESA therapy or the dose requirements of ESA necessary to achieve the target hematocrit in dialysis patients. Thus, their use cannot be recommended as adjunctive treatment for the management of anemia in ESA-treated dialysis patients.

References

[1] Pfeffer MA, Burdmann EA, Chen CY, et al. A trial of darbepoetin alfa in type 2 diabetes and chronic kidney disease. N Engl J Med 2009;361:2019—32.

[2] Steinbrook R. Medicare and erythropoietin. N Engl J Med 2007;356:4—6.

[3] Singh AK, Szczech L, Tang KL, Barnhart H, Sapp S, Wolfson M. Reddan, D: Correction of anemia with epoetin alfa in chronic kidney disease. N Engl J Med 2006;355:2085—98.

[4] Hutchinson FN, Jones WJ. A cost-effectiveness analysis of anemia screening before erythropoietin in patients with end-stage renal disease. Am J Kidney Dis 1997;29:651—7.

[5] Mehrotra R, Berman N, Alistwani A, Kopple JD. Improvement of nutritional status after initiation of maintenance hemodialysis. Am J Kidney Dis 2002;40:133—42.

[6] Moore LW, Acchiardo S, Sargent JA, Burk L. Incidence, causes, and treatment of iron deficiency in haemodialysis patients. J Ren Nutr 1992;3:105—12.

[7] Bergmann M, Grutzmacher P, Heuser J, Kaltwasser JP. Iron metabolism under rEPO therapy in patients on maintenance hemodialysis. Int J Artif Organs 1990;13:109—12.

[8] National Kidney Foundation. KDOQI Clinical Practice Guidelines and Clinical Practice Recommendations for Anemia in Chronic Kidney Disease. Am J Kidney Dis 2006;47:S1—S145.

[9] Horl WH, Jacobs C, Macdougall IC, Valderrabano F, Parrondo I, Thompson K, et al. European best practice guidelines 14—16: inadequate response to epoetin. Nephrol Dial Transplant 2000;15(Suppl. 4):43—50.

[10] Allegra V, Mengozzi G, Vasile A. Iron deficiency in maintenance hemodialysis patients: assessment of diagnosis criteria and of three different iron treatments. Nephron 1991;57:175—82.

[11] Fishbane S, Frei GL, Maesaka J. Reduction in recombinant human erythropoietin doses by the use of chronic intravenous iron supplementation. Am J Kidney Dis 1995;26:41—6.

[12] Wingard RL, Parker RA, Ismail N, Hakim RM. Efficacy of oral iron therapy in patients receiving recombinant human erythropoietin. Am J Kidney Dis 1995;25:433—9.

[13] Macdougall IC, Tucker B, Thompson J, Tomson CR, Baker LR, Raine AE. A randomized controlled study of iron supplementation in patients treated with erythropoietin. Kidney Int 1996;50:1694—9.

[14] Sunder-Plassmann G, Horl WH. Importance of iron supply for erythropoietin therapy. Nephrol Dial Transplant 1995;10:2070—6.

[15] Charytan C, Levin N, Al-Saloum M, Hafeez T, Gagnon S, Van Wyck DB. Efficacy and safety of iron sucrose for iron deficiency in patients with dialysis-associated anemia: North American clinical trial. Am J Kidney Dis 2001;37:300—7.

[16] Schwenk MH. Ferumoxytol: a new intravenous iron preparation for the treatment of iron deficiency anemia in patients with chronic kidney disease. Pharmacotherapy 2010;30:70—9.

[17] Moore RA, Gaskell H, Rose P, Allan J. Meta-analysis of efficacy and safety of intravenous ferric carboxymaltose (Ferinject) from clinical trial reports and published trial data. BMC blood disorders 2011;11:4.

[18] Bailie GR. Comparison of rates of reported adverse events associated with i.v. iron products in the United States. American journal of health-system pharmacy: AJHP: official journal of the American Society of Health-System Pharmacists 2012;69:310—20.

[19] Taylor JE, Peat N, Porter C, Morgan AG. Regular low-dose intravenous iron therapy improves response to erythropoietin in haemodialysis patients. Nephrol Dial Transplant 1996;11:1079—83.

[20] Coyne DW, Kapoian T, Suki W, Singh AK, Moran JE, Dahl NV, et al. Ferric gluconate is highly efficacious in anemic hemodialysis patients with high serum ferritin and low transferrin saturation: results of the Dialysis Patients' Response to IV Iron with Elevated Ferritin (DRIVE) Study. J Am Soc Nephrol 2007;18:975—84.

[21] Kapoian T, O'Mara NB, Singh AK, Moran J, Rizkala AR, Geronemus R, et al. Ferric gluconate reduces epoetin requirements in hemodialysis patients with elevated ferritin. J Am Soc Nephrol 2008;19:372—9.

[22] Fishbane S, Lynn RI. The utility of zinc protoporphyrin for predicting the need for intravenous iron therapy in hemodialysis patients. Am J Kidney Dis 1995;25:426—32.

[23] Macdougall IC, Cavill I, Hulme B, Bain B, McGregor E, McKay P, et al. Detection of functional iron deficiency during erythropoietin treatment: a new approach. Bmj 1992;304:225—6.

[24] Schaefer RM, Schaefer L. The hypochromic red cell: a new parameter for monitoring of iron supplementation during rhEPO therapy. J Perinatal Med 1995;23:83—8.

[25] Mittman N, Sreedhara R, Mushnick R, Chattopadhyay J, Zelmanovic D, Vaseghi M, et al. Reticulocyte hemoglobin content predicts functional iron deficiency in hemodialysis patients receiving rHuEPO. Am J Kidney Dis 1997;30:912—22.

[26] Park CH, Valore EV, Waring AJ, Ganz T. Hepcidin, a urinary antimicrobial peptide synthesized in the liver. J Biol Chem 2001;276:7806—10.

[27] Ganz T. Molecular control of iron transport. J Am Soc Nephrol 2007;18:394—400.

[28] Ashby DR, Gale DP, Busbridge M, et al. Plasma hepcidin levels are elevated but responsive to erythropoietin therapy in renal disease. Kidney Int 2009;75:976—81.

[29] Zaritsky J, Young B, Wang HJ, Westerman M, Olbina G, Nemeth E, et al. Hepcidin — a potential novel biomarker for iron status in chronic kidney disease. Clin J Am Soc Nephrol 2009;4:1051—6.

[30] Weiss G, Theurl I, Eder S, Koppelstaetter C, Kurz K, Sonnweber T, et al. Serum hepcidin concentration in chronic haemodialysis patients: associations and effects of dialysis, iron and erythropoietin therapy. Eur J Clin Invest 2009;39:883—90.

[31] Tessitore N, Girelli D, Campostrini N, Bedogna V, Pietro Solero G, Castagna A, et al. Hepcidin is not useful as a biomarker for iron needs in haemodialysis patients on maintenance erythropoiesis-stimulating agents. Nephrol Dial Transplant 2010;25:3996—4002.

[32] Seifert A, von Herrath D, Schaefer K. Iron overload, but not treatment with desferrioxamine favours the development of septicemia in patients on maintenance hemodialysis. Q J Med 1987;65:1015—24.

[33] Hoen B, Kessler M, Hestin D, Mayeux D. Risk factors for bacterial infections in chronic haemodialysis adult patients: a multicentre prospective survey. Nephrol Dial Transplant 1995;10:377—81.

[34] Hoen B, Paul-Dauphin A, Hestin D, Kessler M. EPIBACDIAL: a multicenter prospective study of risk factors for bacteremia in chronic hemodialysis patients. J Am Soc Nephrol 1998;9:869—76.

[35] Kuo KL, Hung SC, Wei YH, Tarng DC. Intravenous iron exacerbates oxidative DNA damage in peripheral blood lymphocytes in chronic hemodialysis patients. J Am Soc Nephrol 2008;19:1817—26.

[36] Tovbin D, Mazor D, Vorobiov M, Chaimovitz C, Meyerstein N. Induction of protein oxidation by intravenous iron in hemodialysis patients: role of inflammation. Am J Kidney Dis 2002;40:1005—12.

[37] Goldberg A. The enzymic formation of haem by the incorporation of iron into protoporphyrin; importance of ascorbic acid, ergothioneine and glutathione. Br J Haematol 1959;5:150—7.

[38] Deicher R, Ziai F, Bieglmayer C, Schillinger M, Horl WH. Low total vitamin C plasma level is a risk factor for cardiovascular morbidity and mortality in hemodialysis patients. J Am Soc Nephrol 2005;16:1811—8.

[39] Singer R, Rhodes HC, Chin G, Kulkarni H, Ferrari P. High prevalence of ascorbate deficiency in an Australian peritoneal dialysis population. Nephrology (Carlton, Vic) 2008;13:17—22.

[40] Finkelstein FO, Juergensen P, Wang S, Santacroce S, Levine M, Kotanko P, et al. Hemoglobin and plasma vitamin C levels in patients on peritoneal dialysis. Perit Dial Int 2011;31:74—9.

[41] Dashti-Khavidaki S, Talasaz AH, Tabeefar H, Hajimahmoodi M, Moghaddam G, Khalili H, et al. Plasma vitamin C concentrations in patients on routine hemodialysis and its relationship to patients' morbidity and mortality. International journal for vitamin and nutrition research Internationale Zeitschrift fur Vitamin- und Ernahrungsforschung J Internat Vitaminol Nutr 2011;81:197—203.

[42] Zhang K, Dong J, Cheng X, Bai W, Guo W, Wu L, et al. Association between vitamin C deficiency and dialysis modalities. Nephrology (Carlton, Vic) 2012;17:452—7.

[43] Coveney N, Polkinghorne KR, Linehan L, Corradini A, Kerr PG. Water-soluble vitamin levels in extended hours hemodialysis. Hemodial Int 2011;15:30—8.

[44] Sezer S, Ozdemir FN, Yakupoglu U, Arat Z, Turan M, Haberal M. Intravenous ascorbic acid administration for erythropoietin-hyporesponsive anemia in iron loaded hemodialysis patients. Artificial Organs 2002;26:366—70.

[45] Deira J, Diego J, Martinez R, Oyarbide A, Gonzalez A, Diaz H, et al. Comparative study of intravenous ascorbic acid versus low-dose desferroxamine in patients on hemodialysis with hyperferritinemia. J Nephrol 2003;16:703—9.

[46] Chan D, Irish A, Dogra G. Efficacy and safety of oral versus intravenous ascorbic acid for anaemia in haemodialysis patients. Nephrology (Carlton, Vic) 2005;10:336—40.

[47] Giancaspro V, Nuzziello M, Pallotta G, Sacchetti A, Petrarulo F. Intravenous ascorbic acid in hemodialysis patients with functional iron deficiency: a clinical trial. J Nephrol 2000;13:444—9.

[48] Keven K, Kutlay S, Nergizoglu G, Erturk S. Randomized, crossover study of the effect of vitamin C on EPO response in hemodialysis patients. Am J Kidney Dis 2003;41:1233—9.

[49] Deved V, Poyah P, James MT, Tonelli M, Manns BJ, Walsh M, et al. Ascorbic acid for anemia management in hemodialysis patients: a systematic review and meta-analysis. Am J Kidney Dis 2009;54:1089—97.

[50] Einerson B, Nathorn C, Kitiyakara C, Sirada M, Thamlikitkul V. The efficacy of ascorbic acid in suboptimal responsive anemic hemodialysis patients receiving erythropoietin: a meta-analysis. J Med Assoc Thailand = Chotmaihet thangphaet 2011;94(Suppl. 1):S134—46.

[51] Tarng DC, Huang TP. A parallel, comparative study of intravenous iron versus intravenous ascorbic acid for erythropoietin-hyporesponsive anaemia in haemodialysis patients with iron overload. Nephrol Dial Transplant 1998;13:2867—72.

[52] Tarng DC, Wei YH, Huang TP, Kuo BI, Yang WC. Intravenous ascorbic acid as an adjuvant therapy for recombinant erythropoietin in hemodialysis patients with hyperferritinemia. Kidney Int 1999;55:2477—86.

[53] Pru C, Eaton J, Kjellstrand C. Vitamin C intoxication and hyperoxalemia in chronic hemodialysis patients. Nephron 1985;39:112—6.

[54] Alkhunaizi AM, Chan L. Secondary oxalosis: a cause of delayed recovery of renal function in the setting of acute renal failure. J Am Soc Nephrol 1996;7:2320—6.

[55] Rao DS, Shih MS, Mohini R. Effect of serum parathyroid hormone and bone marrow fibrosis on the response to erythropoietin in uremia. N Engl J Med 1993;328:171—5.

[56] Zingraff J, Drueke T, Marie P, Man NK, Jungers P, Bordier P. Anemia and secondary hyperparathyroidism. Arch Intern Med 1978;138:1650—2.

[57] Barbour GL. Effect of parathyroidectomy on anemia in chronic renal failure. Arch Intern Med 1979;139:889—91.

[58] Urena P, Eckardt KU, Sarfati E, Zingraff J, Zins B, Roullet JB, et al. Serum erythropoietin and erythropoiesis in primary and secondary hyperparathyroidism: effect of parathyroidectomy. Nephron 1991;59:384—93.

[59] Battistella M, Richardson RM, Bargman JM, Chan CT. Improved parathyroid hormone control by cinacalcet is associated with reduction in darbepoetin requirement in patients with end-stage renal disease. Clin Nephrol 2011;76:99—103.

[60] Aucella F, Scalzulli RP, Gatta G, Vigilante M, Carella AM, Stallone C. Calcitriol increases burst-forming unit-erythroid proliferation in chronic renal failure. A synergistic effect with r-HuEpo. Nephron Clin Pract 2003;95:c121—7.

[61] Carozzi S, Ramello A, Nasini MG, Schelotto C, Caviglia PM, Cantaluppi A, et al. Ca++ and 1,25(OH)2D3 regulate in vitro and in vivo the response to human recombinant erythropoietin in CAPD patients. Adv Perit Dial 1990;6:312—5.

[62] Holick MF. Vitamin D deficiency. N Engl J Med 2007;357:266—81.

[63] Wolf M, Shah A, Gutierrez O, Ankers E, Monroy M, Tamez H, et al. Vitamin D levels and early mortality among incident hemodialysis patients. Kidney Int 2007;72:1004—13.

[64] Wang AY, Lam CW, Sanderson JE, Wang M, Chan IH, Lui SF, et al. Serum 25-hydroxyvitamin D status and cardiovascular outcomes in chronic peritoneal dialysis patients: a 3-y prospective cohort study. Am J Clin Nutr 2008;87:1631—8.

[65] Shimada T, Hasegawa H, Yamazaki Y, Muto T, Hino R, Takeuchi Y, et al. Yamashita, T: FGF-23 is a potent regulator of vitamin D metabolism and phosphate homeostasis. J Bone Miner Res 2004;19:429—35.

[66] Teng M, Wolf M, Ofsthun MN, Lazarus JM, Hernan MA, Camargo Jr CA. Thadhani, R: Activated injectable vitamin D and hemodialysis survival: a historical cohort study. J Am Soc Nephrol 2005;16:1115—25.

[67] Kumar VA, Kujubu DA, Sim JJ, Rasgon SA, Yang PS. Vitamin D supplementation and recombinant human erythropoietin utilization in vitamin D-deficient hemodialysis patients. J Nephrol 2011;24:98—105.

[68] Albitar S, Genin R, Fen-Chong M, Serveaux MO, Schohn D, Chuet C. High-dose alfacalcidol improves anaemia in patients on haemodialysis. Nephrol Dial Transplant 1997;12:514—8.

[69] Argiles A, Mourad G, Lorho R, Kerr PG, Flavier JL, Canaud B, et al. Medical treatment of severe hyperparathyroidism and its influence on anaemia in end-stage renal failure. Nephrol Dial Transplant 1994;9:1809—12.

[70] Goicoechea M, Vazquez MI, Ruiz MA, Gomez-Campdera F, Perez-Garcia R, Valderrabano F. Intravenous calcitriol improves anaemia and reduces the need for erythropoietin in haemodialysis patients. Nephron 1998;78:23—7.

[71] Capuano A, Serio V, Pota A, Memoli B, Andreucci VE. Beneficial effects of better control of secondary hyperparathyroidism with paricalcitol in chronic dialysis patients. J Nephrol 2009;22:59—68.

[72] Fellah H, Feki M, Taieb SH, Hammami B, Boubaker K, Lacour B, et al. Vitamin A, E, B12, and folic acid in end-stage renal disease Tunisian patients: status and predictive value for overall mortality and cardiovascular events. Clinical laboratory 2011;57:939—46.

[73] Lasseur C, Parrot F, Delmas Y, Level C, Ged C, Redonnet-Vernhet I, et al. Impact of high-flux/high-efficiency dialysis on folate and homocysteine metabolism. J Nephrol 2001;14:32—5.

[74] Leblanc M, Pichette V, Geadah D, Ouimet D. Folic acid and pyridoxal-5′-phosphate losses during high-efficiency hemodialysis in patients without hydrosoluble vitamin supplementation. J Ren Nutr 2000;10:196—201.

[75] Boeschoten EW, Schrijver J, Krediet RT, Schreurs WH, Arisz L. Deficiencies of vitamins in CAPD patients: the effect of supplementation. Nephrol Dial Transplant 1988;3:187—93.

[76] Westhuyzen J, Matherson K, Tracey R, Fleming SJ. Effect of withdrawal of folic acid supplementation in maintenance hemodialysis patients. Clin Nephrol 1993;40:96—9.

[77] Bamonti-Catena F, Buccianti G, Porcella A, Valenti G, Como G, Finazzi S, et al. Folate measurements in patients on regular hemodialysis treatment. Am J Kidney Dis 1999;33:492—7.

[78] Tremblay R, Bonnardeaux A, Geadah D, Busque L, Lebrun M, Ouimet D, et al. Hyperhomocysteinemia in hemodialysis patients: effects of 12-month supplementation with hydrosoluble vitamins. Kidney Int 2000;58:851—8.

[79] Billion S, Tribout B, Cadet E, Queinnec C, Rochette J, Wheatley P, et al. Hyperhomocysteinaemia, folate and vitamin B12 in unsupplemented haemodialysis patients: effect of oral therapy with folic acid and vitamin B12. Nephrol Dial Transplant 2002;17:455—61.

[80] Bamgbola OF, Kaskel F. Role of folate deficiency on erythropoietin resistance in pediatric and adolescent patients on chronic dialysis. Pediatr Nephrol 2005;20:1622—9.

[81] Breen CP, Macdougall IC. Correction of epoetin-resistant megaloblastic anaemia following vitamin B(12) and folate administration. Nephron 1999;83:374—5.

[82] Schiffl H, Lang SM. Folic acid deficiency modifies the haematopoietic response to recombinant human erythropoietin in maintenance dialysis patients. Nephrol Dial Transplant 2006;21:133—7.

[83] Pronai W, Riegler-Keil M, Silberbauer K, Stockenhuber F. Folic acid supplementation improves erythropoietin response. Nephron 1995;71:395—400.

[84] Ono K, Hisasue Y. Is folate supplementation necessary in hemodialysis patients on erythropoietin therapy. Clin Nephrol 1992;38:290—2.

[85] Horl WH. Is there a role for adjuvant therapy in patients being treated with epoetin? Nephrol Dial Transplant 1999;14(Suppl. 2):50—60.

[86] Kopple JD, Mercurio K, Blumenkrantz MJ, Jones MR, Tallos J, Roberts C, et al. Daily requirement for pyridoxine supplements in chronic renal failure. Kidney Int 1981;19:694—704.

[87] Blumberg A, Hanck A. Sander, G: Vitamin nutrition in patients on continuous ambulatory peritoneal dialysis (CAPD). Clin Nephrol 1983;20:244—50.

[88] Kasama R, Koch T, Canals-Navas C, Pitone JM. Vitamin B6 and hemodialysis: the impact of high-flux/high-efficiency dialysis and review of the literature. Am J Kidney Dis 1996;27:680—6.

[89] Mydlik M, Derzsiova K. Erythrocyte vitamins B1, B2 and B6 and erythropoietin. Am J Nephrol 1993;13:464—6.

[90] Mydlik M, Derzsiova K, Zemberova E. Metabolism of vitamin B6 and its requirement in chronic renal failure. Kidney Int Suppl 1997;62:S56—9.

[91] Toriyama T, Matsuo S, Fukatsu A, Takahashi H, Sato K, Mimuro N, et al. Effects of high-dose vitamin B6 therapy on microcytic and hypochromic anemia in hemodialysis patients. Nihon Jinzo Gakkai shi 1993;35:975—80.

[92] Weissgarten J, Modai D, Oz D, Chen Levy Z, Cohn M, Marcus O, et al. Vitamin B(6) therapy does not improve hematocrit in hemodialysis patients supplemented with iron and erythropoietin. Nephron 2001;87:328—32.

[93] Descombes E, Hanck AB, Fellay G. Water soluble vitamins in chronic hemodialysis patients and need for supplementation. Kidney Int 1993;43:1319—28.

[94] Zachee P, Chew SL, Daelemans R, Lins RL. Erythropoietin resistance due to vitamin B12 deficiency. Case report and retrospective analysis of B12 levels after erythropoietin treatment. Am J Nephrol 1992;12:188—91.

[95] De Vecchi AF, Bamonti-Catena F, Finazzi S, Patrosso C, Taioli E, Novembrino C, et al. Homocysteine, vitamin B12, serum and erythrocyte folate in peritoneal dialysis patients. Clin Nephrol 2001;55:313—7.

[96] Su VC, Shalansky K, Jastrzebski J, Martyn A, Li G, Yeung CK, et al. Zalunardo, N: Parenteral vitamin B12 in macrocytic hemodialysis patients reduced MMA levels but did not change mean red cell volume or hemoglobin. Clin Nephrol 2011;75:336—45.

[97] Rosenmund A, Binswanger U, Straub PW. Oxidative injury to erythrocytes, cell rigidity, and splenic hemolysis in hemodialyzed uremic patients. Ann Intern Med 1975;82:460—5.

[98] Zachee P, Ferrant A, Daelemans R, Coolen L, Goossens W, Lins RL, et al. Oxidative injury to erythrocytes, cell rigidity and splenic hemolysis in hemodialyzed patients before and during erythropoietin treatment. Nephron 1993;65:288—93.

[99] Kooistra MP, Struyvenberg A, van Es A. The response to recombinant human erythropoietin in patients with the anemia of end-stage renal disease is correlated with serum carnitine levels. Nephron 1991;57:127—8.

[100] Matsumura M, Hatakeyama S, Koni I, Mabuchi H, Muramoto H. Correlation between serum carnitine levels and erythrocyte osmotic fragility in hemodialysis patients. Nephron 1996;72:574—8.

[101] Nikolaos S, George A, Telemachos T, Maria S, Yannis M, Konstantinos M. Effect of L-carnitine supplementation on red blood cells deformability in hemodialysis patients. Renal Failure 2000;22:73–80.

[102] Labonia WD. L-carnitine effects on anemia in hemodialyzed patients treated with erythropoietin. Am J Kidney Dis 1995;26:757–64.

[103] Hurot JM, Cucherat M, Haugh M, Fouque D. Effects of L-carnitine supplementation in maintenance hemodialysis patients: a systematic review. J Am Soc Nephrol 2002;13:708–14.

[104] Hedayati SS. Dialysis-related carnitine disorder. Seminars in Dialysis 2006;19:323–8.

[105] Bellinghieri G, Savica V, Mallamace A, Di Stefano C, Consolo F, Spagnoli LG, et al. Correlation between increased serum and tissue L-carnitine levels and improved muscle symptoms in hemodialyzed patients. Am J Clin Nutr 1983;38:523–31.

[106] Rathod R, Baig MS, Khandelwal PN, Kulkarni SG, Gade PR, Siddiqui S. Results of a single blind, randomized, placebo-controlled clinical trial to study the effect of intravenous L-carnitine supplementation on health-related quality of life in Indian patients on maintenance hemodialysis. Indian J Med Sci 2006;60:143–53.

[107] Kurtz A, Jelkmann W, Bauer C. A new candidate for the regulation of erythropoiesis. Insulin-like growth factor I. FEBS Lett 1982;149:105–8.

[108] Akahane K, Tojo A, Urabe A, Takaku F. Pure erythropoietic colony and burst formations in serum-free culture and their enhancement by insulin-like growth factor I. Exp Hematol 1987;15:797–802.

[109] Claustres M, Chatelain P, Sultan C. Insulin-like growth factor I stimulates human erythroid colony formation in vitro. J Clin Endocrinol Metab 1987;65:78–82.

[110] Merchav S, Tatarsky I, Hochberg Z. Enhancement of erythropoiesis in vitro by human growth hormone is mediated by insulin-like growth factor I. Br J Haematol 1988;70:267–71.

[111] Kurtz A, Zapf J, Eckardt KU, Clemons G, Froesch ER, Bauer C. Insulin-like growth factor I stimulates erythropoiesis in hypophysectomized rats. Proc Natl Acad Sci USA 1988;85:7825–9.

[112] Brox AG, Zhang F, Guyda H, Gagnon RF. Subtherapeutic erythropoietin and insulin-like growth factor-1 correct the anemia of chronic renal failure in the mouse. Kidney Int 1996;50:937–43.

[113] Sohmiya M, Kato Y. Human growth hormone and insulin-like growth factor-I inhibit erythropoietin secretion from the kidneys of adult rats. J Endocrinol 2005;184:199–207.

[114] Sohmiya M, Kato Y. Effect of long-term administration of recombinant human growth hormone (rhGH) on plasma erythropoietin (EPO) and haemoglobin levels in anaemic patients with adult GH deficiency. Clin Endocrinol (Oxf) 2001;55:749–54.

[115] Sohmiya M, Ishikawa K, Kato Y. Stimulation of erythropoietin secretion by continuous subcutaneous infusion of recombinant human GH in anemic patients with chronic renal failure. Eur J Endocrinol 1998;138:302–6.

[116] Shih LY, Huang JY, Lee CT. Insulin-like growth factor I plays a role in regulating erythropoiesis in patients with end-stage renal disease and erythrocytosis. J Am Soc Nephrol 1999;10:315–22.

[117] Brox AG, Mangel J, Hanley JA, St Louis G, Mongrain S, Gagnon RF. Erythrocytosis after renal transplantation represents an abnormality of insulin-like growth factor-I and its binding proteins. Transplantation 1998;66:1053–8.

26

Nutritional and Non-nutritional Management of the Nephrotic Syndrome

Alessio Molfino[1,2,3], Burl R. Don[1], George A. Kaysen[1]

[1]Department of Internal Medicine, Division of Nephrology, University of California, Davis, USA
[2]Clinical Nutrition, Department of Internal Medicine, University of Rome "Tor Vergata", Rome, Italy
[3]Department of Clinical Medicine, Sapienza University of Rome, Rome, Italy

INTRODUCTION

The nephrotic syndrome is a consequence of the urinary loss of albumin and other plasma proteins of similar size and is characterized by hypoalbuminemia, hyperlipidemia and edema formation [1–4]. While albumin is the principal protein found in the urine, comprising between 75% and 90% of urinary protein, many other proteins are lost as well. These include transferrin, ceruloplasmin, and the binding proteins for vitamin D [5]. Albumin is the principal zinc carrying protein in plasma. Thus iron, zinc, copper, and a key metabolite that regulates calcium metabolism may all be lost in the urine in significant amounts with the nephrotic syndrome [6–8].

Lipoprotein metabolism is also greatly disturbed, either as a consequence of urinary protein loss [9], or as a consequence of hypoalbuminemia per se. Hyperlipidemia in the nephrotic syndrome is characterized by increased triglyceride levels, increased levels of low density lipoprotein (LDL) [10] and either a normal or reduced level of high density lipoprotein [11]. The atherogenic lipoprotein Lp(a) is also increased as a consequence of increased synthetic rate [12]. Thus disordered lipid metabolism imposes at least the potential for atherogenic risk to this patient population.

What role, if any, does dietary management play in the management of the nephrotic syndrome? The major rationale(s) for changing a patient's diet is to blunt manifestations of the syndrome, such as edema, to replace nutrients lost in the urine, or reduce risks either of progression of renal disease as might be caused by a high protein diet or of atherosclerosis that might be a consequence of altered lipid metabolism. It might also be possible that specific allergens contained in food may cause renal disease in some patients [13–17]. In this case dietary modification might prove curative.

The principal physiologic role of the kidney is to maintain internal solute balance within narrow limits despite wide differences in the intake of water, minerals, electrolytes, protein, and other nutrients. Fulfillment of this role requires renal function to change in response to variations in diet. Clearly the kidney must be able to quickly respond to changes in water, sodium or potassium ingestion; however, changes in dietary protein also cause functional adaptations in the kidney.

Renal blood flow, glomerular filtration rate (GFR) [18–20] and the permselective properties of the glomerular capillary [21–24] increase quickly following an augmentation in dietary protein intake. Renal hypertrophy also occurs [25–27]. Ingestion of protein results in the release of a cascade of hormones and vasoactive substances, including growth hormone [28], insulin [28], glucagon [29], kinins [30], prostaglandins [31], dopamine [32,33] and insulin-like growth factor-1 (IGF-1) [34,35]. In addition, the renin-angiotensin system has been implicated as one of the mediators of protein-induced hyperfiltration [36]. Dietary protein intake stimulates renin secretion [24] and the secondary formation of angiotensin II will, by its effect on efferent arteriolar vasoconstriction, increase intraglomerular capillary pressure and GFR [37]. The potent vasodilator, nitric oxide (NO) has also been proposed as a potential mediator of protein-induced hyperfiltration. NO is formed by the vascular endothelium from the guanidino group of arginine by the action of the enzyme nitric oxide synthase. Endothelial-derived NO plays a role in maintaining both afferent and efferent arteriolar vasodilation

FIGURE 26.1 Dietary protein augmentation causes increased secretion of glucagon by the pancreas, alters activity of the renin angiotensin axis, increases release of nitric oxide and augments renal prostaglandin synthesis [31]. These, and possibly other hormones, increase renal blood flow, glomerular filtration rate (GFR) and under some circumstances, increase hydraulic pressure across the glomerular capillary. These processes combine to decrease the selectivity of the glomerular capillary and increase proteinuria. Pharmacologic intervention that blocks either kinin, angiotensin II (Ang II) or aldosterone prevents the increase in proteinuria [21,45,48,69,114].

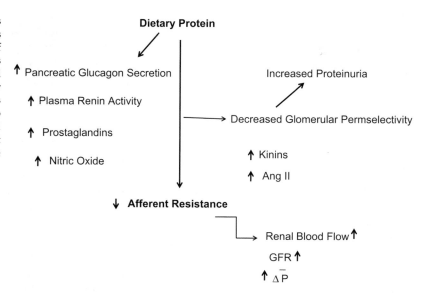

[38—40]. It is not surprising, therefore that the expression of a variety of renal diseases can be modified by changes in dietary protein (Figure 26.1).

DIETARY PROTEIN

In superficial ways, the nephrotic syndrome is similar to the type of protein-energy malnutrition known as Kwashiorkor. In both cases albumin concentration is reduced, plasma volume is expanded, and albumin pools shift from the extravascular to the vascular compartment. Metabolic abnormalities in the nephrotic syndrome include depletion of plasma [22,23,41—44] and tissue protein pools [45—47]. However, in the case of protein malnutrition it is possible to correct all of the manifestations by providing the needed protein and calories, while this is not the case in the nephrotic syndrome. Although average values for proteinuria are approximately 6 to 8 grams per day [22,42,48,49], approximately the amount contained in a hen's egg, simply increasing dietary protein by much more than that amount is of little demonstrable benefit. In fact, dietary protein supplementation causes a greater defect in the filtration barrier of the glomerular capillary [23,24] resulting in increased urinary protein losses (Figure 26.1). Kasiske et al. in a meta-analysis found that dietary protein restriction reduced the rate of decline in estimated glomerular filtration rate by only 0.53 mL/min/yr, although adjustments were not made for the degree of compliance to the prescribed diets. The effect of protein restriction was less in randomized versus nonrandomized trials. Interestingly, diabetic patients presented a relatively greater benefit versus nondiabetics, even though the number of diabetic patients was small and the duration of follow-up short

in most trials. Similarly, none of the baseline patient characteristics, such as the level of renal function or the degree of proteinuria, influenced the magnitude of the effect of a reduced-protein diet [50].

ALBUMIN HOMEOSTASIS IN THE NEPHROTIC SYNDROME

Albumin is the most abundant protein in plasma. The most notable change in plasma protein composition in the nephrotic syndrome is a decrease in plasma albumin concentrations. In nephrotic patients, the primary causes of hypoalbuminemia are urinary losses of albumin and an inappropriate increase in the fractional catabolic rate of albumin [51,52]. Although the albumin synthetic rate is increased in the nephrotic syndrome, it is insufficient to replace the losses of albumin due to urinary excretion and catabolism. Additionally, since the basal synthetic rate of albumin is approximately 10—14 grams per day, urinary losses in the average range for a nephrotic patient of 5 grams per day represent 30% of the total daily synthetic rate. Furthermore, if albumin concentrations were not reduced the urine losses would be even greater assuming a constant renal clearance, putting a further challenge on the capacity of the liver to increase albumin synthesis in response to external loss. In experiments that we conducted, when albumin synthesis was increased by dietary protein supplementation, urinary albumin excretion increased as did the absolute and fractional catabolic rate of albumin, while serum albumin concentrations did not [22]. The lack of an increase in albumin concentrations was in part a consequence of increased renal albumin clearance, as well as an increase in the fractional catabolic rate of albumin, but also in part a consequence of the limits of hepatic albumin synthesis.

It should also be recognized that total body protein synthesis does not increase in the nephrotic syndrome [53], so the protein lost in the urine is essentially supplied by reduced protein synthesis elsewhere, including in skeletal muscle may lead to wasting.

Dietary Protein and Renal Hemodyamics

Protein supplementation is followed rather promptly by an increase in both renal and splanchnic blood flow, by an increase in GFR in both humans [28] and animals [20,54–56], and by increased permeability of the glomerular capillary to protein. As a consequence, urinary albumin excretion increases when patients or animals with the nephrotic syndrome are fed a high protein diet [22,23,57–59], although a component of increased albuminuria may be a consequence of the added dietary acid load associated with protein intake acting through an endothelin mediated mechanism. [60,61]. The increase in albuminuria is not a consequence of increased plasma albumin levels. Plasma albumin levels either remain the same, or decrease following dietary protein augmentation, and in the rat plasma albumin invariably increases when dietary protein is restricted [21,23,45,62]. The fractional rate of albumin catabolism (the fraction of the plasma pool catabolized per unit time) also increases in nephrotic patients fed a high protein diet [22]. It may be more informative to look at fractional excretion of a specific protein rather than total excretion in order to estimate both the magnitude of the injury to the filtration barrier as well as to provide prognostic information [63]. Augmentation of dietary protein intake has two separate effects. One effect is an increase in albumin synthetic rate and the second is an increase in the fractional renal excretion. The latter predominates. It is unknown whether the increased fractional rate of protein catabolism is a direct effect of dietary protein intake on the albumin catabolic rate in catabolic sites throughout the body, or instead is a consequence of increased renal filtration of albumin followed by increased uptake and catabolism in the kidney of a greater amount of filtered albumin that occurs in patients eating a high protein diet. However, either way, the increased fractional rate of albumin catabolism, like the increase fractional renal clearance, will reduce albumin levels and negate the positive effect of increased albumin synthesis.

In this light, several studies investigated the molecular mechanisms underlying protein reabsorption in the proximal tubule. Megalin was the first receptor to be studied. It binds a variety of filtered molecules and is able to mediate endocytosis in the cytoplasmic tail.

Cubulin is a peripheral membrane protein and is thereby dependent on megalin to assure internalization of its ligands. Besides, megalin, cubulin also interacts on the apical membrane with another protein named amionless. The association between amionless and cubulin is mediated through the epidermal growth-factor-like repeats in cubulin [64].

In physiological conditions all filtered proteins are internalized by the receptor complex megalin/cubulin/amnionless, and the proteins are degraded within lysosomes. Normally low molecular weight proteins are filtered, reabsorbed and catabolized proximally. Even proteins as large as albumin are filtered and reabsorbed, but the fractional clearance is quite low, on the order of 10^{-4}. When glomerular permselectivity is altered, the fractional clearance of larger proteins is increased and the reabsorptive capacity of the proximal tubular cells is overwhelmed. Even the uptake of proteins normally catabolized by the proximal tubule completely, such as beta-2 microglobulin, lysozyme [65], N-acetyl-beta-D-glucosaminidase (NAG) or apo A I appear in the urine even though their glomerular clearance is unlikely to be increased. Protein accumulation in lysosomes, due to increased protein internalization, is thought to mediate inflammation and fibrosis, eventually leading to renal failure [64].

Thus, dietary protein augmentation causes three independent processes that may change plasma albumin concentration in proteinuric subjects: [1] an increase in the rate of albumin synthesis tending to increase albumin mass; [2] an increase in the fractional rate of albumin catabolism, tending to decrease albumin mass; and [3] an increase in urinary loss, also tending to deplete albumin pools. There are two possible mechanisms whereby increasing dietary protein intake worsens proteinuria. First, dietary protein intakes increases glomerular capillary hydraulic pressure which will facilitate greater protein passage across the glomerular capillary wall, and second, dietary protein may alter the permselectivity of the glomerular basement pore structure favoring larger pores. Chan et al. [37] demonstrated that dietary protein increases glomerular ultrafiltration pressure in nephrotic patients but did not alter glomerular permselectivity. This would suggest that glomerular porosity is not affected by dietary protein and that increased capillary pressure is the culprit for worsening of proteinuria. Rosenberg et al. [62], however, did show that dietary protein intake did alter glomerular permselectivity in patients with proteinuria and renal insufficiency. Thus, it may be that dietary protein worsens proteinuria both by increased glomerular pressures and by greater porosity of the glomerular basement membrane. In summary, proteinuria worsens and serum albumin concentrations may actually decrease in both nephrotic patients [22] and animals [23] following dietary protein augmentation.

The physiologic effects of amino acids on renal hemodynamics appears to depend upon the specific amino acids fed or infused. Infusion of branched chain amino acids, for example, fails to increase GFR or renal blood flow in normal rats [66] or humans [28], whereas infusion of arginine causes marked changes in renal hemodynamics [54], but not necessarily a change in urinary protein excretion. The renal hemodynamic response to dietary protein may therefore depend on specific amino acids in the proteins, rather than simply solute or nitrogen intake.

Since the increase in GFR and renal blood flow can be prevented by somatostatin [56], it is hypothesized that changes in renal function induced by protein or amino acid administration, are in part, hormonally mediated. Dietary protein augmentation causes an increased secretion of glucagon [20], corticosteroids [67,68], dopamine [33], and alters expression of the renin-angiotensin system [24], which, in turn, stimulates prostaglandin synthesis [31]. Increased pancreatic glucagon secretion seems to be necessary for the increase in GFR and renal blood flow [20] that follows dietary protein augmentation, however infusion of even large amounts of glucagon exerts no effect on urinary albumin excretion [62]. Paller and Hostetter demonstrated that high protein diets augment expression of the renin-angiotensin system in the rat [24] and that dietary protein augmentation resulted in altered glomerular permselectivity in nephrotic humans [57]. This observation has also been noted in patients [48]. There is, however, some conflicting data on the effect of a low protein diet on renal renin secretion. Martinez-Maldonado et al. suggest that renal Ang-II activity is increased during dietary protein restriction [36,67] and contributes to renal vasoconstriction and reduced GFR. This observation has not been corroborated by other studies, and most clinical and experimental studies suggest that protein administration increases plasma renin activity [24,48,57,69]. It is generally agreed that dietary protein intake leads to activation of the renin-angiotensin system, increased renal blood flow and GFR, and worsening of proteinuria in patients with pre-existing proteinuria. Moreover, it is well appreciated that inhibition of the renin-angiotensin system with angiotensin converting enzyme (ACE) inhibitors can blunt or prevent the proteinuric effect of dietary protein in experimental renal diseases [21,70,71] and in nephrotic patients [48,49].

The hormonal response to the infusion of amino acids, like the renal hemodynamic changes, is dependent, in part, upon the specific amino acids infused. Infusion of either a mixture of amino acids or arginine causes a prompt increase in the secretion both of growth hormone and glucagon, whereas infusion of branched chain amino acids do not [28,72]. In correlating the changes in GFR with an amino acid infusion, the plasma levels of insulin, growth hormone and glucagon all increase in response to the infusion, but only changes in glucagon exhibited a significant temporal relationship with changes in GFR [28].

A potential mediator of arginine-induced renal vasodilation may be NO, inasmuch as arginine is the substrate for NO production. In experimental animals however, arginine supplementation actually amliorates both proteinuria and hyperfiltration in diabetic rats, and has no effect on urinary albumin excretion in rats with passive Heymann nephritis [73]. Thus, like the protein-renin interaction outlined above, there are conflicting data regarding the relationship between arginine, its effect on renal hemodynamics, and how that is then translated into alterations in permselectivity.

DIETARY PROTEIN AND RENAL INJURY

By increasing the filtered load of protein, dietary protein supplementation may worsen renal injury. It is becoming more appreciated that proteinuria may be directly damaging to the renal interstitium [74] (Table 26.1). Several proteins, including albumin [75] and transferrin [76], have been implicated. Glomerular damage and the concomitant increased glomerular permeability results in a marked increase in protein filtration and initially in augmented proximal tubular reabsorption of protein. Filtered proteins are reabsorbed, carrying iron [77,78], complement components [79] and biologically active lipids [80] into the renal interstitial space causing injury. Consequently, tubular protein overload occurs leading to tubular cell injury leading to interstitial fibrosis [81]. This process probably involves the induction of cytokines and such other pro-inflammatory molecules as monocyte chemoattractant protein-1, osteopontin and platelet-derived growth factor [82]. The trafficking and deposition of excess filtered protein

TABLE 26.1 Adverse Effects of Proteinuria

Increased Tubular Reabsorption of Protein

Increased tubular exposure to filtered components of the complement cascade		Recruitment of macrophages
Increased tubular exposure to reabsorbed iron		Increased TGF β
		Increased PDGF
Increased tubular exposure to biologically active lipids		
Increased tubular exposure to filtered growth factors		

may be a link between the initial glomerular injury and the subsequent development of tubulointerstitial disease. The resulting tubulointerstitial disease is a better predictor of the glomerular filtration rate and long-term prognosis than is the severity of glomerular damage in almost all chronic progressive glomerular diseases, including IgA nephropathy, membranous nephropathy, membranoproliferative glomerulonephritis, and lupus nephritis [83–85]. Furthermore, diets that are high in protein also generate more acid, inducing the kidney to increase ammoniagenesis. Accelerated rates of renal ammonia production that result from increased dietary acid loads which accompany high protein diets may also lead to renal injury, possibly by the activation of complement [85,86]. Higher hydrogen ion concentrations enhance generation of endothelin-1 in the kidney, which also promotes progressive renal injury as well as increasing proteinuria [60,61] (see Chapter 18). The reduction in urinary protein excretion that follows dietary protein restriction potentially can have a salutary effect on progressive renal injury through any or all of these mechanisms. Thus, any process that reduces urinary protein losses should be encouraged.

Dietary protein restriction also reduces the synthesis and/or gene expression of several proteins thought to play a role in progression of renal injury, such as transforming growth factor β (TGF β) [87], platelet derived growth factor (PDGF) [88] and fibrinogen [89]. Whether decreased expression of these genes is a direct consequence of dietary protein restriction or instead a consequence of secondary effects of a protein restricted diet, such as decreased proteinuria with reduced contact of the interstitium to filtered plasma constituents, or reduced renal ammoniagenesis is unknown (Table 26.1). In nephrotic patients, the rate of fibrinogen synthesis is increased in proportion to the increased synthesis of albumin [90] and hyperfibrinogenemia may contribute to increased thrombosis associated with the nephrotic syndrome. Moreover, hyperfibrinogenemia may accelerate the progression of renal disease [91]. It is interesting to note that dietary protein restriction reduces the synthesis of both albumin and fibrinogen in nephrotic patients, however the serum levels of albumin tends to increase whereas serum fibrinogen levels decrease [90]. Thus, dietary protein restriction appears to have a favorable effect on both albumin and fibrinogen metabolism in nephrotic patients.

Several studies suggest that the composition of dietary protein may be as important as the absolute nitrogen content. In experimental studies in rats, dietary protein augmentation with a mixture of certain amino acids causes a prompt increase in urinary albumin excretion [62], while other amino acids, specifically branch chain amino acids, arginine, proline, glutamine, glutamate, aspartate or asparagine, are devoid of any effect on proteinuria [73]. Studies by D'Amico et al. [92] and Walser [93] suggest that dietary protein composition may also be of importance in humans with renal disease. D'Amico et al. found that when patients with the nephrotic syndrome were fed a vegetarian soy diet urinary protein excretion decreased as did blood lipid levels [92]. The diet was also low in fat (28% of calories) and of low protein content (0.71 g/kg normal body weight). The salutary effects of soy diets in nephrotic patients may be a consequence of the amino composition in those diets, although differences in lipid composition or in protein absorption may also explain the apparent benefit of these diets as well. In a subsequent study, fish oil was added to the vegetarian soy diet. However, the addition of fish oil did not give any additional benefit [94]. Walser has shown that supplementing a very low protein diet (0.3 g/kg/day) with essential amino acids or ketoacids not only reduced proteinuria in patients with the nephrotic syndrome, but also maintained or improved glomerular filtration rate. In fact, this regimen may induce a prolonged remission, even if the patients resume ingesting a normal diet. As noted by the investigators, the mechanism for this response is not known [95].

EFFECTS OF THE NEPHROTIC SYNDROME ON SOLID TISSUE PROTEINS

While it is more difficult to quantitate the losses of tissue protein, marked muscle wasting [47,96], sometimes obscured by edema, has been described in patients with continuous massive proteinuria. Rats with Heymann nephritis gain weight at a rate significantly less than normal rats [45]. While increasing dietary protein from 8.5% casein to 40% causes a significant increase in growth velocity in normal rats, dietary protein augmentation causes significantly less improvement in growth rate in rats with Heymann nephritis. In fact, nephrotic rats fed 40% protein gain weight significantly more slowly than do normal rats fed 8.5% protein [45], even though the difference in protein intake between 8.5% and 40% is many times greater than the urinary protein lost in either nephrotic group. When dietary protein is increased from 8.5% to 40% protein, total carcass (muscle) protein pools are increased in normal rats. In contrast, none of the increase in weight of nephrotic rats fed 40% protein is found in muscle, but instead is in viscera, namely liver and kidney [45]. Most of the increased protein nitrogen consumed when high protein diets are fed to these animals is excreted in the urine as urea [62,97].

Nephrotic rats have a reduced rate of muscle protein synthesis [46] and an increased rate of hepatic protein synthesis, providing a mechanism for growth impairment in these animals. Total body protein synthesis is the same in nephrotic and healthy rats [98], yet the nephrotic animals must replace the vast amounts of protein lost in the urine, which they do through increased hepatic protein synthesis [46]. In part, amino acid oxidation is reduced in nephrotic animals in response to the urinary protein losses [98]. It is unknown whether this represents an alteration in muscle metabolism [47,99].

These observations have supported the notion that dietary protein augmentation does not replete protein pools that have been depleted in nephrotic patients or animals, but in addition, high protein diets are detrimental in that they cause progressive renal injury in a variety of experimental renal diseases in animals [100] and in humans [101–103]. Since a high dietary protein intake is of no benefit in nephrotic patients or animals, a high protein diet, or completely unrestricted diet with regard to protein intake is not recommended.

The long term safety of a low protein diet is uncertain. Using leucine turnover rates as a marker of protein breakdown, Lim et al. [104] noted that nephrotic patients maintained positive nitrogen balance and had lower rates of protein degradation on a modestly restricted protein diet (0.9 g/kg/day) over a period of 35 days. Similarly, Maroni et al. [105] demonstrated that nephrotic patients ingesting 0.8 g/kg/day over a period of 24 days maintained positive nitrogen balance. The principal compensatory response to dietary protein restriction was a decrease in amino acid oxidation. In addition, the investigators noted an inverse correlation between leucine oxidation and the degree of proteinuria, suggesting that proteinuria is the stimulus to conserve dietary essential amino acids. Thus, modest protein restriction may be safe and an effective therapy in reducing proteinuria. However, there are no data on the effect of long-term restriction of protein to amounts much less than 0.8 g/kg/day in nephrotic patients. It is, therefore, probably not justifiable to place patients who are heavily proteinuric on diets that contain less than 0.8 g/kg/day except on an experimental basis.

Urinary urea excretion should be monitored to assure that patients are not eating more (or less) protein than recommended, and that proteinuria decreases (and plasma albumin and protein concentration do not decrease) when protein intake is restricted. Dietary protein intake can be estimated because, under steady state conditions, protein intake is only slightly more than the protein nitrogen appearance (PNA or PCR). Dietary protein intake generally exceeds PNA by about 3 to 7 g protein/day due to the unmeasured nitrogen losses through skin, respiration, etc (see Chapter 33). If total body urea pools do not change in any 24 hour period (i.e., serum urea nitrogen (SUN) is neither decreasing

nor increasing), it is possible to estimate the amount of protein that has been eaten by the formula:

$$\text{Protein nitrogen appearance} = (10.7 + 24 \text{ hour urinary urea excretion}/0.14) \text{ g/day} + \text{urinary protein excretion}$$

If there is variance from the prescribed diet, an accurate dietary intake history should be obtained and the diet adjusted accordingly.

It is still not known whether specific protein sources are clinically superior to others. The amino acid composition of the protein may turn out to be as important as the quantity of protein in the diet, but no specific recommendations can be made at this time. Clearly it is unlikely to be harmful to place patients on a largely vegetarian diet, considering the low fat content and the excellent results reported by D'Amico [92].

DIETARY PROTEINS AS POTENTIAL ALLERGENS RESPONSIBLE FOR RENAL DISEASE

The etiologic agents responsible for many diseases that cause the nephrotic syndrome are unknown. In some patients with minimal change nephrotic syndrome or patients with mesangial proliferation, exposure to specific dietary proteins, such as cow's milk has been implicated as causal [13–17,106]. Bovine serum albumin and casein have also been identified as an allergen in a patient with immune complex glomerulonephritis. In these cases, clinical remission followed removal of the offending agent from the diet. Lagrue et al. systematically evaluated 42 patients with steroid resistant nephrotic syndrome and ultimately seven of their patients entered remission following removal of offending antigens from their diet. Interpretation of these data is made difficult because these studies were not randomized prospective trials, and proteinuria may spontaneously remit without treatment in the nephrotic syndrome [15]. There is an association of gluten enteropathy IgA deposition in the glomeruli and the development of IgA nephropathy, and this may be due to an allergic reaction to gluten in the diet [107]. Overall, it is unclear what fraction of patients with the nephrotic syndrome have food allergy as a causative factor. Nevertheless, the possibility that food allergy might be responsible for the development of specific renal diseases is rarely considered by most clinicians and may be of over looked importance.

DIETARY FAT

Hyperlipidemia is common in the nephrotic syndrome and is a consequence of both increased synthesis and decreased catabolism of lipids and apolipoproteins [108–110]. The characteristic disorders in blood lipid composition in nephrotic patients are an increase in the low density lipoprotein (LDL), very low density lipoprotein (VLDL) [10] and/or intermediate density lipoprotein (IDL) fractions, but no change [10] or a decrease in high density lipoproteins (HDL) [11] resulting in an increased LDL/HDL cholesterol ratio. The IDL fraction probably rises as VLDL and chylomicron remnants which are atherogenic [111]. The atherogenic lipoprotein Lp(a) also increases in patients with the nephrotic syndrome [12]. All of these changes in the lipid profile in the nephrotic syndrome are characteristic of those which are associated with accelerated atherogenesis in other clinical settings.

In both nephrotic patients and rats, VLDL levels are increased predominantly because of decreased VLDL clearance, catabolism or delipidation [9,112,113]. One determinant of VLDL catabolism is endothelial bound lipoprotein lipase (LPL). LPL is synthesized in mesenchymal tissue such as adipose tissue, and muscle cells, is then secreted and is initially bound to the surface of mesenchymal tissue [114]. The endothelial bound pool is reduced in the nephrotic syndrome [109] and also in hereditary analbuminemia, suggesting that it is hypoalbuminemia rather than proteinuria that causes the depletion in this important lipase pool [115]. While hereditary analbuminemia does increase lipid levels, the degree of hyperlipidemia is far less than seen in the nephrotic syndrome, both in humans and in experimental models of renal disease in the rat. These findings suggest that an additional factor, most likely proteinuria, contributes substantially to hyperlipidemia in the nephrotic syndrome. We postulated that the combined decrease in endothelial bound LPL and altered VLDL structure together led to the profound defect in clearance of triglyceride rich lipoproteins as well as the massive increase in triglyceride levels seen in the nephrotic syndrome.

Supporting this hypothesis is the observation [116] that reduction in urinary protein excretion in patients with the nephrotic syndrome leads to a decrease in serum lipid levels even if serum albumin concentration is not increased. The clinical message from these observations is that all efforts must be targeted at reducing proteinuria.

Although diminished catabolism may be the major mechanism underlying the elevations in VLDL, increases in LDL appear to be primarily due to increased hepatic synthesis in nephrotic patients. It has been clearly demonstrated that the synthesis of LDL apolipoprotein B 100 is increased in patients with the nephrotic syndrome [113]. It is not clear what the stimulus might be for augmentation in apo B 100 synthesis. In addition to increased synthesis, decreased hepatic uptake of LDL particles may account, in part, for elevations of this lipoprotein [117]. There is conflicting data as to whether clearance of LDL is reduced in nephrotic syndrome, however, a recent study has noted decreased expression of the LDL receptor in nephrotic rats suggesting a mechanism for impaired clearance of this lipoprotein [118].

Serum total HDL levels are usually normal or decreased in nephrotic humans [119], whereas it is increased in nephrotic rats [120]. Although HDL levels may be normal, there appears to be a greater percentage of immature HDL_3 in the circulation of nephrotic patients [121]. This may be due to the fact that there is impaired maturation of HDL due to a defect in the activity of the enzyme lethicin:cholesterol acyltransferase which promotes the accumulation of cholesterol on the developing HDL particle.

Lipoprotein (a) (Lp(a)) is a specialized form of LDL in which a single molecule of apolipoprotein (a) is linked covalently to the apo B 100 moiety via a disulfide bridge [122]. The apolipoprotein (a) chain contains domains or kringles, and the structure consists of a single kringle V domain with multiple kringle IV repeats [123]. The structure of apolipoprotein (a) is quite homologous to plasmin but lacks proteolytic activity [124]. Synthesis of the apo B 100 moiety associated with Lp(a) may be regulated entirely separately from the pool of apo B 100 that is necessary for secretion of VLDL or LDL. The number of kringle IV repeats and consequently the size of apo (a) in Lp(a) is genetically determined [125]. In addition, the synthetic rates and plasma levels of Lp(a) vary inversely with the molecular weight of the isoform encoded [126]. Individuals having the largest apo (a) subtypes are most common and have the lowest plasma concentration of Lp(a). Other genetic factors may play a role in establishing Lp(a) levels as well as the number of kringle IV domains expressed [125]. However, dietary alterations or the use of lipid lowering agents has no effect on Lp(a) levels in patients.

Serum Lp(a) levels are increased in nephrotic patients [127,128] regardless of the isoform expressed. The elevated Lp(a) levels result from increased synthesis alone [128], whereas the increased levels of the other apo B lipoproteins (VLDL, IDL, LDL) in nephrotic patients is due predominantly to decreased catabolism. During remission of the nephrotic syndrome, Lp(a) levels decrease.

THE EFFECT OF ALTERED GLOMERULAR PERMSELECTIVITY ON LIPID METABOLISM

Hyperlipidemia is found in rats with hereditary analbuminemia [9,52,129]. These animals have a reduced plasma oncotic pressure and only trace amounts of albumin in their plasma. The genetic disorder is a seven nucleotide deletion isolated to the MN intron of the albumin gene creating a splicing defect during albumin mRNA processing [130]. While this finding would suggest that reduced plasma oncotic pressure or reduced plasma albumin concentration alone is the signal to induce the lipid abnormalities described above, the catabolism of both VLDL and chylomicrons is normal in these animals [9]. A severe defect in catabolism of both of these lipoproteins follows the onset of proteinuria [116] suggesting that proteinuria plays a role in the pathogenesis of disordered lipid metabolism independent of the serum albumin levels or oncotic pressure. Supporting this hypothesis are the observations that reducing albuminuria by administering angiotensin converting enzyme (ACE) inhibitors or dietary protein restriction reduces blood lipid levels [9,116,131] even if neither plasma albumin concentration nor plasma oncotic pressure are increased. The mechanism by which proteinuria is able to induce a reduction in the catabolism of VLDL is through an alteration in VLDL structure that decreases its binding to LpL. The specific link between VLDL structural changes and urinary protein losses remains to be elucidated.

CARDIOVASCULAR EFFECTS OF HYPERLIPIDEMIA IN THE NEPHROTIC SYNDROME

Accelerated atherosclerosis occurs in patients with proteinuria and hyperlipidemia and is probably responsible for the sharply increased incidence of cardiovascular disease and stroke [132,133]. One study reported an 85-fold increase in the incidence of ischemic heart disease in nephrotic patients [134]. This is not surprising when one considers that serum HDL, specifically the HDL_2 fraction, is reduced [11,121] while serum low density lipoprotein (LDL), intermediate density lipoprotein (IDL) and very low density lipoprotein (VLDL) fractions are increased. It is not yet known what the biological significance is of the increased levels of serum Lp(a) seen in the nephrotic syndrome. Lp(a) is a powerful atherosclerotic risk factor when it occurs genetically [135]. However, these high Lp(a) concentrations occur in combination with the low molecular weight isoform. Thus, it is difficult to know whether it is the concentration or the specific isoform of Lp(a) present that promotes atherogenesis. Recently studies suggest that the low molecular weight isoform per se may confer atherosclerotic risk [136]. It remains to be determined whether the elevated serum levels of Lp(a) in nephrotic patients contribute to the increased rate of atherosclerosis seen in this population. While the plasma concentration of most intermediate sized proteins is reduced, the serum concentrations of many larger proteins, such as fibrinogen and prothrombin [137], are increased and potentially may play a role in the hypercoagulable state associated with this syndrome [138] and contribute to atherosclerosis. Hyperlipidemia, therefore, is a serious consequence of proteinuria and should be addressed to protect patients from atherosclerosis. Hyperlipidemia may also contribute to progression of the renal disease [139,140], and may even initiate renal injury [141,142].

THROMBOEMBOLIC COMPLICATIONS

Patients with the nephrotic syndrome present an increased risk for thromboembolic events. The use of diuretics, intravascular volume reduction, protein C and protein S deficiencies and antiphospholipid antibodies are relevant contributing factors [143]. The deep veins of the lower limb are the most common sites of thrombosis in adults affected by nephrotic syndrome. Renal vein thrombosis is uncommon, but pulmonary embolism can occur and is most likely to be due to deep venous thrombosis. A retrospective study analyzing diagnostic codes of patients at the time of their hospital discharge showed that deep vein thrombosis occurred in 1.5% and renal vein thrombosis in 0.5% of patients affected by nephrotic syndrome [144].

Another large retrospective cohort study assessed the risk of venous thromboembolism and arterial thromboembolism in patients with nephrotic syndrome. The high risk of asymptomatic venous thromboembolism and arterial thromboembolism were remarkably elevated within the first 6 months of presentation of the nephrotic syndrome. The ratio of proteinuria to serum albumin predicted venous thromboembolism, whereas estimated GFR and multiple classic risk factors for atherosclerosis were predictors of arterial thromboembolism [145].

Currently, there are no randomized control trials that have examined the clinical indications for prophylactic anticoagulant therapy or for how long such therapy should be given. General factors such as the presence of edema, immobility and a previous history of thromboembolic events have to be considered by physicians to initiate an anticoagulant therapy.

EFFECTS OF LIPIDS ON RENAL DISEASE

It is generally accepted that both qualitative and quantitative alterations in blood lipids cause macrovascular disease, and hyperlipidemia caused by the nephrotic syndrome is no less dangerous than hyperlipidemia due to other causes. In the process of atherogenesis, lipid laden macrophages accumulate in the vessel wall, followed by intimal hyperplasia, and ultimately by atherosclerosis. Recent work from several laboratories [139,141,146] suggests that similar changes may occur in the microvasculature of the kidney, specifically the glomerular mesangium. Al Shebeb et al. [141] found that focal glomerular sclerosis occurred in guinea pigs fed a high cholesterol diet for 70 days. The animals developed proteinuria and hematuria. A high cholesterol diet also caused albuminuria, accelerated focal glomerulosclerosis, and increased glomerular capillary pressure in rats by [139].

The obese Zucker rat develops spontaneous hyperlipidemia, proteinuria and progressive glomerulosclerosis. These processes can be attenuated by cholesterol lowering drugs [139,147]. It is interesting to note that glomerular capillary pressure and single nephron GFR (SNGFR) are within the normal range, suggesting that hyperfiltration does not mediate the glomerular injury caused by hyperlipidemia [139]. Diamond et al. [146] found that rats with the nephrotic syndrome induced by puromycin aminonuleoside (PAN) had more proteinuria and a lower GFR when fed a high cholesterol diet as compared to nephrotic rats eating a regular diet. The glomeruli in rats fed a high cholesterol diet were more sclerotic and had mesangial cell proliferation and foam cells. Lowering plasma cholesterol by administration of cholestyramine resin attenuated both acute and chronic proteinuria in these animals [139]. It has been hypothesized that increased blood lipid levels, either from dietary cholesterol or secondary to hyperlipidemia caused by the renal disease, may play an important role in intensifying the rate at which established renal diseases progress [139,140] and may even initiate glomerular injury [141,142]. These changes could be mediated either hemodynamically or after the direct injury that follows the uptake of lipids by the glomerulus.

The oxidation of circulating lipids may play a role in progressive renal injury. Glomerular macrophages endocytose LDL both through specific LDL receptors and through the nonspecific scavenger system. It is known that hyperlipidemia activates mesangial cells (which have LDL receptors). This leads to the stimulation of mesangial cell proliferation and to increased production of macrophage chemotactic factors, fibronectin (a component of the extracellular matrix), and reactive oxygen species [148–150]. Both increased mesangial lipid deposition and enhanced expression of LDL-receptors on mesangial and epithelial cells have been demonstrated in patients with chronic glomerular diseases. Unregulated absorption of oxidized LDL may then lead to an uncontrolled increase in intracellular cholesterol [151] because oxidized lipids bypass the protective mechanism regulating LDL uptake. After endocytosis, cholesterol is esterified by acetyl Co-A cholesterol acyl transferase (ACAT) to form the insoluble cholesterol oleate ester [151]. This process results in creation of foam cells in the glomerulus analogous to that of early atherosclerosis in blood vessels. Thus, the oxidative state of lipids may also play a role in their nephrotoxicity; hence, antioxidant drugs might prove protective.

These studies in animals are supported in part by further, albeit uncontrolled, observations in patients in which reducing lipid levels with a HMG CoA reductase inhibitor reduces proteinuria or slows the rate of progressive injury [152]. Hypercholesterolemia is also a separate independent risk factor for progression of renal injury in diabetic patients [153].

Lipids represent a wide variety of substances, including steroids, saturated and unsaturated fatty acids, phospholipids and other compounds, many of which are either directly biologically active or are precursors of important biologically active metabolites. Much attention has been focused on the effect of polyunsaturated fatty acids on renal hemodynamics and on the manifestations of renal injury.

POLYUNSATURATED FATTY ACIDS

Prostaglandins and thromboxane are metabolic products of the metabolism of polyunsaturated fatty acids. They include both vasoconstrictors, such as thromboxane A_2, and vasodilators, such as PGE_2 or PGI_2, and they exert important hemodynamic effects. The effects of oxidized lipoproteins may also be mediated by these autocoids [154].

Eicosanoids are derived from polyunsaturated fatty acids (PUFA) in the diet because PUFA cannot be synthesized by mammals. Thus, eicosanoid metabolism can be manipulated nutritionally. Lipids derived from marine sources are enriched with omega-3 PUFA (e.g. eicosapentaenoic acid) while those derived from vegetable oils are enriched with omega-6 PUFA (e.g. arachidonic acid). Eicosapentaenoic acid competes with arachidonic acid as a substrate for cyclooxygenase and lipooxygenase. Cyclooxygenase converts arachidonic acid and eicosapentaenoic acid to the diene (e.g. PGI_2, TXA_2) and triene metabolites (e.g. PGI_3, TXA_3) respectively [155,156]. Lipooxygenase converts arachidonic acid and eicosapentaenoic acid to the four and five series of leukotrienes, respectively [157,158]. Thromboxane A_2 (TXA_2), an arachidonic acid metabolite, is a potent vasoconstrictor, while TXA_3, a metabolite of eicosapentaenoic acid, is biologically inert [159]. In contrast, the vasodilators PGI_2 and PGI_3 are equipotent [155].

Alterations in the generation of both vasodilatory prostaglandins (PGE_2, PGI_2) and vasoconstricting cyclooxygenase metabolites (TXA_2) can occur during renal injury or during physiologic stress, such as plasma volume contraction. While changes in eicosanoid metabolism can support the GFR adaption to renal injury or plasma volume contraction, they may also play a pathogenic role. Because of the differences in biological activity of their vasoconstrictive and vasodilatory metabolites, substitution of eicosapentaenoic acid for arachidonic acid in the diet may alter the expression of renal injury.

The effect of dietary PUFA, particularly fish oil, has been studied in a variety of experimental models of renal disease including the nephrotic syndrome [160–162]. In adriamycin-induced nephrosis in the rat, Ito et al. [163] found that plasma cholesterol and triglycerides, proteinuria, and plasma creatinine were significantly lower in rats fed fish oil than in rats fed beef tallow. Glomerular hyalinosis and endothelial swelling were also less in the fish oil-fed rats and were correlated with the changes in plasma triglycerides and cholesterol.

In a subsequent study of the same model, dietary fish oil induced a dose-dependent, reduction in glomerular synthesis of dienoic eicosanoids, PGE_2, 6-keto-$PGF_1\alpha$ (a stable metabolite of PGI_2) and TXB_2, a stable product of TXA_2. Fish oil also decreased the generation of TXB_2 from platelets. In studies of rats with nephrotic syndrome induced by adriamycin, Barcelli et al. [164] reported that dietary fish oil (a source of omega-3 PUFA), evening primrose oil (a source of omega-6 PUFA) or a mixture of these two PUFAs reduced plasma triglyceride and cholesterol levels compared to rats fed beef tallow. The fatty acid composition of the kidney was different in each dietary group, but neither the magnitude of proteinuria nor changes in plasma creatinine were affected by dietary fish oil. In another model of progressive renal injury in the rat, partial renal ablation, Scharschmidt found that diets supplemented with fish oil accelerated the course of renal injury [161] and caused increased mortality.

In studies involving human subjects, Gentile et al. [94] added 5 grams of fish oil per day to the diet of patients with the nephrotic syndrome who had been maintained on a soy vegetarian diet. These investigators found no beneficial effect of the fish oil on either proteinuria or on blood lipids when compared to patients maintained on the soy diet without fish oil supplementation. In contrast, Hall et al. [165] found that 15 grams of fish oil per day caused a decrease in total triglycerides and in LDL triglycerides and an increase in LDL cholesterol. Donadio et al. [166] treated 55 patients with IgA nephropathy and proteinuria with 12 grams of fish oil per day in a prospective randomized placebo controlled study. They found a significant reduction in the rate of progression of renal disease using a 50% increase in serum creatinine concentration as a study end point. However, there was no significant effect on proteinuria or blood pressure. These studies suggest that while alterations in dietary PUFA may alter some manifestations of the nephrotic state; the effects are dependent upon the model being investigated and the possible therapeutic value of PUFA should still be viewed with caution. These agents may be neither predictable nor salutary for all patients with renal disease.

Harrs et al. [167] reported that a diet entirely devoid of essential fatty acids provided renal protection by inhibiting macrophage function. While vasoactive lipids probably do play a role in altering the course of a variety of renal diseases, the effects of specific alterations in the composition and amounts of dietary PUFAs on the course of renal diseases in humans are not completely known. For this reason, there is no strong reason at this time to recommend the dietary supplements to patients with the nephrotic syndrome, with the possible exception of heavily proteinuric patients with IgA nephropathy [168]. Even here the value of using fish oil remains questionable.

DERANGEMENTS IN DIVALENT CATION METABOLISM IN THE NEPHROTIC SYNDROME

Some abnormalities in divalent cations can be directly traced to the urinary loss of proteins that either carry divalent cations or in some way regulate their metabolism. Transferrin, a glycoprotein whose principal function is to transport iron [169], is lost in the urine, [170,171] providing a potential mechanism for a microcytic hypochromic anemia found uncommonly in nephrotic patients [166,167]. Transferrin turnover rate is also increased in patients with the nephrotic syndrome [41,172]. Reduced plasma iron in the presence of a hypochromic microcytic anemia may result from urinary iron loss in nephrotic patients.

Complicating this paradigm are the observations of Alfrey et al. [77,78] suggesting that increased delivery of iron to the renal interstitium by filtered transferrin, a protein that binds up to two moles of iron per mole of protein, may be of importance in causing the interstitial inflammation that ultimately destroys the kidney. The decision therefore to provide iron supplementation to these patients may not be a trivial one.

Anemia may also be a consequence of the urinary loss of another glycoprotein that is of a size likely to pass the glomerular filtration barrier in the nephrotic syndrome, erythropoietin [173–175]. Indeed, plasma levels of this protein are reduced in both nephrotic patients [173] and rats [174], and it doesn't appear that synthesis of erythropoietin is increased in response to its urinary loss [174]. There are no prospective randomized studies of the effect of administration of either iron (potentially harmful) or erythropoietin (expensive and inconvenient) to anemic patients with the nephrotic syndrome to guide clinical practice.

Copper, like iron, is also bound to a circulating plasma protein, ceruloplasmin. While the urinary loss of this 151 kDa protein may cause a decrease in blood copper [6,8], it results in no clinically recognized manifestations [176]. The most important zinc-binding protein is albumin, with the greatest losses occurring in the nephrotic syndrome. Documented zinc deficiency is probably a consequence of both reduced intestinal absorption of zinc in conjunction with excessive urinary loss [177]. The effect of proteinuria on zinc metabolism has been largely ignored and it is not known to what extent zinc depletion plays a role in the clinical manifestations of the nephrotic syndrome.

Hypocalcemia is well recognized in nephrotic patients [178–181], and includes reduced serum ionized as well as total calcium. Hypocalcemia does not result entirely from a reduction in the fraction of calcium bound to albumin since plasma vitamin D is reduced [5,178,182,183], and the decrease in serum calcium concentration correlates with urinary albumin excretion [178]. Plasma albumin and vitamin D concentrations correlate closely. Vitamin D binding protein is present in the urine of nephrotic patients [5,183], and serum vitamin D levels normalize when proteinuria resolves [183,184]. Labeled vitamin D appears rapidly in the urine of nephrotic subjects [185], suggesting that urinary vitamin D loss is the cause of hypovitaminosis D in these patients. Hypovitaminosis D is not the result of loss of renal mass, since plasma vitamin D levels are also low in nephrotic patients with normal renal function [178–180]. The hypovitaminosis D of the nephrotic syndrome may result in rickets, especially in children [181,185]. Nephrotic patients malabsorb calcium [178], a defect that can be corrected by exogenously administered vitamin D [185]. It is not known whether synthesis of vitamin D binding protein is altered in response to its urinary loss or whether it is modulated by dietary protein intake. Unlike many of the other manifestations of the nephrotic syndrome, hypovitaminosis D can be managed with replacement therapy.

DERANGEMENTS IN SALT AND WATER METABOLISM IN THE NEPHROTIC SYNDROME (VOLUME HOMEOSTASIS)

Edema formation is one of the most bothersome symptoms of the nephrotic syndrome. There are two basic steps in edema formation: [1] there is an alteration in capillary hemodynamics that favors movement of fluid from the vascular space into the interstitium and [2] there is a pathologic retention of salt and water. The classic model of edema formation in the nephrotic syndrome indicated that a decrease in plasma albumin concentration would inevitably lead to a decrease in the difference between interstitial and plasma oncotic pressure (delta oncotic pressure) and lead to plasma volume contraction (Figure 26.2). Ultimately, edema occurs when the amount of fluid filtered into the interstitium exceeds maximal lymph flow, decreasing the circulatory volume due to the plasma ultrafiltrate left behind in the interstitium [186]. One would predict that plasma volume contraction would activate the renin angiotensin aldosterone axis and lead to secondary (via plasma volume depletion) renal sodium retention - the so called "underfill" edema. Since plasma volume contraction also causes an increase in vasopressin secretion one would anticipate that water would also be retained leading to hyponatremia (as seen in other edema forming states, specifically congestive heart failure and liver disease).

The classic or "undefill" model of edema formation in the nephrotic syndrome has been challenged by a number of observations. It is important to note that when one looks at Starling forces, it is the transcapillary oncotic pressure gradient between the vascular and interstitial compartment that drives fluid movement and not simply the plasma oncotic pressure. In the setting of the nephrotic syndrome, with the fall in plasma albumin concentration and oncotic pressure, there is a concomitant fall in interstitial oncotic pressure [187]. Thus, there are probably only minor changes in the transcapillary oncotic gradient, and hypoalbuminemia is not the primary step in edema formation. In patients with minimal change disease going into remission with corticosteroid treatment, the maximum recovery diuresis occurs before there has been a substantial increase in plasma albumin concentrations [188]. Dorhout-Mees and co workers [3] found that both plasma volume and blood volume decreased in individual patients with minimal-change nephrotic syndrome when they entered remission, providing strong evidence that even (adult) patients with

FIGURE 26.2 Primary edema formation with renal sodium retention. The Plasma Underfill Hypothesis: Hypoalbuminemia leads to increased transudation of fluid into the interstitium resulting in plasma-volume contraction with secondary activation of the renin-angiotensin-aldosterone axis and subsequent renal sodium retention. Because a normal plasma volume cannot be maintained in the presence of hypoalbuminemia, a positive feedback cycle occurs. The reabsorbed salt and water also enter the interstitial space. Edema formation is a direct consequence of hypoalbuminemia, and salt and water retention is a consequence of the plasma-volume contraction that results.

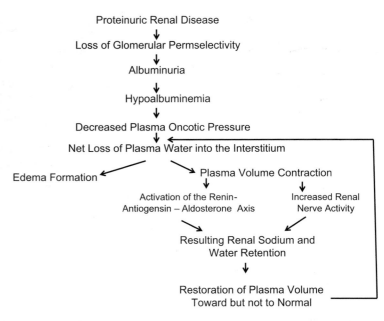

minimal-change nephrotic syndrome were apparently plasma volume expanded during their "nephrotic" phase. Furthermore, they found no correlation between plasma volume and renin activity, or between plasma albumin and blood volume [189]. The lack of a relationship between plasma renin activity and blood volume, or between plasma albumin and blood volume characterized both patients with minimal-change nephrotic syndrome and patients with other kidney diseases. The two groups were indistinguishable [189]. These observations raised important questions about the proposed mechanism of edema formation in the nephrotic syndrome.

An alternative explanation to the "underfill" model of edema formation proposes that renal disease induces primary sodium and water retention leading to plasma volume expansion and increased capillary hydrostatic pressure. The sodium avidity is intrinsic to the nephrotic kidney itself and is unrelated to systemic volume needs. Strong evidence for this hypothesis is provided by studies using unilateral proteinuric renal disease. In unilateral kidney models of the nephrotic syndrome, impaired sodium excretion is intrinsic to the nephrotic kidney and does not reflect plasma volume regulation. In one such study, Perico et al. [190] demonstrated an inability of the proteinuric kidney to excrete fluid or sodium in response to infused atrial natriuretic peptide (ANP) even though GFR increased similarly in both the proteinuric and normal contralateral kidney. Ichikawa et al. demonstrated that the proteinuric kidney avidly reabsorbed filtered salt in the distal part of the nephron in PAN induced nephrotic syndrome in the rat, whereas the normal contralateral kidney did not [191]. Clearly, both the normal kidney and the contralateral proteinuric

kidney were exposed to the same oncotic pressure and circulating hormones.

Both experimental and human studies have suggested relative resistance to ANP. This defect may be due, in part, to increased phosphodiesterase activity in the nephrotic kidney leading to more rapid degradation of cyclic GMP, which is the second messenger for ANP. Valentin et al. [192] found that the normal increase in urinary cyclic GMP that follows saline infusion was blunted in nephrotic rats because of increased phosphodiesterase in the inner medullary collecting duct cells. Treatment with a phosphodiesterase inhibitor reverses this defect and restores the normal natriuretic response to volume expansion. Thus, an increase in phosphodiesterase activity in the nephrotic syndrome was proposed to accelerate hydrolysis of cGMP resulting in impaired natriuresis. These observations provide a cellular basis for the observations of Perico et al. [190] and Ichikawa et al. [191]. The proteinuric kidney avidly reabsorbs filtered salt in the distal nephron and is not responsive to increased ANP that should normally cause a natriuresis when plasma volume is expanded [191]. In addition, there is increased activity of the sodium-potassium ATPase pump in the cortical collecting duct in nephrotic rats [193].

In the setting of primary renal sodium retention, the systemic capillary bed is faced with increased hydrostatic pressure at the very time that defense mechanisms normally employed to counteract edema formation, (increased lymphatic flow and decreased interstitial protein concentration), have already been maximized. Hence, edema results from the combined effect of primary renal salt and water retention coupled with urinary losses of proteins of intermediate weight,

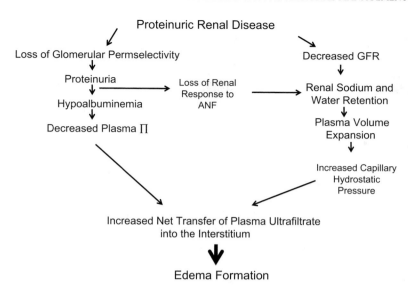

FIGURE 26.3 Primary renal sodium retention with edema formation. The Plasma Overfill Hypothesis: Renal salt and water retention occur as a result of the renal disease or protein losses themselves causing plasma volume expansion. This produces increased capillary hydrostatic pressure, which in conjunction with the increased transcapillary flux of fluid resulting from hypoalbuminemia, causes edema. Edema formation is not a direct consequence of reduced oncotic pressure alone. Renal salt and water retention is also a consequence of an unresponsiveness of the kidney to atrial natriuretic peptide (ANP).

thereby causing a decrease in both plasma and interstitial oncotic pressure (Figure 26.3). These processes deprive the lymphatic system of the capacity to respond to increased hydrostatic pressure. Since sodium retention is frequently, at least in part, a direct result of the renal disease itself and not a consequence of plasma volume contraction, dietary sodium restriction is indicated. Clinically significant hyponatremia is unlikely to occur in nephrotic patients in the absence of diuretic use, and is not often encountered in patients with this syndrome.

The relative roles of primary sodium retention versus the "underfill" pathophysiology in the development of edema in the nephrotic syndrome are not clear. Their relative contributions to edema may vary depending on the underlying cause for the renal disease. Based on their studies in nephrotic patients, Meltzer et al. [4] proposed that nephrotic patients with edema could be divided into two groups. One group was termed "nephrotic" and was made up predominantly of those with minimal change with low plasma volume and high plasma renin. The cause of their edema would fit more with the "underfill" model. The other patients were classified as "nephritic" and comprised those with glomerulonephritis or diabetes. These patients had normal or expanded plasma volume and reduced plasma renin activity, despite a profound reduction in plasma oncotic pressure. Patients with an elevated intravascular volume tend to have lower GFRs (<50%) and higher serum albumin concentrations. Patients with so-called "underfill" edema, tend to have normal GFRs and more severe hypoalbuminemia, the prototype of this being minimal change disease. Many of the studies evaluating the overflow versus primary sodium retention models have been conflicting, and it is possible that either or both mechanisms may be operational in

a given patient depending on his underlying renal disease and other factors.

It is possible for patients with the nephrotic syndrome to become plasma volume contracted. This must be detected, guarded against and treated. It is, however, impossible to predict the plasma volume of a nephrotic patient by measuring plasma protein or albumin concentration or by measuring plasma renin activity [189]. It is important, therefore, to estimate the intravascular volume state of each patient individually by measuring orthostatic blood pressure, observing neck vein distention and evaluating the SUN relative to serum creatinine. Patients who show no evidence of plasma volume contraction should respond to the gentle use of diuretics. Patients who have plasma volume contraction should not be treated with diuretics, but their volume deficit should be treated by bed rest, support hose, or even fluid replacement if necessary.

RECOMMENDATIONS FOR NUTRITIONAL AND NON-NUTRITIONAL TREATMENT OF THE NEPHROTIC SYNDROME

The treatment of the nephrotic syndrome begins with identifying the specific cause of the proteinuria and treatment of the underlying disorder if possible. There are, however, general nutritional and non-nutritional management issues in patients with the nephrotic syndrome per se.

Proteinuria

Reducing proteinuria should be a primary objective in the treatment of the nephrotic syndrome. As detailed in this chapter, proteinuria may contribute to further renal damage by promoting tubulo-interstitial inflammation and fibrosis. The notion here is that "proteinuria begets more proteinuria". Moreover, reducing proteinuria improves the hyperlipidemia and edema of the nephrotic syndrome. Although the nephrotic syndrome results from the loss of plasma proteins into the urine, high protein diets are ineffective in correcting the metabolic consequences of urinary protein loss. Furthermore, diets rich in protein increase proteinuria and may accelerate the course of a variety of renal diseases. Thus, dietary supplements to provide high protein intakes should be avoided. As detailed in this chapter, dietary protein restriction not only reduces proteinuria but preserves serum albumin concentration. Moreover, modest protein restriction (0.8 g/kg/day) has been shown to maintain nitrogen balance. The studies utilizing an extremely low protein diet (0.3 g/kg/day) supplemented with essential amino acids are provocative but need to be verified by larger controlled trials. The safest recommendation would be to prescribe a diet containing 0.8−1.0 g/kg/day of protein and 35 kcal/kg/day which is low in fat and high in complex carbohydrates but restricted in sodium chloride. Based on the studies with soy protein, vegetarian diets may be especially useful. Modest protein restriction may also be beneficial in attenuating the progression of the primary renal disease by its effects on reducing intraglomerular pressure and possibly other mechanisms. Whether it is necessary to replace large urinary protein losses in targeting net protein intake is an area of uncertainty. If a patient with massive proteinuria fails to exhibit a major reduction in urinary protein excretion after dietary protein has been restricted and pharmacologic therapy (i.e. ACEi, ARB) has been implemented, and urinary protein excretion remains high and serum albumin remains low, it may be prudent to replace average urinary protein losses above about 10 g/day in addition to the 0.8 g/kg protein intake target.

Angiotensin converting enzyme inhibitors [194,195] or angiotensin II receptor antagonists have become the mainstay of treatment as a result of evidence from randomized controlled trials and meta-analyses [196,197]. An interesting role in proteinuria management has been recently attributed to the aldosterone receptor antagonists. In particular, the effect of spironolactone administration in patients with persistent proteinuria on long-term angiotensin-converting enzyme inhibitor therapy with or without an angiotensin II receptor blocker was investigated in a double-blind, placebo-controlled study. A significant reduction in proteinuria among patients given spironolactone was observed [198]. In another study, Tylicki et al. showed that an aldosterone receptor antagonist in addition to double renin-angiotensin blockade was able to reduce proteinuria and slow the progression of the disease in nondiabetic patients with chronic kidney disease [199]. In an acute animal model of the nephrotic syndrome, Fukuda et al. showed that blockers of mineralcorticoid receptors and angiotensin II receptors decreased proteinuria and preserved expression of glomerular podocyte protein independently of blood pressure levels [200].

Thus, proteinuria can be ameliorated with the use of blockers of the renin-angiotensin-aldosterone system without modification in blood pressure. Treatment with combinations of these blockers reduces proteinuria more effectively than single drug therapy alone. The use of these agents must be associated with regular monitoring of serum electrolytes, particularly serum potassium, which may increase to hazardous levels, and sodium which may decrease. The full antiproteinuric effect of these blockers can take several months to become evident. Independently of these blockers, blood pressure lowering will also reduce proteinuria. Unfortunately, these treatments usually will not eradicate proteinuria in patients with substantial proteinuria. However, as indicated above, even a reduction in proteinuria may have major beneficial effects including slowing of the rate of progression of renal failure and reduction in serum lipid levels.

Hyperlipidemia

Hyperlipidemia in the nephrotic syndrome poses the danger of accelerated atherosclerosis and progressive renal injury. Reductions in plasma lipid levels have been accomplished using such therapies as a low-fat diet [92] and fish oil supplements [165]. Dietary therapy with a low fat diet, however, is generally of only minimal benefit, and there is no long-term experience with the use of a low fat diet in the treatment of the hyperlipidemia of the nephrotic syndrome. In addition, there is no compelling reason to prescribe unsaturated fatty acid supplements (such as fish oil) until results from controlled studies are available. It is best to ingest low cholesterol and saturated fatty acid diets. It has been shown that reducing proteinuria, using drugs such as ACE inhibitors, lowers blood lipid levels in nephrotic animals [9] and humans [201]. Keilani et al. [201] demonstrated a 10−20% decrease in the plasma levels of total and LDL-cholesterol and Lp(a) with the use of an ACE inhibitor. The magnitude of these changes appears to be related to the degree of reduction in proteinuria. The angiotensin II receptor antagonist, losartan, appears to have a similar beneficial effect on the lipid profile in nephrotic patients [202]. Thus, therapy directed at reducing the increased renal clearance of macromolecules has a salutary effect on improving the hyperlipidemia associated with the nephrotic syndrome.

A study conducted on patients with idiopathic nephrotic syndrome indicated that the addition of 20 mg/day of fluvastatin to the basic therapy was associated with a 40% reduction in cholesterol levels, 60% reduction in proteinuria and 60% increase in serum albumin levels [203]. Similar results were obtained by Valdivesio et al. after administering 10 mg/day of atorvastatin to 10 dyslipidemic patients who had hypoalbuminemia and proteinuria >3.5 g/24 h [204]. Rayner et al. [205] showed that, in patients with the nephrotic syndrome, the use of a low-lipid diet without pharmaceutical treatment led to a minimal reduction in plasma cholesterol levels, a limited reduction in urinary protein excretion, and normalization of serum albumin levels.

Lipid lowering agents, such as statins [206], probucol [207,208] or gemfibrozil [209] may prove useful in reducing blood lipid levels in these patients [210−212]. The long term benefits of treatment remain unproven but may include a reduction in cardiovascular risk and preservation of residual renal function. Use of these agents may engender some morbidity, such as rhabdomyolysis with statins [213], especially when given in combination with gemfibrozil [214], and hepatoxicity. It is noteworthy that many nephrotic patients go into remission with treatment of the underlying disease. Thus identifying and treating the underlying cause of nephrotic syndrome and thereby reducing proteinuria will improve or resolve the dyslipidaemia. Similarly, pharmacologic intervention with angiotensin converting enzyme inhibitors or ARBs that are successful in reducing urinary protein loss will similarly effect a reduction in blood lipid levels.

Antioxidants

Increased levels of oxidative stress markers have been found in sera and urine of nephrotic children [215] and in animal models of the nephrotic syndrome [216,217]. In children it was shown that primary nephrotic syndrome is associated with oxidative stress even during remission. This stress may modulate the response to corticosteroids [218]. Pedraza-Chaverri et al. showed that proteinuria, hypoproteinemia, renal dysfunction and ultrastructural alterations were higher in nephrotic rats fed a deficient diet of antioxidants in contrast to rats treated with vitamin E and selenium [219]. In other studies, after treatment of nephrotic animals with antioxidants, such as catalase or α-tocopherol, a significant reduction of the proteinuria was observed [220−222]. More recently Granquvist et al. described an increase in the plasma antioxidant capacity combined with decreased oxidation of proteins in sera from nephrotic rats. These findings indicate a downregulation of different antioxidative enzymes in nephrotic kidneys. This observation suggests that oxidative damage to glomerular cells may contribute to the progressive renal injury in the nephrotic syndrome [223]. In conclusion, the use of antioxidant medicines in the nephrotic syndrome appears useful, but large clinical trials to ascertain their effectiveness and safety in nephrotic patients are still lacking.

Edema

No randomized trials are available concerning the management of edema in patients with the nephrotic syndrome. The aim of medical treatment is to induce a negative sodium and water balance. Mandatory is to limit patients' dietary sodium intake (<3 g/day), restrict their fluid intake (maximum 1.5 liters/day), and take diuretics. It is recommended to reverse the edema slowly, with a maximum weight loss of 0.5−1 kg/day. Diuresis with substantial reduction in body sodium and water can cause electrolyte disturbances, acute renal failure, and, as a result of hemoconcentration, thromboembolism [224], as already discussed. Loop diuretics, such as furosemide, are generally preferred. Medicinal absorption may be affected by edema of the intestinal wall, so high doses of intravenous diuretics are often used for refractory cases. Commonly used diuretics are mostly protein bound so their effectiveness may be affected when large amounts of proteinuria are present. Thiazide diuretics or potassium sparing diuretics are often added to improve diuresis because of their synergism for distal inhibition of sodium reabsorption. Intravenous albumin administration also has been used to improve diuresis. It probably acts by increasing delivery of the diuretic to its site of action and by expanding plasma volume. Intravenous albumin is often used in hypotensive patients in whom conventional treatment is failing. However, its use is not supported by research data, and it can have harmful effects, such as hypertension, and pulmonary edema [225].

Acknowledgements

This work was supported in part by a grant from the National Institutes of Health 1-RO1 DK 42297-01 and in part by the research service of the United States Department of Veterans Affairs.

References

[1] Earley LC, Farland M. Nephrotic syndrome. In: Strauss MB, Welt LG, editors. Diseases of the kidney. 3rd ed. Boston Little Brown Co; 1979. p. 765−813.
[2] Earley LE, Havel RJ, Hopper J, Graus H. Nephrotic Syndrome. Calif Med 1971;115:23−41.

[3] Dorhoot- Mees EJ, Roos JC, Boer P, Yoe OH, Simatupang TA. Observations on edema formation in the nephrotic syndrome in adults with minimal lesions. Am J Med 1979;67:378—84.

[4] Meltzer JI, Keim HJ, Laragh JH, Sealey JE, Jan KM, Chien S. Nephrotic syndrome Vasoconstriction and hypervolemia types indicated by renin sodium profiling. Ann Int Med 1979;67:2001. 387—384.

[5] Barragry JM, France MW, Carter ND, Auton JA, Beer M, Boucher BJ, et al. Vitamin D metabolism in nephrotic syndrome. Lancet 1977;2:629—32.

[6] Pedraza-Chaverri J, Torres-Rodriguez GA, Cruz C, Mainero A, Tapia E, Ibarra-Rubio ME, et al. Copper and zinc metabolism in aminonucleoside-induced nephrotic syndrome. Nephron 1994; 6:87—92.

[7] Perrone L, Gialanella G, Giordano V, La Manna A, Moro R, Di Toro R. Impaired zinc metabolic status in children affected by idiopathic nephrotic syndrome. European Journal of Pediatrics 1990;149:438—40.

[8] Stec J, Podracka L, Pavkovcekova O, Kollar J. Zinc and copper metabolism in nephrotic syndrome. Nephron 1990;56:186—7.

[9] Davies RW, Staprans I, Hutchison FN, Kaysen GA. Proteinuria not altered albumin metabolism affects hyperlipidemia in the nephrotic rat. J Clin Invest 1990;86:600—5.

[10] Joven J, Villabona C, Vilella E, Masana L, Albertí R, Vallés M. Abnormalities of lipoprotein metabolism in patients with the nephrotic syndrome. N Engl J Med 1990;323:579—84.

[11] Gherardi E, Rota E, Calandra S, Genova R, Tamborino A. Relationship among the concentrations of serum lipoproteins and changes in their chemical composition in patients with untreated nephrotic syndrome. Eur J Clin Invest 1977;7: 563—70.

[12] Wanner C, Rader D, Bartens W, Kramer J, Brewer HB, Schollmeyer P, et al. Elevated plasma lipoprotein a in patients with the nephrotic syndrome. Ann Intern Med 1993;119:263—9.

[13] Sieniawska M, Szymanik-Grzelak H, Kowalewska M, Wasik M, Koleska D. The role of cow's milk protein intolerance in steroid-resistant nephrotic syndrome. Acta Paediatrica 1992;81: 1007—12.

[14] Laurent J, Lagrue G. Dietary manipulation for idiopathic nephrotic syndrome. A new approach to therapy. Allergy 1989;44:599—603.

[15] Lagrue G, Laurent J, Rostoker G. Food allergy and idiopathic nephrotic syndrome. Kidney Internat 1989;(Suppl. 27):S147—51.

[16] Laurent J, Rostoker G, Robeva R, Bruneau C, Lagrue G. Is adult idiopathic nephrotic syndrome food allergy Value of oligoantigenic diets. Nephron 1987;47(1):7—11.

[17] Lagrue G, Heslan JM, Belghiti D, Sainte-Laudy J, Laurent J. Basophil sensitization for food allergens in idiopathic nephrotic syndrome. Nephron 1986;42:123—7.

[18] Bergstrom J, Ahlberg M, Alvestrand A. Influence of protein intake on renal hemodynamics and plasma hormone concentrations in normal subjects. Acta Med Scand 1985;217:189—96.

[19] Lee KE, Summerill RA. Glomerular filtration rate following administration of individual amino acids in conscious dogs. Q J Exp Physiol 1982;67:459—65.

[20] Premen AJ, Hall JE, Smith MJ. Postprandial regulation of renal hemodynamics role of pancreatic glucagon. Am J Physiol, 248 Renal Fluid Electrolyte Physiol 1985;17:F656—62.

[21] Hutchison FN, Martin VI, Jones Jr H, Kaysen GA. Differing actions of dietary protein and enalapril on renal function and proteinuria. Am J Physiol, 258 Renal Fluid Electrolyte Physiol 1990;27:F126—32.

[22] Kaysen GA, Gambertoglio J, Jiminez I, Jones H, Hutchison FN. Effect of dietary protein intake on albumin homeostasis in nephrotic patients. Kidney Int 1986;29:572—7.

[23] Kaysen GA, Kirkpatrick WG, Couser WG. Albumin homeostasis in the nephrotic rat nutritional considerations. Am J Physiol, 247 Renal Fluid Electrolyte Physiol 1984;16:F192—202.

[24] Paller MS, Hostetter TH. Dietary protein increases plasma renin and reduces pressor reactivity to angiotensin II. Am J Physiol, 251 Renal Fluid Electrolyte Physiol 1986;20:F34—9.

[25] Fine L. The biology of renal hypertrophy. Kidney Int 1986;29: 619—34.

[26] Kaysen GA, Rosenthal C, Hutchison FN. GFR increases before renal mass or ODC activity increase in rats fed high protein diets. Kidney Int 1989;36:441—6.

[27] Kenner CH, Evan AP, Blomgren AP, Aronoff GR, Luft FC. Effect of protein intake on renal function and structure in partially nephrectomized rats. Kidney Int 1985;27:739—50.

[28] Wada L, Don BR, Schambelan M. Hormonal mediators of amino-acid induced glomerular hyperfiltration in humans. Am J Physiol, 260 Renal Fluid Electrolyte Physiol 1991;29:F797—2.

[29] Woods LL. Mechanisms of renal hemodynamic regulation in response to protein feeding. Kidney Int 1993;44:659—75.

[30] Jaffa AA, Vio CP, Silva RH, et al. Evidence for renal kinins as mediators of amino acid-induced hyperperfusion and hyperfiltration in the rat. J Clin Invest 1992;89:1460—8.

[31] Don BR, Blake S, Hutchison FN, Kaysen GA, Schambelan M. Dietary protein intake modulates glomerular eicosanoid production in the rat. Am J Physiol Renal Fluid Electrolyte Physiol 1989;25:F516—23.

[32] El Sayed AA, Haylor J, El Nahas AM. Mediators of the direct effects of amino acids on the rat kidney. Clin Sci 1991;81:427—32.

[33] Williams M, Young JB, Rosa RM, Gunn S, Epstein FH, Landsberg L. Effect of protein ingestion on urinary dopamine excretion. Evidence for the functional importance of renal decarboxylation of circulating 3 4-dihydroxyphenylalanine in man. J Clin Invest 1986;78:687—1693.

[34] Straus DS, Takemoto CD. Effect of dietary protein deprivation on insulin-like growth factor IGF I and II IGF binding protein-2 and serum albumin gene expression in rat. Endocrinology 1990;127:1849—60.

[35] Lemozy S, Pucilowska JB, Underwood LE. Reduction of insulin-like growth factor-I IGF-I in protein-restricted rats is associated with differential regulation of IGF-binding protein messenger ribonucleic acids in liver and kidney and peptides in liver and serum. Endocrinology 1994;135:617—23.

[36] Martinez-Maldonado M, Benabe JE, Wilcox JN, Wang S, Luo C. Renal renin angiotensinogen and angiotensin I-converting-enzyme gene expression influence of dietary protein. Am J Physiol 1993;264:F981—8.

[37] Chan YM, Cheng M-LL, Keil LC, Myers BD. Functional response of healthy and diseased glomeruli to a large protein meal. J Clin Invest 1988;81:245—54.

[38] Palmer RMJ, Ferrige AG, Moncada S. Nitric oxide release accounts for the biological activity of endothelium-derived relaxing factor. Nature 327 524-525 1989. Tolins JP Raij L. Effects of amino acid infusion on renal hemodynamics. Hypertension 1991;17:1045—51.

[39] Tolins JP, Raij L. Effects of amino acid infusion on renal hemodynamics. Hypertension 1991;17:1045—51.

[40] Ito S, Juncos LA, Nushiro N, Johnson CS, Carretero OA. Endothelium-Derived relaxing factor modulates endothelin action in afferent arterioles. Hypertension 1991;17:1052—6.

[41] Gitlin D, Janeway CA, Farr LE. Studies on the metabolism of plasma proteins in nephrotic syndrome. I. Albumin gamma globulin and iron-binding globulin. J Clin Invest 1956;35:44—55.

[42] Jensen H, Rossing N, Anderson SB, Jarnum S. Albumin metabolism in the nephrotic syndrome in adults. Clin Sci 1967;33:445—57.

[43] Kaitz AL. Albumin metabolism in nephrotic adults. J Lab & Clin Med 1959;53:186—94.

[44] Yssing M, Jensen H, Jarnum S. Albumin metabolism and gastrointestinal protein loss in children with nephrotic syndrome. Acta Paediat Scand 1969;58:109—15.

[45] Kaysen GA, Davies RW, Hutchison FN. Effect of dietary protein intake and angiotensin converting enzyme inhibition in Heymann nephritis. Kidney Int 1989;36:S154—62.

[46] Kaysen GA, Carstensen A, Martin VI. Muscle protein synthesis is impaired in nephrotic rats. Mineral and Electrolyte Metabolism 1992;18:228—32.

[47] Keutmann EH, Bassett SH. Dietary protein in hemorrhagic Bright's disease. II. The effect of diet on serum proteins proteinuria and tissue proteins. J Clin Invest 1935;14:871—88.

[48] Don BR, Kaysen GA, Hutchison FN, Schambelan M. The effect of angiotensin-converting enzyme inhibition and dietary protein restriction in the treatment of proteinuria. Am J Kid Dis 1991;17:10—7.

[49] Heeg JE, de Jong PE, van der Hem GK, de Zeeuw D. Angiotensin II does not acutely reverse the reduction of proteinuria by long-term ACE inhibition. Kidney Int 1991;40:734—41.

[50] Kasiske BL, Lakatua JDA, Ma JZ, Louis TA. A meta-analysis of effects of dietary protein restriction on the rate of decline in renal function. Am J Kidney Dis 1998;31:954—61.

[51] Kaysen GA. Albumin turnover in renal disease. Miner Electrolyte Metab 1998;24:55—63.

[52] Ando S, Kon K, Tanaka Y, Nagase S, Nagai YJ. Characterization of hyperlipidemia in Nagase Analbuminemia Rat NAR. Biochem 1980;87:1859—92.

[53] de Sain-Van Der Velden MG, de Meer K, Kulik W, Melissant CF, Rabelink TJ, Berger R, et al. Nephrotic proteinuria has no net effect on total body protein synthesis: measurements with (13) C valine. Am J Kidney Dis 2000;35:1149—54.

[54] Blainey JD. High protein diets in the treatment of the nephrotic syndrome. Clin Sci 1954;13:567—81.

[55] Kirsch R, Frith L, Black E, Hoffenberg R. Regulation of albumin synthesis and catabolism by alteration of dietary protein Nature 1968;217:578—9.

[56] Rothschild MA, Oratz M, Evans CD, Schreiber SS. Albumin Synthesis. In: Rosemoer M, Oratz M, Rothschild A, editors. Albumin Structure Function and Uses. New York: Permagon Press; 1977. p. 227—55.

[57] Hirschberg RR, Zipser RD, Slomowitz LA, Kopple JD. Glucagon and prostaglandins are mediators of amino acid-induced rise in renal hemodynamics. Kidney Int 1988;33:1147—55.

[58] Hirschberg R, Kopple JD. Role of growth hormone in the amino acid-induced acute rise in renal function in man. Kidney Int 1987;32:382—7.

[59] Premen AJ. Potential mechanisms mediating postprandial renal hyperemia and hyperfiltration. FASEB J 1988;2:131—7.

[60] Phisitkul S, Hacker C, Simoni J, Tran RM, Wesson DE. Dietary protein causes a decline in the glomerular filtration rate of the remnant kidney mediated by metabolic acidosis and endothelin receptors. Kidney Int 2008;73:192—9.

[61] Wesson DE, Simoni J, Prabhakar S. Endothelin-induced increased nitric oxide mediates augmented distal nephron acidification as a result of dietary protein. J Am Soc Nephrol 2006;17:406—13.

[62] Rosenberg ME, Swanson JE, Thomas BL, Hostetter TH. Glomerular and hormonal responses to dietary protein intake in human renal disease. Am J Physiol 1987;253:F1083—90.

[63] Kaysen GA, Jones Jr H, Martin V, Hutchison FN. A low protein diet restricts albumin synthesis in nephrotic rats. J Clin Invest 1989;83:1623—9.

[64] Moestrup SK, Nielsen LB. The role of the kidney in lipid metabolism. Curr Opin Lipidol 2005;16:301—6.

[65] Hutchison FN, Kaysen GA. Albuminuria causes lysozymuria in rats with Heymann nephritis. Kidney Int 1988;33:787—91.

[66] Kaysen GA, al-Bander H, Martin VI, Jones Jr H, Hutchison FN. Branched-chain amino acids augment neither albuminuria nor albumin synthesis in nephrotic rats. Am J Physiol 1991;260: R177—84.

[67] McQuarrie EP, Shakerdi L, Jardine AG, Fox JG, Mackinnon B. Fractional excretions of albumin and IgG are the best predictors of progression in primary glomerulonephritis. Nephrol Dial Transplant 2010. Epub ahead of print.

[68] Nielsen R, Christensen EI. Proteinuria and events beyond the slit. Pediatr Nephrol 2010;25:813—22.

[69] Claris-Appiani A, Assael BM, Tirelli AS, Marra G, Cavanna G. Lack of glomerular hemodynamic stimulation after infusion of branch-chain amino acids. Kidney Int 1988;33:91—4.

[70] Anderson KE, Rosner W, Khan MS, New MI, Pang S, Wissel PS, et al. Diet-hormone interactions Protein carbohydrate ratio alters reciprocally the plasma levels of testosterone and cortisol and their respective binding globulins in man. Life Sci 1987;40:1761—8.

[71] Ishizuka B, Quigley ME, Yen SSC. Pituitary hormone release in response to food ingestion: Evidence for neuroendocrine signals from gut to brain. J C E & M 1983;57:1111—6.

[72] Benabe JE, Wang S, Wilcox JN, Martinez-Maldonado M. Modulation of angiotensin II receptor and its mRNA in normal rat by low-protein feeding. Am J Physiol 1993;265:F660—9.

[73] Kaysen GA, Martin VI, Jones Jr H. Arginine augments neither albuminuria nor albumin synthesis caused by high-protein diets in nephrosis. Am J Physiol 263 Renal Fluid Electrolyte Physiol 1992;32:F907—17.

[74] Eddy AA, McCulloch L, Liu E, Adams J. A relationship between proteinuria and acute tubulointerstitial disease in rats with experimental nephrotic syndrome. Am J Pathol 1991;138: 1111—23.

[75] Thomas ME, Schreiner GF. Contribution of proteinuria to progressive renal injury Consequences of tubular uptake of fatty acid bearing albumin. Am J Nephrol 1993;13:385—98.

[76] Cooper MA, Buddington B, Miller NL, Alfrey AC. Urinary iron speciation in nephrotic syndrome. Am J Kidney Dis 1995;25:314—9.

[77] Alfrey AC. Role of iron and oxygen radicals in the progression of chronic renal failure. Am J Kidney Dis 1994;23:183—7.

[78] Alfrey AC, Hammond WS. Renal iron handling in the nephrotic syndrome. Kidney Int 1990;37:1409—13.

[79] Nath KA, Hostetter MK, Hostetter TH. Increased ammonia-genesis as a determinant of progressive renal injury. Am J Kidney Dis 1991;17:654—7.

[80] Thomas ME, Schreiner Jr GF. Contribution of proteinuria to progressive renal injury consequences of tubular uptake of fatty acid bearing albumin. Am J Nephrol 1993;13:385—98.

[81] Abbate M, Zoja C, Corna D, Capitanio M, Bertani T, Remuzzi G. In progressive nephropathies overload of tubular cells with filtered proteins translates glomerular permeability dysfunction into cellular signals of interstitial inflammation. J Am Soc Nephrol 1998;9:1213—24.

[82] Burton CJ, Combe C, Walls J, Harris KP. Secretion of chemokines by human tubular epithelial cells in response to proteins. Nephrol Dial Transplant 1999;14:2628—33.

[83] Nath KD. Tubulointerstitial changes as a major determinant in the progression of renal damage. Am J Kidney Dis 1992;20:1—17.

[84] Alexopoulos E, Seron D, Hartley RB, Cameron JS. Lupus nephritis Correlation of interstitial cells with glomerular function. Kidney Int 1990;37:100—9.

[85] Clark EC, Nath KA, Hostetter MK, Hostetter TH. Role of ammonia in tubulointerstitial injury. Mineral and Electrolyte Metabolism 1990;16:315—1321.

[86] Agarwal A, Nath KA. Effect of proteinuria on renal interstitium effect of products of nitrogen metabolism. Am J Nephrol 1993;13:376−84.

[87] Eddy AA. Protein restriction reduces transforming growth factor-beta and interstitial fibrosis in nephrotic syndrome. Am J Physiol 1994;266:F884−93.

[88] Fukui M, Nakamura T, Ebihara I, Nagaoka I, Tomino Y, Koide H. Low-protein diet attenuates increased gene expression of platelet-derived growth factor and transforming growth factor-beta in experimental glomerular sclerosis. J Lab Clin Med 1993;121:224−34.

[89] Giordano M, De Feo P, Lucidid P, DePascale E, Giordano G, Cirillo D, et al. Effects of dietary protein restriction on fibrinogen and albumin metabolism in nephrotic patients. Kidney Int 2001;60:235−42.

[90] de Sain van der Velden MGM, Kaysen GA, De Meer K, Stellard F, Voorbij HA, Reijngoud DJ, et al. Proportionate increase of fibrinogen and albumin synthesis in nephrotic patients measurement with stable isotopes. Kidney Int 1998;53:181−8.

[91] Vaziri ND, Gonzales E, Barton CH, Nguyen Q, Arquilla M. Factor XIII and its substrates fibronectin fibrinogen and alpha 2-antiplasmina in plasma and urine of patients with nephrosis. J Lab Clin Med 1991;117:152−6.

[92] D'Amico G, Gentile MG, Manna G, Fellin G, Ciceri R, Cofano F, et al. Effect of vegetarian soy diet on hyperlipidaemia in nephrotic syndrome. Lancet 1992;339:1131−4.

[93] Walser M. Does prolonged protein restriction preceding dialysis lead to protein malnutrition at the onset of dialysis? Kidney Int 1993;44:1139−44.

[94] Gentile MG, Fellin G, Cofano F, Delle Fave A, Manna G, Ciceri R, et al. Treatment of proteinuric patients with a vegetarian soy diet and fish oil. Clinical Nephrology 1993;40(6):315−20.

[95] Walser M, Hill S, Tomalis EA. Treatment of nephrotic adults with a supplemented very low protein diet. Am J Kidney Dis 1996;28:354−64.

[96] Peters JP, Bulger HA. The relation of albuminuria to protein requirement in nephritis. Arch Int Med 1926;37:153−85.

[97] Al-Bander H, Kaysen GA. Ineffectiveness of dietary protein augmentation in the management of the nephrotic syndrome. Pediatric Nephrology 1991;5:482−6.

[98] Choi EJ, Bailey J, May RC, Masud T, Maroni BJ. Metabolic responses to nephrosis effect of a low-protein diet. Am J Physiol 1994;266:F432−8.

[99] Katoh T, Takahashi K, Klahr S, Reyes AA, Badr KF. Dietary supplementation with L-arginine ameliorates glomerular hypertension in rats with subtotal nephrectomy. J Am Soc Neph 1994;4:1690−4.

[100] Klahr S, Buerhert J, Purkerson ML. Role of dietary factors in the progression of chronic renal disease. Kidney Int 1983;24:579−87.

[101] Evanoff G, Thompson C, Brown H, Weinman E. Prolonged dietary protein restriction in diabetic nephropathy. Arch Intern Med 1989;149:1129−33.

[102] Jireidine KF, Hogg RJ, van Renen MJ, Southwood TR, Henning PH, Cobiac L, et al. Evaluation of long-term aggressive dietary management of chronic renal failure in children. Pediatr Nephrol 1990;4:1−10.

[103] Zeller K, Whittaker E, Sullivan L, Raskin P, Jacobson HR. Effect of restricting dietary protein on the progression of renal failure in patients with insulin dependent diabetes mellitus. N Engl J Med 1991;324:78−84.

[104] Lim VS, Wolfson M, Yarasheski KE, Flanigan MJ, Kopple JD. Leucine turnover in patients with the nephrotic syndrome evidence suggesting body protein conservation. J Am Soc Nephrol 1998;9:1067−73.

[105] Maroni BJ, Staffeld C, Young VR, Manatunga A, Tom K. Mechanisms permitting nephrotic patients to achieve nitrogen equilibrium with a protein-restricted diet. J Clin Invest 1997;99: 2479−87.

[106] McCrory WW, Becker CG, Cunningham-Rundles C, Klein RF, Mouradian J, Reisman L. Immune complex glomerulopathy in a child with food hypersensitivity. Kidney Int 1986;30:592−8.

[107] Coppo R, Amore A, Roccatello D. Dietary antigens and primary immunoglobulin A nephropathy. J Am Soc Nephrol 1992;2: S173−80.

[108] Marsh JB. Lipoprotein metabolism in experimental nephrosis. J Lipid Res 1984;25:1619−23.

[109] Garber DW, Gottlieb BA, Marsh JB, Sparks CE. Catabolism of very low density lipo-proteins in experimental nephrosis. J Clin Invest 1984;74:1375−83.

[110] Staprans I, Felts JM, Couser WG. Glycosaminoglycans and chylomicron metabolism in control and nephrotic rats. Metabolism 1987;36:496−501.

[111] Chung BH, Segrest JP, Smith K, Griffin FM, Brouillette CG. Lipolytic surface remnants of triglyceride-rich lipoproteins are cytotoxic to macrophages but not in the presence of high density lipoprotein A possible mechanism of atherogenesis. J Clin Invest 1989;83:1363−74.

[112] Demant T, Mathes C, Gutlich K, Bedynek A, Steinhauer HB, Bosch T, et al. A simultaneous study of the metabolism of apolipoprotein B and albumin in nephrotic patients. Kidney Int 1998;54:2064−80.

[113] de Sain-van der Velden MG, Kaysen GA, Barrett HA, Stellaard F, Gadellaa MM, Voorbij HA, et al. Increased VLDL in nephrotic patients results from a decreased catabolism while increased LDL results from increased synthesis. Kidney Int 1998;53:994−1001.

[114] Blanchette-Mackie EJ, Masuno H, Dwyer NK, Olivecrona T, Scow RO. Lipoprotein lipase in myocytes and capillary endothelium of heart immunocytochemical study. Am J Physiol 1989;256:E818−28.

[115] Shearer GC, Stevenson FT, Atkinson DN, Jones H, Staprans I, Kaysen GA. Hypoalbuminemia and proteinuria contribute separately to reduced lipoprotein lipase in the nephrotic syndrome. Kidney Int 2001;59:179−89.

[116] Kaysen GA, Don B, Schambelan M. Proteinuria albumin synthesis and hyperlipidemia in the nephrotic syndrome. Nephrol Dial Transplant 1991;6:141−9.

[117] Warwick GL, Packard CJ, Demant T, Bedford DK, Boulton-Jones M, Shepard J. Metabolism of B-containing lipoproteins in subject with nephrotic-range proteinuria. Kidney Int 1991;40:129−38.

[118] Vaziri ND, Liang KH. Down regulation of hepatic LDL receptor in experimental nephrosis. Kidney Int 1996;50:887−93.

[119] Appel G. Lipid abnormalities in renal disease. Kidney Int 1991;39:169−83.

[120] Sun X, Jones Jr H, Joles JA, van Tol A, Kaysen GA. Apolipoprotein gene expression in analbuminemic rats and in rats with Heymann nephritis. Am J Physiol 1992;262:F755−61.

[121] Mils E, Rosseneu M, Daneels R, Schurgers M, Boelaert J. Lipoprotein distribution and composition in the human nephrotic syndrome. Atherosclerosis 1985;54:225−37.

[122] Steyrer E, Durovic S, Frank S, Giessauf W, Burger A, Dieplinger H, et al. The role of lecithin cholesterol acyltransferase for lipoprotein a assembly. Structural integrity of low density lipoproteins is a prerequisite for Lp a formation in human plasma. J Clin Invest 1994;94:2330−40.

[123] McLean JW, Tomlinson JE, Kuang WJ, Eaton DL, Chen EY, Fless GM, et al. cDNA sequence of human apolipoprotein a is homologous to plasminogen. Nature 1987;330:132−7.

[124] Loscalzo J, Weinfeld M, Fless GM, Scanu AM. Lipoprotein a fibrin binding and plasminogen activation. Arteriosclerosis 1990;10:240−5.

[125] Kraft HG, Lingenhel A, Pang RW, Delport R, Trommsdorff M, Vermaak H, et al. Frequency distributions of apolipoprotein a kringle IV repeat alleles and their effects on lipoprotein a levels in Caucasian Asian and African populations the distribution of null alleles is non-random. European Journal of Human Genetics 1996;4:74−87.

[126] Gavish D, Azrolan N, Breslow J. Plasma Lp a concentration is inversely correlated with the ratio of kringle IV kringle V encoding domains in the apo a gene. J Clin Invest 1989;84: 2021−7.

[127] Wanner C, Rader D, Bartens W, Kramer J, Brewer HB, Schollmeyer P, et al. Elevated plasma lipoprotein a in patients with the nephrotic syndrome. Ann Intern Med 1993;119:263−9.

[128] de Sain-Van Der Velden MG, Reijngoud DJ, Kaysen GA, Gadellaa MM, Voorbij H, Stellaard F, et al. Evidence for increased synthesis of Lipoprotein a in the nephrotic syndrome. J Am Soc Nephrol 1998;9:1474−81.

[129] Takahashi M, Kusumi K, Shumiya S, Nagase S. Plasma lipid concentrations and enzyme activities in Nagase Analbuminemia Rats. NAR Exp Anim 1983;32:39−46.

[130] Esumi H, Takahashi Y, Sekiya T, Sata S, Nagase S, Sugimura T. Presence of albumin mRNA precursors in nuclei of analbuminemic rat liver lacking cytoplasmic albumin mRNA. Proc Natl Acad Sci 1982;79:734−8.

[131] Kaysen GA, Davies RW. Reduction in proteinuria attenuates Hyperlipidemia in the nephrotic syndrome. J Am Soc Neph 1990;1:S75−9.

[132] Mallick NP, Short CD. The nephrotic syndrome and ischaemic heart disease. Nephron 1981;27:54−7.

[133] Wheeler DC, Bernard DB. Lipid abnormalities in the nephrotic syndrome Causes consequences and treatment. Am J Kidney Dis 1994;23:331−46.

[134] Berlyne GM, Mallick NP. Ischemic heart disease as a complication of nephrotic syndrome. Lancet 1969;2:399−400.

[135] Schreiner PJ, Heiss G, Tyroler HA, Morrisett JD, Davis CE, Smith R. Race and gender differences in the association of Lp a with carotid artery wall thickness. The Atherosclerosis Risk in Communities ARIC Study. Arteriosclerosis Thrombosis and Vascular Biology 1996;16:471−8.

[136] Sechi LA, Kronenberg F, De Carli S, Falleti E, Zingaro L, Catena C, et al. Association of serum lipoprotein a levels and apolipoprotein a size polymorphism with target-organ damage in arterial hypertension. JAMA 1997;277:1689−95.

[137] Girot R, Jaubert F, Leon M, Bellon B, Aiach M, Josso F, et al. Albumin fibrinogen prothrombin and antithrombin III variations in blood urines and liver in rat nephrotic syndrome Heymann nephritis. Thromb Haemostas 1983;49:13−7.

[138] Llach F. Nephrotic syndrome: hypercoagulability, renal vein thrombosis and other thromboembolic complications. In: Brenner BM, Stein JH, editors. Contemporary issues in nephrology 9 Nephrotic Syndrome. New York: Churchill Livingstone; 1982. p. 121−44.

[139] Schmitz PG, Kasiske BL, O'Donnell MP, Keane WF. Lipids and progressive renal injury. Seminar in Nephrology 1989;9:354−69.

[140] Wellman KF, Volk BW. Renal changes in experimental hypercholesterolemia in normal and subdiabetic rabbits I. Short term studies. Lab Invest 1970;22:36−48.

[141] Al-Shebeb T, Frohlich J, Magil AB. Glomerular disease in hypercholesterolemic guinea pigs A pathogenetic study. Kidney Int 1988;33:498−507.

[142] Drevon CA, Hoving T. The effects of cholesterol fat feeding on lipid levels and morphological structures in liver kidney and spleen in guinea pigs. Acta Pathol Micro Immunol Scand 1977;85:1−18.

[143] Hull RP, Goldsmith DJA. Nephrotic syndrome in adults. BMJ 2008;336:1185−9.

[144] Kayali F, Najjar R, Aswad F, Matta F, Stein PD. Venous thromboembolism in patients hospitalized with nephrotic syndrome. Am J Med 2008;121:226−30.

[145] Mahmoodi BK, ten Kate MK, Waanders F, Veeger NJ, Brouwer JL, Vogt L, et al. High absolute risks and predictors of venous and arterial thromboembolic events in patients with nephrotic syndrome: results from a large retrospective cohort study. Circulation 2008;117:224−30.

[146] Diamond JR, Karnovsky MJ. Exacerbation of chronic aminonucleoside nephrosis by dietary cholesterol supplementation. Kidney Int 1987;31:671−7.

[147] Kasiske BL, O'Donnell MP, Garvis WJ, Keane WF. Pharmacologic treatment of hyperlipidemia reduces glomerular injury in rat 5 6 nephrectomy model of chronic renal failure. Circ Res 1988;62:367−74.

[148] Keane WF. Lipids and the kidney. Kidney Int 1994;46:910−20.

[149] Rovin BH, Tan LC. LDL stimulates mesangial fibronectin production and chemoattractant expression. Kidney Int 1993;43: 218−25.

[150] Keane WF, O'Donnell MP, Kasiske BL, Kim Y. Oxidative modification of low-density lipoproteins by mesangial cells. J Am Soc Nephrol 1993;4:187−94.

[151] Grone HJ, Walli AK, Grone E, Kramer A, Clemens MR, Seidel D. Receptor mediated uptake of apo B and apo E rich lipoproteins by human glomerular epithelial cells. Kidney Int 1990;37:1449−59.

[152] Rabelink AJ, Hene RJ, Erkelens DW, Joles JA, Koomans HA. Partial remission of nephrotic syndrome in patients on long-term simvastatin. Lancet 1990;335:1045−6.

[153] Ravid M, Brosh D, Ravid-Safran D, Levy Z, Rachmani R. Main risk factors for nephropathy in type 2 diabetes mellitus are plasma cholesterol levels mean blood pressure and hyperglycemia. Arch Intern Med 1998;158:998−1004.

[154] Kaplan R, Aynedjian HS, Schlondorff D, Bank N. Renal vasoconstriction caused by short-term cholesterol feeding ins corrected by thromboxane antagonist or probucol. J Clin Invest 1990;86:1707−14.

[155] Culp BR, Titus BG, Lands WEM. Inhibition of prostaglandin biosynthesis by eicosapentaenoic acid. Prostaglandin Med 1979;3:269−78.

[156] Zoja C, Benigni A, Verroust P, Ronco P, Bertani T, Remuzzi G. Indomethacin reduces proteinuria in passive Heymann nephritis in rats. Kidney Int 1987;31:1335−43.

[157] Remuzzi G, Imberti L, Rossini M, Morelli C, Carminati C, Cattaneo GM, et al. Increased glomerular thromboxane synthesis as a possible cause of proteinuria in experimental nephrosis. J Clin Invest 1985;75:94−101.

[158] Spector AA, Kaduce TL, Figard PH, Norton KC, Hoak JC, Czervionke RL. Eicosapentaenoic acid and prostaglandin production by cultured human endothelial cells. J Lipid Res 1983;24:1595−604.

[159] Needleman P, Raz A, Minkes MS, Ferrendelli JA, Sprecher H. Triene Prostaglandins prostacyclin and thromboxane biosynthesis and unique biological properties. Proc Natl Acad Sci 1979;76:944−8.

[160] Prickett JD, Robinson DR, Steinberg AD. Dietary enrichment with the polyunsaturated fatty acids eicosapentaenoic acid prevents proteinuria and prolong survival in NZB x NZW f1 mice. J Clin Invest 1981;68:556−9.

[161] Scharschmidt LA, Gibbons NB, McGarry L, Berger P, Axelord M, Janis R, et al. Effects of dietary fish oil on renal

insufficiency in rats with subtotal nephrectomy. Kidney Int 1987;32:700—9.

[162] Sinclair HM. Essential fatty acids in perspective. Hum Nutr Clin Nutr 1984;38:245—60.

[163] Ito Y, Yamashita W, Barcelli U, Pollak V. Dietary fat in experimental nephrotic syndrome Beneficial effects of fish oil on serum lipids and indirectly on the kidney. Life Sci 1987;40:2317—24.

[164] Barcelli UO, Beach DC, Thompson M, Weiss M, Pollak VE. A diet containing n-3 and n-6 fatty acids favorably alters the renal phospholipids Eicosanoid synthesis and plasma lipids in nephrotic rats. Lipids 1988;23:1059—63.

[165] Hall AV, Parbtani A, Clark WF, Spanner E, Huff MW, Philbrick DJ, et al. Omega-3 fatty acid supplementation in primary nephrotic syndrome effects on plasma lipids and coagulopathy. J Am Soc Nephrol 1992;36:1321—9.

[166] Donadio Jr JV, Bergstralh EJ, Offord KP, Spencer DC, Holley K. A controlled trial of fish oil in IgA nephropathy. New Engl J Med 1994;331:1194—9.

[167] Harrs KPG, Lefkowith JB, Klahr S, Schreiner GF. Essential fatty acid deficiency ameliorates acute renal dysfunction in the rat after the administration of the aminonucleoside of puromycin. J Clin Invest 1990;86:1115—23.

[168] de Jong G, van Dijk JP, van Eijk HG. The biology of transferrin. Clin Chim Acta 1990;190:1—46.

[169] Ellis D. Anemia in the course of the nephrotic syndrome secondary to transferrin depletion. J Pediatr 1977;90:953—5.

[170] Rifkind D, Kravetz HM, Knight V, Schade AL. Urinary excretion of iron-binding protein in the nephrotic syndrome. N Eng J Med 1961;265:115—8.

[171] Jensen H, Bro-Jorgensen K, Jarnum S, Olesen H, Yssing M. Transferrin metabolism in the nephrotic syndrome and in protein-losing gastroenteropathy. Scandinavian. J Clin Lab Invest 1968;21:293—304.

[172] Vaziri ND, Kaupke CJ, Barton CH, Gonzales E. Plasma concentration and urinary excretion of erythropoietin in adult nephrotic syndrome. Am J Med 1992;92:35—40.

[173] Zhou XJ, Vaziri ND. Erythropoietin metabolism and pharmacokinetics in experimental nephrosis. Am J Physiol 1992;263:F812—5.

[174] Vaziri ND. Erythropoietin and transferrin metabolism in nephrotic syndrome. Am J Kidney Dis 2001;38:1—8.

[175] Cartwright GE, Gubler CJ, Wintrobe MM. Studies on copper metabolism Copper and iron metabolism in the nephrotic syndrome. J Clin Invest 1954;33:685—98.

[176] Reichel M, Mauro TM, Ziboh VA, Huntley AC, Fletcher MP. Acrodermatitis enteropathica in a patient with the acquired immune deficiency syndrome. Arch Derm 1992;128:415—7.

[177] Goldstein DA, Haldimann B, Sherman D, Norman AW, Massry SG. Vitamin D metabolites and calcium metabolism in patients with nephrotic syndrome and normal renal function. J Clin Endocrinol Metab 1981;53:116—21.

[178] Emerson Jr K, Beckman WW. Calcium metabolism in nephrosis. I. A description of an abnormality in calcium metabolism in children with nephrosis. J Clin Invest 1945;24:564—72.

[179] Lim P, Jacob E, Chio LF, Pwee HS. Serum ionized calcium in nephrotic syndrome. Q J Med 1976;45:421—6.

[180] Stickler GB, Hayles AB, Power MH, Ulrich JA. Renal tubular dysfunction complicating the nephrotic syndrome. Pediatrics 1960;26:75—85.

[181] Goldstein DA, Oda Y, Kurokawa K, Massry SG. Blood levels of 25-hydroxy-vitamin D in nephrotic syndrome. Studies in 26 patients. Ann Intern Med 1977;87:664—7.

[182] Haddad Jr JG, Walgate J. Radioimmunoassay of the binding protein for vitamin D and its metabolites in human serum:

[183] Concentrations in normal subjects and patients with disorders of mineral homeostasis. J Clin Invest 1976;58:1217—22.

[183] Goldstein DA, Haldimann B, Sherman D, Norman AW, Massry SG. Vitamin D metabolites and calcium metabolism in patients with nephrotic syndrome and normal renal function. J Clin Endocrinol Metab 1981;53:116—21.

[184] Emerson Jr K, Beckman WW. Calcium metabolism in nephrosis. I. A description of an abnormality in calcium metabolism in children with nephrosis. J Clin Invest 1945;24:564—72.

[185] Lim P, Jacob E, Chio LF, Pwee HS. Serum ionized calcium in nephrotic syndrome. Q J Med 1976;45:421—6.

[186] Kaysen GA, Myers BD, Couser WG, Rabkin R, Felts JM. Mechanisms and consequences of proteinuria. Lab Invest 1986;54:479—98.

[187] Koomans HA, Kortlandt W, Geers AB, Dorhout Mees EJ. Lowered protein content of tissue fluid in patients with the nephrotic syndrome Observations during disease and recovery. Nephron 1985;40:391—5.

[188] Koomans HA, Boer WH, Dorhout Mees EJ. Renal function during recovery from minimal lesions nephrotic syndrome. Nephron 1987;47:173—8.

[189] Geers AB, Koomans HA, Roos JC, Boer P, Dorhout-Mees EJ. Functional relationships in the nephrotic syndrome. Kidney Int 1984;26:324—30.

[190] Perico N, Delaini F, Lupini C, Benigni A, Galbusera M, Boccardo P, et al. Blunted excretory response to atrial natriuretic peptide in experimental nephrosis. Kidney Int 1989;36:57—64.

[191] Ichikawa I, Rennke HG, Hoyer JR, Badr KF, Schol N, Troy JL, et al. Role for intrarenal mechanisms in the impaired salt excretion of experimental nephrotic syndrome. J Clin Invest 1983;71:91—104.

[192] Valentin JP, Qiu C, Muldowney WP, Ying WZ, Gardner DG, Humphreys MH. Cellular basis for blunted volume expansion natriuresis in experimental nephrotic syndrome. J Clin Invest 1992;90:1302—12.

[193] Feraille E, Vogt B, Rousselot M, Bartlet-Bas C, Cheval L, Doucet A, et al. Mechanisms of enhanced Na-K-ATPase activity in cortical collecting duct from rats with nephrotic syndrome. J Clin Invest 1993;91:1295—300.

[194] Lewis EJ, Hunsicker LG, Bain RP, Rohde RD. The effect of angiotensin-converting enzyme inhibition on diabetic nephropathy. N Engl J Med 1993;329:1456—62.

[195] Maschio G, Albert D, Janin G, Locatelli F, Mann JF, Motolese M, et al. Effect of the angiotensin-converting-enzyme inhibitor benazepril on the progression of chronic renal insufficiency. N Engl J Med 1996;334:939—45.

[196] Parving H-H, Lehnert H, Brochner-Mortensen J, Gomis R, Andersen S, Arner P. The effect of irbesartan on the development of diabetic nephropathy in patients with type 2 diabetes. N Engl J Med 2001;345:870—8.

[197] Brenner BM, Cooper ME, DeZeeuw D, Keane WF, Mitch WE, Parving H-H, et al. Effects of losartan on renal and cardiovascular outcomes in patients with type 2 diabetes and nephropathy. N Engl J Med 2001;345:861—9.

[198] Chrysostomou A, Pedagogos E, MacGregor L, Becker GJ. Double-blind, placebo-controlled study on the effect of the aldosterone receptor antagonist spironolactone in patients who have persistent proteinuria and are no long-term angiotensin-converting enzyme inhibitor therapy, with or without an angiotensin II receptor blocker. Clin J Am Soc Nephrol 2006;1:256—62.

[199] Tylicki L, Rutkowski P, Renke M, Larczynski W, Aleksandrowicz E, Lysiak-Szydlowska W, et al. Triple pharmacological blockade of the renin-angiotensin-aldosteron system in nondiabetic CKD: An open-label crossover randomized controlled trial. Am J Kid Dis 2008;52:486—93.

[200] Fukuda A, Fujimoto S, Iwatsubo S, Kawachi H, Kitamura K. Effects of mineralcorticoid and angiotensin II receptor blockers on proteinuria and glomerular podocyte protein expression in a model of minimal change nephrotic syndrome. Nephrology 2010;15:321—6.

[201] Keilani T, Schleuter WA, Levin ML, Batlle DC. Improvement of lipid abnormalities associated with proteinuria using fosinopril an angiotensin-converting enzyme inhibitor. Ann Intern Med 1993;118:246—354.

[202] de Zeeuw D, Gansevoort RT, Dullaart RP, de Jong PE. Angiotensin II antagonism improves the lipoprotein profile in patients with nephrotic syndrome. J Hypertens 1995; 13(Suppl. 1):S53.

[203] Gheit OA, Sobh MA, Mohamed Kel-S, El-Baz MA, El-Husseini F, Gazarin SS, et al. Impact of treatment of dyslipidemia on renal function, fat deposits and scarring in patients with persistent nephrotic syndrome. Nephron 2002; 91:612—9.

[204] Valdivesio P, Moliz M, Valera A, Corrales MA, Sanchez-Chaparro MA, Gonzalez-Santos P. Atorvastatin in dislipidemia of the nephrotic syndrome. Nephrology 2003;8:61—4.

[205] Rayner BL, Byrne MJ, van Zyl Smit R. A prospective clinical trial comparing the treatment of diopathic membranous nephropathy and nephrotic syndrome with simvastatin, and diet, versus diet alone. Clin Nephrol 1996;46:219—24.

[206] Laquaniti A, Bolignano D, Donato V, Bono C, Fazio MR, Buemi M. Alterations of lipid metabolism in chronic nephropathies: mechanisms, diagnosis and treatment. Kidney Blood Press Res 2010;33:100—10.

[207] Lida H, Izumino K, Asaka M, Fujita M, Nishino A, Sasayama S. Effect of probucol on hyperlipidemia in patients with nephrotic syndrome. Nephron 1987;47:280—3.

[208] Valeri A, Gelfand J, Blum C, Appel GB. Treatment of the hyperlipidemia of the nephrotic syndrome a controlled trial. Am J Kidney Dis 1986;8:388—96.

[209] Groggel GC, Cheung AK, Ellis-Benigni K, Wilson DE. Treatment of nephrotic hyperlipoproteinemia with gemfibrozil. Kidney Int 1989;36:266—71.

[210] Rabelink AJ, Hené RJ, Erkelens DW, Joles JA, Koomans HA. Effects of simvastatin and cholestyramine on lipoprotein profile in hyperlipidaemia of nephrotic syndrome. Lancet, II 1988: 1335—8.

[211] Kasiske BL, Velosa JA, Halstenson CE, LaBelle P, Langendorfer A, Keane WF. The effects of lovastatin in hyperlipidemic patients with the nephrotic syndrome. Am J Kidney Dis 1990;15:8—15.

[212] Golper TA, Illingworth DR, Morris CD, Bennett WM. Lovastatin in the treatment of multifactorial hyperlipidemia associated with proteinuria. Am J Kid Dis 1989;13:312—20.

[213] Corpier CL, Jones PH, Suki WN, Lederer ED, Quinones MA, Schmidt SW, et al. Rhabdomyolysis and renal injury with lovastatin use. Report of two cases in cardiac transplant recipients. JAMA 1988;260:239—41.

[214] Marais GE, Larson KK. Rhabdomyolysis and acute renal failure induced by combination lovastatin and gemfibrozil therapy. Ann Intern Med 1990;112:228—30.

[215] Candiano G, Musante L, Petretto A, Bruschi M, Santucci L, Urbani A, et al. Proteomics of plasma and urine in primary nephrotic syndrome in children. Contrib Nephrol 2008;160:17—28.

[216] Gwinner W, Landmesser U, Brandes RP, Kubat B, Plasger J, Eberhard O, et al. Reactive oxygen species and antioxidant defense in puromycin aminonucleoside glomerulopathy. J Am Soc Nephrol 1997;8:1722—31.

[217] Rincon J, Romero M, Viera N, Pedreanez A, Mosquera J. Increased oxidative stress and apoptosis in acute puromycin aminonucleoside nephrosis. Int J Exp Pathol 2004;85:25—33.

[218] Bakr A, Hassan SA, Shoker M, Zaki M, Hassan R. Oxidant stress in primary nephrotic syndrome: does it modulate the response to corticosteroids? Pediatr Nephrol 2009;24:2375—80.

[219] Pedraza-Chaverri J, Arevalo AE, Hernandez-Pando R, Larriva-Sahd J. Effect of dietary antioxidants on puromycin aminonucleoside nephrotic syndrome. Int J Biochem Cell Biol 1995;27:683—91.

[220] Beaman M, Birtwistle R, Howie AJ, Michael J, Adu D. The role of superoxide anion and hydrogen peroxide in glomerular injury induced by puromycin aminonucleoside in rats. Clin Sci (Lond) 1987;73:329—32.

[221] Diamond JR, Bonventre JV, Karnovsky MJ. A role for oxygen free radicals in aminonucleoside nephrosis. Kidney Int 1986;29: 478—83.

[222] Ricardo SD, Bertram JF, Ryan GB. Antioxidants protect podocyte foot process in puromycin aminonucleoside-treated rats. J Am Soc Nephrol 1994;4:1974—86.

[223] Granqvist A, Nilsson UA, Ebefors K, Haraldsson B, Nystrom J. Impaired glomerular and tubular antioxidative defense mechanisms in nephrotic syndrome. Am J Physiol Renal Physiol 2010;299:F898—904.

[224] Hull RP, Goldsmith DJA. Nephrotic syndrome in adults. BMJ 2008;336:1185—9.

[225] Dorhout Mees EJ. Does it make sense to administer albumin to the patient with nephrotic oedema? Nephrol Dial Transplant 1996;11:1224—6.

27

Nutrition and Blood Pressure

Joel D. Kopple

Los Angeles Biomedical Research Institute at Harbor-UCLA Medical Center, David Geffen School of Medicine at UCLA
and UCLA Fielding School of Public Health, Los Angeles, California, USA

INTRODUCTION

Hypertension is one of the most common chronic diseases. It is currently estimated that approximately 50 million people in the United States and about one billion people worldwide have hypertension [1,2]. The degree of severity of high blood pressure and hypertension has been classified by the Joint National Committee (JNC) on Prevention, Detection, Evaluation, and Treatment of High Blood Pressure: the JNC 7 report as indicated in Table 27.1 [2]. The widespread concern over the high prevalence of hypertension is due to compelling evidence that it is a major cause of morbidity and mortality [3–5]. Moreover, lifestyle clearly plays a major role in the pathogenesis and current high prevalence of hypertension. Hence, to the extent that hypertension is caused or intensified by unhealthy lifestyles, including unhealthy diets, it should, in theory, be preventable or treatable by modifying people's behavior. Overweight and obesity, particularly visceral obesity, low birth weight, high sodium chloride intakes, and increased or reduced intake of a number of other nutrients have been associated with increased blood pressure (BP) [6,7–10]. In the past several decades, overweight and obesity have increased to epidemic proportions in industrialized countries, and the prevalence of these conditions is increasing rapidly in the developing world [10,11]. Worldwide, approximately 1.4 billion adults are estimated to be overweight or obese [12], and the number of such individuals appears to be increasing. Thus, the effects on blood pressure of obesity, energy intake and excessive or deficient intakes of other nutrients has become a subject of great importance. Table 27.2 lists nutritional factors that may affect BP. This chapter will review the relationships between BP and obesity and energy intake and then between BP and the intake of other nutrients.

OBESITY AND ENERGY INTAKE

Body Mass and Obesity

In adults, normal or desirable body weight has been described as a body mass index (BMI, defined as weight in kg divided by height in meters squared) from 18.5 to 24.9 kg/m^2. Overweight is defined as a BMI of 25.0–29.9 kg/m^2, and obesity as a BMI of 30 kg/m^2 or greater. Morbid obesity has been defined as a BMI above 35.0 kg/m^2 [11]. Obesity has also been classified as Class I (BMI, 30–34.9 kg/m^2), Class II (BMI, 35.0–39.9 kg/m^2) and Class III (BMI, ≥40.0 kg/m^2). Overweight and obesity are considered to occur at a lower BMI in Asian peoples, because the direct association of these variables with increased risk for adverse cardiovascular outcomes, including hypertension, occurs at lower weights-for-height than in Caucasians [13,14].

Scientific evidence strongly links obesity with elevated BP. Obesity, by itself, appears to directly increase BP, and obese individuals are more likely to have elevated BP than nonobese subjects [10,14,15]. Even among older adults, a higher BMI is associated with an increased risk for hypertension. In a study of adult family medicine patients, the prevalence of pre-hypertension (systolic BP (SBP) 120–139 mmHg; diastolic BP (SBP) 80–89 mmHg) increases significantly as the BMI rises from overweight to obese to morbidly obese [16]. Gain in BMI or in body fat is associated with increased risk of developing hypertension [17]. In obese people, a low dietary energy intake that induces weight loss reduces blood pressure [18,19]. BP has been correlated with both fat cell size and number [15]. Obese individuals may have larger adipocytes with altered metabolic activity that may produce bioactive molecules that predispose to hypertension (e.g., leptin, angiotensinogen, free fatty acids, reactive oxygen species) as discussed in the following

TABLE 27.1 Classification of Blood Pressure (BP) for Adults

BP Classification	Systolic BP (mmHg)	Diastolic BP (mmHg)
Normal	<120	<80
Prehypertension	120–139	80–89
Stage 1 Hypertension	140–159	90–99
Stage 2 Hypertension	≥160	≥100

This classification is based on the average of two or more properly measured, seated, blood pressure readings performed on each of two or more office visits. *Reprinted from The Seventh Report of the Joint National Committee on Prevention, Detection, Evaluation, and Treatment of High Blood Pressure. JAMA 2003;289:2560–72, U.S. Department of Health and Human Services, National*

TABLE 27.2 Nutritional Factors that May Affect Blood Pressure*

Nutritional Factor	Effect of Increased Nutrient Intake or Nutritional Status on Blood Pressure
Obesity	Increase[†]
Energy intake	May increase
Fat intake	May increase
PUFA intake**	May decrease
Fructose, glucose intake	Increase
Protein, certain amino acid intakes	May decrease
Sodium intake	Increase[†]
Potassium intake	Decrease
Magnesium intake	May decrease
Calcium intake	Little or no intake[††]
Dietary fiber	May decrease
Alcohol intake	Increase
Green coffee bean extract	Decrease
Regular coffee (+) or (−) caffeine	Decrease
Green, Oolong or black tea	Decrease
Dark chocolate	May decrease
Liquid dairy products (milk, yogurt)	Decrease
DASH/Mediterranean diets	Decrease

For some of the nutrients listed, they have been shown to either reduce the risk of developing hypertension or of lowering blood pressure but the evidence that they do both is not clear.
[†]*Obesity and high sodium intakes have the greatest blood pressure increasing effects.*
**PUFA; polyunsaturated fatty acids.*
[††]*Blood pressure effects of calcium are unclear. It is possible that calcium supplements may reduce blood pressure only in people who have low calcium intakes.*

paragraphs [20–22]. The adipose tissue of obese individuals may exhibit enhanced infiltration of macrophages into adipose tissue, which engenders an inflammatory state [20].

Obesity can also be classified according to the waist circumference or the waist:hip ratio. These measurements reflect the amount of abdominal visceral fat mass which is considered to be the fat which is more closely associated with the adverse effects of excess body fat. The waist circumference and waist:hip ratio are independent risk factors for the development of hypertension, diabetes mellitus and cardiovascular and total mortality [23,24]. An abdominal (waist) circumference 102 cm or greater in men and 88 cm or greater in women is considered to indicate abdominal obesity [24]. The ratio of the circumference of the waist to the hip correlates directly with both SBP and DBP (i.e., the male fat distribution is correlated with the blood pressure level) [8,15]. Moreover, the combination of abdominal obesity and truncal obesity (ratio of the subscapular to triceps skinfold thicknesses of 2.24 or greater in men and 1.32 or greater in women) is associated with an increased risk of hypertension. The risk of hypertension associated with this altered fat distribution varies according to race and ethnicity [25,26] and even lower waist circumferences are associated with increased cardiovascular risk in certain Asian populations (e.g., greater than 87 cm and greater than 83 cm in Japanese men and women, respectively [27]). These racial/ethnic differences concerning the quantity and location of body fat and hypertension are consistent with the results of several studies indicating that there is a gene-obesity interaction in the pathogenesis of hypertension in some people [28,29].

Mechanisms by Which Increased Body Fat Causes High Blood Pressure

Overweight and obesity are associated with many physiological and metabolic changes that promote hypertension, as indicated in Table 27.3, and that have recently been reviewed [20,30–32]. One such alteration is elevated activity of the renin-angiotensin-aldosterone system (RAAS) [15,33]. Obesity is associated with increased plasma angiotensinogen, renin, aldosterone and angiotensin converting enzyme (ACE) levels and urinary aldosterone [34,35]. Plasma renin activity (PRA), relative to the intake of sodium chloride, may be disproportionately high [15,19]. PRA and plasma aldosterone levels decrease when obese individuals lose weight, and this decrease is independent of changes in the sodium intake [15]. In experimental animal models, adipocytes release factors that stimulate the release of aldosterone and other compounds that may

TABLE 27.3 Mechanisms of Hypertension in Obesity

1. Activation of the renin-angiotensin-aldosterone system (RAAS):
   (a) Increased serum angiotensinogen, renin, aldosterone and ACE levels are found in obesity.
   (b) Plasma renin activity, relative to sodium chloride intake, is increased in obese subjects.
   (c) Adipose tissue releases factors that stimulate the release of aldosterone and other mineralcorticoid compounds.
2. Obese individuals often have increased sodium intake.
3. Activation of the sympathetic nervous system (SNS):
   (a) Glucose ingestion increases plasma norepinephrine.
   (b) Obese subjects have higher supine plasma epinephrine, norepinephrine and PRA and greater norepinephrine response to upright posture and handgrip exercise.
   (c) Weight loss leads to more normal plasma hormone levels.
4. Thyroid hormone. Overeating increases triiodothyronine production. T3 increases beta-adrenaline receptors.
5. Insulin resistance (causes increased renal NaCl reabsorption, SNS overactivity, proliferation of vascular smooth muscle cells).
6. Obesity-associated chronic kidney disease (e.g., from focal segmental glomerulosclerosis, diabetic nephropathy).
7. Release from adipose tissue of leptin, resistin (antagonizes insulin), proinflammatory cytokines (C- reactive protein [CRP], tumor necrosis factor-alpha [TNFα], interleuken-6 [IL-6], nonesterified fatty acids [NEFA]), reactive oxygen species. Rat studies indicate that these compounds may activate the mineralcorticoid receptor.
8. Endothelin-1 (causes vasoconstriction, may impair nitric oxide synthesis capacity).
9. Nonesterified fatty acids (NEFA) Excessive nutrient intake may increase portal venous delivery of unsaturated NEFA that are associated with increased blood pressure.
10. Increased leptin levels, which may promote SNS activity.
11. Low adiponectin levels in obesity. Low adiponectin is associated HTN, low nitric oxide production, and endothelial dysfunction.
12. Obstructive sleep apnea (may increase SNS activity, cause endothelial dysfunction and enhance RAAS activity, and may be associated with low adiponectin levels.

Reprinted with permission from the Annual Review of Nutrition [269].

activate the mineralcorticoid receptor and promote sodium retention [36].

Obese people who do not have heart failure or chronic kidney disease (CKD) and nonobese people with higher BMIs may have lower levels of serum or plasma pro-brain natriuretic peptide as well as the saliuretic compound, brain natriuretic peptide [32,37—40]. Subcutaneous adipose tissue in obese hypertensive individuals display a reduced ratio of the mRNA level for the natriuretic peptide membrane receptor, guanylyl cyclase type-A, which is activated by natriuretic peptides, as compared to the mRNA level for the natriuretic peptide clearance receptor, which clears these peptides [32,39,40]. These data suggest that in obesity there may be reduced synthesis of the natriuretic peptide membrane receptor and increased synthesis of the receptor that clears the natriuretic peptide from plasma. These findings may explain why the natriuretic and diuretic response to atrial natriuretic peptide may be reduced in obesity [41].

Sympathetic nervous system (SNS) activity may be increased in both the metabolic syndrome and obesity [15,19,42]. Insulin resistance with hyperinsulinemia and increased plasma leptin, which is common in obesity, increase SNS activity [19,42—45]. Obese subjects have higher supine plasma epinephrine, norepinephrine and PRA, increased urinary norepinephrine and a greater norepinephrine response to upright posture and isometric hand-grip exercise [19]. Weight reduction in these individuals reduces these hormones to more normal plasma levels [19]. Glucose ingestion increases plasma norepinephrine, and may raise plasma thyroid hormone. Overeating may enhance triiodothyronine production from thyroxine, and greater triiodothyronine levels may increase beta-adrenaline receptors [42,46]. In this regard, in a cross-sectional study, intake of sugar-sweetened beverages was directly related with SBP and DBP [47]. There was a direct relationship of dietary fructose and glucose with SBP and DBP in people with higher dietary sodium intakes [47]. The PREMIER Trial (see below) also indicated that reduced intake of sugar-sweetened beverages was associated with decreased BP [48].

Obesity predisposes to obstructive sleep apnea [42,49,50]. Persons with increased episodes of apnea or hypopnea during sleep are at increased risk for developing hypertension [51]. Obstructive sleep apnea is associated with insulin resistance, increased SNS activity, endothelial dysfunction, enhanced RAAS activity, increased plasma leptin and low serum adiponectin [42,49,52,53]. These associations may explain why obstructive sleep apnea associated hypertension can be resistant to pharmacological therapy. When obstructive sleep apnea is treated effectively, there is commonly a reduction in SNS activity and a decrease in both daytime and nocturnal BP and in the refractoriness of hypertension to treatment [54,55].

Obesity may also predispose to hypertension by promoting renal sodium retention through insulin resistance. Insulin promotes the intracellular transport of glucose by stimulating insulin receptor substrate-1 (IRS-1). Obesity induces IRS-1 resistance to the actions of insulin, and this appears to be a cause of the hyperglycemia and elevated insulin levels that occur in obesity. On the other hand, insulin stimulation of sodium reabsorption in the proximal tubules appears to be mediated primarily by stimulating insulin receptor substrate-2 (IRS-2) [30,56]. In isolated renal proximal tubules obtained from knock-out mice for IRS-1, insulin still induces sodium reabsorption, presumably by activating IRS-2 [56]. However, insulin stimulation of sodium reabsorption is significantly reduced in knock-out mice for IRS-2 [56]. Thus the high circulating levels of insulin in obesity, which is in part due to IRS-1 resistance to insulin, may overly stimulate IRS-2 activity and thereby enhance renal tubular sodium reabsorption, sodium retention, salt sensitive hypertension and edema. Weight loss reduces resistance to insulin [57].

Obesity increases the risk of CKD due primarily to diabetes mellitus, hypertension, and focal and segmental glomerulosclerosis. These former two conditions often lead to diabetic nephropathy and/or hypertensive nephrosclerosis [31]. As discussed in Chapters 26, 27 and 29, obesity also promotes proteinuria and accelerates the progression of many types of renal disease. CKD, in turn, may predispose to sodium retention and hypertension.

Obesity may be associated with increased plasma leptin levels and resistance to leptin [42,43], abnormal plasma levels of coagulation factors, increased reactive oxygen species, inflammation and endothelial dysfunction which may also contribute to hypertension [21,42,58−60]. Weight loss in overweight and obese adults improves conduit and resistance artery endothelial function and reduces plasma leptin [57]. Evidence, somewhat conflicting, suggests that increased leptin may contribute to SNS activation, sodium retention and vascular resistance [31,43,61,62]. Adipose tissue releases leptin, resistin (which antagonizes the actions of insulin), such proinflammatory cytokines as tumor necrosis factor alpha (TNFα), nonesterified fatty acids (NEFA), and reactive oxygen species [30]. Studies in rats suggest that these latter compounds may activate the mineralcorticoid receptor [30]. Endothelin-1 released from adipose tissue causes vasoconstriction and may impair nitric oxide synthesis. Excessive nutrient intake may also increase portal venous delivery of NEFAs which may elevate blood pressure (see above). Serum adiponectin levels are reduced in obesity, and low adiponectin is associated with low nitric oxide production, endothelial dysfunction and hypertension.

It has been proposed that obesity also induces dysfunction of the microvasculature by the release from adipose tissue of inflammatory cytokines, free fatty acids, and other vasoactive compounds [63]. These processes lead to obesity-associated altered physiology and rarefaction of the microcirculation. The consequences may be increased microvascular resistance and impaired delivery of insulin and glucose to target tissues (e.g., skeletal muscle). These disorders may result in insulin resistance, glucose intolerance, possibly salt sensitivity, and increased risk of type 2 diabetes mellitus, hypertension and cardiovascular disease [63].

As is evident, many of the foregoing processes may work additively to promote hypertension and particularly salt-sensitive hypertension in overweight and obese people. For example, the combination of hyperreninemia, hyperaldosteronism, other compounds with mineralcorticoid-like actions, hyperinsulinemia, increased SNS

activity, CKD, a propensity to retain sodium, and polyphagia with excessive sodium intake may cause sodium chloride sensitive hypertension [31,56,64,65]. Insulin resistance also may predispose to both increased activity of the renin-angiotensin system [33] and inflammation [66]. Increased SNS activity in association with increased endothelin-1 and other factors elaborated with obesity may promote endothelial and vascular dysfunction [31]. The metabolic actions of adipocytes appear to contribute importantly to many of these processes.

Obese individuals are at increased risk for the metabolic syndrome. The Adult Treatment Panel III (ATP) of the National Cholesterol Education Program defines the metabolic syndrome as the presence of at least three of the following constellation of characteristics [67,68]: an increased abdominal waist circumference (greater than 40 inches in men; greater than 35 inches in women), elevated BP (130/85 mmHg or greater), hypertriglyceridemia (150 mg/dL or greater), low serum high-density lipoprotein cholesterol (less than 40 mg/dL in men and less than 50 mg/dL in women), and a fasting blood glucose of 110 mg/dL or greater. Other expert groups have defined the metabolic syndrome somewhat differently, but the essence of these other definitions of the metabolic syndrome is similar to what is described here [67].

People with the metabolic syndrome are likely to have hypertension (which can be considered a part of the metabolic syndrome) and are prone to develop diabetes mellitus, particularly of the type 2 variety. They are also at high risk for cardiovascular, cerebral-vascular, and peripheral vascular disease. As a result of this association with vascular disease, some investigators have expanded the concept of the metabolic syndrome to include other cardiovascular risk factors, and particularly those risk factors associated with inflammation, CKD or cardiovascular disease [7]. Emerging evidence indicates that the metabolic syndrome, which includes obesity as one of its characteristics, is also associated with increased production of aldosterone and activation of the mineralcorticoid receptor, and that these changes may promote inflammation, oxidative stress and insulin resistance [69]. The usefulness of the concept of the metabolic syndrome has recently been challenged because, it is argued, the hazard ratios for morbidity and mortality associated with the metabolic syndrome may be no greater than the sum of the hazard ratios of the individual components of the syndrome [70].

Some observers have described a direct association between BMI, obesity, weight gain, increased waist circumference, diabetes mellitus, nephrolithiasis and hypertension [71−76]. Both calcium oxalate and uric acid stones, as well as elevated serum urate and altered urate metabolism, have been associated with an increased prevalence of obesity, diabetes mellitus and hypertension [71,72,74—76]. Several causes for these interrelationships have been proposed [73,75,76], but the exact mechanisms have not been clearly established. People who are psychologically depressed are also at greater risk for hypertension. This latter relationship may be due, in part, to the greater likelihood that depressed people will have a high BMI [77].

High energy intakes, independent of obesity, also seem to engender hypertension in obese individuals. Dornfeld and coworkers studied the BP of obese patients during and after treatment with a protein-sparing modified fast [78]. During this treatment, BP fell quickly and profoundly, even before much weight was lost. When the low energy formula diets were discontinued and regular foods were reintroduced into their diet, many of these individuals began to ingest excessive quantities of energy and regained weight. Interestingly, for a given body weight, the patients' SBPs and DBPs were significantly greater when these same patients were ingesting excessive energy intakes and gaining weight as compared to when they were at the same body weight but eating a calorie deficient diet and losing weight. The excessive energy intake could be the cause of the greater BPs for a given body weight during weight gain as compared to weight loss. However, possible contributions to this elevated BP from metabolic processes associated with new fat deposition or from the excessive intake of other nutrients, such as sodium and chloride, cannot be excluded.

Among obese, normotensive individuals, short-term weight gain, weight loss, or weight gain followed by weight loss, as compared to those whose weight was stable, was associated with an increased risk of developing hypertension within two years [79]. The reduction in BP that occurs with weight reduction does not appear to be due exclusively to reduction in energy intake and fat mass. Obese individuals often have increased dietary sodium intake [80], which may also promote hypertension (see below). As indicated above, hyperinsulinemia and possibly alterations in the physiology and anatomy of the microcirculation, which are often present in obesity, tend to increase renal tubular sodium reabsorption. However, Reisin et al. provided evidence that in obese, hypertensive individuals, ingestion of low calorie diets and weight loss, independent of a reduction in dietary sodium intake, can lower BP [18]. These investigators placed obese patients on an energy-restricted, weight reduction diet. Each day each individual was fed an amount of sodium equal to the sodium content in his previous 24-hour urinary output. Even though the total body sodium content fell little if at all in these patients, they experienced a substantial fall in mean BP as they lost weight [18].

The foregoing considerations indicate that there are multifactorial causes for hypertension in overweight and obese people. Reduced dietary energy intake and weight loss in obese people probably reduces hypertension by a number of mechanisms. It is important to keep in mind that very obese individuals may have a falsely elevated BP when it is measured with a normal sized blood pressure cuff. For accurate BP measurements, the cuff size should be increased for individuals with large arm circumferences and reduced for people with small arm circumferences.

Excess Fat in Neonates and Children and Low Birth Weights

Overweight children are at increased risk for hypertension as they become older. Obese children develop substantially increased numbers of adipocytes in their bodies that persist into adulthood, and this is considered to be a factor contributing to the difficulty in attaining normal fat mass in obese adult patients who were obese in childhood. On the other hand, children with low birth weights are also at greater risk for developing hypertension. This latter phenomenon was observed in the Helsinki study [81]. The low birth weights are often due to maternal malnutrition or to impaired ability to deliver the nutrients to the fetus; e.g., due to disorders in the placenta or reduced blood flow through the umbilical artery. [82] Low birth weight children often gain excessive weight by the end of the first 10 or 15 years of life, and presumably their increased body mass may contribute to their increased risk of developing hypertension [81]. It has also been postulated that low birth weight children often have a smaller number of nephrons in their kidneys, and this may predispose them to sodium chloride retention and, hence, hypertension [81]. Other metabolic derangements in low birth weight or high birth weight babies may predispose to the metabolic syndrome, obesity and hypertension [82—85].

Fetal Undernutrition

The Dutch Famine, which led to undernutrition of mothers and newborn infants in the Netherlands near the end of World War II, is an example of the long-term effects of fetal undernutrition on the propensity for obesity and hypertension [86]. Fetuses whose mothers were subjected to prenatal famine while the fetuses were in the second and, to a lesser extent, the third trimester of pregnancy in the Netherlands between November, 1944 and May, 1945, tended to be born with low birth weights. They were shown to be more likely to become overweight in childhood and to have a high prevalence of obesity, hypertension and diabetes mellitus, among other disorders, when they aged into their 50s and 60s [86].

INDIVIDUAL NUTRIENTS, MISCELLANEOUS SUBSTANCES AND BLOOD PRESSURE

Sodium Chloride

There is abundant evidence for a direct relation between sodium chloride intake and BP [42,58–60, 64,87,88]. Sodium chloride intake correlates directly with BP across population groups. The association of sodium chloride intake and BP increases with age, BP level, renal insufficiency, and among individuals with a family history of hypertension. The International Study of Salt and Blood Pressure (INTERSALT) indicated that in about 10,000 adults, aged 20–59 years old, who were evaluated at 52 centers in 32 countries, 24-hour urine sodium excretion was significantly and positively associated with the median SBP and DBP, the upward slope of SBP and DBP that occurs with age, and the prevalence of elevated BP [87,89]. Other cross-sectional population-based studies describe a direct relationship between 24-hour urinary sodium and systolic blood pressure, even after multivariant adjustments [90].

Even in normal adults, salt intake affects extracellular volume which, in turn, can affect the risk of hypertension; a reduction of dietary salt intake from 160 to 80 mEq/day reduces their body weight and extracellular volume by 1–1.5 L [91]. The chloride salt of sodium appears to have a substantially greater effect on raising BP than does sodium bicarbonate [92]. Among individuals of similar age and BP level, the pressor response to high sodium intakes varies greatly. The BP of some individuals rises with high sodium chloride intakes, whereas in other individuals, the BP does not appear to be affected by the sodium chloride intake [93]. Sodium chloride sensitivity can be diagnosed by a reduction in BP associated with low sodium chloride intake and/or an increase in BP with sodium chloride loading. It has been estimated that approximately 30–50% of hypertensive persons and a smaller percentage of nonhypertensive persons are sodium chloride sensitive. A limitation of these studies is that the testing for sodium chloride sensitivity with salt loading is generally carried out for only a few weeks or less. It is possible that a person in whom BP does not increase during several weeks of sodium chloride loading, and therefore is classified as sodium chloride resistant, might be predisposed to hypertension if he chronically ingests large quantities of sodium chloride for many months or years. Also,

people who are not determined to be sodium chloride sensitive in these short-term studies can subsequently develop diseases that render them sodium chloride sensitive; for example, CKD or obesity. These matters are of substantial concern because the dietary sodium intakes in many societies are quite high and also because there is a high prevalence of hypertension among adults worldwide, particularly as people age. Reduction in sodium intake may be particularly effective in lowering BP in individuals who are older, obese, African-Americans, possibly in females, and who have CKD, higher SBPs or a greater SBP response to the cold pressor test [88,94].

Several meta-analyses have examined the effects of salt reduction on BP [88,95–100]. Whereas, most meta-analyses report that there is a fall in BP in response to a lower sodium chloride intake, some do not [95,96]. This discrepancy may be due to the inclusion in these latter studies of acute salt loads or short-term periods of salt restriction, sometimes lasting for only five days. Large and abrupt reductions in salt intake can increase sympathetic tone, plasma renin activity and angiotensin II levels [99,101]. When only studies of four or more weeks' duration were included in the meta-analysis, modest restriction of salt intake (i.e., a reduction to 78 mmol or 4.6 g of NaCl) was shown to be associated with lowering of BP [101]. Simply following a "no added salt diet" may reduce SBP and DBP by an average of 12.1 and 6.8 mmHg during the day and 11.1 and 5.9 mmHg at night [102]. This "no added salt diet" is defined as no added salt to foods and no intake of salty foods; salt intake should be below 5 g/day with a urinary sodium excretion below 100 mEq/24 hours. An extensive Cochrane review of randomized studies of high-sodium vs. low-sodium diets indicated that high sodium diets slightly, but significantly decreased blood pressure by 1% in normotensive and 3.5% in hypertensive people [88]. This latter meta-analysis also described highly significant increases in plasma renin, aldosterone, noradrenaline, adrenaline, cholesterol and triglycerides with sodium restriction [88].

Obesity appears to increase the sensitivity of BP to sodium chloride intake in adolescents, possibly because of the hyperinsulinemia, hyperaldosteronism and enhanced sympathetic nervous system activity that are commonly found in obese individuals [64]. Weight loss in these individuals appears to decrease their salt sensitivity. Patients with essential hypertension have higher urinary free cortisol excretion [103]. Such hypertensive individuals who had higher urinary free cortisol excretion were found to have a lower reduction in SBP and mean arterial pressure in response to reduced sodium intake [103]. Moreover, baseline plasma renin concentrations, obtained at the onset of an eight-week study, were inversely related with the magnitude of salt sensitivity, whereas the baseline plasma N-terminal atrial natriuretic peptide levels correlated directly with this phenomenon [104].

There is direct evidence for a genetic link for the association between hypertension and sodium intake and possibly obesity. In people who were 60 years of age or older, there was a linear increase in SBP and DBP with sodium loading [105]. This increase in BP with sodium loading was greatest in individuals with isolated systolic hypertension. The change in DBP in response to sodium loading varied in accordance to the type of gene polymorphism of the angiotensinogen gene, but not with regard to polymorphisms of the angiotensin converting enzyme gene [105]. Obese hypertensives who were homozygous (TT genotype) or heterozygous (TC+CC genotype) for the T-786 endothelial nitric oxide synthase (eNOS) gene were studied [106]. The metabolic product of this enzyme, endothelial-derived nitric oxide (NOx), is a vasodilator. The heterozygous obese hypertensive patients with the TC+CC genotype, as compared to the homogyzous TT genotype patients, had a greater increase in diastolic and mean arterial BP, and a significant decrease in renal plasma flow and glomerular filtration rate in response to sodium loading [106]. Moreover, with sodium loading, the TT genotype has a significantly greater increase in plasma NOx, whereas the TC+CC genotype had a borderline significant increase (p = 0.051) in urinary NOx excretion.

BP in individuals with stage 4 (GFR 15–29 mL/min/1.73 m^2) or stage 5 (GFR <15 mL/min/1.73 m^2) CKD may be particularly sensitive to sodium or volume expansion [107,108]. Shaldon reported that in a 23-year-old male with chronic renal failure who was fed a salt restricted diet for eight weeks, BP fell from 230/145 mmHg to 135/90 mmHg, and there was a reduction in headache, nausea, vomiting and papilledema and improvement in vision [109]. The reduction in BP may continue for months after the removal of body NaCl by dietary restriction and dialysis ultrafiltration. The authors speculate that this delayed response may be due to the decrease in non-osmotically active sodium which is possibly bound in proteoglycans and glycosaminoglycans in the interstitial matrix that lines the intimal surfaces of blood vessels [110]. A growing body of evidence suggests that high sodium intakes may promote more rapid progression of chronic kidney failure, possibly by an increase in oxidative stress, albuminuria and BP, and alterations in glomerular hemodynamics [110,111]. Some authorities have postulated that salt sensitive hypertension may be caused by subtle injuries to the kidney. Such injuries may be associated with both renal microstructural and physiological abnormalities [112]. These disorders may cause an impaired ability to excrete a sodium load and the consequent development of volume expansion with attendant hypertension.

Potassium

Epidemiological and clinical studies concerning potassium intake support the thesis that potassium supplements (e.g., 60–120 mEq/day) lower BP, but results of randomized, prospective trials have yielded conflicting results. However, in a meta-analysis of 19 clinical trials involving 586 hypertensives, Cappuccio and MacGregor reported that oral potassium supplements significantly lowered both SBP and DBP by −5.9 mmHg (95 % CI, −6.6 to −5.2) and by −3.4 mmHg (−4.0 to −2.8), respectively, in subjects with essential hypertension [77]. In the meta-analysis of Whelton and co-workers, potassium supplementation was associated with a significant reduction in mean SBP and DBP of −3.11 mmHg (−1.91 to −4.31 mmHg) and −1.97 mmHg (−0.52 to −3.42 mmHg), respectively [113].

Potassium deficiency, even of a mild nature, may induce renal sodium retention, increase BP and engender salt sensitivity [114–116]. Mu and associates presented evidence that supplements of potassium and calcium may prevent hypertension in adolescents by promoting urinary sodium excretion [117]. Pere and co-workers fed a high-sodium diet and administered cyclosporine A to eight week old spontaneously hypertensive rats [118]. The animals developed hypertension and renal injury associated with renal dopaminergic deficiency [118]. A combined dietary supplement of magnesium and potassium prevented hypertension in these rats. Potassium deficient diets are particularly common in African Americans and have been associated with the high prevalence of hypertension and sodium chloride sensitivity in these individuals.

Potassium intake may lower elevated BP by a number of mechanisms [119]. As indicated above, potassium intake may increase renal sodium excretion. Potassium may modulate baroreflex sensitivity, directly cause vasodilation, or reduce cardiovascular reactivity to norepinephrine or angiotensin II. A supplement of potassium, 217 mg/day, and magnesium, 71 mg/day, for four weeks increased small artery compliance and reduced BP in patients with essential hypertension [120]. Thus, it has been recommended that a substantial potassium intake should be maintained to prevent or treat hypertension, particularly in subjects who are unable to reduce their sodium intake and in those who are salt sensitive or who have a family history of hypertension [119]. Nowson and coworkers reported that a reduction in sodium intake to about 70 mmol/day and an increase in dietary potassium to 85 mmol/day can maintain a lower BP and reduce the burden of cardiovascular disease [121].

The Dietary Reference Intakes propose that an adequate potassium intake is 4.7 g (120 mmol) per day which should lower BP and reduce the BP raising effects of sodium chloride [122]. In this regard, an increase in dietary potassium intake to 120 mmol/day abolished or suppressed the frequency or severity of salt sensitivity in normotensive African American men to the levels found in normotensive white men [116]. Also, a randomized, double-blind, prospective controlled trial of potassium supplementation, 80 mmol/day, or placebo for 21 days in normotensive or mildly hypertensive African Americans ingesting a low, 32–35 mmol/day, potassium diet significantly reduced their SBP and DBP [123]. A somewhat longer-term, six-week, randomized, double-blind placebo controlled trial in mostly normotensive adults of European descent that provided only 24 mmol/day of supplemental KCl also showed that this modest potassium dose significantly lowered mean arterial BP, SBP and DBP [124].

Calcium

There is considerable controversy as to whether high calcium intakes lower BP. McCarron and co-workers conducted a series of studies suggesting that calcium supplementation lowers BP [125]. Indeed, they and others found an inverse correlation across populations and ethnic groups between the mean dietary calcium intake and BP levels [125–127]. The Nurses' Health Study initially found an inverse relationship between dietary calcium and BP after the first four years of follow-up [128]. With longer follow-up, no independent relationship between dietary calcium intake and BP could be demonstrated [129]. Cappuccio and coworkers carried out a meta-analysis of 23 observational studies and reported an inverse relationship between calcium intake (determined from dietary diaries and food frequency questionnaires) and BP [130]. However the effect was rather small, and there was evidence of publication bias and heterogeneity of data across the investigations.

Bucher and associates performed a meta-analysis of 33 randomized clinical trials of dietary calcium supplementation involving 2412 individuals with or without hypertension [131]. They described for the entire group a small but significant reduction in SBP of −1.27 mmHg (95% CI, -2.25 to −0.29 mmHg; p = 0.01) but no change in DBP (0.24 mmHg; 95 % CI, −0.92 to 0.44 mmHg; p = 0.49). In six of these studies in which participants were classified according to whether they were hypertensive or not, there was a significant fall in SBP and DBP in the hypertensive individuals but not in the normotensives [131]. Allender and co-workers carried out

a meta-analysis of 22 randomized clinical trials in 1231 individuals [132]. In this meta-analysis, calcium supplementation was associated with a statistically significant, but not very clinically important reduction, in SBP, −0.89 mmHg (95% CI, −3.18 to 0.18 mmHg) and in DBP, 0.18 mmHg (95% CI, −0.75 to 0.40 mmHg). Griffith et al., in a large meta-analysis on the effects of supplemental calcium on BP, reported a reduction in SBP of −1.44 mmHg (95% CI, −2.20 to −0.68, p < 0.001) and in DBP of −0.84 mmHg (95% CI, −1.44 to −0.24, p < 0.001) [133]. Subjects in these studies were given calcium supplements of 400 to 2000 mg/day [129–133]. Calcium supplements that resulted in a median total daily calcium intake of about 1 g/day did not affect SBP or DBP in normotensive individuals [132–135]. In three small studies, the supplemental calcium intake diminished the rise in BP response to a high sodium intake [134–136].

It has been suggested that the discrepancies in the published results concerning the effects of calcium intake on BP may be related to the possibility that a low calcium diet predisposes to hypertension, whereas in individuals who are already eating adequate calcium, higher intakes of calcium have little or no BP lowering effect [131–133]. In this regard, Pan and coworkers gave calcium supplements to individuals with mild or moderate hypertension who lived in areas of China where there is both a higher prevalence of hypertension and a high salt and low calcium content of the diet. They reported that after 35 days of treatment with calcium lactate supplements that provided 800 mg of calcium per day, there was a reduction in SBP and DBP of −4.7 (p = 0.027) and −2.2 (p = 0.074) mmHg, respectively. Moreover, it was reported that calcium supplements reduced BP in normotensive individuals as well [135]. Further studies will be needed to resolve this question of a possible BP lowering effect of calcium that may be largely or entirely limited to calcium-deficient individuals. It is possible that the higher calcium intake in the DASH combination diet and in low fat and fluid dairy products contributed to the BP lowering effects of these regimens (see DASH diet below).

Fish Oil

There are two meta-analyses of controlled clinical trials of the use of omega-3 fatty acids [137,138]. In the study of Appel and coworkers concerning 11 trials that enrolled 728 normotensive individuals [137], omega-3 PUFA supplements led to a significant reduction in SBP and in DBP in only two and one of these trials, respectively. In six studies involving 291 untreated mildly hypertensive individuals, reductions in SBP and DBP were observed in two and four of the trials, respectively [137]. The weighted, pooled reductions in

SBP and DBP in the normotensive individuals averaged −1.0 (95% CI, −2.0 to 0.0) and −0.5 (95% CI, −1.2 to +0.2) mmHg. In the trials of untreated hypertensive persons, the weighted, pooled decreases in SBP and DBP averaged −5.5 (−8.1 to −2.9) and −3.5 (−5.0 to −2.1) mmHg. The doses of omega-3 PUFA used in these studies tended to be rather high, usually 3 g/d or greater [137].

Morris et al. evaluated 31 placebo-controlled clinical trials involving 1356 subjects and showed, with fish oil use, a mean reduction in SBP of −3.0 mmHg (95% CI, −4.5, −1.5 mmHg) and in DBP of −1.5 mmHg (95%CI, −2.2, −0.8 mmHg) with a statistically significant dose-response relationship [138]. There was a dose response relationship between fish oil dose and SBP and DBP reduction. The decrease in SBP and DBP was statistically significant in the hypertensive patients but not in the normotensive subjects, although the fish oil dose used was slightly higher in the hypertensives (5.6 g/d) as compared to the normotensives (4.2 g/d) [138]. These meta-analyses indicate that in people who are assigned to a relatively high omega-3 fatty acid intake, there is a statistically significant reduction in BP in hypertensive individuals, and little or no effect in normotensive persons.

More recently, a randomized prospective double-blind clinical trial, in a 2 × 2 design, compared the effects on BP of daily doses of n-3 polyunsaturated fatty acids (n-3 PUFA), 1200 mg, a combination of three B vitamins (5-methyl-tetrahydrofolate 560 μg, vitamin B_6 3 mg, and vitamin B_{12} 20 μg), both of these treatments combined, or placebo [139]. The n-3 PUFA provided EPA and DHA in a 2:1 ratio. The B vitamins were given, in part, to assess the effect of lowering plasma homocysteine on BP. A total of 2501 men and women with a history of cardiovascular disease were studied for 5 years. At baseline, their mean SBP and DBP (mmHg) averaged in the low 130s and 80s, respectively, with a mean number of 1.7 antihypertensive medications taken per subject. There was no effect of the n-3 PUFA, the three B vitamins, or the combination of both of these supplements on SBP, DBP or mean BP in these individuals. It is possible that a higher n-3 PUFA dose than was used in this trial might have been more effective.

The mechanism by which fish oil may lower BP in hypertensive patients is not clear. It may be related to enhanced elaboration of prostaglandins which, in turn, may increase sodium and water excretion, promote vasodilation, and/or inhibit the release of thromboxane (a vasoconstrictor). Also, it is possible that prostaglandins may regulate renin release or decrease responsiveness to vasopressor hormones. The preponderance of studies with fish oil were of short duration (less than 3 months). Longer term studies will be necessary to determine whether fish oil has a sustained anti-hypertensive effect in hypertensive persons and also to assess the optimal fish oil dose for BP lowering. There are a number of side effects with fish oil intake, including most commonly eructation and a bad or fishy taste [137,138]. The higher percentage of polyunsaturated fatty acids in the DASH Combination Diet might have also contributed to the reduced BP with this diet (see below).

Magnesium

Whether magnesium supplements lowers BP in hypertensive individuals is controversial. Some studies show that magnesium reduces BP [140], whereas other studies do not [141]. The antihypertensive effects of magnesium supplementation are small in many of the studies that suggest such an effect. In one meta-analysis of 20 randomized clinical trials of magnesium supplementation in hypertensive persons (14 trials) and normotensive individuals (six trials) 1220 persons were evaluated [140]. The dose of magnesium supplements ranged from 10 to 40 mmol/d with a median intake of 15.4 mmol/d. The pooled net estimates of BP effects showed only a small reduction in SBP, −0.6 mmHg (95%CI, −2.2 to +1.0, p = 0.051), and DBP, −0.8 mmHg (95%CI, −2.1 to +0.5, p = 0.142), with magnesium supplements. There was no significant fall in SBP (p = 0.06) or DBP (p = 0.17) when analysis was restricted to the 14 hypertensive trials. There appeared to be a dose-dependent effect of magnesium with an average reduction in SBP of −4.3 mmHg (95%CI, −6.3 to −2.2, p < 0.001) and in DBP of −2.3 mmHg (95%CI, −4.9 to 0.0, p < 0.09) for each 10 mmol/day (~240 mg/day) increase in magnesium intake [140]. Larger intakes of magnesium, i.e., 500 to 1000 mg/day, may be more likely to lower blood pressure [142]. However, many people with hypertension have CKD with reduced ability to excrete magnesium, and they may be at risk for hypermagnesemia with large magnesium supplements. It is suggested that magnesium may have a more pronounced BP lowering effect when it is provided with a high potassium and low sodium intake [142]. Magnesium may exert its BP lowering effects by decreasing intracellular sodium and cytoplasmic free calcium [143]. The combined intake of magnesium and taurine may lower SBP and DBP possibly because both chemicals decrease intracellular calcium and sodium [143,144].

Protein and Amino Acids

Epidemiological studies indicate an inverse relationship between protein intake and BP [145]. A small number of clinical trials indicate that supplements of soybean protein may decrease SBP or DBP [145—147]. A larger scale, randomized double-blind, controlled trial was carried out in 302 adults in China in which subjects were assigned to receive either 40 g/day of supplemental soybean protein or 40 g/day of complex carbohydrates [146]. All participants had prehypertension or stage 1 hypertension with an initial untreated SBP of 130—159 mmHg and/or DBP of 80—99. During the 12 weeks of treatment, SBP and DBP fell in both groups but deceased significantly more in the soybean protein treated group. The greater decrease in BP in the soybean protein treated participants over the complex carbohydrate treated group was by −4.31 (95% CI, −2.11 to −6.51) mmHg systolic and −2.76 (95% CI, −1.35 to −4.16) mmHg diastolic at 12 weeks of intervention. In a subgroup analysis there were significantly greater decreases in SBP (−7.88 mmHg) and DBP (−5.27 mmHg) in the soybean protein vs. the carbohydrate treated subjects who had stage 1 hypertension [146]. The prehypertensive individuals showed a trend, not significant, for a reduction in SBP and DBP. This study did not examine whether it was the protein or the isoflavones in the soybean that reduced the BP.

Several potential mechanisms have been suggested to explain how soybean protein may reduce BP [146]. Soybean protein contains substantial amounts of arginine, which can be converted to nitric oxide, a potent vasodilator [148]. Intravenous injection of arginine reduces peripheral vascular resistance and decreases BP in humans [149]. Glutamic acid, which is high in vegetable proteins, may have special blood pressure lowering effects [150]. Digestion of proteins derived from foods may release bioactive peptides that inhibit angiotensin converting enzyme and that probably have other antihypertensive actions [151]. Proteins derived from milk are particularly likely to yield these peptides [151]. This may contribute to the antihypertensive effects of the DASH diet (see below). Protein may also increase urinary excretion of sodium, water, and free dopamine [152,153]. A dopamine mediated natriuresis engendered by ingested protein may lower BP [153]. Soybean protein may also increase insulin sensitivity and glucose tolerance [154]; since insulin resistance and consequent hyperinsulinemia may predispose to hypertension (see above), this latter effect of soybean protein may decrease BP [155].

An epidemiological study of 3588 Dutch adults followed for up to 10 years reported that greater ingestion of grain protein was associated with a small decrease in the incidence of hypertension; HR = 0.85; 95% CI, 0.73 to 1.00; $p_{trend} = 0.04$ for the risk of new onset hypertension between the upper and lower tertiles of protein intake from grain [156]. No association was found between the development of hypertension and the intake of either animal or dairy protein in this study. Large protein supplements may not be indicated for individuals who have diseases that render them protein intolerant, such as CKD, acute kidney injury or liver failure. As indicated above, the combination of increased taurine and magnesium intakes may lower BP [144].

Fiber

Dietary fiber is considered part of a healthy diet that may exert protective effects on the gastrointestinal tract and cardiovascular system. Streppel and coworkers carried out a meta-analysis showing that increasing dietary fiber intake in Western populations, where the usual fiber intake is well below recommended levels, may help to prevent hypertension [154]. In another meta-analysis, Whelton and co-workers reported that increased intake of dietary fiber may reduce BP in hypertensive patients; in normotensive individuals, there was a smaller, less conclusive reduction in BP [155]. A randomized, controlled trial in hypertensive individuals indicated that dietary protein and fiber had significant, additive effects on lowering both 24-hour and awake SBP [147]. It is possible that some of the antihypertensive effects of dietary sodium restriction may involve changes in the intake of such other nutrients as fiber. Sciarrone and associates report that reduction in sodium intake may decrease the dietary content of both fats and fiber, which might independently affect BP and lipid metabolism [157]. In a more recent rather small scale study, overweight and obese adults were randomly assigned to ingest their usual diet with placebo, their usual diet with 21 g/day of psyllium fiber, or a healthy diet with placebo and without supplemental fiber [158]. In the 57 subjects who completed the 12- week study, those who were fed psyllium did not demonstrate a sustained reduction in either SBP or DBP as compared to the control group.

Alcohol

Excessive alcohol intake often increases BP. However, these effects are generally transient, and BP usually falls rapidly when individuals stop drinking alcohol [159]. A time dependent association between alcohol consumption and BP levels was reported by Moreira in experimental studies of free-living individuals. In contrast to these findings, the frequency of alcohol consumption and type of beverage ingested were not found to be independently associated with BP levels [160]. Subjects of African ancestry who consumed large amounts of alcohol showed a high risk of developing hypertension [161]. In hypertensive individuals, heavy alcohol consumption leads to a significant increase in the risk of cerebral hemorrhage, suggesting a synergistic effect of alcohol and hypertension [162]. On the other hand, light alcohol consumption significantly reduces the risk for stroke. In the North American free-living population, the consumption of alcohol in amounts greater than 210 g per week is an independent risk factor for hypertension, whereas consumption of low to moderate amounts appears to be associated with higher risk of hypertension in black men but not in white men or black or white women [163]. In Chinese males, a higher intake of alcohol is associated with a higher risk for isolated systolic hypertension, both systolic and diastolic hypertension, and isolated diastolic hypertension [164].

The mechanisms involved in alcohol-generating hypertension appear to include the effects of vasoconstriction, modification of smooth muscles, and calcium movement [165]. Zilkens and coworkers studied 24 healthy men who underwent four regimens, in random order, for four weeks each: (i) abstinence from all alcohol and grape products or a daily intake of: (ii) 375 mL of red wine containing 39 g alcohol; (iii) 375 mL of de-alcoholized red wine; or (iv) 1125 mL of beer providing 41 g alcohol. Daily consumption of about 40 grams of alcohol either as red wine or beer resulted in a similar mild increase in 24-hour SBP and awake SBP and 24-hour heart rate, whereas de-alcoholized red wine did not lower BP. The red wine, beer and de-alcoholized red wine did not affect vascular function (i.e., flow-mediated vasodilation). These observations suggest that in men it is the alcohol in red wine and beer that increases SBP and that nonalcoholic components of red wine do not mitigate the BP elevating effects of alcohol [166]. Notwithstanding evidence that alcohol intake, particularly in larger amounts, is associated with increased BP, there are abundant epidemiological data indicating that alcoholic drinks, and perhaps particularly red wine, may reduce the risk of death from cardiovascular disease. The mechanisms for this protective effect are not completely understood and may involve the actions of alcohol per se and possibly also the effects of the antioxidant and vasodilator phenolic compounds.

Vitamin D

Vitamin D deficiency (deficiency of 25-hydroxycholecalciferol [25(OH)D] is reported to occur in almost 50% of the world's population [167]. Vitamin D insufficiency is often defined as serum 25(OH)D 20−30 ng/mL (50−75 nmol/L), and vitamin D deficiency is defined as 25[OH]D below 20 ng/mL (<50 nmol/L) [167]. Approximately 80−90% of the body's vitamin D levels are considered to come from the effects of sunlight on the skin [167], and the high risk of vitamin D deficiency is considered to be due reduced outdoor activities, the desire to avoid sun exposure, air pollutants, living at high latitudes, dark skin, frequent use of

sunscreens, and the impaired ability of older people to produce vitamin D in the skin in response to sunlight. Knock out mice for the vitamin D receptor or the 1α-hydroxylase enzyme develop high renin hypertension and cardiac hypertrophy hypertension [168,169]. In hypertensive patients, there may be an inverse relationship between plasma renin activity and 1,25(OH)2D levels [170]. Studies at the cellular and molecular level, indicate that 1,25 [OH]2D is a negative regulator of renin gene expression by binding of the vitamin D receptor to the transcription factor cAMP-response element-binding protein [171]. 1,25[OH]2D also suppresses vascular endothelial and smooth muscle cell tissue factor, thrombospondin and plasminogen activator inhibirtor-1 and increases synthesis of vascular endothelial growth factor, prostaglandin and hepatic thrombomodulin [172]. These effects would appear to be cardioprotective, inhibitory of thrombosis, and promotive of fibrinolysis [172,173].

Epidemiological and other studies also suggest that, in addition to bone mineral and divalent ion metabolism, vitamin D may also reduce insulin resistance and have vascular protective, renoprotective and anti-inflammatory effects [174−177]. Hence, vitamin D may not only reduce blood pressure but may also prevent or ameliorate a number of the vascular and renal complications of hypertension. On the other hand, excessive vitamin D intake with toxicity (serum 25[OH]D >150 ng/mL, >374.4 nmol/L) may induce hypercalcemia, arterial stiffness, hypertension and progressive renal failure [167].

Some, but not all epidemiological cross-sectional studies describe an inverse relation between serum 1,25[OH]2D and especially 25[OH]D levels and SBP or DBP [172,173]. Clinical trials of vitamin D supplementation on BP are less consistent. One double-blind trial of 1200 mg calcium/day alone or with 800 IU vitamin D/day in elderly vitamin D deficient women showed significant reductions in SBP and DBP in both groups, but with a significantly greater reduction in SBP, by −7.4 mmHg, in the vitamin D treated group [178]. Most, but not all, of the other trials of vitamin D supplements on SBP or DBP were negative [173]. However, it has been argued that most of these studies were not primarily or adequately designed to assess the effects of vitamin D on BP, the subjects were not hypertensive or vitamin D deficient, the vitamin D dose might have been too low (e.g., 400 IU/day) or the BPs may not have been measured in a sophisticated fashion [173]. An example is the Women's Health Initiative which conducted the largest randomized clinical trial of vitamin D [179]. This trial, which was carried out for a mean of 7 years, randomized over 32,000 postmenopausal women to receive 400 IU vitamin D plus 1000 mg calcium per day or placebo. There were no significant differences in changes in SBP or DBP or in the incidence of hypertension during the study. Possibly the vitamin D dose was too small.

Supplementation with 1,25[OH]$_2$D or its analogues, paricalcitol or 1α-hydroxyvitamin D, have also given inconsistent results with regard to BP reduction [173]. Some evidence suggests that BP-lowering effects of vitamin D supplements may be more effective in people who are vitamin D deficient. The PRIMO Trial studied 115 patients with stage 3 and 4 CKD and left ventricular hypertrophy and preserved left ventricular ejection fraction who were randomized to receive paricalcitol, 2.0 μg/day and 112 similar patients randomized to placebo for up to 48 weeks [180]. The paricalcitol dose could be reduced down to 1 μg/day if patients became hypercalcemic. 96% of patients were hypertensive. SBP or DBP did not differ significantly during the course of the study. More well designed, adequately powered randomized controlled clinical trials are needed to definitively assess the possible effects of vitamin D on BP.

Chocolate

A randomized, cross-over, short-term (seven day) study was conducted to assess the effect of ingestion of chocolate on BP in 20 patients with grade I essential hypertension who had never received antihypertensive treatment [181]. Eating dark chocolate, but not white chocolate, was associated with a significant lowering of SBP ($-11.9 \pm$ SD9.7 mmHg, $p < 0.0001$) and DBP (-8.1 ± 5.0 mmHg, $p < 0.0001$). The authors suggest that dark chocolate may lower BP by its high flavonol content which induces vasorelaxation. Dark chocolate has also been shown to decrease isolated systolic hypertension in geriatric patients [182] and in one [183] but not in all studies [184,185], in healthy persons.

Coffee

Suzuki et al. showed hypotensive effects of green coffee bean extract and its metabolites in spontaneously hypertensive rats [186]. Kozuma et al. reported a dose-responsive antihypertensive affect of green coffee bean extract given to mildly hypertensive individuals for 28 days [187]. These findings were confirmed by Watanabe and coworkers who studied essential hypertension in rats and humans [188]. The BP lowering effect of green coffee bean extract is attributed to the effects of chlorogenic acid and its metabolites on vascular reactivity [186–189].

Interestingly, roasted coffee extract may not have these antihypertensive effects [186]. Caffeine induced fluctuations in BP by stimulating not well specified cardiovascular mechanisms [190]. Corti studied the acute effects of coffee in volunteers who drank a triple espresso or a decaffeinated triple Espresso or who were infused intravenously with 250 mg of caffeine. The subjects showed an increase in sympathetic nerve activity and BP after receiving the coffee which was independent of whether caffeine was present [191]. An epidemiological study described an association between coffee intake, even as low as one cup per day, and a small increase in SBP and DBP. Coffee drinking was also associated with a small increase in risk of hypertension [192]. A meta-analysis of 11 interventional trials of coffee drinking, 10 of which were randomized, found that it was associated with a mild increase in SBP and DBP [193]. The median coffee intake in the studies was five cups/day. It has been suggested that pregnant women should limit their ingestion of coffee to no more than three cups per day and ingest no more than 300 mg of caffeine per day to reduce the probability of spontaneous abortion or impaired fetal growth and to reduce such cardiovascular disease risk factors as elevated BP and hyperhomocysteinemia [194]. On the other hand, prehypertensive or hypertensive men who were habitual alcohol drinkers demonstrated a reduction in SBP and DBP when they drank more than three cups of coffee per day for four weeks [195].

Tea

The relationship between BP and tea drinking is particularly relevant, because the volume of tea consumption is second only to water intake in the world [196]. The effect of tea on BP may be less consistent than the effects of coffee according to different reports [196]. However, Yang and coworkers report that chronic, moderate consumers of green or oolong tea are less likely to develop hypertension [197]. The effect may be due to flavonoids, which affect endothelial function [198]. Green, oolong and black tea contain a number of flavonoids and other compounds that in animal or human studies engender vasodilatation, protect against endothelial dysfunction, and have anti-oxidant, anti-inflammatory or hypolipidemic effects [196,197,199]. Hodgson et al. studied the acute effects of tea on fasting and postprandial vascular function and BP in humans. They showed that consumption of foods altered the acute beneficial effects of tea on vascular function and blood pressure [200].

A controlled trial was conducted in 95 regular tea drinkers who were randomized to drink three cups/day of black tea or placebo for six months [201]. Mean 24 hour baseline SBP and DBP were 121.4 and 72.9 mmHg. Compared with placebo, at six months, the black tea drinkers sustained a significant decrease in 24 hour ambulatory SBP (-2.0 mmHg, $p = 0.05$) and DBP (-2.1 mmHg, $p = 0.003$). 24 hour ambulatory

SBP and DBP were also significantly lower in the black tea drinking participants at 3 months [201]. Consumption of either sugar-containing or diet cola beverages has been associated with increased risk for hypertension possibly due to their caffeine content [202].

Urate

As indicated in the above discussion of obesity, elevated urate levels may predispose to hypertension. In a double-blind, placebo-controlled, cross-over trial in adolescents with newly diagnosed stage 1 essential hypertension and with serum urate levels of 6.0 mg/dL or greater, short-term treatment with allopurinol, which decreased serum urate levels, lowered BP [203]. Twenty-two of the 30 participants in this study were overweight or obese. Fructose intake predisposes to urate formation. As indicated above, fructose intake is directly correlated with SBP and DBP in people with higher urinary sodium excretion [47].

NUTRITIONAL MANAGEMENT STRATEGIES FOR THE PREVENTION OR TREATMENT OF HYPERTENSION

In addition to increasing or reducing the intake of the above reviewed nutrients that may affect blood pressure, a number of specific nutritional strategies have been developed to prevent or treat hypertension. These are reviewed below.

Prevention and Treatment of Excessive Body Fat

Methods for prevention of excessive fat gain and weight reduction treatments utilizing healthy lifestyles and reduced energy intake or bariatric surgery are discussed in Chapters 27, 28 and 29. The following comments briefly summarize these approaches, particularly with regard to prevention or treatment of hypertension.

Energy Intake and Blood Pressure

Weight loss due to dietary intervention or bariatric surgery in obese, hypertensive persons, with or without diabetes mellitus or chronic kidney disease, is generally associated with a decrease in BP [204–206]. Programs that are designed to lower dietary energy intakes, fat mass and blood pressure generally include a more global health-oriented approach that also emphasizes an overall healthier diet and lifestyle. These programs will be discussed below. The effects of medicine-induced weight loss on hypertension will also briefly discussed [49,204,207,208].

Bariatric Surgery

The clinical experience with bariatric surgery is discussed in detail in Chapter 28. Some types of bariatric surgery appear to be the most reliable and effective methods for reducing fat mass in obese individuals including patients with diabetes mellitus [205,209, 210–212]. In general, weight loss is substantially greater with bariatric surgery than with diet and lifestyle treatments (see below), particularly when the effectiveness of treatment is evaluated over periods of time measured in years rather than just a few months. Moreover, reversal of type 2 diabetes in obese individuals appears to be more common with bariatric surgery, than with diet and lifestyle changes alone and are reported to reach values of 75% with Roux-in-Y gastric bypass and 95% with biliopancreatic diversion [212].

It should be emphasized that successful bariatric surgery programs also include counseling to reduce calorie intake and to adopt a healthier lifestyle. After surgery, the types and volumes of foods that can be ingested by the patient may need to be dramatically changed. There are several types of bariatric surgery, as discussed in Chapter 28. Gastric banding and sleeve gastrectomy are less invasive than some of the other bariatric surgery procedures, and the incidence of serious complications tend to be lower, but weight loss may also be lower than with more extensive surgery (see Chapter 28 [211,212]). Overall, the complication rates with bariatric surgery are not high. However, the numbers of patients studied and the duration of follow-up with bariatric surgery are still rather limited, particularly in randomized controlled trials, and further experience will be necessary before the full therapeutic impact and complication rates of various types of bariatric surgery will be well-defined [210]. Nonetheless, evidence from long-term follow-up suggests that weight loss, reduced glycemia and cardiovascular risk may be sustained for 10 or more years after bariatric surgery [205,209]. Bariatric surgery is becoming an increasingly common option to attain long-term weight reduction for people who are refractory to weight reduction by dietary and lifestyle changes alone (please see Chapters 27, 28 and 29).

HEALTH ENHANCING DIETS AND LIFESTYLES

In the past 25 years, there has been a growing focus on the use of complex, health-enhancing diets to prevent or treat hypertension, usually of the mild to moderately severe variety. The composition of these diets is generally based on evidence that the individual constituents of these diets have preventative or therapeutic effects on hypertension. Much of this evidence is summarized in the first part of this chapter. Experience regarding the effectiveness of and patient-adherence to these diets are discussed below.

The Hypertension Prevention Trial (HPT)

The HPT was a multicenter trial in which 841 adults with DBPs of 78–89 mmHg were randomly assigned to one of four dietary counseling treatments (decreased energy intake, decreased sodium intake, decreased sodium and energy intake, or decreased sodium and increased potassium intake) or to a control group that did not receive dietary counseling [213]. Men and women with lower BMIs (n = 211), were not assigned to the two low energy intake groups. Subjects assigned to one of the four treatments underwent group counseling weekly for the first 10 weeks, then every other week for the next four weeks and finally bimonthly for the duration of study. Phone calls, newsletters and other methods were employed to facilitate training and compliance. People were followed for three years. Attendance at scheduled counseling sessions declined significantly with time. At six months, overnight urine sodium excretion had fallen by 13%, urine potassium increased by 8%, and body weight fell by −7% as compared to changes in the control group. At three years, the reductions in urine sodium and weight, compared to changes in controls, were −10% and −4%, respectively, whereas there was no change in urine potassium. The net reductions in weight in the low energy groups at three years were due in large part to the increase in weight in the control group. BP decreased from baseline in all treatment groups including the controls. The largest net reduction in SBP and DBP occurred in the low energy group alone, −5.1 and −2.4 mmHg and -2.8 and −1.8 mmHg, at 6 months and 3 years, respectively (p < 0.05 for each BP at each time). The sodium reduction groups sustained a significantly lower composite rate of hypertensive events (i.e., SBP ≥ 140 mmHg, DBP ≥ 90 mmHg or intake of antihypertensive medicines); the other treatment groups experienced a nonsignificant trend in this same direction.

The Trials of Hypertension Prevention (TOHP): TOHP Phase I

The TOHP was a multicenter trial involving two phases. TOHP Phase I was a short-term trial designed to test the effect of three different lifestyle interventions and four nutritional supplements on BP control in individuals with high normal DBP. TOHP Phase II was designed to test more long-term, for 36–48 months, those interventions that were demonstrated in TOHP Phase I to lower BP. In phase I, 2182 men and women

with average high normal DBP (80–89 mmHg) and with SBP ≤160 mmHg were randomized in a parallel-controlled fashion to receive weight loss intervention, dietary sodium reduction, stress management or usual care for 18 months [214,215]. Four nutritional supplements were fed in a double-blind, placebo-controlled design. The nutritional supplements were fed in two stages, each of six months duration. In stage 1, participants were fed a supplement providing, each day, 1.0 g calcium, 360 mg magnesium or placebo. After a washout period they entered stage 2, where they were re-randomized to be fed a supplement providing, each day, 6 g fish oil (containing 3.0 g omega-3-fatty acids), 60 mmol potassium or placebo. The weight loss, sodium reduction and stress management groups underwent weekly group counseling sessions for 14, 10 and 8 weeks, respectively and then at semi-monthly or monthly intervals for the rest of the 18 month intervention.

In TOHP Phase I, in a comparison of baseline data to the final measurements, weight reduction produced a weight loss of −3.9 kg (p < 0.01) and a decrease in SBP of −2.9 mmHg (p < 0.01) and DBP of −2.3 mmHg (p < 0.01) [215]; the sodium reduction diet decreased urine sodium excretion by −44 mmol (p < 0.01), SBP by −1.7 mmHg (p < 0.01) and DBP by −2.9 mmHg (p < 0.05). There was no significant decrease in SBP or DBP between the baseline and final measurements with either stress management or the dietary supplements, despite evidence for good compliance. Essentially similar results were observed for the lifestyle interventions at the six-month follow-up, or for the nutritional supplements at the three-month follow-up, except that DBP fell significantly at three months with the potassium supplement [215]. A post-trial follow-up evaluation seven years later of 181 of the subjects indicated that the weight loss group and dietary sodium restriction group displayed a 77% and 35% decrease in the odds ratio of having hypertension, respectively [214].

TOHP Phase II

TOHP Phase II tested whether weight loss, reduced sodium intake or a combination of weight loss and reduced sodium intake will decrease DBP, SBP or the incidence of hypertension (defined as DBP of 90 mmHg or greater, SBP 140 mmHg or greater, and/or the use of antihypertensive medications) in overweight or moderately obese individuals with high normal DBP (83–89 mmHg) and SBP below 140 mmHg at entry into the study [216–219]. A total of 2382 men and women who were 110 to 165 % above desirable body weight were randomly assigned to these three treatment arms or to a usual care group in a two by two factorial design where they were assigned to weight loss or no weight loss and sodium reduction or no sodium reduction. Subjects were followed for three to four years. Patients participated in group meetings and received individual counseling during this time which initially was intensive and then became less frequent as the study progressed. Body weight, urinary sodium and BP were measured every six months, and at 18 and 36 months, BP was measured over a series of three visits separated from each other by 7–10 days.

In the two weight reduction groups combined, mean body weight loss was −4.1 kg, −2.2 kg and −0.3 kg at 6, 18 and 36 months, respectively [217,218]. The usual care group displayed a progressive weight gain that reached +1.8 kg at 36 months. The decrease in weight in the weight loss groups, calculated as the difference between the weight change in the two weight loss groups combined and the weight change in the usual care group, was significantly negative at each of these three time points. Mean SBP and DBP decreased by −6.0/−5.5, −3.6/−4.5 and −0.8/−3.2 mmHg, respectively, in the two weight loss groups combined at 6, 18 and 36 months. The reduction in SBP and DBP were each significantly greater in the two weight loss groups combined as compared to the usual care group at these three time points.

Urinary sodium excretion decreased by −64.3, −45.4 and −34.1 mmol/day with the two dietary sodium reduction groups combined at 6, 18 and 36 months, respectively. In the usual care group, urinary sodium decreased by −27.6, −16.8 and −10.5 mmol/day at these three time points [217]. The fall in urinary sodium excretion in the two sodium reduction groups, calculated as the difference between the decrease in urinary sodium in the two sodium reduction groups combined and the decrease in urinary sodium in the usual care group, was significantly greater at 6, 18 and 36 months. The decrease in mean SBP and DBP in the two sodium reduction groups combined was −5.1/−4.4, −3.8/−4.4 and −0.7/−3.0 mmHg, respectively, at these three time points. In the two sodium reduction groups combined, as compared to the usual care group, the reduction in SBP was significantly greater at all three time points, whereas the reduction in DBP was significantly greater only at 6 and 18 months.

Throughout the 48 months of the TOHP Phase II clinical trial, the incidence of hypertension, defined as SBP ≥140 mmHg or DBP ≥90 mmHg or the use of antihypertensive medicines, was less, and usually statistically significantly less, in the two weight loss groups combined, in the two sodium reduction groups combined and in the weight loss and sodium reduction intervention group as compared to the usual care group (average relative risks, 0.78–0.82). Those subjects who displayed greater and sustained weight loss had the greatest reduction in BP and the lowest risk ratio for hypertension. The effects of weight loss and decreased

sodium chloride intake combined were not additive. After six months of treatment, the two interventions were less effective in maintaining both weight loss and low sodium intake, and, possibly for these reasons, the reduction in BP was also attenuated [217–219]. The results of the HPT, TOHP Phase I and TOHP Phase II trials demonstrate that in overweight or moderately obese individuals, dietary modifications that reduce body weight and dietary sodium intake will reduce BP, but that weight loss, reduced sodium intake, and the decreased BP are difficult to sustain for 2–3 years or longer.

The Dietary Approaches to Stop Hypertension (DASH) Diet

The DASH study provides much relevant information concerning appropriate dietary therapy to control BP [220]. The DASH study was a multicenter study that compared a "control" typical American diet (low in fruits, vegetables, dairy products, essential minerals and fiber and high in saturated and total fat) to a diet rich in fruits and vegetables and also to a combination diet rich in fruits, vegetables and low fat dairy products and with a reduced saturated and total fatty acid content. The study was conducted in 459 adults with a mean age of 44 years, SBPs less than 160 mmHg and DBPs of 80–95 mmHg. About 65% of the study subjects were racial minorities, especially African-American.

The control diet was fed to all subjects for three weeks, and individuals were then randomly assigned to remain on this diet or to ingest the diet rich in fruits and vegetables or the combination diet for an additional eight weeks. All meals were prepared for the participants in a research kitchen, and five meals per week were ingested on the study site. The study used food rather than nonfood sources of calcium. As can be seen from Table 27.4, the control diet was low in calcium, potassium and magnesium. The sodium content of all diets was similar. Baseline SBPs and DBPs averaged 131.3 ± SD 10.8 mmHg and 84.7 ± 4.7 mmHg, respectively. Hence, many individuals had only high-normal or normal BPs.

After the subjects commenced their experimental diets, there was a rapid, significant and sustained fall in SBP and DBP with both the fruits and vegetables diet and the combination diet [221]. SBP and DBP fell more with the fruits and vegetables diet than with the control diet, by −2.8 (97.5% CI, −4.7 to −0.9) mmHg (p < 0.001) and −1.1 (97.5% CI, −2.4 to −0.3) mmHg (p = 0.07), respectively. SBP and DBP also decreased more with the combination diet than the fruits and vegetables diet, by −2.7 (97.5% CI, −4.6 to −0.9) mmHg (p = 0.001) and −1.9 −3.3 to −0.6) mmHg (p = 0.002). These

TABLE 27.4   Key Nutrients in the DASH and DASH-Sodium Diets and the Western Control Diet[*,†]

Nutrients	Western Control Diet	DASH Combination Diet
Fat (% of total kcal)	37	27
saturated	16	6
monounsaturated	13	13
polyunsaturated	8	8
Carbohydrate (% of total kcal)	48	55
Protein (% of total kcal)	15	18
Cholesterol (mg/day)	300	150
Fiber (g/day)	9	31
Potassium (mg/day)	1700	4700
Magnesium (mg/day)	165	500
Calcium (mg/day)	450	1240
Sodium (mg/day)**	3000 (130 mmol/day)	3000 (130 mmol/day)

Adapted from [220].

†*Values are for diets designed to provide an energy level of 2100 kcal/day.*

**For the DASH-Sodium trial, the prescribed daily sodium intakes were 150 mmol (high intake, 3.45 g), 100 mmol (intermediate intake, 2.30 g) and 50 mmol (low intake, 1.15 g) [221].*

declines in BP with both experimental diets occurred within 2–3 weeks and essentially persisted throughout the rest of the 8-week study period. Thus, this study indicates that a diet high in fruits and vegetables significantly reduces BP and that the addition of about three daily servings of dairy products, predominantly low-fat milk, in association with a reduced saturated and total fat intake, approximately doubled the degree of BP reduction observed with the fruits and vegetables diet. It should be emphasized that these two experimental diets were only studied for eight weeks in this trial, and the long-term effects of these two diets were not investigated.

The DASH Low Sodium Diet

It is also noteworthy that the DASH diet was neither a low sodium diet or a weight reduction diet. The DASH-Sodium Trial was therefore carried out to examine whether a restricted sodium intake would have an additional BP-lowering effect in people ingesting the DASH combination diet [221]. The DASH-Sodium Trial was a multicenter study in which three different dietary sodium intakes were prescribed: a high sodium diet, 3.45 g Na/day – roughly a typical

USA sodium intake; an intermediate sodium diet, 2.3 g Na/day – a currently recommended intake; and a low sodium intake, 1.15 g Na/day. A total of 412 individuals were studied in four clinical centers [221]. Acceptance criteria included adults 22 years or older who had average SBPs of 120 to 159 mmHg or who had DBPs of 80 to 95 mmHg. Subjects first underwent a two week-run-in period with a high sodium Western diet. They were then randomly assigned to the DASH combination diet or to the Western diet. Both diet groups were fed each of the three levels of sodium intake for 30 days each in a randomized crossover design [221]. The primary and secondary end points of the study were the SBPs and DBPs with the three different sodium intakes. Statistical analyses were performed by intention-to-treat methods.

The results indicated that with the control Western diet, the intermediate sodium intake, as compared to the high intake, was associated with a reduction in SBP of −2.1 (95% CI, −3.4 to −0.8) mmHg (p < 0.001) and a reduction in DBP of −1.1 (95% CI, −1.9 to −0.2) mmHg (p < 0.01). When those individuals fed the DASH diet were fed the intermediate sodium diet, as compared to the high sodium diet, there was also a reduction in SBP and DBP of −1.3 (95% CI, −2.6 to 0.0) mmHg (p < 0.05) and −0.6 (−1.5 to 0.2) (p = NS), respectively. A comparison of the low vs. the intermediate sodium intakes with the control Western diet indicated a further reduction in SBP of −4.6 (−5.9 to −3.2) mmHg (p < 0.01) and −2.4 (−3.3 to −1.5) mmHg (p < 0.001). The SBPs and DBPs with the DASH Diet were also further reduced with the low as compared to the intermediate sodium intake, by −1.7 (−3.0 to −0.4) mmHg (p < 0.01) and −1.0 (−1.9 to −0.1) mmHg (p < 0.01), respectively [221].

These BP reductions with the DASH low sodium diet were in addition to the BP lowering effects of the DASH diet itself. At each level of sodium intake, the SBPs and DBPs were significantly lower with the DASH diet as compared to the control diet except for the DBP with the low sodium diet. With the low sodium intake, the mean DBP with the DASH diet was lower than with the Western diet, but not significantly so. The BP lowering effects of low sodium intakes were greater in the subjects who were hypertensive than in those who were normotensive; this was observed in the individuals assigned to the control Western diet as well as in those assigned to the DASH diet. A greater reduction in BP was observed in black subjects at intermediate and low levels of sodium intake as compared to white participants. However, the DASH diet with reduced sodium intake lowered BP in many other hypertensive subgroups as well and also in nonhypertensive patients who were older than 45 years or 45 years of age or younger [222].

What is in the DASH Diet that Lowers Blood Pressure?

The answer to this question is not clear, but the following potential factors have been identified.

Nitrate

Webb and coworkers described a possible role for nitrate in the BP lowering effects of the DASH diet. This latter diet is high in vegetables [223,224], and vegetables contain substantial amounts of nitrate (NO_3). Ingested nitrate is absorbed from the stomach and small intestine into the circulation where some nitrate is secreted into saliva and converted to nitrite (NO_2) by the action of bacteria on the tongue. This nitrite is than swallowed where gastric acid converts the nitrite to the vasodilator nitric oxide (NO). In one study, healthy volunteers were randomized to drink either beetroot juice, a rich source of inorganic nitrate, or water in a crossover design. After drinking beetroot juice, plasma nitrate and nitrite rose, and SBP and DBP fell by -10.4 and -8.0 mmHg, respectively [223]. The volunteers repeated this activity, but also spit out their saliva continuously for several hours so that the nitrite would not be swallowed and thereby exposed to gastric acid. During this time, plasma nitrate again rose, but there was no rise in plasma nitrite, and SBP was significantly higher as compared to when they were allowed to swallow. Ingesting the beetroot juice and swallowing saliva also reduced endothelial dysfunction as indicated by protection against suppression of the flow mediated dilation of the brachial artery following ischemia/reperfusion. Finally, swallowing beetroot juice also inhibited aggregation of platelets that were exposed to ADP or collagen.

Dairy Products

A recent systematic review and meta-analysis reported that ingestion of dairy foods reduces the development of elevated blood pressure, but it is the low fat dairy foods that accounts for this effect [225]. Lowering of the development of elevated blood pressure was also associated with increased intake of fluid dairy foods (milk or yogurt) but not cheese.

The Mediterranean Diet

This diet, which is high in fruits, vegetables and olive oil, has been associated epidemiologically with reduced cardiovascular disease and mortality [226,227]. Such diets also seem to improve vascular function, with a greater forearm blood flow in response to a vasodilator challenge [228]. As indicated in the DASH study, a high fruits and vegetables diet may reduce blood pressure [220]. This antihypertensive effect may be partly due to the associated higher intake of olive oil [229]. The BP lowering effects of nitrate [22,224], glutamic acid, which is present in higher amounts in vegetable proteins [150], and PUFA in olive oil may contribute to the antihypertensive effects of these high fruits and vegetables diets.

The PREMIER Clinical Trial

Modifications have been made to the DASH lower sodium diet to add a weight loss component and other interventions [222]. In the PREMIER Clinical Trial, 810 participants individuals with BPs above the optimal level, including those with prehypertension or stage 1 hypertension (SBP 120—159 mmHg; DBP, 80—95 mmHg), can make multiple lifestyle changes during this period of time that lower BP and reduce their risk factors for cardiovascular disease [58,230]. Subjects, who were mostly overweight or obese, were randomly assigned to one of three treatment groups: (1) one 30 minute counseling session on diet and physical activity plus educational materials, but no counseling on behavioral changes (i.e., advice only); (2) an intensive behavioral intervention to achieve a set of established (EST) healthy lifestyle goals, including weight loss, dietary sodium reduction, increased physical activity and limited alcohol intake; or (3) the EST intervention with the DASH combination diet (EST+DASH) [230]. Groups 2 and 3 were scheduled to have 18 counseling sessions over the six months of the trial.

The PREMIER Trial results indicated that both the EST and the EST+DASH interventions lowered SBP to a similar degree and significantly more than the advice only group. After subtracting the BP changes in the advice only group, the EST intervention and the DASH diet plus EST intervention groups showed significant reductions at six months in SBP and DBP of $-3.7/-1.7$ and $-4.3/-2.6$ mmHg, respectively. The prevalence of hypertension at six months was similar in the two intervention groups and significantly lower than in the advice only group. However, in the subgroup of patients with the metabolic syndrome, the EST lowering effect on SBP was not significantly greater than advice only, whereas EST+DASH had a similar effect in those with and without this syndrome [231]. Moreover, the EST+DASH regimen after six months lowered SBP equally effectively in prehypertension and stage-1 hypertension patients who did or did not have the metabolic syndrome, whereas the EST regimen alone did not lower SBP as effectively in individuals who had the metabolic syndrome [231].

Compliance to the treatment regimens was fairly good, and the EST and EST+DASH interventions also differed significantly from the advice only group with regard to greater weight loss, increased physical fitness, and reduced serum total cholesterol and insulin resistance [58,231]; they showed a trend toward lower urine sodium that was significant only in the EST group. The DASH diet also decreased the prevalence of the metabolic syndrome in other studies [232,233]. The benefits of these dietary and lifestyle interventions have been sufficiently impressive so that they have been incorporated into the recommendations for the prevention and treatment of hypertension by many national advisory groups and are included in the Therapeutic Lifestyle Changes of the JNC [2]. These groups now commonly recommend a DASH-low sodium type of diet along with recommendations similar to the EST lifestyle changes described above [2,234–236].

Effect of Dietary Sources of Fuel on Blood Pressure

Since the DASH diet provides less fat and more protein, is it possible that these differences in fuel composition contribute to its BP lowering effects? As indicated above, amino acids and peptides derived from ingested proteins may have blood pressure lowering effects [97,145,147–149,152–155,237]. The OmniHeart study examined the relative contribution of diets providing relatively high amounts of carbohydrates, proteins or monounsaturated fatty acids to BP changes [9,220]. Adults with prehypertension or untreated stage 1 hypertension were randomly assigned to receive each of these three diets in a crossover design. The high protein diet increased protein intake to 25% of total energy intake, and the high monounsaturated diet increased fat to 37% of total energy intake. The carbohydrate content in these latter two diets was 48% of total calories, as compared to 58% of total calories with the high carbohydrate diet which is similar to the composition of the DASH diet. Weight was kept stable by adjusting total energy intake. The higher protein diet and the higher monounsaturated fat diet were each more effective at lowering BP as compared to the high carbohydrate diet. Whether this was due to the lower carbohydrate intake or the higher protein or fat intake is not clear. However, these findings are consistent with observational studies indicating that higher protein or fat intakes are associated with a lower death rate from coronary heart disease and greater survival [238,239]. A meta-analysis of 10 studies comparing the effects of high carbohydrate vs. high cis-monounsaturated fat diets also indicated that the high carbohydrate diets were associated with slightly, but significantly higher SBPs (mean difference, 2.6 mmHg (95% CI, 0.4 to 4.7) and DBP (mean difference, 1.8 mmHg (95% CI, 0.01 to 3.6) [240]. The same trends were noted when the analysis was restricted to crossover studies, but the results

were no longer statistically significant. As indicated above, intake of sugar-sweetened beverages and, in people who had high urinary sodium, fructose and glucose were directly correlated with SBP and DBP [47,48].

It is pertinent that higher protein diets have also been associated, short-term, with improved serum glucose and possibly other metabolic benefits in patients with type 2 diabetes mellitus [241,242]. It is not yet clear whether these higher protein diets are safe for long-term use, and they may be contraindicated in people with early CKD, as they are in persons with more advanced CKD, because of the potential risk of accelerating progressive kidney failure and also, in the latter condition, by engendering uremic toxicity. More research into these questions would be helpful.

LONG-TERM ADHERENCE AND BLOOD PRESSURE RESPONSES TO HEALTH ENHANCING LIFESTYLES

Longer Term Experience with the Previously Described Clinical Trials

Many studies have examined or are now examining the longer term responses to healthy diet recommendations. As indicated above, the Hypertension Prevention Trial (HPT) and Trials of Hypertension Prevention (TOHP Phase I and Phase II) in which patients were counseled on weight reduction and/or sodium reduction diets for up to four years, indicated that there was a progressive loss of adherence to these dietary intakes [213,217–219]. TOHP Phase I also indicated a reduced odds ratio of hypertension seven years after the onset of the trial, and the THP and TOHP Phase II trials also demonstrated that some antihypertensive effect remained three or four years after the onset of the trial [213,217–219].

In the PREMIER Clinical Trial, participants were followed for an additional 12 months during which the advice only group underwent one additional 30-minute counseling session and received educational materials; the established (EST) intervention and EST intervention+DASH diet groups attended monthly group sessions and three individual counseling sessions, and were asked to keep food diaries, monitor their dietary energy and sodium intake and record the minutes of physical activity. At 18 months after the onset of the Premier Trial, the EST intervention and EST intervention+Dash diet groups, in comparison to the advice only group, each showed greater weight losses of −2.2 kg and −2.7 kg, respectively (p < 0.01 for each group), and significantly lower energy intakes [243]. 25% of both EST intervention groups attained the target weight loss goal of −6.8 kg. Urinary sodium excretion was also significantly lower in both intervention groups as compared to the advice only group, by −12.8 mmol Na and −18.9 mmol Na, respectively. Compared to the advice only group, the odds ratio for hypertension was 0.83 and 0.77 in the EST and EST+Dash groups at 18 months and was significantly lower only in the EST+DASH group. Among people who were hypertensive at baseline, the odds ratio for remaining hypertensive was significantly lower in both intervention groups as compared to the advice group. However, the change in blood pressure levels at 18 months was not different among the three groups.

A randomized, controlled trial conducted in Turkey involved 70 mildly hypertensive overweight or obese men and women, of whom 60 completed the trial [244]. Subjects were counseled repetitively for three months to follow lifestyle changes similar to those of the EST+DASH study. Six months after the onset of study, the interventional group showed improvements in body weight, BP, serum lipids and lifestyle patterns.

Other Studies on Diet, Adherence and Blood Pressure

Folsom et al. employed a DASH diet index score to evaluate the long-term effects of complying with the DASH diet by nonhypertensive participants in the Iowa Women's Health Study [245]. Adjusting for age and energy intake, they found that greater adherence to the DASH diet was associated with a lower incidence of hypertension and cardiovascular mortality, but these associations were not statistically significant after adjustment for other risk factors. However, these women were assessed while they ingested their usual intakes, and they did not undergo specific training and follow-up regarding adherence to the DASH diet.

The Women's Health Initiative (WHI) Dietary Modification Trial evaluated the effect of intensive behavioral modification to ingest a diet of increased fruits, vegetables and whole grains and reduced fat on BP and other clinical outcomes, including cardiovascular events [247]. 48,835 postmenopausal women were randomized to this treatment or to receive dietary educational materials and followed for a mean of 8.1 years. The primary aim of this study was to assess reduction in the incidence of breast and colorectal cancer. The diet was not specifically designed to lower sodium or energy intake, although there was a small decrease in energy intake and body weight in the treatment vs. the control group. Although intake of all dietary components changed in the prescribed direction, SBP did not change significantly, and there was a significant but very modest

(−0.31 mmHg) reduction in DBP. Moreover, there was no reduction in the incidence of coronary heart disease, stroke or all cardiovascular events with this diet.

In the DEW-IT study, a nine-week intensive healthy lifestyle modification intervention, that included a low-energy version of the DASH diet, vs. a nonactive intervention arm was evaluated in 44 overweight and obese hypertensive patients [205]. Although there was significantly greater weight loss with the lifestyle intervention at the end of the two-month period, at one year of follow-up, the weight loss group had regained almost all of their lost weight and their weight change was not different from the nonintervention group.

The ADAPT study evaluated changes in lifestyle and clinical characteristics in 241 overweight or obese hypertensive adults after they were randomized to usual care or an intensive program of lifestyle counseling [247,248]. At four months and one year, there was significantly greater weight loss associated with a more healthy dietary intake in the lifestyle changes group. Ambulatory BP was lower at four months after starting counseling but not at one year [247,249]. Three years after completion of the program the relative improvements in the lifestyles group, as compared to usual care, were limited to increased physical activity, some dietary intakes, and a minor decrease in serum cholesterol but no difference in weight loss, BP, changes in antihypertensive medications or other risk factors. Other programs also report that initial weight losses are not maintained long-term [250]. However, Viera et al. evaluated adults who had participated in a survey and who indicated that they were told they were hypertensive [251]. Those adults who also stated that they were advised on lifestyle changes were significantly more likely to describe healthy changes in lifestyle (e.g., changed eating habits including reduced salt and alcohol intake or exercise) than those who did not recall being advised on lifestyle changes. It is emphasized that these data were obtained from participant reports.

CHALLENGES TO DIET AND LIFESTYLE APPROACHES FOR PREVENTING AND TREATING HYPERTENSION

A number of other researchers report rather mediocre long-term (i.e., more than 6−24 months) adherence to the foregoing diets. Adherence to diet prescription and weight loss, although often statistically significant from baseline or control diets, were often small [243,252]. For example, many obese patients have 15, 25 or more kg of excess body fat. Dietary weight reduction programs are often considered rather successful if the participant loses 5 or 6 kg over the long-term. It is possible, of course, that a disproportionately healthy value may be obtained with these rather modest fat losses by obese patients.

Different ethnic groups may have difficulty adhering to different components of the DASH diet [253,254]. Examination of the NHANES data for the years 1999–2004 indicate that only 19.4 ± 1.2(SEM)% of 4386 people with known hypertension had a diet consistent with the DASH diet [255]. These values are substantially lower than the proportion of known hypertensives who were accordant with the DASH diet (26.7 ± 1.1%) in the NHANES data for 1988–1994 [255]. Indeed, recent NHANES data indicate that adherence to healthy lifestyles appears to be diminishing in the United States [256]. Although at least most of these patients probably had not actually been [intensively] trained in the importance of or the preparation of the DASH diet, the principles of the DASH diet have been recommended by the JNC for many years [257,258]. However, large numbers of Americans are now counseled in healthy lifestyle modifications, although some population groups are still not as commonly counseled, particularly the young and people with low cardiovascular risk factors [231].

Thus, the results regarding compliance to the DASH or other dietary prescriptions to reduce BP or cardiovascular events are somewhat conflicting. As pointed out by Logan [259], there are several possible explanations for the differences in compliance to these diets. The DASH trial was short-term, and all food was prepared in research kitchens and provided to the subjects at no cost. Moreover, on weekdays either lunch or supper meals were eaten in a research unit [29,67]. In contrast, in other studies, the food had to be purchased and prepared by the participants. When food must be purchased and prepared for long or indefinite periods of time by the consumer who is not participating in an intensively controlled research protocol, compliance may fall.

Another concern is the labor costs of long-term counseling by healthcare workers in order to maintain adherence to healthy lifestyles and diets. In this regard, people who are not trained to be professional healthcare workers (e.g., dietitians, nurses) can be trained rather quickly to become effective lifestyle coaches [260]. Long-term remote counseling for weight reduction by telephone, a program-specific web site and email was examined as a strategy for effectively promoting weight reduction at greater efficiency and less cost [261]. Primary care providers played a supportive role in the program but were not directly involved in the interventions. In this latter trial, one group of obese participants received exclusively remote but frequent counseling; another group received a combination of in-center person-to person counseling plus three remote counseling sessions. A third group served as controls. At 24 months, weight loss averaged −0.8 kg in the control

group, −4.8 kg in the group receiving remote counseling (p < 0.001 vs. controls), and 5.1 kg in the group receiving direct person plus remote counseling (p < 0.001 vs. controls). Thus, a combination of employing trained lay people as counsellors plus the use of remote counseling may substantially reduce the costs of diet and lifestyle induced weight loss programs, especially if the techniques for weight reduction can be made more effective.

The long-term, multi-year, effects of strict compliance to the DASH or DASH-sodium diets also are not yet known, although it seems reasonable to believe that these diets and lifestyle changes will be healthy indefinitely [262]. It also is not entirely clear that these diets are similarly effective for all racial and ethnic groups. In both DASH studies, the potassium content of the control diet was below the 25th percentile of the estimated usual potassium intake in the United States [259]. Moreover, most of the DASH study patients were African American [220], a population whose BP is particularly potassium sensitive and who may require a high potassium intake in the range of the DASH diet to avoid sodium sensitivity induced by potassium deficiency [116]. Thus, these results may not be as applicable to non-African Americans or to people who are already ingesting higher potassium diets. On the other hand the large scale, observational, multi-year Nurses' Health Study II, indicated that those individuals who followed a low-risk diet and low-risk lifestyle had a lower self-reported incidence of hypertension [263]. It is relevant and encouraging that the demonstrated BP lowering effects of healthy dietary regimens and lifestyles coupled with difficulty in adherence has provided a commercial incentive to develop functional foods and nutraceuticals that may provide recommend nutrients [264]. Hopefully, these products will enhance the ability of people to follow recommended guidelines.

Exercise

Exercise training and its physiological, metabolic and clinical consequences are discussed more fully in Chapter 43. Some but not all studies of exercise and BP suggest that regular exercise training may reduce BP. Exercise, particularly when combined with a low fat intake, may lower serum cholesterol [265,266]. Exercise may also accelerate weight reduction in obese individuals who are ingesting a low calorie diet [267]. A cohort of 3148 healthy adults underwent studies of cardiorespiratory fitness, determined by treadmill exercise, which was measured over a six-year interval of time [17]. Improvement in cardiorespiratory fitness was associated with a reduction in the incidence of hypertension, the metabolic syndrome and hypercholesterolemia. A gain in the percent body fat or BMI was each associated with an increased incidence of hypertension, metabolic syndrome and hypercholesterolemia.

It is important to remember that the increase in BP that occurs when normal people exercise may be greatly exaggerated in hypertensive individuals. Thus, BP should be monitored carefully in hypertensive persons who are embarking on exercise training until it is ascertained that dangerous levels of hypertension do not occur [265]. Aerobic exercise training and resistance training were reported to decrease BP in pre-hypertensive and stage-1 hypertensive individuals [265,266]. Two mechanisms by which regular physical exercise may lower BP include reduction in oxidative stress and amelioration of insulin resistance and its consequent hyperinsulinemia [265]. In the presence of oxidative stress, 8-Iso-PGF2α, a potent vasoconstrictor, is produced [265]. Insulin resistance with hyperinsulinemia impairs NO synthesis, which will predispose to hypertension.

Anorexigenic Medicines

Meta-analysis indicates that the drugs orlistat and sibutramine are effective at inducing weight loss more effectively than placebo treatment, on average by roughly 4 kg [268]. The effect of these drugs on BP is more nuanced. Selective CB_1 receptor blockade with higher doses of rimonabant in obese patients is reported to both induce weight loss and modestly reduce BP [207]. This reduction in blood pressure may be due solely to the effect of the weight loss [49]. Orlistat also lowers BP [49,204,207,208]. In the meta-analysis, there was a statistically significant weighted SBP and DBP reduction with orlistat of −2.5 and −1.9 mmHg, respectively [268]. In contrast, sibutramine was associated with increased SBP [204] or DBP [268].

CONCLUSIONS AND RECOMMENDATIONS

Many studies indicate that nutritional intake and nutritional status have a major effect on the probability of developing hypertension and on the severity of hypertension in the general population. Appropriate dietary management may prevent the onset of hypertension or eradicate or improve mild hypertension and can be a useful adjunct to pharmacological therapy for the treatment of more severe established hypertension. Key elements that prevent or ameliorate hypertension include prevention of obesity, the low sodium DASH combination diet, adequate potassium intake, and possibly sufficient intake of fish oil and magnesium. Some evidence indicates that regular exercise may reduce resting BP; exercise, of course, has other health

TABLE 27.5 A Suggested Dietary Approach to Prevent or Treat Hypertension*,†

1. Maintain desirable body weight
2. Use the DASH combination diet (a diet high in fruits, vegetables and low fat dairy products and low in saturated and total fat)
3. Limit daily NaCl consumption to 5.85 g/day or lower
4. Maintain adequate potassium and magnesium intake
5. Recommended calcium intake for noncalcium stone formers (about 1000 mg/day for persons aged 19–50 years and 1200 mg/day for persons ≥50 years)
6. For individuals who drink alcohol, no more than two drinks (3–4 units) per day
7. Consider a high omega-3 fatty acid diet (i.e., about 3–6 g/day of fish oil per day)

*For any person with a chronic illness, each of these recommendations should be reviewed with his physician to ensure that it is compatible with medical management.
†Regular (approximately daily) exercise activity is also recommended.
Reproduced with permission [270].

enhancing advantages. A dietary approach to either prevent or treat hypertension is indicated in Table 27.5. For patients who have a major elevation in BP, it is very uncommon for their hypertension to respond adequately to dietary management alone. These individuals will almost certainly also require medicines to control their hypertension, but dietary control may still improve the ease with which elevated blood pressure may be managed.

Individuals who are obese or have other dietary habits that may predispose to hypertension (e.g., high sodium chloride intake) should be encouraged to inaugurate appropriate dietary therapy. If the BP is substantially elevated, a reasonable approach would be to start pharmacological anti-hypertensive therapy concomitantly with dietary management. If the patient is committed to dietary therapy of hypertension, he may do the following. Once the BP has stabilized at the target level, attempts may be made to gradually withdraw the antihypertensive medicines while maintaining strict dietary management. Exercise training should be encouraged, but only after careful medical evaluation of the cardiovascular and hemodynamic responses, including the rise in blood pressure, in response to exercise of persons who have hypertension, who are older, or who have major underlying illnesses, such as heart disease or kidney failure.

KEY POINTS

1. Obesity is one of the main nutritional predisposing factors to hypertension.
2. The many mechanisms by which obesity and excessive energy intake predispose to hypertension include increased activity of the RAAS, probably a rise in nonaldosterone mediated mineralcorticoid

activity, increased SNS activity, insulin resistance, salt sensitive hypertension, excess salt intake and the reduced kidney function which is often present in obese individuals.

3. High sodium chloride intake is the other main nutritional predisposing factor to hypertension.

4. Increasing potassium intake, particularly in people with potassium-deficient intakes, may lower BP.

5. Higher intakes of PUFA, protein and possibly certain amino acids, vitamin D and green coffee bean extract, may lower BP.

6. Some evidence suggests that dark chocolate, but not white chocolate, and oolong, green and black tea may reduce the risk of hypertension.

7. Evidence suggests that dietary excessive energy intake, sugar sweetened beverages, fructose and glucose may raise BP.

8. Large alcohol intakes may increase the risk of hypertension and acutely and chronically raise BP. Low alcohol intakes may raise BP in African-American men but not in white men or women or African-American women.

9. Certain diets and lifestyle changes, including regular exercise, appear to lower blood pressure in people with prehypertension or mild hypertension or to prevent the development of hypertension.

10. The DASH low sodium diet, which is high in fruits and vegetables, low fat dairy products, potassium, magnesium, calcium and fiber and low in saturated fatty acids, total fat and sodium, is such a diet.

11. Long-term adherence to healthy, BP lowering diets is difficult for many people to attain, and methods for obtaining long-term adherence to such diets and healthy lifestyles continue to be investigated.

12. Bariatric surgical procedures in association with counseling for healthy lifestyle changes appear at present to be the most effective and reliable methods for long-term, major reductions in body fat.

References

[1] Kearney PM, et al. Global burden of hypertension: analysis of worldwide data. Lancet 2005;365:217—23, http://dx.doi.org/10.1016/S0140-6736(05)17741-1.

[2] Chobanian AV, et al. The Seventh Report of the Joint National Committee on Prevention, Detection, Evaluation, and Treatment of High Blood Pressure: the JNC 7 report. JAMA 2003;289:2560—72.

[3] MacMahon S, et al. Blood pressure, stroke, and coronary heart disease. Part 1, Prolonged differences in blood pressure: prospective observational studies corrected for the regression dilution bias. Lancet 1990;335:765—74.

[4] Stamler J, Stamler R, Neaton JD. Blood pressure, systolic and diastolic, and cardiovascular risks. US population data. Arch Intern Med 1993;153:598—615.

[5] Klag MJ, et al. Blood pressure and end-stage renal disease in men. N Engl J Med 1996;334:13—8.

[6] Zhang X, et al. Total and abdominal obesity among rural Chinese women and the association with hypertension. Nutrition 2012;28:46—52, http://dx.doi.org/10.1016/j.nut.2011.02.004.

[7] Govindarajan G, Whaley-Connell A, Mugo M, Stump C, Sowers JR. The cardiometabolic syndrome as a cardiovascular risk factor. Am J Med Sci 2005;330:311—8.

[8] Narkiewicz K. Diagnosis and management of hypertension in obesity. Obes Rev 2006;7:155—62.

[9] Appel LJ, et al. Dietary approaches to prevent and treat hypertension: a scientific statement from the American Heart Association. Hypertension 2006;47:296—308.

[10] Ford ES, Zhao G, Li C, Pearson WS, Mokdad AH. Trends in obesity and abdominal obesity among hypertensive and non-hypertensive adults in the United States. Am J Hypertens 2008;21:1124—8.

[11] Friedrich MJ. Epidemic of obesity expands its spread to developing countries. Jama 2002;287:1382—6.

[12] Kelly T, Yang W, Chen CS, Reynolds K, He J. Global burden of obesity in 2005 and projections to 2030. Int J Obes (Lond) 2008;32:1431—7, http://dx.doi.org/ijo2008102 [pii] 10.1038/ijo.2008.102.

[13] Jafar TH, Chaturvedi N, Pappas G. Prevalence of overweight and obesity and their association with hypertension and diabetes mellitus in an Indo-Asian population. CMAJ 2006;175:1071—7.

[14] Nguyen TT, Adair LS, He K, Popkin BM. Optimal cutoff values for overweight: using body mass index to predict incidence of hypertension in 18- to 65-year-old Chinese adults. J Nutr 2008;138:1377—82.

[15] Dornfeld LP, Maxwell MH, Waks A, Tuck M. Mechanisms of hypertension in obesity. Kidney Int 1987;(Suppl. 22):S254—8.

[16] Rohrer JE, Anderson GJ, Furst JW. Obesity and pre-hypertension in family medicine: implications for quality improvement. BMC Health Serv Res 2007;7:212, http://dx.doi.org/1472-6963-7-212 [pii] 10.1186/1472-6963-7-212.

[17] Lee DC, et al. Changes in fitness and fatness on the development of cardiovascular disease risk factors hypertension, metabolic syndrome, and hypercholesterolemia. J Am Coll Cardiol 2012;59:665—72, http://dx.doi.org/10.1016/j.jacc.2011.11.013.

[18] Reisin E, et al. Effect of weight loss without salt restriction on the reduction of blood pressure in overweight hypertensive patients. N Engl J Med 1978;298:1—6.

[19] Scherrer U, et al. Body fat and sympathetic nerve activity in healthy subjects. Circulation 1994;89:2634—40.

[20] Pausova Z. From big fat cells to high blood pressure: a pathway to obesity-associated hypertension. Curr Opin Nephrol Hypertens 2006;15:173—8.

[21] Furukawa S, et al. Increased oxidative stress in obesity and its impact on metabolic syndrome. J Clin Invest 2004;114:1752—61.

[22] Touyz RM. Reactive oxygen species, vascular oxidative stress, and redox signaling in hypertension: what is the clinical significance? Hypertension 2004;44:248—52.

[23] Pouliot MC, et al. Waist circumference and abdominal sagittal diameter: best simple anthropometric indexes of abdominal visceral adipose tissue accumulation and related cardiovascular risk in men and women. Am J Cardiol 1994;73:460—8.

[24] Lean ME, Han TS, Morrison CE. Waist circumference as a measure for indicating need for weight management. BMJ 1995;311:158—61.

[25] Canoy D, et al. Fat distribution, body mass index and blood pressure in 22,090 men and women in the Norfolk cohort of the

European Prospective Investigation into Cancer and Nutrition (EPIC-Norfolk) study. J Hypertens 2004;22:2067–74.

[26] Huxley R, et al. Ethnic comparisons of the cross-sectional relationships between measures of body size with diabetes and hypertension. Obes Rev 2008;9(Suppl. 1):53–61.

[27] Narisawa S, et al. Appropriate waist circumference cutoff values for persons with multiple cardiovascular risk factors in Japan: a large cross-sectional study. J Epidemiol 2008;18:37–42.

[28] Pausova Z, et al. Genome-wide scan for linkage to obesity-associated hypertension in French Canadians. Hypertension 2005;46:1280–5.

[29] Danoviz ME, Pereira AC, Mill JG, Krieger JE. Hypertension, obesity and GNB 3 gene variants. Clin Exp Pharmacol Physiol 2006;33:248–52.

[30] Fujita T. Aldosterone in salt-sensitive hypertension and metabolic syndrome. J Mol Med 2008;86:729–34.

[31] Kurukulasuriya LR, Stas S, Lastra G, Manrique C, Sowers JR. Hypertension in obesity. Endocrinol Metab Clin North Am 2008;37:647–62. ix.

[32] Sarzani R, Salvi F, Dessi-Fulgheri P, Rappelli A. Renin-angiotensin system, natriuretic peptides, obesity, metabolic syndrome, and hypertension: an integrated view in humans. J Hypertens 2008;26:831–43.

[33] Sharma AM, Engeli S, Pischon T. New developments in mechanisms of obesity-induced hypertension: role of adipose tissue. Curr Hypertens Rep 2001;3:152–6.

[34] Cooper R, et al. ACE, angiotensinogen and obesity: a potential pathway leading to hypertension. J Hum Hypertens 1997;11:107–11.

[35] Rossi GP, et al. Body mass index predicts plasma aldosterone concentrations in overweight-obese primary hypertensive patients. J Clin Endocrinol Metab 2008;93:2566–71.

[36] Fujita T. Aldosterone and CKD in metabolic syndrome. Curr Hypertens Rep 2008;10:421–3.

[37] Olsen MH, et al. N-terminal pro brain natriuretic peptide is inversely related to metabolic cardiovascular risk factors and the metabolic syndrome. Hypertension 2005;46:660–6.

[38] St Peter JV, Hartley GG, Murakami MM, Apple FS. B-type natriuretic peptide (BNP) and N-terminal pro-BNP in obese patients without heart failure: relationship to body mass index and gastric bypass surgery. Clin Chem 2006;52:680–5.

[39] Dessi-Fulgheri P, et al. Plasma atrial natriuretic peptide and natriuretic peptide receptor gene expression in adipose tissue of normotensive and hypertensive obese patients. J Hypertens 1997;15:1695–9.

[40] Wang TJ, et al. Impact of obesity on plasma natriuretic peptide levels. Circulation 2004;109:594–600.

[41] De Pergola G, et al. Reduced effectiveness of atrial natriuretic factor in pre-menopausal obese women. Int J Obes Relat Metab Disord 1994;18:93–7.

[42] Kaaja RJ, Poyhonen-Alho MK. Insulin resistance and sympathetic overactivity in women. J Hypertens 2006;24:131–41.

[43] Beltowski J. Role of leptin in blood pressure regulation and arterial hypertension. J Hypertens 2006;24:789–801.

[44] Landsberg L. Insulin-mediated sympathetic stimulation: role in the pathogenesis of obesity-related hypertension (or, how insulin affects blood pressure, and why). J Hypertens 2001;19:523–8.

[45] Modan M, et al. Hyperinsulinemia. A link between hypertension obesity and glucose intolerance. J Clin Invest 1985;75:809–17.

[46] Katzeff HL. Increasing age impairs the thyroid hormone response to overfeeding. Proc Soc Exp Biol Med 1990;194:198–203.

[47] Brown IJ, et al. Sugar-sweetened beverage, sugar intake of individuals, and their blood pressure: international study of macro/micronutrients and blood pressure. Hypertension 2011;57:695–701, http://dx.doi.org/10.1161/HYPERTENSION AHA.110.165456.

[48] Chen L, et al. Reducing consumption of sugar-sweetened beverages is associated with reduced blood pressure: a prospective study among United States adults. Circulation 2010;121:2398–406, http://dx.doi.org/10.1161/CIRCULATION AHA.109.911164.

[49] Grassi G, et al. Obstructive sleep apnea-dependent and -independent adrenergic activation in obesity. Hypertension 2005;46:321–5.

[50] Shamsuzzaman AS, Gersh BJ, Somers VK. Obstructive sleep apnea: implications for cardiac and vascular disease. Jama 2003;290:1906–14.

[51] Peppard PE, Young T, Palta M, Skatrud J. Prospective study of the association between sleep-disordered breathing and hypertension. N Engl J Med 2000;342:1378–84.

[52] Phillips BG, Kato M, Narkiewicz K, Choe I, Somers VK. Increases in leptin levels, sympathetic drive, and weight gain in obstructive sleep apnea. Am J Physiol Heart Circ Physiol 2000;279:H234–7.

[53] Ip MS, et al. Obstructive sleep apnea is independently associated with insulin resistance. Am J Respir Crit Care Med 2002;165:670–6.

[54] Baguet JP, Narkiewicz K, Mallion JM. Update on Hypertension Management: obstructive sleep apnea and hypertension. J Hypertens 2006;24:205–8.

[55] Narkiewicz K, et al. Nocturnal continuous positive airway pressure decreases daytime sympathetic traffic in obstructive sleep apnea. Circulation 1999;100:2332–5.

[56] Zheng Y, et al. Roles of insulin receptor substrates in insulin-induced stimulation of renal proximal bicarbonate absorption. J Am Soc Nephrol 2005;16:2288–95.

[57] Pierce GL, et al. Weight loss alone improves conduit and resistance artery endothelial function in young and older overweight/obese adults. Hypertension 2008;52:72–9.

[58] Appel LJ, et al. Effects of comprehensive lifestyle modification on blood pressure control: main results of the PREMIER clinical trial. JAMA 2003;289:2083–93.

[59] Brook RD, Bard RL, Rubenfire M, Ridker PM, Rajagopalan S. Usefulness of visceral obesity (waist/hip ratio) in predicting vascular endothelial function in healthy overweight adults. Am J Cardiol 2001;88:1264–9.

[60] Sharma AM. Adipose tissue: a mediator of cardiovascular risk. Int J Obes Relat Metab Disord 2002;26(Suppl. 4):S5–7.

[61] Patel SB, Reams GP, Spear RM, Freeman RH, Villarreal D. Leptin: linking obesity, the metabolic syndrome, and cardiovascular disease. Curr Hypertens Rep 2008;10:131–7.

[62] Haynes WG, Morgan DA, Walsh SA, Mark AL, Sivitz WI. Receptor-mediated regional sympathetic nerve activation by leptin. J Clin Invest 1997;100:270–8.

[63] De Boer MP, et al. Microvascular dysfunction: a potential mechanism in the pathogenesis of obesity-associated insulin resistance and hypertension. Microcirculation 2012;19:5–18, http://dx.doi.org/10.1111/j.1549-8719.2011.00130.x.

[64] Rocchini AP, et al. The effect of weight loss on the sensitivity of blood pressure to sodium in obese adolescents. N Engl J Med 1989;321:580–5.

[65] Wofford MR, Hall JE. Pathophysiology and treatment of obesity hypertension. Curr Pharm Des 2004;10:3621–37.

[66] Festa A, et al. Chronic subclinical inflammation as part of the insulin resistance syndrome: the Insulin Resistance Atherosclerosis Study (IRAS). Circulation 2000;102:42–7.

[67] Hafidh S, Senkottaiyan N, Villarreal D, Alpert MA. Management of the metabolic syndrome. Am J Med Sci 2005;330:343–51.

[68] Third Report of the National Cholesterol Education Program (NCEP) Expert Panel on Detection, Evaluation, and Treatment of High Blood Cholesterol in Adults (Adult Treatment Panel III) final report. Circulation 2002;106:3143—421.

[69] Tirosh A, Garg R, Adler GK. Mineralocorticoid receptor antagonists and the metabolic syndrome. Curr Hypertens Rep 2010;12:252—7, http://dx.doi.org/10.1007/s11906-010-0126-2.

[70] Kahn R, Buse J, Ferrannini E, Stern M. The metabolic syndrome. Lancet 2005;366:1921—2. author reply 1923-1924.

[71] Curhan GC, Willett WC, Rimm EB, Speizer FE, Stampfer MJ. Body size and risk of kidney stones. J Am Soc Nephrol 1998;9:1645—52.

[72] Hamano S, et al. Kidney stone disease and risk factors for coronary heart disease. Int J Urol 2005;12:859—63.

[73] Taylor EN, Stampfer MJ, Curhan GC. Diabetes mellitus and the risk of nephrolithiasis. Kidney Int 2005;68:1230—5.

[74] Taylor EN, Stampfer MJ, Curhan GC. Obesity, weight gain, and the risk of kidney stones. JAMA 2005;293:455—62.

[75] Obligado SH, Goldfarb DS. The association of nephrolithiasis with hypertension and obesity: a review. Am J Hypertens 2008;21:257—64.

[76] Feig DI, Kang DH, Johnson RJ. Uric acid and cardiovascular risk. N Engl J Med 2008;359:1811—21.

[77] Kabir AA, Whelton PK, Khan MM, Gustat J, Chen W. Association of symptoms of depression and obesity with hypertension: the Bogalusa Heart Study. Am J Hypertens 2006;19:639—45.

[78] Dornfeld LP, Maxwell MH, Waks AU, Schroth P, Tuck ML. Obesity and hypertension: long-term effects of weight reduction on blood pressure. Int J Obes 1985;9:381—9.

[79] Schulz M, et al. Associations of short-term weight changes and weight cycling with incidence of essential hypertension in the EPIC-Potsdam Study. J Hum Hypertens 2005;19:61—7.

[80] Taylor EN, Curhan GC. Body size and 24-hour urine composition. Am J Kidney Dis 2006;48:905—15.

[81] Eriksson J, Forsen T, Tuomilehto J, Osmond C, Barker D. Fetal and childhood growth and hypertension in adult life. Hypertension 2000;36:790—4.

[82] Barker DJ, Bagby SP, Hanson MA. Mechanisms of disease: in utero programming in the pathogenesis of hypertension. Nat Clin Pract Nephrol 2006;2:700—7, http://dx.doi.org/10.1038/ncpneph0344.

[83] Power C, Elliott J. Cohort profile: 1958 British birth cohort (National Child Development Study). Int J Epidemiol 2006;35:34—41.

[84] Barker DJ. The fetal and infant origins of disease. Eur J Clin Invest 1995;25:457—63.

[85] Cottrell EC, Ozanne SE. Developmental programming of energy balance and the metabolic syndrome. Proc Nutr Soc 2007;66:198—206.

[86] Stein AD, Zybert PA, van der Pal-de Bruin K, Lumey LH. Exposure to famine during gestation, size at birth, and blood pressure at age 59 y: evidence from the Dutch Famine. Eur J Epidemiol 2006;21:759—65, http://dx.doi.org/10.1007/s10654-006-9065-2.

[87] Intersalt: an international study of electrolyte excretion and blood pressure. Results for 24 hour urinary sodium and potassium excretion. Intersalt Cooperative Research Group. Brit J Med 1988;297:319—28.

[88] Graudal NA, Hubeck-Graudal T, Jurgens G. Effects of low-sodium diet vs. high-sodium diet on blood pressure, renin, aldosterone, catecholamines, cholesterol, and triglyceride (Cochrane Review). Am J Hypertens 2012;25:1—15, http://dx.doi.org/10.1038/ajh.2011.210.

[89] Stamler J. The INTERSALT Study: background, methods, findings, and implications. Am J Clin Nutr 1997;65:626S—42S.

[90] Stolarz-Skrzypek K, et al. Fatal and nonfatal outcomes, incidence of hypertension, and blood pressure changes in relation to urinary sodium excretion. JAMA 2011;305:1777—85, http://dx.doi.org/10.1001/jama.2011.574.

[91] Antonios TF, MacGregor GA. Salt — more adverse effects. Lancet 1996;348:250—1.

[92] de Brito-Ashurst I, Varagunam M, Raftery MJ, Yaqoob MM. Bicarbonate supplementation slows progression of CKD and improves nutritional status. J Am Soc Nephrol 2009;20:2075—84.

[93] Kotchen TA, McCarron DA. Dietary electrolytes and blood pressure: a statement for healthcare professionals from the American Heart Association Nutrition Committee. Circulation 1998;98:613—7.

[94] Montasser ME, et al. Determinants of blood pressure response to low-salt intake in a healthy adult population. J Clin Hypertens (Greenwich) 2011;13:795—800, http://dx.doi.org/10.1111/j.1751-7176.2011.00523.x.

[95] Graudal NA, Galloe AM, Garred P. Effects of sodium restriction on blood pressure, renin, aldosterone, catecholamines, cholesterols, and triglyceride: a meta-analysis. JAMA 1998;279:1383—91.

[96] Altura BM, Altura BT, Gebrewold A, Ising H, Gunther T. Magnesium deficiency and hypertension: correlation between magnesium-deficient diets and microcirculatory changes in situ. Science 1984;223:1315—7.

[97] Cutler JA, Follmann D, Allender PS. Randomized trials of sodium reduction: an overview. Am J Clin Nutr 1997;65:643S—51S.

[98] Cutler JA, Follmann D, Elliott P, Suh I. An overview of randomized trials of sodium reduction and blood pressure. Hypertension 1991;17:I27—33.

[99] He FJ, MacGregor GA. Effect of modest salt reduction on blood pressure: a meta-analysis of randomized trials. Implications for public health. J Hum Hypertens 2002;16:761—70.

[100] Law MR, Frost CD, Wald NJ. By how much does dietary salt reduction lower blood pressure? III — Analysis of data from trials of salt reduction. BMJ 1991;302:819—24.

[101] Midgley JP, Matthew AG, Greenwood CM, Logan AG. Effect of reduced dietary sodium on blood pressure: a meta-analysis of randomized controlled trials. Jama 1996;275:1590—7.

[102] Kojuri J, Rahimi R. Effect of "no added salt diet" on blood pressure control and 24 hour urinary sodium excretion in mild to moderate hypertension. BMC Cardiovasc Disord 2007;7:34.

[103] Chamarthi B, et al. Urinary free cortisol: an intermediate phenotype and a potential genetic marker for a salt-resistant subset of essential hypertension. J Clin Endocrinol Metab 2007;92:1340—6.

[104] Melander O, et al. Moderate salt restriction effectively lowers blood pressure and degree of salt sensitivity is related to baseline concentration of renin and N-terminal atrial natriuretic peptide in plasma. J Hypertens 2007;25:619—27.

[105] Johnson AG, Nguyen TV, Davis D. Blood pressure is linked to salt intake and modulated by the angiotensinogen gene in normotensive and hypertensive elderly subjects. J Hypertens 2001;19:1053—60.

[106] Dengel DR, Brown MD, Ferrell RE, Reynolds TH, Supiano MA. A preliminary study on T-786C endothelial nitric oxide synthase gene and renal hemodynamic and blood pressure responses to dietary sodium. Physiol Res 2007;56:393—401.

[107] De Nicola L, et al. Italian audit on therapy of hypertension in chronic kidney disease: the TABLE-CKD study. Semin Nephrol 2005;25:425—30.

[108] Sanders PW. Assessment and treatment of hypertension in dialysis: the case for salt restriction. Semin Dial 2007;20:408—11.

[109] Shaldon S. Dietary salt restriction and drug-free treatment of hypertension in ESRD patients: a largely abandoned therapy. Nephrol Dial Transplant 2002;17:1163—5.

[110] Shaldon S. An explanation for the "lag phenomenon" in drug-free control of hypertension by dietary salt restriction in patients with chronic kidney disease on hemodialysis. Clin Nephrol 2006;66:1—2.

[111] Jones-Burton C, et al. An in-depth review of the evidence linking dietary salt intake and progression of chronic kidney disease. Am J Nephrol 2006;26:268—75.

[112] Johnson RJ, Herrera-Acosta J, Schreiner GF, Rodriguez-Iturbe B. Subtle acquired renal injury as a mechanism of salt-sensitive hypertension. N Engl J Med 2002;346:913—23.

[113] Whelton PK, et al. Effects of oral potassium on blood pressure. Meta-analysis of randomized controlled clinical trials. Jama 1997;277:1624—32.

[114] Krishna GG, Chusid P, Hoeldtke RD. Mild potassium depletion provokes renal sodium retention. J Lab Clin Med 1987;109:724—30.

[115] Gallen IW, et al. On the mechanism of the effects of potassium restriction on blood pressure and renal sodium retention. Am J Kidney Dis 1998;31:19—27.

[116] Morris Jr RC, Sebastian A, Forman A, Tanaka M, Schmidlin O. Normotensive salt sensitivity: effects of race and dietary potassium. Hypertension 1999;33:18—23.

[117] Mu JJ, et al. [Long-term observation in effects of potassium and calcium supplementation on arterial blood pressure and sodium metabolism in adolescents with higher blood pressure]. Zhonghua Yu Fang Yi Xue Za Zhi 2003;37:90—2.

[118] Pere AK, et al. Dietary potassium and magnesium supplementation in cyclosporine-induced hypertension and nephrotoxicity. Kidney Int 2000;58:2462—72.

[119] Barri YM, Wingo CS. The effects of potassium depletion and supplementation on blood pressure: a clinical review. Am J Med Sci 1997;314:37—40.

[120] Wu G, et al. Potassium magnesium supplementation for four weeks improves small distal artery compliance and reduces blood pressure in patients with essential hypertension. Clin Exp Hypertens 2006;28:489—97.

[121] Nowson CA, Morgan TO, Gibbons C. Decreasing dietary sodium while following a self-selected potassium-rich diet reduces blood pressure. J Nutr 2003;133:4118—23.

[122] Institute of Medicine(IOM). Dietary reference intakes for water, potassium, sodium chloride, and sulphate. Washington, DC: National Academic Press; 2004. 1—20.

[123] Brancati FL, Appel LJ, Seidler AJ, Whelton PK. Effect of potassium supplementation on blood pressure in African Americans on a low-potassium diet. A randomized, double-blind, placebo-controlled trial. Arch Intern Med 1996;156:61—7.

[124] Naismith DJ, Braschi A. The effect of low-dose potassium supplementation on blood pressure in apparently healthy volunteers. Br J Nutr 2003;90:53—60.

[125] McCarron DA. Epidemiological evidence and clinical trials of dietary calcium's effect on blood pressure. Contrib Nephrol 1991;90:2—10.

[126] McCarron DA, Metz JA, Hatton DC. Mineral intake and blood pressure in African Americans. Am J Clin Nutr 1998;68:517—8.

[127] McCarron DA, Reusser ME. Are low intakes of calcium and potassium important causes of cardiovascular disease? Am J Hypertens 2001;14:206S—12S.

[128] Witteman JC, et al. A prospective study of nutritional factors and hypertension among US women. Circulation 1989;80:1320—7.

[129] Ascherio A, et al. Prospective study of nutritional factors, blood pressure, and hypertension among US women. Hypertension 1996;27:1065—72.

[130] Cappuccio FP, et al. Epidemiologic association between dietary calcium intake and blood pressure: a meta-analysis of published data. Am J Epidemiol 1995;142:935—45.

[131] Bucher HC, et al. Effects of dietary calcium supplementation on blood pressure. A meta-analysis of randomized controlled trials. JAMA 1996;275:1016—22.

[132] Allender PS, et al. Dietary calcium and blood pressure: a meta-analysis of randomized clinical trials. Ann Intern Med 1996;124:825—31.

[133] Griffith LE, Guyatt GH, Cook RJ, Bucher HC, Cook DJ. The influence of dietary and nondietary calcium supplementation on blood pressure: an updated metaanalysis of randomized controlled trials. Am J Hypertens 1999;12:84—92.

[134] Saito K, Sano H, Furuta Y, Fukuzaki H. Effect of oral calcium on blood pressure response in salt-loaded borderline hypertensive patients. Hypertension 1989;13:219—26.

[135] Zemel MB, Gualdoni SM, Soewers JR. Sodium excretion and plasma renin activity in normotensive and hypertensive black adults affected by dietary calcium and sodium. Journal of Hypertension 1986;4:S343—5.

[136] Rich GM, McCullough M, Olmedo A, Malarick C, Moore TJ. Blood pressure and renal blood flow responses to dietary calcium and sodium intake in humans. Am J Hypertens 1991;4:642S—5S.

[137] Appel LJ, Miller 3rd ER, Seidler AJ, Whelton PK. Does supplementation of diet with 'fish oil' reduce blood pressure? A meta-analysis of controlled clinical trials. Arch Intern Med 1993;153:1429—38.

[138] Morris MC, Sacks F, Rosner B. Does fish oil lower blood pressure? A meta-analysis of controlled trials. Circulation 1993;88:523—33.

[139] Szabo de Edelenyi F, et al. Effect of B-vitamins and n-3 PUFA supplementation for 5 years on blood pressure in patients with CVD. Br J Nutr 2012;107:921—7, http://dx.doi.org/10.1017/S0007114511003692.

[140] Jee SH, et al. The effect of magnesium supplementation on blood pressure: a meta-analysis of randomized clinical trials. Am J Hypertens 2002;15:691—6.

[141] Cappuccio FP, et al. Lack of effect of oral magnesium on high blood pressure: a double blind study. Br Med J (Clin Res Ed) 1985;291:235—8.

[142] Houston M. The role of magnesium in hypertension and cardiovascular disease. J Clin Hypertens (Greenwich) 2011;13:843—7, http://dx.doi.org/10.1111/j.1751-7176.2011.00538.x.

[143] McCarty MF. Complementary vascular-protective actions of magnesium and taurine: a rationale for magnesium taurate. Med Hypotheses 1996;46:89—100.

[144] Yamori Y, Taguchi T, Mori H, Mori M. Low cardiovascular risks in the middle aged males and females excreting greater 24-hour urinary taurine and magnesium in 41 WHO-CARDIAC study populations in the world. J Biomed Sci 2010;17(Suppl. 1):S21, http://dx.doi.org/10.1186/1423-0127-17-S1-S21.

[145] Obarzanek E, Velletri PA, Cutler JA. Dietary protein and blood pressure. Jama 1996;275:1598—603.

[146] He J, et al. Effect of soybean protein on blood pressure: a randomized, controlled trial. Ann Intern Med 2005;143:1—9.

[147] Burke V, et al. Dietary protein and soluble fiber reduce ambulatory blood pressure in treated hypertensives. Hypertension 2001;38:821—6.

[148] Nakaki T, Hishikawa K, Suzuki H, Saruta T, Kato R. L-arginine-induced hypotension. Lancet 1990;336:696.

[149] Hishikawa K, et al. Effect of systemic L-arginine administration on hemodynamics and nitric oxide release in man. Jpn Heart J 1992;33:41—8.

[150] Stamler J, et al. Glutamic acid, the main dietary amino acid, and blood pressure: the INTERMAP Study (International Collaborative Study of Macronutrients, Micronutrients and Blood Pressure). Circulation 2009;120:221—8, http://dx.doi.org/CIRCULATION AHA.108.839241.

[151] Saito T. Antihypertensive peptides derived from bovine casein and whey proteins. Adv Exp Med Biol 2008;606:295—317, http://dx.doi.org/10.1007/978-0-387-74087-4_12.

[152] Williams M, et al. Effect of protein ingestion on urinary dopamine excretion. Evidence for the functional importance of renal decarboxylation of circulating 3,4-dihydroxyphenylalanine in man. J Clin Invest 1986;78:1687—93.

[153] Kuchel O. Differential catecholamine responses to protein intake in healthy and hypertensive subjects. Am J Physiol 1998;275:R1164—73.

[154] Lavigne C, Marette A, Jacques H. Cod and soy proteins compared with casein improve glucose tolerance and insulin sensitivity in rats. Am J Physiol Endocrinol Metab 2000;278: E491—500.

[155] Whelton SP, et al. Effect of dietary fiber intake on blood pressure: a meta-analysis of randomized, controlled clinical trials. J Hypertens 2005;23:475—81.

[156] Altorf-van der Kuil W, Engberink MF, Geleijnse JM, Boer JM, Verschuren WM. Sources of dietary protein and risk of hypertension in a general Dutch population. Br J Nutr:1—7, http://dx.doi.org/10.1017/s0007114512000049 2012.

[157] Sciarrone SE, Rouse IL, Rogers P, Beilin LJ. A factorial study of fat and fibre changes and sodium restriction on blood pressure of human hypertensive subjects. Clin Exp Pharmacol Physiol 1990;17:197—201.

[158] Pal S, Khossousi A, Binns C, Dhaliwal S, Radavelli-Bagatini S. The effects of 12-week psyllium fibre supplementation or healthy diet on blood pressure and arterial stiffness in overweight and obese individuals. Br J Nutr 2012;107:725—34, http://dx.doi.org/10.1017/S0007114511003497.

[159] MacGregor GA. Nutrition and blood pressure. Nutr Metab Cardiovasc Dis 1999;9:6—15.

[160] Moreira LB, Fuchs FD, Moraes RS, Bredemeier M, Duncan BB. Alcohol intake and blood pressure: the importance of time elapsed since last drink. J Hypertens 1998;16:175—80.

[161] Steffens AA, et al. Incidence of hypertension by alcohol consumption: is it modified by race? J Hypertens 2006;24: 1489—92.

[162] Kiyohara Y, Kato I, Iwamoto H, Nakayama K, Fujishima M. The impact of alcohol and hypertension on stroke incidence in a general Japanese population. The Hisayama Study. Stroke 1995;26:368—72.

[163] Fuchs FD, Chambless LE, Whelton PK, Nieto FJ, Heiss G. Alcohol consumption and the incidence of hypertension: The Atherosclerosis Risk in Communities Study. Hypertension 2001;37:1242—50.

[164] Wildman RP, et al. Alcohol intake and hypertension subtypes in Chinese men. J Hypertens 2005;23:737—43.

[165] Leuenberger V, Gache P, Sutter K, Rieder Nakhle A. High blood pressure and alcohol consumption. Rev Med Suisse 2006;2:2041—2. 2044—2046.

[166] Zilkens RR, et al. Red wine and beer elevate blood pressure in normotensive men. Hypertension 2005;45:874—9.

[167] Holick MF. Vitamin D deficiency. N Engl J Med 2007;357: 266—81.

[168] Xiang W, et al. Cardiac hypertrophy in vitamin D receptor knockout mice: role of the systemic and cardiac renin-angiotensin systems. Am J Physiol Endocrinol Metab 2005;288: E125—32.

[169] Zhou C, et al. Calcium-independent and 1,25(OH)2D3-dependent regulation of the renin-angiotensin system in 1alpha-hydroxylase knockout mice. Kidney Int 2008;74:170—9.

[170] Resnick LM, Muller FB, Laragh JH. Calcium-regulating hormones in essential hypertension. Relation to plasma renin activity and sodium metabolism. Ann Intern Med 1986;105: 649—54.

[171] Yuan W, et al. 1,25-dihydroxyvitamin D3 suppresses renin gene transcription by blocking the activity of the cyclic AMP response element in the renin gene promoter. J Biol Chem 2007;282:29821—30.

[172] Bouillon R. Vitamin D as potential baseline therapy for blood pressure control. Am J Hypertens 2009;22:816.

[173] Pilz S, Tomaschitz A, Ritz E, Pieber TR. Vitamin D status and arterial hypertension: a systematic review. Nat Rev Cardiol 2009;6:621—30.

[174] Pittas AG, Lau J, Hu FB, Dawson-Hughes B. The role of vitamin D and calcium in type 2 diabetes. A systematic review and meta-analysis. J Clin Endocrinol Metab 2007;92:2017—29.

[175] Kuhlmann A, et al. 1,25-Dihydroxyvitamin D3 decreases podocyte loss and podocyte hypertrophy in the subtotally nephrectomized rat. Am J Physiol Renal Physiol 2004;286: F526—33.

[176] Hariharan S, et al. Effect of 1,25-dihydroxyvitamin D3 on mesangial cell proliferation. J Lab Clin Med 1991;117:423—9.

[177] Talmor Y, Bernheim J, Klein O, Green J, Rashid G. Calcitriol blunts pro-atherosclerotic parameters through NFkappaB and p38 in vitro. Eur J Clin Invest 2008;38:548—54.

[178] Pfeifer M, Begerow B, Minne HW, Nachtigall D, Hansen C. Effects of a short-term vitamin D(3) and calcium supplementation on blood pressure and parathyroid hormone levels in elderly women. J Clin Endocrinol Metab 2001;86: 1633—7.

[179] Margolis KL, et al. Effect of calcium and vitamin D supplementation on blood pressure: the Women's Health Initiative Randomized Trial. Hypertension 2008;52:847—55.

[180] Thadhani R, et al. Vitamin D therapy and cardiac structure and function in patients with chronic kidney disease: the PRIMO randomized controlled trial. JAMA 2012;307:674—84, http://dx.doi.org/10.1001/jama.2012.120.

[181] Grassi D, et al. Cocoa reduces blood pressure and insulin resistance and improves endothelium-dependent vasodilation in hypertensives. Hypertension 2005;46:398—405.

[182] Taubert D, Berkels R, Roesen R, Klaus W. Chocolate and blood pressure in elderly individuals with isolated systolic hypertension. JAMA 2003;290:1029—30.

[183] Grassi D, Lippi C, Necozione S, Desideri G, Ferri C. Short-term administration of dark chocolate is followed by a significant increase in insulin sensitivity and a decrease in blood pressure in healthy persons. Am J Clin Nutr 2005;81:611—4.

[184] Fisher ND, Hughes M, Gerhard-Herman M, Hollenberg NK. Flavanol-rich cocoa induces nitric-oxide-dependent vasodilation in healthy humans. J Hypertens 2003;21:2281—6.

[185] Engler MB, et al. Flavonoid-rich dark chocolate improves endothelial function and increases plasma epicatechin concentrations in healthy adults. J Am Coll Nutr 2004;23:197—204.

[186] Suzuki A, Kagawa D, Ochiai R, Tokimitsu I, Saito I. Green coffee bean extract and its metabolites have a hypotensive effect in spontaneously hypertensive rats. Hypertens Res 2002;25: 99—107.

[187] Kozuma K, Tsuchiya S, Kohori J, Hase T, Tokimitsu I. Antihypertensive effect of green coffee bean extract on mildly hypertensive subjects. Hypertens Res 2005;28:711–8.

[188] Watanabe T, et al. The blood pressure-lowering effect and safety of chlorogenic acid from green coffee bean extract in essential hypertension. Clin Exp Hypertens 2006;28:439–49.

[189] Ochiai R, et al. Green coffee bean extract improves human vasoreactivity. Hypertens Res 2004;27:731–7.

[190] Papaioannou TG, Vlachopoulos C, Ioakeimidis N, Alexopoulos N, Stefanadis C. Nonlinear dynamics of blood pressure variability after caffeine consumption. Clin Med Res 2006;4:114–8.

[191] Corti R, et al. Coffee acutely increases sympathetic nerve activity and blood pressure independently of caffeine content: role of habitual versus nonhabitual drinking. Circulation 2002;106:2935–40.

[192] Klag MJ, et al. Coffee intake and risk of hypertension: the Johns Hopkins precursors study. Arch Intern Med 2002;162:657–62.

[193] Jee SH, He J, Whelton PK, Suh I, Klag MJ. The effect of chronic coffee drinking on blood pressure: a meta-analysis of controlled clinical trials. Hypertension 1999;33:647–52.

[194] Higdon JV, Frei B. Coffee and health: a review of recent human research. Crit Rev Food Sci Nutr 2006;46:101–23.

[195] Funatsu K, Yamashita T, Nakamura H. Effect of coffee intake on blood pressure in male habitual alcohol drinkers. Hypertens Res 2005;28:521–7.

[196] Yung LM, et al. Tea polyphenols benefit vascular function. Inflammopharmacology 2008;16:230–4.

[197] Yang CS, Hong J, Hou Z, Sang S. Green tea polyphenols: antioxidative and prooxidative effects. J Nutr 2004;134:3181S.

[198] Hodgson JM. Effects of tea and tea flavonoids on endothelial function and blood pressure: a brief review. Clin Exp Pharmacol Physiol 2006;33:838–41.

[199] Hodgson JM, Puddey IB, Burke V, Watts GF, Beilin LJ. Regular ingestion of black tea improves brachial artery vasodilator function. Clin Sci (Lond) 2002;102:195–201.

[200] Hodgson JM, Burke V, Puddey IB. Acute effects of tea on fasting and postprandial vascular function and blood pressure in humans. J Hypertens 2005;23:47–54.

[201] Hodgson JM, et al. Effects of black tea on blood pressure: a randomized controlled trial. Arch Intern Med 2012;172:186–8, http://dx.doi.org/10.1001/archinte.172.2.186.

[202] Winkelmayer WC, Stampfer MJ, Willett WC, Curhan GC. Habitual caffeine intake and the risk of hypertension in women. Jama 2005;294:2330–5.

[203] Feig DI, Soletsky B, Johnson RJ. Effect of allopurinol on blood pressure of adolescents with newly diagnosed essential hypertension: a randomized trial. Jama 2008;300:924–32.

[204] Horvath K, et al. Long-term effects of weight-reducing interventions in hypertensive patients: systematic review and meta-analysis. Arch Intern Med 2008;168:571–80, http://dx.doi.org/10.1001/archinte.168.6.571.

[205] Sjostrom L, et al. Lifestyle, diabetes, and cardiovascular risk factors 10 years after bariatric surgery. N Engl J Med 2004;351:2683–93, http://dx.doi.org/10.1056/NEJMoa035622.

[206] Navaneethan SD, et al. Weight loss interventions in chronic kidney disease: a systematic review and meta-analysis. Clin J Am Soc Nephrol 2009;4:1565–74, http://dx.doi.org/10.2215/CJN.02250409.

[207] Grassi G, et al. Blood pressure lowering effects of rimonabant in obesity-related hypertension. J Neuroendocrinol 2008;20(Suppl. 1):63–8.

[208] Mark AL. Weight reduction for treatment of obesity-associated hypertension: nuances and challenges. Curr Hypertens Rep 2007;9:368–72.

[209] Sjostrom L, et al. Bariatric surgery and long-term cardiovascular events. JAMA 2012;307:56–65, http://dx.doi.org/10.1001/jama.2011.1914.

[210] Zimmet P, Alberti KG. Surgery or medical therapy for obese patients with type 2 diabetes? N Engl J Med 2012;366:1635–6, http://dx.doi.org/10.1056/NEJMe1202443.

[211] Schauer PR, et al. Bariatric surgery versus intensive medical therapy in obese patients with diabetes. N Engl J Med 2012;366:1567–76, http://dx.doi.org/10.1056/NEJMoa1200225.

[212] Mingrone G, et al. Bariatric surgery versus conventional medical therapy for type 2 diabetes. N Engl J Med 2012;366:1577–85, http://dx.doi.org/10.1056/NEJMoa1200111.

[213] The Hypertension Prevention Trial: three-year effects of dietary changes on blood pressure. Hypertension Prevention Trial Research Group. Arch Intern Med 1990;150:153–62.

[214] Satterfield S, et al. Trials of hypertension prevention. Phase I design. Ann Epidemiol 1991;1:455–71.

[215] The effects of nonpharmacologic interventions on blood pressure of persons with high normal levels. Results of the Trials of Hypertension Prevention. Phase I. JAMA 1992;267:1213–20.

[216] Hebert PR, et al. Design of a multicenter trial to evaluate long-term lifestyle intervention in adults with high-normal blood pressure levels. Trials of Hypertension Prevention (phase II). Trials of Hypertension Prevention (TOHP) Collaborative Research Group. Ann Epidemiol 1995;5:130–9.

[217] Effects of weight loss and sodium reduction intervention on blood pressure and hypertension incidence in overweight people with high-normal blood pressure. The Trials of Hypertension Prevention, phase II. The Trials of Hypertension Prevention Collaborative Research Group. Arch Intern Med 1997;157:657–67.

[218] Stevens VJ, et al. Long-term weight loss and changes in blood pressure: results of the Trials of Hypertension Prevention, phase II. Ann Intern Med 2001;134:1–11.

[219] Kumanyika SK, et al. Sodium reduction for hypertension prevention in overweight adults: further results from the Trials of Hypertension Prevention Phase II. J Hum Hypertens 2005;19:33–45.

[220] Appel LJ, et al. A clinical trial of the effects of dietary patterns on blood pressure. DASH Collaborative Research Group. N Engl J Med 1997;336:1117–24.

[221] Sacks FM, et al. Effects on blood pressure of reduced dietary sodium and the Dietary Approaches to Stop Hypertension (DASH) diet. DASH-Sodium Collaborative Research Group. N Engl J Med 2001;344:3–10.

[222] Vollmer WM, et al. Effects of diet and sodium intake on blood pressure: subgroup analysis of the DASH-sodium trial. Ann Intern Med 2001;135:1019–28.

[223] Webb AJ, et al. Acute blood pressure lowering, vasoprotective, and antiplatelet properties of dietary nitrate via bioconversion to nitrite. Hypertension 2008;51:784–90.

[224] Hord NG, Tang Y, Bryan NS. Food sources of nitrates and nitrites: the physiologic context for potential health benefits. Am J Clin Nutr 2009;90:1–10, http://dx.doi.org/10.3945/ajcn.2008.27131 [pii] 10.3945/ajcn.2008.27131.

[225] Ralston RA, Lee JH, Truby H, Palermo CE, Walker KZ. A systematic review and meta-analysis of elevated blood pressure and consumption of dairy foods. J Hum Hypertens 2012;26:3–13, http://dx.doi.org/10.1038/jhh.2011.3.

[226] Dauchet L, Amouyel P, Hercberg S, Dallongeville J. Fruit and vegetable consumption and risk of coronary heart disease: a meta-analysis of cohort studies. J Nutr 2006;136:2588–93, http://dx.doi.org/136/10/2588 [pii].

[227] He FJ, Nowson CA, MacGregor GA. Fruit and vegetable consumption and stroke: meta-analysis of cohort studies. Lancet 2006;367:320−6, http://dx.doi.org/S0140-6736(06)68069-0 [pii] 10.1016/S0140-6736(06)68069-0.

[228] McCall DO, et al. Dietary intake of fruits and vegetables improves microvascular function in hypertensive subjects in a dose-dependent manner. Circulation 2009;119:2153−60, http://dx.doi.org/CIRCULATIONAHA.108.831297 [pii] 10.1161/CIRCULATIONAHA.108.831297.

[229] Nunez-Cordoba JM, et al. Role of vegetables and fruits in Mediterranean diets to prevent hypertension. Eur J Clin Nutr 2009;63:605−12, http://dx.doi.org/ejcn200822 [pii] 10.1038/ejcn.2008.22.

[230] Funk KL, et al. PREMIER − a trial of lifestyle interventions for blood pressure control: intervention design and rationale. Health Promot Pract 2008;9:271−80.

[231] Lien LF, et al. Effects of PREMIER lifestyle modifications on participants with and without the metabolic syndrome. Hypertension 2007;50:609−16.

[232] Azadbakht L, Mirmiran P, Esmaillzadeh A, Azizi T, Azizi F. Beneficial effects of a Dietary Approaches to Stop Hypertension eating plan on features of the metabolic syndrome. Diabetes Care 2005;28:2823−31.

[233] Esposito K, Giugliano D. Beneficial effects of a Dietary Approaches to Stop Hypertension eating plan on features of the metabolic syndrome. Diabetes Care 2006;29:954. author reply 954-955.

[234] Whelton PK, et al. Primary prevention of hypertension: clinical and public health advisory from The National High Blood Pressure Education Program. Jama 2002;288:1882−8.

[235] US Department of Health and Human Services and the US Department of Agriculture. Dietary Guidelines for Americans; 2005.

[236] Khan NA, et al. The 2006 Canadian Hypertension Education Program recommendations for the management of hypertension: Part II − Therapy. Can J Cardiol 2006;22:583−93.

[237] He J, et al. Effect of soybean protein on blood pressure: a randomized, controlled trial. Ann Intern Med 2005;143:1−9, http://dx.doi.org/143/1/1 [pii].

[238] Hu FB, et al. Dietary fat intake and the risk of coronary heart disease in women. N Engl J Med 1997;337:1491−9.

[239] Kelemen LE, Kushi LH, Jacobs Jr DR, Cerhan JR. Associations of dietary protein with disease and mortality in a prospective study of postmenopausal women. Am J Epidemiol 2005;161:239−49.

[240] Shah M, Adams-Huet B, Garg A. Effect of high-carbohydrate or high-cis-monounsaturated fat diets on blood pressure: a meta-analysis of intervention trials. Am J Clin Nutr 2007;85:1251−6.

[241] Nuttall FQ, Schweim K, Hoover H, Gannon MC. Metabolic effect of a LoBAG30 diet in men with type 2 diabetes. Am J Physiol Endocrinol Metab 2006;291:E786−91, http://dx.doi.org/00011.2006 [pii] 10.1152/ajpendo.00011.2006.

[242] Kennedy RL, Chokkalingam K, Farshchi HR. Nutrition in patients with Type 2 diabetes: are low-carbohydrate diets effective, safe or desirable? Diabet Med 2005;22:821−32, http://dx.doi.org/DME1594 [pii] 10.1111/j.1464-5491.2005.01594.x.

[243] Elmer PJ, et al. Effects of comprehensive lifestyle modification on diet, weight, physical fitness, and blood pressure control: 18-month results of a randomized trial. Ann Intern Med 2006;144:485−95.

[244] Cakir H, Pinar R. Randomized controlled trial on lifestyle modification in hypertensive patients. West J Nurs Res 2006;28:190−209. discussion 210-195.

[245] Folsom AR, Parker ED, Harnack LJ. Degree of concordance with DASH diet guidelines and incidence of hypertension and fatal cardiovascular disease. Am J Hypertens 2007;20:225−32.

[246] Howard BV, et al. Low-fat dietary pattern and risk of cardiovascular disease: the Women's Health Initiative Randomized Controlled Dietary Modification Trial. Jama 2006;295:655−66.

[247] Burke V, et al. Effects of a lifestyle programme on ambulatory blood pressure and drug dosage in treated hypertensive patients: a randomized controlled trial. J Hypertens 2005;23:1241−9.

[248] Burke V, et al. Changes in cognitive measures associated with a lifestyle program for treated hypertensives: a randomized controlled trial (ADAPT). Health Educ Res 2008;23:202−17.

[249] Burke V, Mansour J, Beilin LJ, Mori TA. Long-term follow-up of participants in a health promotion program for treated hypertensives (ADAPT). Nutr Metab Cardiovasc Dis 2008;18:198−206.

[250] Jeffery RW, et al. Long-term maintenance of weight loss: current status. Health Psychol 2000;19:5−16.

[251] Viera AJ, Kshirsagar AV, Hinderliter AL. Lifestyle modifications to lower or control high blood pressure: is advice associated with action? The behavioral risk factor surveillance survey. J Clin Hypertens (Greenwich) 2008;10:105−11.

[252] Knowler WC, et al. 10-year follow-up of diabetes incidence and weight loss in the Diabetes Prevention Program Outcomes Study. Lancet 2009;374:1677−86, http://dx.doi.org/10.1016/S0140-6736(09)61457-4.

[253] Gao SK, et al. Suboptimal nutritional intake for hypertension control in 4 ethnic groups. Arch Intern Med 2009;169:702−7, http://dx.doi.org/169/7/702 [pii] 10.1001/archinternmed.2009.17.

[254] Bertoni AG, et al. A multilevel assessment of barriers to adoption of Dietary Approaches to Stop Hypertension (DASH) among African Americans of low socioeconomic status. J Health Care Poor Underserved 2011;22:1205−20, http://dx.doi.org/10.1353/hpu.2011.0142.

[255] Mellen PB, Gao SK, Vitolins MZ, Goff Jr DC. Deteriorating dietary habits among adults with hypertension: DASH dietary accordance, NHANES 1988-1994 and 1999-2004. Arch Intern Med 2008;168:308−14.

[256] King DE, Mainous 3rd AG, Carnemolla M, Everett CJ. Adherence to healthy lifestyle habits in US adults, 1988-2006. Am J Med 2009;122:528−34, http://dx.doi.org/S0002-9343(08)01207-2 [pii] 10.1016/j.amjmed.2008.11.013.

[257] The Sixth report of the Joint National Committee on Prevention, Detection, Evaluation, and Treatment of High Blood Pressure. Arch Intern Med 1997;157:2413−46.

[258] Chobanian AV, et al. Seventh Report of the Joint National Committee on Prevention, Detection, Evaluation, and Treatment of High Blood Pressure. Hypertension 2003;42:1206−52.

[259] Logan AGDASH. Diet: time for a critical appraisal? Am J Hypertens 2007;20:223−4.

[260] Wadden TA, et al. A two-year randomized trial of obesity treatment in primary care practice. N Engl J Med 2011;365:1969−79, http://dx.doi.org/10.1056/NEJMoa1109220.

[261] Appel LJ, et al. Comparative effectiveness of weight-loss interventions in clinical practice. N Engl J Med 2011;365:1959−68, http://dx.doi.org/10.1056/NEJMoa1108660.

[262] Kotchen TA. Does the DASH diet improve clinical outcomes in hypertensive patients? Am J Hypertens 2009;22:350, http://dx.doi.org/ajh200915 [pii] 10.1038/ajh.2009.15.

[263] Forman JP, Stampfer MJ, Curhan GC. Diet and lifestyle risk factors associated with incident hypertension in women. Jama 2009;302:401−11, http://dx.doi.org/302/4/401 [pii] 0.1001/jama.2009.1060.

[264] Chen ZY, et al. Anti-hypertensive nutraceuticals and functional foods. J Agric Food Chem 2009;57:4485—99, http://dx.doi.org/10.1021/jf900803r.

[265] Collier SR, et al. Effect of 4 weeks of aerobic or resistance exercise training on arterial stiffness, blood flow and blood pressure in pre- and stage-1 hypertensives. J Hum Hypertens 2008;22:678—86.

[266] Mann M. Prognostic significance of systolic blood pressure during exercise stress testing. Am J Cardiol 2008;101:1518. author reply 1518—1519.

[267] Henson LC, Poole DC, Donahoe CP, Heber D. Effects of exercise training on resting energy expenditure during caloric restriction. Am J Clin Nutr 1987;46:893—9.

[268] Siebenhofer A, et al. Long-term effects of weight-reducing drugs in hypertensive patients. Cochrane Database Syst Rev CD007654, http://dx.doi.org/10.1002/14651858.CD007654.pub2 2009.

[269] Savica V, Bellinghieri G, Kopple JD. The effect of nutrition on blood pressure. Annu Rev Nutr 2010;30:365—401, http://dx.doi.org/10.1146/annurev-nutr-010510-103954.

28

Effect of Obesity and the Metabolic Syndrome on Incident Kidney Disease and the Progression to Chronic Kidney Failure

Alex Chang[1], Holly Kramer[1,2]

[1]Loyola University Medical Center, Department of Medicine, Division of Nephrology and Hypertension, Maywood, IL, USA
[2]Department of Preventive Medicine and Epidemiology, Maywood, IL, USA

INTRODUCTION

Over the last half of the 20th century, substantial gains were made in life expectancy for both sexes and all racial/ethnic groups in the United States. These life year gains were largely the result of population reduction in average blood pressure and serum cholesterol levels through diet and medicinal interventions. Due to the obesity epidemic, it is likely that reversals in life expectancy will occur over the next decade because there has been no major downward shift in the mean body mass index (BMI) of the U.S. population [1]. The obesity epidemic affects nearly every region of the world; the International Obesity Task Force estimates that approximately one billion adults are currently overweight, as defined as a BMI between $25-29.9$ kg/m^2, and another 475 million adults are obese, as defined as a BMI ≥ 30 kg/m^2 [2]. When using the Asian-specific BMI cut-point to define obesity (>28 kg/m^2), the number of obese individuals increases to 600 million [2]. In Western countries such as the United States, only 1/3 of Americans have a BMI within the ideal range (BMI $18.5-24.9$ kg/m^2) [3]. Obesity trends in adults with end-stage kidney disease (ESKD) parallel those in the general population [4,5]. During years $1995-2002$, the mean BMI among patients starting dialysis increased from 25.7 to 27.5 kg/m^2 [5]. The percentage of patients starting dialysis with a BMI>35 kg/m^2 (stage II obesity) increased from 9.4% to 15.4% during this time frame [5]. Similarly, the percentage of obese (BMI≥ 30 kg/m^2) patients listed for kidney transplantation also increased from 11.6% to 25.1% between the years 1987 and 2001 [4].

Abdominal adiposity, in particular, appears to be the primary driver for the cluster of clinical traits (insulin resistance (IR), hypertension, and dyslipidemia) known as the metabolic syndrome, which now affects one in four U.S. adults [6,7]. Obesity places an individual at increased risk for hypertension and diabetes [8], which probably cause the majority of chronic kidney disease (CKD) and ESKD in industrialized societies [9]. Possible mechanisms underlying obesity-induced renal injury are explored in this chapter. While the majority of obesity-associated CKD may be attributable to hypertension and diabetes, some obese individuals develop substantial proteinuria and progressive kidney disease with biopsy findings of glomerulomegaly, usually with focal segmental glomerulosclerosis (FSGS) and foot process fusion [10–12]. Moreover, glomerulosclerosis of varying degrees has been reported in morbidly obese individuals who do not have clinically apparent kidney disease [13].

The increasing prevalence of obesity world-wide will probably cause the prevalence of all stages of CKD to rise. Intentional weight loss appears to improve certain manifestations of kidney disease, but the long-term effects of weight loss on the course of CKD remain poorly explored [13–21]. The weight loss which occurs after bariatric surgery for obesity management in the morbidly obese is accompanied by improvement in all elements of the metabolic syndrome, as well as decreases in absolute (not indexed for body surface area) glomerular filtration rate (GFR), effective renal plasma flow (RPF) and urine protein excretion [17,22,23]. Additional studies on the effects of lifestyle behaviors on the incidence and progression of kidney disease are urgently needed in order to curtail the adverse effects of obesity on the kidney.

This chapter will discuss the definitions of obesity and metabolic syndrome, the association between obesity, the metabolic syndrome and CKD, and potential mechanisms which connect obesity and the metabolic syndrome with kidney disease. The benefits of weight loss in these conditions will also be reviewed.

DEFINITIONS OF OBESITY/METABOLIC SYNDROME

Body Mass Index (BMI)

The Metropolitan Life Insurance Company created weight-for-height tables using data from adults who purchased life insurance from 1935 to 1954 and described desirable body weights associated with the lowest mortality risk [24]. The World Health Organization (WHO) has since formally defined BMI categories (see Table 28.1) including obesity stages: I (BMI 30.0–34.9 kg/m^2), II (BMI 35.0–39.9 kg/m^2), and III ($\geq$40 kg/m^2) [25]. Among young and middle-aged adults in the general population, life expectancy is shorter among individuals with a BMI $\geq$35 kg/m^2 compared to the nonobese [26,27]. BMI includes fat mass and fat-free mass and does not provide information about body composition or regional adiposity. As a result, BMI categories may not be as accurate for capturing mortality risk in such populations as the elderly, certain racial/ethnic groups, and some disease states associated with wasting such as CKD or ESKD [28,29]. This likely reflects the fact that differences in

TABLE 28.1 Classification of Underweight, Overweight, and Obesity by BMI and Waist Circumference*

BMI	(kg/m^2)
Underweight	<18.5
Normal (Desirable)	18.5–24.9
Overweight	25.0–29.9
Class I Obesity	30.0–34.9
Class II Obesity	35.0–39.9
Class III Obesity	$\geq$40
Waist Circumference	**(cm)**
Decreased risk	Men $\leq$102 Women $\leq$88
Increased risk[§]	Men >102 Women >88

* Adapted from World Health Organization 1998 guidelines for obesity classification [25].
[§] >87 cm and >83 cm in Japanese men and women, respectively [33].

BMI may be due to differences in muscle mass, which may strongly influence mortality risk.

Abdominal Obesity

Although abdominal fat can be measured directly by dual-energy X-ray absorptiometry, computed tomography, or magnetic resonance imaging, waist circumference can be easily and reliably measured without the use of expensive instruments [30,31]. Clinically, abdominal obesity is defined as a waist circumference $\geq$102 cm in men and $\geq$88 cm in women because these thresholds discerned obese from nonobese adults with a high waist:hip ratio in a Scottish population (Table 28.1) [32]. Waist circumference thresholds for abdominal adiposity may differ by racial/ethnic groups and are considered to be lower for Asian men and women (>87 cm and >83 cm in Japanese men and women) [33]. Individuals with abdominal obesity are more likely to have hypertension, diabetes, dyslipidemia, and cardiovascular disease than individuals without abdominal obesity, even after adjusting for BMI [34,35]. Furthermore, a direct association between waist circumference and mortality risk has been noted in many racial/ethnic group groups and in adults with all stages of CKD regardless of BMI [36–39]. Many studies show that in ESKD patients, in contrast to normal people, an increasing BMI is associated with reduced mortality rates [40]. The same phenomenon appears to occur in the less advanced stages of CKD [37,38,41]. Among 5805 adults with stage 1–4 CKD, those with a BMI $\geq$30 kg/m^2 had a lower risk of mortality during 4 years of follow-up compared to those with a BMI between 25–29.9 kg/m^2 (Figure 28.1). In contrast, mortality among individuals in the highest waist circumference category ($\geq$108 cm in women and >122 cm in men) was two-fold higher than those with waist circumference <80 cm in women and <94 cm in men (Figure 28.2) [37]. Similar findings have been reported in adults with ESKD [39]. These findings suggest that waist circumference should be used in conjunction with BMI to best identify individuals who might benefit from weight loss interventions in the CKD population.

Metabolic Syndrome

In 1998, the clustering of metabolic risk factors, including obesity, dyslipidemia, hypertension, and hyperglycemia, was labeled as "Syndrome X" which was later renamed the metabolic syndrome [42]. There have been several variations of this definition including one from the World Health Organization which included increased urine albumin concentration as one of the defining traits [43]. The Third Report of the Expert

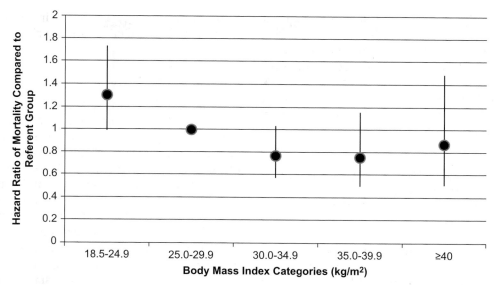

FIGURE 28.1 Hazard ratios for mortality by BMI (Figure 28.1) or waist circumference groups (Figure 28.2) among REGARDS participants with stages 1–4 chronic kidney disease. All hazard ratios are adjusted for age, sex, race, coronary heart disease, stroke, cancer, hypertension, diabetes, smoking status, educational attainment, household income, health insurance, urine albumin-creatinine ratio, eGFR, systolic blood pressure, HDL, LDL, and adjusted for either waist circumference *(1)* or BMI *(2)*. *Adapted from Kramer et al. [37].*

Panel on Detection, Evaluation and Treatment of High Blood Cholesterol in Adults (Adult Treatment Panel III, or ATP III) from the National Cholesterol Education Program (NCEP) defined metabolic syndrome as the presence of at least 3 of the following five criteria: central obesity (waist circumference in men >102 cm and in women >88cm), hypertriglyceridemia (≥150 mg/dL), low HDL cholesterol (men <40 mg/dL, women, <50 mg/dL), elevated fasting glucose (≥110 mg/dL), and

hypertension (≥130/85 mmHg) [6]. It remains controversial whether metabolic syndrome is more than just the sum of its parts. Certainly each of the traits confers an increased risk of cardiovascular events [44], and is linked with abdominal adiposity.

Abdominal adiposity leads to insulin resistance which underlies all of the elements of the metabolic syndrome (see Figure 28.3) [45] Adipocytes serve a role in storing energy efficiently in times of caloric

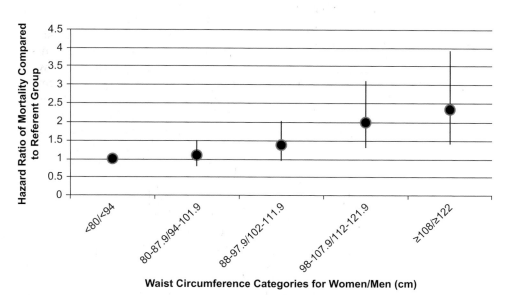

FIGURE 28.2 Hazard ratios for mortality by BMI (Figure 28.1) or waist circumference groups (Figure 28.2) among REGARDS participants with stages 1–4 chronic kidney disease. All hazard ratios are adjusted for age, sex, race, coronary heart disease, stroke, cancer, hypertension, diabetes, smoking status, educational attainment, household income, health insurance, urine albumin-creatinine ratio, eGFR, systolic blood pressure, HDL, LDL, and adjusted for either waist circumference *(1)* or BMI *(2)*. *Adapted from Kramer et al. [37].*

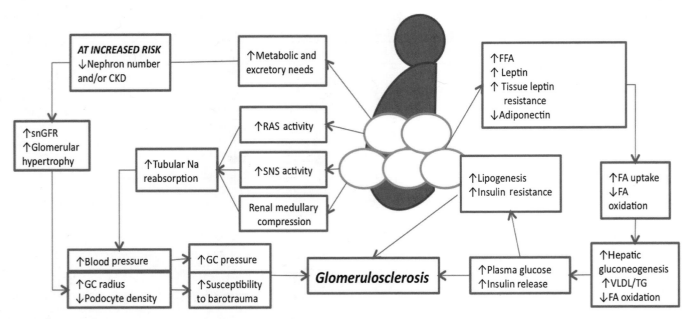

FIGURE 28.3   In obesity/the metabolic syndrome, free fatty acid delivery to the portal circulation is increased leading to increased synthesis of triglycerides TGs and atherogenic VLDLs. Leptin levels increase but tissue resistance develops. Adiponectin levels are reduced which increases hepatic gluconeogenesis and plasma glucose and insulin levels. Lipogenesis is thus augmented and cytosolic fatty acid levels increase resulting in insulin resistance. Blood pressure increases due to increased renal tubular sodium reabsorption. Autoregulation is impaired and higher blood pressures are transmitted to a glomerulus susceptible to barotrauma. Abbreviations: snGFR, single nephron glomerular filtration rate; GC, glomerulocapillary; RAS, renal-angiotensin system; SNS, sympathetic nervous system; FFA, free fatty acid; FA, fatty acid; VLDL, very-low-density lipoprotein; TG, triglycerides. This figure is reproduced in color in the color plate section.

excess; this stored energy, in turn, can be released in times of starvation [46]. Adipocytes also protect nonadipocytes from the negative effects of lipid overload including lipid overload-induced apoptosis [46]. Beyond simply storing energy, adipocytes produce numerous bioactive molecules, including leptin and adiponectin, which appear to protect against some of the adverse consequences of excess calorie intake. With abdominal obesity, adiponectin levels are low despite the fact that adiponectin is secreted by adipocytes. Adiponectin sensitizes tissues to insulin by inhibiting liver enzymes and peroxisome proliferator-activated receptor-α which promote gluconeogenesis [47] and increase cellular glucose uptake [48], respectively. Adiponectin stimulates fatty acid oxidation in peripheral tissues, and may play a role in endothelial dysfunction, because adiponectin knockout mice show heightened inflammatory response to endothelial injury [49–51]. The effects of adiponectin are mediated through activation of AMP protein kinase (AMPK), a key regulator of cellular energy via phosphorylation [52]. Activation of AMPK switches cells from ATP consumption to active ATP production and fatty acid and glucose oxidation. AMPK also acts on the hypothalamus, interacting with leptin and ghrelin to influence satiety. Activation of AMPK is also a critical step for translocation of GLUT4 into skeletal muscle and other organs for glucose transport [53,54]. Thus, a decrease in AMPK activity will lead

to energy storage. Since adiponectin stimulates AMPK phosphorylation, it comes as no surprise that low levels of adiponectin are found with the metabolic syndrome, abdominal obesity, diabetes mellitus, and cardiovascular disease [55].

Leptin acts centrally in the central nervous system by decreasing appetite and increasing energy expenditure through stimulation of the sympathetic nervous system and also promoting oxidation of muscle fatty acids [55]. Leptin deficiency may result in extreme hyperphagia and obesity, while recombinant leptin replacement may produce weight loss in states of leptin deficiency [56]. Due to tissue resistance to leptin in the obese state, fatty acids accumulate in the cytosol of adipocytes [57]. Visceral adipocytes are particularly important because they secrete free fatty acids directly into the portal circulation which augments synthesis of triglycerides and very low-density lipoproteins (VLDLs) which are very atherogenic [45]. Due to hepatic insulin resistance, hepatic gluconeogenesis is promoted instead of glycogen synthesis. This leads to a compensatory increase in serum insulin levels. This phenomenon was demonstrated in a dramatic fashion in dogs fed an iso-caloric moderate-fat diet that developed a doubling of trunk adiposity with little weight change [58]. After 12 weeks of this moderate-fat diet, hepatic gluconeogenesis remained insuppressible by insulin [58].

OBESITY AND METABOLIC SYNDROME AS RISK FACTORS FOR INCIDENT CKD

Many epidemiologic studies have found associations between obesity, the metabolic syndrome and CKD. In a cross-sectional analysis of the third National Health and Nutrition Examination Study (NHANES III), individuals with the metabolic syndrome had over twice the odds of having an estimated GFR (eGFR) <60 mL/min/m^2 (95% CI, 1.68–4.03) as compared to individuals without the metabolic syndrome. Individuals with the metabolic syndrome were also more likely to have microalbuminuria (OR 1.89; 95% CI, 1.34–2.67) [59]. The prevalence of CKD increased progressively with the higher the number of metabolic syndrome traits [59]. These findings have been supported by several prospective studies which showed a heightened risk of incident CKD among individuals with metabolic syndrome traits compared to individuals without these traits [60–62]. Although the presence of any of the metabolic syndrome traits heightens the risk of incident CKD, these associations are not strong [60,61,63].

Modest associations are also noted between overweight and obesity (defined by BMI) and incident CKD defined by an eGFR <60 mL/min/1.73 m^2 [64,65]. For example, after 18 years of follow-up among participants of the Framingham Offspring Study, odds of incident CKD (eGFR<60 mL/min/m^2) increased by 21% (95% CI 1.06–1.39) for every 1 standard deviation unit increment in BMI after controlling for age, diabetes, smoking, and baseline estimated GFR [66]. In contrast, associations between obesity and risk of ESKD are very robust. The largest study which focused on ESKD utilized data from 320,252 adults enrolled in the Kaiser Permanente health system who volunteered for a screening health checkup between 1964 and 1985 and were followed until death, dialysis, or through 31 December 2000. The adults who had a baseline BMI ≥40 kg/m^2 had a 600% higher risk of ESKD as compared to those with a baseline BMI in the desirable range (18.5–24.9 kg/m^2) [67]. Controlling for baseline blood pressure and presence of diabetes attenuated these associations somewhat, but overall the associations remained strong.

OBESITY AND METABOLIC SYNDROME AS RISK FACTORS FOR PROGRESSION OF CKD

Studies of the effects of obesity and metabolic syndrome on progression of CKD have been limited. One study examined the effect of excessive weight (defined as BMI ≥25 kg/m^2) in 162 patients with biopsy-proven IgA nephropathy and serum creatinine of 1.1 ± 0.5 mg/dL (median 1.0 mg/dL; range 0.6 to 4.6 mg/dL) [66]. Mean follow-up was 46 ± 35 months after biopsy, and incident CKD was defined as a follow-up serum creatinine >1.5 mg/dL in men and >1.2 mg/dL in women, with a 24 hour creatinine clearance <80 mL/min/1.73m^2 [68]. The presence of excessive weight at the time of renal biopsy was significantly correlated with the severity of histologic findings on biopsy and risk of incident hypertension. Among 842 participants in the African African-American Study of Kidney Disease and Hypertension (which was restricted to individuals with hypertensive kidney disease), 41.7% met the criteria for metabolic syndrome at baseline [69]. These individuals had greater levels of proteinuria as compared to study participants without metabolic syndrome. The presence of the metabolic syndrome was associated with a 31% relative increase in the risk for the composite outcome of a 50% decline in GFR as compared to the baseline GFR, the initiation of dialysis or death. However, the association was no longer significant after accounting for baseline urine protein excretion [69]. Thus, individuals with the metabolic syndrome and kidney disease may progress to ESKD faster than those without the metabolic syndrome. This faster progression may explain why obesity is so strongly associated with ESKD and yet is weakly associated with earlier stages of CKD.

PATHOPHYSIOLOGY OF OBESITY ON THE KIDNEY

Glomerular Hyperfiltration — Physiologic or Maladaptive?

Obesity often leads to increases in both fat and muscle mass, and a high daily energy intake is needed to maintain the obese state. Thus, obesity not only reflects a larger body size, but usually a higher intake of protein and total calories as well as other nutrients. Single nephron GFR must increase to keep pace with the higher metabolic/excretory needs in the obese state [22,70]. Nephron number actually varies substantially, ranging from 230,000 to 1.8 million in one multi-ethnic study of 67 autopsy cases from Australia and the United States [71]. Studies in humans show higher absolute GFR and effective RPF among obese individuals compared to nonobese individuals. After adjusting for body surface area, these differences in GFR and effective RPF are no longer evident [22,72]. In humans, both GFR and RPF can increase substantially through alteration of the afferent and efferent arteriolar resistance and expansion of glomerular capillary surface area without necessarily heightening glomerular capillary pressure [70].

However, an absolute increase in GFR should result in an increase in single nephron GFR, since nephron number does not increase with weight gain. Consequentially, individuals with low nephron number may be at particular risk for higher intracapillary glomerular pressure and subsequent glomerulosclerosis if they gain substantial weight [73,74].

Increased Susceptibility to Barotrauma

Glomerular hypertrophy also occurs as GFR increases in the obese state. GFR is typically indexed to body surface area (BSA), because GFR and RPF are proportional to kidney size, and kidney size tends to be proportional to body size in humans. However, BSA calculated by the Du Bois formula may be inaccurate in the severely obese patient. Hence, factoring GFR by BSA, estimated from formulas or nomograms in obese individuals, may lead to an underestimate of the GFR adjusted for BSA [75]. In a dog model of obesity induced by feeding a high-fat diet for 24 weeks, the absolute GFR was markedly increased, by 38%, and RPF was increased by 61%, while plasma renin and insulin concentrations were more than doubled [76]. Renal structural and functional damage occurred after just 7 to 9 weeks of high-fat feeding. Biopsy findings included expansion of Bowman's capsule, glomerular cell proliferation, thickened glomerular and basement membranes, and increased mesangial matrix [76].

Autopsy data demonstrate that body size alone is not strongly correlated with the extent of glomerulosclerosis but is positively and directly correlated with the glomerular diameter [10]. This glomerular hypertrophy could lead to kidney injury by increasing glomerular capillary wall tension [70]. The radius of the glomerular capillary wall must increase with glomerular hypertrophy and will lead to increased glomerular capillary wall tension in accordance with La Place's law: Tension = Pressure*Radius/Wall Thickness.

Another theory that may explain obesity-induced glomerulosclerosis shifts the focus to the glomerular podocyte, which provides structural support against increased glomerulocapillary pressure [77]. Podocytes have limited ability to replicate, and with glomerular hypertrophy in the obese state, podocyte density may become relatively decreased [7–80]. Wiggins et al. studied podocyte changes in Fischer 344 rats which develop proteinuria and glomerulosclerosis on an ad libitum diet [81]. The ad libitum-fed rats demonstrated increase in podocyte number and size that was proportional to the increase in glomerular volume at 6 months. By 17 months, these ad libitum-fed rats no longer increased their podocyte number, and it was podocyte hypertrophy that increased in proportion to the greater glomerular volume. Levels of desmin mRNA were

increased at this stage, suggesting podocyte stress. Eventually, these rats were unable to maintain increases in podocyte mass that were proportional to increases in glomerular mass, and consequently developed proteinuria and glomerulosclerosis. Podocyte abnormalities including decreased podocyte density and increased foot process width have been described in a series of 46 Chinese patients with obesity-related glomerulopathy [82]. It has been hypothesized that these podocyte adaptations to glomerular hypertrophy lead to detachment of the foot processes from the basement membrane and subsequent proteinuria [81].

Obesity-Related Glomerulopathy

The relationship between obesity, proteinuria and progressive kidney disease with characteristic biopsy findings of glomerulomegaly, with or without FSGS, has been noted since the 1970s [10,11]. FSGS associated with obesity tends to be less severe than idiopathic FSGS with less proteinuria, hypoalbuminemia, edema, and lower risk of progression to ESKD [12]; this is consistent with secondary forms of FSGS [83]. As most biopsy studies include obese patients who had kidney biopsies for specific indications (i.e. proteinuria, decreased renal function) [12,82], they may not capture more subtle findings that could be present but not clinically evident in obese individuals.

One interesting study compared 95 extremely obese individuals (BMI range 40–94 kg/m^2) without overt renal disease who underwent renal biopsy at the time of bariatric surgery with 40 normal-weight healthy controls who were undergoing protocol biopsies (i.e., while undergoing nephrectomy or donating a kidney) [13]. In the extremely obese group, mean age was 41.8 ± 10.1 years; mean BMI was 53.6 ± 9.2 kg/m^2, and diabetes, hypertension and impaired fasting glucose were noted in 59%, 14% and 38% of the individuals, respectively. Timed urine collections were used to calculate creatinine clearance, proteinuria, and albuminuria. Among the 95 individuals, 31 had creatinine clearance >140 mL/min, 43 had increased urine albumin excretion. FSGS was present in only five of these extremely obese individuals. However, more subtle findings such as increased mesangial matrix, podocyte hypertrophy, mesangial cell proliferation, and glomerulomegaly were present in a substantial number of the extremely obese group and were rarely present in the normal weight individuals (77% in the obese group vs. 5% in the normal weight group, p < 0.001) [13]. These observations suggest that obesity may cause mild renal damage without overt clinical findings and that glomerulomegaly is a fairly consistent finding in kidney biopsy specimens among morbidly obese individuals.

Obesity and Blood Pressure

Obesity may also influence CKD progression due to its influence on the traditional risk factors for progression, including hypertension. The prevalence of hypertension is dramatically higher among younger age individuals (<60 years old) who have a higher BMI [84]. Weight gain is strongly associated with an increased risk of incident hypertension. Several mechanisms have been proposed to explain how obesity increases blood pressure and are discussed in detail in Chapter 27. These include increased activity of the sympathetic nervous system (SNS), activation of the renin-angiotensin system (RAS), and altered intrarenal physical forces [85,86]. Increased SNS activity with obesity occurs in a number of tissues, including the kidney, which raises blood pressure due to heightened sodium reabsorption. Renal denervation in dogs fed a high-fat diet substantially attenuated the increase in blood pressure and the sodium retention associated with weight gain, suggesting an important role for the SNS in obesity-related hypertension [87]. Leptin has also been proposed to play a role in the hypertension associated with obesity. Chronic infusion of leptin into rats increases SNS activity and blood pressure [88]. Obese mice deficient in leptin do not develop hypertension as compared to obese wild-type leptin (control) mice [89].

Excess RAS activity may also mediate the obesity related increases in blood pressure. This seems counterintuitive given that obesity impairs natriuresis and thus is a volume expanded state. However, angiotensinogen, the precursor to angiotensin II, is produced by visceral adipocytes, and plasma angiotensinogen levels correlate directly with the degree of visceral adiposity [90]. Moreover, higher RAS activity and aldosterone levels have been noted in obese adults with and without hypertension [91–93]. Excess angiotensin II and aldosterone augment sodium reabsorption and further inhibit natriuresis. Intake of other nutrients may strongly influence blood pressure and should also be considered. In a community based survey of adults living in Maywood, IL, a predominantly African-American community outside of Chicago, sodium intake was determined by the average of three 24-hour urine collections. Sodium intake increased as BMI rose, and individuals with a BMI ≥ 35 kg/m^2 consumed >13 grams of sodium per day [94]. Sodium intake and the ratio of sodium to potassium intake were significantly and positively associated with higher systolic blood pressure even after adjustment for BMI [94].

Insulin Resistance and CKD

The metabolic syndrome, which occurs in the majority of individuals with obesity, and especially severe obesity (BMI >35 kg/m^2), may also contribute to kidney disease risk. It is fairly well established that kidney disease is frequently accompanied by insulin resistance regardless of the CKD etiology. The temporality of this association may be difficult to discern in many patients, especially given the high prevalence of overweight, obesity and physical inactivity among patients with CKD. A Japanese study used the hyperinsulinemic euglycemic clamp technique to measure insulin sensitivity in 45 nonobese adults with diabetes and varying degrees of albuminuria and decreased renal function [95]. Individuals with an elevated serum creatinine >2.0 mg/dL were roughly one-half as sensitive to insulin compared to the adults with normal renal function and normoalbuminuria [95]. Studies in populations without diabetes have also demonstrated reduced insulin sensitivity in people with CKD in the absence of diabetes as compared to people without CKD or diabetes [96].

Insulin resistance and elevated insulin concentrations appear to have proliferative effects on renal glomerular and mesangial cells and impair endothelial nitric oxide release leading to endothelial dysfunction. Evidence is largely based on in vitro studies showing the induction of glomerular hypertrophy and vasodilation by increased insulin levels [97,98]. It is likely that insulin does not induce pathologic changes in the glomerulus by itself but rather participates in the orchestration of multiple factors that induce podocyte enlargement, mesangial expansion and subsequent glomerular sclerosis.

Adiponectin and the Podocyte

Multiple cross-sectional studies have demonstrated an association between abdominal obesity and increased urine albumin excretion [99–102]. This association may in part be mediated by lower levels of adiponectin due to obesity. Adiponectin receptors are present on podocytes, and adiponectin null mice demonstrate effacement of podocyte foot processes and albuminuria. Adiponectin repletion ameliorates podocyte effacement [103]. The important role that adiponectin plays in glomerular adaptation to obesity was demonstrated in an elegant study that performed 5/6 nephrectomies on adiponectin knock-out mice and wild-type mice. The adiponectin knock-out demonstrated stronger expression of vascular cell adhesion molecule-1, tumor necrosis factor-alpha and NADPH oxidase compared to the wild-type mice with normal adiponectin expression. Urine albumin excretion in the adiponectin knock-out mice was also higher. Treatment of the knockout mice with adiponectin reduced albuminuria, the inflammatory markers and NADPH oxidase to levels commensurate with the wild-type mice. Glomerular hypertrophy and tubulointerstitial fibrosis were also ameliorated with adiponectin treatment in the adiponectin knock-out mice [104].

Lipotoxicity

Hyperlipidemia and lipotoxicity have long been suspected to play a direct role in renal damage. Animal models, such as the obese Zucker rat model, have shown that hyperlipidemia is associated with early podocyte damage and glomerular macrophage infiltration [105,106]. Moreover, direct proximal tubular injury caused by lipotoxicity was demonstrated in a mouse model where free fatty acids bound to albumin caused severe tubulointerstitial injury [107]. Therapy with lipid-lowering agents decreases the development of proteinuria and glomerulosclerosis in the obese Zucker rat [106]. Statin therapy in human interventional studies has also been shown to reduce proteinuria in most studies [108]. Despite this possible benefit, there is little evidence that statin therapy delays the progression of kidney failure. The Study of Heart and Renal Protection (SHARP) study was designed to examine the effect of ezetimibe and simvastatin on individuals with CKD. A total of 6347 individuals with CKD not on dialysis and 3023 patients undergoing maintenance dialysis were enrolled [109]. While the lipid-lowering therapy was successful in reducing the primary outcome of major atherosclerotic events, there was no effect of statins on the secondary outcome of progression to CKD in the nondialysis CKD participants. About one-third of the nondialyzed participants in the treatment and placebo groups progressed to ESKD.

Other agents, such as omega-3 polyunsaturated fatty acids, that might improve lipid profiles have been not been studied extensively in kidney disease. Potential mechanisms by which omega-3 polyunsaturated fatty acids could influence kidney disease include lowering blood pressure and serum triglyceride levels and promoting anti-inflammatory and endothelial-protective effects [110]. A meta-analysis of 17 trials including 626 participants with CKD found that omega-3 fatty acid supplementation resulted in decreased urinary protein excretion [111]. However, no effect of omega-3 fatty acids on eGFR was found in this meta-analysis. Adequately powered randomized controlled trials are still needed to determine whether omega-3 polyunsaturated fatty acids could provide long-standing benefits.

EFFECT OF WEIGHT LOSS INTERVENTIONS ON KIDNEY DISEASE

Many independent groups showed over 20 years ago that calorie restriction retards renal injury in animal models of subtotal nephrectomy. These models included the spontaneously hypertensive rat that is subjected to uninephrectomy [112–115]. The effects of calorie restriction in these models were noted even in the setting of a liberal protein intake. Thus, the high calorie intake that is needed to obtain and then sustain the obese state may itself influence CKD progression. While lifestyle modification lowers BP, and decreases the risk of diabetes [116,117], few studies have examined lifestyle modification for the treatment of established kidney disease and modulation of kidney disease progression. Morales and coworkers studied the effects of weight loss in 30 overweight and obese patients (BMI >27 kg/m^2) with proteinuria and diabetic and nondiabetic kidney diseases [17]. Individuals were randomized to receive either a diet providing 500 kcal/day or a usual diet. Protein intake was 1.0 to 1.2 g/kg/d in both groups. After five months, mean weight loss in the diet group was 4.1% ± 3% of baseline weight, and proteinuria in this group decreased from a mean of 2.8 g/day to 1.9 gm/day. Both the mean BMI and proteinuria increased in the control group (p < 0.05). While modest weight reduction over the short duration of this study decreased urine protein excretion, GFR did not change significantly [17].

More drastic weight loss has been best examined in the studies of surgical interventions. One such study examined weight loss after gastroplasty in extremely obese individuals (BMI range 38.1–61.3 kg/m^2) who did not have overt renal disease [14]. Absolute GFR and effective RPF, determined by inulin and p-amminohippuric acid clearances, respectively, were 61% and 32% higher in the extremely obese than in the nonobese healthy control group. Approximately 12–17 months after gastric bypass, mean BMI had decreased from 48 to 32.1 kg/m^2 and absolute GFR decreased by 24% while RPF decreased by 13%. Despite the fact that these individuals remained obese, urinary albumin excretion decreased from 16 μg/min to 5 μg/min. Systolic blood pressure, fasting glucose and insulin levels also decreased substantially [14]. Decreases in urine protein excretion have been reported in other groups of morbidly obese patients without established kidney disease who undergo bariatric surgery for obesity management [16]. Since insulin sensitivity improves after gastric bypass surgery, long-term benefits in kidney function might be anticipated. Given the effects of calorie restriction on glomerulosclerosis in the remnant kidney model [113–115], the effects of weight loss on kidney disease progression may be a function of calorie intake. This is supported by the improvements in parameters of kidney disease with only mild weight loss in morbidly obese individuals [14].

CONCLUSION

BMI reflects both muscle and fat mass. Thus, measures for defining obesity in adults with kidney disease should incorporate both BMI and waist circumference to determine which patients might benefit from weight reduction. Obesity and the metabolic syndrome heighten the risk for developing CKD and for more rapid progression of CKD. This association may be mediated by lower adiponectin levels which promote insulin resistance and reduce the stability of podocytes. Weight loss should be encouraged in patients with CKD. Abdominal obesity and bariatric surgery should be considered for the severely obese individuals with CKD who fail lifestyle interventions.

References

[1] U.S. Department of Health and Human Services. The Surgeon General's vision for a healthy and fit nation, Office of the Surgeon General. Public Health Service. retrieved 8/18/ 2011 from, www.surgeongeneral.gov; 2010.

[2] International Obesity Taskforce. Obesity the Global Epidemic. retrieved 8/18/2011 from www.iaso.org/iotf/obesity/obesitytheglobalepidemic/.

[3] Flegal KM, Carroll MD, Ogden CL, Curtin LR. Prevalence and trends in obesity among US adults, 1999-2008. JAMA 2010;303(3):235−41, http://dx.doi.org/10.1001/jama.2009.2014.

[4] Friedman AN, Miskulin DC, Rosenberg IH, Levey AS. Demographics and trends in overweight and obesity in patients at time of kidney transplantation. Am J Kidney Dis 2003;41(2):480−7, http://dx.doi.org/10.1053/ajkd.2003.50059.

[5] Kramer HJ, Saranathan A, Luke A, et al. Increasing body mass index and obesity in the incident ESRD population. J Am Soc Nephrol 2006;17(5):1453−9, http://dx.doi.org/10.1681/ASN.2005111241.

[6] National Cholesterol Education Program (NCEP) Expert Panel on Detection. Evaluation, and Treatment of High Blood Cholesterol in Adults (Adult Treatment Panel III). Third report of the National Cholesterol Education Program (NCEP) Expert Panel on Detection, Evaluation, and Treatment of High Blood Cholesterol in Adults (Adult Treatment Panel III) final report. Circulation 2002;106(25):3143−421.

[7] Ford ES, Giles WH, Dietz WH. Prevalence of the metabolic syndrome among US adults: Findings from the Third National Health and Nutrition Examination Survey. JAMA 2002;287(3):356−9.

[8] Must A, Spadano J, Coakley EH, Field AE, Colditz G, Dietz WH. The disease burden associated with overweight and obesity. JAMA 1999;282(16):1523−9.

[9] U S Renal Data System, USRDS. 2010 Annual Data Report: Atlas of chronic kidney disease and end-stage renal disease in the United States. Bethesda, MD: National Institutes of Health, National Institute of Diabetes and Digestive and Kidney Diseases; 2010.

[10] Kasiske BL, Napier J. Glomerular sclerosis in patients with massive obesity. Am J Nephrol 1985;5(1):45−50.

[11] Weisinger JR, Kempson RL, Eldridge FL, Swenson RS. The nephrotic syndrome: A complication of massive obesity. Ann Intern Med 1974;81(4):440−7.

[12] Kambham N, Markowitz GS, Valeri AM, Lin J, D'Agati VD. Obesity-related glomerulopathy: An emerging epidemic. Kidney Int 2001;59(4):1498−509, http://dx.doi.org/10.1046/j.1523-1755.2001.0590041498.x.

[13] Serra A, Romero R, Lopez D, et al. Renal injury in the extremely obese patients with normal renal function. Kidney Int 2008;73(8):947−55, http://dx.doi.org/10.1038/sj.ki.5002796.

[14] Chagnac A, Weinstein T, Herman M, Hirsh J, Gafter U, Ori Y. The effects of weight loss on renal function in patients with severe obesity. J Am Soc Nephrol 2003;14(6):1480−6.

[15] Praga M. Synergy of low nephron number and obesity: A new focus on hyperfiltration nephropathy. Nephrol Dial Transplant 2005;20(12):2594−7, http://dx.doi.org/10.1093/ndt/gfi201.

[16] Navarro-Diaz M, Serra A, Romero R, et al. Effect of drastic weight loss after bariatric surgery on renal parameters in extremely obese patients: Long-term follow-up. J Am Soc Nephrol 2006;17(12 Suppl. 3):S213−7, http://dx.doi.org/10.1681/ASN.2006080917.

[17] Morales E, Valero MA, Leon M, Hernandez E, Praga M. Beneficial effects of weight loss in overweight patients with chronic proteinuric nephropathies. American Journal of Kidney Diseases 2003;41(2):319−27.

[18] Agrawal V, Khan I, Rai B, et al. The effect of weight loss after bariatric surgery on albuminuria. Clin Nephrol 2008;70(3):194−202.

[19] Solerte SB, Fioravanti M, Schifino N, Ferrari E. Effects of diet-therapy on urinary protein excretion albuminuria and renal haemodynamic function in obese diabetic patients with overt nephropathy. Int J Obes 1989;13(2):203−11.

[20] Nicholson AS, Sklar M, Barnard ND, Gore S, Sullivan R, Browning S. Toward improved management of NIDDM: A randomized, controlled, pilot intervention using a lowfat, vegetarian diet. Prev Med 1999;29(2):87−91.

[21] Saiki A, Nagayama D, Ohhira M, et al. Effect of weight loss using formula diet on renal function in obese patients with diabetic nephropathy. Int J Obes 2005;29(9):1115−20.

[22] Chagnac A, Weinstein T, Korzets A, Ramadan E, Hirsch J, Gafter U. Glomerular hemodynamics in severe obesity. Am J Physiol Renal Physiol 2000;278(5):F817−22.

[23] Praga M, Hernandez E, Andres A, Leon M, Ruilope LM, Rodicio JL. Effects of body-weight loss and captopril treatment on proteinuria associated with obesity. Nephron 1995;70(1):35−41.

[24] Kuczmarski RJ, Flegal KM. Criteria for definition of overweight in transition: Background and recommendations for the United States. Am J Clin Nutr 2000;72(5):1074−81.

[25] Obesity. Preventing and managing the global epidemic. Geneva: Report of a WHO consultation on obesity; June 3-5, 1997. 1998.

[26] Flegal KM, Graubard BI, Williamson DF, Gail MH. Cause-specific excess deaths associated with underweight, overweight, and obesity. JAMA 2007;298(17):2028−37, http://dx.doi.org/10.1001/jama.298.17.2028.

[27] Prospective studies collaboration. body-mass index and cause-specific mortality in 900,000 adults: Collaborative analyses of 57 prospective studies. Lancet 2009;373:1083−96.

[28] Stevens J, Plankey MW, Williamson DF, et al. The body mass index-mortality relationship in white and African American women. Obes Res. 1998;6(4):268−77.

[29] Kalantar-Zadeh K, Ikizler TA, Block G, Avram MM, Kopple JD. Malnutrition-inflammation complex syndrome in dialysis patients: Causes and consequences. Am J Kidney Dis 2003;42(5):864−81.

[30] Rankinen T, Kim SY, Perusse L, Despres JP, Bouchard C. The prediction of abdominal visceral fat level from body

composition and anthropometry: ROC analysis. Int J Obes Relat Metab Disord 1999;23(8):801—9.

[31] Pouliot MC, Despres JP, Lemieux S, et al. Waist circumference and abdominal sagittal diameter: Best simple anthropometric indexes of abdominal visceral adipose tissue accumulation and related cardiovascular risk in men and women. Am J Cardiol 1994;73(7):460—8.

[32] Lean ME, Han TS, Morrison CE. Waist circumference as a measure for indicating need for weight management. BMJ 1995;311(6998):158—61.

[33] Narisawa S, Nakamura K, Kato K, Yamada K, Sasaki J, Yamamoto M. Appropriate waist circumference cutoff values for persons with multiple cardiovascular risk factors in Japan: A large cross-sectional study. Journal of Epidemiology 2008;18: 37—42.

[34] Janssen I, Katzmarzyk PT, Ross R. Body mass index, waist circumference, and health risk: Evidence in support of current national institutes of health guidelines. Arch Intern Med 2002;162(18):2074—9.

[35] Balkau B, Deanfield JE, Despres JP, et al. International Day for the Evaluation of Abdominal Obesity (IDEA): A study of waist circumference, cardiovascular disease, and diabetes mellitus in 168,000 primary care patients in 63 countries. Circulation 2007;116(17):1942—51, http://dx.doi.org/10.1161/CIRCULATION AHA.106.676379.

[36] Koster A, Leitzmann MF, Schatzkin A, et al. Waist circumference and mortality. Am J Epidemiol 2008;167(12):1465—75, http://dx.doi.org/10.1093/aje/kwn079.

[37] Kramer H, Shoham D, McClure LA, et al. Association of waist circumference and body mass index with all-cause mortality in CKD: The REGARDS (Reasons for Geographic and Racial Differences in Stroke) study. Am J Kidney Dis 2011;58(2):177—85, http://dx.doi.org/10.1053/j.ajkd.2011.02.390.

[38] Elsayed EF, Sarnak MJ, Tighiouart H, et al. Waist-to-hip ratio, body mass index, and subsequent kidney disease and death. Am J Kidney Dis 2008;52(1):29—38, http://dx.doi.org/10.1053/j.ajkd.2008.02.363.

[39] Postorino M, Marino C, Tripepi G, Zoccali C. CREDIT (Calabria Registry of Dialysis and Transplantation) Working Group. Abdominal obesity and all-cause and cardiovascular mortality in end-stage renal disease. J Am Coll Cardiol 2009;53(15):1265—72, http://dx.doi.org/10.1016/j.jacc.2008.12.040.

[40] Johansen KL, Young B, Kaysen GA, Chertow GM. Association of body size with outcomes among patients beginning dialysis. Am J Clin Nutr 2004;80(2):324—32.

[41] Kwan BC, Murtaugh MA, Beddhu S. Associations of body size with metabolic syndrome and mortality in moderate chronic kidney disease. Clin J Am Soc Nephrol 2007;2(5):992—8, http://dx.doi.org/10.2215/CJN.04221206.

[42] Reaven GM. Banting lecture 1988. role of insulin resistance in human disease. Diabetes 1988;37(12):1595—607.

[43] Abuaisha B, Kumar S, Malik R, Boulton AJ. Relationship of elevated urinary albumin excretion to components of the metabolic syndrome in non-insulin-dependent diabetes mellitus. Diabetes Research & Clinical Practice 1998;39(2):93—9.

[44] Grundy SM, Brewer Jr HB, Cleeman JI, et al. Definition of metabolic syndrome: Report of the National Heart, Lung, and Blood Institute/American Heart Association Conference on Scientific Issues Related to Definition. Circulation 2004;109(3):433—8, http://dx.doi.org/10.1161/01.CIR.0000111245.75752.C6.

[45] Bagby SP. Obesity-initiated metabolic syndrome and the kidney: A recipe for chronic kidney disease? J Am Soc Nephrol 2004;15(11):2775—91, http://dx.doi.org/10.1097/01.ASN.00001 41965.28037.EE.

[46] Unger RH. Minireview: Weapons of lean body mass destruction: The role of ectopic lipids in the metabolic syndrome. Endocrinology 2003;144(12):5159—65, http://dx.doi.org/10.1210/en.2003-0870.

[47] Berg AH, Combs TP, Du X, Brownlee M, Scherer PE. The adipocyte-secreted protein Acrp30 enhances hepatic insulin action. Nat Med 2001;7(8):947—53.

[48] Kadowaki T, Yamauchi T, Kubota N, Hara K, Ueki K, Tobe K. Adiponectin and adiponectin receptors in insulin resistance, diabetes, and the metabolic syndrome. J Clin Invest 2006;116(7): 1784—92.

[49] Kubota N, Terauchi Y, Yamauchi T, et al. Disruption of adiponectin causes insulin resistance and neointimal formation. J Biol Chem. 2002;277(29):25863—6, http://dx.doi.org/10.1074/jbc.C200251200.

[50] Matsuzawa Y, Funahashi T, Kihara S, Shimomura I. Adiponectin and metabolic syndrome. Arterioscler Thromb Vasc Biol. 2004;24(1):29—33, http://dx.doi.org/10.1161/01.ATV.0000099786.99623.EF.

[51] Yamauchi T, Kamon J, Minokoshi Y, et al. Adiponectin stimulates glucose utilization and fatty-acid oxidation by activating AMP-activated protein kinase. Nat Med 2002;8(11): 1288—95.

[52] Yamauchi T, Kamon J, Minokoshi Y, et al. Adiponectin stimulates glucose utilization and fatty-acid oxidation by activating AMP-activated protein kinase. Nat Med 2002;8(11):1288—95.

[53] Holmes BF, Kurth-Kraczek EJ, Winder WW. Chronic activation of 5'-AMP-activated protein kinase increases GLUT-4, hexokinase, and glycogen in muscle. J Appl Physiol 1999;87(5): 1990—5.

[54] Kurth-Kraczek EJ, Hirshman MF, Goodyear LJ, Winder WW. 5' AMP-activated protein kinase activation causes GLUT4 translocation in skeletal muscle. Diabetes 1999;48(8):1667—71.

[55] Havel PJ. Update on adipocyte hormones: Regulation of energy balance and carbohydrate/lipid metabolism. Diabetes 2004;53(Suppl. 1):S143—51.

[56] Farooqi IS, Jebb SA, Langmack G, et al. Effects of recombinant leptin therapy in a child with congenital leptin deficiency. N Engl J Med 1999;341(12):879—84, http://dx.doi.org/10.1056/NEJM199909163411204.

[57] Sharma K, Considine RV. The ob protein (leptin) and the kidney. Kidney Int 1998;53(6):1483—7, http://dx.doi.org/10.1046/j.1523-1755.1998.00929.x.

[58] Kim SP, Ellmerer M, Van Citters GW, Bergman RN. Primacy of hepatic insulin resistance in the development of the metabolic syndrome induced by an isocaloric moderate-fat diet in the dog. Diabetes 2003;52(10):2453—60.

[59] Chen J, Muntner P, Hamm LL, et al. The metabolic syndrome and chronic kidney disease in U.S. adults. Ann Intern Med 2004;140(3):167—74.

[60] Muntner P, Coresh J, Smith JC, Eckfeldt J, Klag MJ. Plasma lipids and risk of developing renal dysfunction: The atherosclerosis risk in communities study. Kidney Int 2000;58(1):293—301, http://dx.doi.org/10.1046/j.1523-1755.2000.00165.x.

[61] Fox CS, Larson MG, Leip EP, Meigs JB, Wilson PW, Levy D. Glycemic status and development of kidney disease: The Framingham Heart Study. Diabetes Care 2005;28(10):2436—40.

[62] Kurella M, Lo JC, Chertow GM. Metabolic syndrome and the risk for chronic kidney disease among nondiabetic adults. J Am Soc Nephrol 2005;16(7):2134—40, http://dx.doi.org/10.1681/ASN.2005010106.

[63] Chen J, Muntner P, Hamm LL, et al. Insulin resistance and risk of chronic kidney disease in nondiabetic US adults. J Am Soc Nephrol 2003;14(2):469—77.

[64] Gelber RP, Kurth T, Kausz AT, et al. Association between body mass index and CKD in apparently healthy men. Am J Kidney Dis 2005;46(5):871—80, http://dx.doi.org/10.1053/j.ajkd.2005. 08.015.

[65] Kramer H, Luke A, Bidani A, Cao G, Cooper R, McGee D. Obesity and prevalent and incident CKD: The Hypertension Detection and Follow-up Program. Am J Kidney Dis 2005;46(4):587—94, http://dx.doi.org/10.1053/j.ajkd.2005.06. 007.

[66] Fox CS, Larson MG, Leip EP, Culleton B, Wilson PW, Levy D. Predictors of new-onset kidney disease in a community-based population. JAMA 2004;291(7):844—50, http://dx.doi.org/ 10.1001/jama.291.7.844.

[67] Hsu CY, McCulloch CE, Iribarren C, Darbinian J, Go AS. Body mass index and risk for end-stage renal disease. Ann Intern Med 2006;144(1):21—8.

[68] Bonnet F, Deprele C, Sassolas A, et al. Excessive body weight as a new independent risk factor for clinical and pathological progression in primary IgA nephritis. Am J Kidney Dis 2001;37(4):720—7.

[69] Lea J, Cheek D, Thornley-Brown D, et al. Metabolic syndrome, proteinuria, and the risk of progressive CKD in hypertensive African Americans. Am J Kidney Dis 2008;51(5):732—40, http:// dx.doi.org/10.1053/j.ajkd.2008.01.013.

[70] Griffin KA, Kramer H, Bidani AK. Adverse renal consequences of obesity. Am J Physiol Renal Physiol 2008;294(4):F685—96, http://dx.doi.org/10.1152/ajprenal.00324.2007.

[71] Hoy WE, Douglas-Denton RN, Hughson MD, Cass A, Johnson K, Bertram JF. A stereological study of glomerular number and volume: Preliminary findings in a multiracial study of kidneys at autopsy. Kidney Int Suppl 2003; 83(83):S31—7.

[72] Wuerzner G, Pruijm M, Maillard M, et al. Marked association between obesity and glomerular hyperfiltration: A cross-sectional study in an African population. Am.. J. Kidney Dis 2010.

[73] Hostetter TH, Rennke HG, Brenner BM. The case for intrarenal hypertension in the initiation and progression of diabetic and other glomerulopathies. Am J Med 1982;72(3):375—80.

[74] Luyckx VA, Brenner BM. Low birth weight, nephron number, and kidney disease. Kidney Int Suppl 2005;97(97):S68—77, http://dx.doi.org/10.1111/j.1523-1755.2005.09712.x.

[75] Delanaye P, Radermecker RP, Rorive M, Depas G, Krzesinski JM. Indexing glomerular filtration rate for body surface area in obese patients is misleading: Concept and example. Nephrol Dial Transplant 2005;20(10):2024—8, http:// dx.doi.org/10.1093/ndt/gfh983.

[76] Henegar JR, Bigler SA, Henegar LK, Tyagi SC, Hall JE. Functional and structural changes in the kidney in the early stages of obesity. J Am Soc Nephrol 2001;12(6):1211—7.

[77] Kriz W, Elger M, Mundel P, Lemley KV. Structure-stabilizing forces in the glomerular tuft. J Am Soc Nephrol 1995;5(10): 1731—9.

[78] Miller PL, Rennke HG, Meyer TW. Glomerular hypertrophy accelerates hypertensive glomerular injury in rats. Am J Physiol 1991;261(3 Pt 2):F459—65.

[79] Wiggins RC. The spectrum of podocytopathies: A unifying view of glomerular diseases. Kidney Int 2007;71(12):1205—14, http:// dx.doi.org/10.1038/sj.ki.5002222.

[80] Pavenstadt H, Kriz W, Kretzler M. Cell biology of the glomerular podocyte. Physiol Rev 2003;83(1):253—307, http://dx.doi. org/10.1152/physrev.00020.2002.

[81] Wiggins JE, Goyal M, Sanden SK, et al. Podocyte hypertrophy, "adaptation," and "decompensation" associated with glomerular enlargement and glomerulosclerosis in the aging rat: Prevention by calorie restriction. Journal of the American Society of Nephrology 2005;16(10):2953—66.

[82] Chen HM, Liu ZH, Zeng CH, Li SJ, Wang QW, Li LS. Podocyte lesions in patients with obesity-related glomerulopathy. Am J Kidney Dis 2006;48(5):772—9, http://dx.doi.org/10.1053/j.ajkd. 2006.07.025.

[83] Rennke HG, Klein PS. Pathogenesis and significance of non-primary focal and segmental glomerulosclerosis. American Journal of Kidney Diseases 1989;13(6):443—56.

[84] Brown CD, Higgins M, Donato KA, et al. Body mass index and the prevalence of hypertension and dyslipidemia. Obes Res. 2000;8(9):605—19.

[85] Hall JE, Kuo JJ, da Silva AA, de Paula RB, Liu J, Tallam L. Obesity-associated hypertension and kidney disease. Curr Opin Nephrol Hypertens 2003;12(2):195—200, http://dx.doi.org/ 10.1097/01.mnh.0000058795.51455.3f.

[86] Hall JE, Jones DW, Kuo JJ, da Silva A, Tallam LS, Liu J. Impact of the obesity epidemic on hypertension and renal disease. Curr Hypertens Rep 2003;5(5):386—92.

[87] Kassab S, Kato T, Wilkins FC, Chen R, Hall JE, Granger JP. Renal denervation attenuates the sodium retention and hypertension associated with obesity. Hypertension 1995;25(4 Pt 2):893—7.

[88] Shek EW, Brands MW, Hall JE. Chronic leptin infusion increases arterial pressure. Hypertension 1998;31(1 Pt 2):409—14.

[89] Mark AL, Shaffer RA, Correia ML, Morgan DA, Sigmund CD, Haynes WG. Contrasting blood pressure effects of obesity in leptin-deficient ob/ob mice and agouti yellow obese mice. J Hypertens 1999;17(12 Pt 2):1949—53.

[90] Cooper R, Forrester T, Ogunbiyi O, Muffinda J. Angiotensinogen levels and obesity in four black populations. ICSHIB investigators. J Hypertens 1998;16(5):571—5.

[91] Licata G, Scaglione R, Ganguzza A, et al. Central obesity and hypertension. relationship between fasting serum insulin, plasma renin activity, and diastolic blood pressure in young obese subjects. Am J Hypertens 1994;7(4 Pt 1):314—20.

[92] Schorr U, Blaschke K, Turan S, Distler A, Sharma AM. Relationship between angiotensinogen, leptin and blood pressure levels in young normotensive men. J Hypertens 1998;16(10):1475—80.

[93] Granger JP, West D, Scott J. Abnormal pressure natriuresis in the dog model of obesity-induced hypertension. Hypertension 1994;23(Suppl. 1):8—11.

[94] Tayo B, Luke A, McKenzie CA, et al. Patterns of sodium and potassium excretion and blood pressure in the African diaspora. J Human Hypertens http://dx.doi.org/10.1038/jhh.2011. 39; 2011.

[95] Emoto M, Nishizawa Y, Maekawa K, et al. Insulin resistance in non-obese, non-insulin-dependent diabetic patients with diabetic nephropathy. Metabolism 1997;46(9):1013—8.

[96] Kobayashi S, Maesato K, Moriya H, Ohtake T, Ikeda T. Insulin resistance in patients with chronic kidney disease. Am J Kidney Dis 2005;45(2):275—80.

[97] Abrass CK, Raugi GJ, Gabourel LS, Lovett DH. Insulin and insulin-like growth factor I binding to cultured rat glomerular mesangial cells. Endocrinology 1988;123(5):2432—9.

[98] Pete G, Hu Y, Walsh M, Sowers J, Dunbar JC. Insulin-like growth factor-I decreases mean blood pressure and selectively increases regional blood flow in normal rats. Proc Soc Exp Biol Med 1996;213(2):187—92.

[99] Kramer H, Reboussin D, Bertoni AG, et al. Obesity and albuminuria among adults with type 2 diabetes: The look AHEAD (action for health in diabetes) study. Diabetes Care 2009;32(5):851—3.

[100] Kawar B, Bello AK, El Nahas AM. High prevalence of microalbuminuria in the overweight and obese population: Data from

a UK population screening programme. Nephron 2009;112(3): 205–12.

[101] Chen B, Yang D, Chen Y, Xu W, Ye B, Ni Z. The prevalence of microalbuminuria and its relationships with the components of metabolic syndrome in the general population of China. Clinica Chimica Acta 2010;411(9-10):705–9.

[102] Thoenes M, Reil JC, Khan BV, et al. Abdominal obesity is associated with microalbuminuria and an elevated cardiovascular risk profile in patients with hypertension. Vasc Health & Risk Manage 2009;5(4):577–85.

[103] Sharma K, Ramachandrarao S, Qiu G, et al. Adiponectin regulates albuminuria and podocyte function in mice. J Clin Invest 2008;118(5):1645–56.

[104] Ohashi K, Iwatani H, Kihara S, et al. Exacerbation of albuminuria and renal fibrosis in subtotal renal ablation model of adiponectin-knockout mice. Arteriosclerosis, Thrombosis & Vasc Biol. 2007;27(9):1910–7.

[105] Coimbra TM, Janssen U, Grone HJ, et al. Early events leading to renal injury in obese zucker (fatty) rats with type II diabetes. Kidney Int 2000;57(1):167–82, http://dx.doi.org/10.1046/j.1523-1755.2000.00836.x.

[106] Kasiske BL, O'Donnell MP, Keane WF. The zucker rat model of obesity, insulin resistance, hyperlipidemia, and renal injury. Hypertension 1992;19(Suppl. 1):I110–5.

[107] Kamijo A, Kimura K, Sugaya T, et al. Urinary free fatty acids bound to albumin aggravate tubulointerstitial damage. Kidney Int 2002;62(5):1628–37, http://dx.doi.org/10.1046/j.1523-1755.2002.00618.x.

[108] Douglas K, O'Malley PG, Jackson JL. Meta-analysis: The effect of statins on albuminuria. Ann Intern Med 2006;145(2):117–24.

[109] Baigent C, Landray MJ, Reith C, et al. The effects of lowering LDL cholesterol with simvastatin plus ezetimibe in patients with chronic kidney disease (study of heart and renal protection): A randomised placebo-controlled trial. Lancet 2011;377(9784): 2181–92, http://dx.doi.org/10.1016/S0140-6736(11)60739-3.

[110] Fassett RG, Gobe GC, Peake JM, Coombes JS. Omega-3 polyunsaturated fatty acids in the treatment of kidney disease. Am J Kidney Dis 2010;56(4):728–42.

[111] Miller 3rd ER, Juraschek SP, Appel LJ, et al. The effect of n-3 long-chain polyunsaturated fatty acid supplementation on urine protein excretion and kidney function: Meta-analysis of clinical trials. Am J Clin Nutr 2009;89(6):1937–45, http://dx.doi.org/10.3945/ajcn.2008.26867.

[112] Reisin E, Azar S, DeBoisblanc BP, Guzman MA, Lohmann T. Low calorie unrestricted protein diet attenuates renal injury in hypertensive rats. Hypertension 1993;21(6 Pt 2):971–4.

[113] Tapp DC, Wortham WG, Addison JF, Hammonds DN, Barnes JL, Venkatachalam MA. Food restriction retards body growth and prevents end-stage renal pathology in remnant kidneys of rats regardless of protein intake. Lab Invest 1989;60(2):184–95.

[114] Kobayashi S, Venkatachalam MA. Differential effects of calorie restriction on glomeruli and tubules of the remnant kidney. Kidney Int 1992;42(3):710–7.

[115] Gumprecht LA, Long CR, Soper KA, Smith PF, Haschek-Hock WM, Keenan KP. The early effects of dietary restriction on the pathogenesis of chronic renal disease in Sprague-Dawley rats at 12 months. Toxicol Pathol 1993;21(6):528–37.

[116] Orchard TJ, Temprosa M, Goldberg R, et al. The effect of metformin and intensive lifestyle intervention on the metabolic syndrome: The Diabetes Prevention Program Randomized Trial. Ann Intern Med 2005;142(8):611–9.

[117] Elmer PJ, Obarzanek E, Vollmer WM, et al. Effects of comprehensive lifestyle modification on diet, weight, physical fitness, and blood pressure control: 18-month results of a randomized trial. Ann Intern Med 2006;144(7):485–95.

29

Nutritional and Metabolic Management of Obesity and the Metabolic Syndrome in the Patient with Chronic Kidney Disease

Mark E. Williams[1], Greta Magerowski[2], George L. Blackburn[2]

[1]Joslin Diabetes Center, Department of Medicine, Harvard Medical School, Boston, MA, USA
[2]Center for the Study of Nutrition Medicine, Department of Surgery, Beth Israel Deaconess Medical Center, Boston, MA, USA

INTRODUCTION

Obesity has reached epidemic proportions globally, affecting industrialized as well as developing nations. With more than 1 billion adults overweight [1] — at least 300 million of them obese — the condition is a major contributor to the worldwide burden of chronic disease and disability. In the last three decades, obesity rates have doubled. Today, approximately 10% of males and 14% of females in every country with available data [2] are obese.

In the United States, the lifetime risk of becoming overweight (BMI 25.0–29.9) is 50%, and that of becoming obese (BMI 30.0–39.9) is 25% [3]. In total, 65% of the population is above ideal body weight [4], and 32% are obese. By 2020, an estimated three out of four Americans will be overweight, and if trends continue, 50% of all men will be obese by 2030 [5]. According to the Centers for Disease Control and Prevention (CDC), obesity rates in all states exceed 20%, and in 12 states, are greater than 30%. Recent data from the National Health and Nutrition Examination Survey (NHANES) (2007–2008) indicate a prevalence of obesity of 34% among adults, with 6% of the population considered extremely obese (BMI >40) [6]. This increase is occurring in all age groups, races, and genders, although minorities are disproportionately affected. If trends continue, an estimated 165 million Americans will be obese by 2030 [5].

Energy balance is determined by calorie intake and physical activity. A failure to match calorie intake and energy output is the basic cause of obesity, but societal changes and a worldwide transition in nutritional intake are driving the epidemic. Modern lifestyles encourage overconsumption of calories while discouraging physical activity or energy expenditure [7]. In the U.S., mass-produced convenience foods — rich in sugar, salt, and fat — along with decreased energy requirements for daily living, account for the rise in American weight since 1970 [8].

Data show that in the general population, mortality risk increases exponentially with obesity [9] (Figure 29.1A), and that the association includes greater risk of death from all causes [10]. In developed and developing nations, being overweight is the sixth most important risk factor contributing to the overall burden of disease [11]. Overweight and obesity pose a major risk for serious diet-related chronic diseases, including chronic kidney disease (CKD) [12], diabetes, hypertension, hyperlipidemia, stroke, obstructive sleep apnea/hypoventilation, cancer, nonalcoholic fatty liver disease, nonalcoholic steatohepatitis, and congestive heart failure [13].

Medical complications associated with obesity make it a leading cause of death in the U.S. [14]. For every five-point rise in BMI, the risk of esophageal cancer in males increases by 52%, while that for colon cancer rises by 24%; for obese females, the risk of both endometrial and gall bladder cancer increases by 59%, and the risk for breast cancer in postmenopausal women is increased by 12%. Birth defects have also been linked to maternal obesity.

While average life expectancy in the U.S. is higher than ever, the number of years Americans can expect

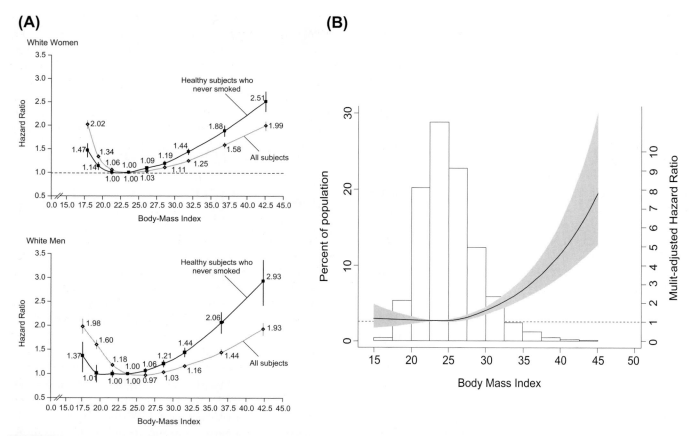

FIGURE 29.1 (A) Estimated hazard ratios for death from any cause according to body mass index in a pooled analysis of almost 1.5 million U.S. adults. Hazard ratios, shown with 95% confidence intervals for white women (A) and white men (B), increased with progressively higher and lower levels of body mass index. *(From Ref. [9].)* (B) Multi-adjusted hazard ratio for treated end-stage renal disease or chronic kidney disease by body mass index in 75,000 adults in Norway. Distributions of body mass index in the study population are shown. Hazard ratios for body mass index curve increased especially in the obese range. *(From Ref. [30].)*

to live free of type 2 diabetes is decreasing. Between the 1980s and the 2000s, obese individuals experienced the greatest decreases in diabetes-free life expectancy. Men lost an estimated 5.6 years; women, 2.5 years [15]. Trends indicate that by 2030, the healthcare burden will be increased by an estimated eight million more cases of diabetes, a leading cause of morbidity in later life.

Health care expenditures are significantly greater for the overweight or obese patient. In addition to the individual toll in morbidity and mortality, obesity imposes a growing burden on the healthcare system as a whole. It accounts for up to 10% of Medicare and 17% of Medicaid expenditures in individual states. National obesity-related costs are approximately $150 billion a year [16]. Obese individuals face widespread stigma and discrimination. They also tend to earn less income and marry less frequently than their nonobese counterparts. Despite these and other adverse consequences of obesity, there are those who claim that warnings about the obesity epidemic are exaggerated [17].

OBESITY-RELATED CHRONIC KIDNEY DISEASE (CKD)

An accumulating body of experimental and clinical evidence implicates obesity as an important cause of CKD. In addition to being closely linked to diabetes and hypertension, it is a top risk factor for CKD, and contributes to the increasing incidence and prevalence of the disease [18]. Despite adjustments for blood pressure and diabetes, Hsu et al. found that even moderate obesity nearly doubles the risk of advanced CKD [19]. A recent report estimated that up to one-third of kidney disease in the U.S. is related to obesity [20]. It has been over 10 years since epidemiologic data linking obesity and CKD, independent of diabetes, hypertension, and other proximate causes, began to appear [21–23]. Since then, the number of reports of CKD in obese patients without pre-existing renal disease have continued to increase [24]. Hsu et al. observed a nearly doubled risk for CKD in moderately obese individuals even after adjustment for blood pressure and diabetes.

Anthropometric data from a nationwide, population-based, case-control study on incident, moderately severe CKD in Sweden, showed a parallel rise in obesity and CKD with or without end-stage renal disease (ESRD) [25]. Eligible cases were all native Swedes aged 18–74 years whose initial and ongoing serum creatinine levels exceeded 3.4 mg/dL (males) or 2.8 mg/dL (females). Approximately 1000 patients and case control subjects were randomly enrolled from the database. Logistic regression models with adjustments for several cofactors were used to estimate the relative risk for CKD as it related to BMI. The relative risk for all major subtypes of CKD was two- to three-fold higher for overweight (BMI $\geq$ 25 kg/m^2) and obese (BMI $\geq$ 30 kg/m^2) individuals. Analyses confined to strata without hypertension or diabetes showed that risk in subjects who were overweight at age 20 was three-fold higher than that in their normal-weight peers. For those with a maximum lifetime BMI > 35 kg/m^2, the increase in risk was less significant, possibly because their obesity was usually of shorter duration.

Overweight and obesity have also been identified as strong risk factors for ESRD in the U.S. Hsu et al. matched USRDS registry data with that from a large, integrated health care delivery system in northern California in which patients volunteered for health screening [19]. In multivariable models that included adjustments for hypertension, diabetes, age, race, proteinuria, serum creatinine, and other factors, higher BMI was a risk factor for ESRD. Compared with normal-weight individuals, the relative risk of ESRD rose from 1.87 to 7.07 as weight increased from overweight to extreme obesity. A smaller study from Japan, with a follow-up period of 17 years, also found that BMI was associated with a modest risk of ESRD in men, but not women [26]. Obesity is associated with faster loss of renal function in IgA nephropathy [21] and during kidney transplant rejection [27]. Another small study on the rate of CKD progression and the risk of decline in kidney function, found that baseline BMI was strongly and independently associated with a steeper slope of decline in glomerular filtration rate (GFR) [28]. During seven years of follow-up in a moderately large community-based population of older adults ($\geq$65 years), DeBoer et al. found that obesity was associated with a decrease in GFR estimated by the Modification of Diet in Renal Disease (MDRD) study equation (MDRD Study equation) [29]. The association was stronger in those with impaired baseline GFR (<60 mL/min/1.73 m^2). However, adjustments for diabetes, hypertension, and C-reactive protein (a marker of inflammation) attenuated the relationship.

More recently, the relations among blood pressure, body weight, risk of CKD, and survival outcomes were evaluated in nearly 75,000 individuals followed for two decades in the Health Study in Nord-Trondelag (HUNT I), a population-based study in Norway [30] (Figure 29.1B). No lower threshold existed for treated ESRD or CKD-related death, but the risk for both conditions increased above a BMI of 25 kg/m^2. For individuals with a BMI >30 kg/m^2, the hazard ratio rose sharply. The role of obesity in CKD has been documented in studies involving dietary interventions and/or bariatric surgery, and renin-angiotensin (RAS) blockade [31,32].

OBESITY-RELATED GLOMERULOPATHY

Weisinger et al. initially reported the association between obesity and glomerulopathy in a small series of patients; the glomerulopathy was manifested as a specific form of glomerulomegaly, with or without secondary focal glomerulosclerosis and, in some cases, with heavy proteinuria [33]. That study focused on severe obesity. However, recent data indicate that obesity-related glomerulopathy (ORG) can occur even with less severe degrees of obesity. In a large, renal biopsy-based clinicopathologic study on ORG, Kambham et al. described a progressive increase in the incidence of ORG from 0.2% in 1986–1990 to 2.0% in 1996–2000; mean BMI ranged from 30.9 to 62.7 kg/m^2 The increase in ORG coincided with a sharp increase in the prevalence of obesity, as described in epidemiologic data for the general population [34].

Early histopathological changes in kidneys of severely obese patients with no clinical evidence of nephropathy were recently reported in patients undergoing bariatric surgery. These changes included glomerulomegaly and histological lesions resembling those of early diabetic nephropathy [35]. Although there is overlap in the clinical and pathological features of focal glomerulosclerosis, ORG has a lower incidence of nephrotic proteinuria and nephritic syndrome, more selective proteinuria, slower progression to kidney failure, a greater prevalence of glomerulomegaly, a lower percentage of glomeruli affected by segmental sclerosis, and milder foot process fusion [34] as compared to focal glomerulosclerosis. Reduced podocyte density and numbers, mesangial expansion, and abnormalities of the renal interstitium have also been reported [37].

Renal functional abnormalities include renal hyperperfusion and increased filtration fraction. Similar to the range of histologic abnormalities in ORG, a stepwise increase in glomerular filtration occurs in parallel with BMI; this has been attributed to glomerulomegaly and extracellular volume expansion. Wuerzner et al. found that glomerular hyperfiltration (>140 mL/min) associated with higher effective renal plasma flow — a condition similar to an early phase of diabetic nephropathy — was three times more likely to be present in obese subjects than in lean ones [38]. The effects of obesity on renal function in animal models also suggest such alterations as increased glomerular filtration and renal blood flow [39]. Whether glomerular hyperfiltration predicts "overt" ORG in obesity has not been studied. However, obesity may pose a hemodynamic risk to kidneys via glomerular hypertension akin to that reported in other forms of CKD. Several elements of the renin-angiotensin system are activated in obesity [32].

The precise mechanisms of structure and function changes that link obesity and CKD are incompletely understood. Traditional and nontraditional mechanisms are considered to be significant causal factors in CKD secondary to obesity [40] (Figure 29.2). Commonly cited mediators include features of the metabolic syndrome; insulin resistance; oxidative stress; increased chronic inflammatory markers and cytokines; excessive aldosterone concentration and/or

mineralocorticoid receptor stimulation by cortisol (due to reduced 11-B-hydroxy-steroid dehydrogenase 2 activity) [41]; aldosterone-independent, salt-dependent stimulation of the mineralocorticoid receptor through Rac1GTPase [42]; diminished nephron number relative to actual body mass; and, impaired renal hemodynamics that may be related to activation of the renin-angiotensin system. Risk factors in the metabolic syndrome may share common mechanisms that lead to CKD. In an analysis of over 100,000 adults in the Taiwan Longitudinal Health Check-Up-Based Population Database, Sun et al. found that the risk of incident CKD increased progressively with the number of metabolic syndrome components [43]. Chen et al. examined the relation between HOMA-insulin resistance and CKD risk in nondiabetic U.S. adults who participated in the Third National Health and Nutrition Examination Survey (NHANES III) [44]. After adjustment for confounding variables, the prevalence of CKD became progressively higher as levels of HOMA-IR and serum insulin values increased. Tissue insensitivity to insulin

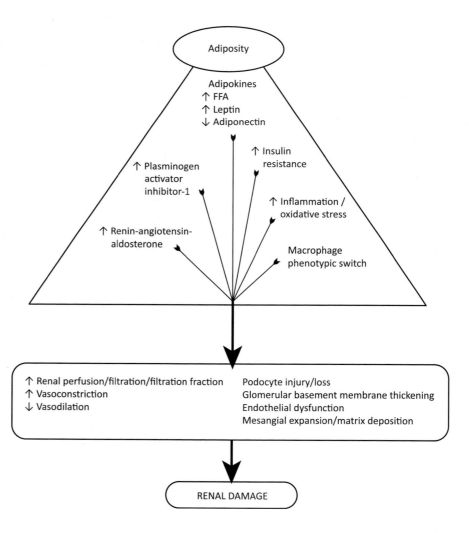

FIGURE 29.2 Mechanisms of obesity-related kidney disease. Construct emphasizes adipose tissue as source of multiple mediators which impact on kidney structure and function. *(From Ref. [40].)*

was the primary cause of insulin resistance in patients with CKD.

MEASURING GFR

Although obesity is characterized by hyperfiltration, its significance in predicting CKD in the obese population has not been studied. The mechanism by which obesity becomes a determinant of kidney function is not well-understood. Gerchman et al. found that excessive weight gain in adults may raise renal plasma flow and hyperfiltration without an increase in nephron number [45]. However, interpretation of eGFR data in obese individuals is controversial. Disputes revolve around which formula best approximates the GFR in the obese patient. Available measures for GFR estimation may include size variables, allow for standardization of results to a "normal" body size, do both, or do neither. No consensus exists as to whether or how parameters of kidney function should be normalized to body surface area (BSA).

The adjustment may be a vestige of the 19th century, when physiologic variables (e.g., metabolic rate or GFR) were indexed to BSA to adjust for differences in body size [46]. Measurements of creatinine clearances from people of different sizes (insofar as results were not adjusted for weight, BSA or BMI) were often indexed to a BSA of 1.73 m^2. This convention "downsized" GFR measurements from obese individuals.

The derived Cockroft and Gault equation [47] included body weight as a key variable, raising concerns that the equation grossly overestimated GFR in obese individuals [48]. Wuerzner et al. measured insulin clearance in 301 Seychelle Islands residents of African descent who had a family history of hypertension [49]. The prevalence of hyperfiltration, defined as measured insulin clearance >140 mL/min, increased progressively with BMI categories of normal, overweight, and obese. GFR was elevated to a greater extent than renal plasma flow, suggesting an increase in filtration fraction with increasing body fat mass. The association of obesity with hyperfiltration was eliminated when GFRs were indexed to BSA. The adjustment of inulin-based GFR for BSA led to underestimation of GFR [50].

In comparison, MDRD and CKD-EPI estimating equations are intrinsically BSA-adjusted [46] in overweight populations (mean BSA is approximately 1.9 m^2). This eliminates the need for further indexing of GFR to BSA. For equations which estimate the GFR and which do not include size as a variable, indexing of GFR to 1.73 m^2 BSA leads to a systematic underestimation of GFR in obese patients, since their BSA exceeds this value [45,51].

Nair et al. found that the four-variable MDRD equation underestimated GFR in obese individuals with CKD and type 2 diabetes [52]. As a result, validation of eGFR equations in obese individuals has yet to be achieved [53]. However, recent evidence suggests that the CKD-EPI equation provides the best overall accuracy of GFR estimation in obese individuals [54]. In a recent a cross-sectional study of Japanese-American men and women without diabetes, Gerchman et al. used creatinine clearance to evaluate whether the association between obesity and GFR was related to body fat distribution [45]. The results suggest that BMI rather than body fat distribution determines GFR.

METABOLIC SYNDROME

As obesity has increased around the globe, the worldwide prevalence of metabolic syndrome (or insulin resistance) has also risen sharply. Almost a quarter of U.S. residents tested as part of NHANES III had the metabolic syndrome [55]. Cross-sectional surveys report that one-third of U.S. adults [56] and up to 60% of overweight and obese youth [57] have the metabolic syndrome.

The association between obesity and the metabolic disorders that constitute this multifactorial syndrome has been known for many years [58]. Over the past decade, different definitions of the metabolic syndrome have been used. Essential components include insulin resistance, hyperglycemia (glucose intolerance, impaired glucose tolerance, or overt diabetes), hypertension, dyslipidemia (elevated triglycerides or reduced HDL) and abdominal obesity (waist circumference ≥102 cm in males or 88 cm in females [59] or elevated BMI (>30 kg/m^2). Although definitions vary, the diagnosis of metabolic syndrome commonly requires the presence of at least three of these factors. Insulin resistance and abdominal obesity are the more common features [60]. The links between elevated insulin concentrations and the phenotypic traits of the metabolic syndrome continue to be explored. For example, hyperuricemia and elevated proinflammatory/prothrombotic factors are not uncommonly found in people with the metabolic syndrome.

Metabolic syndrome consists of key risk factors for the development of cardiovascular disease and type 2 diabetes and is widely used to identify patients at increased risk for cardiovascular disease, i.e., the primary clinical outcome of metabolic syndrome. Individuals who have metabolic syndrome but no diabetes have a greater risk of cardiovascular disease than those with diabetes but no metabolic syndrome [61]. Next to glucose tolerance alone, the syndrome is strongly associated with type 2 diabetes, and is used to identify individuals at risk for the disease [62].

Like obesity, metabolic syndrome is an accurate predictor of CKD. A number of U.S. studies indicate that it is an independent risk factor for CKD [63]. In NHANES III, CKD was present in 1.2% of subjects without the metabolic syndrome and 6.0% of those with it [64]. The multivariate-adjusted odds ratios of CKD and microalbuminuria in those with metabolic syndrome compared to those without it were 2.60 and 1.89, respectively (Figure 29.3). Even mildly elevated blood pressure or increased serum glucose are associated with an increased risk for CKD and microalbuminuria. According to the WHO classification, microalbuminuria is also a clinical feature of the metabolic syndrome [59].

Hoechner et al. reported that nondiabetic Native Americans with three or more symptoms of the metabolic syndrome had more than a twofold risk of microalbuminuria [58]. In a recent meta-analysis of 11 studies involving 30,146 individuals, the odds ratio for the development of CKD was 1.55 in those who had the metabolic syndrome [60]. Independent of elevated blood pressure and fasting blood glucose, the estimated risk for CKD increased in line with the number of metabolic syndrome components present. On the other hand, population-based studies show inconsistent evidence of an association between insulin levels and microalbuminuria in nondiabetic or prediabetic individuals [65].

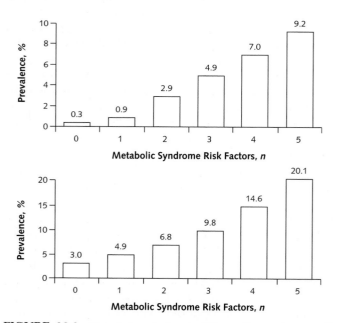

FIGURE 29.3 Prevalence of chronic kidney disease (top panel) and microalbuminuria (bottom panel) according to number of components of the metabolic syndrome present. Participants 20 years of age or older were studied in the chronic kidney disease (n = 6217) and microalbuminuria (n = 6125) analyses of the cross-sectional Third National Health and Nutrition Examination Survey. *(From Ref. [64].)*

TREATMENT OF OBESITY AND OBESITY-RELATED KIDNEY DISEASE

RAS Blockade

The effects of renoprotective therapies in overweight and obese individuals, including those with metabolic syndrome, have yet to be fully elucidated. Evidence from in vitro and clinical studies over the past decade indicates that an overactive renin-angiotensin system (RAS) is associated with both obesity and the metabolic syndrome [66]. The RAS is of particular relevance in obesity-related kidney disease [32]. High plasma renin, angiotensinogen, angiotensin-converting enzyme, and aldosterone levels are frequently present in obese individuals. Components of the RAS are expressed in adipose tissue. In vitro, angiotensin II induces adipogenesis (differentiation into adipocytes) and lipogenesis (triglyceride storage in adipocytes) [40]. Mice lacking renin have only half the adipose tissue weight of wild-type mice. Animal models with targeted inactivation of RAS genes show improved insulin sensitivity and protection from insulin resistance induced by a high fat diet [67]. Clinical trials indicate that angiotensin converting enzyme (ACE) inhibitors and receptor blockers improve insulin sensitivity [67].

Molecular sieving experiments in obese subjects show that obesity significantly alters renal hemodynamics, causing an increase in filtration fraction [40], a known effect of angiotensin. The Ramipril Efficacy in Nephropathy (REIN) Study was a double-blind, randomized, placebo-controlled trial that tested the nephroprotective properties of the ACE inhibitor, ramipril. In one of the few clinical studies to address the role of RAS blockade in obese patients, Mallamaci et al. performed a secondary post hoc analysis of REIN data [32]. Approximately 30% of participants were overweight, and an additional 14% were obese. Renal endpoints of either ESRD or doubling of the serum creatinine were higher in obese patients than in others. Ramipril reduced the rate of renal events regardless of BMI, but the benefit was greatest in the obese cohort (the reduction in the incidence rate for ESRD was 86%; for the two combined endpoints, it was 79%). Proteinuria was also reduced (Figure 29.4). Prospective studies specific to obese patients are needed.

Weight Loss

An extensive body of evidence from clinical efficacy trials indicates that weight loss can be achieved through lifestyle modification, particularly with intensive in-person interventions in highly selected participants [68]. Intensive weight loss from a diet low in calories, fat, and sodium may improve glycemia, hypertension

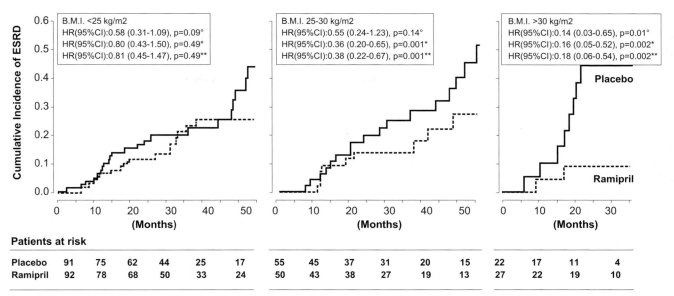

° Crude.
* Calculated in a model including treatment (Ramipril versus placebo), BMI classes, BMI*treatment interaction term, gender, baseline systolic blood pressure, albumin, hemoglobin, urinary protein and GFR.
** Shrinkage corrected.

FIGURE 29.4 Interaction between body mass index and efficacy of the ACE inhibition with ramipril in chronic kidney disease patients. Effect modification of body mass index on the efficacy of ramipril on the incidence rate of ESRD is shown is a post-hoc analysis from the Ramipril Efficacy in Nephropathy (REIN) trial. *(From Ref. [32].)*

and cardiovascular risk [69]. For example, general lifestyle modification incorporating diets reduced in calories along with increased physical activity is not only central to diabetes management; effective programs are now known to be successful in the primary prevention of type 2 diabetes mellitus in high-risk individuals. The largest and most rigorous randomized trial, the Diabetes Prevention Program (DPP) [70], assigned 3234 overweight middle-aged adults with prediabetes to one of three interventions: placebo, metformin 850 mg twice per day, or intensive lifestyle intervention aimed at 7% weight loss combined with moderate-intensity exercise. The diet and exercise combination led to 58% risk reduction in the incidence of diabetes compared to placebo. Weight loss was the most important factor, with a 16% risk reduction for diabetes per kilogram weight loss [71]. The diabetes incidence was reduced by 31% with metformin. In the subsequent Diabetes Prevention Program Outcomes Study (DPPOS) [72], 88% of DPP participants were followed for an additional 5.7 years. All three DPP groups were offered a less rigorous lifestyle modification regimen than in the DPP study. The incidence of diabetes in the original DPP placebo and metformin groups now fell into the same range as the original lifestyle group, indicating that primary prevention of diabetes could persist for at least 10 years, and indicated that both lifestyle and metformin interventions, with similar mean weight loss of 2–2.5 kg over the full study period, could be effective. Whether primary

prevention of diabetes reduces cardiovascular endpoints or mortality remains unresolved. Other studies have established the benefit of higher quantities of physical activity on obesity [73]. For obese patients with elevated blood pressure, the addition of exercise and weight loss to the DASH diet produces additional blood pressure lowering over the diet alone [74]. Weight loss may also have renal benefits, including reductions in blood pressure and proteinuria, that may prevent or retard further decline in kidney function. However, weight loss surgery appears to be the most effective and durable treatment [vide infra and please see Chapter 28] for ameliorating obesity-related comorbidities.

A recent meta-analysis identified six studies (four observational; two randomized, prospective) on the impact of nonsurgical weight loss (diet, exercise, and/ or anti-obesity agents) in patients with preexisting CKD [75], and included 174 patients followed for over four weeks to 12 months. Mean follow-up was 7.4 months. Causes of CKD, based on clinical diagnosis, included obesity-related glomerulopathy, diabetic nephropathy, hypertension, glomerulonephritis, and undefined proteinuria. Dietary interventions generally involved hypocaloric diets with no protein restriction. Parameters of renal outcome included 24-hour urine protein excretion and estimated creatinine clearance using the Cockroft–Gault formula, adjusted in some cases for body surface area. Nonsurgical weight loss led to a mean difference in BMI of 3.67 kg/m² compared to baseline, and was associated with decreases in systolic blood pressure of approximately 9 mmHg, and in proteinuria of 1.31 g/24 hours (Figure 29.5). Renal function remained stable during follow-up. The analysis did not adjust for the use of renoprotective medications. The authors concluded that improvements in proteinuria, although not associated with change in GFR during this short term follow-up, were achieved in CKD patients with nonsurgical interventions.

Other studies indicated that modest weight loss by calorie restriction in the absence of changes in dietary protein can also significantly reduce proteinuria [76]. This may occur within weeks of initiating the diet, when only a small fraction of weight loss has occurred [77]; the mechanism might involve lower adiponectin and higher fetuin-A levels. The independent role of changes in dietary protein is relevant because continuous intake of a high-protein diet could exacerbate glomerular hyperfiltration. Friedman et al. [78] analyzed the effects of short-term high protein (170 g/day) and low protein (50 g/day) diets in 17 obese individuals. Independent of sodium or calorie intake, the high protein diet was associated with a modest increase in GFR and urinary protein excretion. The pathophysiologic mechanisms responsible for these changes continue to be evaluated.

Shen et al. used a diet and exercise intervention in a physician-supervised weight loss program to evaluate the relationship between body weight reduction and proteinuria in 63 patients with obesity-related, biopsy-proven glomerulopathy [79]. Weight loss through lifestyle modification was associated with a 35% decrease in urinary protein excretion after six months and

a 51% reduction after 24 months. No correlation was seen between changes in body weight and alterations in GFR. However, it should be noted that in this study, almost a quarter of patients had poor adherence and were lost to follow-up. Of the remainder, less than half showed continued weight reduction at 24 months. Weight loss surgery may be an option for obese and severely obese individuals with obesity-related comobidities or CKD who fail to lose weight through lifestyle modification.

BARIATRIC SURGERY (SEE ALSO CHAPTER 28)

Indications

Indications for weight loss surgery are changing as rapidly as are the technologies and techniques used to perform the procedures. Once limited by the National Institutes of Health to individuals with a BMI >40 kg/m² or >35 kg/m² with obesity-related comorbidities [80], bariatric surgery has expanded into the metabolic realm and is now being used to treat or resolve diabetes in those with a BMI <35 kg/m² [81], and to reduce GFR, albuminuria, and blood pressure in patients with chronic kidney disease [75].

Among just the people who are severely obese, the American Heart Association recently projected that over 30 million adults may qualify for weight loss surgery in the near future [82]. For these individuals, this option provides durable and, in some cases, probably lifesaving long-term weight loss.

Study or Subgroup	After weight loss			Before weight loss			Weight	Mean Difference IV, Random, 95% CI	Mean Difference IV, Random, 95% CI
	Mean	SD	Total	Mean	SD	Total			
1.13.1 Observational studies									
Saiki 2005	1.5	1.28	22	3.27	2.63	22	19.6%	-1.77 (-2.99, -0.55)	
Solerte 1989	0.62	0.3	24	1.28	0.51	24	34.9%	5.50 (-0.90, -0.42)	
Subtotal (95% CI)			46			46	54.5%	-1.05 (-2.08, -0.01)	
Heterogeneity: Tau²=0.41; Chi²=3.05, df=1 (P=0.03); I² = 67%									
Test for overall effect: Z=1.98 (P=0.05)									
1.13.2 Randomized studies									
Morales 2003	1.9	1.4	20	2.8	1.4	20	25.3%	-0.90 (-1.73, -0.03)	
Praga 1995	0.4	0.6	9	2.9	1.7	9	20.2%	-2.50 (-3.68, -1.32)	
Subtotal (95% CI)			29			29	45.5%	-1.65 (-3.21, -0.08)	
Heterogeneity: Tau²=0.00; Chi²=0.04, df=1 (P=0.85); I² = 0%									
Test for overall effect: Z=0.33 (P=0.74)									
Total (95% CI)			75			75	100.0%	-1.31 (-2.11, -0.51)	
Heterogeneity: Tau²=0.46; Chi²=11.77, df=3 (P=0.008); I² = 75%									
Test for overall effect: Z=1.10 (P=0.27)									
Test for Subgroup differences: Chi²=4.12, df=1 (P=0.04); I² = 75.7%									

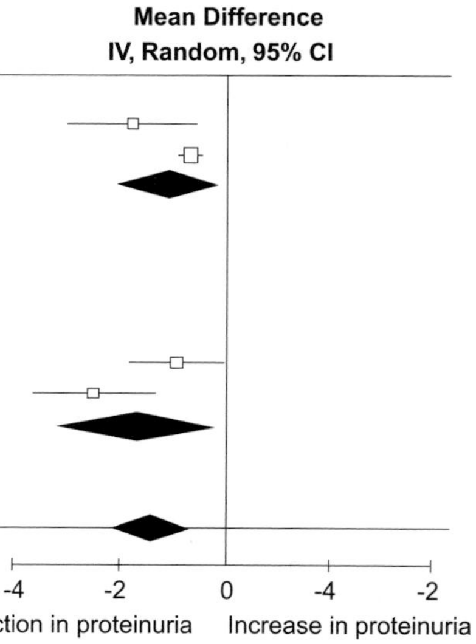

-4 -2 0 -4 -2
Reduction in proteinuria   Increase in proteinuria

FIGURE 29.5 Effect of nonsurgical interventions (diet, exercise, and/or antiobesity agents) on urinary protein excretion in adult patients with nondialysis-dependent chronic kidney disease. From a meta-analysis that included 75 patients from four studies, and a mean follow-up of 7.4 months. *(From Ref. [75].)*

Obesity is a chronic disease that is subject to relapse. The dearth of medical treatments and effective lifestyle interventions make weight loss surgery the only safe, well-established, and effective treatment for severe obesity and its related comorbidities. It results in metabolic changes that alter gut hormones in ways that enable patients to lose more weight than is possible through other means [83].

Numerous types of laparoscopic surgical procedures are available and are discussed in more detail in Chapter 28. The right one for any given patient depends on a variety of factors and individual risks and benefits. Some approaches, such as gastric bypass, result in greater weight loss than gastric banding, but are surgically complex and require more extensive lifestyle changes [84].

Mechanisms of Action

Weight loss surgery works in one of two ways — gastric restriction (Figure 29.6) or malabsorption (Figure 29.7). The former involves the creation of a small neogastric pouch and gastric outlet; the latter rearranges the small intestine to reduce nutrient absorption. Patients lose greater amounts of weight with malabsorptive procedures [84], but are at increased risk for complications that include nutrient and/or protein deficiencies, oxalate kidney stones, and metabolic bone disease. Patients with adjustable gastric bands are at risk for band slippage and eventual erosion.

Dramatic improvement of diabetes before significant weight loss suggests that gastric bypass alters the entero-hypothalamic-endocrine axis [85—87]. One meta-analysis found that surgery resolved diabetes mellitus in 78.1% of severely obese patients, and reduced or resolved it in 86.6% of them [81].

A number of obesity-related comorbidities improve with weight loss. This may be due to changes to the hormonal milieu of the gut. Gastrointestinal tract peptides that play a role in appetite regulation include ghrelin, neuropeptide Y, peptide YY, glucagon-like peptide 1, pancreatic polypeptide, and oxyntomodulin. However, many of their underlying mechanisms still remain unclear.

Complications

Complications are typically divided into three categories depending on time relative to surgery: intraoperative, early, or late (Table 29.1; see Chapter 28). Intraoperative complications include splenic injury, bowel ischemia, and trocar injury. These can result from technical difficulties during operations; for example, when thick subcutaneous tissue impedes visualization and fine movements in the abdominal cavity.

Early phase complications vary by type of surgery (see Chapter 28). Overall, the mortality rates of the most common weight loss surgeries (Roux-en-Y gastric bypass (RYGB) and gastric banding) are between 0% and 2.5% [88]. Late phase complications develop slowly from the altered state of the digestive tract. Decreased gallbladder emptying, disruption of hepatic branches of the vagus nerve, or changes in mucin production, calcium concentration, or the bile salt/cholesterol ratio can result in gallstones. Although common in weight loss surgery patients, these can generally be prevented with ursodiol, also known as **ursodeoxycholic acid**,

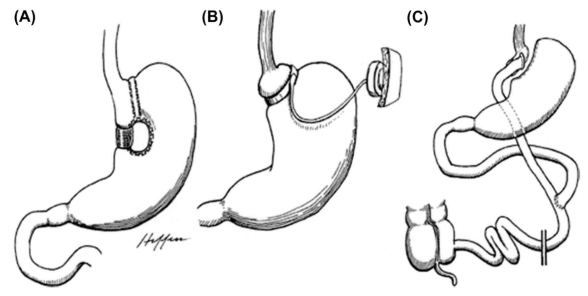

(A)   **(B)**   **(C)**

FIGURE 29.6   Weight loss surgery by gastric restriction.

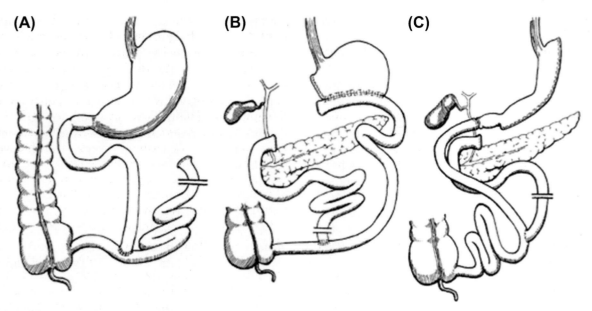

FIGURE 29.7 Weight loss surgery by malabsorption.

TABLE 29.1 Potential Benefits of Weight Loss Surgery

Benefits of Weight Loss Surgery
Increased life expectancy (Christou et al., 2004)
Decreased risk of cardiovascular event (Blackburn and Mun, 2005)
Resolution of diabetes (Blackburn, 2005; Buchwald et al., 2009; Clements et al., 2004; Schauer et al., 2003)
Resolution of hypertension (Buchwald et al., 2004)
Resolution of dyslipidemia (Buchwald et al., 2004)
Resolution of sleep apnea (Buchwald et al., 2004)
Resolution of GERD (Tolonen et al., 2006)
Resolution of polycystic ovarian syndrome (Escobar-Morreale et al., 2005)
Resolution of urinary stress incontinence (Burgio et al., 2007)
Improvement of osteoarthritis (Abu-Abeid et al., 2005)
Improvement of venous stasis disease
Improvement of nonalcoholic fatty liver disease (Klein et al., 2006)
Increased fertility (Gerrits et al., 2003)
Decreased complications from pregnancy and childbirth (Cnattingius et al., 1998; Deitel et al., 1988)
Improved quality of life (Buchwald, 2005)
Improved outcomes from non-bariatric operations
Decreased cancer risk (Blackburn and Mun, 2005)

Adapted from ref. [129].

which reduces cholesterol absorption and is used to prevent the formation of gallstones.

Many severely obese individuals have nutritional deficiencies that can be exacerbated after malabsorptive procedures [89]. These may also develop in restrictive surgery patients from poor eating habits or food intolerance. For these reasons, postoperative dietary monitoring is necessary for all patients.

Neurologic complications occur in 5% to 16% of weight loss surgery patients [90]. Many symptoms are related to malnutrition, and can include encephalopathy, optic neuropathy, posterolateral myelopathy, acute polyradiculopathy, and polyneuropathy. In addition, patients may suffer from psychological illnesses before and after surgery. Although weight loss tends to have a positive effect on these disorders, multidisciplinary care should include mental health assessments. Inadequate postoperative weight loss or weight regain can reduce quality of life and affect mental health.

Matlaga et al. identified urolithiasis in 7.65% of RYGB patients compared to 4.63% in controls [91]. In adults without stones, hyperoxaluria can occur at an increased rate after both RYGB and biliopancreatic diversion with duodenal switch [92,93]. As a complication of RYGB, oxalate nephropathy can lead to chronic kidney disease or end-stage renal failure [94]. Purely restrictive procedures do not increase urinary oxalate excretion compared to controls [95].

One retrospective study found a correlation between the stage of chronic kidney disease and incidence of complications in 27,736 patients who underwent weight loss surgery [96]. Ultimately, improvement of hypertension, blood pressure, weight, creatinine, and proteinuria may outweigh operative risks for patients with chronic kidney disease, especially those who require renal transplant [97,98].

Dumping syndrome is another side effect that occurs in up to 50% of RYGB patients. Dumping shortly after meals is considered early; that which takes place hours afterwards, is considered late. This complication occurs when hyperosmotic foods enter the jejunum, causing distention and intestinal contractility. Dumping syndrome is treated with dietary changes that include more complex carbohydrates, fiber, and protein-rich foods.

Metabolic Effects

Weight loss surgery can cause malnutrition by affecting total vitamin intake as well as the body's ability to absorb specific nutrients and vitamins. Common nutritional deficiencies include B_{12}, folate, iron, thiamin, protein, calcium, zinc, and vitamins A, D, E and K. These will be discussed in more detail later. Malabsorptive procedures that impede the body's ability to absorb key nutrients can lead to serious complications, such as osteopenia. Patients may require larger intakes of vitamin D and fat soluble vitamins to offset impaired absorption in their digestive tracts and prevent hypovitaminosis.

B_{12} deficiency affects 25% to 75% of gastric bypass patients due to lack of stomach acid and limited intrinsic factor [99–101]. Hence, patients with malabsorptive procedures cannot maintain adequate levels of B_{12} with oral supplementation alone, and must have parenteral supplementation to prevent deficiency [100].

Stores of water-soluble vitamins are limited. Therefore, patients with postoperative vomiting are especially susceptible to folate, thiamin, and B_1 deficiencies, and require supplementation to replace lost nutrients [99,102]. Maintaining adequate levels of B_{12} and folate prevents increasing homocysteine levels in patients with, or at risk for, metabolic syndrome [103].

Multidisciplinary Postoperative Management

Weight loss surgery requires lifelong follow-up to minimize complications and maximize outcomes. A multidisciplinary team is needed to address and avoid problems that may arise. In that potential complications of weight loss surgery vary greatly, interdisciplinary communication provides an optimal way to assess patient needs. For effective support, the team should include consulting specialists (e.g., in mental health, nutrition, exercise) as well as the primary care clinician.

Long-Term Benefits

Weight-loss surgery has many unique benefits (Table 29.1). Unlike other interventions, it can reset energy equilibrium, affect gut hormones and peptides, and help offset obesogenic environmental influences by inducing changes in the weight regulation centers of the brain. The most obvious benefit is weight loss; this alone reduces a number of weight-related comorbidities, including hypertension [104], dyslipidemia [104], sleep apnea [104], GERD [105], weight-related osteoarthritis [106], nonalcoholic fatty liver disease [107], urinary stress incontinence [108], polycystic ovary syndrome [109], and infertility [110]. Postsurgical weight loss can also normalize blood pressure. Data show lower diastolic blood pressure and greater weight loss among bariatric surgery patients than among those who lose weight through other means [88].

As mentioned earlier, metabolic changes after weight loss surgery resolve type 2 diabetes before significant weight loss [81,85–87]. Because glucostatic mechanisms are affected, surgical treatment can be effective for patients with BMI $\leq$ 35. Compared to diet and normalized-to-equivalent weight loss, it increases insulin sensitivity as well as secretion. Two randomized controlled trials comparing surgical and medical treatment of diabetes found that bariatric surgery produced lower glycated hemoglobin levels at 12 months [111] and produced a higher rate of diabetes remission, 75% for RYGB compared to no remission in the medical therapy group [112]. While these studies provide strong evidence for dramatic short-term improvement of diabetes, long-term benefits and complications of surgery in diabetic patients must be determined to fully assess the effectiveness of surgery compared to medical therapy [113].

Excluding the duodenum from nutrient passage produces short-term improvements in glycemia [114]. In this way, gastric bypass surgery may achieve an 80% remission of type 2 diabetes compared to roughly 50% with restrictive procedures [115]. However, the former increases risk of hospitalization for hypoglycemia two to seven times compared to a reference population [116], whereas gastric banding carries no such risk.

Overall, weight loss surgery reduces numerous obesity-related risks, including those of cardiovascular events and certain cancers [117]. It also lessens complications during pregnancy and childbirth [118,119], and makes it easier to perform future operations unrelated to weight loss. It improves depression and quality of life [120], and increases life expectancy. In a study of 1035 weight loss surgery patients and 5746 matched controls, mortality in the former was 0.68% while that in the latter was 6.17% over a 5-year period [121].

As noted above, for patients with chronic kidney disease, obesity is associated with elevations in GFR and proteinuria [78]. Weight loss surgery normalizes GFR and reduces proteinuria and systolic blood pressure. It also reduces GFR, microalbuminuria, and blood pressure in individuals with glomerular hyperfiltration [75], but leaves creatinine levels unaffected [122].

Weight loss through bariatric surgery may eliminate the need for dialysis and transplantation in some CKD patients [123], or at least stabilize serum creatinine in those with impaired renal function [122]. Further, reduced BMI may enable patients to meet inclusion criteria for kidney transplants. However, special postoperative care may be required to meet the nutritional requirements of kidney transplant patients who undergo weight loss surgery [124].

The use of bariatric surgery in patients with chronic kidney disease involves a complex combination of benefits and potential risks for the patient. Obesity itself is a risk factor for developing chronic kidney disease; thus, bariatric surgery often corrects the underlying problem as well as a number of parameters related to kidney function including insulin resistance and adiponectin, tumor necrosis factor-α, interleukin-18, and C-reactive protein [125]. Likewise, bariatric surgery improves a number of conditions that directly impact kidney function including dislipidemia, hypertension, urinary albumin excretion, markers of atherosclerosis, and quality of life and leads to improvement of parameters used to measure kidney function including glomerular filtration rate, especially in diabetic patients [125].

However, bariatric surgery also poses risks for the development or progression of kidney disease. The risk of stone formation is greater due to increased urinary oxalate and calcium oxalate supersaturation and decreased urinary volume and citrate levels (see Chapter 28). After bariatric surgery, intraluminal fatty acids bind to calcium which prevents the formation of calcium oxalate, leading to hyperoxaluria and urinary calculus [125]. A higher incidence of hyperoxaluria is noted in both stone formers and non-stone formers following roux-en-y gastric bypass [126] but not gastric banding [127]. Roux-en-y gastric bypass can lead to oxalate nephropathy and chronic kidney disease, especially in patients with previous renal insufficiency [125].

Further research is necessary to determine if reversal of bariatric surgery corrects renal problems and ways to manage or prevent hyperoxaluria after surgery [125]. The benefits of treating diabetic nephropathy must be weighed against the potential for the development of hyperoxaluria [127] and the safety and efficiency of surgery for patients with renal failure to maximize their health outcomes [128,129].

METABOLIC SYNDROME

Therapeutic lifestyle change, emphasizing weight reduction, is first-line therapy for metabolic syndrome [59]. Whether treatment of components of the syndrome (with the exception of hypertension) can impact CKD incidence and progression remains unknown. Accumulating evidence suggests that therapy with mineralocorticoid receptor antagonists may be beneficial in preventing cardiovascular disease and CKD in patients with metabolic syndrome [130].

Sowers et al. reviewed the emerging role of aldosterone in patients with resistant hypertension and metabolic syndrome [41]. Inappropriate aldosterone secretion as well as glucocorticoid signaling through mineralocorticoid receptors in extrarenal tissues may promote the development of insulin resistance and hypertension in patients with metabolic syndrome [131]. Blocking mineralocorticoid activation may attenuate vascular and renal injury as well as improve insulin release and glucose utilization. Clinical trials show benefits of mineralocorticoid receptor antagonists in heart failure, hypertension, and diabetic nephropathy [130]. Large, multicenter, randomized trials are needed to evaluate its effects in metabolic syndrome.

References

[1] Haslam DW. A long look at obesity. Lancet 2010;376:85—6.

[2] McAllister EJ, Dhurandhar NV, Keith SC, et al. Ten putative contributors to the obesity epidemic. Crit Rev Food Sci Nutr 2009;49:868—913.

[3] Vasan RS, Pencina MJ, Cabain M, et al. Estimated risks for developing obesity in the Framingham Hear Study. Annals Int Med 2005;143:473—9.

[4] Ogden CL, Yanovski SZ, Carroll MD, et al. The epidemiology of obesity Gastroenterology 2007;132:2087—102.

[5] Deitz WH. Reversing the tide of obesity. Lancet 2011;378:744—5.

[6] Flegal KM, Carroll MD, Ogden CL, et al. Prevalence and trends in obesity among US adults, 1999—2998. JAMA 2010;303:3335—41.

[7] Abrass CK. Overview: Obesity: What does it have to do with kidney disease? J Am Soc Nephrol 2004;15:2768—72.

[8] Hall KD, Sacks G, Chandramohan D, et al. Quantification of the effect of energy imbalance on bodyweight. Lancet 2011;378:826—37.

[9] deGonzalez AB, Hartge P, Cerhan JR, et al. Body-Mass Index and mortality among 1.46 million white adults. NEJM 2010;363:2211—9.

[10] Calle EE, Thun MJ, Petrelli JM, et al. Body-mass index and mortality in a prospective cohort of U.S. adults. N Engl J Med 1999;341:1097—105.

[11] King D. The future challenge of obesity. Lancet 2011;378:743—4.

[12] Szczech LA, Harmon W, Hostetter TH, et al. World Kidney Day 2009: Problems and challenges in the emerging epidemic of kidney disease. J Am Soc Nephrol 2009;20:453—64.

[13] Yach D, Stuckler D, Brownell KD. Epidemiologic and economic consequences of the global epidemics of obesity and diabetes. Nature Med 2006;12:62—6.

[14] Alison DB, Fontaine KR, Manson JE, et al. Annual deaths attributable to obesity in the United States. JAMA 1999;282: 1530—8.

[15] Cunningham SA, Riosmena F, Wang J, et al. Decreases in diabetes-free life expectancy in the U.S. and the role of obesity. Diabetes Care 2011;34:2225—30.

[16] Finkelstein EA, Trogdon JG, Cohen JW, et al. Annual medical spending attributable to obesity: payer- and service-specific estimates. Health Aff (Millwood) 2009;28:822—31. Epub 2009 July 27.

[17] Farrell AE. Fat shame: stigma and the fat body in american culture. New York: NYU Press; 2011.

[18] Ritz E. Obesity and CKD: How to assess the risk? Am J Kidney Dis 2008;52:1—6.

[19] Hsu C-Y, McCulloch CE, Iribarren C, et al. Body mass index and risk for end-stage renal disease. Ann Int Med 2006;144:21—8.

[20] Wang Y, Chen X, Song Y, et al. Association between obesity and kidney disease: a systematic review and meta-analysis. Kidney Int 2008;73:19—33.

[21] Bonnet F, Deprele C, Sassolas A, et al. Excessive body weight as a new independent risk factor for clinical and pathological progression in primary IgA nephritis. Am J Kidney Dis 2001;37:720—7.

[22] Cirillo M, Senigalliesi L, Laurenzi M, et al. Microalbuminuria in nondiabetic adults: Relation of blood pressure, body mass index, plasma cholesterol levels, and smoking: The Gubbio Population Study. Arch Intern Med 1998;158:1933—9.

[23] Tozawa M, Iseki K, Iseki C, et al. Influence of smoking and obesity on the development of proteinuria. Kidney Int 2002;62: 956—62.

[24] Praga M. Obesity: A neglected culprit in renal disease. Nephrol Dial Transplant 2002;17:1157—9.

[25] Ejerblad E, Fored CM, Lindblad P, et al. Obesity and risk for chronic renal failure. J Am Soc Nephrol 2006;17: 1695—702.

[26] Iseki K, Ikemiya Y, Kinjo K, et al. Body mass index and the risk of development of end-stage renal disease in a screened cohort. Kidney Int 2004;65:1870—6.

[27] Meier-Kriesche H, Arndorfer JA, Kaplan B. The impact of body mass index on renal transplant outcomes: a significant independent risk factor for graft failure and patient death. Transplantation 2002;73:70—4.

[28] Othman M, Kawar B, Meguid El Nahas A. Influence of obesity on progression of non-diabetic chronic kidney disease: a retrospective study. Nephron Clin Pract 2009;114:c16—23.

[29] DeBoer IH, Katz R, Fried LF, et al. Obesity and change in estimated GFR among older adults. Am J Kidney Dis 2009;54: 1043—51.

[30] Munkhaugen J, Lydersen S, Wideroe T-E, et al. Prehypertension, obesity, and risk of kidney disease: a 20-year follow-up of the HUNT I Study in Norway. Am J Kidney Dis 2009;54:638—46.

[31] Ritz E. Metabolic syndrome and kidney disease. Blood Purif 2008;26:59—62.

[32] Mallamaci F, Ruggenenti P, Perna A, et al. ACE inhibition is renoprotective among obese patients with proteinuria. J Am Soc Nephrol 2011;22:1122—8.

[33] Weisinger JR, Kempson RL, Eldridge FL, et al. The nephritic syndrome: a complication of massive obesity. Ann Intern Med 1974;81:440—7.

[34] Kambham N, Markowitz GS, Valeria AM, et al. Obesity-related glomerulopathy: An emerging epidemic. Kidney Int 2001;59: 1498—509.

[35] Goumenos DS, Kawar B, El Nahas M, et al. Early histologic changes in the kidney of people with morbid obesity. Nephrol Dial Transplant 2009;24:3732—8.

[36] Chen HM, Liu ZH, Zeng CH, et al. Podocyte lesions in patients with obesity-related glomerulopathy. Am J Kidney Dis 2006;58: 772—9.

[37] Ritz E, Koleganova N, Piecha G. Is there an obesity-related glomerulopathy? Curr Opin Hypertens 2010;20:44—9.

[38] Wuerzner G, Pruijm M, Maillard M, et al. Marked association between obesity and glomerular hyperfiltration: a cross-sectional study in an African population. Am J Kidney Dis 2001;37:164—78.

[39] Chagnac A, Weinstein T, Korzets A, et al. Glomerular hemodynamics in severe obesity. Am J Physiol Renal Physiol 2000;278:F817—22.

[40] Hunley TE, Ma L-J, Kon V. Scope and mechanisms of obesity-related renal disease. Curr Opin Nephrol Hypertens 2010; 19:227—34.

[41] Sowers JR, Whaley-Connell A, Epstein M. Narrative review: the emerging clinical implications of the role of aldosterone in the metabolic syndrome and resistant hypertension. Ann Intern Med 2009;150:776—83.

[42] Shibata S, Nagase M, Yoshida S, et al. Modification of mineralocorticoid receptor function by Rac1GTPase: implication in proteinuric kidney disease. Nat Med 2008;14:1370—6.

[43] Sun F, Tao Q, Zhan S. Metabolic syndrome and the development of chronic kidney disease among 118,924 non-diabetic Taiwanese in a retrospective cohort. Nephrology 2010;1:84—92.

[44] Chen J, Muntner P, Hamm LL, et al. Insulin resistance and risk of chronic kidney disease in nondiabetic US adults. J Am Soc Nephrol 2003;14:469—77.

[45] Gerchman F, Tong J, Ultzschneider KM, et al. Body mass index is associated with increased creatinine clearance by a mechanism independent of body fat distribution. J Clin Endo Metab 2009;94:3781—8.

[46] Botev R, Mallie J-P, Wetzels JFM, et al. The clinician and estimation of glomerular filtration rate by creatinine-based formulas: current limitations and quo vadis. Clin J Am Soc Nephrol 2011;6:937—50.

[47] Cockcroft DW, Gault MH. Prediction of creatinine clearance from serum creatinine. Nephron 1976;1:31—41.

[48] Milic R, Colombini A, Lombardi G, et-al. Estimation of glomerular filtration rate by MDRD equation in athletes: role of body surface area. Eur J App Physiol http://dx.doi.org/10.1007/s00421-011-1969-1.

[49] Wuerzner G, Pruijm M, Maillard M, et al. Marked association between obesity and glomerular hyperfiltration: a cross-sectional study in an African population. Am J Kidney Dis 2010;56:303—12.

[50] Delanaye P, Radermecker RP, Rorive M, et al. Indexing glomerular filtration rate for body surface area in obese patients is misleading: concept and example. Nephrol Dial Transp 2005;20:2024—8.

[51] Wuerzner G, Bochud M, Giusti V, et al. Measurement of glomerular filtration rate in obese patients: pitfalls and potential consequences on drug therapy. Obes Facts 2011;4:238—43.

[52] Nair S, Mishra V, Hayden K, et al. The four-variable modification of diet in renal disease formula underestimates glomerular filtration rate in obese type 2 diabetic individuals with chronic kidney disease. Diabetologia 2011;54:1304—11.

[53] Praditpornsilpa K, Townamchai N, Chaiwatanarat T, et al. The need for robust validation for MDRD-based glomerular filtration rate estimation in various CKD populations. Nephrol Dial Transplant 2011;26:2780—5.

[54] Michels WM, Grootendorst DC, Verduijn M, et al. Performance of the Cockroft-Gault, MDRD, and new CKD-EPI formulas in relation to GFR, age, and body size. Clin J Am Soc Nephrol 2010;5:1003—9.

[55] Ford ES, Giles WH, Dietz WH. Prevalence of the metabolic syndrome among U.S. adults: findings from the third National Health and Nutrition Examination Survey. JAMA 2002;287. 356—350.

[56] Ervin RB. Prevalence of metabolic syndrome among adults 20 years of age and over, by sex, age, race and ethnicity, and body mass index: United States, 2003—2006. National Health Statistics Report, no 13. Hyattsville MD: National Center for Health Statistics; 2009.

[57] Taylor AM, Peeters PH, Norat T, et al. An update on the prevalence of metabolic syndrome in children and adolescents. Int J Petiatr Ob 2010;5:202—8.

[58] Hoehner CM, Greenlund KJ, Rith-Najarian S, et al. Association of the insulin resistance syndrome and microalbuminuria among nondiabetic native Americans. The Inter-Tribal Heart Project. J Am Soc Nephrol 2002;13:1626—34.

[59] Grundy SM, Brewer HB, Cleeman JI, et al. Definition of metabolic syndrome: Report of the National Heart, Lung, and Blood Institute/American Heart Association Conference on Scientific Issues Related to Definition. Circulation 2004;109:433—8.

[60] Thomas G, Ar Sehgal, Kashyap SR, et al. Metabolic syndrome and kidney disease: a systematic review and meta-analysis. Clin J Am Soc Nephrol 2011;6:2634—2373.

[61] Alexander CM, Landsman PB, Teutsch SM, et al. NCEP-defined metabolic syndrome, diabetes, and prevalence of coronary heart disease among HHANES III participants age 50 years and older. Diabetes 003;52:1210

[62] Lorenzo C, Wiliams K, Hunt KJ, et al. The National Cholesterol Education Program-Adult Treatment Panel III, International Diabetes Federation, and World Health Organization definitions of the metabolic syndrome as predictors of incident cardiovascular disease and diabetes. Diabetes Care 2007;30:8.

[63] Kurella M, Lo JC, Chertow GM, et al. Metabolic syndrome and the risk for chronic kidney disease among nondiabetic adults. J Am Soc Nephrol 2005;16:2134—40.

[64] Chen J, Muntner P, Hamm LL, et al. The metabolic syndrome and chronic kidney disease in U.S. adults. Ann Intern Med 2004;140:167—74.

[65] Haffner SM, Gonzales C, Valdez RA, et al. Is microalbuminuria part of the prediabetic state? The Mexico City Diabetes Study. Diabetologia 1993;36:1002—6.

[66] Wang C-H, Li F, Takahashi N. The renin-angiotensin system and the metabolic syndrome. Open Hypertens J 2010;3:1—13.

[67] Kalupahana NS, Moustaid-Moussa N. The renin-angiotensin system: a link between obesity, inflammation, and insulin resistance. Obes Rev 2011:1467.

[68] Appel LJ, Clark JM, Yeh H-C, et al. Comparative effectiveness of weight-loss interventions in clinical practice. NEJM 2011;365:1959—68.

[69] Bakris G, Vassalotti J, Ritz E, et al. National Kidney Foundation consensus conference on cardiovascular and kidney diseases and diabetes risk: an integrated therapeutic approach to reduce events. Kidney Int 2010;78:726—36.

[70] Diabetes Prevention Program Research Group. Reduction in the incidence of type 2 diabetes with lifestyle intervention or metformin. N Engl J Med 2002;346:393—403.

[71] Hamman RF, Wing RR, Edelstein SL, et al. Effect of weight loss with lifestyle intervention on risk of diabetes. Diabetes Care 2006;29:2102—7.

[72] Diabetes Prevention Program Research Group. 10-year follow-up of diabetes incidence and weight loss in the Diabetes Prevention Program Outcomes Study. Lancet 2009;374:1677—86.

[73] Patrick K, Norman GJ, Calfas KJ, et al. Diet, physical activity, and sedentary behaviors as risk factors for overweight in adolescence. Arch Pediatr Adolesc Med 2004;158:385—90.

[74] Blumenthal JA, Babyak MA, Hinderliter AK, et al. Effects of the DASH diet alone and in combination with exercise and weight loss on blood pressure and cardiovascular biomarkers in men and women with high blood pressure. The ENCORE Study. Arch Intern Med 2010;170:126—35.

[75] Navaneethan SD, Yehnert H, Moustarah F, et al. Weight loss interventions in chronic kidney disease: A systematic review and meta-analysis. Clin J Am Soc Nephr 2009;4:1565—74.

[76] Morales E, Valero MA, Leon M, et al. Beneficial effects of weight loss in overweight patients with chronic proteinuric nephropathies. Am J Kidney Dis 2003;41:319—27.

[77] Praga M, Morales E. Obesity-related renal damage: changing diet to avoid progression. Kidney Int 2010;78:633—5.

[78] Friedman AN, Zhangsheng Y, Be Juliar, et al. Independent influence of dietary protein on markers of kidney function and disease in obesity. Kidney Int 2010;78:693—7.

[79] Shen W-w, Chen H-m, Chen H, et al. Obesity-related glomerulopathy: body mass index and proteinuria. Clin J Am Soc Nephrol 2010;5:1401—9.

[80] NIH conference. Gastrointestinal surgery for severe obesity. Consensus Development Conference Panel. Ann Intern Med 1991;115:956—61.

[81] Buchwald H, Estok R, Fahrbach K, et al. Weight and type 2 diabetes after bariatric surgery: systematic review and meta-analysis. Am J Med 2009;122:248—56. e245.

[82] Poirier P, Cornier MA, Mazzone T, et al. Bariatric surgery and cardiovascular risk factors a scientific statement form the American Heart Association. Circulation 2011;123:1683—701.

[83] Sjostrom L, Narbro K, Sjostrom CD, et al. Effects of bariatric surgery on mortality in Swedish obese subjects. N Engl J Med 2007;357(8):741—52.

[84] Mun EC, Blackburn GL, Matthews JB. Current status of medical and surgical therapy for obesity. Gastroenterology 2001;120:669—81.

[85] ASMBS. Updated position statement on sleeve gastrectomy as a bariatric procedure, http://asmbs.org/; [accessed 1.11.11].

[86] Blackburn GL. Solutions in weight control: lessons from gastric surgery. Am J Clin Nutr 2005;82:248S—52S.

[87] Schauer PR, Burguera B, Ikramuddin S, et al. Effect of laparoscopic Roux-en Y gastric bypass on type 2 diabetes mellitus. Ann Surg 2003;238:467—84. discussion 484—465.

[88] Maggard MA, Shugarman LR, Suttorp M, et al. Meta-analysis: surgical treatment of obesity. Ann Intern Med 2005;142:547—59.

[89] Alvarez-Leite JI. Nutrient deficiencies secondary to bariatric surgery. Curr Opin Clin Nutr Metab Care 2004;7(5):569—75.

[90] Abarbanel JM, Berginer VM, Osimani A, et al. Neurologic complications after gastric restriction surgery for morbid obesity. Neurology 1987;37:196—200.

[91] Matlaga BR, Shore AD, Magnuson T, et al. Effect of gastric bypass surgery on kidney stone disease. J Urol 2009;181(6):2573—7.

[92] Patel BN, Passman CM, Fernandez A, et al. Prevalence of hyperoxaluria after bariatric surgery. J Urol 2009;181(1):161—6.

[93] Lieske JC, Kumar R, Collazo-Clavell ML. Nephrolithiasis after bariatric surgery for obesity. Semin Nephrol 2008;28(2):163—73.

[94] Nasr SH, D'Agati VD, Said SM, et al. Oxalate nephropathy complicating Roux-en-Y Gastric Bypass: an underrecognized cause of irreversible renal failure. Clin J Am Soc Nephrol 2008;3(6):1676—83.

[95] Semins MJ, Asplin JR, Steele K, et al. The effect of restrictive bariatric surgery on urinary stone risk factors. Urology 2010;76(4):826—9.

[96] Turgeon NA, Perez S, Mondestin M, et al. The impact of renal function on outcomes of bariatric surgery. J Am Soc Nephrol 2011. Epub 2012 March 1.

[97] Blackburn GL, Magerowski G. The impact of renal function on outcomes of bariatric surgery. J Am Soc Nephrol. Epub 2012 April 12.

[98] Currie A, Chetwood A, Ahmed AR. Bariatric surgery and renal function. Obes Surg 2011;21(4):528—39.

[99] Halverson JD. Micronutrient deficiencies after gastric bypass for morbid obesity. Am Surg 1986;52:594—8.

[100] Rhode BM, Arseneau P, Cooper BA, et al. Vitamin B-12 deficiency after gastric surgery for obesity. Am J Clin Nutr 1996;63(1):103—9.

[101] Schilling RF, Gohdes PN, Hardie GH. Vitamin B12 deficiency after gastric bypass surgery for obesity. Ann Intern Med 1984; 101(4):501—2.

[102] Halverson JD. Metabolic risk of obesity surgery and long-term follow-up. Am J Clin Nutr 1992;55:602S—5S.

[103] Brolin RE, Gorman JH, Gorman RC, et al. Are vitamin B12 and folate deficiency clinically important after roux-en-Y gastric bypass? J Gastrointest Surg 1998;2:436—42.

[104] Buchwald H, Avidor Y, Braunwald E, et al. Bariatric surgery: a systematic review and meta-analysis. JAMA 2004;292:1724—37.

[105] Tolonen P, Victorzon M, Niemi R, et al. Does gastric banding for morbid obesity reduce or increase gastroesophageal reflux? Obes Surg 2006;16:1469—74.

[106] Abu-Abeid S, Wishnitzer N, Szold A, et al. The influence of surgically-induced weight loss on the knee joint. Obes Surg 2005;15:1437—42.

[107] Klein S, Mittendorfer B, Eagon JC, et al. Gastric bypass surgery improves metabolic and hepatic abnormalities associated with nonalcoholic fatty liver disease. Gastroenterology 2006;130: 1564—72.

[108] Burgio KL, Richter HE, Clements RH, et al. Changes in urinary and fecal incontinence symptoms with weight loss surgery in morbidly obese women. Obstet Gynecol 2007;110:1034—40.

[109] Escobar-Morreale HF, Botella-Carretero JI, Alvarez-Blasco F, et al. The polycystic ovary syndrome associated with morbid obesity may resolve after weight loss induced by bariatric surgery. J Clin Endocrinol Metab 2005;90:6364—9.

[110] Gerrits EG, Ceulemans R, van Hee R, et al. Contraceptive treatment after biliopancreatic diversion needs consensus. Obes Surg 2003;13:378—82.

[111] Schauer PR, Kashyap SR, Wolski K, et al. Bariatric Surgery versus Intensive Medical Therapy in Obese Patients with Diabetes. N Engl J Med 2012;336:1567—76.

[112] Mingrone G, Panunzi S, De Gaetano A, et al. Bariatric Surgery versus Conventional Medical Therapy for Type 2 Diabetes. N Engl J Med 2012;336:1577—85.

[113] Zimmet P, Alberti KG. Surgery or medical therapy for obese patients with type 2 diabetes? N Engl J Med. Epub 2012 March 26.

[114] Plum L, Ahmed L, Febres G, et al. Comparison of glucostatic parameters after hypocaloric diet or bariatric surgery and equivalent weight loss. Obesity 2011;19(11):2149—57.

[115] Lee WJ, Chong K, Ser KH, et al. Gastric bypass vs. sleeve gastrectomy for type 2 diabetes mellitus: a randomized controlled trial. Arch Surg 2011;146:143—8.

[116] Patti ME, Goldfine AB. Hypoglycaemia following gastric bypass surgery — diabetes remission in the extreme? Diabetologia 2010;53(11):2276—9.

[117] Blackburn GL, Mun EC. Therapy insight: weight-loss surgery and major cardiovascular risk factors. Nat Clin Pract Cardiovasc Med 2005;2:585—91.

[118] Cnattingius S, Bergstrom R, Lipworth L, et al. Prepregnancy weight and the risk of adverse pregnancy outcomes. N Engl J Med 1998;338:147—52.

[119] Deitel M, Stone E, Kassam HA, et al. Gynecologic-obstetric changes after loss of massive excess weight following bariatric surgery. J Am Coll Nutr 1988;7:147—53.

[120] Buchwald H. The future of bariatric surgery. Obes Surg 2005;15:598—605.

[121] Christou NV, Sampalis JS, Liberman M, et al. Surgery decreases long-term mortality, morbidity, and health care use in morbidly obese patients. Ann Surg 2004;240:416—23; discussion 423—414.

[122] Schuster DP, Teodorescu M, Mikami D, et al. Effect of bariatric surgery on normal and abnormal renal function. Surg Obes Relat Dis 2011;7:459—64.

[123] Tafti BA, Haghdoost M, Alvarez L, et al. Recovery of renal function in a dialysis-dependent patient following gastric bypass surgery. Obes Surg 2009;19:1335—9.

[124] Lightner AL, Lau J, Obayashi P, et al. Potential nutritional conflicts in bariatric and renal transplant patients. Obes Surg 2011;21:1965—70.

[125] Ahmed MH, Byrne CD. Bariatric surgery and renal function: a precarious balance between benefit and harm. Nephrol Dial Transplant 2010;25(10):3142—7.

[126] Canales BK, Asmar A, Canales MT. Gastric bypass in patients with chronic kidney disease. Nephrol Dial Transplant 2010;25(12):4116—7; author reply 4117—8.

[127] Cohen P. Bariatric surgery for diabetic nephropathy. Nephrol Dial Transplant 2011;26(5):1755; author reply 1755—6.

[128] Gore JL. Obesity and renal transplantation: is bariatric surgery the answer? Transplantation 2009;87(8):1115.

[129] Lim RB, Blackburn GL, Jones DB. Benchmarking best practices in weight loss surgery. Curr Probl Surg 2010;47(2):79—174.

[130] Tirosh A, Garg R, Adler GK. Mineralocorticoid receptor antagonists and the metabolic syndrome. Curr Hypertens Rep 2010;12(4): 252—7.

[131] deKloet AD, Krause Woods EG, Woods SC. The renin-angiotensin system and the metabolic syndrome. Physiol Behav 2010;100(5):525—34.

Bariatric Surgery and Renal Disease

J. Bikhchandani, R.A. Forse

Creighton University Medical Center, Department of Surgery, Omaha, Nebraska, USA

MAGNITUDE OF PROBLEM

The World Health Organization has reported that 1.7 billion people worldwide are overweight or obese [1]. In fact it is has been predicted that there are now more people at risk for obesity on the planet than at risk for starvation. There is an epidemic of obesity in the United States with two-thirds of the population being overweight and 50% of them being obese, that is with a body mass index (BMI) greater than 30 [2]. In the year 2000, 21 states reported that more than 15% of their population belonged to the obese category [3], while by 2007 48 states reported up to 15%. Some states in the middle of the country reported 35% of their population being obese. Obesity has now also affected the pediatric population and is a growing concern representing its own serious epidemic [4]. A BMI of over 40 kg/m^2 defines morbid obesity and is sometimes referred to as severe or stage 3 obesity as it is associated with obesity related co-morbidities, and a significantly increased mortality. About 5% of the U.S. population or more than 23 million people are morbidly obese [5]. Morbid obesity with its increased morbidity has a mortality rate of over 280,000 deaths per year across the United States [3].

PATHOGENESIS OF OBESITY

The pathophysiology of obesity is multifactorial and includes genetic, environmental, behavioral and psychological factors [6]. Several studies have reported a genetic predisposition to obesity and that is why usually more than one member of the family is found to be obese [7]. The severity of obesity corresponds more with the natural parents than with adoptive parents [8,9]. Monozygotic twins have more similar weights than dizygotic twins, even if they grow up in different environments [10]. However genetic factors alone cannot account for the exponential increase in the number of obese individuals [11]. Lifestyle factors like declining rates of physical activity and increase in the consumption of high calorie foods play a role [12,13]. Obese individuals either have lack of satiety even with large portions of food, or eat multiple times in a day, leading to increased calorie intake. The basal or resting energy expenditure (REE) also appears to play a role as it has been found to be lower in morbidly obese individuals [14]. Postprandial increases in the REE appear to be less in obese patients than in thin patients and there are some data suggesting that these differences are related to the levels and expression of uncoupling proteins. Ghrelin is a peptide secreted by the stomach which increases in response to fasting and decreases postprandially. Ghrelin levels are lower in obese individuals, do not get suppressed by food intake and appear to be a related factor in terms of etiology [15]. The adipocyte hormone leptin stimulates hypothalamic anorexigenic neuropeptides to inhibit food intake and there are some obese patients who have increased serum levels of leptin with possible resistance to leptin effects on food intake [16]. As with so many chronic human diseases, obesity is multi-factorial and the impact of each factor is not clearly defined. What has made the approach to treating obesity even more complex is the evidence that medical therapy of medical co-morbidities may aggravate the primary problem. For example the more aggressive approach to blood glucose control results in an increase in body weight, negating the benefit of glucose control and therefore resulting in no decrease in cardiac mortality.

CLINICAL MANIFESTATIONS

Obesity results in significant medical problems which are either related to the metabolic changes (diabetes, dyslipidemia, atherosclerosis, PCOS) or the direct effect (accelerated degenerative arthritis, hernias, sleep apnea) of the obesity. The clustering of insulin resistance with dysglycemia, dyslipidemia, hypertension and central obesity represent the metabolic syndrome [17]. The syndrome is associated with accelerated cardiovascular disease and early death. Patients with morbid obesity almost always develop the metabolic syndrome due to impaired glucose tolerance, systemic hyperinsulinemia, impaired hepatic uptake of insulin and insulin resistance in the tissues. There are several other medical co-morbidities associated with obesity (Table 30.1). Morbidly obese patients have increased circulating blood volume, increased cardiac output, left ventricular dilation, and compensatory eccentric left ventricular hypertrophy as well as systolic and diastolic dysfunction [18]. Obesity cardiomyopathy is the form of congestive heart failure resulting from the compensatory structural cardiac changes associated with obesity [19]. This structural re-modeling predisposes to arrhythmias [20] and there is an increased risk of coronary atherosclerosis with high BMI [21]. Respiratory insufficiency of obesity includes obesity hypoventilation syndrome or obstructive sleep apnea or both. Morbidly obese patients also have a restrictive pulmonary defect from heavy chest walls, decreased expiratory volumes, chronic hypoxemia and poor ventilatory response to hypercarbia. Chronic hypoxemia leads to pulmonary artery vasoconstriction. This can cause secondary pulmonary hypertension and subsequent right-sided heart failure [22]. Obstructive sleep apnea patients have severe daytime somnolence, frequent nocturnal awakening, loud snoring, and morning headaches. The prevalence of obstructive sleep apnea in morbidly obese patients is as high as 71% [23]. Severe obstructive sleep apnea syndrome can be associated with prolonged sinus arrest, premature ventricular contractions and sudden death. Morbidly obese patients become resistant to insulin because of downregulation of insulin receptors and develop type 2 diabetes [22]. Insulin resistance is also thought to be responsible for the alterations in fatty acid metabolism particularly in the liver resulting in nonalcoholic steatohepatitis (NASH). NASH in conjunction with the obesity epidemic is now thought to equal hepatitis C as the cause of hepatic cirrhosis. Obese patients have an increased risk for deep venous thrombosis and pulmonary embolism from altered endothelium, venous stasis and accentuated by raised intra-abdominal pressure. Early degenerative arthritis of weight-bearing joints is common due to the enormous weight causing wear and tear.

MEDICAL THERAPY

The primary focus of all obesity management is lifestyle changes. Emphasis is placed on reducing the caloric intake particularly fat intake while increasing activity. There are a number of programs offered to achieve weight loss, i.e. commerical diets, protein-sparing diets and behavioral therapies. Although many people can lose some weight through dietary manipulation, only 5% to 10% of patients with severe obesity can obtain and sustain significant weight reduction [24]. There is no dietary approach to date that has achieved the long-term success needed to treat morbidly obese [25]. Several weight reduction medications have been used without much success (Table 30.2) [26]. Some of the newer drugs target reducing fat absorption including Orlistat, a pancreatic lipase inhibitor, but there are problems with compliance [27]. Another drug Sibutramine has been used as an appetite suppressant. These agents provide only modest weight loss of up to 5% above placebo. Weight returns once these medications are stopped despite attempts at concurrent diet and life style changes. In terms of overall disease control and treatment these results are inadequate therapy for patients with morbid obesity.

TABLE 30.1 Co-Morbidities Associated with Morbid Obesity

- Coronary artery disease
- Hypertension
- Hyperlipidemia
- Diabetes mellitus
- Hepatic steatosis
- Obstructive sleep apnea
- Degenerative osteoarthritis
- Cardiomyopathy
- Deep venous thrombosis, venous stasis and ulcers
- Pulmonary hypertension, heart failure
- Hypoventilation syndrome of obesity
- Gastroesophageal reflux disease
- Gallstone disease
- Stress urinary incontinence

TABLE 30.2 Anti-Obesity Medications

Drug	Mechanism of Action
Orlistat	Lipase inhibitor, decreases fat absorption
Sibutramine	Inhibits reuptake of serotonin and Noradrenaline
Fenfluramine	Serotonin agonist
Phentermine	Amphetamine related appetite suppressant
Dexfenfluramine	Serotonin agonist
Diethylpropion	Sympathomimetic appetite suppressant
Ephedrine	Sympathomimetic appetite suppressant

ROLE OF BARIATRIC SURGERY IN TREATMENT OF MORBID OBESITY

There has been an exponential rise in bariatric surgery over the last decade with the epidemic of obesity and the advent of laparoscopic techniques. In 1991, the National Institutes of Health Consensus Conference for severe obesity recommended bariatric surgery for a BMI of 40 or higher, or a BMI of 35 or higher in a patient with a high-risk weight related co-morbidities including severe sleep apnea, cardiovascular disease including obesity-related cardiomyopathy, or severe diabetes mellitus [28]. It was recommended that these patients should have tried medical therapy for obesity; they should be psychologically stable and not dependent on alcohol or illicit drugs. Another essential factor which must be confirmed prior to offering surgery is to ensure the patient's motivation for losing weight. Patients must be willing to change their lifestyle drastically to achieve weight reduction and maintain it. It is important for patients to realize that bariatric surgery is just a means to make their path to a healthier lifestyle easier. Specific contraindications to bariatric surgery are few. They include cognitive impairment limiting the patient's ability to understand the procedure and its implications. Other contraindications include severe medical illness like unstable coronary artery disease, or advanced liver disease with portal hypertension [11].

Bariatric procedures reduce caloric intake by altering the anatomy of alimentary tract. These operations are broadly categorized as either restrictive or malabsorptive. Restrictive procedures limit oral intake by creating a small gastric reservoir. Malabsorptive procedures bypass varying portions of the small intestine and impair nutrient absorption. Restrictive procedures include gastric stapling (gastroplasty), adjustable gastric banding (wrapping a synthetic, inflatable band around the stomach to create a small pouch with a narrow outlet), or gastric resection termed a sleeve gastrectomy. Gastric bypass or the biliopancreatic diversion, are the other two main procedures which cause weight reduction by both restricting caloric consumption through gastric volume reduction and by inhibiting nutrient absorption. In 2005, the number of bariatric procedures performed in the United States was 171,000; a ten times rise since 1994 [29]. Laparoscopic gastric banding, laparoscopic Roux-en-Y gastric bypass and open gastric bypass are the three main techniques which account for more than 90% of bariatric procedures performed across the world [29]. The sleeve gastrectomy is newest procedure to be accepted and its application is increasing.

SURGICAL TECHNIQUES OF BARIATRIC SURGERY (See Figure 30.1)

Laparoscopic Adjustable Gastric Band

An adjustable gastric band is the most popular restrictive surgery performed today. In the United States, there are two brands of adjustable gastric bands available — LAP-Band and Realize Band. Both are similar in principle but differ primarily in the design of the subcutaneous port. Pars flaccida technique for placement of gastric band has now become a standard. The first step is division of the gastrohepatic ligament, sparing the anterior branch of vagus nerve and exposure of the the right crus of diaphragm. A retrogastric tunnel is then carefully created connecting the point between the right crus of diaphragm to the angle of His. The narrow end of the band (already placed intra-peritoneally) is grasped by the tunneler and pulled through the tunnel from the greater curvature to the lesser curvature side of the stomach. This end is passed through the locking mechanism of the band. The locked band is adjusted to lie on the lesser curvature side of the stomach. A 5-mm grasper is inserted between the band and stomach to ensure that it is not too tight. The anterior gastric wall is imbricated over the band with interrupted, nonabsorbable sutures securing it 1 cm below the gastro-esophageal junction. The tubing of the band is pulled through the 15-mm trocar site and connected to the access port. The port is sutured to the fascia. The benefits of this surgery include the limitation of food intake, very few complications, less vitamin deficiencies, very infrequent protein malnutrition and it is reversible. The disadvantages include moderate weight loss, band slippage and gastric prolapse, band erosions, esophageal motility problems, and late weight regain.

Laparoscopic Sleeve Gastrectomy

Sleeve gastrectomy is another recently popularized restrictive bariatric surgery. Its role as an independent bariatric surgical procedure has been under intense research lately as an alternative to gastric banding due to the frequent band related complications [30]. The technique involves placing a 30–40 F orogastric calibration tube to facilitate creation of a sleeve out of the stomach using a linear endo-stapler starting from 6 cm proximal to the pylorus reaching close to but not up to the gastroesophageal junction. The procedure produces a long tube-like stomach with both a functional esophago-gastric sphincter and pylorus intake. In reducing the stomach there is a reduction in the amount of ghrelin which may help to reduce appetite. The benefits include

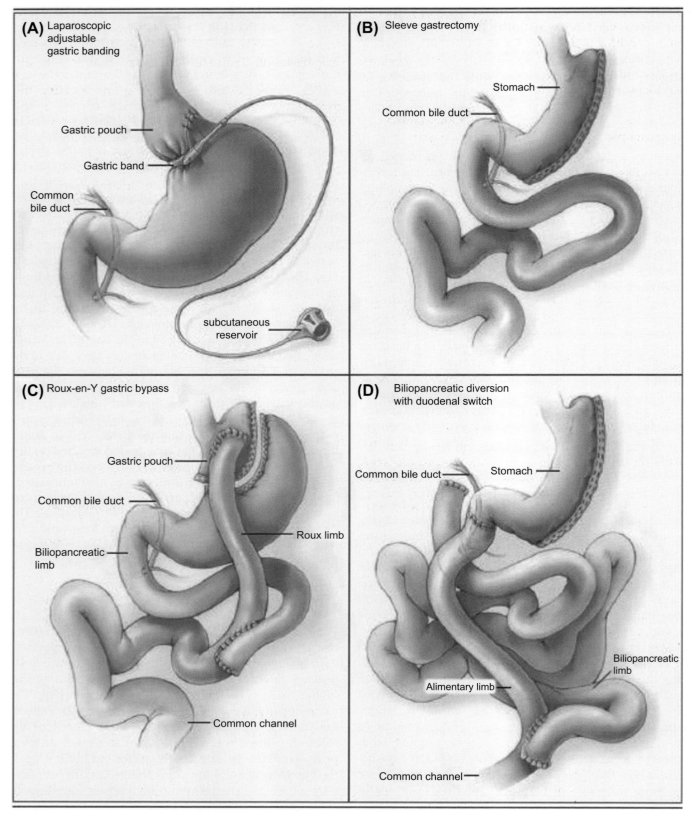

FIGURE 30.1   Bariatric procedures: (A) Adjustable gastric banding; (B) Sleeve gastrectomy; (C) Roux-n-Y gastric bypass; (D) Biliopancreatic diversion with duodenal switch. This figure is reproduced in color in the color plate section.

limitation of food intake, few complications, less vitamin deficiencies, very infrequent malnutrition and a reduction in ghrelin and appetite. The disadvantages include leaks, fistulas, esophageal motility problems, it is irreversible and it is a new procedure with limited long-term follow-up.

Laparoscopic Roux-en-Y Gastric Bypass

The first open gastric bypass was described by Mason and Ito in 1969 which involved anastomosing a loop of jejunum to the gastric pouch. This operation never got widely accepted due to significant bile reflux. The technique was therefore modified to a Roux-en-Y gastric bypass which solved the reflux issues and is now the most commonly performed bariatric surgery in the country. It is a procedure that has both a restrictive component to it due to the small gastric pouch as well as a malabsorptive component from the bypassed length of proximal jejunum. Jejunum is divided using endoscopic stapler at 40 cm from the ligament of Treitz. Approximately 80 to 150 cm length of the jejunum is run from this point of division onwards and moved into the supracolic compartment (Roux limb) either through a retrocolic or antecolic route. A stapled jejunojenunostomy is then performed to re-create bowel continuity. The next step involves formation of a 15 to 30 mL gastric pouch. Peritoneum between the spleen and the gastroesophageal junction is divided. The gastrohepatic ligament is divided to open the lesser sac and multiple stapler firings are done to form a gastric pouch using the proximal part of the lesser curvature side of stomach. The newly created gastric pouch is then anastomosed to the proximal part of Roux limb (gastrojejunostomy) using a circular stapler. All mesenteric defects are closed to prevent internal hernias in future. The advantages of this operation include significant limitation of food intake, few hepatic and renal malabsorptive complications, limited diarrhea, infrequent protein malnutrition, satisfactory weight loss and it is reversible. Disadvantages include marginal ulceration, infrequent gastrogastric fistulas, cholelithiasis, anemia, some vitamin deficiencies, and some late weight regain.

Biliopancreatic Diversion with Duodenal Switch

Biliopancreatic diversion works primarily on the principle of malabsorption. The anatomy of the small intestinal tract is completely transformed to allow only the last 100 cm of ileum, named as the common channel, to be able to absorb any nutrient. Another 250 cm of bowel is measured proximally from this point on the ileum and divided using staplers. The distal end is moved cephalad to create the proximal anastomosis (alimentary limb) while the proximal end is anatomosed to the previously marked 100 cm point as the biliary limb (using an endostapler). With a 60 French bougie in place, a sleeve is then made out of the stomach using a linear stapler device by dividing and excising the greater curvature side of the stomach starting at the middle of the gastric antrum. The gastric sleeve has a volume of roughly 200 mL. The duodenum is then divided with a stapler just beyond the pylorus. The part of the bowel which has been moved up into the supracolic compartment is then anastomosed to the duodenum using a circular stapler. Appendectomy and cholecystectomy is performed as part of the procedure. All mesenteric defects are closed prior to completion of the procedure. In certain bariatric centers, this operation is performed in two stages [31]. The sleeve gastrectomy is done as the first step to produce weight loss so as to make the second stage technically easier and reduce the overall morbidity and mortality from the procedure. Some surgeons have shown that weight loss after the gastric sleeve formation may be enough, completely avoiding the need for a second step operation [32]. As a result, there have been recent reports of using sleeve gastrectomy as a primary bariatric procedure by itself. In such a case, this would be a purely restrictive operation like gastric banding. The advantages of the BPD-DS include the ability to eat more, fewer hepatic and renal malabsorption complications, excellent weight loss and less late weight regain. Disadvantages include stomal ulcerations, steatorrhea, cholelithiasis, flatus, anemia, significant vitamin deficiencies including metabolic bone disease, and it is irreversible.

OUTCOMES OF BARIATRIC SURGERY

The results of a Cochrane Review published in 2005 and two meta-analyses show that there is an average weight loss of 20 to 50 kg with various bariatric procedures [33–35]. The Swedish Obese Subjects (SOS) trial including 2010 bariatric surgery patients versus 2037 matched controls (nonsurgical) indicate that weight changes were significantly greater in the surgical group [36]. Among 1268 patients followed for 10 years, weight loss was 16.1% in the surgical group while 1.6% was gained in the control group. Weight loss with malabsorptive procedures is higher than with restrictive procedures [34]. There is convincing evidence in the literature to prove that bariatric surgery is effective and plays an important role in curing various medical conditions that are associated with morbid obesity. Following gastric bypass, diabetes has been shown to resolve in 73% of cases while sleep apnea resolves in 75% of patients [22]. Systemic hypertension is cured in

56% of cases. All these effects are long lasting if the weight reduction is sustained. In a meta-analysis by Buchwald et al., 77% of patients with preoperative diabetes no longer required medication after surgery. Similar improvements were seen for patients with hyperlipidemia (83%), hypertension (66%), and sleep apnea (88%) [34]. The SOS data suggest that some of these benefits are less marked at 10 years than at 2 years, although they are still significant [36].

The mortality rates from bariatric surgery have been reported to be 0.1% to 2.0% [37–39]. In the meta-analysis by Buchwald et al., operative mortality was 0.5% for gastric bypass, 0.1% for gastric banding, and 1.1% for malabsorptive procedures [34]. In the SOS trial, postoperative complications occurred in 13% of patients; 6% pulmonary, 1.8% wound complications, bleeding (0.5%) and thromboembolism (0.8%) [36]. The Longitudinal Assessment of Bariatric Surgery 1 (LABS-1) trial, a prospective, multicenter observational study assessed 30-day complication rates of bariatric surgery in 4776 patients and reported a mortality rate of 0.3%, with a complication rate 4.1% [40]. The 30-day cumulative outcome of death, serious complications, reintervention, or prolonged hospitalization was 1.0% after adjustable gastric banding patients versus 4.8% after laparoscopic gastric bypass. Another study based on NSQIP (National Surgical Quality Improvement Project) database reports on the 30-day morbidity and mortality of bariatric surgery as 4.2% and 0.2% respectively [41]. A recently published study shows an interesting finding that the risk of open gastric bypass increases in patients who have preoperative weight gain [42]. This study indirectly highlights the importance of bariatric patients losing some weight preoperatively for improving the surgical outcomes. The various complications of bariatric surgery are enlisted in Table 30.3. Dumping syndrome, manifested as diarrhea, flushing, light-headedness and

palpitations, is common after Roux-en-Y gastric bypass [43]. Deficiencies of iron, calcium, folate, vitamin B_{12} occur frequently after malabsorptive procedures and require regular monitoring with replacement [43,44].

RENAL DISEASE AND MORBID OBESITY

At present there are 20 to 30 million Americans with chronic kidney disease. There will be an estimated 700,000 end stage renal disease patients by 2015 [45]. Obesity has been shown to be an independent risk factor in the development of chronic kidney disease and end-stage renal disease (ESRD) [46,47]. All the manifestations of metabolic syndrome are also risk factors for chronic kidney disease [48,49]. In a population based study which followed 2738 individuals for a mean duration of 18.5 years; having a BMI greater than 30 kg /m^2 increased the risk of developing chronic kidney disease by 23%, odds ratio 1.23 (confidence interval 1.08–1.41) [50]. Incidence of endstage renal disease has also been shown to increase proportionately with rising BMI over a period of 25 years [51]. The risk of ESRD increased with greater than 35 BMI with an odds ratio of 4.39 (confidence intervals 3.38–5.70) [51]. Obesity being an independent modifiable risk factor for renal diseases, bariatric surgery can potentially be used as a therapeutic option to stabilize or prevent progression of kidney disease in morbidly obese individuals.

PATHOGENESIS OF RENAL DISEASE IN OBESITY

Morbidly obese patients are known to have proteinuria and segmental glomerulosclerosis even in the absence of diabetes mellitus [52]. Obesity is independently associated with hyperfiltration and hyperperfusion at the level of the glomerular nephron irrespective of hypertension. Hyperfiltration increases the physical stress on the glomerular wall resulting in proteinuria [53]. Obese patients have high levels of adipocyte-derived cytokine leptin [54]. The kidney is rich in receptors for leptin which promotes expression of prosclerotic TGF-β1 cytokine and subsequent cellular proliferation [55]. This may be one of the causes of renal scarring in obese individuals [56]. Obesity also increases the levels of proinflammatory cytokines like interleukin-6 and C-reactive protein [54]. This generates a proinflammatory state which accelerates the renal fibrosis by enhancing TGF-β1 signaling [57]. All the clinical components of the metabolic syndrome which commonly affect the morbidly obese play an important role in the development of renal impairment. Systemic hypertension is a major cause of renal dysfunction in the obese [58].

TABLE 30.3 Complications of Bariatric Surgery

Complications of Adjustable Gastric Banding	
Postoperative	Wound infection, pulmonary complications, DVT/PE, Nausea/vomiting
Short and long term	Nausea/vomiting, band prolapse, band erosion, esophageal dilation, GERD, dysphagia
Nutritional	B_{12}/iron deficiency
Complications of RNYGB or Biliopancreatic Diversion	
Postoperative	Bleeding, wound infection, anastomotic leak, pulmonary complications, DVT/PE
Short and long term	Dumping, steatorrhoea, marginal ulcer, internal hernias, bowel obstruction, anastomotic stenosis, gallstone formation, hepatic failure, nephrolithiasis
Nutritional	Protein malnutrition, B_{12}/iron/calcium deficiency

Glomerular hypertension causes endothelial dysfunction resulting in microalbuminuria [59]. Obesity also aggravates the effect of hypertension on albuminuria [60]. Other mechanisms that lead to renal injury in obesity include insulin resistance, hypercoagulability and impaired fibrinolysis.

ROLE OF BARIATRIC SURGERY IN CHRONIC KIDNEY DISEASE

Bariatric surgery is known to improve insulin resistance and reduce inflammation. This may be the reason behind the improvement seen in the renal function with surgically induced weight reduction [61]. Weight loss is associated with improvement in glomerular hemodynamics, insulin sensitivity and decreased urinary albumin excretion [62]. Evidence in the literature shows that bariatric surgery improves all the parameters of renal function. In a study of 25 obese patients with chronic kidney disease having mean BMI 49.8 kg/m^2 and mean GFR 47.9 mL/min/1.73 m^2; 12 months post-bariatric surgery, the BMI reduced to 34.5 kg/m^2 while the GFR increased to 61.6 mL/min/1.73 m^2 [63]. A prospective trial including 61 bariatric patients showed that one year after the operation, the glomerular filtration rate and proteinuria improved significantly [64]. In a study of 45 gastric bypass patients with preoperative kidney disease, nine patients had resolution, improvement, or stabilization of their renal function [65]. Two patients who were on dialysis pre-surgery were able to discontinue dialysis. The remaining 34 patients had stable renal function during a follow up for 2–5 years. In a retrospective study of 94 obese adults who had RNYGB; a significant reduction in albuminuria was seen [66]. Several case reports have also showed an improvement in proteinuria after bariatric surgery. Cuda et al. reported on a patient with chronic renal disease with levels of proteinuria reduced from 1.15 grams per 24 hours to 0.27 grams after a gastric bypass [67]. Izzedine et al. have reported that proteinuria was reduced by 99% in a patient after gastric bypass [68].

ROLE OF BARIATRIC SURGERY IN TRANSPLANT CANDIDATES

The number of obese patients awaiting organ transplantation has multiplied with the increasing prevalence of obesity [69]. Morbidly obese patients have higher morbidity and mortality after any major surgery [70]. This trend has also been seen in renal transplant recipients with increased postoperative complications, graft loss, and mortality [71–75]. In a comparative study of obese versus nonobese renal transplant patients,

reduced graft and overall survival at 10 years was seen in the obese group; 58% living with functioning graft versus 72% for normal weight patients [76]. Not surprisingly, the presence of diabetes, hypertension and coronary artery disease was higher in the obese group. Meier-Kriesche et al. analyzed the database of over 50,000 renal transplant recipients (1988–1997) from the United States Renal Data System (USRDS) and showed that the relative risk ratio for graft loss was 1.4 times higher in patients with a BMI >36 kg/m^2, [77]. The best results were found in patients with a BMI of 22–24 kg/m^2. Due to this most transplant centers have set body mass index limits over which patients are not considered eligible for transplant (35 kg/m^2). Bariatric surgery is currently the most effective treatment for morbid obesity and its benefits should be extended to potential kidney transplant candidates. Bariatric surgery can be utilized to make morbidly obese dialysis dependent patients eligible for renal transplant by significant weight loss and improvement in associated co-morbidities [78]. However, performing bariatric procedures on renal failure patients may be associated with added risks. A study on 101 ESRD patients who had bariatric surgery reported comparable weight loss to published trials but higher mortality (3.5%) [79]. Preoperative dependence on dialysis has been shown to be one of the strongest predictors of postoperative complications after bariatric surgery [80]. Nevertheless, there have been recent reports of bariatric procedures being performed safely in chronic renal disease patients. Takata et al. performed LRYGB in seven patients with ESRD without any complications with over 60% weight loss in mean 15 months [81]. All the patients were listed for the renal graft. Safety of bariatric surgery has also been reported in patients who have already had renal transplant [82]. Concerns that malabsorptive surgery may significantly alter the levels of drugs like tacrolimus or cyclosporine have not been substantiated.

BARIATRIC SURGERY AND NEPHROLITHIASIS

Studies have shown that obesity is associated with increased risk of nephrolithiasis due to increased oral intake of calcium, oxalate and purine-rich foods. However, any increase in BMI above and beyond 30 kg/m^2 do not further impact the risk of renal stone formation [83–87]. Obesity is the strongest predictor of stone recurrence in first-time stone formers by multivariate regression analysis [87]. On the contrary, weight loss from bariatric surgery has been shown to promote stone formation and kidney disease. Early bariatric procedures, such as jejuno-ileal bypass, were associated with significant kidney complications [88]. The association with hyperoxaluria was identified as the cause for increased incidence of renal stones and kidney failure. In 1977, this procedure was banned by the US Food and Drug Administration due to its adverse renal effects [89]. Modern bariatric surgery, predominantly RNY gastric bypass, also causes hyperoxaluria with increased risk of renal calculus formation. Park et al. showed that after bariatric surgery, urinary oxalate and calcium oxalate supersaturation was increased [90]. There was also decreased volume of urine and urinary citrate [90]. In a recent study, hyperoxaluria was seen in 74% of patients after RNY gastric bypass [91]. Even in the individuals who did not develop calculi, there was higher prevalence of hyperoxaluria.

Hyperoxaluria after bariatric surgery is most likely from fat malabsorption. Normally calcium conjugates with oxalate to form insoluble calcium oxalate which does not get absorbed. Post-bariatric surgery, patients cannot absorb fatty acids which then sequester the intestinal calcium. This would indirectly cause increased reabsorption of unbound oxalate and hence hyperoxaluria [92,93]. In addition, reduced bile salts absorption after bariatric procedures, increases their concentration in the colon which enhances colonic permeability to oxalate [94]. Therefore there is increased colonic oxalate absorption and subsequent renal excretion with stone formation. Crystalline deposition of calcium oxalate in the renal tubules leads to oxalate nephropathy [92,93]. The prognosis of oxalate nephropathy is poor and may lead to endstage renal disease. Sinha et al. reported that in 60 patients who had bariatric surgery, two developed chronic renal disease with biopsy-proven oxalate nephropathy [95]. Nelson et al. also reported two cases of oxalate nephropathy needing dialysis [96]. Nasr et al. suggested that oxalate nephropathy is an under-recognized complication of RNYGB and there is a higher risk in patients with pre-existing renal disease [97]. In a study including over 9000 patients, 7.65% of RNYGB patients were diagnosed with kidney stones compared with 4.63% of obese controls [98]. As a result, post-bariatric surgery patients had higher chances of requiring shock wave lithotripsy (1.75% versus 0.41%). Logistic regression analysis showed that gastric bypass surgery was a significant predictor of nephrolithiasis. Mole et al. described eight patients who underwent bariatric surgery and developed significant kidney disease due to oxalate nephropathy, three of whom had reversal of bypass prior to endstage renal failure [89].

Maintenance of a low oxalate and high calcium diet is effective in protecting post-gastric bypass patients from hyperoxaluria, nephrolithiasis and oxalate nephropathy [99]. Strict compliance with low fat diets is also very important. Development of renal impairment post-bariatric procedure may necessitate reversal of the bypass. However, to date, the evidence is not clear on whether reversal of gastric bypass would improve renal function, especially if oxalate nephropathy has set in. Patients with restrictive bariatric surgery are known to have a lower urinary oxalate excretion than with malabsorptive procedures. In a study comparing restrictive (sleeve = 4 and banding = 14) versus malabsorptive (gastric bypass = 54) surgery groups, the urinary oxalate excretion was significantly lower in the former during a two-month follow-up period [100]. Gastric banding was not associated with increased risk of kidney stones during a 5-year follow-up [101]. This finding was supported by Penniston [102], who reported that gastric banding was not a significant risk factor for nephrolithiasis. It is well known that RNYGB results in a more effective weight loss than gastric banding, but in a patient with renal impairment there is an argument to pursue a restrictive procedure to prevent risk of oxalate nephropathy in the long term.

OTHER RENAL EFFECTS OF BARIATRIC SURGERY

Persistent metabolic acidosis has been reported after jejunoileal bypass surgery. A Scandinavian study demonstrated the impaired capacity for acidification of urine, categorized as distal renal tubular acidosis [103]. Renal failure secondary to amyloidosis has been reported as a long-term sequela of jejunoileal bypass surgery [104]. Prolonged pneumoperitoneum produced during laparoscopic gastric bypass may cause intraoperative oliguria, but this is usually temporary and does not translate to impaired postoperative renal function [105]. Acute renal failure secondary to rhabdomyolysis is a commonly reported complication after bariatric surgery [106], a problem which is aggravated by the length of the surgical procedure and the size of the patient.

FUTURE RESEARCH

Prospective studies need to evaluate the ability of all types of bariatric surgery to reverse renal impairment in obese kidney disease patients. To date there are data available only after RNY gastric bypass. There is no doubt that there is increasing application of bariatric procedures in patients with chronic kidney disease, but we must keep in mind that this surgery in itself may cause kidney injury from hyperoxaluria in the long term. Further work needs to be done to compare the outcomes in obese chronic kidney disease patients, to determine what degree of renal failure can be suppressed or even reversed. If there is a significant decrease in dialysis requirements and the need for transplantation, then there may be an overall economic impact as well as overall improved survival. The correct timing of performing the bariatric procedure in transplant candidates also needs to be investigated.

References

[1] Deitel M. Overweight and obesity worldwide now estimated to involve 1.7 billion people. Obes Surg 2003;13:329—30.

[2] National Center for Health Statistics NHANES IV Report. Available at www.cdc.gov/nchs/product/pubs/pubd/hestats/obes/obese99.htm2002. [accessed 29.11.2004].

[3] Fontaine KR, Redden DT, Wang C, et al. Years of life lost due to obesity. JAMA 2003;289:187—93.

[4] Ogden CL, Flegal KM, Carroll MD, et al. Prevalence and trends in overweight among US children and adolescents, 1999—2000. JAMA 2002;288:1728—32.

[5] Flegal KM, Carroll MD, Ogden CL, et al. Prevalence and trends in obesity among US adults, 1999-2000. JAMA 2002;288:1723—7.

[6] Cope MB, Allison DB. Obesity: person and population. Obesity 2006;14(Suppl. 4):156S—9S.

[7] Day FR, Loos RJ. Developments in obesity genetics in the era of genome-wide association studies. J Nutrigenet Nutrigenomics 2011;4(4):222—38.

[8] Stunkard AJ, Sorensen TA, Hanis C, et al. An adoptive study of human obesity. New Engl J Med 1986;314:193—8.

[9] Vogler GP, Sorensen TI, Stunkard AJ, et al. Influences of genes and shared family environment on adult body mass index assessed in an adoption study by a comprehensive path model. Int J Obes Relat Metab Disord 1995;19:40—5.

[10] Stunkard AJ, Harris JR, Pedersen NL, et al. The body-mass index of twins who have been reared apart. N Engl J Med 1990;322:1483—7.

[11] Demaria EJ. Bariatric Surgery for morbid obesity. N Engl J Med 2007;24;356(21):2176—83.

[12] Brownson RC, Boehmer TK, Luke DA. Declining rates of physical activity in the United States: what are the contributors? Annu Rev Public Health 2005;26:421—43.

[13] Ledikwe JH, Blanck HM, Khan LK, et al. Dietary energy density is associated with energy intake and weight status in US adults. Am J Clin Nutr 2006;83:1362—8.

[14] van Gemert WG, Westerterp KR, van Acker BA, et al. Energy, substrate and protein metabolism in morbid obesity before, during and after massive weight loss. Int J Obes Relat Metab Disord 2000;24:711—8.

[15] Neary NM, Small CJ, Bloom SR. Gut and mind. Gut 2003;52:918—21.

[16] Jequier E. Leptin signaling, adiposity, and energy balance. Ann N Y Acad Sci 2002;967:379—88.

[17] Ahmed MH, Byrne CD. Metabolic syndrome, diabetes and CHD risk. In: Packard CJ, editor. The Year in Lipid Disorders. Oxford: Clinical Publishing; 2007. p. 3—26.

[18] Wong CY, O'Moore-Sullivan T, et al. Alterations of left ventricular myocardial characteristics associated with obesity. Circulation 2004;110:3081—7.

[19] Alpert MA. Obesity cardiomyopathy: pathophysiology and evolution of the clinical syndrome. Am J Med Sci 2001;321:225—36.

[20] Wang TJ, Parise H, Levy D, et al. Obesity and the risk of new-onset atrial fibrillation. JAMA 2004;292:2471—7.

[21] Huang B, Rodreiguez BL, Burchfiel CM, et al. Associations of adiposity with prevalent coronary heart disease among elderly men: the Honolulu Heart Program. Int J Obes Relat Metab Disord 1997;21:340—8.

[22] DeMaria EJ. Morbid Obesity. In: Greenfield's Surgery: Scientific Principles and Practice. 5th ed. Mulholland MW: Philadelphia: Lippincott Williams & Wilkins; 2010.

[23] Frey WC, Pilcher J. Obstructive sleep-related breathing disorders in patients evaluated for bariatric surgery. Obes Surg 2003;13:676—83.

[24] Fisher BL, Schauer P. Medical and surgical options in the treatment of severe obesity. Am J Surg 2002;184:9S—16S.

[25] NIH Technology Assessment Conference Panel. NIH conference: methods for voluntary weight loss and control. Ann Intern Med 1992;116:942—9.

[26] Stafford RS, Radley DC. National trends in anti-obesity medication use. Arch Int Med 2003;163:1046—50.

[27] Hollander P. Orlistat in the treatment of obesity. Prim Care 2003;30(2):427—40.

[28] Gastrointestinal surgery for severe obesity: National Institutes of Health Consensus Development Conference Statement. Am J Clin Nutr 1992;55(Suppl. 2):615S—9S.

[29] Robinson MK. Surgical treatment of obesity — weighing the facts. NEJM 2009;361:520—1.

[30] Brethauer SA, Hammel JP, Schauer PR. Systematic review of sleeve gastrectomy as staging and primary bariatric procedure. Surg Obes Relat Dis 2009;5:469—75.

[31] Milone L, Strong V, Gagner M. Laparoscopic sleeve gastrectomy is superior to endoscopic intragastric balloon as a first stage procedure for super-obese patients. Obes Surg 2005;15:612—7.

[32] DeMaria EJ, Schauer P, Patterson E, et al. The optimal surgical management of the super-obese patient: The debate. Presented at the annual meeting of the Society of American Gastrointestinal and Endoscopic Surgeons, Hollywood, Florida, USA, April 13—16, 2005. Surg Innov. 2005;12:107—121.

[33] Colquitt J, Clegg A, Loveman E, Royle P, Sidhu MK. Surgery for morbid obesity. Cochrane Database Syst Rev 2005;4: CD003641.

[34] Buchwald H, Avidor Y, Braunwald E, et al. Bariatric surgery: a systematic review and meta-analysis. JAMA 2004;292:1724—37. [Erratum, JAMA 2005;293:1728.].

[35] Maggard MA, Shugarman LR, Suttorp M, et al. Meta-analysis: surgical treatment of obesity. Ann Intern Med 2005;142:547—59.

[36] Sjostrom L, Lindroos AK, Peltonen M, et al. Lifestyle, diabetes, and cardiovascular risk factors 10 years after bariatric surgery. N Engl J Med 2004;351:2683—93.

[37] Flum DR, Dellinger EP. Impact of gastric bypass operation on survival: a population-based analysis. J Am Coll Surg 2004;199:543—51.

[38] Pratt GM, McLees B, Pories WJ. The ASBS Bariatric Surgery Centers of Excellence program: a blueprint for quality improvement. Surg Obes Relat Dis 2006;2:497—503.

[39] Flum DR, Salem L, Elrod JA, Dellinger EP, Cheadle A, Chan L. Early mortality among Medicare beneficiaries undergoing bariatric surgical procedures. JAMA 2005;294:1903—8.

[40] The Longitudinal Assessment of Bariatric Surgery (LABS) Consortium. Perioperative safety in the longitudinal assessment of bariatric surgery. N Engl J Med 2009;361:445—54.

[41] Gupta P, Franck C, Miller WJ, Gupta H, Forse RA. Development and validation of a bariatric surgery morbidity risk calculator using the prospective, multicenter NSQIP dataset. Journal of the American College f Surgeons 2011;212:301—9.

[42] Istfan N, Anderson W, Apovian C, Forse RA. Pre-operative weight gain increases the risk of gastric bypass surgery. surgery for obesity and related diseases 2011;7(2):157—64.

[43] Stocker DJ. Management of the bariatric surgery patient. Endocrinol Metab Clin North Am 2003;32:437—57.

[44] McMahon MM, Sarr MG, Clark MM, et al. Clinical management after bariatric surgery: value of a multidisciplinary approach. Mayo Clin Proc 2006;81(Suppl. 10):S34—45.

[45] Coresh J, Selvin E, Stevens LA, et al. Prevalence of chronic kidney disease in the United States. JAMA 2007;298:2038–47.

[46] Wahba IM, Mak RH. Obesity and obesity-initiated metabolic syndrome: mechanistic links to chronic kidney disease. Clin J Am Soc Nephrol 2007;2(3):550–62.

[47] Wang Y, Chen X, Song Y, et al. Association between obesity and kidney disease: a systematic review and meta-analysis. Kidney Int 2008;73(1):19–33.

[48] Hu FB, Willett WC, Li T, et al. Adiposity as compared with physical activity in predicting mortality among women. N Engl J Med 2004;351(26):2694–703.

[49] Yan LL, Daviglus ML, Liu K, et al. Midlife body mass index and hospitalization and mortality in older age. JAMA 2006;295(2):190–8.

[50] Fox CS. Predictors of new-onset kidney disease in a communitybased population. JAMA 2004;291(7):844–50.

[51] Hsu CY, Iribarren C, McCulloch CE, et al. Risk factors for endstage renal disease: 25-year follow-up. Arch Intern Med 2009;169(4):342–50.

[52] Wesson DE, Kurtzman NA, Frommer JP. Massive obesity and nephritic proteinuria with a normal renal biopsy. Nephron 1985;40:235–7.

[53] Metcalf P, Baker J, Scott A, et al. Albuminuria in people at least 40 years old: effect of obesity, hypertension, and hyperlipidemia. Clin Chem. 1992;38(9):1802–8.

[54] Wisse BE. The inflammatory syndrome: the role of adipose tissue cytokines in metabolic disorders linked to obesity. J Am Soc Nephrol 2004;15(11):2792–800.

[55] Wolf G, Hamann A, Han DC, et al. Leptin stimulates proliferation and TGF-beta expression in renal glomerular endothelial cells: potential role in glomerulosclerosis. Kidney Int 1999;56(3):860–72.

[56] Serradeil-Le Gal C, Raufaste D, Brossard G, et al. Characterization and localization of leptin receptors in the rat kidney. FEBS Lett. 1997;404(2–3):185–91.

[57] Zhang XL, Topley N, Ito T, et al. Interleukin-6 regulation of transforming growth factor (TGF)-beta receptor compartmentalization and turnover enhances TGF-beta1 signaling. J Biol Chem. 2005;280(13):12239–45.

[58] Montani JP, Antic V, Yang Z, et al. Pathways from obesity to hypertension: from the perspective of a vicious triangle. Int J Obes Relat Metab Disord 2002;26(Suppl. 2):S28–38.

[59] Lastra G, Manrique C, Sowers JR. Obesity, cardiometabolic syndrome, and chronic kidney disease: the weight of the evidence. Adv Chronic Kidney Dis 2006;13:365–73.

[60] Ribstein J, Halimi JM, du Cailar G, et al. Renal characteristics and effect of angiotensin suppression in oral contraceptive users. Hypertension 1999;33(1):90–5.

[61] Agnani S, Vachharajani VT, Gupta R, et al. Does treating obesity stabilize chronic kidney disease? BMC Nephrol 2005;6:7.

[62] Cignarelli M, Lamacchia O. Obesity and kidney disease. Nutr Metab Cardiovasc Dis 2007;17:757–62.

[63] Navaneethan SD, Yehnert H. Bariatric surgery and progression of chronic kidney disease. Surg Obes Relat Dis 2009;5:662–5.

[64] Navarro-Díaz M, Serra A, Romero R, et al. Effect of drastic weight loss after bariatric surgery on renal parameters in extremely obese patients: long-term follow-up. J Am Soc Nephrol 2006;17(12 Suppl. 3):S213–7.

[65] Alexander JW, Goodman HR, Hawver LR, et al. Improvement and stabilization of chronic kidney disease after gastric bypass. Surg Obes Relat Dis 2009;5(2):237–41.

[66] Agrawal V, Khan I, Rai B, et al. The effect of weight loss after bariatric surgery on albuminuria. Clin Nephrol 2008;70:194–202.

[67] Cuda SP, Chung MH, Denunzio TM, et al. Reduction of proteinuria after gastric bypass surgery: case presentation and management. Surg Obes Relat Dis 2005;1(1):64–6.

[68] Izzedine H, Coupaye M, Reach I, et al. Gastric bypass and resolution of proteinuria in an obese diabetic patient. Diabet Med 2005;22(12):1761–2.

[69] Friedman AN, Miskulin DC, Rosenberg IH, Levey AS. Demographics and trends in overweight and obesity in patients at time of kidney transplantation. Am J Kidney Dis 2003;41:480–7.

[70] Choban PS, Flancbaum L. The impact of obesity on surgical outcome: a review. J Am Coll Surg 1997;185:593–603.

[71] Pirsch JD, Armbrust MJ, Knechtle SJ, et al. Obesity as a risk factor following renal transplantation. Transplantation 1995;59:631.

[72] Holley JL, Shapiro R, Lopatin WB, Tzakis AG, Hakala TR, Starzl TE. Obesity as a risk factor following cadaveric renal transplantation. Transplantation 1990;49:387–9.

[73] Johnson CP, Kuhn EM, Hariharan S, Hartz AJ, Roza AM, Adams MB. Pre-transplant identification of risk factors that adversely affect length of stay and charges for renal transplantation. Clin Transplant 1999;13:168–75.

[74] Gore JL, Pham PT, Danovitch GM, et al. Obesity and outcome following renal transplantation. Am J Transplant 2006;6:357–63.

[75] Blumke M, Keller E, Eble F, Nausner M, Kriste G. Obesity in kidney transplant patients as a risk factor. Transplant Proc 1993;25:2618.

[76] El-Agroudy AE, Wafa EW, Gheith OE, et al. Weight gain after renal transplantation is a risk factor for patient and graft outcome. Transplantation 2004;77(9):1381–5.

[77] Meier-Kriesche HU, Arndorfer JA, Kaplan B. The impact of body mass index on renal transplant outcomes: a significant independent risk factor for graft failure and patient death. Transplantation 2002;73(1):70–4.

[78] Gore JL. Obesity and renal transplantation: is bariatric surgery the answer? Transplantation 2009;87(8):1115.

[79] Modanlou KA, Muthyala U, Xiao HL, et al. Bariatric surgery among kidney transplant candidates and recipients: analysis of the United States Renal Data System and Literature Review. Transplantation 2009;87(8):1167–73.

[80] Gupta PK, Gupta H, Miller WJ, Forse RA. Determinants of resource utlization in laparoscopic roux-en-y gastric bypass" a multicenter analysis of 6322 patients. Surgical Endoscopy 2011;25(8):2613–25.

[81] Takata MC, Campos GM, Ciovica R, et al. Laparoscopic bariatric surgery improves candidacy in morbidly obese patients awaiting transplantation. Surg Obes Relat Dis 2008;4(2):159–64.

[82] Szomstein S, Rojas R, Rosenthal RJ. Outcomes of laparoscopic bariatric surgery after renal transplant. Obes Surg 2009;20(3):383–5.

[83] Obligado SH, Goldfarb DS. The association of nephrolithiasis with hypertension and obesity: a review. Am J Hypertens 2008;21:257–64.

[84] Negri AL, Spivacow FR, Del Valle EE, et al. Role of overweight and oesity on the urinary excretion of promoters and inhibitors of stone formation in stone formers. Urol Res 2008;36:303–7.

[85] Taylor EN, Stampfer MJ, Curhan GC. Obesity, weight gain, and the risk of kidney stones. JAMA 2005;293:455–62.

[86] Semins MJ, Shore AD, Makary MA, et al. The association of increasing body mass index and kidney stone disease. J Urol 2009;183(2):571–5.

[87] Lee SC, Kim YJ, Kim TH, et al. Impact of obesity in patients with urolithiasis and its prognostic usefulness in stone recurrence. J Urol 2008;179:570–4.

[88] Requarth JA, Burchard KW, Colacchio TA, et al. Long-term morbidity following jejunoileal bypass. The continuing potential need for surgical reversal. Arch Surg 1995;130(3):318–25.

[89] Mole DR, Tomson CR, Mortensen N, et al. Renal complications of jejuno-ileal bypass for obesity. QJM 2001;94(2):69—77.

[90] Park AM, Storm DW, Fulmer BR, et al. A prospective study of risk factors for nephrolithiasis after Roux-en-Y gastric bypass surgery. J Urol 2009;182:2334—9.

[91] Patel BN, Passman CM, Fernandez A, et al. Prevalence of hyperoxaluria after bariatric surgery. J Urol 2009;181:161—6.

[92] Brenner BM, Garcia DL, Anderson S. Glomeruli and blood pressure. Less of one, more the other? Am J Hypertens 1988;1:335—79.

[93] Hales CN, Barker DJ. The thrifty phenotype hypothesis. Br Med Bull 2001;60:5—20.

[94] Maalouf NM, Tondapu P, Guth ES, et al. Hypocitraturia and hyperoxaluria after Roux-en-Y gastric bypass surgery. J Urol 2010;183(3):1026—30.

[95] Sinha MK, Collazo-Clavell ML, Rule A, et al. Hyperoxaluric nephrolithiasis is a complication of Roux-en-Y gastric bypass surgery. Kidney Int 2007;72:100—7.

[96] Nelson WK, Houghton SG, Milliner DS, et al. Enteric hyperoxaluria, nephrolithiasis, and oxalate nephropathy: potentially serious and unappreciated complications of Roux-en-Y gastric bypass. Surg Obes Relat Dis 2005;1:481—5.

[97] Nasr SH, D'Agati VD, Said SM, et al. Oxalate nephropathy complicating Roux-en-Y gastric bypass: an underrecognized cause of irreversible renal failure. Clin J Am Soc Nephrol 2008;3:1676—83.

[98] Matlaga BR, Shore AD, Magnuson T, et al. Effect of gastric bypass surgery on kidney stone disease. J Urol 2009;181:2573—7.

[99] Whitson JM, Stackhouse GB, Stoller ML. Hyperoxaluria after modern bariatric surgery: case series and literature review. Int Urol Nephrol 2010;42(2):369—74.

[100] Semins MJ, Asplin JR, Steele K, et al. The effect of restrictive bariatric surgery on urinary stone risk factors. Urology 2010;76(4):826—9.

[101] Semins MJ, Matlaga BR, Shore AD, et al. The effect of gastric banding on kidney stone disease. Urology 2009;74(4):746—9.

[102] Penniston KL, Kaplon DM, Gould JC, et al. Gastric band placement for obesity is not associated with increased urinary risk of urolithiasis compared to bypass. J Urol 2009;182(5):2340—6.

[103] Schaffalitzky de Muckadell OB, Ladefoged J, Thorup J. Renal tubular acidosis secondary to jejunoileal bypass for morbid obesity. Scand J Gastroenterol 1985;20:823—8.

[104] Korzets Z, Smorjik Y, Zahavi T, et al. Renal AA amyloidosis — a long term sequela of jejuno-ileal bypass. Nephrol Dial Transplant 1998;13:1843—5.

[105] Nguyen NT, Perez RV, Fleming N, et al. Effect of prolonged pneumoperitoneum on intraoperative urine output during laparoscopic gastric bypass. J Am Coll Surg 2002;195:476—83.

[106] de Oliveira LD, Diniz MT, de Fátima HS, Diniz M, et al. Rhabdomyolysis after bariatric surgery by Roux-en-Y gastric bypass: a prospective study. Obes Surg 2009;19:1102—7.

31

Nutritional and Metabolic Management of the Diabetic Patient with Chronic Kidney Disease and Chronic Renal Failure

Mark E. Williams, Robert Stanton

Harvard Medical School, Joslin Diabetes Center, Boston, MA, USA

INTRODUCTION

Diabetes mellitus (DM) continues to be the single largest contributor to the growing prevalence of chronic kidney disease (CKD) worldwide. Diabetic nephropathy affects 10—20% of individuals with DM, the majority of whom have type 2 diabetes. While the risk of incident ESRD attributed to diabetes appears to have stabilized in the US and elsewhere, the incidence of DM as well as its overall prevalence continue to increase. In the U.S., 23% of all adults 60 years and older have DM [1]. It is estimated that the worldwide prevalence of DM will reach about 450 million people by the year 2030 [2].

Albuminuria and estimated glomerular filtration rate (eGFR) are each predictors of ESRD and mortality in diabetic CKD. Because the combination of eGFR and albuminuria predicts outcomes better than either measure alone [3], risk assessment based on CKD staging level is increasingly including albuminuria to add prognostic information. It is clear that early and later phases of diabetic CKD may respond differently to similar therapeutic strategies. Multiple detection, prevention, and interventional studies have resulted in several treatment strategies of proven benefit. Standard guideline-based therapy for diabetic CKD consists of tight glycemic control, intensive management of hypertension, and aggressive use of RAS blockade. Randomized trials have consistently demonstrated the benefit of RAS blockade (particularly with ACEI and ARBs) in slowing progression of CKD in both type 1 and type 2 DM.

Nonetheless, the limitations of RAS blockade in diabetic CKD are evident, as the decline in kidney function despite treatment remains higher than that expected due to aging [4]. Meanwhile, concerns remain about the limitations of tight glycemic control, the use of blockade with combinations of RAS medicines, and disappointing development of newer therapies. With or without standard therapy, significant numbers of patients with DM will continue to progress through the stages of CKD. As diabetic CKD worsens, it becomes more of a systemic disease. When combined, DM and CKD pose a double threat in terms of nutritional and metabolic abnormalities. This chapter presents the pathogenesis and clinical consequences of disorders of nutrition and metabolism in the diabetic CKD patient.

GLUCOSE/INSULIN HOMEOSTASIS

Insulin resistance and glucose intolerance are well-recognized features in patients with CKD.

The cellular mechanisms by which uremia interferes with insulin actions on glucose transport (Figure 31.1) in target tissues remain uncertain. Glucose transport is one of the major activities of insulin and is believed to be rate-limiting for glucose uptake in peripheral tissues. The transport of glucose into cells is mediated by specific glucose transporter proteins. Insulin actions at the cellular level are complex, but are known to include activation of intrinsic tyrosine kinase activities found in the receptor intracellular beta-subunit portion, intracellular responses including generation of messengers for insulin, interiorization of the receptor-insulin complex within the cell, translocation of hexose transporter units into the plasma membrane from intracellular storage sites, and the downstream metabolic effects of the hormone [5].

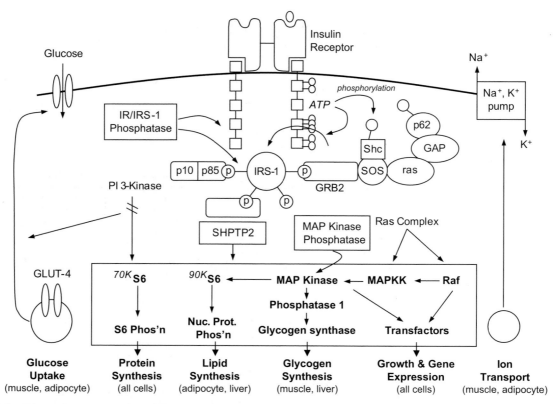

FIGURE 31.1 Schematic representation of the tetrameric insulin receptor and activation of insulin-triggered cellular events in responsive tissues. In activating cellular glucose transport and disposal pathways, insulin first binds to the alpha-subunit of its receptor. Complex effects executed through the insulin signaling pathways and leading to the metabolic actions of insulin are shown.

Even nondiabetic CKD patients may have mild fasting hyperglycemia and decreased glucose tolerance [6]. In fact, in a cross-sectional analysis of participants in the Third National Health and Nutrition Examination Survey, Chen et al. reported that insulin resistance estimated by the homeostasis model assessment (HOMA) was associated with an increased risk of having CKD [7]. Contributing factors to the abnormalities in glucose homeostasis in people with kidney impairment are shown in Figure 31.2. Abnormal insulin metabolism involves reduction in renal insulin clearance which is typically present in advanced CKD, stages 4 and 5 [8]. Some evidence suggests that a reduction in pancreatic insulin secretion also occurs, is related to hyperparathyroidism and vitamin D deficiency, and improves with correction of these disorders [9–10]. In a recent clinical report of 120 CKD stage 2–3 patients (of whom 19 were being treated for diabetes), 42% suffered from vitamin D insufficiency and 41% were moderately deficient [11]. Research on the metabolic profiles of pancreatic islets during progression of chronic renal failure has suggested that glucose-induced insulin secretion is impaired because of alterations in closure of ATP-dependent potassium channels and reduction in glucose-induced calcium signaling [12]. Other recent research has explored the mechanisms and clinical

significance of insulin resistance in CKD. It is commonly understood that insulin resistance is a characteristic feature of uremia, regardless of the cause of renal disease. In insulin-resistant states, insulin-stimulated cellular glucose uptake is impaired; such other insulin actions as suppression of glycogenolysis, gluconeogenesis, lipolysis and fatty acid release, protein catabolism, and cellular potassium and phosphate uptake, may not be similarly impaired [13].

A recent cross-sectional study of 128 diabetic patients from India assessed the degree of insulin resistance (IR) in those with different stages of diabetic kidney disease (microalbuminuria, macroalbuminuria) as compared to those with normoalbuminuria [14]. Insulin resistance was calculated using the HOMA method. There was no significant difference between the study groups with regard to age, body mass index, duration of diabetes, or glycemic control. Mean HOMA IR increased significantly with worsening renal disease (p < 0.0001). In contrast, when 73 nondiabetic CKD patients were evaluated for insulin resistance, HOMA IR did not differ in patients with or without a renal ESRD endpoint, and even after over 24 months of follow-up, the GFR level was not associated with the degree of insulin resistance [15]. In reality, insulin resistance is somewhat variable in kidney disease, as it is in such

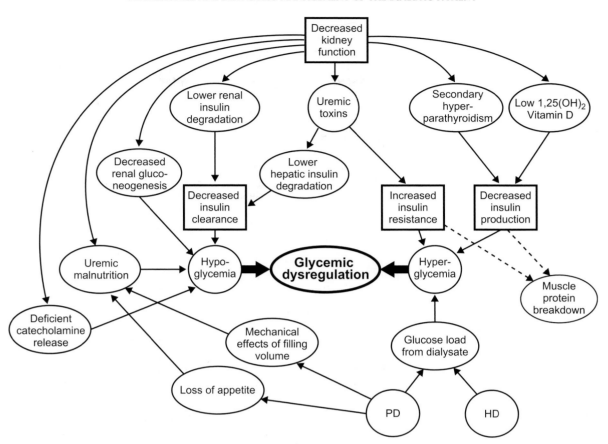

FIGURE 31.2 Overview of glucose/insulin homeostasis in chronic kidney disease/ESRD. Disturbances of glucose metabolism include insulin resistance and glucose intolerance. Several factors contribute to hypoglycemia, which may coexist with hyperglycemia. Abbreviations: PD, peritoneal dialysis; HD, hemodialysis. *(Adapted from Ref [6].)*

other conditions as type 2 diabetes, obesity, or even in normal subjects [16]. Numerous studies suggest that insulin resistance in uremia appears to be restricted to defects in glucose uptake and muscle protein anabolism. The ability of insulin to stimulate peripheral glucose disposal by muscle and adipose tissue is markedly impaired, while hepatic glucose uptake is normal and hepatic glucose production is suppressible in uremia [17]. At least two other insulin-mediated effects, its anti-proteolytic action and translocation of potassium into cells, are not impaired in advanced renal failure [17–18].

Insulin resistance in uremia is an acquired defect in the insulin receptor signaling pathway. Stimulation of glucose transport is one of the major activities of insulin and is believed to be rate-limiting for glucose uptake in peripheral tissues [19]. Central to the biologic actions of insulin, insulin signaling occurs when insulin binds to its receptor, a tyrosine kinase, which then phosphory-lates insulin receptor substrates such as IRS1 [20]. Recruitment of multiple downstream targets such as glycogen synthase protein kinase C, endothelial nitric oxide synthase (eNOS), and others, elicit wide-ranging effects including enhancement of glucose uptake,

glycogenesis, lipogenesis and cellular proliferation [21]. In muscle and adipose tissue, insulin stimulates glucose uptake by promoting translocation of an intra-cellular pool of glucose transporters to the plasma membrane. Physiological studies have shown that kidney tissues are also responsive to insulin. Moreover, insulin resistance in the glomerulus is similar to the insulin resistance found in the endothelium of other vascular tissues. This resistance could contribute to the initiation and progression of glomerular lesions in diabetes, in combination with the abnormal pathophys-iology in the mesangial cells and podocytes [22]. Insulin resistance appears to involve sites distal to the insulin receptor (Figure 31.2), from the generation of intracel-lular messengers for insulin [23] to glucose transport to effects of insulin on one of the intracellular enzymes involved in glucose metabolism itself [24].

The mechanism(s) behind insulin resistance in CKD patients are incompletely understood. The improvement in insulin sensitivity associated with dialysis suggests a role for uremic toxins [25–26]. Recent data suggest that alterations in metabolism with CKD may alter adipose tissue secretion patterns independently of obesity. Released adipokines then become an important source of pro-inflammatory molecules which cause insulin resistance [27]. Plasma adinopectin levels are inversely associated with kidney function, and increased adinopectin concentrations may contribute to insulin resistance [28]. Production of proinflammatory molecules in adipose tissue may also be modulated by oxidative stress [29]. Yet another factor, erythropoietin deficiency, might contribute to insulin resistance. This possibility was suggested by a recent study that showed recombinant erythropoietin-treated hemodialysis patients had lower mean insulin levels and (HOMA IR) levels than those not treated with erythropoietin [30].

The clinical relevance of insulin resistance in the CKD patient is not fully understood. Insulin resistance may contribute to protein-energy wasting, atherosclerosis, and cardiovascular complications in CKD/ESRD patients. One important consequence of insulin resistance is protein-energy wasting [31]. Dialysis patients even without diabetes mellitus or obesity have measurable insulin resistance associated with increased muscle protein breakdown. Muscle protein breakdown in renal failure is at least partly mediated through the ubiquitin-proteasome pathway and is related to suppression of phosphatidylinositol-3 kinase [32,33]. A recent report examined the relationship between HOMA and fasting whole-body and skeletal muscle protein turnover to determine mean skeletal muscle protein synthesis, breakdown, and net balance in nondiabetic chronic hemodialysis patients [34]. An inverse relationship between net skeletal muscle protein balance and HOMA was noted.

Progress in understanding the development of insulin resistance in the kidney was recently reported by Mima et al. [22]. These investigators conducted the first comparative analysis of insulin signaling and cellular actions involving the renal glomerulus and tubules; these processes were evaluated in diabetic, insulin-resistant, and control states. It is known that in diabetes, the actions of insulin on the glomerulus may be blunted [21]. After insulin binds to its receptor, downstream targets recruited include Akt, glycogen synthase kinase 3, Ras, ERK, and protein kinase C. Activation of these targets elicit wide-ranging metabolic effects. Mima et al. [22] characterized dysfunctional insulin signaling in glomeruli and tubules of diabetic and insulin-resistant animals and suggested that some of these alterations may contribute to diabetic glomerulopathy.

Increased attention has been given recently to the contribution of the kidneys to glucose homeostasis through processes that include gluconeogenesis and glucose filtration and resorption [35]. Normally, up to 180 grams of glucose may be filtered each day by the glomerulus, and nearly all of this glucose is reabsorbed in the proximal tubule. This resorption is mediated as secondary active transport through two sodium-dependent glucose transporter (SGLT) proteins. The majority of glucose resorption occurs through sodium D: glucose D-transporter 2 (SGLT2), present in the S1 segment of the proximal tubule [36]. Increased reabsorption of glucose by the kidneys occurs in type 2 diabetes and is a target of recently developed hypoglycemic agents. Various glucoside compounds have been synthesized that have a high affinity for SGLT2 [37]. Because of their ability to prevent glucose reabsorption and increase urinary glucose excretion, SGLT2 inhibitors are being evaluated as an insulin-independent treatment for diabetes [38]. Available information indicates that the administration of SGLT2 inhibitors can induce glucosuria and improve glycemic control in patients with type 2 diabetes without the risk of inducing severe hypoglycemia [39].

VALUE OF GLYCEMIC CONTROL, AND ITS DETERMINATION IN CKD

The currently recommended hemoglobin A1c (HbA1c) targets in the setting of CKD are identical to those for the general diabetic population; i.e., <7% regardless of the absence or presence of CKD [40]. Recent observational studies have been consistent in calling into question this approach, while providing somewhat contrasting results and significant methodological differences [41−43]. These studies indicate that the overall relationship between glycemic control and survival outcomes are weaker in the presence of ESRD (Figure 31.3). In particular, higher HgA1c targets may be preferable in patients with higher levels of comorbidity [44].

HbA1c, used in these observational studies, remains the most widely used index of glycemic control in the diabetic population. For two decades, since the DCCT [45] and UKPDS [46] demonstrated that hemoglobin A1c levels strongly predict the risk of microvascular complications associated with type 1 and type 2 diabetes mellitus, respectively, the glycohemoglobin level has been the primary basis of diabetes management. Indeed, the strength of the association between glycemic control and clinical outcomes is reliant on the relationship between hyperglycemic and elevated Hgb A1c levels. It has recently been proposed that Hgb A1c can be used to report estimated average serum glucose levels (eAG) [47]. Hemoglobin A1c is a minor component of hemoglobin, comprising about 4% of total hemoglobin in normal adult erythrocytes. The hemoglobin A1c level as a marker of hyperglycemia reflects average blood glucose concentration over roughly the three preceding months [48]. Good correlation between Hgb A1c and

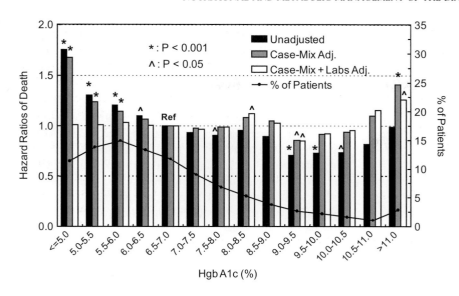

FIGURE 31.3 Relation of glycemic control and hemodialysis survival among 24,875 hemodialysis patients with follow-up of three years, using time-dependent survival models with repeated measures. Data were collected at baseline and every quarter to a maximum of 3 years' follow-up. Extremes of glycemia were weakly associated with survival in the study population. *(Ref. [41].)*

blood glucose levels in patients with preserved kidney function has been reported in the Diabetes Control and Complications Trial [45] and the A1c-Derived Average Glucose (ADAG) Study [49]. The American Diabetes Association recommends using point-of-care A1c testing to guide management with a goal of lowering A1c to below 7% [2].

However, its unreliability has been recognized in a number of clinical conditions [50], particularly hematologic diseases involving anemia or hemolysis, and has been attributed to the analytical, biological, and clinical variability associated with HbA1c. Analytical variability has resolved with introduction of newer assay methods [51]. Nonetheless, biological and clinical variability of HbA1c continue to limit its application to individual patients, even in the general diabetic population. One source of the variability is differential glycation rates, which appear to vary significantly among individuals. The relationship between HgA1c and time-averaged serum glucose levels also varies across racial backgrounds [50].

More recently, discordance from other measures of glycemic control in clinical studies [52] have raised concerns about the validity of A1c in predicting outcomes in the setting of advanced CKD/ESRD. The KDOQI guidelines for diabetic kidney disease acknowledge that data for validating methods for monitoring glycemia in kidney impairment are severely lacking [40]. For example, a recent USRDS report indicated that the prevalence of patients with A1c levels over the 7% target was 63% for stages 1—2 CKD, but fell to 46% in stages 3-4 CKD [53], in whom factors such as anemia, typically due to a reduced erythrocyte life span, administration of erythropoietin, blood transfusions and metabolic acidosis, could affect the reliability of the A1c results [54]. In our large national ESRD database

analysis, the mean hemoglobin A1c value was only 6.77%, and values over 7.0% were found in only 35% of patients [41]. Unlike the high performance liquid chromatography assay previously used in routine laboratory A1c testing, the contemporary immunoturbidimetric assay methodology is not influenced by high serum urea nitrogen levels. Nonetheless, A1c may not optimally represent the glycemic state in advanced kidney disease due to the unique changes in physiology. The most cited influences on A1c variability in kidney patients are anemia and the use of erythrocyte stimulating agents (ESAs). HbA1c indicates the percentage of circulating hemoglobin that has chemically reacted with glucose. Reduced erythrocyte survival in ESRD would be expected to lower hemoglobin A1c levels by reducing the time for exposure to ambient glucose [55]. In addition, the widespread use of ESAs increases the proportion of immature red blood cells in the circulation, with less propensity for glycosylation. One report described a false lowering of A1c with both erythropoietin and darbopoietin analogues in a single patient [56]. As a result, HbA1c levels tend to be lower in diabetic patients with kidney impairment or who are undergoing renal replacement therapy [57]. Peacock et al. measured levels of glycated hemoglobin (HbA1c) and glycated albumin in 307 patients with diabetes, of whom 258 were undergoing maintenance hemodialysis and the remainder were without overt kidney disease [57]. In patients undergoing maintenance hemodialysis, the ratio of glycated albumin to HbA1c were higher, suggesting that the HbA1c significantly underestimated serum glucose levels. A recent study by Chen et al. in patients with CKD stages 3 and 4 reported that the mean measured serum glucose levels were about 5—10% higher than an estimated average glucose calculated from the same HbA1c, in comparison to the serum glucose in patients with normal kidney function [58]. These findings indicate that the HbA1c underestimates mean blood glucose levels in CKD. A recent small study contrasted four-day continuous serum glucose monitoring (CGMS) in type 2 diabetic patients undergoing maintenance hemodialysis (N = 19) with a larger group of type 2 diabetic patients without nephropathy (N = 39) [59]. In all patients, the CGMS results and glucose concentrations according to the glucose meter were similar. Glycated hemoglobin and mean glucose concentrations were strongly correlated in the nondialysis group (r = .71), but were weakly correlated in those undergoing hemodialysis (r = .47). Hemodialysis patients were receiving erythropoiesis stimulating agents, and had lower hemoglobin levels than the comparator group (11.6 vs. 13.6 g/dL, p < .0001). These data also indicate that CGMS is a potential tool for understanding changes in glucose homeostasis related to the dialysis procedure itself [60].

Ongoing identification of sources of variability in HbA1c levels have raised particular concern with regard to relying on this test as the sole measure of glycemia in the diabetic kidney disease population. Fructosamine is increasingly available for the monitoring of diabetes treatment, particularly for short-term control, but does not correlate strongly with fasting serum glucose levels [50], and the need to correct values for total protein or albumin concentrations remains unresolved [61]. Similar to the HbA1c findings, the study by Chen et al. reported that fructosamine levels were also lower than expected for the same glucose concentration in CKD patients, as compared to patients with normal kidney function [58]. Relative to HbA1c, glycated albumin (GA) may more accurately reflect glycemic control in diabetic patients with CKD/ESRD, where HbA1c is particularly unreliable. Albumin undergoes glycation similarly to hemoglobin, and accounts for most of the serum glycated proteins. Because the turnover of serum albumin is shorter, (a half-life of approximately 20 days), it reflects a shorter glucose exposure and a potentially more sensitive metric of glycemia. Although not influenced by dialysis or the age or lifespan of erythrocytes, anemia, or erythropoietin, its precision may be limited in states of abnormal protein turnover, such as from inflammation, hypercatabolic states, peritoneal dialysis, proteinuria, albumin infusions, or gastrointestinal protein losses. Glycated albumin reflects glycemic control for only the 1–2 weeks prior to obtaining the sample [62]. In patients with nephrotic proteinuria, glycated albumin levels may be falsely reduced. Confounders in glycated albumin testing include obesity, smoking, and hyperuricemia, all of which are prevalent in the diabetic CKD population [50]. The case for glycated albumin has been bolstered by an improved assay that is unaffected by changes in serum

albumin. It has also been suggested that glycated albumin in vivo has biologic properties that could actually contribute to the pathogenesis of diabetic vascular or other complications [63], as an Amadori-modified reaction product capable of inducing oxidative stress and enhance pro-inflammatory endothelial responses in the vessel wall. Glycated albumin can be measured using a bromocresol purple method, and calculated as the percentage relative to total albumin. A reference range of about 12% has been determined for nondiabetic American individuals with normal kidney function [57], with a somewhat wider reference interval compared to the more compressed range of measured values for HbA1c.

Glycated albumin was deemed superior to A1c in two recent studies of kidney patients [62–63]. In a large Japanese study of 538 maintenance hemodialysis patients with type 2 diabetes, 828 hemodialysis patients without diabetes, and 365 diabetic patients without significant kidney impairment, Inaba et al. [63] demonstrated significantly lower HgA1c levels relative to blood glucose or to glycated albumin levels in patients undergoing chronic dialysis, as compared to those without kidney impairment. The ratio of glycated albumin to HbA1c (with a previously reported ratio of approximately 3.0), was 2.93 in patients without CKD, and 3.81 in those undergoing chronic dialysis. HbA1c levels were also higher in patients not treated with ESAs. Glycated albumin levels were affected by glucose but not serum albumin levels. In a subsequent US study, the glycated albumin/HbA1c ratio was also significantly higher in ESRD patients (2.72 vs. 2.07) [57]. Analysis of evidence linking serum glycated albumin to diabetic ESRD outcomes is now emerging. Recently, Freedman et al. [64] determined the association between glycated albumin, HgbA1c, and serum glucose levels with outcomes (hospitalization, survival) in diabetic dialysis patients (90% hemodialysis) (Figure 31.4). Quarterly serum glycated albumin levels were measured for up to 2.3 years in 444 prevalent patients. Time-dependent analyses allowed comparisons with available HbA1c and monthly random serum glucose levels. Mean (SD) serum glycated albumin was 21.5 ± 6% and HbA1c was 6.9 ± 1.6%. Increasing glycated albumin, but not HbA1c or serum glucose concentrations, were predictive of hospitalization and survival.

HYPOGLYCEMIA

Increasing attention is being given to the risks of hypoglycemia (<70 mg%) in the diabetic CKD/ESRD population. The American Diabetes Association recommends a goal HbA1c of <7.0% or as close to normal and as safely as possible without unacceptable

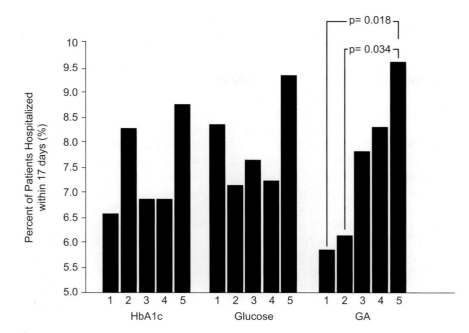

FIGURE 31.4 Relationship between longitudinal measurements of glycated albumin levels and hospitalization rates within 17 days of the measurement in 444 patients with ESRD and diabetes. Higher glycated albumin rates were increased hospitalization and also with poorer survival (not shown). *(Ref. [64].)*

hypoglycemia [2]. However, diabetes itself is characterized by acute glucose fluctuations and general glycemic variability. Therefore, the regimens used for serum glucose control should be associated with a low risk of hypoglycemia. However, with increasing pressure to achieve tight glycemic control targets, hypoglycemia, in many cases iatrogenic, is becoming more prevalent. In general, use of insulin secretagogues, missed meals, advanced age, duration of diabetes, and unawareness of hypoglycemia are factors which increase the risk of hypoglycemia [65]. Although hypoglycemia is associated with more intensive glycemic therapy and causes adverse clinical outcomes in patients with diabetes, published reviews on glycemic control in diabetic CKD patients typically include only token mention of hypoglycemia [6]. Increasing attention is being given to the risks of hypoglycemia (below the fasting reference range of about 70 mg/dL) in the diabetic CKD/ESRD population. The altered glucose metabolism in CKD patients poses not only a problem for blood glucose control, but also increases the risk of hypoglycemia, which may occur in both diabetic and nondiabetic CKD patients, and which then becomes a deterrent to achieving glycemic control at current target levels for patients with diabetes. The greatest risk of harm is in patients with both CKD and diabetes, particularly in the elderly [66], in whom hypoglycemic episodes may be difficult to diagnose.

In settings such as acute myocardial infarction [67] or the intensive care unit [68], enthusiasm for aggressive glycemic control has been tempered by its association with hypoglycemia and worse outcomes. Recent large

studies have shown lack of benefit and sometimes higher risks of morbidity and mortality with tight intensive glycemic control [69]. Adverse consequences of hypoglycemia could partially explain the outcomes from three recent studies, ACCORD [70], ADVANCE [71], and VADT [72], which tried to determine whether diabetes management more aggressive than currently recommended (with a goal of achieving HbA1c levels near 6.0%) would reduce cardiovascular risk in patients with longstanding diabetes. Hypoglycemia occurred more frequently in the intensive therapy arms of all three trials, and in the ACCORD trial, the rate of hypoglycemic episodes requiring medical assistance was three times higher. In ADVANCE, severe hypoglycemia was nearly twice as common in the intensive control group, and half of patients in the low A1c group had at least a minor hypoglycemic event during the study. All three trials failed to demonstrate cardiovascular benefit with such intensive therapy. The ACCORD trial had significantly greater mortality in the intensively treated group and was terminated early because of this higher mortality. This latter group also suffered more hypoglycemia, However, the greater frequency of hypoglycemia in the intensive treatment group was not considered to be the likely explanation for their excess mortality. A subsequent analysis of the ADVANCE trial indicated that severe hypoglycemia was associated with increased macrovascular events and death from a cardiovascular cause [73]. Reports on hypoglycemia and kidney disease have generally been limited to case reports, small series, and reviews [74]. In the ADVANCE trial analysis, higher creatinine levels were an independent risk factor for severe hypoglycemia [73]. In patients with uremia, hypoglycemia is more common than generally appreciated. End-stage renal disease unrelated to diabetes is the second most frequent cause of hypoglycemia in hospitalized patients [74] and has a high mortality rate [75]. However, concomitant illness, malnutrition, or drugs commonly contribute to hypoglycemia in these patients [76]. Only one-half of the cases of renal insufficiency and hypoglycemia were diabetic in one study [77]. Mild cognitive impairment, a common problem, particularly in the elderly ESRD patient, may predispose patients to hypoglycemia. In diabetic ESRD patients, glucose levels may be lower during the intradialytic period, and the risk of hypoglycemia is greater within 24 hours of a hemodialysis treatment [79]. In one survey, one-half of diabetic chronic hemodialysis patients suffered hypoglycemia over a three-month period [79]. In a recent CKD report, the rate of hypoglycemia within diabetes strata was higher in subjects with CKD, and the risk of severe hypoglycemic events was highest in the group with both diabetes and CKD [78]. However, epidemiological data regarding the incidence of hypoglycemia among CKD/ESRD patients and on the association between hypoglycemia and overall clinical outcomes are very limited.

The pathogenesis of hypoglycemia in diabetic CKD patients is complex and coexists with overall disturbances of glucose metabolism in renal failure. As with uremic carbohydrate intolerance, several factors contribute to uremic hypoglycemia (Table 31.1). Anorexia and suboptimal caloric intake lead to reduced glycogen stores. Reduced renal insulin clearance as the GFR falls to 15–20 mL/min/1.73 m^2 results in a prolonged action of insulin. The kidneys are the most important extrahepatic organs for degradation of insulin, and their contribution to insulin removal decreases with declining kidney function. However, insulin levels generally are reported as normal when measured [80]. Oral anti-diabetic therapies which are renally excreted frequently contribute to hypoglycemia. Insulin doses often need to be reduced by as much as half, especially after dialysis has been initiated. Rapid-acting insulin analogues may be less likely to cause hypoglycemia than regular insulin because the pharmacokinetics are less effected by renal failure [81]. The decline in renal mass and impaired kidney function lead to decreased renal gluconeogenesis. During starvation, the kidneys become a major source of glucose production through gluconeogenesis from precursor molecules. Deficient catecholamine release in renal failure leads to an impaired counterregulatory response that would normally defend against hypoglycemia. The protective response of glucagon, epinephrine, cortisol, and growth hormone is known to be impaired in diabetes mellitus [82], and deficiencies in glucagon and catecholamines are known to occur in uremic diabetic patients [83]. A recent case report supports a role for parathyroid hormone in inhibiting insulin secretion in a nondiabetic chronic hemodialysis patient; severe hypoglycemia with endogenous hyperinsulinemia followed parathyroidectomy for severe secondary hyperparathyroidism [84]. Nosocomial hypoglycemia may also occur due to administration of any one of a number of other medications, including b-adrenergic blockers, salicylates, propoxyphene, and sulfonamides [85]. Preliminary findings suggest that the risk of hypoglycemia is especially high in diabetic ESRD patients who have greater glycemic variability [86].

The health consequences of hypoglycemia can be severe. Hypoglycemic unawareness may occur. Signs and symptoms, when they do occur, include cold sweats, agitation, dizziness, disorientation, slurred speech, fatigue, and decreased level of consciousness. The occurrence of hypoglycemia complicated by central pontine myelinolysis and quadriplegia was recently described [87]. Hypoglycemia, particularly when severe, is a powerful stimulant to the sympathetic nervous system and may cause acute secondary adverse cardiovascular outcomes. The adrenergic response may result in chest pain due to coronary vasoconstriction and ischemia, myocardial infarction, serious cardiac arrhythmias including QT prolongation and ventricular arrhythmias, and sudden death [88]. While the DCCT clinical trial showed no adverse effects of intensive therapy, without or with severe hypoglycemia, on cognitive status measured objectively over 18 years of follow-up [89], a recent study among elderly type 2 patients with no prior cognitive impairment showed that episodes of hypoglycemia may be associated with increased risk of dementia [90].

DIABETES/BONE AND MINERAL METABOLISM

Epidemiologic evidence and prospective studies have linked vitamin D deficiency to an increased risk of diverse chronic diseases, including autoimmune and cardiovascular disease, cancer, infectious diseases, and type 2 diabetes mellitus [91]. Epidemiologic data also suggest that a significant proportion of cases of type 2

TABLE 31.1 Factors Contributing to Hypoglycemia

- Poor caloric intake
- Impaired hepatic glycogenolysis
- Defective renal gluconeogenesis
- Diminished counter-regulatory response
- Increased glucose variability
- Medication

diabetes (the most common form of diabetes) may be attributed to modifiable risk factors related to lifestyle and personal habits [92]. Diabetes is a risk factor for bone loss [93]. Diabetes directly impairs osteoblast function which may lead to decreased bone mass and suppression of bone turnover, and impairs bone quality by blunting the secretion of parathyroid hormone. Diabetes also modifies bone collagen through AGE-modification [94—95]. Even when bone density in diabetics appears to be similar to that of nondiabetics, diabetic bone may be more fragile [96].

Vitamin D deficiency and insufficiency have been defined as a serum 25-hydroxyvitamin D <20 ng/mL and 21—29 ng/mL, respectively [91]. Data indicate that patients with diabetes have lower serum concentrations of vitamin D than other patients, [97] as well as lower serum intact parathyroid hormone levels [98]. There is little information regarding why diabetes mellitus is associated with low serum vitamin D levels. Recent animal and human studies have provided confirmation that vitamin D might be a potential risk modifier for diabetes [99]; i.e. there may be an association between diabetes and vitamin D deficiency. A meta-analysis of five observational studies of vitamin D supplementation in children reported a nearly one-third risk reduction of type 1 diabetes in children who reported ever having received vitamin D supplements [100]. In one recent study, a low vitamin D status doubled the risk of newly diagnosed type 2 diabetes in elderly patients, after multiple statistical adjustments [101]. An inverse association between vitamin D status and both type 1 and type 2 diabetes has been suggested by some observational studies, whereas other studies on this subject are inconclusive. Based on published data that vitamin D deficiency is associated with impaired B-cell function and insulin resistance in animal models and humans, Mattilo et al. evaluated longitudinal data from 4097 adults collected from 1978—1980 as part of the Mini-Finland Health Survey [102]. The relative risk of type 2 diabetes between quartiles of vitamin D, after adjustment for confounding factors, was estimated using Cox's model. A significant inverse association was determined between serum 25-OH-D levels and the risk of type 2 diabetes.

To evaluate the association of HbA1c levels with vitamin D status in U.S. adults, Kositsawat et al. analyzed data on 9773 participants in the National Health and Nutrition Examination Survey (NHANES) 2003—2006 [103]. After adjustment for multiple covariates, they observed an inverse relationship between A1c and 25-(OH)-D levels in those individuals who were 35—74 years old. Limited by a single determination of both A1c and vitamin D levels, these cross sectional results nonetheless suggest a metabolic link between vitamin D concentrations and glucose homeostasis. The authors suggest screening patients with elevated A1c levels for vitamin D deficiency. Data that relate vitamin D and the risk of type 2 diabetes are limited by post-hoc analyses and generally inadequate adjustment for confounding variables [104].

The mechanisms by which vitamin D deficiency may cause diabetes mellitus could include increased insulin resistance, decreased insulin secretion, and/or autoimmune/inflammatory damage to pancreatic islet cells [99]. A vitamin D receptor, as well as expressible 1-alpha-hydroxylase, are present in pancreatic beta cells. Potential mechanisms whereby vitamin D might affect glucose metabolism by enhancing insulin sensitivity have been recently reviewed [99]. Vitamin D is thought to have both direct (through activation of the vitamin D receptor) and indirect (via regulation of calcium homeostasis) effects on several mechanisms relevant to glucose homeostasis, which could enhance the risk for diabetes in the presence of vitamin D deficiency. A recent study examined vitamin D status and the relationship between serum 25-(OH)-D concentrations and the components of insulin resistance. Insulin sensitivity/resistance was calculated by the quantitative insulin sensitivity check index. Only 17% of subjects had serum 25-(OH)-D concentrations in the recommended range of $\geq$ 30 ng/mL. Insulin resistance was significantly and inversely correlated with serum vitamin D concentrations [105]. Vitamin D status and insulin resistance (by homeostasis model assessment of insulin resistance, HOMA-IR) were also inversely related in the data obtained from the Third National Health and Nutrition Examination Survey (NHANES III) [106]. Although correcting and preventing vitamin D deficiency might have beneficial effects on diabetes and CKD, no randomized, prospective trials have been conducted to determine the effects of vitamin D supplementation on insulin resistance in CKD patients [107].

In contrast to observational studies, information pooled from vitamin D interventional trials appear to be inconclusive [108]. Might vitamin D have a role in reducing the risk of diabetes? The Women's Health Study, for example, suggested a reduction in the development of type 2 diabetes related to a modest increase in vitamin D intake, but lacked statistical adjustments [109]. Small doses of vitamin D do not appear to affect measurements of fasting glucose or insulin resistance. Vitamin D supplementation in pregnancy or early childhood may reduce the subsequent risk of type 1 diabetes [99]. In a recent study, Marjamaki et al. reported data from the Diabetes Prediction and Prevention Study (DIPP), in which the dietary habits of Finnish women were carefully examined and linked to the onset of autoimmunity in their offspring [110]. There was no correlation between the amount of vitamin D consumed by the mother and the appearance of islet autoantibodies in the blood of their offspring in the first postnatal year.

Longitudinal observational studies suggest an inconsistent association between vitamin D insufficiency and incident type 2 diabetes [99]. Studies addressing administration of high doses of vitamin D or metabolites with diabetes are limited to trials involving small numbers of patients or animal studies [111]. Careful prospective, placebo-controlled, randomized trials to confirm a role of vitamin D supplementation in individuals at risk for diabetes, with measurement of 25-(OH)-D as the exposure variable, will be needed to provide more definitive information.

The active metabolite of vitamin D regulates transcription of multiple gene products, with antiproliferative, prodifferentiative, and immunomodulatory effects. For example, in vitro studies of bone marrow red cell precursor cells demonstrated that 1,25-vitamin D increases epo-receptor expression [112]. One recent study showed that both 25-vitamin D and 1,25-vitamin D deficiency are associated with anemia [113]. In a recent study from Denmark, severe vitamin D deficiency was associated with increased all-cause (HR 1.96) and cardiovascular (HR 1.95) mortality [114] in patients with diabetes. Diabetes itself is known to disturb bone metabolism, chiefly in the form of low bone turnover [115], although the relationship between diabetes and bone disease is complex [96]. Both type 1 and type 2 diabetes are associated with increased bone fragility and a higher risk of fracture. Abnormalities in a number of regulators of bone metabolism have been demonstrated in diabetes that might play a role in the genesis of diabetes-associated osteopenia and reduced osteoblast function. Such abnormalities may include altered vitamin D regulation and relatively low serum parathyroid hormone levels. In cultured bovine parathyroid cells, for example, high glucose levels reversibly suppress parathyroid secretion [116]. Changes in osteoblast phenotype were demonstrated in one recent study, where decreased matrix mineralization was described in bone marrow culture from diabetic mice [117]; this was associated with decreased gene expression of osteocalcin, parathyroid-related protein receptor, the parathyroid receptor, and other factors.

Several studies have demonstrated that calcitriol, paricalcitol, and 1-alpha-D2 effectively suppress serum PTH levels [118]. Tanaka et al. evaluated the impact of diabetes on vitamin D metabolism in predialysis CKD patients by extracting data from over 600 patients (112 of whom had diabetes) in the observational Osaka Vitamin D study [95]. The study reported differences in relevant laboratory measurements (intact parathyroid hormone, 25-hydroxy vitamin D, calcitriol, FGF-23, calcium, and phosphorus) between 112 diabetic and 112 nondiabetic patients matched for gender, age, and eGFR. Bone mineral density and urinary protein excretion were also determined. No enrolled patient

had received vitamin D, bisphosphonates, estrogens, or raloxifene. Mean eGFR was 34.6 mL/min/1.73 m in the diabetic group and 35.6 mL/min/1.73 m in the controls. Corrected serum calcium and serum phosphorus were slightly higher in the diabetes group, while neither PTH nor FGF-23 differed; serum levels of both of these latter hormones increased as kidney function declined. However, diabetic patients had more deficient vitamin D status. Despite similar levels of serum PTH, the diabetes group had lower serum 1,25-D (calcitriol) levels (p < .0001) (Figure 31.5); this difference persisted after multivariate linear regression adjustments for the degree of proteinuria. Low 1,25-D levels in diabetes were related to lower levels of 25-D, its substrate. In diabetic dialysis patients, osteodystrophy is mainly manifested as an aplastic or low-turnover type due to low serum intact PTH concentrations. Serum PTH levels

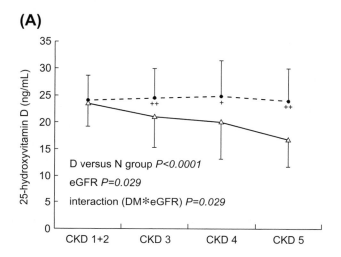

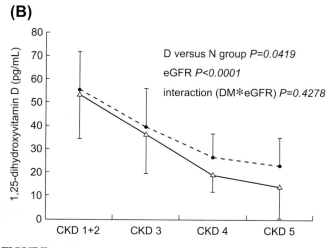

FIGURE 31.5 Impact of diabetes and CKD on vitamin D status in predialysis patients. Differences between the groups was observed in the association between CKD stage and both 25-hydroxy- and 1,25-hydroxy vitamin D. Broken line = nondiabetic, solid line = diabetic. Compared with nondiabetics, diabetic CKD patients had poorer vitamin D status *(Ref. [95].)*

were affected by the degree of glycemic control in one hemodialysis study, with lower PTH levels in those with poor glycemic control [119]. There are currently no data indicating that the needs for other vitamins or for trace elements for the patient with diabetic CKD are different from that of CKD patients without diabetic kidney disease who have the same degree of proteinuria (please see Chapters 20, 21 and 23).

DIETARY PROTEIN INTAKE AND DIABETIC KIDNEY DISEASE

Dietary protein intake has been considered to be an important factor in maintaining kidney health since the last half of the 19th century. There have been many low protein diets proposed for CKD patients which, initially, were usually aimed at limiting the symptoms of patients with near ESRD and/or reducing the affects of azotemia. Some of the early studies were also designed to reduce progression of CKD. An article by Giordano in Kidney International [120] described the work in 1923 of F.M. Allen at the New England Deaconess Hospital. Dr. Allen did studies to determine the feasibility of a very low protein diet initially by feeding a medical student a diet of 4000 calories for 24 days that consisted of carbohydrates and fats (and only 300 mg of protein/day). The urine urea nitrogen excretion dropped from 14.25 g/day to 1.58 g/day. Apparently the medical student stopped the study earlier than Dr. Allen because the student feared for his health and had distaste for the very low protein diet. Dr. Allen followed up that study by administering a diet of 18 grams of protein/day to a 70 kg azotemic patient (0.26 g/kg) for 6 months. The diet successfully lowered nitrogen waste excretion but was extremely hard to maintain.

The contemporary approach to the utility of low protein diets derives primarily from work from the 1970s to 1990s. Low protein diets have been used for two major goals: [1] to slow the decline in glomerular filtration rate (GFR); and [2] to ameliorate signs and symptoms of patients with near ESRD. But are low protein diets effective? Seminal work from this time period was done in Munich-Wistar rats that have their glomeruli near the cortical surface thus making them accessible for micropuncture studies [121−127]. Using tiny glass pipettes, researchers measured glomerular pressures (including transcapillary pressure, ΔP) and glomerular filtration rate as well as afferent renal blood flow, Q_A). The value of this animal model is that very exact, detailed readings could be obtained from single nephrons. As most models of kidney failure take a long time to develop, rat models were designed to accelerate the rate of decline in GFR. These models included various degrees of removal of kidney tissue such as the one and {2/3} nephrectomy model where the rat was left with only {1/3} of one kidney. Other models consisted of altering the protein in the diet and/or making the animals diabetic.

A landmark paper published by Zatz et al. provided a hemodynamic explanation for declining GFR and a pathophysiologic rationale for limiting protein in the diet in patients with diabetic kidney disease [127]. Rats were maintained for 1 year on a 6% protein diet (low protein), 12% protein diet (normal rat diet), or 50% protein diet (high protein). In addition half of the rats were made diabetic. Rats were studied at 2−10 weeks for micropuncture studies and at 11-13 months for pathology. Figure 31.6 shows the essential findings that as protein intake increased there were increases in single nephron GFR (SNGFR) and increases in Q_A and ΔP. Animals that were diabetic had even greater increases in SNGFR, Q_A and ΔP.

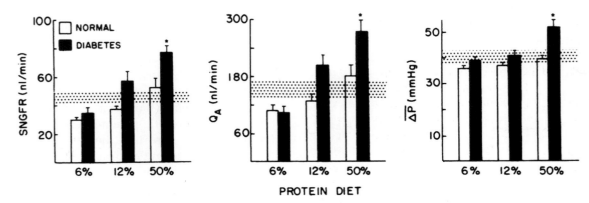

FIGURE 31.6   Munich−Wistar rats were treated with three different diets as noted above and were either nondiabetic or diabetic (by injection of streptoztocin). After 2−10 weeks, micropuncture studies were performed. Both increased dietary protein and diabetes led to increased glomerular flow rates (single nephron glomerular filtration rate-SNGFR), afferent renal arteriole blood flow rate (Q_A), and intraglomerular pressure ($\Delta\Pi$). The combination of high protein and diabetes had the greatest increases in these hemodynamic parameters. *(Ref. [127].)*

And the combination of a high protein diet and diabetes engendered the greatest increase in all of these parameters. Importantly, the rats maintained on the low protein diet (diabetic or not diabetic) showed no changes in these parameters as compared to nondiabetic control rats on a normal 12% diet. Urinary albumin excretion was also studied. The data revealed that the diabetic rats fed a high protein diet developed especially high levels of urinary albumin, whereas the rats fed the low protein diet had normal levels of urinary albumin, whether or not they were diabetic (Figure 31.7). Examination of the kidney pathology consistently revealed a lesion of secondary focal and segmental sclerosis in the rats that had increased glomerular pressures, blood flow, and increased urine albumin levels as compared to the rats with normal glomerular pressures and blood flow. Thus the hypothesis for progression of diabetic kidney disease was proposed, stating that glomerular hyperfiltration/hypertension leads to progressive sclerosis of glomeruli and loss of GFR and interventions that prevent these hemodynamic changes should slow or prevent the decline in GFR. Hence, low protein diets should effectively slow progression by lowering intraglomerular pressures and blood flow rates. These results provided very compelling arguments for human studies to test the value of low protein diets for slowing progression of diabetic kidney disease.

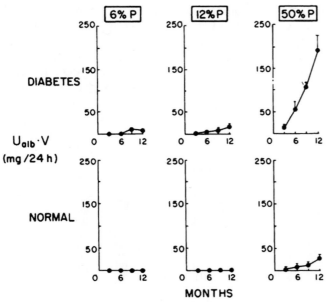

FIGURE 31.7 Munich—Wistar rats were treated with 3 different diets as noted above and were either nondiabetic or diabetic (by injection of streptoztocin). Dietary protein percentages are shown at the top of the graph. Urinary albumin excretion rates were followed over time. The combination of diabetes and 50% protein diet had the greatest effect on increasing urinary albumin excretion rate. (*Ref.* [127].)

Although these physiological studies appear to be convincing, there are concerns as to the interpretation of results, which are as follows. First, the measurements in these models were from a very small number of nephrons and may not reflect hemodynamics in the kidney as a whole. Second, of necessity, the micropuncture studies were a snapshot in time and may reflect only the hemodynamics of that time period but not necessarily reflect the hemodynamics over an extended period of time. Indeed, the micropuncture measurements were done at 2—10 weeks after the creation of diabetes, whereas the increases in urine albumin level did not occur until months later. And the pathology was examined 10—12 months after the micropuncture studies. Moreover, these results indicate that glomerular hyperfiltration per se is deleterious; yet, to date, there is no convincing evidence in humans that prolonged glomeruar hyperfiltration does predict declining GFR. Third, there is the usual concern that animal models do not reflect human disease, nor do they necessarily reflect the response to treatment in humans. Nevertheless, important studies such as Zatz et al. and others have provided the basis for the hypothesis that a critical component of treatment of patients with diabetic kidney disease is to lower the intraglomerular pressures or flows [121—127]. Hence, the presumed efficacy of low protein diets is to lower intraglomerular pressures and flows. Since angiotensin II is the major regulator of intraglomerular pressures by causing vasoconstriction, preferentially in the efferent arteriole, studies have been conducted using inhibitors of angiotensin II. In a subsequent paper, Zatz et al. used the angiotensin converting enzyme (ACE) inhibitor enalapril in the same diabetic rat model that the protein studies were done and showed that enalapril reduced glomerular pressures, lowered urine albuminuria, and ameliorated the deleterious effects of diabetes on rat kidneys [126]. Since then many human studies have proven that agents that block the actions of angiotensin II successfully slow progression of diabetic kidney disease in patients who have increased levels of urine albumin level. These medicines include the ACE inhibitors, angiotensin receptor blockers, and renin inhibitors [128]. Interestingly, for these medicines there is evidence that there is a hemodynamically mediated decrease in GFR that is necessary for optimal efficacy of these agents. For example, in the RENAAL study in which diabetic patients were treated with or without the ARB, losartan, the results demonstrated that the greater the initial decline in GFR in patients treated with losartan, the slower the subsequent rate of decline in GFR [129]. Of note, these studies do not prove that decreases in GFR are mechanistically important for the effect of losartan for slowing the decrease in GFR; this reduction in the decline in GFR may just be a marker of drug effect.

Since the early 1980s there have been many small studies that suggested that low protein diets were effective in slowing progression of diabetic kidney disease. However, the largest and most influential study on the effect of low protein diets on the progression of kidney disease had very few diabetic kidney disease patients. The Modification of Diet in Renal Disease (MDRD) study that was published in 1994 [130] followed two groups (the mean follow up was 2.2 years) — one with GFRs between 25-55 mL/min (585 participants — who were randomly assigned to a "normal" protein diet providing 1.3 g/kg/day or a low protein diet containing 0.58 g/kg/day) and a second group with more advanced kidney disease who had GFRs between 13−24 mL/min (255 participants) and who were randomly assigned to diets providing either 0.58 g/kg/day or 0.26 g/kg/day with supplementation with some essential amino acids and ketoacid analogues of other essential amino acids). The results did not show a beneficial effect of low protein diets on slowing progression of renal disease. There was also a low blood pressure versus normal blood pressure arm of this study. As has been shown by many studies, blood pressure control had a significant effect on slowing a decline in GFR. Only 3% of the participants had diabetes and all of these people had type 2 diabetes as the researchers excluded any patients who were taking insulin. Thus, this study did not adequately determine whether diabetic kidney disease patients would have benefit from a low protein diet. But the negative results of the MDRD led to much decreased enthusiasm for routine use of low protein diets. In 1999, many of the authors of the original study wrote a retrospective review arguing that at best this study was inconclusive and that there were trends toward better outcomes in patients who were assigned to the low protein diet [131]. Moreover, several problems were inadvertently incorporated into the experimental design of the MDRD Study. These are discussed in Chapters 14 and 23 and might account for the inconclusive results of this trial. Thus, it has been argued that a low protein diet should still be considered for patients with CKD. Interestingly the achieved protein diet (as measured by 24-hour urine protein excretion) in the low protein diet group (0.58 g/kg/day) was about 0.77 g/kg/day, almost the same as the recommended protein intake for diabetic patients by the American Diabetes Association of 0.8 g/kg/day [132]. So the argument as to whether diabetic kidney disease patients should be treated with a low protein diet might well be a moot one. However, some workers in this field do recommend substantially lower protein diets for CKD patients (see Chapters 14 and 23).

In 1997, the EURODIAB IDDM trial was published [133]. In this study 2696 type 1 diabetic patients in 30 countries had their dietary history taken and laboratory values measured. The results showed that patients who had <20% of their calories from protein had lower levels of urinary albumin excretion as compared to those patients who reported >20% of their calories from protein. The study appeared to show that as dietary protein increased there was a gradual and significant increase in urine albumin excretion. But the participants with higher urinary albumin excretion also had worse glucose control (as measured by higher glycohemoglobin A1c) and higher blood pressure. In fact, the combination of increased A1c and increased blood pressure was the strongest predictors of high urinary albumin excretion rates, suggesting that protein intake was much less important. Another study published in 2007 from the ERIKA Study group evaluated three diets: very low protein (0.35 g/kg/day), low protein (0.6 g/kg/day), and a free diet (ad libitum protein intake) in patients with stages 4 and 5 CKD [134]. There was significantly lower urinary protein excretion in the very low protein diet group after six months of dietary treatment and not in the other two groups. But it was also noted that the salt intake (as measured by urine sodium content) decreased significantly as protein content in the diet decreased. This suggests the possibility that the decrease in dietary salt intake led to a decline in blood pressure as the main reason for the observed reduction in urine protein level. Indeed, the mean blood pressure in the very low protein group was 143/84 mmHg at the beginning of the study and decreased to 128/78 after six months. The authors concluded that factors other than the amount of protein ingested were responsible for the decrease in urine protein excretion. In 2009, the Cochrane Reviews performed a detailed analysis of randomized controlled trials in patients with diabetic kidney disease [135]. The authors' conclusions were that at that time there was little published evidence that low protein diets were of benefit for CKD patients. The protein content of the low protein diets in the reviewed studies was not very low, between 0.6 and 0.8 g/kg/day, and the sample size of the studies evaluated was often relatively small. Hence, it could be argued that this Cochrane Review of low protein diets for diabetic CKD is not definitive.

None of the studies convincingly showed an effect of low protein diet on slowing progression of kidney disease in patients with diabetic nephropathy. It is our conclusion that at this time there is not convincing evidence that a low protein diet is of benefit in patients with diabetic kidney disease. As the current recommendation for dietary protein for diabetic patients is routinely in the 0.8 to 1.0 g/kg/day range, a low protein diet needs to be less than this. There is not enough evidence for a beneficial effect of protein diets of <0.6 g/kg/day for diabetic patients with CKD, and many studies including the MDRD study suggest that it is difficult to maintain protein diets at 0.6 g/kg/day or lower. On the other hand, the data are insufficient to prove that low protein diets do not retard progression of CKD. Thus, for diabetic CKD patients who are willing to try protein intakes in the range of 0.6 g/kg/day or very low protein diets (about 0.3 g/kg/day) supplemented with ketoacid/essential amino acid mixtures, it can be argued that they should not be discouraged from doing so (please see Chapter 23).

Does the source of the protein make a difference? Again there are only limited studies on this issue. For example, Knight et al. studied changes in estimated GFR in 1135 participants with GFR >80 mL/min and in a second group of 489 participants with GFR between 55 and 80 ml/min from the Nurses Health Study [136]. Only a small percentage of the subjects had diabetes. The groups were subdivided into protein intake that was primarily nondairy animal protein, dairy protein, or vegetable protein. The participants taking the vegetable protein had either no decline or the slowest decline in GFR as compared to the other groups. It is relevant that this study evaluated dietary intake of protein only twice via questionnaires, in 1990 and 1994. Thus, the reliability of the findings is brought into question by the limited frequency of data measurements in the same subjects. Another study (albeit one with only 300 patients) examined whether eating primarily fish protein was beneficial [137]. The authors noted that a high intake of fish protein significantly slowed the development of microalbuminuria in type 1 diabetic patients. These results are interesting but in and of themselves do not present a clear diet plan that should be prescribed for patients with diabetic kidney disease.

Lastly, the onset of end stage kidney disease significantly changes the protein intake recommendations. Protein-energy wasting is a well-documented, important issue in dialysis patients that needs to be properly assessed and treated to prevent significant malnutrition [138]. National Kidney Foundation guidelines recommend an intake of 1.2 g/kg/day for hemodialysis patients and 1.3 g/kg/day for peritoneal dialysis patients [139]. The recommendations for protein intake are higher in dialysis patients than nondialysis patients due to a combination of such factors as increased catabolic rates in dialysis patients, removal of nutrients during dialysis, effects of bioincompatible materials, and others [139]. Moreover, there is a close association of protein wasting with inflammation, strongly suggesting that proper protein intake is needed to limit the inflammatory state of dialysis patients [140]. An interesting retrospective analysis of 53,933 patients undergoing maintenance hemodialysis examined the relationship of mortality and protein intake by evaluating the relation between urea kinetic-based normalized protein nitrogen appearance (nPNA) and all-cause and cardiovascular mortality over a 2-year period [141]. Dialysis patients who ingested <0.8 g/kg/day or >1.4 g/kg/day had significantly higher mortality rates. The best survival was associated with a protein intake of 1.0 to 1.4 g/kg/day. The risks of protein and energy wasting are more pronounced in patients who also have diabetes possibly due to the effects of diabetes on metabolism, decreased effects of insulin and/or insulin resistance as well as to comorbid conditions such as hypertension and vascular disease [142]. Hence, when diabetic patients approach end stage kidney disease (at CKD stage 5), nutritional assessment should be conducted in order to provide optimal protein and calorie intake to prevent wasting and reduce inflammation.

SALT INTAKE AND DIABETIC KIDNEY DISEASE

The link between salt intake and hypertension has been established over many years of research. There is no question that in patients who are salt-sensitive, limiting salt intake will lead to lower blood pressure and as a result improved long term outcomes (please also see Chapter 25). A 2010 Cochrane Review evaluated 818 studies related to reducing salt intake and progression of diabetic nephropathy and concluded that there was strong evidence for limiting sodium chloride intake to at least less than 5–6 grams/day [143]. But the authors noted that there are relatively few well-controlled studies that specifically target salt intake independently of other variables, and that many studies are of short duration or use wide variations in sodium intake. Nevertheless, the current recommendation is to limit sodium chloride intake to help lower blood pressure, as lower blood pressure is clearly beneficial in slowing or even preventing progression of CKD. Moreover, salt intake needs to be limited in patients taking diuretics or the effect of the diuretic will be greatly diminished.

But is there a unique role for salt intake in the progression of diabetic kidney disease? It has been well established that diabetic kidney disease is associated with activation of the renin-angiotensin-aldosterone system (RAAS) [144,145]. Elevated levels of angiotensin II will lead to enhanced proximal reabsorption of sodium and elevated levels of aldosterone will lead to enhance collecting duct reabsorption of sodium. There are very few studies addressing the role of limiting salt intake in patients on specific medications. For example, Bakris and Smith evaluated the role of sodium intake on albumin excretion in diabetic nephropathy patients taking either the dihydropyridine calcium channel blocker, nifedipine or the nondihydropyridine calcium channel blocker, diltiazem [146]. As previously observed, diltiazem led to a decrease in urinary albumin excretion whereas nifedipine did not. And a lower sodium chloride intake enhanced the effects of diltiazem on lowering the urinary albumin excretion. A similar study was done in patients who were treated with the angiotensin receptor blocker, losartan [147]. The authors reported that the achieved mean urinary sodium excretion on a low-sodium diet was 85 and 80 mmol/day in the losartan and placebo groups, respectively. In the losartan group, the additional blood pressure lowering effects when patients ingested a low-sodium diet, as compared to a regular sodium diet, for 24-h systolic, diastolic, and mean arterial blood pressures were 9.7 mmHg, 5.5 mmHg, and 7.3 mmHg, respectively. In the losartan group, the urinary albumin to creatinine ratio decreased significantly on the low-sodium diet as compared to the regular-sodium diet, and it was strongly associated with a decrease in blood pressure. These studies are illustrative of other reports in the literature. At this time, the recommendation is that for hypertensive patients with diabetic kidney disease, it is prudent to limit salt in the diet in order to lower blood pressure and to enhance the effects of various antihypertensive and diuretic medications. Whether there is any role for a low salt diet in normotensive patients with diabetic kidney disease has not been established at this time.

References

[1] National Diabetes Factsheet, www.cdc.gov

[2] American Diabetes Association. Standards of Medical Care in Diabetes-2011. Diabetes Care 2011;34(Suppl. 1):Sll—61.

[3] Berhane AM, Weil EJ, Knowler WC, et al. Albuminuria and estimated glomerular filtration rate as predictors of diabetic end-stage renal disease and death. Clin J Am Soc Nephrol 2011;6:2444—51.

[4] Weber MA, Giles TD. Inhibiting the renin-angiotensin system to prevent cardiovascular diseases: do we need a more comprehensive strategy? Rev Cardiovasc Med 2006;7:45—54.

[5] Mak RHK. Renal disease, insulin resistance, and glucose intolerance. Diabetes Rev 1994;2:19—28.

[6] Kovesdy C, Sharm K, Kalantar-Zadeh K, et al. Glycemic control in diabetic CKD patients: Where do we stand? Am J Kidney Dis 2008;52:766—77.

[7] Chen J, Muntner P, Hamm LL, et al. Insulin resistance and risk of chronic kidney disease in nondiabetic US adults. J Am Soc Nephrol 2003;14:469—77.

[8] Mak RH. Impact of end-stage renal disease and dialysis on glycemic control. Semi Dial 2000;13:4—8.

[9] Akmal M, Massry SG, Goldstein DA, et al. Role of parathyroid hormone in the glucose intolerance of chronic renal failure. J Clin Invest 1985;75:1037—44.

[10] Mak RH. Intravenous 1,25-dihydroxycholecalciferol corrects glucose intolerance in hemodialysis patients. Kidney Int 1992;41:1049—54.

[11] Stefikova K, Spustova V, Krivosikova Z, et al. Insulin resistance and vitamin D deficiency in patients with chronic kidney disease stages 2-3. Physiol Res 2011;60:149—55.

[12] Massry SG. Sequence of cellular events in pancreatic islets leading to impaired insulin secretion in chronic kidney disease. J Ren Nutr 2011;21:92—9.

[13] Graham TE, Kahn BB. Tissue-specific alterations of glucose transport and molecular mechanisms of intertissue communication in obesity and type 2 diabetes. Horm Metab Res 2007;39:717—21.

[14] Viswanathan V, Tilak P, Meerza R, et al. Insulin resistance at different stages of diabetic kidney disease in India. J Assoc Physicians India 2010;58:612—5.

[15] Basturk T, Unsal A. Is insulin resistance a risk factor for the progression of chronic kidney disease? Kidney Blood Press Res 2011;34:111—5.

[16] Fliser D, Pacini G, Engelleiter R, et al. Insulin resistance and hyperinsulinemia are already present in patients with incipient renal disease. Kidney Int 1998;53:1343—7.

[17] Adrogue HJ. Glucose homeostasis and the kidney. Kidney Int 1992;42:1266—71.

[18] Goecke IA, Bonilla S, Marusic ET, et al. Enhanced insulin sensitivity in extrarenal potassium handling in uremic rats. Kidney Int 1991;39:39—43.

[19] Alvestrand A. Carbohydrate and insulin metabolism in renal failure. Kidney Int 1997;52(S62):S48—52.

[20] Goldstein BJ, Mahadev K, Wu X, et al. Redox paradox: insulin action is facilitated by insulin-stimulated reactive oxygen species with multiple potential signaling targets. Diabetes 2005;54:311—21.

[21] Chang G-Y, Park ASD, Susztak K. Tracing the footsteps of glomerular insulin signaling in diabetic kidney disease. Kidney Int 2011;79:802—4.

[22] Mima A, Ohshiro Y, Kitada M, et al. Glomerular-specific protein kinase C-beta-induced insulin receptor substrate-1 dysfunction and insulin resistance in rat models of diabetes and obesity. Kidney Int 2011;79:883—96.

[23] Hager SR. Insulin resistance in uremia. Am J Kidney Dis 1989;14:272—6.

[24] Smith D, DeFronzo RA. Insulin resistance in uremia mediated by ost-binding defects. Kidney Int 1982;22:54—60.

[25] DeFronzo RA, Tobin JD, Rowe JW, et al. Glucose intolerance in uremia. Quantification of pancreatic beta cell sensitivity to glucose and tissue sensitivity to insulin. J Clin Invest 1978;62:425—35.

[26] Schmitz O. Insulin-mediated glucose uptake in nondialyzed uremic insulin-dependent diabetic subjects. Diabetes 1985;34:1152—9.

[27] Manolescu B, Stoian I, Atanasiu V, et al. Review article: The role of adipose tissue in uraemia-related insulin resistance. Nephrology (Carlton) 2008;13:622—8.

[28] Guo LL, Pan Y, Jin HM. Adinopectin is positively associated with insulin resistance in subjects with type 2 diabetic nephropathy and effects of angiotensin II type receptor blocker losartan. Nephrol Dial Transplant 2009;24:1876—83.

[29] Zanetti M, Barazzoni R, Guarnieri G. Inflammation and insulin resistance in uremia. J Ren Nutr 2008;18:70—5.

[30] Khedr E, El-Sharkawy M, Abdulwahab S, et al. Effect of recombinant human erythropoietin on insulin resistance in hemodialysis patients. Hemodialysis Intern 2009;13:340—6.

[31] Siew ED, Ikizler TA. Insulin resistance and protein energy metabolism in patients with advanced chronic kidney disease. Semin Dial 2010;23:378—82.

[32] Ikizler TA. Effects of glucose homeostasis on protein metabolism in patients with advanced chronic kidney disease. J Ren Nutr 2007;17:13–6.

[33] Cusi K, Maezono K, Osman A, et al. Insulin resistance differentially affects the PI 3-kinase-mediated signaling in human muscle. J Clin Invest 2000;105:311–20.

[34] Siew ED, Pupim LB, Majchrzak KM, et al. Insulin resistance is associated with skeletal muscle protein breakdown in non-diabetic chronic hemodialysis patients. Kidney Int 2007;71:146–52.

[35] Mather A, Pollock C. Glucose handling by the kidney. Kidney Int Suppl 2011;120:S1–6.

[36] List JF, Whaley JM. Glucose dynamics and mechanistic implications of SGLT2 inhibitors in animals and humans. Kidney Int Suppl 2011;120:S20–7.

[37] Kinne RK, Castaneda F. SGLT inhibitors as new therapeutic tools in the treatment of diabetes. Hand Exp Pharmacol 2011; 203:105–26.

[38] Jurczak MJ, Lee HY, Birkenfeld AL, et al. SGLT deletion improves glucose homeostasis and preserves pancreatic beta-cell function. Diabetes 2011;60:890–8.

[39] Ahmed MH. The kidneys as an emergent target for the treatment of diabetes mellitus: What we know, thought we knew, and hope to gain. Int J Diabetes Mellitus 2010;2:125–6.

[40] National Kidney Foundation Kidney Disease Outcomes Quality Initiative (NKF-KDOQI). Clinical practice guidelines and clinical practice recommendations for diabetes and chronic kidney disease. Am J Kidney Dis 2007;49:S1–S79.

[41] Williams ME, Lacson Jr E, Teng M, et al. Hemodialyzed type 1 and type II diabetic patients in the US: characteristics, glycemic control, and survival. Kidney Int 2006;70:1503–9.

[42] Kalantar-Zadeh K, Kopple JD, Regidor DL, et al. A1c and survival in maintenance hemodialysis patients. Diabetes Care 2007;30:1049–55.

[43] Williams ME, Lacson Jr E, Wang W, Lazarus JM, Hakim R. Glycemic control and extended hemodialysis survival in patients with diabetes mellitus: Comparative results of traditional and time-dependent Cox model analyses. C J Am Soc Nephr 2010;5:1595–601.

[44] Ix JH. Hemoglobin A1c in hemodialysis patients: should one size fit all? Clin J Am Soc Nephrol 2010;5:1539–41.

[45] Rohlfing CL, Wiedmeyer HM, Little Rr. Defining the relationship between plasma glucose and HbA1c: analysis of glucose profiles and HbA1c in the Diabetic Control and Complications Trial. Diabetes Care 2002;25:275–8.

[46] Stratton IM, Adler AI, Neil HA, et al. Association of glycaemia with macrovascular and microvascular complications of type 2 diabetes (UKPDS 35): prospective observational study. BMJ 2000;321:405–12.

[47] Saudek CK, Brick JC. The clinical use of hemoglobin A1c. J Diabetes Sci Technol 2009;3:629–34.

[48] Dunn PJ, Cole RA, Soeldner JS, et al. Reproducibility of hemoglobin A1c and sensitivity to various degrees of glucose intolerance. Ann Intern Med 1979;91:390–6.

[49] Nathan DM, Kuenen J, Borg R, et al. A1c-Derived Average Glucose Study Group. Translating the A1c assay into estimated average glucose values. Diabetes Care 2008;31:173–1478.

[50] Rubinow KB, Hirsch IB. Reexamining metrics for glucose control. JAMA 2011;305:1132–3.

[51] Holt RIG, Gallen I. Time to move beyond glycosylated haemoglobin. Diabetic Med 2004;21:655–6.

[52] Cohen RM, Smith EP. Frequency of HbA1c discordance in estimating blood glucose control. Curr Opin Clin Nutr Metab Care 2008;11:512–7.

[53] U.S. Renal Data Systems, USRDS 2008 Annual Data Report: Atlas of Chronic Kidney Disease and End-stage Renal Disease in the United States. Bethesda, MD: National Institutes of Health, National Institute of Diabetes and Digestive and Kidney Diseases; 2008.

[54] Feldt-Rasmussen B. Is there a need to optimize glycemic control in hemodialized diabetic patients? Kidney Int 2006;70: 1392–4.

[55] Little RR, Tennill AL, Rohlfing C, et al. Can glycohemoglobin be used to assess glycemic control in patients with chronic renal failure? Clin Chem 2002;48:784–6.

[56] Brown JN, Kemp DW, Brice KR. Class effect of erythropoietin therapy on hemoglobin A (1c) in a patient with diabetes mellitus and chronic kidney disease not undergoing hemodialysis. Pharmacotherapy 2009;29:468–72.

[57] Peacock TP, Shihabi K, Bleyer AJ, et al. Comparison of glycated albumin and hemoglobin A1c levels in diabetic subjects on hemodialysis. Kidney Int 2008;73:1062–8.

[58] Chen H-S, Wu T-E, Lin H-D, et al. Hemoglobin A1c and fructosamine for assessing glycemic control in diabetic patients with CKD stages 3 and 4. Am J Kidney Dis 2010;55:867–74.

[59] Riveline J-P, Teynie J, Belmouaz S, et al. Glycaemic control in type 2 diabetic patients on chronic haemodialysis: use of a continuous glucose monitoring system. Nephrol Dial Transplant 2009;24:2866–71.

[60] Sobngwi E, Ashuntantang G, Ndounia E, et al. Continuous interstitial glucose monitoring in non-diabetic subjects with end-stage renal disease undergoing maintenance haemodialysis. Diabetes Res Clin Pract 2010;90:22–5.

[61] Mehrotra R, Kalantar-Zadeh K, Adler S. Assessment of glycemic control in dialysis patients with diabetes: glycosylated hemoglobin or glycated albumin? Clin J Am Soc Nephrol 2011;7:1520–2.

[62] Abe M, Matsumoto K. Glycated hemoglobin or glycated albumin for assessment of glycemic control in hemodiayzed patients with diabetes? Nature Clin Pract Nephr 2008;4:482–3.

[63] Inaba M, Okuno S, Kumeda Y. Glycated albumin is a better glycemic indicator than glycated hemoglobin values in hemodialysis patients with diabetes: effect of anemia and erythropoietin injection. J Am Soc Nephrol 2007;18:896–903.

[64] Freedman BI, Andries L, Shihabi ZK, et al. Glycated albumin and risk of death and hospitalizations in patients with diabetes on dialysis. Clin J Am Soc Nephrol 2011;6:1635–43.

[65] Amiel SA, Dixon T, Mann R, et al. Hypogycaemia in type 2 diabetes. Diabetes Med 2008;25:245–54.

[66] Munshi MN, Segal AR, Suhl E, et al. Frequent hypoglycemia among elderly patients with poor glycemic control. Arch Int Med 2011;171:362–84.

[67] Kosiborod M, Inzucchi SE, Goyal DA, et al. Relationship between spontaneous and iatrogenic hypoglycemia and mortality in patients hospitalized with acute myocardial infarction. JAMA 2009;301:1556–64.

[68] The NICE-SUGAR Study Investigators. Intensive versus conventional glucose control in critically ill patients. N Engl J Med 1997;360:1283–97.

[69] Skyler JS, Bergenstal R, Bonow RO, et al. American Diabetes Association; American College of Cardiology American Heart Association. Intensive glycemic control and the prevention of cardiovascular events: implications of the ACCORD, ADVANCE, and VA diabetes trials: a position statement of the American Diabetes Association and a scientific statement of the American College of Cardiology Foundation and the American Heart Association. Diabetes Care 2009;32:187–92.

[70] Gerstein HC, Miller ME, Byington RP, et al. Action to Control Cardiovascular Risk in Diabetes (ACCORD) Study Group. Effects of intensive glucose lowering in type 2 diabetes. N Engl J Med 2008;358:2545–59.

[71] Patel A, MacMahon S, Chalmers J, et al. ADVANCE Collaborative Group. Intensive blood glucose control and vascular outcomes in patients with type 2 diabetes. N Engl J Med 2008; 358:2560–71.

[72] Duckworth W, Abraira C, Moritz T, et al. VADT Investigators. Glucose control and vascular complications in veterans with type 2 diabetes. N Engl J Med 2009;360:129–39.

[73] Zoungas S, Chalmers J, Ninomiya T, et al. Association of HbA(1c) levels with vascular complications and death in patients with type 2 diabetes: evidence of glycaemic thresholds. Diabetologia 2011 Dec 21. Epub ahead of print.

[74] Mujais SK, Fadda G. Carbohydrate metabolism in end-stage renal disease. Semin Dial 1989;2:46–53.

[75] Haviv YS, Sharkia M, Safadi R. Hypoglycemia in patients with renal failure. Ren Fail 2000;22:219–23.

[76] Toth EL, Lee DW. Spontaneous/uremic hypoglycemia is not a distinct entity: substantiation from a literature review. Nephron 1991;58:325–9.

[77] Arem R. Hypoglycemia associated with renal failure. Endocrinol Metab Clin North Am 1989;18:103–21.

[78] Moen MF, Zhan M, Hsu VD, et al. Frequency of hypoglycemia and its significance in chronic kidney disease. Clin J Am Soc Nephr 2009;4:1121–7.

[79] Sun CY, Lee CC, Wu MS. Hypoglycemia in diabetic patients undergoing hemodialysis. Ther Apher Dial 2009;13:95–102.

[80] Block MB, Rubinstein AH. Spontaneous hypoglycemia in diabetic patients with renal insufficiency. JAMA 1970;213: 1863–6.

[81] Lubowsky ND, Siegel R, Pittas AG. Management of glycemia in patients with diabetes mellitus and CKD. Am J Kidney Dis 2007;5:865–79.

[82] Cryer PE, Gerich JE. Glucose counterregulation, hypoglycemia, and intensive insulin therapy in diabetes mellitus. N Engl J Med 1985;313:232–41.

[83] Borden G, Reichard GA, Hoeldtke RD, et al. Severe insulin-induced hypoglycemia associated with deficiencies in the release of counterregulatory hormones. N Engl J Med 1981;305: 1200–5.

[84] Nikalji R, Bargman JM. Severe hypoglycemia with endogenous hyperinsulinemia in a nondiabetic hemodialysis patient following parathyroidectomy. Nephrol Dial Transplant 2011;26: 2050–3.

[85] Williams ME. Carbohydrate metabolism in renal failure. In: Kopple JD, Massry SG, editors. Kopple and Massry's Nutritional Management of Renal Disease. 2nd ed. Philadelphia: Lippincott Williams and Wilkins; 2004. p. 25–39.

[86] Williams ME, Lacson Jr E, Wang W, et al. High glucose variability increases risk of all-cause and hypoglycemia-related hospitalization in diabetic chronic hemodialysis patients [Abstract]. J Am Soc Nephrol 2009;20:193A.

[87] Vallurupalli S, Huesmann G, Gregory J, et al. Levofloxacin-associated hypoglycemia complicated by pontine myelinolysis and quadriplegia. Diabet Med 2008;25:856–9.

[88] O'Keefe JH, Abuannadi M, Lavie CJ, et al. Strategies for optimizing glycemic control and cardiovascular prognosis in patients with type 2 diabetes mellitus. Mayo Clin Proc 2011;86: 128–38.

[89] Diabetes Control and Complications Trial Research Group. The effect of intensive treatment of diabetes on the development and progression of long-term complications in insulin-dependent diabetes mellitus. The Diabetes Control and Complications Trial. N Engl J Med 1993;329:977–86.

[90] Whitmer RA, Karter AJ, Yaffe K, et al. Hypoglycemic episodes and risk of dementia in older patients with type 2 diabetes mellitus. JAMA 2009;301:1565–72.

[91] Hollick M. Vitamin D: evolutionary, physiological, and health perspectives. Curr Drug Targets 2011;12:4–18.

[92] Hu FB. Diet, lifestyle, and the risk of type 2 diabetes in women. New Engl J Med 2001;345:790–7.

[93] Binici D, Gunes N. Risk factors leading to reduced bone mineral density in hemodialysis patients with metabolic syndrome. Renal Failure 2010;32:469–74.

[94] Inaba M. Chronic kidney disease (CKD) and bone. Impact of diabetes mellitus on the development of CKD-BMD. Clin Calcium 2009;19:502–7.

[95] Tanaka H, Hamano T, Fujii N, et al. The impact of diabetes mellitus on vitamin D metabolism in predialysis patients. Bone 2009;45:949–55.

[96] Isidro ML, Ruano B. Bone disease in diabetes. Curr Diabetes Rev 2010;6:144–55.

[97] Agarwa R. Vitamin D, proteinuria, diabetic nephropathy, and progression of CKD. Clin J Am Soc Nephrol 2009;4: 1523–8.

[98] Elsurer R, Afsar B, Guner E, et al. Targeting parathyroid hormone levels in diabetic patients with stage 3 to 5 chronic kidney disease: Does metabolic syndrome matter? J Ren Nutr 2010 Jul 20; (Epub ahead of print).

[99] Pittas AG, Dawson-Hughes B. Vitamin D and diabetes. J Steroid Bioch and Mol Biol 2010;121:425–9.

[100] Zipitis CS, Akobeng AK. Vitamin D supplementation in early childhood and risk of type 1 diabetes: a systematic review and meta-analysis. Arch Dis Child 2008;93:512–7.

[101] Dalgard C, Petersen MS, Weihe P, et al. Vitamin D status in relation to glucose metabolism and type 2 diabetes in septuagenarians. Diabetes Care 2011;34:1284–8.

[102] Mattilo C, Knekt P, Mannisto S, et al. Serum 25-OH D concentrations and subsequent risk of diabetes. Diabetes Care 2007;30:2569–70.

[103] Kositsawat J, Freeman VL, Gerber BS, et al. Association of A1c levels with vitamin D status in U.S. adults. Diabetes Care 2010; 33:1236–8.

[104] Thacker TD, Clarke BL. Vitamin D Insufficiency. Mayo Clin Proc 2011;86:50–60.

[105] Stefikova K, Spustova V, Krisosikova Z, et al. Insulin resistance and vitamin D deficiency in patients with chronic kidney disease stage 2–3. Physiol Rev 2011;60:149–15.

[106] Chonchol M, Scragg R. 25-hydroxyvitamin D, insulin resistance, and kidney function in the Third National Health and Nutrition Examination Survey. Kidney Int 2007;71:134–9.

[107] Petchey WG, Hickman IJ, Duncan E, et al. The role of 25-hydroxyvitamin D deficiency in promoting insulin resistance and inflammation in patients with chronic kidney disease: a randomized controlled trial. BMC Nephrol 2009;10:41.

[108] Maxwell CS, Wood RJ. Update on vitamin D and type 2 diabetes. Nutr Rev 2011;69:291–5.

[109] Liu S. Dietary calcium, vitamin D, and the prevalence of metabolic syndrome in middle-aged and older U.S. women. Diabetes Care 2005 2005;28:2926.

[110] Marjamaki L, Niiristos S, Kenward MG, et al. Maternal intake of vitamins during pregnancy and risk of advanced beta cell autoimmunity and type 1 diabetes in offspring. Diabetologia 2010; PMI 20369220.

[111] Mathieu C. Vitamin D and diabetes: the devil is in the D-tails. Diabetologia 2010;53:1545–8.

[112] Alon DB, Chaimovitz C, Dvilansky A, et al. Novel role of 1,25 (OH)(2)D(3) in induction of erythroid progenitor cell proliferation. Exp Hemat 2002;30:403–9.

[113] Patel NM, Gutierrez OM, Andress DL, et al. Vitamin D deficiency and anemia in early chronic kidney disease. Kidney Int 2010;77:715–120.

[114] Joergensen C, Gall MA, Schmedes A, et al. Vitamin D levels and mortality in type 2 diabetes. Diabetes Care 2010;33: 238–2243.

[115] Rosato MT. Bone turnover and Insulin-like growth factor 1 levels increase after improved glycemic control in noninsulin-dependent diabetes mellitus. Calc Tissue Int 1998;63:107.

[116] Sugimoto T, Ritter C, Morrissey J, et al. Effects of high concentrations of glucose on Pth secretion in parathyroid cells. Kidney Int 1990;37:1522–7.

[117] Lozano D, de Castro LF, Daia S, et al. Role of parathyroid hormone-related protein in the decreased osteoblastic function in diabetes-related osteopenia. Endocrinology 2009;150:2027–35.

[118] Wesseling-Perry K, Pereira RC, Sahney S, et al. Calcitriol and doxercalciferol are equivalent in controlling bone turnover, suppressing parathyroid hormone, and increasing fibroblast growth factor-23 in secondary hyperparathyroidism. Kidney Int 2011;79:112–9.

[119] Murakami R, Murakami S, Tsushima R, et al. Glycaemic control and serum intact parathyroid hormone levels in diabetic patients on haemodialysis therapy. Nephrol Dial Transplant 2008;23:315–20.

[120] Giordano C. Protein restriction in chronic renal failure. Kidney Internat 1982;22:401–8.

[121] Dunn BR, Zatz R, Rennke HG, Meyer TW, Anderson S, Brenner BM. Prevention of glomerular capillary hypertension in experimental diabetes mellitus obviates functional and structural glomerular injury. J Hypertens Suppl 1986;4:S251–4.

[122] Hostetter TH, Meyer TW, Rennke HG, Brenner BM. Chronic effects of dietary protein in the rat with intact and reduced renal mass. Kidney Int 1986;30:509–17.

[123] Meyer TW, Anderson S, Rennke HG, Brenner BM. Reversing glomerular hypertension stabilizes established glomerular injury in renal ablation. J Hypertens Suppl 1986;4:S239–41.

[124] Meyer TW, Anderson S, Rennke HG, Brenner BM. Reversing glomerular hypertension stabilizes established glomerular injury. Kidney Int 1987;31:752–9.

[125] Zatz R, Anderson S, Meyer TW, Dunn BR, Rennke HG, Brenner BM. Lowering of arterial blood pressure limits glomerular sclerosis in rats with renal ablation and in experimental diabetes. Kidney Int Suppl 1987;20:S123–9.

[126] Zatz R, Dunn BR, Meyer TW, Anderson S, Rennke HG, Brenner BM. Prevention of diabetic glomerulopathy by pharmacological amelioration of glomerular capillary hypertension. J Clin Invest 1986;77:1925–30.

[127] Zatz R, Meyer TW, Rennke HG, Brenner BM. Predominance of hemodynamic rather than metabolic factors in the pathogenesis of diabetic glomerulopathy. Proc Natl Acad Sci USA 1985;82: 5963–7.

[128] Ruggenenti P, Cravedi P, Remuzzi G. The RAAS in the pathogenesis and treatment of diabetic nephropathy. Nat Rev Nephrol 2010;6:319–30.

[129] Holtkamp FA, de Zeeuw D, Thomas MC, Cooper ME, de Graeff PA, et al. An acute fall in estimated glomerular filtration rate during treatment with losartan predicts a slower decrease in long-term renal function. Kidney Int 2011;80:282–7.

[130] Klahr S. The effects of dietary protein restriction and blood-pressure control on the progression of chronic renal disease. New Engl J Med 1994;330:887–884.

[131] Levey AS, Greene T, Beck GJ, Caggiula AW, Kusek JW, Hunsicker LG, et al. Dietary protein restriction and the progression of chronic renal disease: what have all of the results of the MDRD study shown? Modification of Diet in Renal Disease Study group. J Am Soc Nephrol 1999;10:2426–39.

[132] Association AD. Nutrition Recommendations and Interventions for Diabetes: A position statement of the American Diabetes Association. Diabetes Care 2008;31(Suppl. 1):S61–78.

[133] Toeller M, Buyken A, Heitkamp G, Bramswig S, Mann J, Milne R, et al. Protein intake and urinary albumin excretion rates in the EURODIAB IDDM Complications Study. Diabetologia 1997;40:1219–26.

[134] Bellizzi V, Di Iorio BR, De Nicola L, Minutolo R, Zamboli P, et al. Very low protein diet supplemented with ketoanalogs improves blood pressure control in chronic kidney disease. Kidney Int 2007;71:245–51.

[135] Robertson L, Waugh N, Robertson A. Protein restriction for diabetic renal disease. Cochrane Database Syst Rev 2009; CD002181.

[136] Knight EL, Stampfer MJ, Hankinson SE, Spiegelman D, Curhan GC. The impact of protein intake on renal function decline in women with normal renal function or mild renal insufficiency. Ann Intern Med 2003;138:460–7.

[137] Mollsten AV, Dahlquist GG, Stattin EL, Rudberg S. Higher intakes of fish protein are related to a lower risk of micro-albuminuria in young Swedish type 1 diabetic patients. Diabetes Care 2001;24:805–10.

[138] Kopple JD. Therapeutic approaches to malnutrition in chronic dialysis patients: the different modalities of nutritional support. Am J Kidney Dis 1999;33:180–5.

[139] Kopple JD. The National Kidney Foundation K/DOQI clinical practice guidelines for dietary protein intake for chronic dialysis patients. Am J Kidney Dis 2001;38:S68–73.

[140] Kalantar-Zadeh K, Ikizler TA, Block G, Avram MM, Kopple JD. Malnutrition-inflammation complex syndrome in dialysis patients: causes and consequences. Am J Kidney Dis 2003;42: 864–81.

[141] Shinaberger CS, Kilpatrick RD, Regidor DL, McAllister CJ, Greenland S, Kopple JD, et al. Longitudinal associations between dietary protein intake and survival in hemodialysis patients. Am J Kidney Dis 2006;48:37–49.

[142] Noori N, Kopple JD. Effect of diabetes mellitus on protein-energy wasting and protein wasting in end-stage renal disease. Semin Dial 23:178–184.

[143] Suckling RJ, He FJ, Macgregor GA. Altered dietary salt intake for preventing and treating diabetic kidney disease. Cochrane Database Syst Rev 2011;CD006763.

[144] Berl T. Review: renal protection by inhibition of the renin-angiotensin-aldosterone system. J Renin Angiotensin Aldosterone Syst 2009;10:1–8.

[145] Laight DW. Therapeutic inhibition of the renin angiotensin aldosterone system. Expert Opin Ther Pat 2009;19:753–9.

[146] Bakris GL, Smith A. Effects of sodium intake on albumin excretion in patients with diabetic nephropathy treated with long-acting calcium antagonists. Ann Intern Med 1996;125:201–4.

[147] Houlihan CA, Allen TJ, Baxter AL, Panangiotopoulos S, Casley DJ, Cooper ME, et al. A low-sodium diet potentiates the effects of losartan in type 2 diabetes. Diabetes Care 2002;25:663–71.

Nutritional Management of Maintenance Hemodialysis Patients

Kamyar Kalantar-Zadeh[1], *Joel D. Kopple*[2]

[1]Division of Nephrology and Hypertension, University of California Irvine, School of Medicine, Orange, CA, USA
[2]David Geffen School of Medicine at UCLA, and UCLA Fielding School of Public Health Harbor-UCLA Medical Center, Torrance, CA, USA

INTRODUCTION

Protein-energy wasting (PEW) is a common and strong predictor of poor outcomes in patients undergoing maintenance hemodialysis (MHD) [1,2]. As discussed in detail in Chapter 12, there is a strong association between PEW and greater risk of morbidity and mortality [3–6]. In particular low body weight-for-height or body mass index (BMI), reduced serum cholesterol, albumin and prealbumin (transthyretin), and decreased protein intake have been shown to occur frequently in MHD patients and are also associated with increased risk of morbidity and mortality [7–10]. Other measures that commonly indicate PEW in MHD patients but have not yet been shown to correlate with poor outcome include decreased energy intake, mid-arm muscle circumference [11], skeletal muscle alkali soluble protein, and total body fat, among others [12]. The relationship between outcome and some of these measures, such as low body weight-for-height [8] or BMI [9] and reduced serum cholesterol [10,13,14] in MHD patients are to a substantial degree in opposition to the epidemiological relationships between nutritional measures and outcome that have been observed repeatedly in the general population [15]. This paradoxical reversal of risk factors in MHD patients (the so-called "reverse epidemiology" [7] or obesity paradox [16]) might underscore the importance of nutrition as a predictor for outcome in these individuals, because body weight or serum cholesterol can be increased with appropriate type of nutritional intake. Indeed recent longitudinal studies in large numbers of MHD patients suggest that a gain in post-hemodialysis dry weight over time is associated with greater survival whereas unintentional weight loss harbors increased mortality risk over time (Figure 32.1).

This thesis, i.e. increasing nutritional intake will reduce mortality risk, still needs to be tested in randomized prospective clinical trials.

Inflammation, which is also associated with increased morbidity and mortality in MHD patients, may itself promote malnutrition by engendering both anorexia as well as a catabolic state, while genetic constellation may play a permissive role [17]. It is also possible, but not proven, that PEW may actually predispose to inflammation as well [6]. The findings that measures of inflammation as well as PEM, either independently or combined, predict mortality, and that there may be an interaction between inflammation and PEW have given rise to the concept of the "malnutrition-inflammation complex syndrome" (MICS) [3,6,18,19]. Acidemia, which is also common in individuals with ESRD, including maintenance dialysis patients, may also cause catabolism and contribute to PEW [20]. The fact that mortality of MHD patients still averages about 20% per year in the United States emphasizes the importance of examining the causes of this high mortality in these individuals. The recently completed HEMO Study failed to show an improvement in morbidity or mortality in MHD patients who were treated with a higher dialysis dose (average single-pool Kt/V of 1.71 ± 0.11) vs. a lower dose (average single-pool Kt/V of 1.32 ± 0.09) and/or high flux dialyzer membranes [21]. This suggests the possibility that other factors such as PEW and/or inflammatory diseases may play a more central causal role in the poor outcome of this group of patients.

Nutritional Management of Renal Disease
http://dx.doi.org/10.1016/B978-0-12-391934-2.00032-1

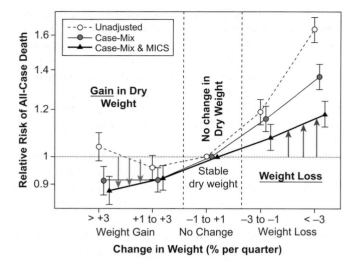

FIGURE 32.1 Association of change in dry weight over 6-months and 5-year mortality in 88,729 MHD patients. *Adapted from Kalantar-Zadeh et al., Mayo Clinic Proceedings, 2010 [16].* This figure is reproduced in color in the color plate section.

PEW is not the only form of malnutrition in MHD patients. It has long been recognized that MHD patients may suffer from deficiency of micronutrients as well. In patients who are not taking vitamin and mineral supplements, deficiencies have been particularly commonly reported for ascorbate, folate, pyridoxine (vitamin B_6) and calcitriol (1,25-dihydroxy-cholecalciferol) [22–26] and iron and zinc [27–29]. Some deficiencies, such as for ascorbate, carotenoids and folate, could play an important role in the development of atherosclerotic cardiovascular diseases [30–32]. Indeed, studies using food frequency questionnaires have found a higher intake of atherogenic diets in MHD patients in association with inadequate ingestion of these antioxidant vitamins [33]. Moreover, management of such important conditions as end-stage renal disease (ESRD) associated anemia and osteodystrophy cannot be achieved without special attention to nutritional intake of such elements as iron, calcium and phosphorus. On the other hand, excessive intake of a number of essential nutrients can be hazardous in renal failure. This is perhaps more commonly shown for sodium, water, potassium, phosphorus, magnesium, calcium, and protein. For instance, excessive intake of calcium-containing foods and, particularly, calcium-containing medications may play a crucial role in the development of coronary artery calcification and the consequent increased rate of cardiovascular events in MHD patients [34,35].

Many factors have been implicated as the cause for malnutrition in both chronic kidney disease (CKD) and ESRD patients; these are described in detail in Chapter 11. The present chapter focuses on the evaluation and management of the nutritional state in MHD patients.

FACTORS ALTERING NUTRIENT INTAKE IN MAINTENANCE HEMODIALYSIS PATIENTS

Appetite is considered to be the gateway to the nutritional state. A diminished appetite occurs commonly in MHD patients and decreases the patient's ability to ingest a sufficient diet [36–38]. Dietary protein intake is often decreased in MHD patients. More strikingly, in almost all studies of nutritional intake, energy intake of individual MHD patients is below that of normal rather sedentary individuals and is also reduced below that recommended for MHD [38] (Chapter 11). A cross-sectional study in 331 MHD patients showed that at least 38% of the MHD patients reported reduced appetite, which was associated with a statistically significant decrease in their protein equivalent of total nitrogen appearance (PNA), also referred to as protein catabolic rate (PCR) [38]. In this study a diminished appetite was also associated with decreased serum levels of such nutritional markers as prealbumin (transthyretin), total cholesterol and total iron binding capacity (TIBC), and increased serum levels of the inflammatory markers, C-reactive protein (CRP), interleukin-6 (IL-6) and tumor necrosis factor alpha (TNF-α). Moreover, MHD patients with a reduced appetite required higher doses of human recombinant erythropoietin and reported a lower quality of life as measured by the SF36 scoring system [38].

In contrast to chronic peritoneal dialysis (CPD) patients who are frequently encouraged to ingest foods that can be high in potassium content, MHD patients often suffer from hyperkalemia, hyperphosphatemia and excess sodium and water gain and therefore are almost invariably asked to reduce intake of foods rich in the above-mentioned components. Such prescribed limitations in the diet of MHD patients may impose additional restrictions on their nutritional intake, even when their appetite is intact. Furthermore, the current interest in advocating anti-atherogenic diets in MHD patients who have a high incidence and prevalence of atherosclerotic diseases may further constrain the ability of MHD patients to eat adequate energy, protein and other nutrients [33]. Dietary treatment of diabetes mellitus, which in MHD patients is both very common (up to 55% of MHD patients in some parts of the United States [39]) and increasing in prevalence, leads to further dietary restriction. Also, many multi-morbid and/or debilitated MHD patients have difficulty in procuring and preparing foods because of insufficient funds to purchase foods or physical or mental disabilities that may impair their capacity to shop, cook, or even ingest food (e.g., emotional depression or lack of dentures). An increased prevalence of metabolic acidemia and other catabolic comorbid conditions may also induce anorexia in MHD patients [36]. Therefore, inadequate nutrient intake in MHD patients may be the most important single factor in the development and maintenance of malnutrition.

LOSS OF NUTRIENTS DURING MAINTENANCE HEMODIALYSIS TREATMENT

Several studies have examined amino acid losses during hemodialysis [40–42]. Kopple et al. showed that free amino acid losses ranged from 4.5 to 7.7 g per hemodialysis in fasting patients who were undergoing dialysis with a Kiil dialyzer for 11 hours [40]; 3.7 g (range, 2.4 to 5.2 g) of bound amino acids (e.g., peptides) were also lost into the dialysate. When patients were fed during the hemodialysis procedure, the free amino acid losses increased to about 5 to 8 g per hemodialysis. These studies were conducted with glucose-free dialysate. When dialysis was carried out with glucose in dialysate, 450 mg/dL (405 mg/dL of anhydrous glucose), free amino acid losses diminished to 3.3 g and 6.0 g in the fasted and nonfasted state, respectively. Gutierrez et al. were unable to confirm that dialysate with glucose suppressed amino acid losses [43]; however, these authors used a standard glucose concentration of 180 mg/dL in the dialysate. These latter investigators used the Baxter cellulose acetate and Gambro GFS plus 20 dialyzers and found 8.3 ± 0.9 SEM g and 7.9 ± 0.4 g of amino acid losses with glucose containing and glucose-free dialysate, respectively.

Wolfson et al [43]. described losses of about 8.2 ± 3.1 g SD of free amino acids during a 5-hour hemodialysis using 1.5 m^2 hollow fiber or 1.0 or 1.5 mL parallel plate dialyzers. When patients were given intravenous infusions of 39.5 g of amino acids and 200 g of D-glucose monohydrate during the hemodialysis, losses increased only slightly, to 12.6 ± 3.6 g. The retention of about 89% of the infused amino acids (68% of the infused amino acids if the amino acid losses during fasting losses are not discounted) was predictable because the plasma amino acid concentrations at the end of the hemodialysis with the amino acid and glucose infusion had increased by 70% over the plasma amino acid levels obtained at the end of a hemodialysis without the infusion of the nutrients. Thus, it was not anticipated that large amounts of the infused amino acids would be removed by hemodialysis.

Ikizler et al. examined amino acid and protein losses in patients undergoing hemodialysis with three different types of dialyzer membranes [42]. The patients ingested a small meal about one hour prior to the hemodialysis procedure. Patients undergoing hemodialysis

with high-flux polysulfone membranes (HF-PS) lost 8.0 ± 2.8 g of amino acid per dialysis session as compared to patients dialyzed with low-flux polymethylmethacrylate membranes, who lost 6.1 ± 1.5 g of amino acids, and those dialyzed with cellulose acetate membranes, who lost 7.1 ± 2.6 g. These small differences in amino acid losses may be due to variations in the dialyzer surface area and blood flow rates, and are probably biologically insignificant.

It should be noted that protein losses during hemodialysis are typically very small. However, several years ago, multiple reuses of high-flux polysulfone (HF-PS) dialyzers after reprocessing of the dialyzers with bleach and formaldehyde resulted in marked increases in protein losses due to increased permeability of these membranes [42,44]. Ikizler et al [42]. found that albumin losses became apparent after the sixth reuse of the HF-PS membrane. These losses increased significantly, from 1.5 ± 1.3 SD g per dialysis session by the fifteenth reuse to 9.3 ± 5.5 g at the twentieth. Kaplan et al. observed similar results [44]. The amino acid losses increased slightly, by 50%, after the sixth reuse in the HF-PS membranes. More recently, polysulfone membranes have been made more resistant to the bleach that is used in the reuse process.

Blood sequestered in the hemodialyzer, clotted or leaking dialyzers, oozing of blood from the needle punctures of the vascular access site, and blood sampling for laboratory testing may contribute to protein losses. Approximately 5 to 10 mL of blood may be trapped in the dialyzer at the end of each dialysis. This could account for another 0.6 to 1.6 g of protein lost per dialysis session [45].

Several investigators have described a high prevalence of acidosis in maintenance hemodialysis patients, as indicated by low predialysis serum bicarbonate concentrations [46–49]. Metabolic acidemia has been shown to promote bone reabsorption and engender protein catabolism [50]. It is therefore important to treat acidemia. The National Kidney Foundation Kidney Disease Outcomes Quality Initiative (K/DOQI) Clinical Practice Guidelines for Nutrition in Chronic Renal Failure recommends that the serum bicarbonate concentration should be maintained at or above 22 mEq/L [51]. Recent information suggests that the serum bicarbonate concentration should be maintained higher [49,52], possibly 24 mEq/L if not greater [50].

It has been argued that the hemodialysis procedure itself may be catabolic. Gutierrez et al [53,54]. demonstrated enhanced release of amino acids from the skeletal muscle of individuals who were sham-dialyzed with Cupraphan dialyzers; no dialysate was used in these studies, and the investigators exclusively examined blood–membrane or blood-tubing interactions. This amino acid release could be abolished by pretreatment with indomethacin, suggesting that prostaglandins were involved in the genesis of the catabolic effects. The data of Borah et al [55]. also suggest that hemodialysis may induce catabolism, although the nitrogen balance studies were short-term and the lack of time for equilibration after changing the dietary protein intake may have inadvertently prejudiced their findings.

It has been argued that the activation of complement and leukocytes by less biocompatible dialyzer membranes may lead to release of such proinflammatory cytokines as TNF-a, IL-1, IL-6, and granulocyte proteases [18,56–58]. Oxidative stress may also play a central role in activation of the inflammatory cascade in MHD patients [59]. The pro-inflammatory cytokines can induce catabolism [60–62]. In recent years, increasing attention has been paid to the role of inflammation as a cause of the hypercatabolic state in MHD patients [6,18,63]. Indeed, some investigators maintain that inflammation plays a primary role in the complex constellation of malnutrition-inflammation-atherosclerosis (hence, called the MIA syndrome [64]), whereas others suggest that anorexia, inadequate nutritional intake and nutrient losses as well as inflammation may predispose to tissue wasting. Inflammation per se appears to promote anorexia, inadequate intake and protein catabolism, whereas PEW might also predispose to inflammation [6], although evidence for this is still preliminary. Thus the term "malnutrition-inflammation complex syndrome" (MICS) may be a more appropriate appellation [65,66]. Recent data also suggest the intriguing possibility that metabolic acidemia may predispose to inflammation [67].

Nutrient losses during MHD are not restricted to protein and amino acids; other macro- and micronutrients may also be lost. Gutierrez et al [43]. found that about 26 g of glucose were removed during a hemodialysis with glucose-free dialysate and about 30 g of glucose were absorbed by the patient when dialysate containing glucose, 180 mg/dL, was used. Wathen et al. obtained similar results [68]. The quantities of water soluble vitamins lost during hemodialysis are not large, because plasma concentrations of the water soluble vitamins are not great and the molecular weights of these compounds are somewhat larger (i.e., greater than many amino acids). Losses are particularly prone to occur for vitamins B_1 (thiamin), B_2 (riboflavin), and B_6 (pyridoxine), ascorbic acid, and folic acid [22,25,26,69–71]. Although vitamin B_{12} is water soluble, its losses during hemodialysis are negligible because it is largely protein bound in plasma. The losses of these vitamins in dialysate are to some extent offset by the marked reduction or absence of urinary vitamin excretion in maintenance dialysis patients. Thus, the removal of water soluble vitamins by hemodialysis is easily

replaceable by food intake and supplements of vitamins. The losses of vitamins during hemodialysis are discussed in more detail in Chapter 24.

IMPORTANCE OF PEW AND DIET AS PATIENTS APPROACH ESRD AND COMMENCE MHD

Data suggest that the nutritional status of both pediatric and adult patients at the onset of maintenance dialysis is a predictor of their nutritional status one or two years later [67,72–75], even though nutritional status may undergo improvement with the advent of dialysis therapy. Thus, to prevent malnutrition in MHD patients, it would seem important to monitor the nutritional status and to endeavor to prevent malnutrition from occurring in patients before MHD is instituted, i.e. during progressive phases of CKD. In this regard, many patients become frankly anorectic, eat poorly, and sustain a deterioration in their nutritional and clinical status prior to the onset of dialysis therapy and particularly between the time when their glomerular filtration rate (GFR) decreases to about 5 to 10 mL/min (CKD stage 5) and the time when they are established on MHD therapy [76]. It follows that steps should be taken to ensure a smooth transition to MHD when the patient has stage 4 or 5 CKD, i.e. estimated GFR less than 30 mL/min [77].

Indeed, the National Kidney Foundation K/DOQI Nutrition Work Group has recommended the following as a nutritional indication for commencing renal replacement therapy in individuals with advanced CKD:

> In patients with chronic renal failure (e.g. GFR <15–20 mL/ min) who are not undergoing maintenance dialysis, if protein-energy malnutrition develops or persists despite vigorous attempts to optimize protein and energy intake and there is no apparent cause for malnutrition other than low nutrient intake, initiation of maintenance dialysis or a renal transplant is recommended [78].

ASSESSMENT OF NUTRITIONAL STATUS IN MHD PATIENTS

Because malnutrition can be insidious in MHD patients, their nutritional status should be assessed when they commence MHD and at monthly intervals thereafter (see Chapter 10 and Tables 32.1 and 32.2). Moreover, due to the strong association between the nutritional state and outcome in MHD patients and because of the high mortality and hospitalization rate in these individuals, many nutritional markers are outcome predictors. For example, serum albumin,

TABLE 32.1 Recommended Measures for Monitoring Nutritional Status of MHD Patients Based on K/DOQI Guidelines

Category	Measure	Minimum Frequency of Measurement
I. Measurements that should be performed routinely in all patients	• Predialysis or stabilized serum albumin • % of usual postdialysis body weight, body mass index (BMI)* and interdialytic weight gain* • % of standard (NHANES II) body weight • Subjective global assessment (SGA) • Dietary interview and/or diary • nPNA (nPCR)	• Monthly • Monthly • Every 4 months • Every 6 months • Every 6 months • Monthly
II. Measures that can be useful to confirm or extend the data obtained from the measures in Category I	• Predialysis or stabilized serum prealbumin (transthyretin) • Skinfold thickness • Mid-arm muscle area, circumference, or diameter • Dual energy X-ray absorptiometry	• As needed • As needed • As needed • As needed

III. Clinically useful measures, which, if low, might suggest the need for a more rigorous examination of protein-energy nutritional status	• Predialysis or stabilized serum
	  − Creatinine
	  − Urea nitrogen
	  − Cholesterol
	• Creatinine index
		
		• As needed
		• As needed
		• As needed

From [78]. Printed with permission.

serum creatinine, and body weight-for-height or BMI are independently associated with survival [79]. Data from the United States Renal Data System (USRDS) and large dialysis organizations confirm these findings,

TABLE 32.2 Additional Recommended Measures for Monitoring Nutritional Status of MHD Patients (see also Table 32.1 for K/DOQI guidelines)

Category	Measure	Minimum Frequency of Measurement
IV. Additional Measures and Tools	• Serum calcium, phosphorus, and Ca-P product	• Monthly
	• Serum potassium	• Monthly
	• Serum bicarbonate, anion gap	• Every 3 months
	• Serum TIBC or transferrin, iron saturation ratio	• Monthly
	• Serum ferritin	• Every 3 months
	• Lipid panel: total cholesterol, triglyceride, LDL and HDL cholesterol	• Every 6 months
	• Serum C-reactive protein*	• Every 3 to 6 months
	• Plasma total homocysteine	• Every 12 months

* Other inflammatory markers in serum that may be increased include interleukin-6 (IL-6), IL-1β), and tumor necrosis factor alpha (TNF-α).

using the serum albumin and BMI (kg/m^2) [80]. In the Canada-USA (CANUSA) Study, both the serum albumin and SGA were independent predictors of death or treatment failure [81]. Chapter 12 includes an outcome-oriented approach to the nutritional assessment of patients with renal failure.

The K/DOQI guidelines include comprehensive recommendations pertaining to the nutritional and dietary assessment of MHD patients. According to these guidelines, nutritional status in MHD patients should be assessed with a combination of valid, complementary measures rather than any single measure alone, since there is no single measure that provides a comprehensive indication of protein-energy nutritional status (Table 32.1). Moreover, measures of energy and protein intake, visceral protein pools, muscle mass, other dimensions of body composition, and functional status identify different aspects of protein-energy nutritional status, and malnutrition may be identified with greater sensitivity and specificity using a combination of factors. The K/DOQI guidelines recommend that nutritional status of MHD patients should be routinely assessed by predialysis or stabilized serum albumin, percent of usual body weight, percent of standard (NHANES II) body weight, SGA, dietary interviews and diaries, and nPNA (nPCR) [77]. Table 32.1 shows a list of parameters and tools to evaluate nutritional status and the assessment intervals as recommended by K/DOQI.

K/DOQI nutritional assessment guidelines include three categories. The first category includes those measurements that should be routinely performed on all MHD patients. Serum albumin should be assessed monthly as should the percent of post-hemodialysis body weight, but percent of standard body weight may be evaluated every 4 months (see Table 32.1). There is no specific recommendation regarding the BMI, but due to the ease of its calculation based on post-hemodialysis dry weight and height (weight in kg divided by height in meters squared) many healthcare workers in dialysis facilities calculate and evaluate the BMI routinely on a monthly to quarterly basis. For routine overall assessment, the conventional version of the Subjective Global Assessment of nutrition (SGA) [82−86] (Chapters 10 and 12) and/or its newer derivatives such as the Malnutrition-Inflammation Score (MIS) [87−89] (Chapters 10 and 12) should be evaluated semiannually. The K/DOQI guidelines recommend calculating nPNA every month.

The second category (Table 32.1) includes those measures that can be useful to confirm or extend data obtained from the measures in Category 1. Serum prealbumin (transthyretin) has a strong association with hospitalization and mortality and, like serum albumin, is a negative acute phase reactant [90−92]. Caliper anthropometry can be used to measure skinfold thicknesses, usually obtained in the biceps, triceps, subscapular and suprailiac areas (an indicator of body fat mass). Midarm muscle circumference (an indicator of skeletal muscle mass) as well as its area and diameter can be measured simultaneously. Anthropometry should be carried out by personnel who have been specifically trained in these techniques and who have accurate and reliable equipment, which is not expensive. Although body composition parameters such as the percentage of body fat can be assessed by such convenient methods as bioelectrical impedance analysis (BIA) [93,94] or near infra-red interactance (NIR) [95], a more objective method of estimating body composition, dual energy X-ray absoptiometry (DEXA) is the recommended technique according to the K/DOQI guidelines [96−99]. Although the availability of these energy-beam based methods (DEXA, BIA, NIR) is increasing, their routine use is still largely limited to the research setting and a few health care center clinical treatment programs. There is not yet evidence that the use of these techniques improves the management or outcome of MHD patients over the generally simpler methods of nutritional assessment indicated in the Category I level of Table 32.1.

The third category includes several clinically useful measures, which, if low, might suggest the need for a more rigorous examination of protein-energy nutritional status. These consist of serum concentrations of creatinine, urea nitrogen and cholesterol as well as the creatinine index (see Table 32.1). The K/DOQI nutritional guidelines do not recommend serum total iron

binding capacity (TIBC), which is a reliable estimator of serum transferrin, because serum TIBC concentrations are influenced by inflammation and iron stores as well as by protein-energy nutritional status [77]. However, recent studies in MHD patients have shown a strong association between serum TIBC and such nutritional markers as SGA and also between TIBC and outcome [100]. Many of the biochemical measurements are influenced by non-nutritional factors. For example, serum albumin is affected by the hydration status as well as by acute illness and inflammation [101,102]. Serum albumin, prealbumin and TIBC are negative acute phase reactants [18,103]. Serum creatinine and urea nitrogen also strongly reflect the dose of dialysis. Notwithstanding these factors, a number of epidemiological studies have clearly demonstrated that these common laboratory measurements are strong predictors of hospitalization and death in MHD patients [14,104−106]. Dietary history can also provide a useful estimate of the patient's intake of protein, energy and other nutrients. However, the services of a trained dietitian or dietetic technician are almost always required to achieve acceptable accuracy. More convenient, self-administered food frequency questionnaires (FFQ) have also been used to compare dietary intake of MHD patients with other individuals [33,107]; but FFQs may not be sufficiently precise, and they tend to underestimate food intake [33]. Their use is essentially limited to epidemiological studies.

The foregoing recommendations are based on K/DOQI guidelines that focus mainly on protein and energy malnutrition [77], More recently, the International Society of Renal Nutrition and Metabolism (ISRNM) has advanced a similar panel of assessment tools to screen for and diagnose PEW [2]. Hence, we propose the ISRNM panels (Table 32.2) for some important nutritional parameters that are not recommended for monitoring in the original K/DOQI panel. In many dialysis facilities, serum concentrations of potassium, calcium and phosphorus are measured routinely on a monthly basis as are iron status indicators including serum ferritin, TIBC and iron saturation ratio. At least biannual measurements of serum lipids including total serum cholesterol and LDL are recommended, because an increasing proportion of MHD patients, particularly those with diabetes mellitus, are hyperlipidemic. On the other hand, a low serum cholesterol is a strong predictor of poor outcome in dialysis patients [13,14]. Although inflammatory markers are not currently measured routinely, we recommend that at least C-reactive protein (CRP) be measured every several months, so that high risk patients with inflammation can be identified [108]. Finally, total plasma homocysteine is a cardiovascular risk factor and also a nutritional marker. Both high [109] as well as low [110−112] plasma homocysteine levels have been associated with poor outcome in MHD patients.

Urea Kinetic, Adequacy of Dialysis, and Nutritional Status

The urea nitrogen appearance (UNA) is used to estimate nitrogen losses and, hence, in the steady state, nitrogen intake. UNA is the quantity of nitrogen that appears in the urine, dialysate, and all other outputs plus the change in body urea nitrogen. The PNA (PCR) expresses total nitrogen appearance in terms of the equivalent amount of protein lost that is represented by the UNA [113,114]. In MHD patients the UNA is directly calculated from urea kinetics by techniques that have been extensively discussed elsewhere [114,115]. PNA can be calculated from the UNA by one of several formulas [113,115,116]. Under steady-state conditions, the UNA can also be used to estimate the dietary nitrogen intake. Because of nitrogen losses through pathways that are difficult to measure (e.g., respiration, sweat, exfoliated skin, hair and nail growth, flatus, blood drawing), the UNA and PNA essentially always underestimate the dietary nitrogen or protein intake under metabolic steady-state conditions. Hence, a different regression equation must be employed to estimate dietary protein intake, as compared to the PNA, from the UNA [113,114]. A fuller discussion of these terms and the methods for calculating these processes in nondialyzed patients and maintenance dialysis patients is given elsewhere [117].

Several studies have shown a correlation between the prescribed dose of hemodialysis as defined by the Kt/V_{urea} and the dietary protein intake as estimated from the PNA [75,118–121]. The direct relationship between Kt/V and PNA has also been observed in CPD patients [118,122,123], although the slope of the relationship is different in the CPD patients as compared to MHD patients [118]. Some studies of MHD patients described a direct correlation between Kt/V and serum albumin levels [121]. However, most of these studies correlating Kt/V and PNA or serum albumin were not prospective or randomized, and conclusions from these studies therefore must be considered tentative. Lindsay et al. [124] showed a direct relation between Kt/V and PNA in a prospective, randomized study in which Kt/V was increased from 0.82 ± 0.19 (SD) to 1.32 ± 0.21 for 3 months in one of the two groups of patients. The PNA rose in the experimental group from an initial value of 0.81 ± 0.08 g/kg/day to 1.02 ± 0.15 ($P = 0.005$), whereas it did not change in the control group. These studies suggest that increasing the dose of hemodialysis from a Kt/V of roughly 0.6 to a Kt/V_{sp} of 1.5–1.6 will increase the dietary protein intake of

MHD patients. Harty et al. have pointed out that in MHD patients the correlation between Kt/V urea and PNA is partly a consequence of mathematical coupling because the two parameters are obtained from the same plasma pre- and postdialysis measurements and are also normalized to body size [125]. However, others have shown that a significant correlation exists between dialysis dose and dietary protein intake even when dialsis dose is not normalized for body size and when dietary protein intake is estimated by dietary histories [126,127].

Epidemiologic studies suggest that decline in dietary protein intake over time, measured by changes in urea kinetic-based normalized PNA (nPNA or nPCR), may be associated with increased mortality risk in MHD patients [75,128]. In a recent longitudinal cohort study in 53,933 MHD patients the relation between nPNA and all-cause and cardiovascular mortality was examined over two years [75]. The best survival was associated with nPNA between 1.0 and 1.4 g/kg/d, whereas nPNA less than 0.8 or greater than 1.4 g/kg/d was associated with greater mortality (Figure 32.2). A decrease in protein intake during the first 6 months in patients with an nPNA in the 0.8- to 1.2-g/kg/d range was associated incrementally with greater death risks in the subsequent 18 months, whereas an increase in nPNA tended to correlate with reduced death risk [75].

It should be emphasized that the correlation between Kt/V_{urea} and PNA, although significant, is not precise, and many patients with a relatively high Kt/V (i.e., ≥ 1.5 for hemodialysis) have a very low PNA and, hence, a reduced dietary protein intake [119–121,124]. This is not surprising because many MHD patients have comorbid conditions that may lead to a reduction

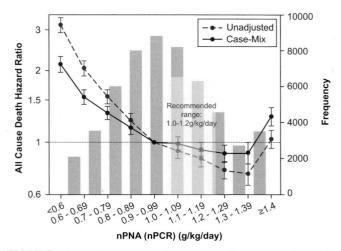

FIGURE 32.2 Association of estimated dietary protein intake (reflected by nPNA or nPCR) and 2-year mortality risk in 53,933 MHD Patients. *Adapted from Shinaberger et al., Am J Kidney Dis 2006; 48:37–49 [75].* This figure is reproduced in color in the color plate section.

in the dietary protein intake independent of their uremic status. Also, patients with severe PEW often have reduced body weight and therefore are more likely to have a higher Kt/V_{urea} even though they may eat poorly [129]. Moreover, there are currently no data as to what extent the Kt/V_{urea} affects the dietary energy intake. A recent prospective study of 122 MHD patients who were adequately dialyzed (i.e., with a delivered average $Kt/V>1.20$ (single pool) over the first 3 months of the cohort, independent of their residual renal function), showed strong associations between normalized PNA (nPNA), measured for three months, and the subsequent 12-month hospitalization and mortality rates [115]. In this latter study, delivered Kt/V ranged from 1.23 to 2.71 (1.77 ± 0.34) and nPNA, from 0.5 to 2.15 (1.13 ± 0.29 g/kg/day). The nPNA and Kt/V did not correlate significantly (r = .09) except when analysis was limited to Kt/V values <1.5 (r = .54) (see Figure 32.3). nPNA and albumin were the only variables with statistically significant correlations with three different measures of hospitalization and mortality [115]. These data are consistent with the possibility that protein intake affects the clinical course of MHD patients even in the setting of an adequate to high dose of dialysis. Moreover, the so-called mathematical coupling between Kt/V and nPCR found in older studies does not appear to occur when Kt/V is greater than 1.50. Studies based on randomized assignments to different protein intakes will be necessary to confirm these conclusions. Current K/DOQI recommendations are to provide MHD patients with a Kt/V_{urea} dose of at least 1.20 [130]; for many dialysis facilities, the Kt/V target is 1.40 or higher. However, the HEMO study failed to show any improvement in hospitalization or mortality with Kt/V (single pool) values of 1.71 ± 0.11 SE as compared to 1.32 ± 0.09 [21], a result that is not consistent with many epidemiological studies based on large sample sizes of five to forty thousand MHD patients [131–134].

ACIDEMIA AND PROTEIN WASTING

Experimental evidence indicates that acidemia may enhance protein catabolism [50,135–143]. In rats, acidemia has been shown to increase the activity of branched chain ketoacid dehydrogenase, which participates in the catabolism of branched chain amino acids [135]. Bergström et al. [141] found a linear correlation between predialysis plasma bicarbonate levels and muscle free valine, suggesting that even transient acidemia may enhance amino acid degradation. Acidemia also increases protein catabolism in skeletal muscle of normal rats and rats with chronic renal failure [137], increases total body protein catabolism, and induces negative nitrogen balance in humans with chronic renal failure [144]. Normal individuals made acutely acidemic, develop reduced albumin synthesis rates and negative nitrogen balance [145]. The acidemia-induced increased proteolysis in skeletal muscle appears to be caused by enhanced activity of the ATP dependent ubiquitin-proteosome pathway [138,140].

Since MHD patients often have low predialysis serum bicarbonate concentrations [46–48,118], acidemia may be common in these patients, at least predialysis. However, low serum bicarbonate is not proof of acidemia; direct measurements of blood pH will provide more definitive information. Nonetheless, the evidence from the foregoing studies that acidemia is harmful appears to be so strong that we currently recommend that bicarbonate supplements be given, when needed, to maintain serum bicarbonate of 24 mEq/L or higher throughout the interdialytic interval unless the low serum bicarbonate levels

FIGURE 32.3 Exploring the association between nPNA and Kt/V_{sp} in 122 MHD patients with a Kt/V_{sp} value >1.20. No significant correlation existed between these two urea kinetic indices despite their known mathematical association (r = .09, p > .20). However, by dividing the patients into two distinct subgroups based on a Kt/V_{sp} cutoff of 1.50, there was a strong, significant correlation between Kt/V and nPNA for the lower Kt/V_{sp} values <1.50 (r = .54, p < .001), whereas there was essentially no correlation at higher Kt/V_{sp} values (r = .03, p > .20). *From [115]. Reprinted with permission.*

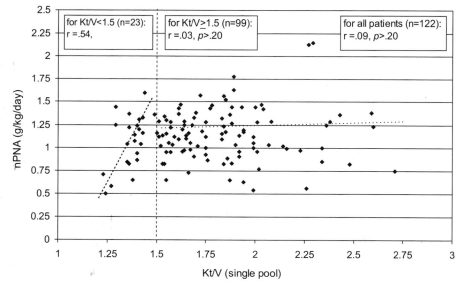

are shown to be associated with a normal blood pH. This value is greater than the National Kidney Foundation K/DOQI guidelines on nutrition [77], but is consistent with more recent experimental findings [146].

GOALS OF NUTRITIONAL MANAGEMENT OF MHD PATIENTS

The goals of dietary therapy and nutritional interventions in MHD patients are: (1) To achieve and maintain good nutritional status; (2) To prevent or retard the development of cardiovascular, cerebrovascular, and peripheral vascular diseases; (3) To prevent or treat hyperparathyroidism and other forms of renal osteodystrophy; and (4) To prevent or ameliorate uremic toxicity and other nutritionally influenced metabolic disorders that occur in renal failure and that are not adequately treated by MHD. Compliance to special diets is often a challenging endeavor for MHD patients and their families. It may require a significant change in their dietary habits as well as their behavioral pattern. They are often required to limit the intake of favorite foods and ingest certain less desirable ones to avoid hyperkalemia or hyperphosphatemia. MHD patients often ingest too little of a required nutrient rather than too much. To enable MHD patients to achieve the desired goals, it is important that patients be educated in the principles of dietary therapy and its targets. Patients and their spouses or other close associates should be instructed in the nutritional content of various foods, as well as the preparation of prescribed diets. Even patients who appear to have no interest in dietary management may benefit from nutritional therapy for several reasons: First, they may decide in the future to follow dietary therapy. Second, even if the patient adheres poorly to the diet, this may provide some health benefits. Finally, nutrition education and encouragement may prevent non-adherent patients from deviating further from good nutrient intake, particularly as they age or are subjected to emotional or physical stress. Chapters 38, 39 and 46 review methods for preparing patients for dietary therapy and maximizing compliance, and indicate some food supplements available for patients with chronic renal failure.

DIETARY NUTRIENT REQUIREMENTS
(See Table 32.3)

Protein Requirements

Surprisingly few studies have assessed the dietary protein requirements for MHD patients [55,147−152]. Moreover, there is not a single randomized prospective clinical trial in which MHD patients were randomly assigned to different levels of dietary protein intake as the independent variable, and the effect of protein intake on morbidity and mortality was examined. The publications that address protein requirements are of two types:

1. Several prospective studies compared the effects of different dietary protein intakes on the nutritional status of the patients; these studies used measures of nutritional status as the indication of a beneficial clinical response. Most of these studies were carried out in hospital research wards or clinical facilities modified for research activities, and the numbers of patients included in each study were small [148,149,151]. It is noteworthy that most of these studies addressing protein requirements in hemodialysis patients were carried out several or more years ago and used dialyzers and dialyzer clearances that are no longer in use [149,151]. The other type of study involved retrospective analyses in larger numbers of patients of the relationships between dietary protein intake, assessed from the nPNA, and morbidity or mortality [75,128,150,153].

2. The National Kidney Foundation K/DOQI guidelines on Nutrition in Chronic Renal Failure recommend a dietary protein intake (DPI) for clinically stable MHD patients of 1.2 g/kg body weight/day; at least 50% of the dietary protein should be of high biological value in order to ensure adequate intake of essential amino acids [78]. These recommendations are based on the level of protein intake that, for the great majority of MHD patients, will maintain neutral or positive nitrogen balance and lead to maintenance or improvement in other such markers of nutritional status as serum albumin [78]. Many MHD patients will maintain protein balance with lower dietary protein intakes [78]. However, this protein intake is considered to be about the minimum level that will maintain neutral or positive nitrogen balance in the great majority, approximately 97%, of clinically stable MHD patients. Hence, it follows that many MHD patients will maintain protein balance with lower dietary protein intakes. Since, a priori, it is generally impossible to ascertain which MHD may maintain protein balance on lower levels of protein intake this quantity of dietary protein is recommended. This is the same type of reasoning that is used for determining the Recommended Dietary Protein Allowances for the general population by both the World Health Organization and the Food and Nutrition Board, National Research Council of the United States National Academy of Sciences [78,154]. The nitrogen balance data on which this recommended protein intake for MHD patients is

TABLE 32.3 Recommended Dietary Nutrient Intake for Adult Patients Undergoing Maintenance Hemodialysis

Macronutrients and Fiber

Dietary protein intake (DPI)[a]	1.2 g/kg body weight/day for clinically stable MHD patients. (At least 50% of the dietary protein should be of high biological value.) $\geq$1.2 to 1.3 g/kg/day for patients who are acutely ill or have more severe protein-energy wasting.
Daily energy intake (DEI)[b]	35 kcal/kg body weight/day for those who are less than 60 years of age and 30 to 35 kcal/kg body weight/day for individuals 60 years or older.
Fat intake[c]	30% of total energy intake
Total fat[c,d]	30% of total energy intake
Saturated fat[c]	Up to 10% of total energy intake
Polyunsaturated − saturated fatty acids[c]	Up to 10% of total calories
Monounsaturated fatty acids[c]	Up to 20% of total calories
Carbohydrate[c,d,e]	Rest of non-protein calories
Total fiber[f]	20−25 g/day

Minerals and Water (range of intake)

Sodium	750 to 2000 mg/day
Potassium	up to 70−80 mEq/day
Phosphorus[g]	10 to 17 mg/kg/day
Calcium[h]	$\leq$1000 mg/day
Magnesium	200 to 300 mg/day
Iron[I]	See text
Zinc	15 mg/day
Water	Usually 750 to 1500 mL/day

Vitamins (including dietary supplements)

Vitamin B_1 (Thiamin)	1.1−1.2 mg/day
Vitamin B_2 (Riboflavin)	1.1−1.3 mg/day
Pantothenic acid	5 mg/day
Biotin	30 µg/day
Niacin	14−16 mg/day
Vitamin B_6 (Pyridoxine)	10 mg/day
Vitamin B_{12}	2.4 µg/day
Vitamin C	75−90 mg/day
Folic Acid[j]	1 to 10 mg/day
Vitamin A	See text

TABLE 32.3 Recommended Dietary Nutrient Intake for Adult Patients Undergoing Maintenance Hemodialysis—cont'd

Macronutrients and Fiber

Vitamin D	See text
Vitamin E[k]	15 IU
Vitamin K[l]	See text

[a, b]According to K/DOQI guidelines [78].

[b]Refers to percent of total energy intake (diet plus dialysate).

[c]Although atherosclerotic vascular disease constitutes a common and serious problem for MHD patients, these recommendations are often hard to adhere to. Moreover, there is no prospective interventional study indicating these dietary modifications are beneficial for MHD patients, although, reasonably, the potential benefits of these modifications seem valuable. They are strongly recommended only if patients adhere closely to more critical aspects of the diet (e.g., sodium, water, potassium, phosphorus, protein and energy intake), and have expressed a particular interest in these modifications or have a specific disorder that may respond to their medications.

[d]Refers to percent of total energy intake; if triglyceride levels are very high, the percentage of fat in the diet may be increased to about 35% of total calories; otherwise, 25−30% of total calories is preferable. Intake of fatty acids should be kept low because they raise LDL cholesterol (see text).

[e]Should be primarily complex carbohydrates.

[f]Less critical to adhere to for the typical MHD patient.

[g]Phosphate binders (aluminum carbonate or hydroxide, or calcium carbonate or acetate) often are needed to maintain normal serum phosphorus levels.

[h]These calcium intakes are commonly ingested because of the use of calcium binders of phosphate. Excess calcium intake must be avoided (see text).

[i]Iron requirements vary according to the dose of administered erythropoietin.

[j]Folic acid 1 mg/day should be routine, but up to 10 mg/day may be given to reduce elevated plasma homocysteine levels.

[k]Vitamin E, 300 or 800 IU day, may be given to reduce oxidative stress and prevent cardiovascular disease, but the value of these supplements is controversial (see text and Chapter 24).

[l]Vitamin K supplements may be needed for patients who are not eating and who receive antibiotics.

based are surprisingly sparse, and more research is clearly indicated in this area. A brief review of the research to date is as follows:

Ginn and co-workers carried out nitrogen balance studies in four men who were undergoing MHD twice weekly [149]. Two of these patients were fed 18 g protein/day and were in severely negative nitrogen balance. The other two patients, who were anephric, were fed higher-protein diets. Their nitrogen balance was positive when they ingested 0.8 g/kg/day of primarily high biologic value protein. Nitrogen balance was sometimes negative with higher protein diets when the protein was of low biologic value. These patients were almost certainly malnourished, and this factor, as well as the reduced (by present standards) frequency of hemodialysis, might have accounted for their positive nitrogen balance with such low (0.8 g/kg/day) protein intakes. In an outpatient study of at least 6 months' duration, Shinaberger and Ginn reported that 10 patients who ingested 0.75 g/kg/day showed improvement in nutritional status [155]. Again many of these patients were malnourished at the onset of study. Also, provision of dialysis only twice weekly could have lowered amino acid and peptide losses into dialysate and reduced the catabolic stress of hemodialysis (see above). These two factors may have increased the patient's ability to develop an anabolic response on this low protein intake. Also, the daily protein intake of these outpatients probably exceeded the prescribed 0.75 g/kg/day.

Kopple et al. carried out nitrogen balance studies on three patients who were living in a metabolic balance unit and were undergoing MHD for 11 hours twice weekly with a Kiil dialyzer [151]. Each patient was fed two isocaloric diets that provided 0.75 or 1.25 g protein/kg/day for about 3 weeks with each diet. The two diets provided, respectively, 0.63 and 0.88 g/kg/day of high biologic value protein. Nitrogen balance, after equilibration and adjusted for unmeasured losses, was negative or neutral with the 0.75 g protein/kg/day diet and strongly positive with the diet providing 1.25 g protein/kg/day. Kopple et al. then carried out an outpatient study in 23 patients who were randomly assigned to receive either diet while they were treated twice weekly with hemodialysis for 10 to 12 hours with Kiil dialyzers. The patients prescribed the lower-protein diet were estimated to have ingested closer to 0.8 to 0.9 g protein/kg/day, whereas the patients receiving the higher-protein prescription ingested about 1.1 to 1.2 g/kg/day of protein. The lower-protein-diet group demonstrated a slight gain in serum albumin and body weight. In contrast, patients prescribed the higher-protein diet demonstrated a statistically significant increase in both serum albumin and body weight. Borah et al. studied five hemodialysis patients given either 0.50 or 1.44 g protein/kg/day under metabolic balance conditions [55]. Each diet was fed for only 7 days. They concluded that the lower protein diet caused negative nitrogen balance, whereas the higher protein intake maintained neutral or positive nitrogen balance.

Slomowitz and co-workers carried out metabolic balance studies in six MHD patients who lived in a clinical research center for 63 to 65 days each and underwent hemodialysis for 4 hours three times weekly with Cuprophan™ or cellulose acetate dialyzers [156]. This study was carried out to assess the dietary energy requirements of the patients (see below), but some of the data obtained may be relevant to the dietary protein needs of MHD patients. These individuals were fed a constant protein diet throughout the study that provided 1.13 ± 0.02 SEM g protein/kg/day. All patients were fed, in random order, three different dietary energy intakes for 21 to 23 days each that provided 25, 35, or 45 kcal/kg/day. Of the six patients, the number that were in neutral or positive nitrogen balance with the 25, 35, and 45 kcal/kg/day intakes were, respectively, one (possibly), four, and six individuals. Since the usual energy intake of clinically stable MHD patients is less than 30 kcal/kg/day [157], these results suggest that for many of the MHD patients who ingest about 25 or even 35 kcal/kg/day, a dietary protein intake of 1.1 g/kg/day may not be sufficiently great to maintain protein balance. The nitrogen balance data with the energy intake of 35 kcal/kg/day and protein intake of 1.1 ± 0.02 SEM g/kg/day are shown in Table 32.4 [156].

TABLE 32.4 Nitrogen Balance Data in Six MHD Patients[a] Ingesting a Diet Providing about 1.13 g Protein/kg/day and about 35 kcal/kg/day

Gender	Age (years)	Body Weight (kg)	Energy Intake per kg Actual Body Weight (kcal/kg/day)	Duration of Study (days)	Stable Period (days)[b]	Nitrogen Intake[c]	Urine Nitrogen	Fecal Nitrogen	Dialysate Nitrogen	Total Nitrogen Output[d]	Adjusted Nitrogen Balance[e]
									(g/day)		
Female	61	60.6	35.8	21	14	11.0	0.78	0.68	7.40	8.86	+2.09
Female	64	73.6	31.3	21	7	11.4	0.20	1.15	9.15	10.50	+0.68
Male	46	73.3	35.6	21	14	13.4	0.84	0.99	10.52	12.35	+1.02
Male	43	58	45.4	21	7	14.0	0	1.60	12.07	13.67	+0.06
Male	24	51.4	41.2	21	14	11.2	0.12	1.14	8.80	10.06	+0.61
Male	42	70.5	34.5	21	7	12.8	0	1.70	11.90	13.75	−1.02
Mean	46.7	64.6	37.3	21	10.5	12.18	0.32	1.21	9.97	11.53	+0.57
SEM	59	3.8	2.1	0	1.6	0.53	0.16	0.16	0.75	0.83	0.42

[a]Balance data were obtained during the stable period, which is the time after patients had stabilized or equilibrated on each diet.
[b]Refers to the period in which nitrogen balance had equilibrated and was no longer changing.
[c]Refers to the measured nitrogen intake minus the nitrogen content of rejected or vomited food.
[d]Sum of urine, fecal, and dialysate nitrogen.
[e]Indicates nitrogen balance adjusted for changes in body urea nitrogen but not unmeasured losses from skin, nails or hair, growth, respiration, or blood drawing.
From [156]. Printed with permission.

Thus, these nitrogen balance studies suggest that some clinically stable MHD will not maintain protein balance with dietary protein intakes of 1.1 g protein/kg/day and, adequate energy intakes (see below). The K/DOQI recommendation, following the general principles used for determining the recommended daily allowances (RDA) (i.e., an intake that should satisfy the nutritional needs of about 97% of the general population) [78,154] therefore proposed, somewhat higher dietary protein intakes. The dietary protein level selected to be the recommended (i.e., safe) amount for stable MHD patients was 1.2 g protein/kg/day. As indicate above, many MHD patients will maintain protein balance with lower protein intakes. However, there is no way to prospectively identify who are these patients. Therefore, safety concerns suggest recommending this higher intake. Moreover, with the current doses of hemodialysis employed, a protein intake of 1.20 g/kg/day will not induce uremic toxicity. Thus, we believe that, until more data are available, the current K/DOQI recommendations are safe and justifiable. Clearly more information concerning protein requirements is needed.

The second type of studies, which are retrospective and observational, provides results that are consistent with these conclusions. Data from the National Cooperative Dialysis Study indicated that patients with a dietary protein intake of less than 0.80 g/kg/day, as estimated by the PNA, had increased morbidity [158]. However, these patients were randomized to a specified midweek predialysis serum urea nitrogen (SUN) and a given range of time for hemodialysis treatment, and, hence, to a given range of dialysis doses. Thus, it could not be conclusively stated that the higher morbidity of these patients was due to lower nutritional intake per se and not due to a decreased Kt/V.

In a retrospective study, Acchiardo and co-workers examined the relationship in 98 nondiabetic patients between dietary protein intake, determined from the PNA (PCR), and frequency of hospitalizations, number of total days hospitalized, and mortality rate during a 12-month period [150]. Patients were divided into four groups based upon their mean PNA: 0.63, 0.93, 1.02, and 1.2 g/kg/day. Both the frequency of hospitalizations and the mortality rate were inversely correlated with dietary protein intake. The frequency and number of days of hospitalization and the mortality rate were particularly likely to be elevated in patients with a PNA of 0.63 g/kg/day. Since the group with the highest PNA averaged 1.2 g/kg/day, it is not known whether an increase in PNA above this level (i.e., an increase in the dietary protein intake necessary to maintain an even greater PNA) would result in any further reduction in morbidity or mortality. A recent study on 122 MHD patients whose equilibrated Kt/V was greater than 1.20 did not show any correlation between nPNA

and Kt/V among those with a Kt/V>1.50 [115] (see Figure 32.3).

Some investigators report that some MHD patients are in nitrogen balance even with a protein intake as low as 0.7 g/kg/day and contend that in stable dialysis patients a safe requirement for protein intake would not be greater than 1 g/kg/day. They suggest that attempts at increasing protein intake beyond this value are not warranted [159,160]. However, given the finding that there is a high incidence of PEW in MHD patients and especially among those with a poor outcome [3,6,161], that metabolic studies clearly indicate that 0.75 g protein/kg/day is nutritionally inadequate for many patients [147], and that 1.1 g protein/kg/day will maintain nitrogen balance in some but not all MHD patients who are ingesting 25 or 35 kcal/kg/day [156], a dietary protein intake of 1.20 g/kg/day has been recommended by K/DOQI guidelines (Table 32.3).

Energy Requirements

Epidemiologic studies in MHD patients suggest that low energy intakes are probably even more common and are more severe than the protein intakes [153, 157,162–167]. The majority of surveys of the energy intake of MHD patients indicates that it is frequently below the recommended energy intake for normal healthy adults engaged in mild physical activity, and that it usually averages about 24–27 kcal/kg/day [166,168]. Indeed, even in the HEMO Study, in which patients were seen periodically by renal dietitians, the energy intake averaged 22.8 ± 8.8 SD kcal/kg adjusted body wt/day [157,169].

The low energy intakes of MHD patients do not reflect a decrease in energy requirements. Studies indicate that under basal metabolic conditions energy expenditure in MHD patients under resting, basal conditions is normal or slightly increased [170–172]. In one study, resting basal energy expenditure in 12 normal subjects and 16 MHD patients was 0.94 ± 0.24 SD and 0.97 ± 0.1 kcal/min/1.73 m^2, respectively; each group was composed of both men and women [170]. Schneeweiss et al. [173] performed indirect calorimetry on 24 normal adults and 86 patients with various forms of chronic renal failure of whom 25 were undergoing MHD. The resting energy expenditure was 1.03 ± 0.04 SEM kcal/min/1.73 m^2 in MHD patients, which was slightly but not statistically increased over values for the control subjects, 0.96 ± 0.02. Neyra et al. [174] measured resting energy expenditure using a whole-room indirect calorimeter (metabolic chamber) after 12-hour fasting in 15 patients with advanced chronic renal failure (CRF), 15 MHD patients, and 10 patients on peritoneal dialysis. Patients undergoing hemodialysis were assessed on a nondialysis day. Resting energy expenditure, adjusted for fat-free mass, was similar in hemodialysis and peritoneal dialysis patients and both were significantly higher than in patients with CKD not on dialysis (p < 0.05). In the non-dialysis dependent CKD patient per se in comparison to the predicted value for normal individuals it was generally about 10% to 20% higher. Thus, the MHD and CPD patients displayed increased resting energy expenditure compared to non-dialyzed CKD patients, who per se have higher energy expenditure than the healthy people [174]. Energy expenditure, in MHD patients, measured by indirect calorimetry, when sitting quietly, with physical activity, and after a defined meal appears to be similar to that of normal individuals [170]. On the other hand, energy expenditure in MHD patients with elevated serum CRP levels or during a MHD treatment may also be increased [174].

In the study by Slomowitz et al. [156], in which nitrogen balance studies were carried out on six clinically stable MHD patients and who were prescribed, in random order, constant protein diets providing 25, 35, or 45 kcal/kg/day [156], both change in body weight and nitrogen balance correlated directly with the dietary energy intake. The grand mean of the nitrogen balances, after equilibration on each diet, was significantly negative with the 25 kcal/kg/day diet, neutral with the 35 kcal/kg/day diet, and significantly positive with the 45 kcal/kg/day intake. Changes in body weight, mid-arm muscle circumference, and estimated body fat also correlated directly and significantly with dietary energy intake, and these parameters tended to increase with the highest energy intake and fall with the lowest intake. Indeed, one can assess from the regression equations of these outcome measures the level of energy intake at which nitrogen balance and anthropometric parameters were neither increasing nor decreasing. This value, which can be construed to indicate the level of energy intake at which patients neither are in positive nor negative energy balance, is about 32 to 38 kcal/kg/day, depending on the nitrogen balance or body composition parameter in question [156]. For an unchanging nitrogen balance, adjusted for estimated unmeasured nitrogen losses (i.e., through respiration, skin and integumentary structures, flatus, and semen or menses), the energy intake value was about 38 kcal/kg/day.

The findings of low body fat and decreased skinfold thicknesses in MHD patients, which have been noted in several studies [163,165,166], seem to support the thesis that the usual energy intakes of these individuals are inadequate for their needs. Moreover, analysis of the altered risk factor patterns of MHD patients indicate that those who have a larger body mass for a given height tend to survive longer [7]. Based upon the foregoing studies, and particularly the energy expenditure

measurements and nitrogen balance studies, the National Kidney Foundation K/DOQI Nutrition Workgroup developed the following guideline: "the recommended daily energy intake for MHD or CPD patients is 35 kcal/kg body weight/day for those who are less than 60 years of age and 30 to 35 kcal/kg body weight/day for individuals 60 years or older" [78]. This recommendation is based on the findings that: (1) Energy expenditure of MHD patients is similar to or possibly slightly greater than that of normal, healthy individuals who are involved in mild physician activity [174]. (2) Metabolic balance studies of people undergoing MHD indicate that a total daily energy intake of about 35 kcal/kg/day induces neutral nitrogen balance and is adequate to maintain serum albumin and anthropometric indices [156]. (3) Because individuals 60 years of age or older tend to be more sedentary, a total energy intake of 30 to 35 kcal/kg is acceptable [78]. Individuals involved in vigorous physical activity may require greater energy intakes. These recommendations are similar to the recommended dietary allowances for sedentary healthy adults by the Food and Nutrition Board of the National Research Council [154].

The daily energy intake from the diet may be increased or reduced according to the net glucose balance across the hemodialyzer. However, the amount of glucose lost or taken up from hemodialysate generally is quite small. Gutierrez et al. [43] described average glucose losses of about 26 g per hemodialysis when glucose-free dialysate was used and a glucose uptake of about 30 g per hemodialysis when dialysate containing 180 mg/dL of glucose was employed. The calorie balance across the dialyzer under these two conditions would be about −88 kcal/and +102 kcal, respectively (i.e., based on a factor of 3.4 kcal per g of dextrose monohydrate). It should be remembered that these energy accruals or losses only occur three times per week for the typical MHD patient. Thus, under most conditions, and unlike the situation with CPD, the dietary energy intake for MHD patients usually does not have to be modified for a standard dialysis treatment. However, with the addition of larger glucose concentrations in hemodialysate or if hemodialysis treatments are conducted more frequently or for longer periods of time, the contribution of dialysis treatments to energy balance could be greater.

Lipids and Hemodialysis

The abnormalities in lipid metabolism and the causes for these disorders in patients with chronic renal failure are discussed in Chapter 3. Lipid disorders in this population constitute a highly significant problem because they are so prevalent, they involve so many of the traditional risk factors for vascular disease, and cardiovascular deaths account for one-half of the mortality of patients undergoing MHD [175,176]. The growing numbers of diabetic patients who develop ESRD who are particularly likely to have lipid disorders, and who have an especially high incidence of cardiovascular, cerebrovascular and peripheral vascular diseases have added to the severity of the problem. However, the paradoxical risk factor reversal that is observed in many epidemiological studies in MHD patients with large sample sizes, indicates that a low total serum cholesterol level poses at least as great a mortality risk as severe hypercholesterolemia [7,13] (Chapter 12). As serum total cholesterol decreases below roughly 200–250 mg/dL, the relative risk of death in MHD patients increases [10,13]. Nevertheless, despite the association between a low serum cholesterol level and poor outcome in MHD patients, students of lipid metabolism in renal failure generally have concluded that until more data are available, it is still advantageous, to create the same serum lipid pattern and dietary lipid intake that is recommended for the general population (see Chapter 3).

Dyslipidemia is more prevalent in ESRD patients than in the general population [177,178]. In MHD patients, hypertriglyceridemia and low serum concentrations of high-density lipoprotein (HDL) are frequently observed [179–183]. Moreover, very low-density lipoprotein (VLDL) cholesterol is usually increased, but serum low density lipoprotein (LDL) and total cholesterol levels are usually within the normal range or even lower than that seen in the general population [184–186]. Increased serum apolipoprotein B containing triglyceride-rich lipoprotein particles containing C-III and (a) or lipoproteinBc particles are often observed in MHD patients [187–189]. A defect in postprandial chylomicron remnant clearance has been described [181,190]. Moreover, there is a high incidence of type IV hyperlipidemia among ESRD patients [187,190]. All serum HDL cholesterol fractions are often decreased, possibly secondary to reduced LCAT activity. Serum HDL 3, which is not a major risk factor for reduced adverse cardiovascular events, is relatively spared. In contrast, there is a greater reduction in the larger HDL 2 fraction, which has a stronger association with a low incidence of cardiovascular morbidity and mortality. The antiatherogenic HDL-associated Apo A-I and Apo A-II are also diminished in sera. Lp (a) levels are often elevated. Lipoprotein lipase (LPL) activities in serum and liver are decreased. The serum levels of oxidized lipids and thiobarbituric acid reactive substances (TBARS) are elevated in CKD and MHD patients. There is some speculation as to whether the hemodialysis procedure increases lipid oxidation; the data of Schettler et al. suggest that this is not the case [191].

In contrast to the moderate prevalence of hypercholesterolemia, hypertriglyceridemia is common in MHD patients [192] (see Chapter 3). MHD patients should be evaluated for systemic causes of hypertriglyceridemia, including diabetes mellitus and hypothyroidism. Dietary therapy, because of its greater safety, in general, is employed when the serum triglyceride concentrations are about 1.25 to 1.50 times the upper limit of normal values. Under these circumstances, patients should be urged to reduce ethanol intake to no more than one drink per day. Attempts should be made to lower the intake of purified sugars and saturated fat. If dietary therapy does not lower serum triglyceride concentrations sufficiently, and if serum triglycerides, after a 10-hour fast, remain above about 500 mg/dL, triglyceride lowering medications are generally prescribed. Medical therapy can be given concurrently with a lipid-lowering diet to lower hypertriglyceridemia [193–195]. Gemfibrozil and fibric acid derivatives such as clofibrate are effective agents for lowering serum triglyceride levels. However, there is a risk of myositis, cholelithiasis, and other disorders with these medicines, and the doses of these medicines should be decreased in hemodialysis patients [196–199].

There is currently no consensus as to the exact lipid composition of the diet for MHD patients. The National Cholesterol Education Program (NCEP) Expert Panel has recommended the *Therapeutic Lifestyle Changes* (TLC) diet in all individuals with LDL cholesterol of 100 to 129 mg/dL or triglycerides higher than 180 mg/dL [200]. Table 32.5 shows the nutrient composition of the TLC diet. Its essential features are: (1) Reduced intakes of saturated fats (<7% of total calories) and cholesterol (<200 mg/day); (2) Sources of total calories in the diet should include up to 10% for polyunsaturated fats, up to 20% from monounsaturated fats, 25–35% from all fat sources, and the rest from protein and carbohydrate. Dietary protein should be modified from the TLC diet to provide 1.20 g protein/kg/day, and dietary carbohydrate should be modified accordingly so as to maintain desirable energy intake; (3) Such therapeutic options for enhancing LDL lowering as ingesting plant stanols/sterols (2 g/day) and increased viscous (soluble) fiber (20–30 g/day); (4) Attainment and maintenance of desirable body weight and physical activity to consume approximately 200 kcal/day [200] (see Chapters 3 and 45).

These guidelines for the treatment of hypercholesterolemia are based on the same principles as for the general population. The TLC diet is a health-enhancing diet and, in general, all individuals in the population-at-large should be encouraged to adhere to it. MHD patients are considered to be at high risk for coronary artery disease and stroke, and the target for their serum LDL-cholesterol is to maintain it below 100 mg/dL. This sometimes can be attained by the TLC diet, but often

TABLE 32.5 Nutrient composition of the Therapeutic Lifestyle Changes (TLC) Diet

Nutrient	Recommended Intake
Saturated fat*	<7% of total calories
Polyunsaturated fat	Up to 10% of total calories
Monounsaturated fat	Up to 20% of total calories
Total fat	25–35% of total calories
Carbohydrate[†,‡]	50–60% of total calories
Fiber	20–30 g/d
Protein[‡]	Approximately 15% of total calories
Cholesterol	<200 mg/d
Total calories**	Balance energy intake and expenditure to maintain desirable body weight/prevent weight gain

*Trans *fatty acids are another LDL-raising fat that should be kept at a low intake.*
[†]*Carbohydrates should be derived predominantly from foods rich in complex carbohydrates including grains, especially whole grains, fruits, and vegetables.*
[‡]*Dietary content of protein and, hence carbohydrate, should be modified according to the specific needs of the MHD (i.e., 1.20 g protein/kg/day). (see text)*
**Daily energy expenditure should include at least moderate physical activity (contributing approximately 200 kcal/day).*
From [200]. Printed with permission.

pharmacological therapy must be given in association with dietary therapy to attain target LDL-cholesterol levels (see also Chapters 3 and 9) [200]. Hydroxymethyl-glutaryl Coenzyme A reductase inhibitors, also known as statins, and fibric acid derivatives, such as clofibrate, have been used successfully to treat hypercholesterol-emia. The recently described anti-inflammatory characteristics of statins may play a major role in improving outcome in MHD patients [201–204]. Some statins also have a modest HDL-cholesterol raising effect [205]. It is important to note that there are racial/ethnic disparities in MHD patients in nutritional status, dietary intake and inflammation, and that they may account for racial survival disparities. In a cohort study of 799 MHD patients [206]. In case-mix-adjusted analyses, dietary intakes in Blacks versus Whites were higher in energy (+293 ± 119 cal/day) and fat (+18 ± 5 g/day), but lower in fiber (−2.9 ± 1.3 g/day) than Whites [206]. It should be emphasized that although these modifications to develop a more healthy lipid pattern appear reasonable, there are currently no data as to whether these changes will reduce morbidity and mortality in MHD patients. Clearly, more research is needed in this area.

Sodium and Water

Sodium and its most prevalent anion, chloride, are the most abundant extracellular solutes, and hence extracellular fluid volume and plasma volume are largely regulated by salt (sodium chloride) balance [207]. Fecal sodium excretion usually amounts to 1 to 3 mmol/day, and in individuals who are not actively sweating, integumentary sodium losses are generally less than 3–4 mEq/day. Hence, in health, it is renal sodium excretion that maintains sodium balance across wide variations in sodium intake. As GFR falls, the fractional excretion of sodium (FeNa) increases for a given sodium intake so that sodium excretion usually remains equal to sodium intake [208–210]. However, when the GFR falls below approximately 15 mL/min the increase in FeNa often does not fully compensate for the fall in the GFR and filtered sodium load, and even a typical or moderately high dietary sodium intake (e.g., 120–200 mmol/day) may lead to sodium retention. Within the first several weeks or months after MHD therapy is inaugurated, the GFR usually decreases to less than 1 or 2 mL/min, and by 12 months of MHD most patients are oliguric or anuric [211]. In these latter cases, sodium balance is largely dictated by the intake and removal by dialysis of sodium.

MHD patients must be counseled against ingesting high sodium diets (Chapter 22). Excessive sodium intake may lead to a large interdialytic weight gain, hypertension, edema, large left ventricular mass, and congestive heart failure [212]. When patients gain large volumes of sodium and water during the interdialytic interval, the rapid removal of this fluid during the brief period of the hemodialysis treatment may cause sudden decreases in blood volume and hence engender hypotension, angina, arrhythmias, or muscle cramps. Shaldon [213, 214] and Tomson [215] both emphasized the importance of restricting dietary sodium intake in MHD patients to achieve medication-free control of blood pressure and to limit interdialytic fluid gain. To that end, it has been contended that longer hours of MHD treatment achieve better blood pressure control by a greater effectiveness at reducing total body sodium and water [216,217]. However, excess intradialytic sodium gain is not always due to dietary indiscretion, since some medications can be major sources of sodium, such as some combined analgesics in effervescent form (e.g. co-codamol; a combination of codeine and paracetamol used especially in Europe) [218]. This preparation is soluble because there are 18 mmol of sodium bicarbonate in each tablet. If a patient takes 6 to 8 tablets per day, the sodium intake from this medicine can drive the intake of an extra 800 mL of water per day to maintain a normal extracellular sodium concentration.

It is not clear whether MHD patients with a high interdialytic weight gain have a higher risk of death [215]. The largest study examining this issue reached the opposite finding: Those MHD patients with low interdialytic weight gain are at highest risk of dying, although very high interdialytic weight gains were also associated with a modest increase in risk [215]. The most likely explanation for this finding is that low interdialytic weight gain is associated with poor nutritional intake and therefore may be associated with serious co-morbid disease. This explanation was supported by a study showing that low interdialytic weight gain was associated with PEW, which per se is an important predictor of poor outcome in MHD patients [219]. In another smaller study, high interdialytic weight gain was associated with increased mortality in diabetic, but not in nondiabetic, MHD patients [220]. A number of investigations indicate that high interdialytic weight gain may contribute to hypertension [221−224], but most studies show no such relationship [225−228] or show it only in a subset of "volume-responsive" patients [219,229]. This lack of a relationship is less surprising than it may seem, because it is the change in plasma volume, not in total extracellular volume or total body water, which is likely to result in changes in blood pressure during dialysis [230]. Nonetheless, given the high morbidity associated with excessive intake of sodium and water and with the consequent increased interdialytic weight gain and the very high frequency of hypertension and need for antihypertensive medications in MHD patients, dietary salt and water restriction appear to be strongly indicated.

In a large epidemiologic study 2-year mortality was examined in 34,107 MHD patients across the United States who had an average weight gain of at least 0.5 kg above their end-dialysis dry weight by the time the subsequent hemodialysis treatment started [231]. The 3-month averaged interdialytic weight gain was divided into eight categories of 0.5-kg increments (up to > or = 4.0 kg). Eighty-six percent of patients gained >1.5 kg between two dialysis sessions. In unadjusted analyses, higher weight gain was associated with better nutritional status (higher protein intake, serum albumin, and body mass index) and tended to be linked to greater survival [231]. However, after multivariate adjustment for demographics and surrogates of malnutrition-inflammation complex, higher weight-gain increments were associated with increased risk of all-cause and cardiovascular death (Figure 32.4). Hence, in MHD patients, greater fluid retention between two subsequent hemodialysis treatment sessions is associated with higher risk of all-cause and cardiovascular death [231]. The mechanisms by which fluid retention influences cardiovascular survival in hemodialysis may be similar to those in patients with heart failure and warrant further research.

A sodium intake of 1000 to 1500 mg per day (43 to 64.5 mmol/day, or 2.54 to 3.82 g/day of sodium chloride or salt) is recommended for MHD patients [215,232]. This level of sodium intake may be difficult to follow for many patients, but it still remains a recommended

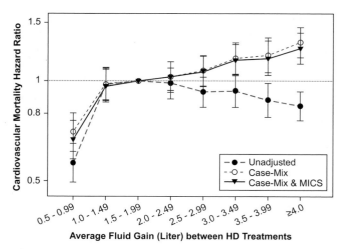

FIGURE 32.4 Association of fluid gain between two consecutive hemodialysis treatment sessions and 2-year cardiovascular mortality in 34,107 MHD patients. *Adapted from Kalantar-Zadeh et al., Circulation 2009 [231].* This figure is reproduced in color in the color plate section.

target. Precooked, processed, and canned foods usually have high sodium content, and the intake of these foods should be minimized. Salt substitutes prepared from herbs often can satisfy a patient's desire for sodium. Salt substitutes composed of potassium chloride generally contain 13 mEq of potassium per packet and may induce hyperkalemia in MHD patients.

Excessive water intake can contribute to the problems described above [232]. Whereas sodium balance is a key regulator of extracellular fluid volume, the cell volume is regulated by plasma tonicity, which in turn is regulated by water balance. Thirst and the renal excretion of water are the two major regulators of water homeostasis [233,234]. Although the ability of the kidney to excrete or retain large amounts of free water is severely reduced in patients with advanced stages of CKD, thirst and the consequent amount of water ingested will generally maintain plasma sodium concentrations within or slightly below the normal range. When sodium intake is adequately restricted and if patients are not hyperglycemic, individuals will often automatically adjust their water intake to appropriate levels. However, perturbations of thirst may interfere with this homeostatic mechanism. Since MHD patients are usually oliguric or anuric, a separate prescription for water intake is usually indicated to prevent fluid overload, excessive interdialytic weight gain and hyponatremia [215]. In general, the water intake for MHD patients should not exceed 750 to 1500 mL per day, including the water ingested in food, unless the patient has a urine output substantially above the oliguric range.

Potassium

Normally, the kidney excretes at least 80% to 90% of the total daily potassium intake, which is usually between 50 to 150 mEq/day (about 2 to 6 g/day) but may vary more widely. About 7 to 10 mEq per day of potassium are normally excreted in the feces; in patients with advanced CKD, fecal potassium excretion rises to about 14 to 25 mEq/day [235–239]. Normally, in the nephron, almost all filtered potassium is reabsorbed, and urinary potassium is largely derived from tubular secretion. As with sodium, when the GFR falls, the fractional excretion of potassium increases [238]. These adaptive responses increase the magnitude by which renal failure can progress before the urinary potassium excretion is no longer sufficient to prevent potassium retention and hyperkalemia. An early response to an increase in the extracellular potassium is to shift potassium inside the cell [240]. Factors that inhibit this transcellular potassium shift or that promote movement of potassium extracellularly may exacerbate the tendency to hyperkalemia in MHD patients. These include insulin deficiency, metabolic acidemia, hypercatabolic states, and treatment with β-blockers or rennin, angiotensin or aldosterone antagonists; these conditions are not infrequently present in a typical multi-morbid patient with chronic renal failure [136,241,242].

In epidemiologic studies, higher serum potassium >5.3 mEq/L is associated with increased death risk in MHD patients [243]. In a recent study of 224 MHD patients mortality predictability of dietary potassium intake from reported food items estimated using the Block Food Frequency Questionnaire at the start of the cohort was examined in a 5-year (2001–2006) cohort [244]. MHD patients with higher potassium intake had greater dietary energy, protein, and phosphorus intakes and higher predialysis serum potassium and phosphorus levels. Greater dietary potassium intake was associated with significantly increased death risk in unadjusted models and after incremental adjustments for case-mix, nutritional factors (including 3-month averaged predialysis serum creatinine, potassium, and phosphorus levels; body mass index; normalized protein nitrogen appearance; and energy, protein, and phosphorus intake) and inflammatory marker levels [244]. In general, a diet providing no more than about 70 mmol/day (roughly 3 g/day) of potassium should be prescribed for MHD patients, although for persistently hyperkalemic patients lower amounts may be required [238]. This restricted intake of potassium is well tolerated by most but not all MHD patients. Because severe hyperkalemia, e.g., serum potassium greater than 7.0 mmol/L, may precipitate fatal arrhythmias, MHD patients should receive detailed instructions concerning the potassium content of various foods and are instructed to avoid or strictly regulate the intake of potassium-rich foods. Constipation should be avoided or treated promptly because of the importance of fecal potassium losses to the body potassium economy in

these individuals [236]. In the past, patients with elevated serum potassium were invariably dialyzed with very low-potassium dialysate containing 0 to 1.0 mmol K/L. This practice has raised the question of a possible contribution of post-dialysis hypokalemia to sudden cardiac death syndrome observed in MHD patients [245]. Karnik et al. examined the records of 400 reported cardiac arrests over a nine-month period in a nationally representative cohort of 77,000 MHD patients dialyzed at outpatient facilities of a for-profit dialysis company in North America [246]. They found that cardiac arrest patients were nearly twice as likely to have been dialyzed with a dialysate containing 0 or 1.0 mEq/L potassium on the day of the cardiac arrest (17.1 vs. 8.8%). Hence, the current trend is to avoid the use of very low potassium dialysate and to employ longer dialysis hours, averaging 4 hours or more, using dialysate bath with potassium as high as 3.0 or 4.0 mmol/L, if possible. A possible alternative approach might be to use these very low potassium containing dialysates for only the first one-half of the dialysis treatment; the safety of this course of action needs to be tested. For noncompliant MHD patients or those who adhere poorly to their dietary potassium prescription, administration of ion exchange resins, such as sodium polystyrene, by mouth or per rectum, may be considered to enhance potassium excretion on off-dialysis days, especially during long intradialytic breaks and weekends. It should be noted that this ion exchange resin exchanges sodium for potassium; hence, this procedure will increase sodium intake.

Magnesium

As is the case for potassium, the kidney is the major excretory organ for magnesium [247–252]. However, because in most foods the magnesium content is lower than the content of phosphorus or potassium and the net fractional absorption of magnesium by the intestine is less (very roughly, 50% of ingested magnesium [249]), hypermagnesemia is usually a less serious problem than hyperphosphatemia or hyperkalemia. Although mild hypermagnesemia is common in MHD patients, severe hypermagnesemia is rare unless patients ingest magnesium containing antacids or laxatives, such as Maalox, Gelusil, milk of magnesia, or cascara sagrada, or receive large doses of intravenous magnesium [250]. ESRD patients, most of whom were undergoing MHD, have been reported to have increased magnesium content of bone and some soft tissues [247,252,253]. In nondialyzed patients with advanced CKD, the magnesium requirement is about 2 to 4 mg/kg/day (i.e., about 200 mg/day) [249]. Patients who are undergoing hemodialysis with 1.0 mEq/L of magnesium in the dialysate and whose dietary magnesium intakes range between 200 and 300 mg/day generally maintain normal or only slightly elevated serum magnesium levels.

Calcium

The normal dietary calcium requirement for nonpregnant, nonlactating adults is 800 to 1200 mg per day [154]. Vitamin D deficiency and resistance to the actions of vitamin D on bone and in the intestinal tract may increase the dietary calcium requirements of patients with chronic renal failure including those undergoing MHD [248,254] (Chapters 19). Foods rich in calcium are often rich in phosphorus; thus MHD patients usually should not ingest these foods in large amounts [249]. With the widespread use of calcium containing phosphate binders, oral calcium intake is not uncommonly 1.0 to 1.5 g/day or greater [255]. Indeed, daily calcium intakes from a combination of calcium containing phosphate binders and foods can be excessive, equaling or exceeding 3.0 g/day. Since the net intestinal absorption of calcium increases with high-calcium diets [249], these latter calcium intakes may engender continuing positive calcium balance and lead to hypercalcemia and calcium deposition in soft tissues (see below). Therefore, to avoid hypercalcemia and calcification, a hemodialysate bath containing 1.25 or 1.5 mmol/L (5.0 to 6.0 mg/dL) of calcium is currently used for most MHD patients if they are taking calcium containing phosphate binders.

Concerns have been raised about the contributing role of ingested calcium to the development of coronary artery calcification and atherosclerotic plaques in MHD patients [35,256–260]. As indicated above, a major source of excessive calcium intake in MHD patients is from calcium containing phosphorus-binders such as calcium carbonate or calcium gluconate [255]. Several studies comparing MHD patients receiving the non-calcium containing binder sevelamer hydrochloride with those taking calcium containing binders showed significantly less progression of vascular and coronary calcification in the former patients [34,261,262], although concerns have been expressed regarding the increased incidence of metabolic acidosis due to ingestion of the large amounts of sevelamer HCl which are often required to treat hyperphosphatemia [263]. These considerations suggest that control of serum phosphorous may be more safely achieved by using binders that do not contain calcium. If calcium containing phosphate binders are not used, the recommended dietary calcium intake for typical MHD patients is about 1200 mg/day. If serum phosphorous cannot be controlled without the additional use of calcium containing binders, then dietary calcium intake from foods should be reduced to below 1.0 g calcium/day, and

hemodialysate containing less than 3.5 mEq/L of calcium should be used.

In large epidemiologic studies, both high (>10.5 mg/dL) and low (<8.0 mg/dL) serum calcium levels are associated with increased mortality risks in MHD patients [264]. Patients who are receiving calcium salts or 1,25-dihydroxyvitamin D should be monitored for hypercalcemia. Hypercalcemia can cause hypertension, pruritus, restlessness, metastatic calcification and calciphylaxis, particularly if the serum calcium–phosphorus product exceeds 70. Thus, the goal is to maintain the morning fasting serum calcium–phosphorus product well below this level and certainly below 60 (see Chapters 19 and 20).

Phosphorus

In general, hemodialysis is not a highly efficient method for removing excessive phosphorus. On average, approximately 250 mg of phosphorus are removed during each hemodialysis session depending on the predialysis serum phosphorus concentrations and the dialysis dose [265]. The typical American diet provides about 1500 to 1700 mg/day of phosphorus [154]. There is net absorption of roughly 60% of ingested phosphorus from the gastrointestinal tract [154,235,240, 248,249]. Thus, the quantity of phosphorus removed by hemodialysis is below that required to avoid severe hyperphosphatemia in most patients. Hence, MHD patients must decrease phosphorus intake and intestinal phosphorus absorption in order to prevent hyperphosphatemia.

It is recommended that MHD patients should be prescribed not more than 10 to 17 mg/kg/day of phosphorus [249,266,267]. The dietary phosphorus content usually is directly related to the quantity of protein, dairy products, and certain cola drinks in the diet [249,266]. However, in recent years there have been increasing attention in the added inorganic phosphorus in form of preservatives [268]. Very low phosphorus diets (e.g., less than 800 mg/day) are often unpalatable to the patient, particularly when the dietary protein intake is high (e.g., about 1.2 g/kg/day or greater). For these reasons, intestinal phosphorus binders are almost invariably required, in addition to dietary phosphorus restriction, in order to reduce intestinal phosphorus absorption and prevent severe hyperphosphatemia. Both hyperphosphatemia [269] and hypophosphatemia [14] are associated with poor outcome in MHD patients. In a large epidemiologic study, MHD patients who ingested more dietary protein (reflected by increase in nPNA or nPCR over 6 months) but lowered serum phosphorus levels had the best survival as compared to those who had a rise in both protein intake and serum phosphorus [128]. Mortality was even higher in those who lowered their protein intake and decreased serum phosphorus level [128].

Since aluminum containing binders such as aluminum hydroxide or aluminum carbonate led to serious side effects (low-turnover bone disease, refractory anemia, and dementia [270–274]), calcium-containing binders were frequently employed. These include calcium carbonate (40% calcium), calcium acetate (25% calcium), and calcium citrate (21% calcium). More recently, calcium-free binders such as sevelamer hydrochloride are frequently prescribed [259]. However, aluminum carbonate or hydroxide due to its superior potency can still be used on a short-term basis or in lower doses in association with other phosphate binders, especially when serum phosphorus levels are very high (>8 mg/dL) or when the product of the serum calcium and phosphorus approaches 70. This is recommended because calcium based phosphorus binders may increase the risk of calcium phosphate deposition, particularly when serum phosphorus is very high [269,275]. Because citrate enhances the absorption of aluminum [276–278], calcium citrate should not be given with aluminum containing phosphate binders. Calcium acetate is a more effective phosphate binder on a weight basis (presumably it is effective at a wider pH range than calcium carbonate) and may be less often associated with hypercalcemia [276,277]. However, some research indicates that the incidence of hypercalcemia is similar with both calcium acetate and calcium carbonate, and gastrointestinal symptoms such as nausea, bloating, or constipation may be more common with calcium acetate [279,280]. Moreover, calcium containing binders are associated with a higher incidence of coronary artery calcification [35,256]. Large doses of calcium binders have also been implicated in adynamic bone disease [281,282].

Sevelamer hydrochloride and other calcium-free binders appear to be less often associated with the foregoing adverse effects. Indeed, some preliminary studies indicate a significantly lower incidence of hypercalcemia and coronary artery calcification with sevelamer HCl [34]. However, due to its hydrochloride content, sevelamer HCl can cause hyperchloremic acidosis [263,283]. This is especially likely to occur when sevelamer HCl is used in higher doses, up to 4 to 7 g given three times per day [263]. A sevelamer phosphate binder that is not bound to hydrochloride but bicarbonate has also been developed, which does not cause metabolic acidosis.

Lanthanum carbonate and trivalent iron-containing compounds are emerging noncalcium containing phosphate binder that are approximately as potent as calcium binders [284–287]. Lanthanum carbonate does not cause metabolic acidosis. Although individuals taking lanthanum carbonate may display a rise in serum or tissue lanthanum values, the rise appears to be small and, so far, has not been associated with adverse side effects [285–287].

Vitamin D

Vitamin D is discussed in Chapters 19 and 21 and is addressed only briefly here. The enzyme, 1α-hydroxylase, which is present in the proximal tubule, converts 25-hydroxycholecalciferol to 1,25-dihydroxycholecalciferol (1,25-dihydroxyvitamin D), the most active form of vitamin D. Therefore, MHD patients are almost invariably deficient in this most active vitamin D analog unless they take supplements or an analogue of this compound. [288,289]. 1,25-dihydroxycholecalciferol has pleiotropic actions. It facilitates calcium and phosphorus absorption from the gastrointestinal tract. It is a strong inhibitor of the production and secretion of parathyroid hormone (PTH). It inhibits PTH mRNA transcription 288 and also inhibits parathyroid cell hyperplasia [290,291]. It also enhances the actions of PTH on bone and may act directly on bone as suggested by the presence of vitamin D receptors on osteoblasts and osteoclasts [292]. Thus in chronic renal failure, vitamin D deficiency, coupled with the impaired ability to excrete phosphorus, results in low serum calcium levels and hyperparathyroidism.

Vitamin D supplements, including native (nutritional) D and active D e.g. 1,25-dihydroxycholecalciferol (calcitriol) [293], are routinely used in MHD patients, which may enhance calcium absorption, prevent or treat hyperparathyroidism and improve bone metabolism. 1,25-dihydroxycholecalciferol derivatives are commercially available in several oral and intravenous preparations [294–297]. To replace low vitamin D levels, MHD patients may be given 0.25 to 1.0 μg/day of calcitriol as an oral dose or, as is a more common practice, intravenously with each hemodialysis session. To treat or prevent hyperparathyroidism, larger doses may be used, which may lead to hypercalcemia (see Chapters 19 and 21). Some newer generations of vitamin D analogues, such as paracalcitol, are reported to cause less hypercalcemia and, hence, have a better safety profile as a suppressant of hyperparathyroidism [298]. Occasionally, patients with refractory secondary or tertiary hyperparathyroidism may not respond to these medications and will require parathyroidectomy. After parathyoidectomy, many MHD patients, may require high doses of calcium and vitamin D, especially during the first weeks to months post-operatively due to the hungry bone syndrome [299,300]; after several months, this increased need for calcium and vitamin D tends to abate, presumably because bone has now become repleted with calcium.

For most MHD patients who do not have refractory hyperparathyroidism, 0.5 to 3.0 μg of calcitriol intravenously with each hemodialysis treatment or 0.25 to 3.0 μg by mouth every other day, three times per week can be given [301,302]. The equivalent dose of 1-alpha-D_2 or D_3 including doxercalciferil and paracalcitol are usually higher and is in the ranges of 2 to 10 μg intravenously with each hemodialysis session [299,300]. The relevant merits and disadvantages of oral and intravenous therapy for the treatment of hyperparathyroidism and a comparison among different forms of active vitamin D are discussed in detail in Chapters 19 and 21. Patients who are given supplemental 1,25-dihydroxycholecalciferol should be routinely monitored for hypercalcemia and hyperphosphatemia. As discussed above, an increasing number of reports indicate the possibility of an increased rate of coronary artery calcification with higher serum calcium concentrations [35,256,262,275]; hence, a more conservative approach to vitamin D and calcium therapy, may be warranted with the possible utilization of lower dialysate calcium concentrations and with more reliance on medicines, including vitamin D analogues, that are less potent at raising serum calcium levels.

Other Vitamins

MHD patients are at increased risk for deficiencies of certain other vitamins [25,26,69,303–306], particularly the water soluble vitamins folic acid and B and C. Vitamin metabolism and needs are described in more detail in Chapter 24. The causes for vitamin deficiencies in MHD patients include: (1) reduced overall food intake due to anorexia or MICS (see above and Chapters 11 and 38); (2) prescription of low-phosphorus, low-potassium diets that restricts intake of such nutritionally valuable foods as fresh fruits and vegetables, dairy products and other items that are high in vitamins [33]; (3) altered metabolism, as is the case for pyridoxine and possibly folate [305,307]; (4) impaired synthesis (e.g., 1,25-dihydroxyvitamin D) (see Chapters 19 and 21); (5) resistance to the actions of vitamins (e.g., vitamin D and possibly folate); (6) decreased intestinal absorption (e.g., decreased intestinal absorption of riboflavin, folate, and vitamin D have been described in rats with chronic renal insufficiency) (see Chapters 19, 21 and 24); and (7) dialysate losses of water soluble vitamins [22,26,308].

In some studies, MHD patients who did not receive vitamin supplements did not develop signs of vitamin deficiency when followed for up to one year [308,309]. Based on these findings, some authors have questioned the need for vitamin supplementation for MHD patients [309]. It is also true that many studies that suggest a need for vitamin supplements were carried out in the 1960s and early 1970s, when there was perhaps a higher incidence of malnutrition in MHD patients [308].

Nevertheless, recent reports continue to show that many MHD patients ingest a vitamin intake that provides less than the recommended dietary allowances [22,33,310], and that there is a small but persistent prevalence of deficiencies for some water soluble vitamins as well as for 1,25-dihydroxyvitamin D [22,70,293,311]. Many medicines that are likely to be taken by MHD patients may also interfere with vitamin function or metabolism (see Chapter 24). At present, it does not seem feasible to identify, a priori, those patients who will develop vitamin deficiencies. The frequent illnesses sustained by many MHD patients may also render their vitamin intake temporarily inadequate for their needs. Since the intake of water soluble vitamins at the proposed levels appears to be safe, we propose that these vitamins be supplemented.

A study comparing food intake of 30 MHD patients with 30 normal individuals (matched for age, gender and race) by means of a food frequency questionnaire found that MHD patients consumed significantly lower amounts of potassium, vitamin C, and dietary fiber as well as lower amounts of some carotenoids including cryptoxanthin and lycopene [33]. The lower vitamin C, fiber, and carotenoid intake of MHD patients may be atherogenic and may also be due to the prescribed restrictions in potassium and phosphorus in MHD patients. These dietary restrictions may lead to reduced fruit, vegetable and milk intake, leaving meat and fats as the main source of calories. The low energy intake of MHD patients (see Chapters 11 and 38) often impels dietitians to recommend a higher fat diet. These factors could contribute to atherosclerosis and increased cardiovascular morbidity and mortality in these patients. This hypothesis needs to be evaluated in future studies.

Several reports indicate that vitamin C supplementation may promote intestinal iron absorption and reduce the incidence of iron deficiency anemia among MHD patients (Chapters 24 and 25) [312–316]. Serum homocysteine concentrations, a cardiovascular risk factor, are significantly increased in MHD patients and pharmacological doses of folic acid can lower plasma total homocysteine levels. Generally, maximum homocysteine-lowering effects of folic acid occurs with doses of 5 to 10 mg/day [32,317]. However, studies in which advanced CKD and MHD patients were randomized to receive pharmacological doses of folic acid, pyridoxine HCl (vitamin B_6), and vitamin B_{12} or placebo did not show improvement in cardiovascular or total mortality with the vitamin supplements [318].

Erythrocyte or serum levels of riboflavin (vitamin B_2), thiamin (vitamin B_1), pantothenic acid, and biotin are usually normal in MHD patients. Case reports of Wernicke's encephalopathy in MHD and CPD patients due to thiamin deficiency are occasionally described [319,320]. Niacin levels are usually within the normal range in MHD patients [308,309,321,322], although many years ago Lasker et al. reported low niacin levels [323]. Pyridoxine (vitamin B_6) is removed by hemodialysis and this factor, and possibly also altered vitamin B_6 metabolism, accounts for an increased daily requirement for this vitamin, about 10 mg of pyridoxine HCl per day [324,325]. Vitamin B_6 participates in the metabolism of homocysteine, although pyridoxine supplements have not been consistently shown to decrease plasma homocysteine in CRF patients (see Chapter 24).

The lipid soluble vitamins are D, K, A and E. Vitamin K levels are usually normal in MHD patients [308]. Administration of a pharmacological dose of vitamin K_2 (45 mg/day orally) for one year was found to prevent loss of bone mass in MHD patients with bone disease characterized by low bone turnover [326]. Moreover, an inverse relationship between the frequency of bone fractures and plasma phylloquinone levels was reported in MHD patients [327]. Also, in the same study, serum PTH was high (>300 ng/L) in patients with low plasma phylloquinone (vitamin K_1) concentrations who also had an abnormally high incidence of an apolipoprotein E phenotype [328]. On the other hand, several reports described a relationship between high plasma vitamin K levels and ectopic soft tissue calcification in MHD patients [329–331]. Since MHD patients generally do not have evidence for vitamin K deficiency, vitamin K supplements are not recommended for routine use [332]. However, patients may be at increased risk for vitamin K deficiency if they are not eating, are not given vitamin K by parenteral administration, and are receiving antibiotics that suppress the intestinal bacteria that synthesize vitamin K. Under these conditions, vitamin K supplements should be given.

Serum vitamin A concentrations are generally increased in MHD patients, especially among long term dialysis survivors [333–335]. MHD patients who are binephrectomized are reported to have higher serum retinol levels than other MHD patients; this probably reflects the loss of the renal contribution to the degradation of retinal binding protein (RBP), the carrier protein for vitamin A [336,337]. Hemodialysis treatment does not change vitamin A levels [338,339]; indeed losses of vitamin A into dialysate would not be expected because of the relatively large size of the vitamin A-RBP-transthyretin (prealbumin) complex. However, β-carotene, ubiquinol and lycopene have been found to be lower in MHD patients than in individuals without renal insufficiency, and β-carotene and ubiquinol fall further after a single HD [340].

An individual's lipid metabolism may also affect serum vitamin A levels. In 72 MHD patients, Werb et al. [338] showed a positive correlation between plasma vitamin A levels and both serum total cholesterol and triglycerides. The hematocrit also has been found to correlate with the plasma vitamin A/RBP ratio in MHD patients, which is consistent with the evidence that vitamin A may promote erythropoiesis (see Chapters 3 and 24) [341]. Patients with advanced chronic renal failure appear to be particularly vulnerable to vitamin A toxicity. Hypercalcemia and elevated serum alkaline phosphatase levels have been described in MHD patients ingesting as little as 7500 to 15,000 units/day of vitamin A [338,342]. Therefore, it is recommended that the daily vitamin A intake from foods and supplements combined should not exceed the recommended dietary allowance of 800 to 1000 μg/day [338–341].

Serum vitamin E (α-tocopherol) levels in MHD patients are reported to be low [343–345], normal [346] or increased [332]. Significant amounts of α-tocopherol are not removed by the dialysis procedure [344,345]. In 10 long-term MHD survivors treated with MHD for an average of 274 ± 35 (SD) months, Chazot et al. found that serum vitamin E levels were abnormally high but not different from 10 age-and-gender-matched patients who were treated with MHD for 51 ± 29 months [347]. There are contradictory results with regard to RBC tocopherol concentrations in MHD patients [343,346]. These findings may reflect either increased consumption of tocopherol, possibly due to oxidative stress, or a defect in the HDL-mediated transfer of tocopherol from plasma to the RBC membrane. Cohen et al. [348] showed that RBC tocopherol concentrations were low in MHD patients who had sustained hemolysis caused by a high chloramine concentration in the water, and rose after the hemolytic condition was corrected by removal of the chloramine [348].

Since MHD patients not infrequently suffer from oxidant stress (see Chapters 5 and 6), several studies have examined the effects on oxidant stress of vitamin E supplementation given orally, during HD treatment utilizing vitamin E-coated dialyzer membranes, or through dialysate (hemolipodialysis). In the SPACE study, a double-blind, prospective clinical trial of 196 MHD patients randomized to receive oral vitamin E, 800 IU/day, or placebo MHD patients assigned to vitamin E treatment had a reduction in subsequent cardiovascular events (RR = 0.46) and myocardial infarction (RR = 0.30) [349]. A number of other studies of vitamin E supplementation in MHD patients as well as in the general population have not always confirmed that such supplements reduce morbidity or mortality [350,351]. Nonetheless, since chronic renal failure is clearly associated with increased oxidant stress and increased cardiovascular risk, and since vitamin E appears to be rather safe and may be beneficial, it is not unreasonable to consider prescribing a supplement of 15 IU/day of vitamin E.

Table 32.3 gives the dietary recommendations for various vitamins for MHD patients. The recommended dietary allowances are proposed for each of the water soluble vitamins and for vitamin A except for higher doses of pyridoxine HCl (10 mg/day, 8.2 mg/day of pyridoxine) and folic acid (about 1 mg/day). Vitamin C is recommended only at the daily allowance levels (70 mg/day) because of the risk of increased oxalate formation at higher intakes [352,353]. Vitamin E supplements appear safe; data concerning their effectiveness is equivocal, vitamin E supplements are therefore considered optional.

Trace Elements

Trace element nutrition in chronic renal failure is discussed in more detail in Chapter 23, and the nutritional requirements in MHD patients are briefly reviewed here. The advent of sophisticated analytic methodology allows for fairly accurate measurements of trace element levels [306]. However, the blood and tissue levels of these elements may be affected by many factors, some of which are independent of the nutritional status for the trace elements. These factors include dietary intake, renal excretory function, environmental and occupational exposure, duration of renal failure, the concentrations in fresh dialysate, and possibly the mode of dialytic therapy [354–363]. Also, many trace elements are highly protein bound. It is possible that uremia may be associated with altered serum binding protein levels or increased serum concentrations of compounds that compete for binding sites on these proteins; such factors may also alter serum trace element concentrations independently of the body burden or nutritional needs for these elements. Malnutrition or possibly inflammation leading to low serum proteins, may be one of the causes of low serum zinc, manganese and nickel [364].

Because many trace elements are present in trace amounts in the plasma and are protein bound, losses during hemodialysis may be minimal [365–367]. Bromide and zinc, however, are removed during hemodialysis because a substantial proportion of the serum concentrations are not protein bound and because the concentrations in the fresh dialysate inflow are quite low [368]. Conversely, the presence in the dialysate of even minute quantities of certain trace elements may lead to uptake by the body because of the avidity with which plasma binding proteins bind to some trace elements. This phenomenon has been observed for lead, copper, and zinc [367,369].

Serum zinc levels are often low, but erythrocyte zinc is often high normal or elevated [27,247,370–374]. Low serum zinc may be related to removal by dialysis [368] and inadequate dietary intake. Although serum zinc tends to rise at the end of dialysis, this can be attributed

entirely to the rise in concentration of carrier proteins due to hemoconcentration (see Chapter 23). Some reports indicate that dysgeusia and impotence in males, may be ameliorated with zinc supplements [375–378]; however, other studies have not confirmed these findings [379]. Until more definitive studies are conducted concerning dietary zinc requirements, the current recommendation is that hemodialysis patients should receive the recommended dietary allowance for zinc, which is 15 mg/day. Intestinal zinc absorption is not affected by vitamin D metabolites [380].

Iron deficiency is common in MHD patients (see Chapter 25). The causes include occult intestinal blood loss, sequestration of blood in the dialyzer at the termination of a hemodialysis procedure, binding of iron to the dialyzer membrane, and frequent blood drawing [314,381]. Treatment with recombinant human erythropoietin (EPO) may reduce the non-hemoglobin bound iron stores by enhancing erythropoiesis unless adequate iron supplementation is given. Malnutrition or inflammation, independently or in combination (i.e., the malnutrition-inflammation complex syndrome (MICS) see above), may lead to a state of refractory anemia and increase the dose of EPO [382] that is needed to attain the target range of hemoglobin of 10 to 12 g/dL [383]. Iron deficiency can be determined by measuring serum iron and total iron binding capacity (TIBC), calculating their ratio, known as transferrin saturation, and assessing serum ferritin levels. However, serum TIBC is affected by nutritional status and inflammation (i.e., it is a negative acute phase reactant), and its serum level is generally decreased in these conditions [85,384]. Hence, in MHD patients with PEW, the transferrin saturation may be erroneously normal to high if the denominator (TIBC) is decreased [384]. Serum ferritin is a positive acute phase reactant and may increase due to non-iron related factors, such as the MICS [385–387]. Oral iron can be prescribed in the form of ferrous sulfate, fumarate, gluconate, or lactate. However, ingestion of oral iron compounds usually does not lead to sufficient uptake of iron for MHD patients, and they are generally given iron intravenously in the form of iron dextran, gluconate and sucrose (saccharide) as well as several other iron compounds [314,388]. Some versions of iron dextran seems to be more often associated with adverse reactions [388,389], and iron gluconate and iron sucrose as well as newer compounds appear safe due to their lower rate of generation of free radicals [390].

Little is known concerning the nutritional requirements or tolerance for other trace elements in MHD patients. It is assumed that the trace quantities in foods and drinking water will satisfy the nutritional needs for these elements. On the other hand, the finding that serum selenium is low in dialysis patients has raised concerns that the dietary intake of selenium may not be adequate [391,392]. This question is particularly relevant because selenium is an anti-oxidant and a component of the defense system against oxidative damage of tissues, which may be increased in renal failure [393–395]. More research is clearly needed concerning the optimal intake for trace elements for chronic dialysis patients.

Carnitine

Carnitine is a naturally occurring compound that is essential for life and that is ingested in foods as well as synthesized in the body by the liver and kidneys. Carnitine facilitates the transfer of long chain (>10 carbon) fatty acids into skeletal muscle mitochondria [396]. Since fatty acids are the major fuel source for muscle during both rest and mild to moderate exercise, carnitine is considered necessary for normal muscle function. In MHD patients, serum total carnitine levels are often normal, free carnitine is below normal, and acylcarnitine (fatty acid-carnitine esters) levels are elevated [397,398]. Free carnitine levels in skeletal muscle are often but not always low in MHD patients [78,399,400].

A number of studies have reported that carnitine supplementation in renal failure may increase blood hemoglobin levels or reduce erythropoietin requirements; decrease such intradialytic symptoms as hypotension and muscle cramps; decrease hyperlipidemia; increase skeletal muscle exercise capacity; improve sense of well-being and reduce postdialysis asthenia and malaise [349,401–403]. One randomized, double-blind prospective clinical trial reported that L-carnitine decreased predialysis serum urea, creatinine, and phosphorus concentrations and increased midarm muscle circumference. Interpretation of these data must be qualified because a number of the outcome measures that showed improvement are imprecise or difficult to quantitate. Also, although several studies showing benefits were randomized, prospective, and blinded (particularly the improvement in hemoglobin levels or reduction in erythropoietin needs, increase in exercise capacity, improvement in global well-being, and intra- and postdialytic symptoms), other studies showing benefits were not prospective, randomized, or blinded. Moreover, some randomized blinded studies did not confirm such benefits or did so only in post-hoc analyses. The studies with regard to serum triglyceride levels are particularly conflictive. Some clinical trials show improvement in serum lipid profiles with L-carnitine treatment [404–406], whereas other clinical trials indicate no benefit [407,408] and some studies described a rise in serum triglycerides [398,409].

As a result of these outcomes, many nephrologists remain unconvinced of the therapeutic value of L-carnitine supplementation. On the other hand, a number of blinded prospective studies did show benefits, and L-carnitine appears to be quite a safe compound. The K/DOQI Nutrition Work Group concluded that there are insufficient data to support the routine use of L-carnitine for maintenance dialysis patients [78]. The K/DOQI guideline adds that:

> Although the administration of L-carnitine may improve subjective symptoms such as malaise, muscle weakness, intradialytic cramps and hypotension, and quality of life in selected MHD patients, the totality of evidence is insufficient to recommend its routine provision for any proposed clinical disorder without prior evaluation and attempts at standard therapy. The most promising of proposed applications is treatment of erythropoietin-resistant anemia [78,403].

Until more definitive data become available, one approach would be to use L-carnitine in the following clinical situations and only when all standard medical therapies have provided no benefit and when there is reason to believe that the medical condition is not irreversible (e.g., Weakness associated with disseminated carcinomatosis could be considered irreversible).

1. Anemia resistant to erythropoietin, iron, and vitamin therapy and with no evident cause.
2. Intradialytic hypotension or muscle cramps.
3. Impaired skeletal muscle exercise capacity.
4. Postdialysis asthenia or malaise.

A thorough medical evaluation for other treatable causes should be conducted before instituting carnitine therapy. The optimal dosage and route of therapy for L-carnitine are unresolved. Gastrointestinal absorption of carnitine in maintenance dialysis patients is not known and may be erratic. The United States Center for MediCare and MedicAid Services (CMS) has recently approved coverage for use of leucocarnitine for maintenance dialysis patients if they have low plasma free carnitine (<40 micromoles/L) and either erythropoietin-resistance anemia or hypotension occurring during hemodialysis treatment [410,411]. Continued coverage will not be given if improvement is not demonstrated within six months of starting treatment. L-carnitine, 10 to 20 mg/kg, intravenously, three times per week after the end of each hemodialysis or 5 to 10 mg/kg/day orally may be employed.

MANAGEMENT OF PEW IN MHD PATIENTS

When MHD patients display evidence for PEW or appear to be at high risk for developing PEW or pure protein-energy malnutrition, the following steps may be implemented to prevent or treat malnutrition:

1. Perform a medical and social history, physical examination, psychologic evaluation, and a nutritional assessment as indicated in Tables 32.1 and 32.2.
2. Identify the causes of the declining nutritional status. This assessment should include evaluating dietary protein and energy intake (e.g., UNA and dietary interviews and diaries) and the presence of acute illnesses, exacerbation of established comorbid illnesses or non-specific inflammation (e.g., an isolated increase in serum CRP), and acidemia. The causes for acidemia or reduced food intake should be investigated (e.g., anorexia from inadequate dialysis, psychological depression, poor dentition, poverty, inadequate social/family support).
3. Assess the patient's nutritional requirements.
4. Counsel the patient and spouse or significant others concerning the appropriate nutritional intake for the patient and strategies for attaining it.
5. If, despite dietary counseling, the nutrient intake remains inadequate for the patient's needs, the following maneuvers may be employed.
    (i) Frequent high protein/high energy meals and oral supplements including during hemodialysis treatment [152] (see Chapter 39).
    (ii) Tube feeding (see Chapter 39).
    (iii) Intradialytic parenteral nutrition (see Chapter 40).
    (iv) Daily parenteral nutrition.

Several studies have shown that oral nutritional supplements in association with dietary counseling can improve the nutritional status of MHD patients [172,412,413]. A recent study by Ikizler et al. showed a nutritional benefit from one can of supplement given thrice weekly during each dialysis session [172]. In the authors' experience, when malnourished MHD patients are given oral nutritional supplements, roughly, 20 to 40% of such individuals will take them on a continuing basis for several months or more. However, MHD patients commonly have modest financial resources, and when MHD patients must purchase the nutritional supplements, the long-term compliance rate is much lower. Tube feeding may be a more effective, less expensive method for nourishing malnourished adult dialysis patients, as it has been shown to be for the pediatric dialysis population (see Chapters 35 and 39). There is a need for studies to examine the benefits and potential risks of tube feeding. Tube feeding may be particularly effective for patients with PEW who are anorexic or noncompliant or may have disorders of motility of the upper gastrointestinal tract.

Several newer methods for the treatment of PEW in MHD patients have been investigated. These include appetite stimulants, particularly with megestrol acetate (see Chapter 38) [37,414,415]. This progestational agent has been shown to improve appetite and food intake and increase water-free body weight in patients with carcinomatosis or AIDS [416,417]. However, some evidence from these latter patients suggests that the water-free weight gain is due to accrual of body fat rather than protein [418]. There are currently no adequate experimental data indicating whether megestrol acetate will improve appetite in anorectic and protein-energy wasted MHD patients.

The feasibility of administering amino acids supplements to the patient by hemodialysate was examined by Chazot et al. (see Chapter 40) [419]. Six clinically stable postabsorptive men underwent hemodialysis on three separate occasions with hemodialysate containing either no amino acids or one or three times the postabsorptive plasma amino acid concentrations. The patients lost 9.3 ± 2.7 g of amino acid when dialyzed with dialysate containing no amino acids. However, there was a net amino acid uptake of 1.5 ± 3.6 g and 37.1 ± 14.8 g when they were treated with dialysate containing one or three times, respectively, the plasma concentrations of amino acids [419]. Further studies will be necessary to demonstrate whether this treatment can be used to improve the nutritional or clinical status of MHD patients with inadequate nutritional intake or PEM.

Finally, a number of studies have examined the possible benefits of recombinant human growth hormone (rhGH) or recombinant human insulin-like growth factor-I (rhIGF-I) to improve nutritional status of malnourished MHD or CPD patients (see Chapter 41) [420–425]. Although patients with advanced chronic renal failure display resistance to both rhGH and rhIGF-I, pharmacological doses of these agents still exert their effects on anabolism, growth and hyperfiltration. Recombinant human growth hormone may promote protein synthesis, decrease protein degradation, and improve nitrogen balance in nonrenal failure patients with catabolic stress [425]. It has been used to enhance growth in children with chronic renal failure and to maintain or increase the GFR in patients with Stage 5 chronic kidney disease and kidney transplantation [426–430]. (Chapter 35)

rhGH has also been used to treat PEW in adult patients with chronic renal failure (see Chapter 41). Several small, short-term trials have been carried out in chronic renal failure patients to treat PEW with rhGH. Zeigler et al [431]. treated five outpatients undergoing MHD with rhGH for 2 weeks. The patients were prescribed a fixed protein and calorie diet. The SUN fell by 20–25% when patients received rhGH, 5 to 10 mg subcutaneously after each hemodialysis. Shulman et al. [432] treated seven malnourished MHD patients with intradialytic parenteral nutrition for 12 weeks. During the last 6 weeks, when patients also received rhGH, 5 mg subcutaneously, with each dialysis, there was a decrease in the PNA, from 0.81 ± 0.04 to 0.67 ± 0.03 g/kg/day and an increase in the serum albumin levels.

Kopple studied six MHD patients with PEW in a General Clinical Research Center for up to 35 days [433]. After a baseline period of 14 to 21 days, patients were administered 0.05 mg rhGH/kg body weight/day for 17 ± SEM 2 days. During the study, patients 3 and 4 experienced acute illness with a reduction in protein and energy intake. Predialysis serum urea nitrogen fell markedly in patients 1, 2, 5, and 6, and less so in patients 3 and 4. Nitrogen balance was also markedly positive in patients 1, 2, 5, and 6, but much less so in patients 3 and 4 [433].

rhIGF-I also promotes positive nitrogen balance and decreases SUN in CPD and MHD patients [421]. Side effects with rhGH injections include hyperglycemia and acromegaly [427,434]. Treatment with rhIGF-I of critically ill intensive care unit patients is reported to increase mortality [435] and should not be done. RhIGF-I, at doses currently employed, may cause hypoglycemia and, uncommonly, cardiac arrhythmias and transient alterations in mental status. At present neither of these agents has been approved by the United States Food and Drug Administration for treatment of PEW or low GFR in CRF or maintenance dialysis patients. rhGH has been approved for treatment of impaired growth in children with chronic renal failure. A recent phase 3 study to examine the use of growth hormone in dialysis patients was discontinued prematurely for logistic and/or financial reasons (see Chapter 41)

TREATMENT OF ACUTE CATABOLIC ILLNESS

When MHD patients sustain superimposed catabolic illnesses, their intolerance for water, nitrogenous products, and many minerals and vitamins dictates that nutritional support must be extensively modified and carefully controlled. The high incidence of malnutrition in MHD patients and the close association between nutritional status and morbidity and mortality also suggest that it may be beneficial to provide nutritional support during acute illness if the patient's nutritional intake falls below his or her nutritional needs. The principles and techniques for nutritional support for MHD patients generally are similar to the methods for nutritional support for patients with acute renal failure and are discussed in Chapter 36. Nutritional management during treatment of the renal failure patient with continuous renal replacement therapy is discussed in Chapter 37.

DAILY OR LONG DURATION HEMODIALYSIS AND NUTRITIONAL STATUS

Several new approaches to standard hemodialysis therapy are currently either employed or are being examined in a small number of dialysis facilities. These include longer-duration and/or more frequent hemodialysis sessions [436–440]. Long-duration hemodialysis is generally carried out for about 6 to 8 hours thrice-weekly using lower blood flow rates of 200 to 250 mL/min [228]. Short daily hemodialysis is characterized by 5 or 6 treatments per week, each lasting about 1.5 to 2.5 hours, using conventional blood and dialysate flow rates [440,441]. Nocturnal hemodialysis is performed 5 to 7 times per week; each treatment usually lasts 6 to 8 hours, with blood flow rates of about 200 to 300 mL/min and dialysate flows of approximately 200 to 300 mL/min [441,442]. With each of these treatments, biocompatible hemodialysis membranes, often high flux, are generally employed. An increasing number of centers are experimenting with the latter two treatment schedules [443,444].

Preliminary data from studies evaluating the effects of daily and nocturnal hemodialysis on nutritional status suggest a number of benefits. With both short daily hemodialysis and nocturnal hemodialysis the patient has less restrictions on dietary intake [436,437, 445,446]. Also, with long-duration, short daily and nocturnal dialyses, the patients' spontaneous dietary energy and protein intake appears to increase [347, 436–439]. This latter observation is supported by a rise in their dry weight, edema-free, fat-free body mass, or serum albumin levels [347,436,437,445,446]. There is often a striking lowering of the predialysis serum phosphorus concentrations that occurs with nocturnal hemodialysis [443]. The reduced anorexia and nutritional improvement may be due to reduced uremic toxicity and also possibly the enhanced sense of well being, less dietetic constraints, and fewer drug prescriptions that are commonly reported with this more intensive hemodialysis treatment regimen. These more intensive hemodialysis treatments are also reported to result in tighter blood pressure control, regression of left ventricular hypertrophy, correction of anemia, and improved quality of life [228,447]. It is not clear whether these biological and clinical improvements are mainly the results of the greater frequency of dialysis treatments or higher weekly clearance doses of dialysis. Prospective clinical trials are required to delineate the full potential of these therapies on nutritional status as well the differences between them.

There are little data on the nutritional needs of patients undergoing daily and/or longer duration hemodialyses. Energy, protein, mineral and vitamin needs are probably as described in Table 32.3. Exceptions to this may be the dietary potassium and phosphorus needs which may be increased [436,437,445,446]. On the other hand, with more frequent or higher weekly doses of hemodialysis there is probably increased tolerance for higher intakes of protein, water, sodium, potassium, phosphorus, magnesium and the potentially more hazardous water soluble (i.e., dialyzable) vitamins, such as ascorbic acid [347,436,437,445,446]. As in all MHD patients, with more frequent and/or higher weekly doses of hemodialysis, the nutrient intake, nutritional status and serum mineral levels of the individual should be monitored closely.

References

[1] Kovesdy CP, Kalantar-Zadeh K. Why is protein-energy wasting associated with mortality in chronic kidney disease? Seminars in Nephrology 2009;29:3–14.

[2] Fouque D, Kalantar-Zadeh K, Kopple J, et al. A proposed nomenclature and diagnostic criteria for protein-energy wasting in acute and chronic kidney disease. Kidney Int 2008;73:391–8.

[3] Kalantar-Zadeh K, Kopple JD, Block G, et al. A malnutrition-inflammation score is correlated with morbidity and mortality in maintenance hemodialysis patients. Am J Kidney Dis 2001;38:1251–63.

[4] Ritz E, Vallance P, Nowicki M. The effect of malnutrition on cardiovascular mortality in dialysis patients: is L-arginine the answer? Nephrol Dial Transplant 1994;9:129–30.

[5] Stenvinkel P, Heimburger O, Paultre F, et al. Strong association between malnutrition, inflammation, and atherosclerosis in chronic renal failure. Kidney Int 1999;55:1899–911.

[6] Kalantar-Zadeh K, Kopple JD. Relative contributions of nutrition and inflammation to clinical outcome in dialysis patients. Am J Kidney Dis 2001;38:1343–50.

[7] Kalantar-Zadeh K, Block G, Humphreys MH, et al. Reverse epidemiology of cardiovascular risk factors in maintenance dialysis patients. Kidney Int 2003;63:793–808.

[8] Kopple JD, Zhu X, Lew NL, et al. Body weight-for-height relationships predict mortality in maintenance hemodialysis patients. Kidney Int 1999;56:1136–48.

[9] Kalantar-Zadeh K, Kopple JD, Kilpatrick RD, et al. Association of morbid obesity and weight change over time with cardiovascular survival in hemodialysis population. Am J Kidney Dis 2005;46:489–500.

[10] Kilpatrick RD, McAllister CJ, Kovesdy CP, et al. Association between serum lipids and survival in hemodialysis patients and impact of race. J Am Soc Nephrol 2007;18:293–303.

[11] Noori N, Kopple JD, Kovesdy CP, et al. Mid-arm muscle circumference and quality of life and survival in maintenance hemodialysis patients. Clin J Am Soc Nephrol: CJASN 2010;5:2258–68.

[12] Kalantar-Zadeh K, Kuwae N, Wu DY, et al. Associations of body fat and its changes over time with quality of life and prospective mortality in hemodialysis patients. Am J Clin Nutr 2006;83:202–10.

[13] Iseki K, Yamazato M, Tozawa M, et al. Hypocholesterolemia is a significant predictor of death in a cohort of chronic hemodialysis patients. Kidney Int 2002;61:1887–93.

[14] Lowrie EG, Lew NL. Death risk in hemodialysis patients: the predictive value of commonly measured variables and an evaluation of death rate differences between facilities. Am J Kidney Dis 1990;15:458–82.

[15] Calle EE, Thun MJ, Petrelli JM, et al. Body-mass index and mortality in a prospective cohort of U.S. adults. N Engl J Med 1999;341:1097–105.

[16] Kalantar-Zadeh K, Streja E, Kovesdy CP, et al. The obesity paradox and mortality associated with surrogates of body size and muscle mass in patients receiving hemodialysis. Mayo Clinic proceedings Mayo Clinic 2010;85:991–1001.

[17] Kovesdy CP, Kalantar-Zadeh K. Do genes allow inflammation to kill or not to kill? J Am Soc Nephrol 2009;20:1429–31.

[18] Kalantar-Zadeh K, Kopple J. Inflammation in renal failure. UpToDate, vol. 10.2. UpToDate, Boston Inc; 2002.

[19] Stenvinkel P, Heimburger O, Paultre F, et al. Strong association between malnutrition, inflammation, and atherosclerosis in chronic renal failure. Kidney Int 1999;55:1899–911.

[20] Kalantar-Zadeh K, Mehrotra R, Fouque D, et al. Metabolic acidosis and malnutrition-inflammation complex syndrome in chronic renal failure. Semin Dial 2004;17:455–65.

[21] Eknoyan G, Beck GJ, Cheung AK, et al. Effect of dialysis dose and membrane flux in maintenance hemodialysis. N Engl J Med 2002;347:2010–9.

[22] Descombes E, Hanck AB, Fellay G. Water soluble vitamins in chronic hemodialysis patients and need for supplementation. Kidney Int 1993;43:1319–28.

[23] Moriwaki K, Kanno Y, Nakamoto H, et al. Vitamin B6 deficiency in elderly patients on chronic peritoneal dialysis. Adv Perit Dial 2000;16:308–12.

[24] Yonemura K, Fujimoto T, Fujigaki Y, et al. Vitamin D deficiency is implicated in reduced serum albumin concentrations in patients with end-stage renal disease. Am J Kidney Dis 2000;36:337–44.

[25] Sullivan JF, Eisenstein AB. Ascorbic acid depletion during hemodialysis. Jama 1972;220:1697–9.

[26] Sullivan JF, Eisenstein AB. Ascorbic acid depletion in patients undergoing chronic hemodialysis. Am J Clin Nutr 1970;23:1339–46.

[27] Erten Y, Kayatas M, Sezer S, et al. Zinc deficiency: prevalence and causes in hemodialysis patients and effect on cellular immune response. Transplant Proc 1998;30:850–1.

[28] Mahajan SK, Prasad AS, Rabbani P, et al. Zinc deficiency: a reversible complication of uremia. Am J Clin Nutr 1982;36:1177–83.

[29] Blendis LM, Ampil M, Wilson DR, et al. The importance of dietary protein in the zinc deficiency of uremia. Am J Clin Nutr 1981;34:2658–61.

[30] Carr AC, Zhu BZ, Frei B. Potential antiatherogenic mechanisms of ascorbate (vitamin C) and alpha-tocopherol (vitamin E). Circ Res 2000;87:349–54.

[31] Jialal I, Grundy SM. Effect of combined supplementation with alpha-tocopherol, ascorbate, and beta carotene on low-density lipoprotein oxidation. Circulation 1993;88:2780–6.

[32] Arnadottir M, Brattstrom L, Simonsen O, et al. The effect of high-dose pyridoxine and folic acid supplementation on serum lipid and plasma homocysteine concentrations in dialysis patients. Clin Nephrol 1993;40:236–40.

[33] Kalantar-Zadeh K, Kopple JD, Deepak S, et al. Food intake characteristics of hemodialysis patients as obtained by food frequency questionnaire. J Ren Nutr 2002;12:17–31.

[34] Chertow GM, Burke SK, Raggi P. Sevelamer attenuates the progression of coronary and aortic calcification in hemodialysis patients. Kidney Int 2002;62:245−52.

[35] Raggi P, Boulay A, Chasan-Taber S, et al. Cardiac calcification in adult hemodialysis patients. A link between end-stage renal disease and cardiovascular disease? J Am Coll Cardiol 2002;39:695−701.

[36] Bergstrom J. Regulation of appetite in chronic renal failure. Miner Electrolyte Metab 1999;25:291−7.

[37] Yeh S, Wu SY, Levine DM, et al. Quality of life and stimulation of weight gain after treatment with megestrol acetate: correlation between cytokine levels and nutritional status, appetite in geriatric patients with wasting syndrome. J Nutr Health Aging 2000;4:246−51.

[38] Kalantar-Zadeh K, Block G, McAllister CJ, et al. Appetite and inflammation, nutrition, anemia and clinical outcome in hemodialysis patients. Am J Clin Nutr 2004;80:299−307.

[39] Ricks J, Molnar MZ, Kovesdy CP, et al. Glycemic control and cardiovascular mortality in hemodialysis patients with diabetes: a 6-year cohort study. Diabetes 2012;61:708−15.

[40] Kopple JD, Swendseid ME, Shinaberger JH, et al. The free and bound amino acids removed by hemodialysis. Trans Am Soc Artif Intern Organs 1973;19:309−13.

[41] Wolfson M, Jones MR, Kopple JD. Amino acid losses during hemodialysis with infusion of amino acids and glucose. Kidney Internat 1982;21:500−6.

[42] Ikizler TA, Flakoll PJ, Parker RA, et al. Amino acid and albumin losses during hemodialysis. Kidney Internat 1994;46:830−7.

[43] Gutierrez A, Bergström J, Alvestrand A. Hemodialysis-associated protein catabolism with and without glucose in the dialysis fluid. Kidney Internat 1994;46:814−22.

[44] Kaplan AA, Halley SE, Lapkin RA, et al. Dialysate protein losses with bleach processed polysulphone dialyzers. Kidney Internat 1995;47:573−8.

[45] Vanherweghem JL, Drukker W, Schwarz A. Clinical significance of blood-device interaction in hemodialysis. A review. Int J Artif Organs 1987;10:219−32.

[46] Oster JR, Lopez RA, Silverstein FJ, et al. The anion gap of patients receiving bicarbonate maintenance hemodialysis. ASAIO Trans 1989;35:800−4.

[47] Tolchin N, Roberts JL, Hayashi J, et al. Metabolic consequences of high mass-transfer hemodialysis. Kidney Int 1977;11:366−78.

[48] Ward RA, Wathen RL, Williams TE, et al. Hemodialysate composition and intradialytic metabolic, acid-base and potassium changes. Kidney Int 1987;32:129−35.

[49] Wu DY, Shinaberger CS, Regidor DL, et al. Association between serum bicarbonate and death in hemodialysis patients: Is it better to be acidotic or alkalotic? Clin J Am Soc Neph 2006;1:70−8.

[50] Wu DY, Shinaberger CS, Regidor DL, et al. Association between serum bicarbonate and death in hemodialysis patients: is it better to be acidotic or alkalotic? Clin J Am Soc Nephrol: CJASN 2006;1:70−8.

[51] (DOQI) NKFKDOQI. Clinical practice guidelines for nutrition in chronic renal failure. Am J Kidney Dis 2000;35(Suppl. 2).

[52] Kovacic V, Roguljic L. Metabolic acidosis of chronically hemodialyzed patients. Am J Nephrol 2003;23:158−64.

[53] Gutierrez A, Alvestrand A, Wahren J, et al. Effect of in vivo contact between blood and dialysis membranes on protein catabolism in humans. Kidney Int 1990;38:487−94.

[54] Gutierrez A, Bergstrom J, Alvestrand A. Protein catabolism in sham-hemodialysis: the effect of different membranes. Clin Nephrol 1992;38:20−9.

[55] Borah MF, Schonfeld PY, Gotch FA, et al. Nitrogen balance during intermittent dialysis therapy of uremia. Kidney Int 1978;14:491−500.

[56] Heidland A, Horl WH, Heller N, et al. Proteolytic enzymes and catabolism: enhanced release of granulocyte proteinases in uremic intoxication and during hemodialysis. Kidney Int Suppl 1983;16:S27−36.

[57] Baracos V, Rodemann HP, Dinarello CA, et al. Stimulation of muscle protein degradation and prostaglandin E2 release by leukocytic pyrogen (interleukin-1). A mechanism for the increased degradation of muscle proteins during fever. N Engl J Med 1983;308:553−8.

[58] Stenvinkel P, Alvestrand A. Inflammation in end-stage renal disease: sources, consequences, and therapy. Semin Dial 2002;15:329−37.

[59] Himmelfarb J, Stenvinkel P, Ikizler TA, et al. The elephant in uremia: oxidant stress as a unifying concept of cardiovascular disease in uremia. Kidney Int 2002;62:1524−38.

[60] Nawabi MD, Block KP, Chakrabarti MC, et al. Administration of endotoxin, tumor necrosis factor, or interleukin 1 to rats activates skeletal muscle branched-chain alpha-keto acid dehydrogenase. J Clin Invest 1990;85:256−63.

[61] Flores EA, Bistrian BR, Pomposelli JJ, et al. Infusion of tumor necrosis factor/cachectin promotes muscle catabolism in the rat. A synergistic effect with interleukin 1. J Clin Invest 1989;83:1614−22.

[62] Perlmutter DH, Dinarello CA, Punsal PI, et al. Cachetin/tumor necrosis factor regulates hepatic acute-phase gene expression. J Clin Inves 1986;78:1349−55.

[63] Stenvinkel P. Malnutrition and chronic inflammation as risk factors for cardiovascular disease in chronic renal failure. Blood Purif 2001;19:143−51.

[64] Stenvinkel P, Heimburger O, Lindholm B, et al. Are there two types of malnutrition in chronic renal failure? Evidence for relationships between malnutrition, inflammation and atherosclerosis (MIA syndrome). Nephrol Dial Transplant 2000;15:953−60.

[65] Kalantar-Zadeh K, Ikizler TA, Block G, et al. Malnutrition-inflammation complex syndrome in dialysis patients: causes and consequences. Am J Kidney Dis 2003;42:864−81.

[66] Kalantar-Zadeh K, Kopple JD, Humphreys MH, et al. Comparing outcome predictability of markers of malnutrition-inflammation complex syndrome in haemodialysis patients. Nephrol Dial Transplant 2004;19:1507−19.

[67] Mehrotra R, Kopple JD. Nutritional Management of Maintenance Dialysis Patients: Why aren't we doing better?. In: McCormick DB, Bier DM, Cousins RJ, editors. Annual Review of Nutrition, vol. 21. Palo Ato, CA: Annual Reviews; 2001. p. 343−80.

[68] Wathen RL, Keshaviah P, Hommeyer P, et al. The metabolic effects of hemodialysis with and without glucose in the dialysate. Am J Clin Nutr 1978;31:1870−5.

[69] Marumo F, Kamata K, Okubo M. Deranged concentrations of water-soluble vitamins in the blood of undialyzed and dialyzed patients with chronic renal failure. Int J Artif Organs 1986;9:17−24.

[70] Stone WJ, Warnock LG, Wagner C. Vitamin B6 deficiency in uremia. Am J Clin Nutr 1975;28:950−7.

[71] Dobbelstein H, Korner WF, Mempel W, et al. Vitamin B6 deficiency in uremia and its implications for the depression of immune responses. Kidney Int 1974;5:233−9.

[72] Jansen MAM, Korevaar JC, Dekker FW, et al. Renal function and nutritional status at the start of dialysis treatment. J Am Soc Nephrol 2001;12:157−63.

[73] Kopple JD, Massry SG, editors. Nutritional management of renal disease. William and Wilkins; Baltimore: 1996. p. 479−531. pp.

[74] Mailloux LU, Napolitano B, Bellucci AG, et al. The impact of co-morbid risk factors at the start of dialysis upon the survival of ESRD patients. ASAIO J 1996;42:164−9.

[75] Shinaberger CS, Kilpatrick RD, Regidor DL, et al. Longitudinal associations between dietary protein intake and survival in hemodialysis patients. Am J Kidney Dis 2006;48:37—49.

[76] Kopple JD. Nutrition in Renal Failure. Causes of Catabolism and Wasting in Acute or Chronic Renal Failure. In: Robinson RR, editor. Nephrology. Proceedings of the IXth International Congress of Nephrology, vol. 2. New York: Springer-Verlag; 1984. p. 1498—515.

[77] National Kidney Foundation I, Kidney-Dialysis Outcome Quality Initiative. K/DOQI clinical practice guidelines for chronic kidney disease: evaluation, classification, and stratification. Am J Kidney Dis 2002:39.

[78] National Kidney Foundation I, Kidney-Dialysis Outcome Quality Initiative. Clinical Practice Guidelines for nutrition in chronic renal failure. Am J Kidney Dis 2000;35:S1—S140.

[79] Lowrie EG, Huang WH, Lew NL. Death risk predictors among peritoneal dialysis and hemodialysis patients. Am J Kidney Dis 1995;26:220—8.

[80] Kalantar-Zadeh K, Kilpatrick RD, Kuwae N, et al. Revisiting mortality predictability of serum albumin in the dialysis population: time dependency, longitudinal changes and population-attributable fraction. Nephrol Dial Transplant 2005;20:1880—8.

[81] Canada-USA Peritoneal Dialysis Study Group. Adequacy of dialysis and nutrition in continuous peritoneal dialysis: association with clinical outcomes. J Am Soc Nephrol 1996;7:198—207.

[82] Enia G, Sicuso C, Alati G, et al. Subjective global assessment of nutrition in dialysis patients. Nephrol Dial Transplant 1993;8:1094—8.

[83] Hirsch S, de Obaldia N, Petermann M, et al. Subjective global assessment of nutritional status: further validation. Nutrition 1991;7:35—7; discussion 37—38.

[84] Detsky AS, McLaughlin JR, Baker JP, et al. What is subjective global assessment of nutritional status? JPEN J Parenter Enteral Nutr 1987;11:8—13.

[85] Kalantar-Zadeh K, Kleiner M, Dunne E, et al. Total iron-binding capacity-estimated transferrin correlates with the nutritional subjective global assessment in hemodialysis patients. Am J Kidney Dis 1998;31:263—72.

[86] McCann L. Using subjective global assessment to identify malnutrition in the ESRD patient. Nephrol News Issues 1999;13:18—9.

[87] Kalantar-Zadeh K, Kleiner M, Dunne E, et al. A modified quantitative subjective global assessment of nutrition for dialysis patients. Nephrol Dial Transplant 1999;14:1732—8.

[88] Kalantar-Zadeh K, Block G, McAllister C, et al. Association between self-reported appetite and markers of inflammation, nutrition, anemia and quality of life in hemodialysis patients [in press] 2003.

[89] Rambod M, Bross R, Zitterkoph J, et al. Association of Malnutrition-Inflammation Score with quality of life and mortality in hemodialysis patients: a 5-year prospective cohort study. Am J Kidney Dis 2009;53:298—309.

[90] Kopple JD, Mehrotra R, Suppasyndh O, et al. Observations with regard to the National Kidney Foundation K/DOQI clinical practice guidelines concerning serum transthyretin in chronic renal failure. Clin Chem Lab Med 2002;40:1308—12.

[91] Chertow GM, Ackert K, Lew NL, et al. Prealbumin is as important as albumin in the nutritional assessment of hemodialysis patients. Kidney Int 2000;58:2512—7.

[92] Rambod M, Kovesdy CP, Bross R, et al. Association of serum prealbumin and its changes over time with clinical outcomes and survival in patients receiving hemodialysis. Am J Clin Nutr 2008;88:1485—94.

[93] Chertow GM, Jacobs D, Lazarus J, Lew N, Lowrie E. Phase angle predicts survival in hemodialysis patients. J Renal Nutrition 1997;7:204—7.

[94] Chertow GM, Lowrie EG, Wilmore DW, et al. Nutritional assessment with bioelectrical impedance analysis in maintenance hemodialysis patients. J Am Soc Nephrol 1995;6:75—81.

[95] Kalantar-Zadeh K, Dunne E, Nixon K, et al. Near infra-red interactance for nutritional assessment of dialysis patients. Nephrol Dial Transplant 1999;14:169—75.

[96] Chertow GM. Estimates of body composition as intermediate outcome variables: are DEXA and BIA ready for prime time? J Ren Nutr 1999;9:138—41.

[97] Dumler F. Use of bioelectric impedance analysis and dual-energy X-ray absorptiometry for monitoring the nutritional status of dialysis patients. Asaio J 1997;43:256—60.

[98] Noori N, Kovesdy CP, Dukkipati R, et al. Survival predictability of lean and fat mass in men and women undergoing maintenance hemodialysis. Am J Clin Nutr 2010;92:1060—70.

[99] Noori N, Kovesdy CP, Bross R, et al. Novel equations to estimate lean body mass in maintenance hemodialysis patients. Am J Kidney Dis 2011;57:130—9.

[100] Bross R, Zitterkoph J, Pithia J, et al. Association of serum total iron-binding capacity and its changes over time with nutritional and clinical outcomes in hemodialysis patients. Am J Nephrol 2009;29:571—81.

[101] Kaysen GA, Rathore V, Shearer GC, et al. Mechanisms of hypoalbuminemia in hemodialysis patients. Kidney Int 1995;48:510—6.

[102] Kaysen GA, Chertow GM, Adhikarla R, et al. Inflammation and dietary protein intake exert competing effects on serum albumin and creatinine in hemodialysis patients. Kidney Int 2001;60:333—40.

[103] Kaysen GA. The microinflammatory state in uremia: causes and potential consequences. J Am Soc Nephrol 2001;12:1549—57.

[104] Owen Jr WF, Lew NL, Liu Y, et al. The urea reduction ratio and serum albumin concentration as predictors of mortality in patients undergoing hemodialysis. N Engl J Med 1993;329:1001—6.

[105] Leavey SF, McCullough K, Hecking E, et al. Body mass index and mortality in 'healthier' as compared with 'sicker' haemodialysis patients: results from the Dialysis Outcomes and Practice Patterns Study (DOPPS). Nephrol Dial Transplant 2001;16:2386—94.

[106] Leavey SF, Strawderman RL, Jones CA, et al. Simple nutritional indicators as independent predictors of mortality in hemodialysis patients. Am J Kidney Dis 1998;31:997—1006.

[107] Bross R, Noori N, Kovesdy CP, et al. Dietary assessment of individuals with chronic kidney disease. Semin Dial 2010;23:359—64.

[108] Bergstrom J. Inflammation, malnutrition, cardiovascular disease and mortality in end-stage renal disease. Pol Arch Med Wewn 2000;104:641—3.

[109] Wilcken DE, Dudman NP, Tyrrell PA, et al. Folic acid lowers elevated plasma homocysteine in chronic renal insufficiency: possible implications for prevention of vascular disease. Metabolism 1988;37:697—701.

[110] Suliman ME, Lindholm B, Barany P, et al. Hyperhomocysteinemia in chronic renal failure patients: relation to nutritional status and cardiovascular disease. Clin Chem Lab Med 2001;39:734—8.

[111] Wrone EM, Zehnder JL, Hornberger JM, et al. An MTHFR variant, homocysteine, and cardiovascular comorbidity in renal disease. Kidney Int 2001;60:1106—13.

[112] Kalantar-Zadeh K, Block G, Humphreys MH, et al. A low, rather than a high, total plasma homocysteine is an indicator of

poor outcome in hemodialysis patients. J Am Soc Nephrol 2004;15:442—53.

[113] Daugirdas JT. The post: pre dialysis plasma urea nitrogen ratio to estimate K.t/V and NPCR: validation. Int J Artif Organs 1989;12:420—7.

[114] Sargent J, Gotch F, Borah M, et al. Urea kinetics: a guide to nutritional management of renal failure. Am J Clin Nutr 1978;31:1696—702.

[115] Kalantar-Zadeh K, Supasyndh O, Lehn RS, et al. Normalized protein nitrogen appearance is correlated with hospitalization and mortality in hemodialysis patients with Kt/V greater than 1.20. J Ren Nutr 2003;13:15—25.

[116] Keshaviah PR, Emerson PF, Nolph KD. Timely initiation of dialysis: a urea kinetic approach. Am J Kidney Dis 1999;33:344—8.

[117] Kopple JD, Jones MR, Keshaviah PR, et al. A proposed glossary for dialysis kinetics. Am J Kidney Dis 1995;26:963—81.

[118] Bergstrom J. Nutrition and adequacy of dialysis in hemodialysis patients. Kidney Int Suppl 1993;41:S261—7.

[119] Lindsay RM, Spanner E. A hypothesis: the protein catabolic rate is dependent upon the type and amount of treatment in dialyzed uremic patients. Am J Kidney Dis 1989;13:382—9.

[120] Hakim RM, Breyer J, Ismail N, et al. Effects of dose of dialysis on morbidity and mortality. Am J Kidney Dis 1994;23:661—9.

[121] Yang CS, Chen SW, Chiang CH, et al. Effects of increasing dialysis dose on serum albumin and mortality in hemodialysis patients. Am J Kidney Dis 1996;27:380—6.

[122] Nolph KD. What's new in peritoneal dialysis—an overview. Kidney Int Suppl 1992;38:S148—52.

[123] Lysaght MJ, Pollock CA, Hallet MD, et al. The relevance of urea kinetic modeling to CAPD. ASAIO Trans 1989;35:784—90.

[124] Lindsay R, Spanner E, Heienheim P, et al. Which comes first, Kt/V or PCR - chicken or egg? Kidney Int 1992;42(Suppl. 3):S32—7.

[125] Harty JC, Boulton H, Curwell J, et al. The normalized protein catabolic rate is a flawed marker of nutrition in CAPD patients. Kidney Int 1994;45:103—9.

[126] Nolph KD, Moore HL, Prowant B, et al. Cross sectional assessment of weekly urea and creatinine clearances and indices of nutrition in continuous ambulatory peritoneal dialysis patients. Perit Dial Int 1993;13:178—83.

[127] Bergstrom J, Furst P, Alvestrand A, et al. Protein and energy intake, nitrogen balance and nitrogen losses in patients treated with continuous ambulatory peritoneal dialysis. Kidney Int 1993;44:1048—57.

[128] Shinaberger CS, Greenland S, Kopple JD, et al. Is controlling phosphorus by decreasing dietary protein intake beneficial or harmful in persons with chronic kidney disease? Am J Clin Nutr 2008;88:1511—8.

[129] Miller JE, Kovesdy CP, Nissenson AR, et al. Association of hemodialysis treatment time and dose with mortality and the role of race and sex. Am J Kidney Dis 2010;55:100—12.

[130] National Kidney Foundation I, Kidney-Dialysis Outcome Quality Initiative. K/DOQI Clinical Practice Guidelines: Peritoneal Dialysis Adequacy. Am J Kidney Dis 2001;37(suppl. 1):S65—136.

[131] Port FK, Wolfe RA. How Will the Results of the HEMO Study Impact Dialysis Practice? Semin Dial 2003;16:13—6.

[132] Rayner HC, Pisoni RL, Gillespie BW, et al. Creation, cannulation and survival of arteriovenous fistulae: Data from the Dialysis Outcomes and Practice Patterns Study. Kidney Int 2003;63:323—30.

[133] Konner K, Hulbert-Shearon TE, Roys EC, et al. Tailoring the initial vascular access for dialysis patients. Kidney Int 2002;62:329—38.

[134] Port FK, Ashby VB, Dhingra RK, et al. Dialysis dose and body mass index are strongly associated with survival in hemodialysis patients. J Am Soc Nephrol 2002;13:1061—6.

[135] Straumann E, Keller U, Kury D, et al. Effect of acute acidosis and alkalosis on leucine kinetics in man. Clin Physiol 1992;12:39—51.

[136] Papadoyannakis NJ, Stefanidis CJ, McGeown M. The effect of the correction of metabolic acidosis on nitrogen and potassium balance of patients with chronic renal failure. American Journal of Clinical Nutrition 1984;40:623—7.

[137] May RC, Kelly RA, Mitch WE. Mechanisms for defects in muscle protein metabolism in rats with chronic uremia: the influence of metabolic acidosis. J Clin Invest 1987;79:1099—103.

[138] Mitch WE, Medina R, Grieber S, et al. Metabolic acidosis stimulates muscle protein degradation by activating the adenosine triphosphate-dependent pathway involving ubiquitin and proteasomes. J Clin Invest 1994;93:2127—33.

[139] Bailey JL, Wang X, England BK, et al. The acidosis of chronic renal failure activates muscle proteolysis in rats by augmenting transcription of genes encoding proteins of the ATP-dependent ubiquitin-proteasome pathway. J Clin Invest 1996;97:1447—53.

[140] Price SR, England BK, Bailey JL, et al. Acidosis and glucocorticoids concomitantly increase ubiquitin and proteasome subunit mRNAs in rat muscle. Am J Physiol 1994;267:C955—60.

[141] Bergstrom J, Alvestrand A, Furst P. Plasma and muscle free amino acids in maintenance hemodialysis patients without protein malnutrition. Kidney Int 1990;38:108—14.

[142] Williams AJ, Dittmer ID, McArley A, et al. High bicarbonate dialysate in haemodialysis patients: effects on acidosis and nutritional status. Nephrol Dial Transplant 1997;12:2633—7.

[143] Kalantar-Zadeh K, Mehrotra R, Fouque D, et al. Metabolic acidosis and malnutrition-inflammation complex syndrome in chronic renal failure. Semin Dial 2004;17:455—65.

[144] Williams B, Hattersley J, Layward E, et al. Metabolic acidosis and skeletal muscle adaptation to low protein diets in chronic uremia. Kidney Internat 1991;40:779—86.

[145] Ballmer PE, McNurlan MA, Hulter HN, et al. Chronic metabolic acidosis decreases albumin synthesis and induces negative nitrogen balance in humans. J Clin Invest 1995;95:39—45.

[146] Mehrotra R, Bross R, Wang H, et al. Effect of high-normal compared with low-normal arterial pH on protein balances in automated peritoneal dialysis patients. Am J Clin Nutr 2009;90:1532—40.

[147] Kopple JD, Shinaberger JH, Coburn JW, et al. Optimal dietary protein treatment during chronic hemodialysis. Trans Am Soc Artif Int Org 1969;15:302—8.

[148] Kluthe R, Luttgren FM, Capetianu T, et al. Protein requirements in maintenance hemodialysis patients. Am J Clin Nutr 1978;31:1812—20.

[149] Ginn HE, Frost A, Lacy WW. Nitrogen balance in hemodialysis patients. Am J Clin Nutr 1968;21:385—93.

[150] Acchiardo SR, Moore LW, Latour PA. Malnutrition as the main factor in morbidity and mortality of hemodialysis patients. Kidney Int Suppl 1983;16:S199—203.

[151] Kopple JD, Shinaberger JH, Coburn JW, et al. Optimal dietary protein treatment during chronic hemodialysis. Trans Am Soc Artif Intern Organs 1969;15:302—8.

[152] Kalantar-Zadeh K, Cano NJ, Budde K, et al. Diets and enteral supplements for improving outcomes in chronic kidney disease. Nature reviews Nephrology 2011;7:369—84.

[153] Schoenfeld PY, Henry RR, Laird NM, et al. Assessment of nutritional status of the National Cooperative Dialysis Study population. Kidney Int Suppl 1983;23:S80—8.

[154] Food and Nutrition Board; Dietary Reference Intakes. Washington, DC: National Academy Press; 2001.

[155] Shinaberger JH, Ginn HE. Low protein, high essential amino acid diet for nitrogen equilibrium in chronic dialysis. Am J Clin Nutr 1968;21:618—25.

[156] Slomowitz LA, Monteon FJ, Grosvenor M, et al. Effect of energy intake on nutritional status in maintenance hemodialysis patients. Kidney Int 1989;35:704—11.

[157] Dwyer JT, Cunniff PJ, Maroni BJ, et al. The hemodialysis pilot study: nutrition program and participant characteristics at baseline. The HEMO Study Group. J Ren Nutr 1998;8:11—20.

[158] Gotch FA, Sargent JA. A mechanistic analysis of the National Cooperative Dialysis Study (NCDS). Kidney Int 1985;28:526—34.

[159] Uribarri J. Doqi guidelines for nutrition in long-term peritoneal dialysis patients: a dissenting view. Am J Kidney Dis 2001;37:1313—8.

[160] Lim VS, Flanigan MJ. Protein intake in patients with renal failure: comments on the current NKF-DOQI guidelines for nutrition in chronic renal failure. Semin Dial 2001;14:150—2.

[161] Kopple JD. Nutritional status as a predictor of morbidity and mortality in maintenance dialysis patients. Asaio J 1997;43:246—50.

[162] Bansal VK, Popli S, Pickering J, et al. Protein-calorie malnutrition and cutaneous anergy in hemodialysis maintained patients. Am J Clin Nutr 1980;33:1608—11.

[163] Blumenkrantz MJ, Kopple JD, Gutman RA, et al. Methods for assessing nutritional status of patients with renal failure. Am J Clin Nutr 1980;33:1567—85.

[164] Thunberg BJ, Swamy AP, Cestero RV. Cross-sectional and longitudinal nutritional measurements in maintenance hemodialysis patients. Am J Clin Nutr 1981;34:2005—12.

[165] Young GA, Swanepoel CR, Croft MR, et al. Anthropometry and plasma valine, amino acids and protein in the nutritional assessment of hemodialysis patients. Kidney Int 1982;21:492—9.

[166] Wolfson M, Strong CJ, Minturn D, et al. Nutritional status and lymphocyte function in maintenance hemodialysis patients. Am J Clin Nutr 1984;39:547—55.

[167] Bilbrey GL, Cohen TL. Identification and treatment of protein calorie malnutrition in chronic hemodialysis patients. Dialysis Transplant 1989;18:669—77.

[168] Blumenkrantz MJ, Gahl GM, Kopple JD, et al. Protein losses during peritoneal dialysis. Kidney Internat 1981;19:593—602.

[169] Dwyer JT, Larive B, Leung J, et al. Nutritional status affects quality of life in Hemodialysis (HEMO) Study patients at baseline. J Ren Nutr 2002;12:213—23.

[170] Monteon FJ, Laidlaw SA, Shaib JK, et al. Energy expenditure in patients with chronic renal failure. Kidney Int 1986;30:741—7.

[171] Ikizler TA, Pupim LB, Brouillette JR, et al. Hemodialysis stimulates muscle and whole body protein loss and alters substrate oxidation. Am J Physiol Endocrinol Metab 2002;282:E107—16.

[172] Pupim LB, Flakoll PJ, Brouillette JR, et al. Intradialytic parenteral nutrition improves protein and energy homeostasis in chronic hemodialysis patients. J Clin Invest 2002;110:483—92.

[173] Schneeweiss B, Graninger W, Stockenhuber F, et al. Energy metabolism in acute and chronic renal failure. Am J Clin Nutr 1990;52:596—601.

[174] Neyra R, Chen KY, Sun M, et al. Increased resting energy expenditure in patients with end-stage renal disease. JPEN J Parenter Enteral Nutr 2003;27:36—42.

[175] Keane WF, Collins AJ. Influence of co-morbidity on mortality and morbidity in patients treated with hemodialysis. Am J Kidney Dis 1994;24:1010—8.

[176] United States Renal Data System. US Department of Public Health and Human Services, Public Health Service. Bethesda: National Institutes of Health; 2001.

[177] Kasiske B. Hyperlipidemia in patients with chronic renal disease. Am J Kidney Dis 1998;32:S142—56.

[178] Brunzell JD, Albers JJ, Haas LB, et al. Prevalence of serum lipid abnormalities in chronic hemodialysis. Metabolism 1977;26:903—10.

[179] Pedro-Botet J, Senti M, Rubies-Prat J, et al. When to treat dyslipidaemia of patients with chronic renal failure on haemodialysis? A need to define specific guidelines. Nephrol Dial Transplant 1996;11:308—13.

[180] Lacour B, Roullet JB, Beyne P, et al. Comparison of several atherogenicity indices by the analysis of serum lipoprotein composition in patients with chronic renal failure with or without haemodialysis, and in renal transplant patients. J Clin Chem Clin Biochem 1985;23:805—10.

[181] Cheung AK, Wu LL, Kablitz C, et al. Atherogenic lipids and lipoproteins in hemodialysis patients. Am J Kidney Dis 1993;22:271—6.

[182] Brook JG, Chaimovitz C, Rapoport J, et al. High-density lipoprotein composition in chronic hemodialysis. N Engl J Med 1979;300:1056.

[183] Rapoport J, Aviram M, Chaimovitz C, et al. Defective high-density lipoprotein composition in patients on chronic hemodialysis. A possible mechanism for accelerated atherosclerosis. N Engl J Med 1978;299:1326—9.

[184] Attman PO. Hyperlipoproteinaemia in renal failure: pathogenesis and perspectives for intervention. Nephrol Dial Transplant 1993;8:294—5.

[185] Attman PO, Alaupovic P. Lipid and apolipoprotein profiles of uremic dyslipoproteinemia — relation to renal function and dialysis. Nephron 1991;57:401—10.

[186] Oi K, Hirano T, Sakai S, et al. Role of hepatic lipase in intermediate-density lipoprotein and small, dense low-density lipoprotein formation in hemodialysis patients. Kidney Int Suppl 1999;71:S227—8.

[187] Senti M, Romero R, Pedro-Botet J, et al. Lipoprotein abnormalities in hyperlipidemic and normolipidemic men on hemodialysis with chronic renal failure. Kidney Int 1992;41:1394—9.

[188] Parsy D, Dracon M, Cachera C, et al. Lipoprotein abnormalities in chronic haemodialysis patients. Nephrol Dial Transplant 1988;3:51—6.

[189] Attman PO, Alaupovic P, Tavella M, et al. Abnormal lipid and apolipoprotein composition of major lipoprotein density classes in patients with chronic renal failure. Nephrol Dial Transplant 1996;11:63—9.

[190] Weintraub M, Burstein A, Rassin T, et al. Severe defect in clearing postprandial chylomicron remnants in dialysis patients. Kidney Int 1992;42:1247—52.

[191] Schettler V, Wieland E, Verwiebe R, et al. Plasma lipids are not oxidized during hemodialysis. Nephron 1994;67:42—7.

[192] Turgan C, Feehally J, Bennett S, et al. Accelerated hypertriglyceridemia in patients on continuous ambulatory peritoneal dialysis — a preventable abnormality. Int J Artif Organs 1981;4:158—60.

[193] Breuer HW. Hypertriglyceridemia: a review of clinical relevance and treatment options: focus on cerivastatin. Curr Med Res Opin 2001;17:60—73.

[194] Rosenson RS. Hypertriglyceridemia and coronaryheart disease risk. Cardiol Rev 1999;7:342—8.

[195] Rapp RJ. Hypertriglyceridemia: a review beyond low-density lipoprotein. Cardiol Rev 2002;10:163—72.

[196] Wanner C. Lipids in end-stage renal disease. J Nephrol 2002;15:202—4.

[197] Hendriks F, Kooman JP, van der Sande FM. Massive rhabdomyolysis and life threatening hyperkalaemia in a patient with

the combination of cerivastatin and gemfibrozil. Nephrol Dial Transplant 2001;16:2418−9.

[198] Ozdemir O, Boran M, Gokce V, et al. A case with severe rhabdomyolysis and renal failure associated with cerivastatin-gemfibrozil combination therapy − a case report. Angiology 2000;51:695−7.

[199] Al Shohaib S. Simvastatin-induced rhabdomyolysis in a patient with chronic renal failure. Am J Nephrol 2000;20:212−3.

[200] Executive Summary of The Third Report of The National Cholesterol Education Program (NCEP) Expert Panel on Detection, Evaluation, And Treatment of High Blood Cholesterol In Adults (Adult Treatment Panel III). Jama 2001;285:2486−97.

[201] Chang JW, Yang WS, Min WK, et al. Effects of simvastatin on high-sensitivity C-reactive protein and serum albumin in hemodialysis patients. Am J Kidney Dis 2002;39:1213−7.

[202] Halkin A, Keren G. Potential indications for angiotensin-converting enzyme inhibitors in atherosclerotic vascular disease. Am J Med 2002;112:126−34.

[203] Oda H, Keane WF. Recent advances in statins and the kidney. Kidney Int Suppl 1999;71:S2−5.

[204] Bickel C, Rupprecht HJ, Blankenberg S, et al. Influence of HMG-CoA reductase inhibitors on markers of coagulation, systemic inflammation and soluble cell adhesion. Int J Cardiol 2002;82:25−31.

[205] Ansell BJ, Watson KE, Weiss RE, et al. hsCRP and HDL Effects of Statins Trial (CHEST): Rapid Effect of Statin Therapy on C-Reactive Protein and High-Density Lipoprotein Levels A Clinical Investigation. Heart Dis 2003;5:2−7.

[206] Noori N, Kovesdy CP, Dukkipati R, et al. Racial and ethnic differences in mortality of hemodialysis patients: role of dietary and nutritional status and inflammation. Am J Nephrol 2011;33:157−67.

[207] Alderman MH, Cohen HW. Impact of dietary sodium on cardiovascular disease morbidity and mortality. Curr Hypertens Rep 2002;4:453−7.

[208] Pru C, Kjellstrand CM. On the clinical usefulness of the FENa test in acute renal failure: a critical analysis. Proc Clin Dial Transplant Forum 1980;10:240−7.

[209] Espinel CH. The FENa test. Use in the differential diagnosis of acute renal failure. Jama 1976;236:579−81.

[210] Kahn T, Mohammad G, Stein RM. Alterations in renal tubular sodium and water reabsorption in chronic renal disease in man. Kidney Int 1972;2:164−74.

[211] Jansen MA, Hart AA, Korevaar JC, et al. Predictors of the rate of decline of residual renal function in incident dialysis patients. Kidney Int 2002;62:1046−53.

[212] Maduell F, Navarro V. Dietary salt intake and blood pressure control in haemodialysis patients. Nephrol Dial Transplant 2000;15:2063.

[213] Shaldon S. Dietary salt restriction and drug-free treatment of hypertension in ESRD patients: a largely abandoned therapy. Nephrol Dial Transplant 2002;17:1163−5.

[214] Krautzig S, Janssen U, Koch KM, et al. Dietary salt restriction and reduction of dialysate sodium to control hypertension in maintenance haemodialysis patients. Nephrol Dial Transplant 1998;13:552−3.

[215] Tomson CR. Advising dialysis patients to restrict fluid intake without restricting sodium intake is not based on evidence and is a waste of time. Nephrol Dial Transplant 2001;16:1538−42.

[216] Charra B, Chazot C, Laurent G. Hypertension/hypotension in dialysis. Kidney Int 1999;55:1128.

[217] Charra B, Calemard E, Cuche M, et al. Control of hypertension and prolonged survival on maintenance hemodialysis. Nephron 1983;33:96−9.

[218] Strain WD, Lye M. Chronic pain, bereavement and overdose in a depressed elderly woman. Age Ageing 2002;31:218−9.

[219] Sherman RA, Cody RP, Rogers ME, et al. Interdialytic weight gain and nutritional parameters in chronic hemodialysis patients. Am J Kidney Dis 1995;25:579−83.

[220] Kimmel PL, Varela MP, Peterson RA, et al. Interdialytic weight gain and survival in hemodialysis patients: effects of duration of ESRD and diabetes mellitus. Kidney Int 2000;57:1141−51.

[221] Fishbane S, Youn S, Flaster E, et al. Ankle-arm blood pressure index as a predictor of mortality in hemodialysis patients. Am J Kidney Dis 1996;27:668−72.

[222] Fishbane S, Youn S, Kowalski EJ, et al. Ankle-arm blood pressure index as a marker for atherosclerotic vascular diseases in hemodialysis patients. Am J Kidney Dis 1995;25:34−9.

[223] Ventura JE, Sposito M. Volume sensitivity of blood pressure in end-stage renal disease. Nephrol Dial Transplant 1997;12:485−91.

[224] Rahman M, Dixit A, Donley V, et al. Factors associated with inadequate blood pressure control in hypertensive hemodialysis patients. Am J Kidney Dis 1999;33:498−506.

[225] Luik AJ, Gladziwa U, Kooman JP, et al. Blood pressure changes in relation to interdialytic weight gain. Contrib Nephrol 1994;106:90−3.

[226] Luik AJ, Gladziwa U, Kooman JP, et al. Influence of interdialytic weight gain on blood pressure in hemodialysis patients. Blood Purif 1994;12:259−66.

[227] Kooman JP, Gladziwa U, Bocker G, et al. Blood pressure during the interdialytic period in haemodialysis patients: estimation of representative blood pressure values. Nephrol Dial Transplant 1992;7:917−23.

[228] Chazot C, Charra B, Laurent G, et al. Interdialysis blood pressure control by long haemodialysis sessions. Nephrol Dial Transplant 1995;10:831−7.

[229] Sherman RA, Daniel A, Cody RP. The effect of interdialytic weight gain on predialysis blood pressure. Artif Organs 1993;17:770−4.

[230] Lins LE, Hedenborg G, Jacobson SH, et al. Blood pressure reduction during hemodialysis correlates to intradialytic changes in plasma volume. Clin Nephrol 1992;37:308−13.

[231] Kalantar-Zadeh K, Regidor DL, Kovesdy CP, et al. Fluid retention is associated with cardiovascular mortality in patients undergoing long-term hemodialysis. Circulation 2009;119:671−9.

[232] Geddes CC, Houston M, Pediani L, et al. Excess interdialytic sodium intake is not always dietary. Nephrol Dial Transplant 2003;18:223.

[233] Dominic SC, Ramachandran S, Somiah S, et al. Quenching the thirst in dialysis patients. Nephron 1996;73:597−600.

[234] Shen FH, Sherrard DJ, Scollard D, et al. Thirst, relative hypernatremia, and excessive weight gain in maintenance peritoneal dialysis. Trans Am Soc Artif Intern Organs 1978;24:142−5.

[235] Blumenkrantz MJ, Kopple JD, Moran JK, et al. Metabolic balance studies and dietary protein requirements in patients undergoing continuous ambulatory peritoneal dialysis. Kidney Int 1982;21:849−61.

[236] Martin RS, Panese S, Virginillo M, et al. Increased secretion of potassium in the rectum of humans with chronic renal failure. Am J Kidney Dis 1986;8:105−10.

[237] Sandle GI, Gaiger E, Tapster S, et al. Evidence for large intestinal control of potassium homoeostasis in uraemic patients undergoing long-term dialysis. Clin Sci (Lond) 1987;73:247−52.

[238] Kopple JD, Coburn JW. Metabolic studies of low protein diets in uremia. I. Nitrogen and potassium. Medicine (Baltimore) 1973;52:583−95.

[239] Boddy K, King PC, Lindsay RM, et al. Total body potassium in non-dialysed and dialysed patients with chronic renal failure. Br Med J 1972;1:771–5.

[240] Hsu CY, Chertow GM. Elevations of serum phosphorus and potassium in mild to moderate chronic renal insufficiency. Nephrol Dial Transplant 2002;17:1419–25.

[241] Abbott KC. Ace inhibitors and survival in dialysis patients: effects on serum potassium? Am J Kidney Dis 2003;41:520–1.

[242] Allon M, Shanklin N. Effect of bicarbonate administration on plasma potassium in dialysis patients: interactions with insulin and albuterol. Am J Kidney Dis 1996;28:508–14.

[243] Kovesdy CP, Regidor DL, Mehrotra R, et al. Serum and dialysate potassium concentrations and survival in hemodialysis patients. Clin J Am Soc Nephrol: CJASN 2007;2:999–1007.

[244] Noori N, Kalantar-Zadeh K, Kovesdy CP, et al. Dietary potassium intake and mortality in long-term hemodialysis patients. Am J Kidney Dis 2010;56:338–47.

[245] Dolson GM. Do potassium deficient diets and K+ removal by dialysis contribute to the cardiovascular morbidity and mortality of patients with end stage renal disease? Int J Artif Organs 1997;20:134–5.

[246] Karnik JA, Young BS, Lew NL, et al. Cardiac arrest and sudden death in dialysis units. Kidney Int 2001;60:350–7.

[247] Pietrzak I, Bladek K, Bulikowski W. Comparison of magnesium and zinc levels in blood in end stage renal disease patients treated by hemodialysis or peritoneal dialysis. Magnes Res 2002;15:229–36.

[248] Coburn JW, Hartenbower DL, Brickman AS, et al. Intestinal absorption of calcium, magnesium and phosphorus in chronic renal insufficiency. In: David DS, editor. Perspectives in Hypertension and Nephrology-Calcium Metabolism in Renal Disease. New York: Wiley; 1977. p. 77–109.

[249] Kopple JD, Coburn JW. Metabolic studies of low protein diets in uremia. II. Calcium, phosphorus and magnesium. Medicine (Baltimore) 1973;52:597–607.

[250] Mansouri K, Halsted JA, Gombos EA. Zinc, copper, magnesium and calcium in dialyzed and nondialyzed uremic patients. Arch Intern Med 1970;125:88–93.

[251] Wallach S. Effects of magnesium on skeletal metabolism. Magnes Trace Elem 1990;9:1–14.

[252] Navarro-Gonzalez JF. Magnesium in dialysis patients: serum levels and clinical implications. Clin Nephrol 1998;49:373–8.

[253] Contiguglia SR, Alfrey AC, Miller N, et al. Total-body magnesium excess in chronic renal failure. Lancet 1972;1:1300–2.

[254] Coburn JW, Hartenbower DL, Massry SG. Intestinal absorption of calcium and the effect of renal insufficiency. Kidney Int 1973;4:96–104.

[255] Addison JF, Foulks CJ. Calcium carbonate: An effective phosphorus binder in patients with chronic renal failure. Curr Ther Res 1985;38:241.

[256] Goodman WG, Goldin J, Kuizon BD, et al. Coronary-artery calcification in young adults with end-stage renal disease who are undergoing dialysis. N Engl J Med 2000;342:1478–83.

[257] Chertow GM, Burke SK, Dillon MA, et al. Long-term effects of sevelamer hydrochloride on the calcium x phosphate product and lipid profile of haemodialysis patients. Nephrol Dial Transplant 1999;14:2907–14.

[258] Chertow GM, Dillon M, Burke SK, et al. A randomized trial of sevelamer hydrochloride (RenaGel) with and without supplemental calcium. Strategies for the control of hyperphosphatemia and hyperparathyroidism in hemodialysis patients. Clin Nephrol 1999;51:18–26.

[259] Chertow GM, Dillon MA, Amin N, et al. Sevelamer with and without calcium and vitamin D: observations from a long-term open-label clinical trial. J Ren Nutr 2000;10:125–32.

[260] Chertow GM, Burke SK, Dillon MA, et al. Long-term effects of sevelamer hydrochloride on the calcium x phosphate product and lipid profile of haemodialysis patients. Nephrol Dial Transplant 2000;15:559.

[261] Fournier A, Presne C, Oprisiu R, et al. Oral calcium, sevelamer and vascular calcification in uraemic patients. Nephrol Dial Transplant 2002;17:2276–7.

[262] Reslerova M, Moe SM. Vascular calcification in dialysis patients: pathogenesis and consequences. Am J Kidney Dis 2003;41: S96–9.

[263] Marco MP, Muray S, Betriu A, et al. Treatment with sevelamer decreases bicarbonate levels in hemodialysis patients. Nephron 2002;92:499–500.

[264] Miller JE, Kovesdy CP, Norris KC, et al. Association of cumulatively low or high serum calcium levels with mortality in long-term hemodialysis patients. Am J Nephrol 2010;32:403–13.

[265] Hou SH, Zhao J, Ellman CF, et al. Calcium and phosphorus fluxes during hemodialysis with low calcium dialysate. Am J Kidney Dis 1991;18:217–24.

[266] Lorenzo V, Martin M, Rufino M, et al. Protein intake, control of serum phosphorus, and relatively low levels of parathyroid hormone in elderly hemodialysis patients. Am J Kidney Dis 2001;37:1260–6.

[267] Barsotti G, Morelli E, Giannoni A, et al. Restricted phosphorus and nitrogen intake to slow the progression of chronic renal failure: a controlled trial. Kidney Int Suppl 1983;16:S278–84.

[268] Kalantar-Zadeh K, Gutekunst L, Mehrotra R, et al. Understanding sources of dietary phosphorus in the treatment of patients with chronic kidney disease. Clin J Am Soc Nephrol: CJASN 2010;5:519–30.

[269] Block GA, Port FK. Re-evaluation of risks associated with hyperphosphatemia and hyperparathyroidism in dialysis patients: recommendations for a change in management. Am J Kidney Dis 2000;35:1226–37.

[270] Chazan JA, Lew NL, Lowrie EG. Increased serum aluminum. An independent risk factor for mortality in patients undergoing long-term hemodialysis. Arch Intern Med 1991;151:319–22.

[271] Hercz G, Pei Y, Greenwood C, et al. Aplastic osteodystrophy without aluminum: the role of "suppressed" parathyroid function. Kidney Int 1993;44:860–6.

[272] Malluche HH, Faugere MC. Aluminum-related bone disease. Blood Purif 1988;6:1–15.

[273] Norris KC, Crooks PW, Nebeker HG, et al. Clinical and laboratory features of aluminum-related bone disease: differences between sporadic and "epidemic" forms of the syndrome. Am J Kidney Dis 1985;6:342–7.

[274] Ott SM, Maloney NA, Coburn JW, et al. The prevalence of bone aluminum deposition in renal osteodystrophy and its relation to the response to calcitriol therapy. N Engl J Med 1982;307:709–13.

[275] Ibels LS, Alfrey AC, Huffer WE, et al. Calcification in end-stage kidneys. Am J Med 1981;71:33–7.

[276] Schiller LR, Santa Ana CA, Sheikh MS, et al. Effect of the time of administration of calcium acetate on phosphorus binding. N Engl J Med 1989;320:1110–3.

[277] Sheikh MS, Maguire JA, Emmett M, et al. Reduction of dietary phosphorus absorption by phosphorus binders. A theoretical, in vitro, and in vivo study. J Clin Invest 1989;83:66–73.

[278] Mai ML, Emmett M, Sheikh MS, et al. Calcium acetate, an effective phosphorus binder in patients with renal failure. Kidney Int 1989;36:690–5.

[279] Schaefer K, Scheer J, Asmus G, et al. The treatment of uraemic hyperphosphataemia with calcium acetate and calcium carbonate: a comparative study. Nephrol Dial Transplant 1991;6:170–5.

[280] Pflanz S, Henderson IS, McElduff N, et al. Calcium acetate versus calcium carbonate as phosphate-binding agents in chronic haemodialysis. Nephrol Dial Transplant 1994;9: 1121–4.

[281] Fournier A, Yverneau PH, Hue P, et al. Adynamic bone disease in patients with uremia. Curr Opin Nephrol Hypertens 1994;3:396–410.

[282] Malluche HH, Monier-Faugere MC. Risk of adynamic bone disease in dialyzed patients. Kidney Int Suppl 1992;38:S62–7.

[283] Borras M, Marco MP, Fernandez E. Treatment with sevelamer decreases bicarbonate levels in peritoneal dialysis patients. Perit Dial Int 2002;22:737–8.

[284] Hutchison AJ. Calcitriol, lanthanum carbonate, and other new phosphate binders in the management of renal osteodystrophy. Perit Dial Int 1999;19(Suppl. 2):S408–12.

[285] Cases A. Recent advances in nephrology: highlights from the 35th annual meeting of the american society of nephrology. Drugs Today (Barc) 2002;38:797–805.

[286] Nelson R. Novel phosphate binder is effective in patients on haemodialysis. Lancet 2002;360:1483.

[287] Hergesell O, Ritz E. Phosphate binders on iron basis: a new perspective? Kidney Int Suppl 1999;73:S42–5.

[288] Gray RW, Weber HP, Dominguez JH, et al. The metabolism of vitamin D3 and 25-hydroxyvitamin D3 in normal and anephric humans. J Clin Endocrinol Metab 1974;39:1045–56.

[289] Vaziri ND, Hollander D, Hung EK, et al. Impaired intestinal absorption of vitamin D3 in azotemic rats. Am J Clin Nutr 1983;37:403–6.

[290] Silver J, Russell J, Sherwood LM. Regulation by vitamin D metabolites of messenger ribonucleic acid for preproparathyroid hormone in isolated bovine parathyroid cells. Proc Natl Acad Sci U S A 1985;82:4270–3.

[291] Fukagawa M, Kitaoka M, Fukuda N, et al. Pathogenesis and management of parathyroid hyperplasia in chronic renal failure: role of calcitriol. Miner Electrolyte Metab 1995;21: 97–100.

[292] Bellido T, Girasole G, Passeri G, et al. Demonstration of estrogen and vitamin D receptors in bone marrow-derived stromal cells: up-regulation of the estrogen receptor by 1,25-dihydroxyvitamin-D3. Endocrinology 1993;133:553–62.

[293] Kalantar-Zadeh K, Kovesdy CP. Clinical outcomes with active versus nutritional vitamin D compounds in chronic kidney disease. Clin J Am Soc Nephrol: CJASN 2009;4:1529–39.

[294] Beckerman P, Silver J. Vitamin D and the parathyroid. Am J Med Sci 1999;317:363–9.

[295] Roussanne MC, Duchambon P, Gogusev J, et al. Parathyroid hyperplasia in chronic renal failure: role of calcium, phosphate, and calcitriol. Nephrol Dial Transplant 1999;14(Suppl. 1):68–9.

[296] Dahl NV, Foote EF. Pulse dose oral calcitriol therapy for renal osteodystrophy: literature review and practice recommendations. Anna J 1997;24:550–5.

[297] Salusky IB, Goodman W. Skeletal response to intermittent calcitriol therapy in secondary hyperparathyroidism. Kidney Int Suppl 1996;53:S135–9.

[298] Martin KJ, Gonzalez EA. Vitamin D analogues for the management of secondary hyperparathyroidism. Am J Kidney Dis 2001;38:S34–40.

[299] Kaye M. Hungry bone syndrome after surgical parathyroidectomy. Am J Kidney Dis 1997;30:730–1.

[300] Slatopolsky E, Brown AJ. Vitamin D analogs for the treatment of secondary hyperparathyroidism. Blood Purif 2002;20:109–12.

[301] Slatopolsky E, Brown A, Dusso A. Pathogenesis of secondary hyperparathyroidism. Kidney Int Suppl 1999;73:S14–9.

[302] Slatopolsky E, Weerts C, Thielan J, et al. Marked suppression of secondary hyperparathyroidism by intravenous administration of 1,25-dihydroxy-cholecalciferol in uremic patients. J Clin Invest 1984;74:2136–43.

[303] Hampers CL, Streiff R, Nathan DG, et al. Megaloblastic hematopoiesis in uremia and in patients on long-term hemodialysis. N Engl J Med 1967;276:551–4.

[304] Whitehead VM, Comty CH, Posen GA, et al. Homeostasis of folic acid in patients undergoing maintenance hemodialysis. N Engl J Med 1968;279:970–4.

[305] Jennette JC, Goldman ID. Inhibition of the membrane transport of folates by anions retained in uremia. J Lab Clin Med 1975;86:834–43.

[306] Kalantar-Zadeh K, Kopple JD. Trace elements and vitamins in maintenance dialysis patients. Adv Ren Replace Ther 2003;10:170–82.

[307] Spannuth Jr CL, Warnock LG, Wagner C, et al. Increased plasma clearance of pyridoxal 5'-phosphate in vitamin B6- deficient uremic man. J Lab Clin Med 1977;90:632–7.

[308] Kopple JD, Swendseid ME. Vitamin nutrition in patients undergoing maintenance hemodialysis. Kidney Int Suppl 1975:79–84.

[309] Ramirez G, Chen M, Boyce Jr HW, et al. Longitudinal follow-up of chronic hemodialysis patients without vitamin supplementation. Kidney Int 1986;30:99–106.

[310] Sharman VL, Cunningham J, Goodwin FJ, et al. In: Br Med J, Res Clin, editors. Do patients receiving regular haemodialysis need folic acid supplements? 285;1982. p. 96–7.

[311] Porrini M, Simonetti P, Ciappellano S, et al. Thiamin, riboflavin and pyridoxine status in chronic renal insufficiency. Int J Vitam Nutr Res 1989;59:304–8.

[312] Giancaspro V, Nuzziello M, Pallotta G, et al. Intravenous ascorbic acid in hemodialysis patients with functional iron deficiency: a clinical trial. J Nephrol 2000;13:444–9.

[313] Sezer S, Ozdemir FN, Yakupoglu U, et al. Intravenous ascorbic acid administration for erythropoietin-hyporesponsive anemia in iron loaded hemodialysis patients. Artif Organs 2002;26:366–70.

[314] Van Wyck DB, Bailie G, Aronoff G. Just the FAQs: frequently asked questions about iron and anemia in patients with chronic kidney disease. Am J Kidney Dis 2002;39:426–32.

[315] Tarng DC, Huang TP, Wei YH. Erythropoietin and iron: the role of ascorbic acid. Nephrol Dial Transplant 2001;16(Suppl. 5):35–9.

[316] Petrarulo F, Giancaspro V. Intravenous ascorbic acid in haemodialysis patients with functional iron deficiency. Nephrol Dial Transplant 2000;15:1717–8.

[317] Lasseur C, Parrot F, Delmas Y, et al. Impact of high-flux/high-efficiency dialysis on folate and homocysteine metabolism. J Nephrol 2001;14:32–5.

[318] Jamison RL, Hartigan P, Kaufman JS, et al. Effect of homocysteine lowering on mortality and vascular disease in advanced chronic kidney disease and end-stage renal disease: a randomized controlled trial. Jama 2007;298:1163–70.

[319] Ihara M, Ito T, Yanagihara C, et al. Wernicke's encephalopathy associated with hemodialysis: report of two cases and review of the literature. Clin Neurol Neurosurg 1999;101:118–21.

[320] Jagadha V, Deck JH, Halliday WC, et al. Wernicke's encephalopathy in patients on peritoneal dialysis or hemodialysis. Ann Neurol 1987;21:78–84.

[321] Allman MA, Pang E, Yau DF, et al. Elevated plasma vitamers of vitamin B6 in patients with chronic renal failure on regular haemodialysis. Eur J Clin Nutr 1992;46:679–83.

[322] Allman MA, Truswell AS, Tiller DJ, et al. Vitamin supplementation of patients receiving haemodialysis. Med J Aust 1989;150:130–3.

[323] Lasker N, Harvey A, Baker H. Vitamin levels in hemodialysis and intermittent peritoneal dialysis. Trans Am Soc Artif Intern Organs 1963;9:51.

[324] Teehan BP, Smith LJ, Sigler MH, et al. Plasma pyridoxal-5′-phosphate levels and clinical correlations in chronic hemodialysis patients. Am J Clin Nutr 1978;31:1932–6.

[325] Lacour B, Parry C, Drueke T, et al. Pyridoxal 5′-phosphate deficiency in uremic undialyzed, hemodialyzed, and non-uremic kidney transplant patients. Clin Chim Acta 1983;127:205–15.

[326] Akiba T, Kurihara S, Tachibana K, et al. Vitamin K increased bone mass in hemodialysis patients with low turn over bone disease. J Am Soc Nephrol 1991;2:608.

[327] Kohlmeier M, Saupe J, Shearer MJ, et al. Bone health of adult hemodialysis patients is related to vitamin K status. Kidney Int 1997;51:1218–21.

[328] Kohlmeier M, Saupe J, Schaefer K, et al. Bone fracture history and prospective bone fracture risk of hemodialysis patients are related to apolipoprotein E genotype. Calcif Tissue Int 1998;62:278–81.

[329] Hodges SJ, Akesson K, Vergnaud P, et al. Circulating levels of vitamins K1 and K2 decreased in elderly women with hip fracture. J Bone Miner Res 1993;8:1241–5.

[330] Bitensky L, Hart JP, Catterall A, et al. Circulating vitamin K levels in patients with fractures. J Bone Joint Surg Br 1988;70:663–4.

[331] Soundararajan R, Leehey DJ, Yu AW, et al. Skin necrosis and protein C deficiency associated with vitamin K depletion in a patient with renal failure. Am J Med 1992;93:467–70.

[332] Stein G, Sperschneider H, Koppe S. Vitamin levels in chronic renal failure and need for supplementation. Blood Purif 1985;3:52–62.

[333] Farrington K, Miller P, Varghese Z, et al. In: Br Med J, Res Clin, editors. Vitamin A toxicity and hypercalcaemia in chronic renal failure, 282; 1981. p. 1999–2002.

[334] Smith FR, Goodman DS. The effects of diseases of the liver, thyroid, and kidneys on the transport of vitamin A in human plasma. J Clin Invest 1971;50:2426–36.

[335] Stein G, Schone S, Geinitz D, et al. No tissue level abnormality of vitamin A concentration despite elevated serum vitamin A of uremic patients. Clin Nephrol 1986;25:87–93.

[336] Vahlquist A. Metabolism of the vitamin-A-transporting protein complex: turnover of retinol-binding protein, prealbumin and vitamin A in a primate (Macaca irus). Scand J Clin Lab Invest 1972;30:349–60.

[337] Vahlquist A, Peterson PA. Comparative studies on the vitamin A transporting protein complex in human and cynomolgus plasma. Biochemistry 1972;11:4526–32.

[338] Werb R, Clark WF, Lindsay RM, et al. Serum vitamin A levels and associated abnormalities in patients on regular dialysis treatment. Clin Nephrol 1979;12:63–8.

[339] Werb R. Vitamin A toxicity in hemodialysis patients. Int J Artif Organs 1979;2:178–80.

[340] Ha TK, Sattar N, Talwar D, et al. Abnormal antioxidant vitamin and carotenoid status in chronic renal failure. Qjm 1996;89:765–9.

[341] Ono K, Waki Y, Takeda K, Hypervitaminosis A. a contributing factor to anemia in regular dialysis patients. Nephron 1984;38:44–7.

[342] Yatzidis H, Digenis P, Fountas P. Hypervitaminosis A accompanying advanced chronic renal failure. Br Med J 1975;3:352–3.

[343] Nenov D, Paskalev D, Yankova T, et al. Lipid peroxidation and vitamin E in red blood cells and plasma in hemodialysis patients under rhEPO treatment. Artif Organs 1995;19:436–9.

[344] Hultqvist M, Hegbrant J, Nilsson-Thorell C, et al. Plasma concentrations of vitamin C, vitamin E and/or malondialdehyde as markers of oxygen free radical production during hemodialysis. Clin Nephrol 1997;47:37–46.

[345] De Bevere VO, Nelis HJ, De Leenheer AP, et al. Vitamin E levels in hemodialysis patients. Jama 1982;247:2371.

[346] Roob JM, Khoschsorur G, Tiran A, et al. Vitamin E attenuates oxidative stress induced by intravenous iron in patients on hemodialysis. J Am Soc Nephrol 2000;11:539–49.

[347] Chazot C, Laurent G, Charra B, et al. Malnutrition in long-term haemodialysis survivors. Nephrol Dial Transplant 2001;16:61–9.

[348] Cohen JD, Viljoen M, Clifford D, et al. Plasma vitamin E levels in a chronically hemolyzing group of dialysis patients. Clin Nephrol 1986;25:42–7.

[349] Ahmad S, Robertson HT, Golper TA, et al. Multicenter trial of L-carnitine in maintenance hemodialysis patients. II. Clinical and biochemical effects. Kidney Int 1990;38:912–8.

[350] Lonn E, Yusuf S, Hoogwerf B, et al. Effects of vitamin E on cardiovascular and microvascular outcomes in high-risk patients with diabetes: results of the HOPE study and MICRO-HOPE substudy. Diabetes Care 2002;25:1919–27.

[351] Mann JF, Gerstein HC, Pogue J, et al. Renal insufficiency as a predictor of cardiovascular outcomes and the impact of ramipril: the HOPE randomized trial. Ann Intern Med 2001;134:629–36.

[352] Balcke P, Schmidt P, Zazgornik J, et al. Effect of vitamin B6 administration on elevated plasma oxalic acid levels in haemodialysed patients. Eur J Clin Invest 1982;12:481–3.

[353] Balcke P, Schmidt P, Zazgornik J, et al. Ascorbic acid aggravates secondary hyperoxalemia in patients on chronic hemodialysis. Ann Intern Med 1984;101:344–5.

[354] Zima T, Tesar V, Mestek O, et al. Trace elements in end-stage renal disease. 1. Methodological aspects and the influence of water treatment and dialysis equipment. Blood Purif 1999;17:182–6.

[355] Zima T, Mestek O, Nemecek K, et al. Trace elements in hemodialysis and continuous ambulatory peritoneal dialysis patients. Blood Purif 1998;16:253–60.

[356] Surian M, Bonforte G, Scanziani R, et al. Trace elements and micropollutant anions in the dialysis and reinfusion fluid prepared on-line for haemodiafiltration. Nephrol Dial Transplant 1998;13(Suppl. 5):24–8.

[357] D'Haese PC, De Broe ME. Adequacy of dialysis: trace elements in dialysis fluids. Nephrol Dial Transplant 1996;11(Suppl. 2):92–7.

[358] Hasanoglu E, Altan N, Sindel S, et al. The relationship between erythrocyte superoxide dismutase activity and plasma levels of some trace elements (Al, Cu, Zn) of dialysis patients. Gen Pharmacol 1994;25:107–10.

[359] Jervis RE, Kua BT, Hercz G. Hair trace elements in kidney dialysis patients by INAA. Biol Trace Elem Res 1994;43-45:335–42.

[360] Padovese P, Gallieni M, Brancaccio D, et al. Trace elements in dialysis fluids and assessment of the exposure of patients on regular hemodialysis, hemofiltration and continuous ambulatory peritoneal dialysis. Nephron 1992;61:442–8.

[361] Berlyne GM, Diskin C, Gonick H, et al. Trace elements in dialysis patients. ASAIO Trans 1986;32:662–70.

[362] Thomson NM, Stevens BJ, Humphery TJ, et al. Comparison of trace elements in peritoneal dialysis, hemodialysis, and uremia. Kidney Int 1983;23:9–14.

[363] Sandstead HH. Trace elements in uremia and hemodialysis. Am J Clin Nutr 1980;33:1501–8.

[364] Hosokawa S, Oyamaguchi A, Yoshida O. Trace elements and complications in patients undergoing chronic hemodialysis. Nephron 1990;55:375–9.

[365] Mahler DJ, Walsh JR, Haynie GD. Magnesium, zinc, and copper in dialysis patients. Am J Clin Pathol 1971;56:17–23.

[366] Gallery ED, Blomfield J, Dixon SR. Acute zinc toxicity in hae-modialysis. Br Med J 1972;4:331–3.

[367] Blomfield J, McPherson J, George CR. Active uptake of copper and zinc during haemodialysis. Br Med J 1969;1:141–5.

[368] Van Renterghem D, Cornelis R, Vanholder R. Behaviour of 12 trace elements in serum of uremic patients on hemodiafiltra-tion. J Trace Elem Electrolytes Health Dis 1992;6:169–74.

[369] Blomfield J. Dialysis and lead absorption. Lancet 1973;2:666–7.

[370] Chevalier CA, Liepa G, Murphy MD, et al. The effects of zinc supplementation on serum zinc and cholesterol concentrations in hemodialysis patients. J Ren Nutr 2002;12:183–9.

[371] Jern NA, VanBeber AD, Gorman MA, et al. The effects of zinc supplementation on serum zinc concentration and protein catabolic rate in hemodialysis patients. J Ren Nutr 2000;10:148–53.

[372] Turk S, Bozfakioglu S, Ecder ST, et al. Effects of zinc supple-mentation on the immune system and on antibody response to multivalent influenza vaccine in hemodialysis patients. Int J Artif Organs 1998;21:274–8.

[373] Schabowski J, Ksiazek A, Paprzycki P, et al. Ferrum, copper, zinc and manganese in tissues of patients treated with long-standing hemodialysis programme. Ann Univ Mariae Curie Sklodowska [Med] 1994;49:61–6.

[374] Reid DJ, Barr SI, Leichter J. Effects of folate and zinc supple-mentation on patients undergoing chronic hemodialysis. J Am Diet Assoc 1992;92:574–9.

[375] Mahajan SK, Abraham J, Hessburg T, et al. Zinc metabolism and taste acuity in renal transplant recipients. Kidney Int Suppl 1983;16:S310–4.

[376] Mahajan SK, Bowersox EM, Rye DL, et al. Factors underlying abnormal zinc metabolism in uremia. Kidney Int Suppl 1989;27:S269–73.

[377] Mahajan SK, Prasad AS, Lambujon J, et al. Improvement of uremic hypogeusia by zinc: a double-blind study. Am J Clin Nutr 1980;33:1517–21.

[378] Sprenger KB, Bundschu D, Lewis K, et al. Improvement of uremic neuropathy and hypogeusia by dialysate zinc supple-mentation: a double-blind study. Kidney Int Suppl 1983;16:S315–8.

[379] Rodger RS, Sheldon WL, Watson MJ, et al. Zinc deficiency and hyperprolactinaemia are not reversible causes of sexual dysfunction in uraemia. Nephrol Dial Transplant 1989;4:888–92.

[380] Kiilerich S, Christiansen C, Christensen MS, et al. Zinc metab-olism in patients with chronic renal failure during treatment with 1.25-dihydroxycholecalciferol: a controlled therapeutic trial. Clin Nephrol 1981;15:23–7.

[381] Kalantar-Zadeh K, Hoffken B, Wunsch H, et al. Diagnosis of iron deficiency anemia in renal failure patients during the post-erythropoietin era. Am J Kidney Dis 1995;26:292–9.

[382] Kalantar-Zadeh K, McAllister C, Lehn R, et al. Effect of malnutrition-inflammation complex syndrome on erythropoi-etin hyporesponsiveness in maintenance hemodialysis patients [in review]/[in press?]: 2003.

[383] National Kidney Foundation I, Kidney-Dialysis Outcome Quality Initiative. K/DOQI Clinical Practice Guidelines: Anemia of Chronic Kidney Disease. Am J Kidney Dis 2001;37(Suppl. 1):S182–238.

[384] Kalantar-Zadeh K, Luft FC. Diagnosis of iron deficiency in ESRD patients. Am J Kidney Dis 1997;30:455–6.

[385] Kalantar-Zadeh K, Don BR, Rodriguez RA, et al. Serum ferritin is a marker of morbidity and mortality in hemodialysis patients. Am J Kidney Dis 2001;37:564–72.

[386] Kalantar-Zadeh K, Luft FC, Humphreys MH. Moderately high serum ferritin concentration is not a sign of iron overload in dialysis patients. Kidney Int 1999;56:758–9.

[387] Barany P, Divino Filho JC, Bergstrom J. High C-reactive protein is a strong predictor of resistance to erythropoietin in hemodi-alysis patients. Am J Kidney Dis 1997;29:565–8.

[388] Fishbane S, Maesaka JK. Iron management in end-stage renal disease. Am J Kidney Dis 1997;29:319–33.

[389] Fishbane S, Ungureanu VD, Maesaka JK, et al. The safety of intravenous iron dextran in hemodialysis patients. Am J Kidney Dis 1996;28:529–34.

[390] Coyne DW, Adkinson NF, Nissenson AR, et al. Sodium ferric gluconate complex in hemodialysis patients. II. Adverse reac-tions in iron dextran-sensitive and dextran-tolerant patients. Kidney Int 2003;63:217–24.

[391] Kostakopoulos A, Kotsalos A, Alexopoulos J, et al. Serum selenium levels in healthy adults and its changes in chronic renal failure. Int Urol Nephrol 1990;22:397–401.

[392] Sher L. Role of selenium depletion in the effects of dialysis on mood and behavior. Med Hypotheses 2002;59:89–91.

[393] Dworkin B, Weseley S, Rosenthal WS, et al. Diminished blood selenium levels in renal failure patients on dialysis: correlations with nutritional status. Am J Med Sci 1987;293:6–12.

[394] Hampel G, Schaller KH, Rosenmuller M, et al. Selenium-deficiency as contributing factor to anemia and thrombocyto-penia in dialysis patients. Life Support Syst 1985;3(Suppl. 1):36–40.

[395] Turan B, Delilbasi E, Dalay N, et al. Serum selenium and glutathione-peroxidase activities and their interaction with toxic metals in dialysis and renal transplantation patients. Biol Trace Elem Res 1992;33:95–102.

[396] Bremer J. Carnitine—metabolism and functions. Physiol Rev 1983;63:1420–80.

[397] Vacha GM, Corsi M, Giorcelli G, et al. Serum and muscle L-carnitine levels in hemodialyzed patients, during and after long-term L-carnitine treatment. Curr Ther Res 1985;37:505.

[398] Wanner C, Forstner-Wanner S, Schaeffer G, et al. Serum free carnitine, carnitine esters and lipids in patients on peritoneal dialysis and hemodialysis. Am J Nephrol 1986;6:206–11.

[399] Bellinghieri G, Santoro D, Calvani M, et al. Carnitine and hemodialysis. Am J Kidney Dis 2003;41:S116–22.

[400] Chazot C, Blanc C, Hurot JM, et al. Nutritional effects of carnitine supplementation in hemodialysis patients. Clin Nephrol 2003;59:24–30.

[401] Golper TA, Ahmad S. L-carnitine administration to hemodial-ysis patients: Has its time come? Seminars in Dialysis 1992;5:94–8.

[402] Labonia WD. L-carnitine effects on anemia in hemodialyzed patients treated with erythropoietin. Am J Kidney Dis 1995;26:757–64.

[403] Hurot JM, Cucherat M, Haugh M, et al. Effects of L-carnitine supplementation in maintenance hemodialysis patients: a systematic review. J Am Soc Nephrol 2002;13:708–14.

[404] Guarnieri G, Toigo G, Crapesi L, et al. Carnitine metabolism in chronic renal failure. Kidney Int Suppl 1987;22:S116–27.

[405] Guarnieri GF, Ranieri F, Toigo G, et al. Lipid-lowering effect of carnitine in chronically uremic patients treated with mainte-nance hemodialysis. Am J Clin Nutr 1980;33:1489–92.

[406] Lacour B, Di Giulio S, Chanard J, et al. Carnitine improves lipid anomalies in haemodialysis patients. Lancet 1980;2:763–4.

[407] Bellinghieri G, Savica V, Mallamace A, et al. Correlation between increased serum and tissue L-carnitine levels and improved muscle symptoms in hemodialyzed patients. Am J Clin Nutr 1983;38:523–31.

[408] Brass EP, Adler S, Sietsema KE, et al. Intravenous L-carnitine increases plasma carnitine, reduces fatigue, and may preserve exercise capacity in hemodialysis patients. Am J Kidney Dis 2001;37:1018–28.

[409] Weschler A, Aviram M, Levin M, et al. High dose of L-carnitine increases platelet aggregation and plasma triglyceride levels in uremic patients on hemodialysis. Nephron 1984;38:120−4.

[410] Eknoyan G, Latos DL, Lindberg J. Practice recommendations for the use of L-Carnitine in dialysis-related carnitine disorder National Kidney Foundation Carnitine Consensus Conference. Am J Kidney Dis 2003;41:868−76.

[411] Ahmad S. L-carnitine in dialysis patients. Semin Dial 2001;14:209−17.

[412] Kuhlmann MK, Schmidt F, Kohler H. High protein/energy vs. standard protein/energy nutritional regimen in the treatment of malnourished hemodialysis patients. Miner Electrolyte Metab 1999;25:306−10.

[413] Leon JB, Majerle AD, Soinski JA, et al. Can a nutrition intervention improve albumin levels among hemodialysis patients? A pilot study. J Ren Nutr 2001;11:9−15.

[414] Boccanfuso JA, Hutton M, McAllister B. The effects of megestrol acetate on nutritional parameters in a dialysis population. J Ren Nutr 2000;10:36−43.

[415] Kopple JD. Therapeutic approaches to malnutrition in chronic dialysis patients: the different modalities of nutritional support. Am J Kidney Dis 1999;33:180−5.

[416] Timpone JG, Wright DJ, Li N, et al. The safety and pharmacokinetics of single-agent and combination therapy with megestrol acetate and dronabinol for the treatment of HIV wasting syndrome. The DATRI 004 Study Group. Division of AIDS Treatment Research Initiative. AIDS Res Hum Retroviruses 1997;13:305−15.

[417] Strang P. The effect of megestrol acetate on anorexia, weight loss and cachexia in cancer and AIDS patients (review). Anticancer Res 1997;17:657−62.

[418] Engelson ES, FX PI-S, Kotler DP. Effects of megestrol acetate and testosterone on body composition in castrated male Sprague-Dawley rats. Nutrition 1999;15:465−73.

[419] Chazot C, Shahmir E, Matias B, et al. Dialytic nutrition: provision of amino acids in dialysate during hemodialysis. Kidney Int 1997;52:1663−70.

[420] Fouque D, Peng SC, Kopple JD. Impaired metabolic response to recombinant insulin-like growth factor-1 in dialysis patients. Kidney Int 1995;47:876−83.

[421] Fouque D, Peng SC, Shamir E, et al. Recombinant human insulin-like growth factor-1 induces an anabolic response in malnourished CAPD patients. Kidney Int 2000;57:646−54.

[422] Fouque D, Peng SC, Kopple JD. Impaired metabolic response to recombinant insulin-like growth factor-1 in dialysis patients. Kidney Int 1995;47:876−83.

[423] Fouque D, Peng SC, Kopple JD. Pharmacokinetics of recombinant human insulin-like growth factor-1 in dialysis patients. Kidney Int 1995;47:869−75.

[424] Fouque D, Tayek JA, Kopple JD. Altered mental function during intravenous infusion of recombinant human insulin-like growth factor 1. JPEN J Parenter Enteral Nutr 1995;19:231−3.

[425] Kopple JD, Ding H, Qing DP. Physiology and potential use of insulin-like growth factor 1 in acute and chronic renal failure. Nephrol Dial Transplant 1998;13:34−9.

[426] Fine RN, Stablein D, Cohen AH, et al. Recombinant human growth hormone post-renal transplantation in children: a randomized controlled study of the NAPRTCS. Kidney Int 2002;62:688−96.

[427] Fine RN, Sullivan EK, Tejani A. The impact of recombinant human growth hormone treatment on final adult height. Pediatr Nephrol 2000;14:679−81.

[428] Fine RN, Sullivan EK, Kuntze J, et al. The impact of recombinant human growth hormone treatment during chronic renal insufficiency on renal transplant recipients. J Pediatr 2000;136:376−82.

[429] Ben-Atia I, Fine M, Tandler A, et al. Preparation of recombinant gilthead seabream (Sparus aurata) growth hormone and its use for stimulation of larvae growth by oral administration. Gen Comp Endocrinol 1999;113:155−64.

[430] Fine RN. Growth hormone treatment of children with chronic renal insufficiency, end-stage renal disease and following renal transplantation—update 1997. J Pediatr Endocrinol Metab 1997;10:361−70.

[431] Ziegler TR, Lazarus JM, Young LS, et al. Effects of recombinant human growth hormone in adults receiving maintenance hemodialysis. J Am Soc Nephrol 1991;2:1130−5.

[432] Schulman G, Wingard RL, Hutchison RL, et al. The effects of recombinant human growth hormone and intradialytic parenteral nutrition in malnourished hemodialysis patients. American Journal of Kidney Diseases 1993;21:527−34.

[433] Kopple JD. The rationale for the use of growth hormone or insulin-like growth factor I in adult patients with renal failure. Miner Electrolyte Metab 1992;18:269−75.

[434] Saadeh E, Ikizler TA, Shyr Y, et al. Recombinant human growth hormone in patients with acute renal failure. J Ren Nutr 2001;11:212−9.

[435] Van den Berghe G. Endocrinology in intensive care medicine: new insights and therapeutic consequences. Verh K Acad Geneeskd Belg 2002;64:167−87. discussion 187−168.

[436] McPhatter LL, Lockridge Jr RS. Nutritional advantages of nightly home hemodialysis. Nephrol News Issues 2002;16(31):34−6.

[437] McPhatter LL, Lockridge Jr RS, Albert J, et al. Nightly home hemodialysis: improvement in nutrition and quality of life. Adv Ren Replace Ther 1999;6:358−65.

[438] Pierratos A. Daily hemodialysis: why the renewed interest? Am J Kidney Dis 1998;32:S76−82.

[439] Pierratos A. Nocturnal home haemodialysis: an update on a 5-year experience. Nephrol Dial Transplant 1999;14:2835−40.

[440] Pierratos A. Daily hemodialysis. Curr Opin Nephrol Hypertens 2000;9:637−42.

[441] Lindsay RM, Kortas C. Hemeral (daily) hemodialysis. Adv Ren Replace Ther 2001;8:236−49.

[442] Lacson Jr E, Diaz-Buxo JA. Daily and nocturnal hemodialysis: how do they stack up? Am J Kidney Dis 2001;38:225−39.

[443] Schulman G. Nutrition in daily hemodialysis. Am J Kidney Dis 2003;41:S112−5.

[444] Goffin E, Pirard Y, Francart J, et al. Daily hemodialysis and nutritional status. Kidney Int 2002;61:1909−10.

[445] Galland R, Traeger J, Arkouche W, et al. Short daily hemodialysis rapidly improves nutritional status in hemodialysis patients. Kidney Int 2001;60:1555−60.

[446] Galland R, Traeger J, Arkouche W, et al. Short daily hemodialysis and nutritional status. Am J Kidney Dis 2001;37:S95−8.

[447] Mohr PE, Neumann PJ, Franco SJ, et al. The quality of life and economic implications of daily dialysis. Policy Anal Brief H Ser 1999;1:1−4.

33

Nutritional Management of End-Stage Renal Disease Patients Treated with Peritoneal Dialysis

Sirin Jiwakanon[1], Rajnish Mehrotra[2]

[1]Hatyai Hospital, Hatyai, Songkhla, Thailand [2]Division of Nephrology, Harborview Medical Center, University of Washington, Seattle, WA, USA

INTRODUCTION

Peritoneal dialysis (PD) has been used for the long-term treatment of uremia since the 1960s [1]. The use of this therapy has expanded substantially since the introduction of the concept of "continuous ambulatory PD" (CAPD) by Popovich and Moncrief in 1976 [2]. As of 2008, nearly 11% of an estimated 1.77 million patients undergoing maintenance dialysis worldwide were being treated with PD [3]. Since the first introduction of ambulatory PD, the frequency of treatment-associated complications has substantially diminished, and there has been a significant reduction in patient morbidity and mortality. Over the last decade, improvements in outcomes of patients treated with PD have outpaced those of maintenance hemodialysis patients [4]. Thus, in contemporary cohorts from different parts of the world, the four-, five- and ten-year survival of maintenance hemodialysis and PD patients is remarkably similar [4]. The equivalency of patient survival with maintenance hemodialysis and the lower societal costs with the use of PD in many parts of the world are likely to result in an increasingly larger number of patients utilizing this therapy in the coming years [5]. In this chapter, we present a brief overview of PD followed by a detailed discussion of the effects of the therapy on protein and energy status, lipid metabolism, and body composition, dietary recommendations for PD patients, and protein-energy wasting (PEW) in patients treated with PD.

TYPE OF PERITONEAL DIALYSIS

PD utilizes the peritoneum as a naturally-occurring dialyzer for the removal of solutes and water. In order to accomplish this, dialysate solution is periodically instilled into and drained from the peritoneal cavity through an indwelling PD catheter. Each instillation and drainage is called an "exchange" and can be performed either manually, as in CAPD, or with the assistance of a cycler (automated PD, APD). The therapy is almost invariably performed at home by a patient or a care-giver after a period of training by dialysis unit staff. Furthermore, PD can be either intermittent or continuous, as described below.

Continuous Therapies

With continuous therapies, dialysate is in continuous contact with the peritoneal membrane 24-hours a day, seven days a week. The overwhelming majority of PD patients are treated with some form of continuous therapy.

CONTINUOUS AMBULATORY PERITONEAL DIALYSIS (CAPD) Patients perform three to five exchanges manually every day. The volume of instilled fluid generally varies between 1.5 and 3.0 L, in increments of 500 mL, and the dwell time for each individual exchange varies from 4—10 hours. In developing countries, CAPD is the most common form of PD used by patients.

CONTINUOUS CYCLING PERITONEAL DIALYSIS (CCPD) PD is performed with the assistance of a cycler at night, and the patient has intra-peritoneal dialysate ("wet" abdomen) during the day time. The optimal number of night-time exchanges is often between three and five over a nine-hour period. In a CCPD patient, the day dwell is generally 15-hours long unless it is interrupted by a manual exchange. In many developed countries, CCPD is the most common form of PD used by patients.

TIDAL PERITONEAL DIALYSIS (TPD) PD is performed with the use of a cycler which is programmed such that rather than emptying the abdomen completely at the end of each exchange, a small intra-peritoneal reservoir of dialysate is left at all times. It was initially introduced as a way to increase solute clearances. However, this advantage has not been corroborated in recent clinical trials, and its use is currently limited to patients with infusion pain [6,7].

Intermittent Therapies

Generally, this technique is appropriate only for those patients who have significant residual renal function and can be used to prescribe peritoneal dialysis incrementally — the delivered dose of dialysis is increased as patient's residual renal function declines [8].

INTERMITTENT PERITONEAL DIALYSIS (IPD) In its classic form, PD is not performed every day but only every 2—4 days. During the treatment periods, exchanges are performed at hourly intervals over 10—36 hours at a time, either manually or as APD, either in a health care center or at home. IPD is not appropriate for long-term treatment of uremia and should be reserved only for exceptional circumstances [9,10].

NIGHTLY INTERMITTENT PERITONEAL DIALYSIS (NIPD) PD is performed every night generally with the assistance of a cycler. During the day time, patient's abdomen is "dry". This is the preferred form of intermittent PD when the therapy is being prescribed intermittently in patients with significant residual renal function.

DAYTIME AMBULATORY PERITONEAL DIALYSIS (DAPD) PD is performed either manually or with the assistance of a cycler during the daytime with the abdomen "dry" at night.

PERITONEAL DIALYSIS SOLUTIONS

The composition of the dialysate used for peritoneal dialysis is based upon the need to remove uremic solutes via diffusion from the blood across their concentration gradient, correct metabolic acidosis, ensure adequate ultrafiltration to substitute for loss of urine volume,

and optimize the serum electrolyte concentrations. The peritoneal dialysate, thus, is a solution of selected electrolytes (sodium, calcium, and magnesium) along with a buffer to correct metabolic acidosis (lactate or bicarbonate), and an osmotic or oncotic agent to generate ultrafiltration (dextrose, icodextrin, or amino acids).

CONVENTIONAL GLUCOSE-BASED SOLUTIONS These solutions use lactate as a buffer and dextrose as an osmotic agent. The composition of this solution is listed in Table 33.1. This solution has been used successfully for PD for over three decades. However, the high glucose concentrations, the presence of glucose degradation products generated during heat sterilization, the use of lactate as buffer, and the low pH makes the solution unphysiologic. Glucose, while very effective in generating ultrafiltration during short-exchanges, is not an appropriate osmotic agent for long dwell times (viz, 8—12 hours overnight dwells for CAPD or 14—16 hours day-dwells for CCPD). Studies have raised concern that formulation of conventional PD solutions induces changes in the peritoneal membrane that limit our ability to use it as a dialysis membrane over the long-term in some patients [11]. Furthermore, systemic glucose absorption makes attaining glycemic control more challenging in diabetics and leads to hyperinsulinemia and fat accumulation even in nondiabetics [12,13]. All these reasons have prompted the development of a variety of newer dialysis solutions.

ICODEXTRIN The electrolyte composition, buffer, and pH of this solution are identical to that of the conventional glucose-based solutions. However, instead of glucose, the solution contains icodextrin that generates ultrafiltration by inducing oncotic pressure across

TABLE 33.1 Composition of Conventional Dextrose Based Peritoneal Dialysis Solution

Component	Concentration
pH	5.2
Osmolality (mOsm/kg)	346, 396, or 485
ELECTROLYTES (mEq/L)	
Sodium	132
Potassium	0
Calcium	2.5 or 3.5
Chloride	96—101
Magnesium	0.75
Lactate	35 or 40
OSMOTIC AGENT	
Dextrose (%)	1.5, 2.5, or 4.25
Glucose, mg/dL	1360, 2250, or 3860

the peritoneal membrane. Icodextrin is a glucose polymer produced by the hydrolysis of corn-starch and has an average molecular weight of 16,800 daltons. Unlike glucose, icodextrin is absorbed slowly from the peritoneal cavity via the lymphatics and hence, is best suited to generate ultrafiltration during long dwells. Randomized, controlled trials have demonstrated a reduction in total body water and regression of left-ventricular hypertrophy with the use of icodextrin in lieu of glucose for the long-dwells [14–16]. There is increasing interest in using it as a part of glucose-sparing strategies for both diabetics and nondiabetics [17]. Furthermore, several clinical trials have shown small but significant reductions in total and low-density-lipoprotein cholesterol with icodextrin [14,17,18]. Finally, one observational study has shown a lower risk for death in icodextrin-treated patients [19]. This solution is used for 30–50% of all PD patients in Europe and Japan, but cost considerations has limited the use of this solution to no more than 10% of all patients in the United States. The use is even lower in developing countries.

AMINO ACID SOLUTIONS The electrolyte composition, and buffer of this solution are identical to that of the conventional glucose-based solutions, but it uses a 1.1% mixture of amino acids as an osmotic agent in lieu of glucose. These solutions were introduced as a nutritional supplement for PD patients with protein-energy wasting [20]. However, the clinical trials have produced disappointing results, and these solutions are increasingly being used as part of glucose-sparing regimens [21–23]. This solution is commercially available in Europe and Canada but has not been approved by the Food and Drug Administration for use in the United States.

LOW GLUCOSE DEGRADATION PRODUCT GLUCOSE-BASED SOLUTION This solution has the same electrolyte composition as conventional PD solutions and uses glucose as an osmotic agent. Depending on the manufacturer, the solution contains lactate, bicarbonate, or a combination of lactate and bicarbonate as a buffer. In order to minimize the generation of glucose-degradation products, the solution bag has at least two compartments – one of the compartments contains glucose at very high concentrations at a very low pH, and the second compartment contains the buffer. This arrangement allows the dialysate solution to be sterilized and stored with a minimal degree of chemical degradation of the glucose. The patient breaks the seal between the two compartments prior to instillation of the solution into the peritoneal cavity. This allows for a neutral pH for the solution. Even though such solutions are more biocompatible both *in vitro* and *in vivo*, no consistent clinical benefit has been demonstrated in clinical trials [24–28].

SPECIFIC EFFECTS OF PERITONEAL DIALYSIS ON NUTRITIONAL STATUS AND METABOLISM

The peritoneal dialysis procedure and its complications modify the effect of uremia on nutritional status, metabolism, and body composition. Knowledge of these factors is central to the nutritional management of patients treated with peritoneal dialysis.

NUTRIENT ABSORPTION AND WEIGHT GAIN As discussed above, PD solutions contain one of three different substances to induce ultrafiltration – glucose, icodextrin, or amino acids. Each of them is absorbed during the course of a dwell and contributes to the total nutrient intake of a patient treated with the therapy. The amount of glucose that is absorbed during the course of the day has been reported to vary between 10–180 g/d; the actual amount depends upon the peritoneal dialysis prescription (tonicity and volume of dialysate, duration of dwell) and the peritoneal transport rate for the individual [29]. Thus, the glucose absorption is higher with larger intra-peritoneal dwell volumes, longer dwell times, and in individuals with a fast (or high) peritoneal transport rate. Even though the data are not consistent, it appears that in most patients the glucose absorption in and of itself does not suppress dietary intakes [30]. For an average patient undergoing PD, this glucose absorption can contribute up to 20–30% of total daily energy intake [29–31]. Indeed, the reported total energy intakes of PD patients are significantly higher than those reported for patients treated with maintenance hemodialysis. The higher energy intake has a protein-sparing effect in that it allows individuals to achieve neutral nitrogen balance in the face of lower protein intakes [32]. Icodextrin, a large molecular weight substance, is absorbed more slowly primarily via the diaphragmatic lymphatics; up to one-third of icodextrin is absorbed during a 12-hour dwell [33,34]. It is metabolized by serum amylase into oligosaccahrides, mainly maltose which, in turn, is metabolized to glucose by maltase present in the lysosomes of most cells [33]. Thus, use of icodextrin provides an amount of energy equivalent to that from a 2.5% dextrose solution [35]. Finally, during the course of an exchange with an amino-acid PD solution, the amount of nitrogen gained from the absorption of amino acids exceeds the nitrogen losses (viz., with losses of albumin and peptides – see below) [36]. Thus, irrespective of the solution that is used, there is net absorption of nutrients. This, in turn, needs to be considered when assessing patients treated with PD.

NUTRIENT ABSORPTION WITH PD EXERTS SYSTEMIC EFFECTS Glucose absorption is associated with hyperinsulinemia and may lead to weight gain [37]. Studies suggest that the increase in weight is primarily driven by an increase in fat mass and is more likely to occur in individuals with polymorphism of the uncoupling protein-2 gene which can alter the metabolic rate [38,39]. Alterations in body composition may be less likely for patients treated with icodextrin. Patients using icodextrin for a single long-dwell are less likely to have significant increases in total fat mass, visceral fat area, total weight gain, and waist/hip ratio than those treated exclusively with glucose-based dialysate [38]. This is probably due to the lower absolute rate of peritoneal absorption of icodextrin. Notwithstanding the potential importance of glucose absorption, in a study of a large cohort of patients new to dialysis, significant weight gain was more likely to occur in patients treated with maintenance hemodialysis rather than those with peritoneal dialysis [40]. This suggests that while glucose absorption is a potentially important cause of weight gain in PD patients, amelioration of uremic anorexia may be a more important cause of significant weight gain in patients starting dialysis therapy.

PERITONEAL DIALYSIS AND LIPID METABOLISM

Patients treated with PD have higher serum total cholesterol, low-density lipoprotein cholesterol, triglycerides, apolipoprotein, leptin, and resistin than those treated with maintenance hemodialysis [41]. Although the pathophysiological mechanisms underlying these changes are not clear, it has been suggested that hyperinsulinemia induced by glucose absorption may enhance the hepatic synthesis and secretion of very-low-density-lipoprotein. Moreover, peritoneal protein losses (see below) stimulate the hepatic synthesis of albumin and other liver-derived proteins, including cholesterol-enriched lipoproteins [42−45]. The high prevalence of dyslipidemia in patients treated with PD makes routine monitoring of lipid levels imperative. Treatment with statins (HMG CoA reductase inhibitors) has been shown to be as effective in lowering serum cholesterol levels in patients treated with PD as is seen in the general population [41]. Use of icodextrin for one dwell in the day is associated with a 5% reduction in total cholesterol and may be considered in patients who are only partially responsive to or intolerant of statins [14,17,18].

GASTRIC EMPTYING

Diabetic and nondiabetic patients with chronic kidney disease, including those undergoing maintenance dialysis, have significant prolongation of gastric emptying times [46−49]. Studies suggest that intraperitoneal instillation of dialysate leads to further prolongation of gastric emptying time [50−52]. In patients treated with PD, gastric emptying time is inversely related to anthropometric nutritional markers such as fat-free, edema-free mass and body mass index [53]. Many patients with significantly prolonged gastric emptying times are asymptomatic, except possibly for unrecognized anorexia, and small clinical trials show significant increases in serum albumin in hypoalbuminemic individuals treated with prokinetic agents [54,55]. Thus, a high index of suspicion for delayed gastric emptying is necessary, and in selected patients treated with PD with protein-energy wasting, empiric treatment with prokinetic agents may prove beneficial.

NUTRIENT LOSSES

During each PD exchange, plasma proteins move into the peritoneal cavity along a concentration gradient and are lost from the body when the fluid is drained. This daily peritoneal protein loss varies considerably from patient to patient, and has been estimated to range from 2.0 to 15.0 g/d, with an average of 6.0−8.0 g/d [56−58]. The magnitude of peritoneal losses is similar for patients treated with CAPD or NIPD but may be higher with CCPD [59−61]. The losses have been reported to be higher within the first few weeks of initiation of PD, with the use of hypertonic dialysate, and during episodes of peritonitis [56]. In patients treated with CCPD, the long daytime dwells contribute disproportionately more per unit drain volume to the daily protein losses than the short night-time exchanges; the protein losses at night are directly related to the number of night-time exchanges [59]. The vast majority of protein lost with the peritoneal dialysis procedure is albumin [58]. The other proteins present in significant concentrations in peritoneal dialysate are IgG, IgA, α2-macroglobulin, and β2-microglobulin [62,63]. The clearance of individual proteins decreases with increasing molecular weight [64]. In addition to proteins, about 2.0−4.0 g/d of amino acids are lost daily as well; almost one-third of the total losses are essential amino acids like the branched chain amino acids, valine, leucine and isoleucine [59,65].

In most patients, the clinical import of peritoneal protein losses is not very large. Undoubtedly, protein losses account for about 15% of total nitrogen appearance in the dialysate and account for up to one-third of the increase in dietary protein requirements in patients treated with PD [59,65]. Furthermore, the prevalence of hypoalbuminemia is significantly higher in patients treated with PD than similar patients treated with hemodialysis; this is thought to be primarily as a result of peritoneal protein losses [66]. However, this lower serum albumin does not appear to disadvantage PD patients as for every range of serum albumin, the risk for death is lower in PD patients. Put differently, the level of serum albumin that confers the same level of risk is lower by 0.2−0.3 g/dL in patients treated with PD than those treated with hemodialysis [67]. Finally, several recent studies have demonstrated an association between peritoneal clearance or total peritoneal protein loss and all-cause mortality [61,68]. The basis for this association is unclear but it is unlikely that the higher risk for death is a direct result of peritoneal protein losses. Instead, it is more likely that peritoneal protein clearances serve as a marker of systemic vascular disease. Although it is not certain, it is unlikely that the risk for death can be lowered by adjusting the PD prescription to decrease peritoneal protein losses.

In addition to proteins and amino acids, a large number of other nutrients are lost during peritoneal dialysis; for example, water-soluble vitamins and minerals. Among water-soluble vitamins, daily losses of vitamin C and folic acid can be high, followed by that of vitamins B_2 and B_6 [69]. There is only a small amount of vitamin B_1 lost with PD, and there is virtually no detectable vitamin B_{12} in the dialysate effluent, probably because plasma vitamin B_{12} is largely bound to protein. There is very little, if any, loss of fat-soluble vitamins, like vitamins A, E and K or carotenoids [70,71]. Conversely, PD patients lose vitamin D-binding protein in the dialysate effluent, and the serum levels of 25-hydroxy vitamin D are significantly reduced [72–74]. The blood selenium level is often reduced in patients treated with PD; lower serum concentrations of selenium binding proteins or reduced selenium binding to carrier proteins may play a role. Whether this reduction is also secondary to peritoneal selenium losses is not settled [75–78]. There are no significant losses of such other minerals as zinc, copper, aluminum, iron, or magnesium [75–77,79,80].

EFFECTS OF PERITONEAL SOLUTE TRANSPORT RATE

The rate of transfer of solutes across the peritoneal membrane depends upon the "effective" peritoneal surface area. This is determined largely by the density of peritoneal capillaries. In patients new to PD, the "effective" peritoneal surface is an intrinsic characteristic of an individual and is elucidated using a standardized test, the peritoneal equilibration test [81]. From this test, the ratio of the concentration of creatinine in the dialysate after four hours of dwell to its serum concentration is used to calculate 4-hour dialysate/plasma creatinine concentration. This, in turn, is used to categorize patients into high, high-average, low-average, or low transporters (or fast, fast-average, slow-average, or slow). Earlier studies demonstrated an inverse relationship between peritoneal transport rate and serum albumin levels in CAPD patients [63,82,83]. Furthermore, a large number of studies have shown a direct relationship between peritoneal transport rate and both mortality and need to transfer to hemodialysis in CAPD patients [84]. The higher death risk in the setting of a higher prevalence of hypoalbuminemia was interpreted as a higher prevalence of protein-energy

wasting — attributable, in part, to peritoneal protein losses — in high transporters. This claim was bolstered by some studies showing higher serum levels of acute-phase proteins like C-reactive protein and cytokines like interleukin-6 [85–87]. However, recent evidence does not support the association between peritoneal transport rate and protein-energy wasting in PD patients [88–90]. It is now believed that both the low serum albumin and higher risk for death are secondary to volume overload arising out of use of inappropriately long dwell times as is the case with CAPD in high transporters [90,91]. In general, faster transporters need shorter dwell times because of the more rapid absorption of the osmotic agents in dialysate (e.g., glucose); with long dwell times, they therefore may begin to reabsorb water from the abdominal cavity. Indeed, in patients treated using prescriptions appropriate for their dwell time (APD for high-transporters), there is no demonstrable relationship between peritoneal transport rate and mortality [84]. Moreover, there is no consistent evidence for a higher prevalence of inflammatory markers or other measures of protein-energy wasting with increasing peritoneal transport rate [89,92]. Thus, while peritoneal transport rate is important to consider when selecting an appropriate dialysis prescription, it does not appear to be an important determinant of protein and energy nutritional status of PD patients.

EFFECT OF PERITONITIS

Peritonitis is the single-most important complication of the peritoneal dialysis procedure. Most of the infections are either intra-luminal (secondary to touch contamination when performing the PD exchange) or peri-luminal (colonization and/or infection of the skin where the catheter enters the abdominal wall) [93]. Over the last three decades, advances in connection devices and widespread use of local skin application of antibiotics have substantially decreased the risk of peritonitis [94–96]. Nevertheless, it remains the most common cause for patients to transfer to hemodialysis [93,97,98]. Episodes of peritonitis are associated with peritoneal inflammation and hence, lead to a transient increase in "effective peritoneal surface area" from an increase in vascular permeability [99]. This, in turn, leads to greater protein clearance, and during episodes of peritonitis, substantial amounts of protein can be lost daily (10–25 g/d) [100]. The effect of these enhanced protein losses is compounded by decreased nutrient intake by acutely ill individuals. Thus, episodes of peritonitis are associated with transient decreases in serum albumin, prealbumin (transthyretin), 25-hydroxy vitamin D, and ionized calcium [101,102]. The long-term effects of single or recurrent episodes of peritonitis however, are less clear [102,103]. Several studies have identified protein-energy wasting and/or hypoalbuminemia as a risk factor for peritonitis [104–106]. Conversely, at least one single center study has demonstrated that in some patients, blood levels of acute phase proteins, like C-reactive protein, remain elevated for up to six weeks after resolution of intraperitoneal inflammation [102]. Individuals with persistent systemic inflammation despite apparent clinical resolution of intraperitoneal inflammation have a significantly higher risk for death [102]. Whether such patients have a higher risk for either developing or worsening protein-energy wasting, however, is not known.

IMPORTANCE OF RESIDUAL RENAL FUNCTION Residual renal function is an important contributor to total solute clearance and fluid removal and is inversely associated with death risk of PD patients [107]. A similar inverse association of residual renal function with death risk has been shown for maintenance hemodialysis patients [108]. Thus, residual renal function is important in maintaining overall health of dialysis patients. Consistent with this thesis, several cross-sectional studies have demonstrated higher prevalence and greater severity of protein-energy wasting with decline in residual renal function (lower serum albumin and dietary protein intake, worse subjective global assessment, and higher systemic levels of acute phase proteins) [109–112]. Furthermore, there is a direct relationship between residual renal clearances and energy and protein intakes as well as intake of water-soluble vitamins like thiamine, riboflavin, vitamin B_6, and B_{12}, folic acid, and vitamin C [113].

Given the importance of residual renal function, all attempts should be made to preserve it for as long as possible. Several observational studies have demonstrated that patients treated with PD maintain residual renal function for longer periods of time than those treated with hemodialysis [114–117]. Among patients treated with PD, those with diabetes or cardiovascular comorbidity have a significantly faster decline in residual renal function and thus, are higher-risk for worsening of protein-energy wasting [118–120]. Angiotensin-converting enzyme inhibitors and angiotensin receptor blockers are effective in slowing the rate of decline of renal function even at the extremely low renal clearances seen in patients undergoing dialysis and there is little, if any, risk for hyperkalemia with these drugs in patients treated with PD [121–123]. In the absence of contraindications for use, these drugs should be used for all patients undergoing PD with significant residual renal function. As discussed above, there is no consistent evidence for the benefit of low-glucose degradation product dialysates, when using glucose-based dialysis solutions, on the rate of decline of residual renal function [24–26,28,124].

DIETARY RECOMMENDATIONS FOR ESRD PATIENTS UNDERGOING PERITONEAL DIALYSIS

The dietary recommendations for some key nutrients for patients treated with peritoneal dialysis are summarized in Table 33.2.

ENERGY The energy intake of PD patients represents the sum of intakes from the diet and from dialysate glucose absorption. There are no clinical trials that have evaluated any relevant clinical outcomes of patients randomized to different levels of dietary energy intakes. Thus, the recommendations for energy intake are based upon carefully conducted metabolic studies of patients treated with CAPD; there are scant data for patients treated with APD [32,125,126]. The resting energy expenditure of CAPD patients appears to be similar to that of otherwise healthy adults [127]. Moreover, there is a direct correlation between total energy intake and nitrogen balance in CAPD patients [32,128]. Based upon these data, several expert groups recommend that the total energy intake of PD patients should be the same as that recommended for individuals without kidney disease (individuals <60 years, 35 kcal/kg/day; age >60 years, 30–35 kcal/kg/day) [129]. As discussed earlier, the amount of energy obtained from absorption of nutrients from the dialysate depends upon the peritoneal transport rate and the PD prescription, including the tonicity of dextrose and use of non-glucose based solutions. Daily energy intake from dialysate averages 300–400 kcal and can be estimated from kinetic modeling software. This needs to be accounted for when estimating the dietary energy intakes for individual patients.

PROTEIN Like for energy intake, the recommendation for dietary protein intakes for PD patients is based upon carefully conducted metabolic balance studies. Each of the three metabolic studies concluded that CAPD patients can maintain neutral or positive nitrogen balance at dietary protein intakes of 1.2–1.3 g/kg/d (Table 33.3) [32,125,126]. It is important to note that there are no such studies done for patients treated with APD; recommendations for these patients have been extrapolated from studies done in CAPD patients.

SODIUM AND WATER In early years of PD therapy, it was believed that the continuous nature of therapy would allow for a more liberal intake of salt and water than is generally possible for patients treated with an intermittent therapy like hemodialysis. Studies over the last decade have demonstrated that this is possible perhaps only for as long as patients maintain significant residual renal function. As indicated above,

TABLE 33.2 Recommended Nutrient Intake and Supplementation Requirements for Patients Treated with Peritoneal Dialysis

	Recommendation*	Supplementation Required
Total energy intake	35 kcal/kg/day 30—35 kcal/kg/day for age >60 years	
Total protein intake	1.2—1.3 g/kg/day	
WATER-SOLUBLE VITAMINS		
Vitamin C	60 mg/day	No
Folate	180—200 µg/day	Yes [70, 277]
Thiamin	1.0—1.5 mg/day	Yes
Riboflavin	1.2—1.7 mg/day	Yes
Niacin	15-20 mg NE/day	Yes
Vitamin B_6	5 mg/day	Yes [70,113,278, 279]
Vitamin B_{12}	2 µg/day	No (280)
FAT-SOLUBLE VITAMINS		
Vitamin A	800—1000 µg RE/day	No [155,280]
Vitamin D	5 µg/day	Sometimes to treat secondary hyperparathyroidism
Vitamin E	8—10 mg α-TE/day	No [155,280]
Vitamin K	65—80 µg/day	Data are not sufficient to recommend routine use.
TRACE ELEMENTS AND MACROMINERALS		
Calcium	800 mg/day	No
Phosphorous	800 mg/day	No
Iron	10—15 mg/day	Sometimes to maximize erythropoietin responsiveness [113,281]
Selenium	55—70 µg/day	Sometimes if patient deficient [158]
Zinc	12—15 mg/day	Sometimes if patient deficient [79,113,282]

* The recommendation for protein and energy intakes are based on recommendations by the Kidney Disease Outcome Quality Initiative (KDOQI), and for vitamins, trace elements and mineral based on recommended dietary allowances (RDA) for adult age $\geq$ 25 years [129,283]. See also Chapters 19, 23 and 24.
Note: NE; niacin equivalents, RE; retinol equivalents, TE; tocopherol equivalents.

observational studies indicate that PD patients maintain residual renal function for a significantly longer period of time than those treated with hemodialysis [117,130]. However, a significant proportion of patients treated with long-term PD develop volume expansion [131]. Furthermore, in a double-blind crossover study, administration of a supplement of 60 mEq/d of sodium as chloride was associated with significant increases in

TABLE 33.3 Summary of Metabolic Balance Studies Done in Patients Treated with Peritoneal Dialysis to Determine Protein Requirements*

Author	Participant No.	Study Duration (days)	Protein Intake (g/kg/day)	Total Energy Intake (kcal/kg/day)	Nitrogen Balance (g/day)
Giordano, 1980 [126]	8	14	1.2	39.6—44.9	0/+ in 7
Blumenkrantz, 1982 [125]	8	14—33	0.98 ± 0.03 1.44 ± 0.02	41.3 ± 1.9 42.1 ± 1.2	+0.35 ± 0.83 +2.94 ± 0.54
Bergstrom, 1993 [32]	12 9	6—11	0.76—2.09 0.64—1.69	28—50 25—51	+Correlation with DPI No correlation with DPI

* Adapted from Mehrotra and Kopple, 2001 [284].
Note: DPI, dietary protein intake

blood pressure underscoring the importance of salt and water restriction in PD patients [132]. Paradoxically, there is at least one study that has demonstrated an inverse relationship between dietary sodium intake and mortality of PD patients [133]. This paradoxical finding is most likely a result of the confounding influence of protein-energy wasting as patients with the highest sodium intake had higher intakes of other nutrients and had higher serum albumin, prealbumin, and fat-free edema-free mass [133]. Thus, notwithstanding this paradoxical observation, it is critical to counsel patients that PD treatment requires salt and water restriction as much as it does for those treated with maintenance hemodialysis [134,135].

POTASSIUM PD treatment does allow for a substantially more liberal intake of potassium than is possible either in late stages of chronic kidney disease or among those treated with hemodialysis. Thus, PD may be a more appropriate therapy for patients with a strong desire to eat large amounts of fruits and vegetables. Initiating PD therapy may also allow for either safe continuation or re-institution of inhibitors of the renin-angiotensin-aldosterone system without significant concern for hyperkalemia despite substantial reduction in renal function. The continuous nature of dialysis with dialysate with zero potassium concentration and the transcellular potassium shift from the hyperinsulinemia induced by glucose absorption probably accounts for the greater ability of patients treated with PD to achieve eukalemia. More than one-third of patients treated with PD develop hypokalemia, which is more likely to occur in those treated with prescriptions with large daily dialysate volumes or those with inadequate dietary intakes [104,136]. Indeed, metabolic balance studies in PD patients indicate a significant correlation between potassium and nitrogen balance, and patients with hypokalemia are more likely to have inadequate protein intake and poor nutritional status [104,125,137]. Hypokalemia is also associated with a higher risk of PD-associated peritonitis [104]. Eukalemia can be achieved either by increasing dietary potassium intakes or use of potassium supplements.

PHOSPHORUS AND CALCIUM There are neither clinical trials nor metabolic studies on which to base recommendations for calcium and phosphorus intakes for patients treated with PD. This question has assumed greater significance in the past decade as a large number of studies have demonstrated a consistent association between serum levels of calcium and phosphorus with death risk in dialysis patients, including those treated with PD [138–140]. The findings from these studies have been bolstered by laboratory findings demonstrating the pathophysiologic role of both calcium and phosphorus

in inducing and accelerating active, cell-mediated vascular calcification [141]. Overall, the strength of the findings for death risk is significantly greater for phosphorus than for calcium. This has led to increased interest in maintaining serum calcium and phosphorus levels within pre-defined target ranges. It is important to note that these recommendations are largely based on observational studies and not clinical trials.

Dietary restriction of phosphorus is an important strategy to limit hyperphosphatemia in patients with kidney disease. The typical daily removal of phosphorus with peritoneal dialysis averages about 400 mg with additional excretion by native kidneys [142,143]. Thus, the magnitude of dietary phosphorus restriction that is necessary generally depends upon residual kidney function — the lower the endogenous renal function, the greater the need to limit phosphorus intake. However, one has to cognizant of the challenges in restricting dietary phosphorus excessively. Many protein-rich foods contain significant amounts of phosphorus and an overtly restrictive dietary phosphorus prescription may make it more challenging for patients to achieve recommended levels of protein intake. Thus, it is prudent to limit dietary phosphorus intake to 800–1000 mg/d and use phosphate binders to limit hyperphosphatemia if necessary.

As indicated earlier, there are no high-level data to base recommendations for dietary calcium intakes. There are three important determinants that can potentially modify the tolerable upper limit of calcium in PD patients — dialysate calcium concentration, calcium intake, especially from the use of calcium-based phosphate binders, and use of active vitamin D for the treatment of hyperparathyroidism. The conventional peritoneal dialysis solutions contained 3.5 mEq/L of calcium leading to significant and sustained calcium absorption from dialysate [144]. This potentially accounted for the reports of a higher prevalence of both adynamic bone disease on bone biopsies and hypercalcemia among patients treated with PD in the 1990s compared to similar patients treated with maintenance hemodialysis [145–149]. Over the last decade, low-calcium dialysate (Ca, 2.5 mEq/L) is increasingly being used and in the United States, accounts for over 85% of all peritoneal dialysate prescriptions. Moreover, noncalcium based phosphate binders are increasingly being used. There are no contemporary studies that have included bone biopsies or studied calcium balance and it remains uncertain if adynamic bone disease is more prevalent in contemporary cohorts of PD patients compared with those treated with in-center hemodialysis.

VITAMIN D Hypovitaminosis D, defined as low levels of serum 25-hydroxy vitamin D levels, is common in patients treated with PD. In addition to the mechanisms operative in other populations of patients with chronic kidney disease (inadequate dietary intake, inadequate sun exposure from reduced physical mobility, urinary losses), PD patients lose significant amounts of vitamin D bound to vitamin D binding protein through the peritoneal dialysis procedure [72–74] (see also Chapters 19 and 21). A large number of primarily observational studies have shown an association between serum 25-hydroxy vitamin D levels and insulin resistance, cardiovascular disease, and death [150–152]. Whether correction of hypovitaminosis D improves any clinically relevant outcomes in effectively anephric dialysis patients is currently unknown. At this time, the clinical paradigm is to use active vitamin D (1,25-dihydroxy vitamin D or analogs) only for the treatment of secondary hyperparathyroidism. There are no data to support 25-hydroxy supplementation for dialysis patients although the possibility of benefit cannot be excluded. In the absence of such data, it may be appropriate to use a supplement of 600 units/day of vitamin D as recommended recently in a report from the Institute of Medicine, in addition to the use of active vitamin D for the treatment of secondary hyperparathyroidism.

NEED FOR OTHER VITAMIN SUPPLEMENTS IN PATIENTS TREATED WITH PERITONEAL DIALYSIS Dialysis patients, including those treated with PD, are at risk for developing deficiency of selected vitamins because of both inadequate intake and increased losses with the dialysate [69,70,113,153]. One in five PD patients has demonstrable vitamin K deficiency [154]. Serum or blood levels of vitamin B_1, B_6, C, and folic acid are low in many patients treated with PD. In contrast, levels of vitamin A and E in PD patients are usually high whereas that of B2 and B12 are often normal or increased [69,70,155–157]. The recommended intakes of each of these vitamins for patients treated with PD are summarized in Table 33.2 (see also Chapter 24).

MINERALS AND TRACE ELEMENTS Patients undergoing PD treatment are at higher risk for developing deficiency of trace elements like iron, selenium, and zinc [78,158]. The iron requirements of PD patients treated with erythropoiesis-stimulating agents are higher though less so than for maintenance hemodialysis patients who are treated with these medicines [159]. Inadequate intake and chronic oxidative stress, and not dialysate losses, account for the deficiency of trace elements in patients treated with PD like selenium, zinc, and magnesium [75,78,113,160]. Recommended daily allowances and amounts of supplementary mineral and trace elements needed for patients undergoing PD are listed in Table 33.2 (see also Chapters 19, 22 and 23).

PROTEIN-ENERGY WASTING IN PERITONEAL DIALYSIS PATIENTS

The preferred term for the clinical syndrome in patients with chronic kidney disease (including among those treated with PD) that has often been referred to as malnutrition is protein-energy wasting (PEW) [161]. PEW refers to abnormalities in any one or more of four categories — biochemical criteria (low serum levels of albumin, prealbumin, or cholesterol); reduced body mass (low body weight, reduced body fat, or weight loss); reduced muscle mass (muscle wasting, reduced mid-arm muscle circumference); and low protein or energy intakes [161]. The criteria for the diagnosis of PEW, as it applies to PD patients, are summarized in Table 33.4. A wide variety of these measures used to diagnose PEW are associated with increased death risk, hospitalizations, and other PD-specific complications like peritonitis [104,105,118,162–164]. Whether prevention and/or treatment of PEW ameliorates the risk of any of these complications, however, has yet to be demonstrated. Nevertheless, determining how to diagnose PEW, understand conditions that may be associated with PEW and prevent or treat PEW in patients treated with PD is essential to the overall management of these patients.

Assessment of Protein-Energy Wasting in Patients Treated with Peritoneal Dialysis

Nutritional status should be routinely monitored in patients treated with PD [129]. The general principles of assessment of nutritional status in patients with chronic kidney disease, as discussed in Chapter 10, apply also to patients treated with PD (summarized in Table 33.5). Special considerations for such measures as they pertain to PD patients are summarized below.

DIETARY INTAKE EVALUATION Adequate nutrient intake is essential for patients treated with PD to maintain health. Energy and protein intakes can be assessed by food diaries, 24-hour diet recall, or food frequency questionnaires [129,165,166]. All three of these techniques become more accurate if they are accompanied by dietary interviews and histories. There is still concern, however, that these methods underestimate dietary intakes particularly in overweight patients [165]. As discussed earlier, it is important to add energy obtained from dialysate glucose absorption to the dietary intakes to estimate total energy intakes. Protein intakes can be estimated indirectly as protein equivalent of total nitrogen appearance normalized to body weight (nPNA). Metabolic studies have shown that urea

TABLE 33.4 Criteria for Diagnosis of Protein-Energy Wasting in Patients Undergoing Peritoneal Dialysis*

Characteristic	Criteria
DIETARY INTAKE	
Unintentional low dietary protein intake	<1.0 g/kg/day at least 2 months
Unintentional low dietary energy intake	<25 kcal/kg/day at least 2 months
ANTHROPOMETRIC AND BODY COMPOSITION	
Body mass index	<23 kg/m^2
Unintentional weight loss	≥5% over 3 months or ≥10% over 6 months
Total body fat	<10% of body weight
Muscle wasting	≥5% over 3 months or ≥10% over 6 months
Mid-arm muscle circumference area	≥10% below the mean values of the 50th percentile of reference population
Calculated creatinine appearance	Low
BIOCHEMICAL**	
Serum albumin	<3.8 g/dL (bromcresol green method)
Serum prealbumin	<30 mg/dL
Serum total cholesterol	<100 mg/dL when patients are not taking lipid lowering medicines
SCORING SYSTEM	
Subjective global assessment	Category C
Seven-point subjective global assessment scores	Severe if score 1–3
Malnutrition inflammation score	Score 21–30
Composite nutritional index	Score >10 (moderate to severe protein-energy wasting)
Protein-nutrition index	Score <6 (probable protein-energy wasting)

* Adapted from Fouque, 2007 [161].
** May not be reliable in those with very heavy urinary or gastrointestinal protein losses, liver disease, or taking lipid-lowering agents.

TABLE 33.5 Assessment Tools for Evaluation of Protein-Energy Wasting in Peritoneal Dialysis Patients

NUTRIENT INTAKES

Direct Method

Dietary diaries with dietitian interviews
24-hour diet recall
Food frequency questionnaires with dietitian interviews

Indirect Method

Calculation based on dialysate and urinary urea nitrogen appearance (normalized protein-equivalent of nitrogen appearance)

BODY COMPOSITION

Weight Based Measurement

Body weight
Body mass index
Weight-for-height

Skin and Muscle Anthropometry

Skin fold thickness
Extremity muscle mass

Neutron Activation Analysis

Total body potassium
Total body nitrogen

Energy-Beam-Based Methods

Dual-energy X-ray absorptiometry
Bioelectrical impedance analysis
Near-infra red reactance

MULTI-SLICE CT OF FAT AND MUSCLE MASS

BIOCHEMICAL VALUES

Visceral proteins: serum albumin, prealbumin (transthyretin), transferrin
Somatic proteins and nitrogen surrogates: serum creatinine
Lipid profiles: serum cholesterol, triglycerides, other lipids and lipoproteins
Peripheral blood cell count: lymphocyte count
Inflammatory marker: C-reactive protein, interleukin-6, tumor necrotic factor-alpha

SCORING SYSTEM

Conventional subjective global assessment of nutrition status and its modification
Malnutrition-inflammation score
Composite Nutritional Index
Protein Nutritional Index

nitrogen appearance is strongly correlated with total nitrogen appearance in patients treated with PD [167]. This correlation, in turn, allows for ready estimation of nPNA from 24-hour collections of urine and dialysate in PD patients [167,168]. Several equations have been proposed, but the following equations are recommended [167]:

$$\text{Total nitrogen appearance(g/24hours)}$$
$$= (0.94 \text{ urea nitrogen appearance}) + 5.54$$

and

Dietary nitrogen intake (g/d)

$$= (0.97 \text{ urea nitrogen appearance}) + 6.80$$

BODY COMPOSITION Serial monitoring of body weight and body mass index are the most widely used measures in clinical practice. Other parameters include skin fold thicknesses, mid-arm muscle circumference, mid-arm muscle area, percent of body fat mass, percent of usual body weight, and percent of standard body weight. Handgrip strength is strongly correlated with fat-free, edema-free body mass and is inversely associated with cardiovascular morbidity and all-cause mortality in PD patients [110].

A variety of methods have been used to estimate fat-free, edema-free body mass in PD patients, a measure that correlates well with dietary protein intakes and somatic protein stores [169,170]. While total body potassium and total body nitrogen by neutron activation analysis are precise measures of fat-free, edema-free body mass, they cannot be practically used in day-to-day clinical practice [171]. Dual-energy X-ray absorptiometry (DEXA) provides reliable estimates but involves exposure to small doses of ionizing radiation, and the DEXA instrument is costly and not portable. Bioelectrical impedance (BIA) can easily be performed at the bedside; the instrument is not expensive, and it is the most promising method for measurement of fat-free, edema-free body mass in clinical practice [172–174]. It is not necessary to drain the peritoneal fluid prior to performing BIA. PD creatinine kinetics can also be used but are not as precise as either DEXA or BIA [175].

BIOCHEMICAL VALUES Serum albumin has been the most commonly used marker of nutritional status for patients with kidney disease, including those treated with PD. Serum albumin is strongly associated with patient morbidity and mortality. Even though it is reduced by systemic inflammation, it is associated with a variety of other measures of nutritional status [67,164,176]. As discussed above, serum albumin levels are lower in PD patients compared to those treated with maintenance hemodialysis possibly because of peritoneal protein losses. The serum albumin level in PD patients that is associated with a risk equivalent to that observed in maintenance HD patients is 0.2–0.3 g/dL lower [67]. Serum levels of a variety of other visceral proteins, like prealbumin (transthyretin), transferrin, and retinol-binding protein, are also predictive of patient outcome but are not routinely used in clinical practice [177–179]. It is important to note that the lowest death risk is observed in patients with serum prealbumin greater than 30 mg/dL [178,179].

SCORING SYSTEMS There are several composite measures that are estimated using elements of medical history, physical examination, and/or laboratory measures of nutritional status. Although on one hand, they are potentially superior to single measures, they are more time-consuming to implement in routine clinical practice. These measures include subjective global assessment (SGA), composite nutritional index (CNI), protein-nutritional index, and malnutrition inflammation score (MIS) [180–184]. SGA is the most widely used tool and is predictive of cardiovascular events and death in PD populations [163,185].

Causes of Protein-Energy Wasting

The potential causes of protein-energy wasting in patients treated with PD are summarized in Table 33.6 and briefly discussed below (please see also Chapters 11 and 12).

TABLE 33.6 Causes of Protein-Energy Wasting in Patients Undergoing Peritoneal Dialysis

INADEQUATE NUTRIENT INTAKE
Anorexia **Induced By**
Increased anorexigens like tumor necrotic factor-alpha, interleukin-6, leptin, glucose-dependent insulinotropic peptide, and cholecystokinin Resistance to action of orexigen substances like neuropeptide Y and ghrelin Intraperitoneal instillation of dialysate Prolonged gastric-emptying time and gastroparesis
Poor Oral and Dental Health
Gastrointestinal Abnormalities
Helicobacter pylori **Infection, Mal-Absorption, Mal-Digestion, Pancreatic Dysfunction, Protein Losing Enteropathy**
Co-existing Illnesses, Including Depression
Dementia Poverty
INFLAMMATION
METABOLIC ACIDOSIS
CO-MORBIDITY
Diabetes Mellitus
Cardiovascular Disease, Including Congestive Heart Failure
Infection
Other Co-Existing Conditions
ENDOCRINE DISORDERS
Resistance to Insulin
Resistance to Growth Hormone and Insulin-Like Growth Factor-I
Hypotestosteronemia
Hyperglucagonemia
Hyperparathyroidism

INADEQUATE DIETARY NUTRIENT INTAKE Recommendations for nutrient intakes, including that for energy and protein, are listed in Table 33.2. Low protein intakes are associated with different measures of protein-energy wasting in PD patients (viz., low serum albumin or body weight or a worse composite nutritional index) and are predictive of poorer clinical outcomes, including death [164,170,182]. There are no contemporary studies or surveys of nutrient intakes of PD patients. Earlier studies indicated that more than one-half of all patients treated with PD had inadequate protein and energy intakes [186–188]. However, some of the studies may have underestimated total energy intakes as they did not account for the peritoneal glucose absorption. Thus, while there is compelling evidence to suggest the importance of low nutrient intakes, its contribution to the prevalence of protein-energy wasting in contemporary PD populations is at best uncertain. Assessment of dietary intakes should be performed in every PD patient with protein-energy wasting.

Anorexia is a cardinal manifestation of uremia and is attributable to an increase in anorexigen substances such as tumor necrotic factor-alpha, leptin, glucose-dependent insulinotropic peptide, and cholecystokinin, and/or inadequate response to orexigen substances such as neuropeptide Y and ghrelin [189,190]. Low nutrient intakes in patients treated with PD could be secondary to partial correction of uremic anorexia either from inadequate solute clearances or from loss of residual renal function, poor oral and dental health, elevation of other proinflammatory cytokines, gastrointestinal abnormalities like prolonged gastric emptying time, *Helicobacter pylori* infection, malabsorption, maldigestion, pancreatic dysfunction, and protein losing enteropathy, coexisting illnesses, and depression, dementia and poverty [112,187,189,191–203]. As discussed earlier, instillation of dialysate could lead to further prolongation of gastric emptying time. Many of these causes of anorexia are potentially treatable, and identification and treatment of these conditions have the potential to ameliorate protein-energy wasting.

INFLAMMATION Over the last 15 years, a large body of evidence has accumulated to support the role of systemic inflammation in inducing protein-energy wasting in individuals with chronic kidney disease, including those undergoing maintenance dialysis [153,204,205]. Numerous studies have demonstrated that serum levels of acute phase proteins (like C-reactive protein) and cytokines (like tumor necrosis factor alpha, interleukin 6, and high mobility group box protein-1 (HMGB-1)) are higher in malnourished than in well-nourished PD patients and are associated with low nutrient intakes [77,111,153,205–207]. Inflammation leads to PEW by potentially inducing anorexia

and/or increased catabolism with higher resting energy expenditure [195,206,207]. Visceral proteins like albumin and prealbumin are also negative acute-phase proteins, and decreases in their serum levels in dialysis patients are in part secondary to systemic inflammation [92,111,208–212]. In patients treated with PD, there are a variety of potential pro-inflammatory stimuli; these include the local and systemic effects of bio-incompatible PD solutions, episodes of PD-related infections like peritonitis, extracellular volume expansion, depression, periodontitis, and co-existing illnesses [28,86,102,106,195,213–218]. Uremia is also associated with increased oxidative stress, another pro-inflammatory stimulus, and in patients treated with PD, peritoneal losses of antioxidants, like vitamin C, may contribute to inflammation [77,153,207,219].

METABOLIC ACIDOSIS Progressive loss of renal function is associated with a decrease in net acid excretion, and hence, metabolic acidosis is ubiquitously present in patients with advanced chronic kidney disease. A large body of data in patients with and without kidney disease, including those treated with PD, has shown that metabolic acidemia induces catabolism by activation of the ATP-dependent ubiquitin-proteasome system and increase in activity of branched chain ketoacid dehydrogenase [220–222]. Furthermore, there is evidence to indicate that metabolic acidemia is anti-anabolic and reduces hepatic albumin synthesis [223]. Thus, uncorrected or partially corrected metabolic acidemia can result in negative nitrogen balance and induce protein energy wasting by its catabolic and anti-anabolic effects. Paradoxically, however, observational studies indicate that it is PD patients with higher serum bicarbonate levels that are more likely to have protein-energy wasting and higher death risk [182,224]. These paradoxical associations are a result of the confounding influence of dietary protein intake on serum bicarbonate levels in functionally anephric, dialysis-dependent patients, since protein metabolism is the dominant source of endogenous daily acid production. In patients treated with hemodialysis, the same general phenomenon has been noted; i.e., low serum bicarbonate levels are associated with reduced mortality. If one adjusts for the higher dietary protein intake in these latter individuals, there is a reverse-J-shaped relationship between serum bicarbonate and death risk with the lowest risk for serum bicarbonate between 21 and 27 mEq/L [225]. There is a paucity of high-quality observational studies concerning acidemia and clinical outcome in PD patients. However, juxtaposing these considerations against the large body of experimental evidence and the results of several randomized controlled trials (discussed below) suggests that uncorrected metabolic acidemia is an important contributor to protein-energy wasting in patients treated with PD.

CO-MORBIDITY Generally, end-stage renal disease patients have a high burden of co-existing illnesses that can potentially exacerbate protein-energy wasting by reducing dietary nutrient intake, contributing to systemic inflammation and/or other morbid effects [195,217,226–228]. Among the co-existing conditions, advanced age, diabetes mellitus, vascular disease, and congestive heart failure are the most common and may mediate the worsening of nutritional decline in patients treated with PD [195,227,228]. In the United States, dialysis patients — including those treated with PD — spend an average of 13 days per year in the hospital often secondary to these co-existing illnesses [229]. Acute decompensation, superimposed upon chronic diseases, can lead to further reduction in nutrient intake, decline in functional status, and worsen protein-energy wasting.

ENDOCRINE DISORDERS OF UREMIA Resistance to or decrease in the level of anabolic hormones (insulin, growth hormone, insulin-like growth factor-I, testosterone) and increase in some catabolic hormones (glucagon, parathyroid hormone) may occur with uremia that could contribute to protein-energy wasting in patients treated with PD [230,231]. Insulin resistance worsens with decline in renal function and is thought to exist at a post-insulin receptor level. This is perhaps accentuated by increased serum glucagon levels commonly seen in patients with chronic kidney disease and its attendant glycemic effects. This increase in glucagon levels, also observed in PD patients, appears to be primarily due to decreased hormonal catabolism [232–235]. Some observational studies suggest that patients treated with PD are more likely to have insulin resistance than similar patients treated with hemodialysis [236,237]. The possible reasons for the higher prevalence of insulin resistance in PD patients, however, are not clear. Resistance to growth hormone and insulin-like growth factor-I often occurs with uremia, and evidence seems to suggest a possible association between alternations in ghrelin levels and function — an orexigen — with disordered insulin and growth hormone metabolism [189,231,238]. There is paucity of data on the role of low serum testosterone levels, present in about half of patients with advanced kidney disease, on protein-energy wasting in PD patients [239,240].

Parathyroid hormone levels are commonly increased in dialysis patients, including those treated with PD, and laboratory evidence suggests that the hormone induces skeletal muscle catabolism [241]. However, there is limited direct evidence for the possible role of parathyroid hormone on protein-energy wasting [242].

Management of Protein-Energy Wasting in Patients Treated with Peritoneal Dialysis

Observational studies show that protein-energy wasting is associated with considerable morbidity and higher mortality in patients treated with PD. Thus, even though there is no evidence to date that treatment results in reduction of death risk, it appears prudent to identify potentially reversible causes of protein-energy wasting and to institute treatments that ameliorate the wasting. A summary of potential interventions is listed in Table 33.7.

ENSURE ADEQUATE SPONTANEOUS NUTRIENT INTAKES As discussed above, anorexia is a cardinal manifestation of uremia. Evidence indicates that a significant proportion of patients have protein-energy wasting at the time of initiation of peritoneal dialysis [164,243]. Initiation of dialysis, including peritoneal dialysis, in uremic individuals with advanced chronic kidney disease ameliorates anorexia, and has been shown to result in improvement in a variety of nutritional measures including serum albumin [244,245]. Thus, timely initiation of dialysis is an important tool

TABLE 33.7 Management Strategies for Protein-Energy Wasting in Patients Undergoing Peritoneal Dialysis*

ENSURE ADEQUATE NUTRIENT INTAKES
Adequate Solute Clearances
Timely initiation of dialysis
Achieve recommended small solute clearances (total weekly Kt/V_{urea} >1.7)
Preserve residual renal function
Nutritional Counseling
Prokinetic Agents
Eradication of *Helicobacter pylori*
Appetite Stimulating Agents Like Oral Megestrol Acetate
NUTRITIONAL SUPPLEMENTATION
Oral Nutritional Supplements
Tube Feeding
Intraperitoneal Amino Acid Solutions
CORRECT METABOLIC ACIDEMIA
ANABOLIC HORMONES
Androgenic Steroid: Nandrolone Decanoate, Oxymetholone
Human Growth Hormone
Recombinant Human Insulin-Like Growth Factor-I
POTENTIAL ANTI-INFLAMMATORY THERAPIES
TREATMENT AND PREVENTION OF CO-EXISTING ILLNESSES

* Adapted from Mehrotra, 2003 [196].

in the armamentarium to ensure optimal nutritional health of patients starting PD; indeed adding dialytic clearances in advanced chronic kidney disease patients as their renal function declines has been shown to improve nutritional status.

Several observational studies have demonstrated an association between dialytic clearances and dietary protein intakes (assessed by nPNA) of PD patients. It has now been recognized, however, that the association seen in cross-sectional studies is at least in part a result of mathematical coupling. Moreover, two randomized controlled clinical trials have shown that increasing dialytic small solute clearances within the range achieved in clinical practice does not lead to further improvement in protein intakes or measures of nutritional status in PD patients [246,247]. These data also suggest that PD patients should achieve total solute clearances, as measured by weekly Kt/V_{urea}, of 1.7 and that attaining this minimum Kt/V_{urea} is another important measure to ensure sufficient nutrient intake. Furthermore, several studies have demonstrated an association between residual renal function and nutritional status of PD patients [109,111]. There is no clinical trial evidence to demonstrate that renoprotective strategies also maintain healthy nutritional status or mitigate protein-energy wasting. Associative data, however, are compelling enough to recommend that efforts be made to minimize the rate of decline of residual renal function. Effective renoprotective strategies for PD patients have been discussed in an earlier section.

Periodic nutritional evaluation and counseling are also important in preventing and/or treating protein-energy wasting, and in a small uncontrolled study, this has been shown to result in an increase in skin-fold thicknesses and serum albumin of PD patients [248]. Furthermore, as discussed above, PD patients often have prolongation of gastric emptying time, and treatment with prokinetic agents has been associated with an increase in serum albumin levels in small, uncontrolled studies [54,55]. Hence, a trial of prokinetic agents may be considered in patients with hyopalbuminemia. Similarly, small studies have demonstrated improvement in measures of nutritional status after treatment of *Helicobacter pylori* [203]. Finally, appetite stimulants such as megestrol acetate can enhance food intake and potentially improve nutritional status in PD patients [249,250]. Preliminary studies indicate that ghrelin or its analogs are promising agents to treat anorexia, but there are no preparations that are currently commercially available [251,252].

NUTRITIONAL SUPPLEMENTATION PD patients have been included in at least four randomized, prospective clinical trials to test the efficacy of oral nutrition supplements, and each of them has demonstrated a significant increase in serum albumin levels [253–256]. Thus, increasing nutrient supply with enteral or intraperitoneal supplementation can be used in selected PD patients who are unable or unwilling to increase dietary nutrient intakes [188,257]. Similarly, increasing nutrient supply with enteral tube feeds has been shown to be effective in improving nutritional status of PD patients but is rarely used in adults [257].

There has been a long-standing interest in using amino acid-based peritoneal dialysis solutions for the treatment of protein-energy wasting. Early proof-of-concept studies demonstrated that amino acid solutions result in a net gain in nitrogen, and metabolic balance studies indicated that they induce anabolism in PD patients with protein-energy wasting [20]. However, long-term studies with amino acid solutions have been unable to demonstrate any consistent benefit on measures of nutritional status [22,23,258–260]. This may, in part, be secondary to inadequate provision of energy at the time of administration of the amino acid solutions. Several small metabolic studies have shown greater anabolism when amino acid solutions are used along with adequate energy intake (either large carbohydrate meals or using a mixture of amino acids and glucose in the PD solution) [261,262]. Whether these strategies lead to long-term improvement in nutritional status, however, remains untested. It is, in part, because of lack of long-term data that amino acid solutions have not been approved by the Food and Drug Administration for use in the United States. Furthermore, these solutions are being increasingly used as a glucose-sparing strategy rather than as a nutritional supplement.

CORRECT METABOLIC ACADEMIA There is increasing support for correction of metabolic acidemia for the prevention and treatment of protein-energy wasting in PD patients. At least two randomized control trials have shown that correction of metabolic acidemia either by using a PD solution with a higher lactate concentration or oral bicarbonate supplementation is associated with reduction in hospitalizations, and improvement in a variety of measures of nutritional status (nPNA, body weight, SGA, mid-arm muscle circumference) [263,264]. Furthermore, there is evidence that the entire normal reference range of arterial pH may not be equivalent for health. In a randomized, cross-over study of automated PD patients, an arterial pH of 7.44 was associated with significantly higher net positive nitrogen balance than a pH of 7.37 in seven of eight patients studied [265]. Finally, bicarbonate supplementation has been shown to be associated with a significant slowing in the rate of decline of renal function in CKD patients not undergoing dialysis therapy [266]. Thus, in addition to amelioration of protein-energy wasting, aggressive correction of metabolic acidemia has the potential to slow the rate of loss of residual renal function in PD patients. This can be readily achieved by either increasing the dialysis dose or use of oral bicarbonate supplements.

ANABOLIC HORMONES Anabolic steroids were used for the correction of anemia associated with kidney disease prior to the introduction of erythropoietin. However, there is evidence to support their role for the treatment of protein-energy wasting in PD patients. At least two small randomized controlled clinical trials and one retrospective study have shown that 100–200 mg weekly intramuscular injections of nandrolone decanoate are associated with an increase in body weight, fat-free-edema-free body mass, triceps skin fold thickness, mid-arm circumference, serum levels of visceral proteins (albumin, prealbumin, transferrin), and functional capacity in PD patients [267–269]. Oral administration of another androgenic steroid, oxymetholone (50 mg twice daily), has been shown in one randomized controlled trial to be associated with an increase in body weight and improvement in SGA in PD patients but its use is limited by induction of liver functional abnormalities [270]. Moreover, subcutaneous administration of recombinant human growth hormone (5 mg/d for 7 days or 0.2 IU/kg/d for one month) results in increase in body weight and net decrease in total urea nitrogen appearance, consistent with anabolism [271,272]. Finally, in metabolic balance studies, subcutaneous injections with recombinant human insulin-like growth factor-I (100 μg/kg twice daily) are associated with significantly more positive nitrogen balances in PD patients with protein-energy wasting [273]. Thus, the short-term data with different anabolic hormones are encouraging, and these agents could be considered as third-line agents (after attempts to improve anorexia and nutritional supplementation) in the treatment of protein-energy wasting in PD patients. The need for parenteral administration for many of these agents and their cost limit their widespread use. Moreover, although protein balance does become more positive with these medicines, they have not yet been clearly shown to improve morbidity, mortality or quality of life in PD patients.

POTENTIAL ANTI-INFLAMMATORY THERAPIES Despite the large body of epidemiologic evidence linking markers of inflammation to protein-energy wasting and all-cause and cardiovascular mortality in dialysis patients, including those treated with PD, there is a paucity of demonstrably effective anti-inflammatory therapies. Even though several studies have demonstrated that diets rich in carotenoids and with vitamin E and low doses of vitamin C have antioxidant and anti-inflammatory effects, there is no evidence that these

result in improvement in nutritional status [274–276]. Optimizing dental health, reducing PD-associated peritonitis, and attaining euvolemia have the potential to mitigate systemic inflammation and potentially improve nutritional status of PD patients.

TREATMENT AND PREVENTION OF CO-EXISTING ILLNESSES Given the high burden of co-existing illnesses and their association with a higher prevalence of protein-energy wasting, it appears prudent to optimize management of such illnesses in PD patients.

References

[1] Tenckhoff H, Schechter H. A bacteriologically safe peritoneal access device. Trans Am Soc Artif Intern Organs 1968;14:181–7.

[2] Popovich RP, Moncrief JW, Nolph KD, Ghods AJ, Twardowski ZJ, Pyle WK. Continuous ambulatory peritoneal dialysis. Ann Intern Med 1978;88(4):449–56.

[3] Lameire N, Van Biesen W. Epidemiology of peritoneal dialysis: a story of believers and nonbelievers. Nat Rev Nephrol 2010;6(2):75–82.

[4] Chiu YW, Jiwakanon S, Lukowsky L, Duong U, Kalantar-Zadeh K, Mehrotra R. An update on the comparisons of mortality outcomes of hemodialysis and peritoneal dialysis patients. Semin Nephrol 2011;31(2):152–8.

[5] Just PM, Riella MC, Tschosik EA, Noe LL, Bhattacharyya SK, de Charro F. Economic evaluations of dialysis treatment modalities. Health Policy 2008;86(2-3):163–80.

[6] Aasarod K, Wideroe TE, Flakne SC. A comparison of solute clearance and ultrafiltration volume in peritoneal dialysis with total or fractional (50%) intraperitoneal volume exchange with the same dialysate flow rate. Nephrol Dial Transplant 1997;12(10):2128–32.

[7] Juergensen PH, Murphy AL, Pherson KA, Chorney WS, Kliger AS, Finkelstein FO. Tidal peritoneal dialysis to achieve comfort in chronic peritoneal dialysis patients. Adv Perit Dial 1999;15:125–6.

[8] Mehrotra R, Nolph KD, Gotch F. Early initiation of chronic dialysis: role of incremental dialysis. Perit Dial Int 1997;17(5):426–30.

[9] Woywodt A, Meier M, Kaiser D, Schneider G, Haller H, Hiss M. In-center intermittent peritoneal dialysis: retrospective ten-year single-center experience with thirty consecutive patients. Perit Dial Int 2008;28(5):518–26.

[10] Fourtounas C, Hardalias A, Dousdampanis P, Savidaki E, Vlachojannis JG. Intermittent peritoneal dialysis (IPD): an old but still effective modality for severely disabled ESRD patients. Nephrol Dial Transplant 2009;24(10):3215–8.

[11] Agarwal R, Mehrotra R. End stage renal disease and dialysis. NephSAP 2007;6(3):117–89.

[12] Fortes PC, Mendes JG, Sesiuk K, Marcondes LB, Aita CA, Riella MC, et al. Glycemic and lipidic profile in diabetic patients undergoing dialysis. Arq Bras Endocrinol Metabol 2010;54(9):793–800.

[13] Skubala A, Zywiec J, Zelobowska K, Gumprecht J, Grzeszczak W. Continuous glucose monitoring system in 72-hour glucose profile assessment in patients with end-stage renal disease on maintenance continuous ambulatory peritoneal dialysis. Med Sci Monit 2010;16(2). CR75-83.

[14] Lin A, Qian J, Li X, Yu X, Liu W, Sun Y, et al. Randomized controlled trial of icodextrin versus glucose containing peritoneal dialysis fluid. Clin J Am Soc Nephrol 2009;4(11):1799–804.

[15] Davies SJ, Woodrow G, Donovan K, Plum J, Williams P, Johansson AC, et al. Icodextrin improves the fluid status of peritoneal dialysis patients: results of a double-blind randomized controlled trial. J Am Soc Nephrol 2003;14(9):2338–44.

[16] Konings CJ, Kooman JP, Schonck M, Gladziwa U, Wirtz J, van den Wall Bake AW, et al. Effect of icodextrin on volume status, blood pressure and echocardiographic parameters: a randomized study. Kidney International 2003;63(4):1556–63.

[17] Paniagua R, Ventura MD, Avila-Diaz M, Cisneros A, Vicente-Martinez M, Furlong MD, et al. Icodextrin improves metabolic and fluid management in high and high-average transport diabetic patients. Perit Dial Int 2009;29(4):422–32.

[18] Bredie SJ, Bosch FH, Demacker PN, Stalenhoef AF, van Leusen R. Effects of peritoneal dialysis with an overnight icodextrin dwell on parameters of glucose and lipid metabolism. Perit Dial Int 2001;21(3):275–81.

[19] Han SH, Ahn SV, Yun JY, Tranaeus A, Han DS. Mortality and technique failure in peritoneal dialysis patients using advanced peritoneal dialysis solutions. Am J Kidney Dis 2009;54(4):711–20.

[20] Kopple JD, Bernard D, Messana J, Swartz R, Bergstrom J, Lindholm B, et al. Treatment of malnourished CAPD patients with an amino acid based dialysate. Kidney Int 1995;47(4):1148–57.

[21] Taylor GS, Patel V, Spencer S, Fluck RJ, McIntyre CW. Long-term use of 1.1% amino acid dialysis solution in hypo-albuminemic continuous ambulatory peritoneal dialysis patients. Clin Nephrol 2002;58(6):445–50.

[22] Li FK, Chan LY, Woo JC, Ho SK, Lo WK, Lai KN, et al. A 3-year, prospective, randomized, controlled study on amino acid dialysate in patients on CAPD. Am J Kidney Dis 2003;42(1):173–83.

[23] Dombros NV, Prutis K, Tong M, Anderson GH, Harrison J, Sombolos K, et al. Six-month overnight intraperitoneal amino-acid infusion in continuous ambulatory peritoneal dialysis (CAPD) patients—no effect on nutritional status. Perit Dial Int 1990;10(1):79–84.

[24] Williams JD, Topley N, Craig KJ, Mackenzie RK, Pischetsrieder M, Lage C, et al. The Euro-Balance Trial: the effect of a new biocompatible peritoneal dialysis fluid (balance) on the peritoneal membrane. Kidney Internat 2004;66(1):408–18.

[25] Haag-Weber M, Kramer R, Haake R, Islam MS, Prischl F, Haug U, et al. Low-GDP fluid (Gambrosol trio) attenuates decline of residual renal function in PD patients: a prospective randomized study. Nephrol Dial Transplant 2010;25(7):2288–96.

[26] Fan SL, Pile T, Punzalan S, Raftery MJ, Yaqoob MM. Randomized controlled study of biocompatible peritoneal dialysis solutions: effect on residual renal function. Kidney Internat 2008;73(2):200–6.

[27] Lee HY, Choi HY, Park HC, Seo BJ, Do JY, Yun SR, et al. Changing prescribing practice in CAPD patients in Korea: increased utilization of low GDP solutions improves patient outcome. Nephrology, Dialysis. Transplantation 2006;21(10):2893–9.

[28] Szeto CC, Chow KM, Lam CW, Leung CB, Kwan BC, Chung KY, et al. Clinical biocompatibility of a neutral peritoneal dialysis solution with minimal glucose-degradation products—a 1-year randomized control trial. Nephrol Dial Transplant 2007;22(2):552–9.

[29] Grodstein GP, Blumenkrantz MJ, Kopple JD, Moran JK, Coburn JW. Glucose absorption during continuous ambulatory peritoneal dialysis. Kidney Int 1981;19(4):564–7.

[30] Davies SJ, Russell L, Bryan J, Phillips L, Russell GI. Impact of peritoneal absorption of glucose on appetite, protein catabolism and survival in CAPD patients. Clin Nephrol 1996;45(3):194–8.

[31] Gahl GM, Baeyer HV, Averdunk R, Riedinger H, Borowzak B, Schurig R, et al. Outpatient evaluation of dietary intake and nitrogen removal in continuous ambulatory peritoneal dialysis. Ann Intern Med 1981;94(5):643–6.

[32] Bergstrom J, Furst P, Alvestrand A, Lindholm B. Protein and energy intake, nitrogen balance and nitrogen losses in patients treated with continuous ambulatory peritoneal dialysis. Kidney Int 1993;44(5):1048–57.

[33] Garcia-Lopez E, Anderstam B, Heimburger O, Amici G, Werynski A, Lindholm B. Determination of high and low molecular weight molecules of icodextrin in plasma and dialysate, using gel filtration chromatography, in peritoneal dialysis patients. Perit Dial Int 2005;25(2):181–91.

[34] Moberly JB, Mujais S, Gehr T, Hamburger R, Sprague S, Kucharski A, et al. Pharmacokinetics of icodextrin in peritoneal dialysis patients. Kidney Int Suppl 2002;(81):S23–33.

[35] Burkart J. Metabolic consequences of peritoneal dialysis. Semin Dial 2004;17(6):498–504.

[36] Jones MR, Gehr TW, Burkart JM, Hamburger RJ, Kraus Jr AP, Piraino BM, et al. Replacement of amino acid and protein losses with 1.1% amino acid peritoneal dialysis solution. Perit Dial Int 1998;18(2):210–6.

[37] da Silva DR, Figueiredo AE, Antonello IC. Poli de Figueiredo CE, d'Avila DO. Solutes transport characteristics in peritoneal dialysis: variations in glucose and insulin serum levels. Ren Fail. 2008;30(2):175–9.

[38] Cho KH, Do JY, Park JW, Yoon KW. Effect of icodextrin dialysis solution on body weight and fat accumulation over time in CAPD patients. Nephrol Dial Transplant 2010;25(2):593–9.

[39] Nordfors L, Heimburger O, Lonnqvist F, Lindholm B, Helmrich J, Schalling M, et al. Fat tissue accumulation during peritoneal dialysis is associated with a polymorphism in uncoupling protein 2. Kidney Int 2000;57(4):1713–9.

[40] Lievense H, Kalantar-Zadeh K, Lukowsky L, Duong U, Krishnan M, Nissenson A, et al. Inter-relationship of body size and initial dialysis modality on subsequent transplantation, mortality, and weight gain of ESRD patients 2012;27(9):3631–8.

[41] Shurraw S, Tonelli M. Statins for treatment of dyslipidemia in chronic kidney disease. Perit Dial Int 2006;26(5):523–39.

[42] Kaysen GA, Schoenfeld PY. Albumin homeostasis in patients undergoing continuous ambulatory peritoneal dialysis. Kidney Int 1984;25(1):107–14.

[43] Kagan A, Bar-Khayim Y, Schafer Z, Fainaru M. Kinetics of peritoneal protein loss during CAPD: II. Lipoprotein leakage and its impact on plasma lipid levels. Kidney Int 1990;37(3):980–90.

[44] Ross EA, Shah GM, Kashyap ML. Elevated plasma lipoprotein(a) levels and hypoalbuminemia in peritoneal dialysis patients. Int J Artif Organs 1995;18(12):751–6.

[45] Shoji T, Nishizawa Y, Nishitani H, Yamakawa M, Morii H. Roles of hypoalbuminemia and lipoprotein lipase on hyperlipoproteinemia in continuous ambulatory peritoneal dialysis. Metabolism 1991;40(10):1002–8.

[46] Hubalewska A, Stompor T, Placzkiewicz E, Staszczak A, Huszno B, Sulowicz W, et al. Evaluation of gastric emptying in patients with chronic renal failure on continuous ambulatory peritoneal dialysis using 99mTc-solid meal. Nucl Med Rev Cent East Eur. 2004;7(1):27–30.

[47] Guz G, Bali M, Poyraz NY, Bagdatoglu O, Yegin ZA, Dogan I, et al. Gastric emptying in patients on renal replacement therapy. Ren Fail. 2004;26(6):619–24.

[48] Bird NJ, Streather CP, O'Doherty MJ, Barton IK, Gaunt JI, Nunan TO. Gastric emptying in patients with chronic renal

failure on continuous ambulatory peritoneal dialysis. Nephrol Dial Transplant 1994;9(3):287–90.

[49] Fernstrom A, Hylander B, Gryback P, Jacobsson H, Hellstrom PM. Gastric emptying and electrogastrography in patients on CAPD. Perit Dial Int 1999;19(5):429–37.

[50] Brown-Cartwright D, Smith HJ, Feldman M. Gastric emptying of an indigestible solid in patients with end-stage renal disease on continuous ambulatory peritoneal dialysis. Gastroenterology 1988;95(1):49–51.

[51] Kim DJ, Kang WH, Kim HY, Lee BH, Kim B, Lee SK, et al. The effect of dialysate dwell on gastric emptying time in patients on continuous ambulatory peritoneal dialysis. Perit Dial Int. 1999;19(Suppl. 2):S176–8.

[52] Schoonjans R, Van Vlem B, Vandamme W, Van Vlierberghe H, Van Heddeghem N, Van Biesen W, et al. Gastric emptying of solids in cirrhotic and peritoneal dialysis patients: influence of peritoneal volume load. Eur J Gastroenterol Hepatol 2002;14(4):395–8.

[53] Stompor T, Hubalewska-Hola A, Staszczak A, Sulowicz W, Huszno B, Szybinski Z. Association between gastric emptying rate and nutritional status in patients treated with continuous ambulatory peritoneal dialysis. Perit Dial Int 2002;22(4): 500–5.

[54] Silang R, Regalado M, Cheng TH, Wesson DE. Prokinetic agents increase plasma albumin in hypoalbuminemic chronic dialysis patients with delayed gastric emptying. Am J Kidney Dis 2001;37(2):287–93.

[55] Ross EA, Koo LC. Improved nutrition after the detection and treatment of occult gastroparesis in nondiabetic dialysis patients. Am J Kidney Dis 1998;31(1):62–6.

[56] Blumenkrantz MJ, Gahl GM, Kopple JD, Kamdar AV, Jones MR, Kessel M, et al. Protein losses during peritoneal dialysis. Kidney Int 1981;19(4):593–602.

[57] Lindholm B, Bergstrom J. Protein and amino acid metabolism in patients undergoing continuous ambulatory peritoneal dialysis (CAPD). Clin Nephrol 1988;30(Suppl. 1):S59–63.

[58] Cooper S, Iliescu EA, Morton AR. The relationship between dialysate protein loss and membrane transport status in peritoneal dialysis patients. Adv Perit Dial 2001;17:244–7.

[59] Westra WM, Kopple JD, Krediet RT, Appell M, Mehrotra R. Dietary protein requirements and dialysate protein losses in chronic peritoneal dialysis patients. Perit Dial Int 2007;27(2):192–5.

[60] Cueto-Manzano AM, Gamba G, Correa-Rotter R. Peritoneal protein loss in patients with high peritoneal permeability: comparison between continuous ambulatory peritoneal dialysis and daytime intermittent peritoneal dialysis. Arch Med Res. 2001;32(3):197–201.

[61] Heaf JG, Sarac S, Afzal S. A high peritoneal large pore fluid flux causes hypoalbuminaemia and is a risk factor for death in peritoneal dialysis patients. Nephrol Dial Transplant 2005;20(10):2194–201.

[62] Krediet RT, Zuyderhoudt FM, Boeschoten EW, Arisz L. Peritoneal permeability to proteins in diabetic and non-diabetic continuous ambulatory peritoneal dialysis patients. Nephron 1986;42(2):133–40.

[63] Cueto-Manzano AM, Gamba G, Correa-Rotter R. Quantification and characterization of protein loss in continuous ambulatory peritoneal dialysis. Rev Invest Clin 2000;52(6):611–7.

[64] Zemel D, Krediet RT, Koomen GC, Struijk DG, Arisz L. Day-to-day variability of protein transport used as a method for analyzing peritoneal permeability in CAPD. Perit Dial Int 1991;11(3):217–23.

[65] Kopple JD, Blumenkrantz MJ, Jones MR, Moran JK, Coburn JW. Plasma amino acid levels and amino acid losses during continuous ambulatory peritoneal dialysis. Am J Clin Nutr 1982;36(3):395–402.

[66] Park YK, Kim JH, Kim KJ, Seo AR, Kang EH, Kim SB, et al. A cross-sectional study comparing the nutritional status of peritoneal dialysis and hemodialysis patients in Korea. J Ren Nutr 1999;9(3):149–56.

[67] Mehrotra R, Duong U, Jiwakanon S, Kovesdy CP, Moran J, Kopple JD, et al. Serum albumin as a predictor of mortality in peritoneal dialysis: comparisons with hemodialysis. Am J Kidney Dis 2011.

[68] Perl J, Huckvale K, Chellar M, John B, Davies SJ. Peritoneal protein clearance and not peritoneal membrane transport status predicts survival in a contemporary cohort of peritoneal dialysis patients. Clin J Am Soc Nephrol 2009;4(7):1201–6.

[69] Blumberg A, Hanck A, Sander G. Vitamin nutrition in patients on continuous ambulatory peritoneal dialysis (CAPD). Clin Nephrol 1983;20(5):244–50.

[70] Boeschoten EW, Schrijver J, Krediet RT, Schreurs WH, Arisz L. Deficiencies of vitamins in CAPD patients: the effect of supplementation. Nephrol Dial Transplant 1988;3(2):187–93.

[71] Tsapas G, Magoula I, Paletas K, Concouris L. Effect of peritoneal dialysis on plasma levels of ascorbic acid. Nephron 1983;33(1):34–7.

[72] Sahin G, Kirli I, Sirmagul B, Colak E, Yalcin AU. Loss via peritoneal fluid as a factor for low 25(OH)D3 level in peritoneal dialysis patients. Int Urol Nephrol 2009;41(4):989–96.

[73] Joffe P, Heaf JG. Vitamin D and vitamin-D-binding protein kinetics in patients treated with continuous ambulatory peritoneal dialysis (CAPD). Perit Dial Int 1989;9(4):281–4.

[74] Aloni Y, Shany S, Chaimovitz C. Losses of 25-hydroxyvitamin D in peritoneal fluid: possible mechanism for bone disease in uremic patients treated with chronic ambulatory peritoneal dialysis. Miner Electrolyte Metab 1983;9(2):82–6.

[75] Sriram K, Abraham G. Loss of zinc and selenium does not occur through peritoneal dialysis. Nutrition 2000;16(11-12):1047–51.

[76] Apostolidis NS, Panoussopoulos DG, Stamou KM, Kekis PB, Paradellis TP, Karydas AG, et al. Selenium metabolism in patients on continuous ambulatory peritoneal dialysis. Perit Dial Int 2002;22(3):400–4.

[77] Guo CH, Wang CL, Chen PC, Yang TC. Linkage of some trace elements, peripheral blood lymphocytes, inflammation, and oxidative stress in patients undergoing either hemodialysis or peritoneal dialysis. Perit Dial Int 2011;31(5):583–91.

[78] Pakfetrat M, Malekmakan L, Hasheminasab M. Diminished selenium levels in hemodialysis and continuous ambulatory peritoneal dialysis patients. Biol Trace Elem Res. 2010;137(3): 335–9.

[79] Grzegorzewska AE, Mariak I. Zinc as a marker of nutrition in continuous ambulatory peritoneal dialysis patients. Adv Perit Dial 2001;17:223–9.

[80] Scancar J, Milacic R, Benedik M, Krizaj I. Total metal concentrations in serum of dialysis patients and fractionation of Cu, Rb, Al, Fe and Zn in spent continuous ambulatory peritoneal dialysis fluids. Talanta 2003;59(2):355–64.

[81] Twardowski ZJ, Nolph KD, Khanna R, Prowant BF, Ryan LP, Moore HL, et al. Peritoneal equilibration test. Peritoneal Dialysis Bull. 1987;7:138–47.

[82] Kang DH, Yoon KI, Choi KB, Lee R, Lee HY, Han DS, et al. Relationship of peritoneal membrane transport characteristics to the nutritional status in CAPD patients. Nephrol Dial Transplant 1999;14(7):1715–22.

[83] Churchill DN, Thorpe KE, Nolph KD, Keshaviah PR, Oreopoulos DG, Page D. Increased peritoneal membrane transport is associated with decreased patient and technique

survival for continuous peritoneal dialysis patients. The Canada-USA (CANUSA) Peritoneal Dialysis Study Group. J Am Soc Nephrol 1998;9(7):1285—92.

[84] Brimble KS, Walker M, Margetts PJ, Kundhal KK, Rabbat CG. Meta-analysis: peritoneal membrane transport, mortality, and technique failure in peritoneal dialysis. J Am Soc Nephrol 2006;17(9):2591—8.

[85] Cho JH, Hur IK, Kim CD, Park SH, Ryu HM, Yook JM, et al. Impact of systemic and local peritoneal inflammation on peritoneal solute transport rate in new peritoneal dialysis patients: a 1-year prospective study. Nephrol Dial Transplant 2010;25(6):1964—73.

[86] Pecoits-Filho R, Carvalho MJ, Stenvinkel P, Lindholm B, Heimburger O. Systemic and intraperitoneal interleukin-6 system during the first year of peritoneal dialysis. Perit Dial Int 2006;26(1):53—63.

[87] Fein PA, Fazil I, Rafiq MA, Schloth T, Matza B, Chattopadhyay J, et al. Relationship of peritoneal transport rate and dialysis adequacy with inflammation in peritoneal dialysis patients. Adv Perit Dial 2006;22:2—6.

[88] Rodrigues AS, Almeida M, Fonseca I, Martins M, Carvalho MJ, Silva F, et al. Peritoneal fast transport in incident peritoneal dialysis patients is not consistently associated with systemic inflammation. Nephrol Dial Transplant 2006;21(3):763—9.

[89] Chung SH, Heimburger O, Stenvinkel P, Wang T, Lindholm B. Influence of peritoneal transport rate, inflammation, and fluid removal on nutritional status and clinical outcome in prevalent peritoneal dialysis patients. Perit Dial Int 2003;23(2):174—83.

[90] Konings CJ, Kooman JP, Schonck M, Struijk DG, Gladziwa U, Hoorntje SJ, et al. Fluid status in CAPD patients is related to peritoneal transport and residual renal function: evidence from a longitudinal study. Nephrol Dial Transplant 2003;18(4):797—803.

[91] Yang X, Fang W, Bargman JM, Oreopoulos DG. High peritoneal permeability is not associated with higher mortality or technique failure in patients on automated peritoneal dialysis. Perit Dial Int 2008;28(1):82—92.

[92] Oh KH, Moon JY, Oh J, Kim SG, Hwang YH, Kim S, et al. Baseline peritoneal solute transport rate is not associated with markers of systemic inflammation or comorbidity in incident Korean peritoneal dialysis patients. Nephrol Dial Transplant 2008;23(7):2356—64.

[93] Piraino B. Peritonitis as a complication of peritoneal dialysis. J Am Soc Nephrol 1998;9(10):1956—64.

[94] Mehrotra R, Marwaha T, Berman N, Mason G, Appell M, Kopple JD. Reducing peritonitis rates in a peritoneal dialysis program of indigent ethnic minorities. Perit Dial Int 2003;23(1):83—5.

[95] Bender FH, Bernardini J, Piraino B. Prevention of infectious complications in peritoneal dialysis: best demonstrated practices. Kidney Int Suppl 2006;(103)::S44—54.

[96] Daly CD, Campbell MK, MacLeod AM, Cody DJ, Vale LD, Grant AM, et al. Do the Y-set and double-bag systems reduce the incidence of CAPD peritonitis? A systematic review of randomized controlled trials. Nephrol Dial Transplant 2001;16(2):341—7.

[97] Mujais S, Story K. Peritoneal dialysis in the US: evaluation of outcomes in contemporary cohorts. Kidney Int Suppl 2006;103:S21—6.

[98] Yang CY, Chen TW, Lin YP, Lin CC, Ng YY, Yang WC, et al. Determinants of catheter loss following continuous ambulatory peritoneal dialysis peritonitis. Perit Dial Int 2008;28(4):361—70.

[99] Zemel D, Koomen GC, Hart AA, ten Berge IJ, Struijk DG, Krediet RT. Relationship of TNF-alpha, interleukin-6, and prostaglandins to peritoneal permeability for macromolecules

during longitudinal follow-up of peritonitis in continuous ambulatory peritoneal dialysis. J Lab Clin Med 1993;122(6):686—96.

[100] Bannister DK, Acchiardo SR, Moore LW, Kraus Jr AP. Nutritional effects of peritonitis in continuous ambulatory peritoneal dialysis (CAPD) patients. J Am Diet Assoc. 1987;87(1):53—6.

[101] Lin CY, Huang TP. Enhancement of ionized calcium and 1,25-dihydroxycholecalciferol loss from peritoneal fluid during peritonitis in patients treated with continuous ambulatory peritoneal dialysis. Nephron 1991;59(1):90—5.

[102] Lam MF, Leung JC, Lo WK, Tam S, Chong MC, Lui SL, et al. Hyperleptinaemia and chronic inflammation after peritonitis predicts poor nutritional status and mortality in patients on peritoneal dialysis. Nephrol Dial Transplant 2007;22(5):1445—50.

[103] Ates K, Koc R, Nergizoglu G, Erturk S, Keven K, Sen A, et al. The longitudinal effect of a single peritonitis episode on peritoneal membrane transport in CAPD patients. Perit Dial Int 2000;20(2):220—6.

[104] Chuang YW, Shu KH, Yu TM, Cheng CH, Chen CH. Hypokalaemia: an independent risk factor of Enterobacteriaceae peritonitis in CAPD patients. Nephrol Dial Transplant 2009;24(5):1603—8.

[105] Prasad N, Gupta A, Sharma RK, Sinha A, Kumar R. Impact of nutritional status on peritonitis in CAPD patients. Perit Dial Int 2007;27(1):42—7.

[106] Perez Fontan M, Rodriguez-Carmona A, Garcia-Naveiro R, Rosales M, Villaverde P, Valdes F. Peritonitis-related mortality in patients undergoing chronic peritoneal dialysis. Perit Dial Int 2005;25(3):274—84.

[107] Bargman JM, Thorpe KE, Churchill DN. Relative contribution of residual renal function and peritoneal clearance to adequacy of dialysis: a reanalysis of the CANUSA study. J Am Soc Nephrol 2001;12(10):2158—62.

[108] Shafi T, Jaar BG, Plantinga LC, Fink NE, Sadler JH, Parekh RS, et al. Association of residual urine output with mortality, quality of life, and inflammation in incident hemodialysis patients: the Choices for Healthy Outcomes in Caring for End-stage Renal Disease (CHOICE) Study. Am J Kidney Dis 2010;56(2):348—58.

[109] Shemin D, Bostom AG, Lambert C, Hill C, Kitsen J, Kliger AS. Residual renal function in a large cohort of peritoneal dialysis patients: change over time, impact on mortality and nutrition. Perit Dial Int 2000;20(4):439—44.

[110] Wang AY, Sea MM, Ho ZS, Lui SF, Li PK, Woo J. Evaluation of handgrip strength as a nutritional marker and prognostic indicator in peritoneal dialysis patients. Am J Clin Nutr 2005;81(1):79—86.

[111] Perez-Flores I, Coronel F, Cigarran S, Herrero JA, Calvo N. Relationship between residual renal function, inflammation, and anemia in peritoneal dialysis. Adv Perit Dial 2007;23:140—3.

[112] Young GA, Kopple JD, Lindholm B, Vonesh EF, De Vecchi A, Scalamogna A, et al. Nutritional assessment of continuous ambulatory peritoneal dialysis patients: an international study. Am J Kidney Dis 1991;17(4):462—71.

[113] Wang AY, Sea MM, Ip R, Law MC, Chow KM, Lui SF, et al. Independent effects of residual renal function and dialysis adequacy on dietary micronutrient intakes in patients receiving continuous ambulatory peritoneal dialysis. Am J Clin Nutr 2002;76(3):569—76.

[114] Lysaght MJ, Vonesh EF, Gotch F, Ibels L, Keen M, Lindholm B, et al. The influence of dialysis treatment modality on the decline of remaining renal function. ASAIO Trans. 1991;37(4):598—604.

[115] Moist LM, Port FK, Orzol SM, Young EW, Ostbye T, Wolfe RA, et al. Predictors of loss of residual renal function among new dialysis patients. J Am Soc Nephrol 2000;11(3):556—64.

[116] Lang SM, Bergner A, Topfer M, Schiffl H. Preservation of residual renal function in dialysis patients: effects of dialysis-technique-related factors. Perit Dial Int 2001;21(1):52—7.

[117] Jansen MA, Hart AA, Korevaar JC, Dekker FW, Boeschoten EW, Krediet RT. Predictors of the rate of decline of residual renal function in incident dialysis patients. Kidney Int 2002;62(3):1046—53.

[118] Chung SH, Han DC, Noh H, Jeon JS, Kwon SH, Lindholm B, et al. Risk factors for mortality in diabetic peritoneal dialysis patients. Nephrol Dial Transplant 2010;25(11):3742—8.

[119] Bernardo A, Fonseca I, Rodrigues A, Carvalho MJ, Cabrita A. Predictors of residual renal function loss in peritoneal dialysis: is previous renal transplantation a risk factor? Adv Perit Dial 2009;25:110—4.

[120] Liao CT, Chen YM, Shiao CC, Hu FC, Huang JW, Kao TW, et al. Rate of decline of residual renal function is associated with all-cause mortality and technique failure in patients on long-term peritoneal dialysis. Nephrol Dial Transplant 2009;24(9):2909—14.

[121] Li PK, Chow KM, Wong TY, Leung CB, Szeto CC. Effects of an angiotensin-converting enzyme inhibitor on residual renal function in patients receiving peritoneal dialysis. A random-ized, controlled study. Ann Intern Med 2003;139(2):105—12.

[122] Suzuki H, Kanno Y, Sugahara S, Okada H, Nakamoto H. Effects of an angiotensin II receptor blocker, valsartan, on residual renal function in patients on CAPD. Am J Kidney Dis 2004;43(6):1056—64.

[123] Phakdeekitcharoen B, Leelasa-nguan P. Effects of an ACE inhibitor or angiotensin receptor blocker on potassium in CAPD patients. Am J Kidney Dis 2004;44(4):738—46.

[124] Kim S, Oh J, Kim S, Chung W, Ahn C, Kim SG, et al. Benefits of biocompatible PD fluid for preservation of residual renal function in incident CAPD patients: a 1-year study. Nephrol Dial Transplant 2009;24(9):2899—908.

[125] Blumenkrantz MJ, Kopple JD, Moran JK, Coburn JW. Metabolic balance studies and dietary protein requirements in patients undergoing continuous ambulatory peritoneal dialysis. Kidney Int 1982;21(6):849—61.

[126] Giordano C, De Santo NG, Pluvio M, Di Leo VA, Capodicasa G, Cirillo D, et al. Protein requirement of patients on CAPD: a study on nitrogen balance. Int J Artif Organs 1980;3(1):11—4.

[127] Bazanelli AP, Kamimura MA, da Silva CB, Avesani CM, Lopes MG, Manfredi SR, et al. Resting energy expenditure in peritoneal dialysis patients. Perit Dial Int 2006;26(6):697—704.

[128] Lindholm B, Alvestrand A, Furst P, Karlander SG, Norbeck HE, Ahlberg M, et al. Metabolic effects of continuous ambulatory peritoneal dialysis. Proc Eur Dial Transplant Assoc. 1980;17:283—90.

[129] Clinical practice guidelines for nutrition in chronic renal failure. K/DOQI, National Kidney Foundation. Am J Kidney Dis 2000;35(6 Suppl. 2):S1—140.

[130] Misra M, Vonesh E, Van Stone JC, Moore HL, Prowant B, Nolph KD. Effect of cause and time of dropout on the residual GFR: a comparative analysis of the decline of GFR on dialysis. Kidney Int 2001;59(2):754—63.

[131] Enia G, Mallamaci F, Benedetto FA, Panuccio V, Parlongo S, Cutrupi S, et al. Long-term CAPD patients are volume expanded and display more severe left ventricular hypertrophy than haemodialysis patients. Nephrol Dial Transplant 2001;16(7):1459—64.

[132] Fine A, Fontaine B, Ma M. Commonly prescribed salt intake in continuous ambulatory peritoneal dialysis patients is too restrictive: results of a double-blind crossover study. J Am Soc Nephrol 1997;8(8):1311—4.

[133] Dong J, Li Y, Yang Z, Luo J. Low dietary sodium intake increases the death risk in peritoneal dialysis. Clin J Am Soc Nephrol 2010;5(2):240—7.

[134] Cheng LT, Chen W, Tang W, Wang T. Residual renal function and volume control in peritoneal dialysis patients. Nephron Clin Pract 2006;104(1):c47—54.

[135] Krediet RT. Dry body weight: water and sodium removal targets in PD. Contrib Nephrol 2006;150:104—10.

[136] Newman LN, Weiss MF, Berger J, Priester A, Negrea LA, Cacho CP. The law of unintended consequences in action: increase in incidence of hypokalemia with improved adequacy of dialysis. Adv Perit Dial 2000;16:134—7.

[137] Jung JY, Chang JH, Lee HH, Chung W, Kim S. De novo hypo-kalemia in incident peritoneal dialysis patients: a 1-year observational study. Electrolyte Blood Press 2009;7(2):231—7. 73—8.

[138] Noordzij M, Korevaar JC, Dekker FW, Boeschoten EW, Bos WJ, Krediet RT, et al. Mineral metabolism and mortality in dialysis patients: a reassessment of the K/DOQI guideline. Blood Purif 2008;26(3):231—7.

[139] Noordzij M, Korevaar JC, Bos WJ, Boeschoten EW, Dekker FW, Bossuyt PM, et al. Mineral metabolism and cardiovascular morbidity and mortality risk: peritoneal dialysis patients compared with haemodialysis patients. Nephrol Dial Trans-plant 2006;21(9):2513—20.

[140] Noordzij M, Korevaar JC, Boeschoten EW, Dekker FW, Bos WJ, Krediet RT. The Kidney Disease Outcomes Quality Initiative (K/DOQI) Guideline for Bone Metabolism and Disease in CKD: association with mortality in dialysis patients. Am J Kidney Dis 2005;46(5):925—32.

[141] Moe SM, Chen NX. Mechanisms of vascular calcification in chronic kidney disease. J Am Soc Nephrol 2008;19(2):213—6.

[142] Dong J, Wang H, Wang M. Low prevalence of hyper-phosphatemia independent of residual renal function in peri-toneal dialysis patients. J Ren Nutr 2007;17(6):389—96.

[143] Sedlacek M, Dimaano F, Uribarri J. Relationship between phosphorus and creatinine clearance in peritoneal dialysis: clinical implications. Am J Kidney Dis 2000;36(5):1020—4.

[144] Bender FH, Bernardini J, Piraino B. Calcium mass transfer with dialysate containing 1.25 and 1.75 mmol/L calcium in perito-neal dialysis patients. Am J Kidney Dis 1992;20(4):367—71.

[145] Heaf JG, Lokkegard H. Parathyroid hormone during mainte-nance dialysis: influence of low calcium dialysate, plasma albumin and age. J Nephrol 1998;11(4):203—10.

[146] Couttenye MM, D'Haese PC, Deng JT, Van Hoof VO, Verpooten GA, De Broe ME. High prevalence of adynamic bone disease diagnosed by biochemical markers in a wide sample of the European CAPD population. Nephrol Dial Transplant 1997;12(10):2144—50.

[147] Pasadakis P, Thodis E, Mourvati E, Euthimiadou A, Margaritis D, Manavis J, et al. Evaluation of bone mineral density in CAPD patients with dual energy X-ray absorptiom-etry. Adv Perit Dial 1996;12:245—9.

[148] Hutchison AJ, Whitehouse RW, Freemont AJ, Adams JE, Mawer EB, Gokal R. Histological, radiological, and biochem-ical features of the adynamic bone lesion in continuous ambulatory peritoneal dialysis patients. Am J Nephrol 1994;14(1):19—29.

[149] Pagliari B, Baretta A, De Cristofaro V, Sama F, Cantaluppi A, Martis L, et al. Short-term effects of low-calcium dialysis solu-tions on calcium mass transfer, ionized calcium, and para-thyroid hormone in CAPD patients. Perit Dial Int 1991;11(4):326—9.

[150] Bindal ME, Taskapan H. Hypovitaminosis D and insulin resistance in peritoneal dialysis patients. Int Urol Nephrol 2011;43(2):527–34.

[151] Obineche EN, Saadi H, Benedict S, Pathan JY, Frampton CM, Nicholls MG. Interrelationships between B-type natriuretic peptides and vitamin D in patients on maintenance peritoneal dialysis. Perit Dial Int 2008;28(6):617–21.

[152] Wang AY, Lam CW, Sanderson JE, Wang M, Chan IH, Lui SF, et al. Serum 25-hydroxyvitamin D status and cardiovascular outcomes in chronic peritoneal dialysis patients: a 3-y prospective cohort study. Am J Clin Nutr 2008;87(6):1631–8.

[153] Martin-Del-Campo F, Batis-Ruvalcaba C, Gonzalez-Espinoza L, Rojas-Campos E, Angel JR, Ruiz N, et al. Dietary Micronutrient Intake in Peritoneal Dialysis Patients: Relationship with Nutrition and Inflammation Status. Perit Dial Int 2012;32(2):183–91.

[154] Holden RM, Iliescu E, Morton AR, Booth SL. Vitamin K status of Canadian peritoneal dialysis patients. Perit Dial Int 2008;28(4):415–8.

[155] Mydlik M, Derzsiova K, Valek A, Szabo T, Dandar V, Takac M. Vitamins and continuous ambulatory peritoneal dialysis (CAPD). Int Urol Nephrol 1985;17(3):281–6.

[156] Singer R, Rhodes HC, Chin G, Kulkarni H, Ferrari P. High prevalence of ascorbate deficiency in an Australian peritoneal dialysis population. Nephrology (Carlton) 2008;13(1):17–22.

[157] Zhang K, Liu L, Cheng X, Dong J, Geng Q, Zuo L. Low levels of vitamin C in dialysis patients is associated with decreased prealbumin and increased C-reactive protein. BMC Nephrol 2011;12:18.

[158] Dworkin B, Weseley S, Rosenthal WS, Schwartz EM, Weiss L. Diminished blood selenium levels in renal failure patients on dialysis: correlations with nutritional status. Am J Med Sci 1987;293(1):6–12.

[159] St Peter WL, Obrador GT, Roberts TL, Collins AJ. Trends in intravenous iron use among dialysis patients in the United States. Am J Kidney Dis 2005 1994-2002;46(4):650–60.

[160] Fein P, Suda V, Borawsky C, Kapupara H, Butikis A, Matza B, et al. Relationship of serum magnesium to body composition and inflammation in peritoneal dialysis patients. Adv Perit Dial 2010;26:112–5.

[161] Fouque D, Kalantar-Zadeh K, Kopple J, Cano N, Chauveau P, Cuppari L, et al. A proposed nomenclature and diagnostic criteria for protein-energy wasting in acute and chronic kidney disease. Kidney Int 2008;73(4):391–8.

[162] Afsar B, Sezer S, Ozdemir FN, Celik H, Elsurer R, Haberal M. Malnutrition-inflammation score is a useful tool in peritoneal dialysis patients. Perit Dial Int 2006;26(6):705–11.

[163] Chung SH, Lindholm B, Lee HB. Influence of initial nutritional status on continuous ambulatory peritoneal dialysis patient survival. Perit Dial Int 2000;20(1):19–26.

[164] Leinig CE, Moraes T, Ribeiro S, Riella MC, Olandoski M, Martins C, et al. Predictive value of malnutrition markers for mortality in peritoneal dialysis patients. J Ren Nutr 2011;21(2):176–83.

[165] Bazanelli AP, Kamimura MA, Vasselai P, Draibe SA, Cuppari L. Underreporting of energy intake in peritoneal dialysis patients. J Ren Nutr 2010;20(4):263–9.

[166] Griffiths A, Russell L, Breslin M, Russell G, Davies S. A comparison of two methods of dietary assessment in peritoneal dialysis patients. J Ren Nutr 1999;9(1):26–31.

[167] Kopple JD, Gao XL, Qing DP. Dietary protein, urea nitrogen appearance and total nitrogen appearance in chronic renal failure and CAPD patients. Kidney Int 1997;52(2):486–94.

[168] Bergstrom J, Heimburger O, Lindholm B. Calculation of the protein equivalent of total nitrogen appearance from urea

[169] Dong J, Li YJ, Lu XH, Gan HP, Zuo L, Wang HY. Correlations of lean body mass with nutritional indicators and mortality in patients on peritoneal dialysis. Kidney Int 2008;73(3):334–40.

[170] Dong J, Li Y, Xu Y, Xu R. Daily protein intake and survival in patients on peritoneal dialysis. Nephrol Dial Transplant 2011;26(11):3715–21.

[171] Kerr PG, Strauss BJ, Atkins RC. Assessment of the nutritional state of dialysis patients. Blood Purif 1996;14(5):382–7.

[172] Schmidt R, Dumler F, Cruz C, Lubkowski T, Kilates C. Improved nutritional follow-up of peritoneal dialysis patients with bioelectrical impedance. Adv Perit Dial 1992;8:157–9.

[173] Fein PA, Gundumalla G, Jorden A, Matza B, Chattopadhyay J, Avram MM. Usefulness of bioelectrical impedance analysis in monitoring nutrition status and survival of peritoneal dialysis patients. Adv Perit Dial 2002;18:195–9.

[174] Medici G, Mussi C, Fantuzzi AL, Malavolti M, Albertazzi A, Bedogni G. Accuracy of eight-polar bioelectrical impedance analysis for the assessment of total and appendicular body composition in peritoneal dialysis patients. Eur J Clin Nutr 2005;59(8):932–7.

[175] Borovnicar DJ, Wong KC, Kerr PG, Stroud DB, Xiong DW, Strauss BJ, et al. Total body protein status assessed by different estimates of fat-free mass in adult peritoneal dialysis patients. Eur J Clin Nutr 1996;50(9):607–16.

[176] Enia G, Sicuso C, Alati G, Zoccali C. Subjective global assessment of nutrition in dialysis patients. Nephrol Dial Transplant 1993;8(10):1094–8.

[177] Avram MM, Mittman N, Bonomini L, Chattopadhyay J, Fein P. Markers for survival in dialysis: a seven-year prospective study. Am J Kidney Dis 1995;26(1):209–19.

[178] Sreedhara R, Avram MM, Blanco M, Batish R, Avram MM, Mittman N. Prealbumin is the best nutritional predictor of survival in hemodialysis and peritoneal dialysis. Am J Kidney Dis 1996;28(6):937–42.

[179] Mittman N, Avram MM, Oo KK, Chattopadhyay J. Serum prealbumin predicts survival in hemodialysis and peritoneal dialysis: 10 years of prospective observation. Am J Kidney Dis 2001;38(6):1358–64.

[180] Detsky AS, McLaughlin JR, Baker JP, Johnston N, Whittaker S, Mendelson RA, et al. What is subjective global assessment of nutritional status? JPEN J Parenter Enteral Nutr 1987;11(1):8–13.

[181] Visser R, Dekker FW, Boeschoten EW, Stevens P, Krediet RT. Reliability of the 7-point subjective global assessment scale in assessing nutritional status of dialysis patients. Adv Perit Dial 1999;15:222–5.

[182] Kang DH, Lee R, Lee HY, Han DS, Cho EY, Lee CH, et al. Metabolic acidosis and composite nutritional index (CNI) in CAPD patients. Clin Nephrol 2000;53(2):124–31.

[183] Kalantar-Zadeh K, Kopple JD, Block G, Humphreys MH. A malnutrition-inflammation score is correlated with morbidity and mortality in maintenance hemodialysis patients. Am J Kidney Dis 2001;38(6):1251–63.

[184] Chen KH, Wu CH, Hsu CW, Chen YM, Weng SM, Yang CW, et al. Protein nutrition index as a function of patient survival rate in peritoneal dialysis. Kidney Blood Press Res. 2010;33(3):174–80.

[185] de Mutsert R, Grootendorst DC, Indemans F, Boeschoten EW, Krediet RT, Dekker FW. Association between serum albumin and mortality in dialysis patients is partly explained by inflammation, and not by malnutrition. J Ren Nutr 2009;19(2):127–35.

[186] Chow VC, Yong RM, Li AL, Lee CW, Ho EH, Chan CK, et al. Nutritional requirements and actual dietary intake of continuous ambulatory peritoneal dialysis patients. Perit Dial Int 2003;23(Suppl. 2):S52—4.

[187] Wang AY, Sea MM, Ng K, Kwan M, Lui SF, Woo J. Nutrient intake during peritoneal dialysis at the Prince of Wales Hospital in Hong Kong. Am J Kidney Dis 2007;49(5):682—92.

[188] Boudville N, Rangan A, Moody H. Oral nutritional supplementation increases caloric and protein intake in peritoneal dialysis patients. Am J Kidney Dis 2003;41(3):658—63.

[189] Aguilera A, Cirugeda A, Amair R, Sansone G, Alegre L, Codoceo R, et al. Ghrelin plasma levels and appetite in peritoneal dialysis patients. Adv Perit Dial 2004;20:194—9.

[190] Aguilera A, Codoceo R, Selgas R, Garcia P, Picornell M, Diaz C, et al. Anorexigen (TNF-alpha, cholecystokinin) and orexigen (neuropeptide Y) plasma levels in peritoneal dialysis (PD) patients: their relationship with nutritional parameters. Nephrol Dial Transplant 1998;13(6):1476—83.

[191] Eltas A, Tozoglu U, Keles M, Canakci V. Assessment of oral health in peritoneal dialysis patients with and without diabetes mellitus. Perit Dial Int 2012;31(2):168—72.

[192] Keles M, Seven B, Varoglu E, Uyanik A, Cayir K, Kursad Ayan A, et al. Salivary gland function in continuous ambulatory peritoneal dialysis patients by 99mTc-pertechnetate scintigraphy. Hell J Nucl Med 2010;13(1):26—9.

[193] Bayraktar G, Kurtulus I, Kazancioglu R, Bayramgurler I, Cintan S, Bural C, et al. Oral health and inflammation in patients with end-stage renal failure. Perit Dial Int 2009;29(4):472—9.

[194] Bayraktar G, Kurtulus I, Kazancioglu R, Bayramgurler I, Cintan S, Bural C, et al. Evaluation of periodontal parameters in patients undergoing peritoneal dialysis or hemodialysis. Oral Dis 2008;14(2):185—9.

[195] Wang AY, Sea MM, Tang N, Lam CW, Chan IH, Lui SF, et al. Energy intake and expenditure profile in chronic peritoneal dialysis patients complicated with circulatory congestion. Am J Clin Nutr 2009;90(5):1179—84.

[196] Mehrotra R, Kopple JD. Protein and energy nutrition among adult patients treated with chronic peritoneal dialysis. Adv Ren Replace Ther 2003;10(3):194—212.

[197] Schoonjans R, Van VB, Vandamme W, Van HN, Verdievel H, Vanholder R, et al. Dyspepsia and gastroparesis in chronic renal failure: the role of *Helicobacter pylori*. Clin Nephrol 2002;57(3):201—7.

[198] Wang AY, Sanderson J, Sea MM, Wang M, Lam CW, Li PK, et al. Important factors other than dialysis adequacy associated with inadequate dietary protein and energy intakes in patients receiving maintenance peritoneal dialysis. Am J Clin Nutr 2003;77(4):834—41.

[199] Davies SJ, Russell L, Bryan J, Phillips L, Russell GI. Comorbidity, urea kinetics, and appetite in continuous ambulatory peritoneal dialysis patients: their interrelationship and prediction of survival. Am J Kidney Dis 1995;26(2):353—61.

[200] Hylander B, Barkeling B, Rossner S. Eating behavior in continuous ambulatory peritoneal dialysis and hemodialysis patients. Am J Kidney Dis 1992;20(6):592—7.

[201] Hylander B, Barkeling B, Rossner S. Changes in patients' eating behavior: in the uremic state, on continuous ambulatory peritoneal dialysis treatment, and after transplantation. Am J Kidney Dis 1997;29(5):691—8.

[202] Aguilera A, Bajo MA, Espinoza M, Olveira A, Paiva AM, Codoceo R, et al. Gastrointestinal and pancreatic function in peritoneal dialysis patients: their relationship with malnutrition and peritoneal membrane abnormalities. Am J Kidney Dis 2003;42(4):787—96.

[203] Aguilera A, Codoceo R, Bajo MA, Diez JJ, del Peso G, Pavone M, et al. Helicobacter pylori infection: a new cause of anorexia in peritoneal dialysis patients. Perit Dial Int 2001;21(Suppl. 3):S152—6.

[204] Maruyama Y, Nordfors L, Stenvinkel P, Heimburger O, Barany P, Pecoits-Filho R, et al. Interleukin-1 gene cluster polymorphisms are associated with nutritional status and inflammation in patients with end-stage renal disease. Blood Purif 2005;23(5):384—93.

[205] Zhu N, Yuan W, Zhou Y, Liu J, Bao J, Hao J, et al. High mobility group box protein-1 correlates with microinflammatory state and nutritional status in continuous ambulatory peritoneal dialysis patients. J Artif Organs 2011;14(2):125—32.

[206] Oner-Iyidogan Y, Gurdol F, Kocak H, Oner P, Cetinalp-Demircan P, Caliskan Y, et al. Appetite-regulating hormones in chronic kidney disease patients. J Ren Nutr 2011;21(4):316—21.

[207] Malgorzewicz S, Lichodziejewska-Niemierko M, Aleksandrowicz-Wrona E, Swietlik D, Rutkowski B, Lysiak-Szydlowska W. Adipokines, endothelial dysfunction and nutritional status in peritoneal dialysis patients. Scand J Urol Nephrol 2010;44(6):445—51.

[208] Yeun JY, Kaysen GA. Acute phase proteins and peritoneal dialysate albumin loss are the main determinants of serum albumin in peritoneal dialysis patients. Am J Kidney Dis 1997;30(6):923—7.

[209] Sezer S, Ozdemir FN, Akman B, Arat Z, Anaforoglu I, Haberal M. Predictors of serum albumin level in patients receiving continuous ambulatory peritoneal dialysis. Adv Perit Dial 2001;17:210—4.

[210] Kaysen GA, Yeun J, Depner T. Albumin synthesis, catabolism and distribution in dialysis patients. Miner Electrolyte Metab 1997;23(3-6):218—24.

[211] Avram MM, Fein PA, Paluch MM, Schloth T, Chattopadhyay J. Association between C-reactive protein and clinical outcomes in peritoneal dialysis patients. Adv Perit Dial 2005;21:154—8.

[212] Fein PA, Mittman N, Gadh R, Chattopadhyay J, Blaustein D, Mushnick R, et al. Malnutrition and inflammation in peritoneal dialysis patients. Kidney Int Suppl 2003;(87):S87—91.

[213] Avila-Diaz M, Ventura MD, Valle D, Vicente-Martinez M, Garcia-Gonzalez Z, Cisneros A, et al. Inflammation and extracellular volume expansion are related to sodium and water removal in patients on peritoneal dialysis. Perit Dial Int 2006;26(5):574—80.

[214] Demirci MS, Demirci C, Ozdogan O, Kircelli F, Akcicek F, Basci A, et al. Relations between malnutrition-inflammation-atherosclerosis and volume status. The usefulness of bioimpedance analysis in peritoneal dialysis patients. Nephrol Dial Transplant 2011;26(5):1708—16.

[215] Park SH, Lee EG, Kim IS, Kim YJ, Cho DK, Kim YL. Effect of glucose degradation products on the peritoneal membrane in a chronic inflammatory infusion model of peritoneal dialysis in the rat. Perit Dial Int 2004;24(2):115—22.

[216] Bender TO, Bohm M, Kratochwill K, Vargha R, Riesenhuber A, Witowski J, et al. Peritoneal dialysis fluids can alter HSP expression in human peritoneal mesothelial cells. Nephrol Dial Transplant 2011;26(3):1046—52.

[217] Li ZJ, An X, Mao HP, Wei X, Chen JH, Yang X, et al. Association between depression and malnutrition-inflammation complex syndrome in patients with continuous ambulatory peritoneal dialysis. Int Urol Nephrol 2011.

[218] Szeto CC, Kwan BC, Chow KM, Lai KB, Chung KY, Leung CB, et al. Endotoxemia is related to systemic inflammation and

atherosclerosis in peritoneal dialysis patients. Clin J Am Soc Nephrol 2008;3(2):431–6.

[219] Lee EJ, Myint CC, Tay ME, Yusuf N, Ong CN. Serum ascorbic acid and protein calorie malnutrition in continuous ambulatory peritoneal dialysis patients. Adv Perit Dial 2001;17:219–22.

[220] Mehrotra R, Kopple JD, Wolfson M. Metabolic acidosis in maintenance dialysis patients: clinical considerations. Kidney Int Suppl 2003;(88):S13–25.

[221] Reaich D, Channon SM, Scrimgeour CM, Goodship TH. Ammonium chloride-induced acidosis increases protein breakdown and amino acid oxidation in humans. Am J Physiol 1992;263(4 Pt 1):E735–9.

[222] Pickering WP, Price SR, Bircher G, Marinovic AC, Mitch WE, Walls J. Nutrition in CAPD: serum bicarbonate and the ubiquitin-proteasome system in muscle. Kidney Int 2002;61(4):1286–92.

[223] Ballmer PE, McNurlan MA, Hulter HN, Anderson SE, Garlick PJ, Krapf R. Chronic metabolic acidosis decreases albumin synthesis and induces negative nitrogen balance in humans. J Clin Invest 1995;95(1):39–45.

[224] Kung SC, Morse SA, Bloom E, Raja RM. Acid-base balance and nutrition in peritoneal dialysis. Adv Perit Dial 2001;17:235–7.

[225] Wu DY, Shinaberger CS, Regidor DL, McAllister CJ, Kopple JD, Kalantar-Zadeh K. Association between serum bicarbonate and death in hemodialysis patients: is it better to be acidotic or alkalotic? Clin J Am Soc Nephrol 2006;1(1):70–8.

[226] Prasad N, Gupta A, Sinha A, Sharma RK, Saxena A, Kaul A, et al. Confounding effect of comorbidities and malnutrition on survival of peritoneal dialysis patients. J Ren Nutr 2010;20(6):384–91.

[227] Dong J, Wang T, Wang HY. The impact of new comorbidities on nutritional status in continuous ambulatory peritoneal dialysis patients. Blood Purif 2006;24(5–6):517–23.

[228] Chung SH, Lindholm B, Lee HB. Is malnutrition an independent predictor of mortality in peritoneal dialysis patients? Nephrol Dial Transplant 2003;18(10):2134–40.

[229] United States Renal Data System. US Department of Public Health and Human Services, Public Health Service. Bethesda: National Institutes of Health; 2010.

[230] Lee SW, Park GH, Lee SW, Song JH, Hong KC, Kim MJ. Insulin resistance and muscle wasting in non-diabetic end-stage renal disease patients. Nephrol Dial Transplant 2007;22(9):2554–62.

[231] Kagan A, Altman Y, Zadik Z, Bar-Khayim Y. Insulin-like growth factor-I in patients on CAPD and hemodialysis: relationship to body weight and albumin level. Adv Perit Dial 1995;11:234–8.

[232] Heaton A, Johnston DG, Haigh JW, Ward MK, Alberti KG, Kerr DN. Twenty-four hour hormonal and metabolic profiles in uraemic patients before and during treatment with continuous ambulatory peritoneal dialysis. Clin Sci (Lond) 1985;69(4):449–57.

[233] Armstrong VW, Creutzfeldt W, Ebert R, Fuchs C, Hilgers R, Scheler F. Effect of dialysate glucose load on plasma glucose and glucoregulatory hormones in CAPD patients. Nephron 1985;39(2):141–5.

[234] Sherwin RS, Bastl C, Finkelstein FO, Fisher M, Black H, Hendler R, et al. Influence of uremia and hemodialysis on the turnover and metabolic effects of glucagon. J Clin Invest 1976;57(3):722–31.

[235] Heaton A, Johnston DG, Burrin JM, Orskov H, Ward MK, Alberti KG, et al. Carbohydrate and lipid metabolism during continuous ambulatory peritoneal dialysis (CAPD): the effect of a single dialysis cycle. Clin Sci (Lond) 1983;65(5):539–45.

[236] Taskapan MC, Taskapan H, Sahin I, Keskin L, Atmaca H, Ozyalin F. Serum leptin, resistin, and lipid levels in patients with end stage renal failure with regard to dialysis modality. Ren Fail. 2007;29(2):147–54.

[237] Tuzcu A, Bahceci M, Yilmaz ME, Turgut C, Kara IH. The determination of insulin sensitivity in hemodialysis and continuous ambulatory peritoneal dialysis in nondiabetic patients with end-stage renal disease. Saudi Med J 2005;26(5):786–91.

[238] Perez-Fontan M, Cordido F, Rodriguez-Carmona A, Peteiro J, Garcia-Naveiro R, Garcia-Buela J. Plasma ghrelin levels in patients undergoing haemodialysis and peritoneal dialysis. Nephrol Dial Transplant 2004;19(8):2095–100.

[239] Albaaj F, Sivalingham M, Haynes P, McKinnon G, Foley RN, Waldek S, et al. Prevalence of hypogonadism in male patients with renal failure. Postgrad Med J 2006;82(972):693–6.

[240] Semple CG, Beastall GH, Henderson IS, Thomson JA, Kennedy AC. The pituitary-testicular axis of uraemic subjects on haemodialysis and continuous ambulatory peritoneal dialysis. Acta Endocrinol (Copenh) 1982;101(3):464–7.

[241] Garber AJ. Effects of parathyroid hormone on skeletal muscle protein and amino acid metabolism in the rat. J Clin Invest 1983;71(6):1806–21.

[242] Drechsler C, Krane V, Grootendorst DC, Ritz E, Winkler K, Marz W, et al. The association between parathyroid hormone and mortality in dialysis patients is modified by wasting. Nephrol Dial Transplant 2009;24(10):3151–7.

[243] Prasad N, Gupta A, Sinha A, Sharma RK, Kumar A, Kumar R. Changes in nutritional status on follow-up of an incident cohort of continuous ambulatory peritoneal dialysis patients. J Ren Nutr 2008;18(2):195–201.

[244] McCusker FX, Teehan BP, Thorpe KE, Keshaviah PR, Churchill DN. How much peritoneal dialysis is required for the maintenance of a good nutritional state? Canada-USA (CAN-USA) Peritoneal Dialysis Study Group. Kidney Internat Supplement 1996;56:S56–61.

[245] Mehrotra R, Berman N, Alistwani A, Kopple JD. Improvement of nutritional status after initiation of maintenance hemodialysis. Am J Kidney Dis 2002;40(1):133–42.

[246] Paniagua R, Amato D, Vonesh E, Correa-Rotter R, Ramos A, Moran J, et al. Effects of increased peritoneal clearances on mortality rates in peritoneal dialysis: ADEMEX, a prospective, randomized, controlled trial. J Am Soc Nephrol 2002;13(5):1307–20.

[247] Lo WK, Ho YW, Li CS, Wong KS, Chan TM, Yu AW, et al. Effect of Kt/V on survival and clinical outcome in CAPD patients in a randomized prospective study. Kidney Int 2003;64:649–56.

[248] Martin-Del-Campo F, Gonzalez-Espinoza L, Rojas-Campos E, Ruiz N, Gonzalez J, Pazarin L, et al. Conventional nutritional counselling maintains nutritional status of patients on continuous ambulatory peritoneal dialysis in spite of systemic inflammation and decrease of residual renal function. Nephrology (Carlton) 2009;14(5):493–8.

[249] Costero O, Bajo MA, del Peso G, Gil F, Aguilera A, Ros S, et al. Treatment of anorexia and malnutrition in peritoneal dialysis patients with megestrol acetate. Adv Perit Dial 2004;20:209–12.

[250] Lien YH, Ruffenach SJ. Low dose megestrol increases serum albumin in malnourished dialysis patients. Int J Artif Organs 1996;19(3):147–50.

[251] Ashby DR, Ford HE, Wynne KJ, Wren AM, Murphy KG, Busbridge M, et al. Sustained appetite improvement in malnourished dialysis patients by daily ghrelin treatment. Kidney Int 2009;76(2):199–206.

[252] Wynne K, Giannitsopoulou K, Small CJ, Patterson M, Frost G, Ghatei MA, et al. Subcutaneous ghrelin enhances acute food intake in malnourished patients who receive maintenance peritoneal dialysis: a randomized, placebo-controlled trial. J Am Soc Nephrol 2005;16(7):2111–8.

[253] Gonzalez-Espinoza L, Gutierrez-Chavez J, del Campo FM, Martinez-Ramirez HR, Cortes-Sanabria L, Rojas-Campos E, et al. Randomized, open label, controlled clinical trial of oral administration of an egg albumin-based protein supplement to patients on continuous ambulatory peritoneal dialysis. Perit Dial Int 2005;25(2):173–80.

[254] Moretti HD, Johnson AM, Keeling-Hathaway TJ. Effects of protein supplementation in chronic hemodialysis and peritoneal dialysis patients. J Ren Nutr 2009;19(4):298–303.

[255] Eustace JA, Coresh J, Kutchey C, Te PL, Gimenez LF, Scheel PJ, et al. Randomized double-blind trial of oral essential amino acids for dialysis-associated hypoalbuminemia. Kidney Int 2000;57(6):2527–38.

[256] Aguirre Galindo BA, Prieto Fierro JG, Cano P, Abularach L, Nieves Renteria A, Navarro M, et al. Effect of polymeric diets in patients on continuous ambulatory peritoneal dialysis. Perit Dial Int 2003;23(5):434–9.

[257] Stratton RJ, Bircher G, Fouque D, Stenvinkel P, de Mutsert R, Engfer M, et al. Multinutrient oral supplements and tube feeding in maintenance dialysis: a systematic review and meta-analysis. Am J Kidney Dis 2005;46(3):387–405.

[258] Jones M, Hagen T, Boyle CA, Vonesh E, Hamburger R, Charytan C, et al. Treatment of malnutrition with 1.1% amino acid peritoneal dialysis solution: results of a multicenter outpatient study. Am J Kidney Dis 1998;32(5):761–9.

[259] Grzegorzewska AE, Mariak I, Dobrowolska-Zachwieja A, Szajdak L. Effects of amino acid dialysis solution on the nutrition of continuous ambulatory peritoneal dialysis patients. Perit Dial Int 1999;19(5):462–70.

[260] Dervisoglu E, Ozdemir O, Yilmaz A. Commencing peritoneal dialysis with 1.1% amino acid solution does not influence biochemical nutritional parameters in incident CAPD patients. Ren Fail 2010;32(6):653–8.

[261] Tjiong HL, van den Berg JW, Wattimena JL, Rietveld T, van Dijk LJ, van der Wiel AM, et al. Dialysate as food: combined amino acid and glucose dialysate improves protein anabolism in renal failure patients on automated peritoneal dialysis. J Am Soc Nephrol 2005;16(5):1486–93.

[262] Tjiong HL, Rietveld T, Wattimena JL, van den Berg JW, Kahriman D, van der Steen J, et al. Peritoneal dialysis with solutions containing amino acids plus glucose promotes protein synthesis during oral feeding. Clin J Am Soc Nephrol 2007;2(1): 74–80.

[263] Stein A, Moorhouse J, Iles-Smith H, Baker F, Johnstone J, James G, et al. Role of an improvement in acid-base status and nutrition in CAPD patients. Kidney Int 1997;52(4): 1089–95.

[264] Szeto CC, Wong TY, Chow KM, Leung CB, Li PK. Oral sodium bicarbonate for the treatment of metabolic acidosis in peritoneal dialysis patients: a randomized placebo-control trial. J Am Soc Nephrol 2003;14(8):2119–26.

[265] Mehrotra R, Bross R, Wang H, Appell M, Tso L, Kopple JD. Effect of high-normal compared with low-normal arterial pH on protein balances in automated peritoneal dialysis patients. Am J Clin Nutr 2009;90(6):1532–40.

[266] de Brito-Ashurst I, Varagunam M, Raftery MJ, Yaqoob MM. Bicarbonate supplementation slows progression of CKD and improves nutritional status. Journal of the Am Soc Nephrol 2009;20(9):2075–84.

[267] Dombros NV, Digenis GE, Soliman G, Oreopoulos DG. Anabolic steroids in the treatment of malnourished CAPD patients: a retrospective study. Perit Dial Int 1994;14(4): 344–7.

[268] Navarro JF, Mora C, Macia M, Garcia J. Randomized prospective comparison between erythropoietin and androgens in CAPD patients. Kidney Int 2002;61(4):1537–44.

[269] Navarro JF, Mora-Fernandez C, Rivero A, Macia M, Gallego E, Chahin J, et al. Androgens for the treatment of anemia in peritoneal dialysis patients. Adv Perit Dial 1998;14:232–5.

[270] Aramwit P, Palapinyo S, Wiwatniwong S, Supasyndh O. The efficacy of oxymetholone in combination with erythropoietin on hematologic parameters and muscle mass in CAPD patients. Int J Clin Pharmacol Ther 2010;48(12):803–13.

[271] Ikizler TA, Wingard RL, Breyer JA, Schulman G, Parker RA, Hakim RM. Short-term effects of recombinant human growth hormone in CAPD patients. Kidney Int 1994;46(4): 1178–83.

[272] Iglesias P, Diez JJ, Fernandez-Reyes MJ, Aguilera A, Burgues S, Martinez-Ara J, et al. Recombinant human growth hormone therapy in malnourished dialysis patients: a randomized controlled study. Am J Kidney Dis 1998;32(3):454–63.

[273] Fouque D, Peng SC, Shamir E, Kopple JD. Recombinant human insulin-like growth factor-1 induces an anabolic response in malnourished CAPD patients. Kidney Int 2000;57(2):646–54.

[274] Sundl I, Roob JM, Meinitzer A, Tiran B, Khoschsorur G, Haditsch B, et al. Antioxidant status of patients on peritoneal dialysis: associations with inflammation and glycoxidative stress. Perit Dial Int 2009;29(1):89–101.

[275] Mydlik M, Derzsiova K, Racz O, Sipulova A, Lovasova E. Antioxidant therapy by oral vitamin E and vitamin E-coated dialyzer in CAPD and haemodialysis patients. Prague Med Rep 2006;107(3):354–64.

[276] Uzum A, Toprak O, Gumustas MK, Ciftci S, Sen S. Effect of vitamin E therapy on oxidative stress and erythrocyte osmotic fragility in patients on peritoneal dialysis and hemodialysis. J Nephrol 2006;19(6):739–45.

[277] de Vecchi AF, Novembrino C, Patrosso MC, Cresseri D, Ippolito S, Rosina M, et al. Effect of incremental doses of folate on homocysteine and metabolically related vitamin concentrations in nondiabetic patients on peritoneal dialysis. Asaio J 2003;49(6):655–9.

[278] Kopple JD, Mercurio K, Blumenkrantz MJ, Jones MR, Tallos J, Roberts C, et al. Daily requirement for pyridoxine supplements in chronic renal failure. Kidney Int 1981;19(5):694–704.

[279] Ross EA, Shah GM, Reynolds RD, Sabo A, Pichon M. Vitamin B6 requirements of patients on chronic peritoneal dialysis. Kidney Int 1989;36(4):702–6.

[280] Stein G, Sperschneider H, Koppe S. Vitamin levels in chronic renal failure and need for supplementation. Blood Purif 1985;3(1–3):52–62.

[281] Grabe DW. Update on clinical practice recommendations and new therapeutic modalities for treating anemia in patients with chronic kidney disease. Am J Health Syst Pharm 2007;64(13 Suppl. 8):S8–14. quiz S23–5.

[282] Arreola F, Paniagua R, Perez A, Diaz-Bensussen S, Junco E, Villalpando S, et al. Effect of zinc treatment on serum thyroid hormones in uremic patients under peritoneal dialysis. Horm Metab Res. 1993;25(10):539–42.

[283] National Research Council. Recommended dietary allowances. 10th ed. Washington. DC: National Academy Press; 1989.

[284] Mehrotra R, Kopple JD. Nutritional management of maintenance dialysis patients: why aren't we doing better? Annu Rev Nutr 2001;21:343–79.

Nutritional Management of Kidney Transplant Recipients

Maria Chan¹, Steve Chadban²

¹The St George Hospital and University of New South Wales, New South Wales, Australia
²Royal Prince Alfred Hospital and University of Sydney, New South Wales, Australia

INTRODUCTION

Successful kidney transplantation largely corrects the metabolic abnormalities associated with uremia and dialysis in patients with end-stage kidney disease (ESKD). However, side effects of immunosuppressive medication and the change of lifestyle after transplantation introduce a new set of metabolic abnormalities which, together with pre-existing co-morbidities, significantly impact on short and long-term health outcomes for kidney transplant recipients (KTR).

Nutritional challenges change over time posttransplant (Figure 34.1). Fasting and immobilization related to surgery, delayed graft function necessitating ongoing dialysis, wound complications, gut disturbances and other events that may occur in the first weeks and months after transplantation may contribute to undernutrition generally or isolated nutrient deficiency. Individualized management is frequently required, including supplemental feeding in selected cases. Once kidney function is restored and surgical recovery is complete, dietary attention to avoid excessive weight gain is frequently required as the effects of steroids, resolution of uremia and relative dietary freedom as compared to dialysis all contribute to enhanced appetite and over-eating. Diabetes is common, both pre-existing and new-onset diabetes after transplantation, and specific advice is required to achieve glycemic control. Consumption of contaminated food poses greater threats to the KTR than it does to members of the general population and avoidance requires specific nutrition education. In the longer term, nutrition requirements may change again as long-term complications such as cardiovascular disease, cancer and kidney transplant dysfunction or failure increase in prevalence, all requiring individualized dietary strategies.

In clinical practice, a comprehensive and structured care process should be established to integrate medical and nutrition management of the transplant recipients. In 2006, a working group of transplant physicians and renal dieticians undertook a comprehensive review of existing literature to develop evidence based practice guidelines on the nutritional management of adult kidney transplant recipients [1]. These guidelines were subject to expert panel reviews and public consultation by renal clinicians and consumers before receiving final endorsement by two authorities in Australia — The Caring for Australasians with Renal Impairment (CARI) guidelines group [2] and the Dietitians Association of Australia (DAA) evidence based practice guidelines [3]. To complement the guidelines, an executive summary and a set of patient education resources were developed to facilitate translation of the guidelines into practice.

This chapter builds upon these guidelines by updating the literature on key nutrition problems faced in the management of KTRs. We discuss the epidemiology and the contribution of diet to each problem, and the potential role of nutrition intervention. We discuss what is known, what needs to be known and what can be done in terms of nutrition management for each condition. We conclude with a general, practical approach to the nutrition management of KTRs.

ANEMIA

Anemia is defined as hemoglobin (Hb) concentration of 12 g/dL or less in women and 13 g/dL or less in men. It is common in both nondialysed and dialysed patients with end-stage kidney disease (ESKD). Treatment with erythropoiesis stimulating agents is recommended to

Kidney function

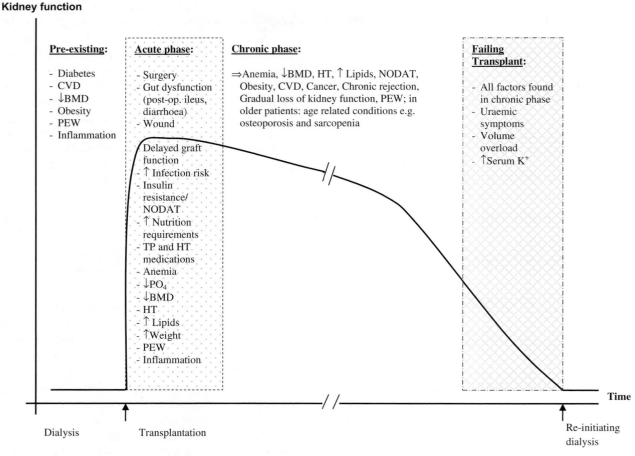

FIGURE 34.1   Schematic diagram showing nutritional and related factors affecting kidney transplant recipients.

achieve target hemoglobin concentrations within the range of 11.0 to 12.0 g/dL [4]. Posttransplant anemia (PTA) is common both early and late after transplantation [5–9] and is an independent risk factor for cardiovascular death, graft failure and all-cause mortality [10,11]. Successful kidney transplantation leads to an increase in erythropoietin (EPO) production and for the majority of KTRs, this corrects anemia over an 8–10 week period [5]. However, approximately 30% of KTRs remain anemic. Impaired kidney transplant function is the dominant cause of PTA, however other transplant-related factors are also contributory [12] including blood losses, bone marrow suppression by immunosuppressant medication, inflammation [13,14], and antihypertensive therapy using angiotensin-converting enzyme inhibitors (ACEi) [15] and angiotensin II receptor blockers (ARB) [16]. From a nutritional perspective, both generalized protein–energy malnutrition [14,17,18] and specific nutrient deficiencies, such as iron, folate and vitamin B_{12} [8,19–23], may be contributory to posttransplant anemia. Whilst nutrient deficiency may be an aggravating factor, impaired kidney function and medications appear to be the main causes [24,25] and there is little evidence to suggest dietary

intervention alone would correct anemia after transplant. It is suggested that all adult kidney transplant recipients should be monitored for anemia and, when present, it is appropriate to assess nutritional status and use pharmacological doses of nutrients in conjunction with dietary interventions to correct anemia if required [26]. As part of a healthy balanced diet, adequate food consumption to meet the recommended daily intake (RDI) [27] of iron, folate, vitamins B_6 and B_{12} is recommended to enable adequate hemoglobin synthesis. Supplementation of nutrients e.g. iron at pharmacological oral doses, appears to be safe and is recommended by the Kidney Disease Improving Global Outcomes (KDIGO) for anemia [28].

BONE DISEASE

Metabolic bone disease is highly prevalent among patients with end-stage kidney disease. After transplantation, immobility, steroids and other immunosuppressants, and the effects of residual hyperparathyroidism may exacerbate existing abnormalities [29]. A rapid decline in bone mineral density (BMD) may occur during the early posttransplant phase [30] and may continue during the first 2 years posttransplant [31,32]. Nutritional status is relevant in that calcium deficiency [33], a low body weight [34], low body mass index (BMI) and low 25 hydroxy vitamin D levels have been found to correlate with low BMD posttransplant [35]. Low BMD posttransplant has been associated with significantly elevated rates of fracture as compared to the general population [36], with 22.5% of patients developing a fracture within 5 years [37]. Related to metabolic bone disease, KTRs are also at high risk of vascular calcification [38].

There are no published data examining the role of diet per se in preventing and managing bone disease in adult KRTs. However, intervention studies administering pharmacological doses of vitamin D or analogue, with or without calcium [35,39–42] or bisphosphonates [43] were found to be effective in preventing bone loss and reducing the risk of bone fracture. Typical doses of vitamin D and calcium supplementation ranged from 0.25 to 0.5 µg/d and 500 to 1500 mg/d respectively. Some of these findings are further supported by the Cochrane systematic review which included twenty four trials (1299 patients) [44] examining the effects of bisphosphonates, vitamin D or calcitonin. In summary, none of the individual agents reduced fracture risk compared to placebo. However, combination therapy was associated with a reduction in the relative risk (RR) of fracture (RR 0.51, 95% CI 0.27 to 0.99). For improvement in BMD, bisphosphonates (any route) and vitamin D both had a beneficial effect at the lumbar spine and neck of femoral, whereas calcitonin provide improvement at the lumbar spine only. Bisphosphonates have greater efficacy to prevent BMD loss when compared with vitamin D sterols. Across all RCTs, supplementation appeared safe and adverse effects were seldom reported. The optimal route, timing, dosages and duration of these interventions remain unknown. A weakness common to most studies is the failure to assess or mandate dietary intake of calcium. There is little evidence that calcium supplementation alone is effective in maintaining BMD or reducing bone fracture risk, however, dietary supplementation with 500 mg elemental calcium daily may provide effective suppression of PTH [45].

The primary management goal is to minimize BMD loss, particularly during the early posttransplant phase. The need for and dose of medications and supplements should be determined on an individual basis with ongoing monitoring. CARI guidelines recommend a vitamin D (or analogue) supplement at a dose of 0.25–0.5 µg calcitriol (1,25-dihydroxyvitamin D) daily [46] and to combine with calcium supplementation. KDIGO [47] and Kidney Disease Outcomes Quality Initiative (K/DOQI) [48] guidelines for post-renal transplantation bone disease management provide comprehensive treatment algorithm for the supplementation of vitamin D (or analogue) and calcium and use of bisphosphonates including a recommended monitoring schedule for serum calcium, phosphorus and PTH.

Although there are no studies to suggest the efficacy of dietary intervention alone in the management of MBD posttransplant, recipients are encouraged to consume an adequate diet to meet the RDIs [27,49] for age and gender with respect to calcium (1000–1300 mg/day) and vitamin D (5–15 µg/day assuming limited sun exposure to prevent the development of skin cancer), with consideration given to supplementation if dietary intake is assessed to be inadequate.

DIABETES MELLITUS

New-onset diabetes after transplantation (NODAT), is a complex metabolic disorder which develops in an additional 10–40% of KTRs during the first year post-transplantation [50–52], differing according to patient factors, immunosuppressive regimen and method of diagnosis. Whilst many studies have reported incidence defined by use of insulin or oral hypoglycemic agents, current consensus recommends the diagnosis be made in accordance with American Diabetes Association criteria, similar to the non-transplant patients. The DIRECT trial [53] applied such criteria, including a protocolized oral glucose tolerance test at month 3 posttransplant, to patients receiving either tacrolimus or cyclosporine together with mycophenolate and maintenance prednisone and reported an incidence of NODAT of 33.6% for tacrolimus treated patients and 26.0 %, P = 0.046 for those randomized to cyclosporine. In addition to NODAT, pre-existing diabetes is typically the cause of kidney failure in 10–20% of those who receive a kidney transplant, thus the total prevalence of diabetes may approach 50% among KTRs. The prevalence of the metabolic syndrome posttransplant is even greater [51,54].

Pre-existing diabetes, NODAT and, to a lesser extent, impaired fasting glucose and impaired glucose tolerance, all have clear prognostic implications, with the key impact being an increase in risk of cardiovascular morbidity and mortality and overall mortality after transplant [55,56]. The pathogenesis of NODAT involves both insulin resistance and insulin deficiency. From a dietary perspective, pretransplant obesity and impaired glucose tolerance are key risk factors for the development of NODAT. Whilst studies are yet to demonstrate that a diet and exercise program to achieve weight loss pretransplant can prevent NODAT, in the authors opinion this would seem to be a reasonable strategy and warrants study. Dietary management posttransplant to either avoid NODAT or manage NODAT should it develop is again relatively unstudied but likely to be crucial. Early posttransplant, whilst sufficient nutrition is required to facilitate wound headlining and surgical recovery, efforts are also required to aid control of diabetes if present through prescription of a healthy, balanced, low-GI diet designed to avoid weight gain. Specifically, patients should be advised to consume approximately 50% carbohydrate-containing foods which are rich in dietary fiber and of low glycemic index (from whole grain cereals and grain products, fruits, vegetables and legumes); total energy as fat should be less than 30% with less than 10% energy as total saturated fat [57–60]. For patients nondiabetic prior to transplant, dietary assessment and advice designed to minimize undesirable weight gain to minimize risk of developing obesity and diabetes is logical, though as yet unproven.

DYSLIPIDEMIA

According to the National Kidney Foundation KDOQI [61] and the Adult Treatment Panel III [62] definitions, dyslipidemia is the presence of one or more of the following: total serum cholesterol, ≥ 200 mg/dL; LDL-cholesterol ≥ 130 mg/dL; triglycerides, ≥ 150 mg/dL; HDL-cholesterol ≤ 40 mg/dL. Dyslipidemia is common after renal transplantation affecting approximately 60% of patients, both early and late posttransplant [63]. A typical lipid profile of transplant recipients includes elevated total serum cholesterol and low-density lipoprotein cholesterol (LDL-C), with variable high-density lipoprotein cholesterol (HDL-C) and triglycerides [63–65].

While dyslipidemia and CVD are often present at the time of transplantation, immunosuppressive medications including calcineurin inhibitors, the mTOR-inhibitors sirolimus and everolimus, and corticosteroids, lifestyle factors, weight gain, physical inactivity combine to exacerbate pre-existing and promote development of de novo dyslipidemia posttransplantation [66]. Dyslipidemia is positively associated with atherosclerotic cardiovascular disease [67] and with cardiovascular death posttransplant [63]. A number of intervention studies have examined the safety and efficacy of dietary management in kidney transplant patients with dyslipidemia. In a small, single center, randomized controlled trial the effects of a modified Mediterranean diet (n = 21) were compared with a control group (n = 20) over a six-month study period [68]. The modified Mediterranean diet was carbohydrate rich, low glycemic index (GI), and vitamin E rich, including whole grain products, nuts and seeds, fruit and vegetables, moderate protein serves and olive oil (monounsaturated fats) with energy derived 15% from protein, 47% carbohydrates

(CHO) and 38% fat; whereas the isocaloric diet of the control group was a standard low fat diet of a typical of Central European dietary pattern, significantly higher GI with energy distribution 17% from protein, 26% fat and 57% CHO. Lipid lowering medication was not permitted and immunosuppressive therapy was unchanged throughout the study period. No significant differences in weight, BMI or body fat were observed, however a decrease in total cholesterol from 230 to 210 mg/dL or 5.9 to 5.4 mmol/L (P < 0.02) and triglycerides, from 194 to 152 mg/dL, or 2.5 to1.7 mmol/L (P < 0.0007) was achieved. The effect was apparent two months after the study commenced and persisted throughout the study period [69]. The results were similar to those achieved in non-transplant populations. In a twelve month prospective intervention study [70], 46 patients recruited within their first year post kidney transplant were advised to consume a diet according to the American Heart Association (AHA) Step One Diet [71]. The diet plan featured energy >25 kcal/kg IBW/day, ~55% energy from CHO, <30% energy from fat, cholesterol <300 mg/d, protein ~0.8 g/kg IBW/d and <4.5 g/d of salt. Patients were also advised to increase their physical activity levels to include exercise for 30 minutes per day for 5 days per week. At three months after the diet commenced, patients were divided into a compliant group (group diet, n = 25) in which patients had been at least 90% compliant with the prescribed diet as assessed by a detailed food-frequency questionnaire; the control group (n = 21) consisted of the remaining "non-compliant" patients. At the end of the study period, the diet group showed a significant reduction in body weight (10.4% in male), BMI (11.4% in male), serum cholesterol (male:female ~25%:20%) and glucose (male:female 17%:9%), whereas all these parameters deteriorated in the control group. Triglycerides remained unchanged in either group.

Other intervention studies in KTRs have been pseudo-randomized controlled [72] or uncontrolled [73–75] but also support the lipid lowering benefit of regimens in line with the Mediterranean style diet and American Heart Association (AHA) Step One diet [76]. In a case-control observational study of stable KTRs (n = 15) with moderate hypercholesterolemia, a 5-week substitution of 25 g of animal protein with 25 g of soy protein (mean 26 ± 8 g/day) in their usual diet showed a significant decrease in total cholesterol (254 ± 22 to 231 ± 31 mg/dL, P < 0.05) and LDL cholesterol (165 ± 20 vs. 143 ± 20 mg/dL, P < 0.01) while no significant change was found in HDL cholesterol and triglycerides [77].

In summary, the dietary recommendations for post-transplantation dyslipidemia are in line with national dietary guidelines for healthy adults [58,62] and renal guidelines [78] that a diet should be high in wholegrain, plant foods (including fruit, vegetables and legumes rich in phytosterols), of low glycemic index, high in dietary fiber (soluble and insoluble) and rich in sources of vitamin E and monounsaturated fats. Overweight/ obese patients should lose weight through an energy controlled diet combined with an increase in exercise.

HYPERTENSION

Hypertension (HT) is common after renal transplantation, present in 50% to 80% of patients. HT is a risk factor for chronic allograft injury, premature graft failure and cardiovascular morbidity and mortality [79–81]. Risk factors for posttransplant HT include male sex, age, donor age, the presence of diabetes, weight gain, body mass index and delayed graft function; other contributing factors are immunosuppressant medications used e.g. calcineurin inhibitors and prednisone. Blood pressure target is <130/80 mmHg for adult patients and pharmacological interventions are often necessary [82].

Studies of dietary intervention to lower blood pressure in this population are limited in the literature which consists of a number of small RCTs and uncontrolled intervention studies.

The efficacy of sodium restriction to lower blood pressure in general and non-transplant populations has been well studied [83,84]. However, sodium restriction remains controversial in KTRs. One observational study, in which patients (n = 244) were given dietary counseling in accordance with the Dietary Approaches to Stop Hypertension (DASH) guidelines, found no correlation between systolic (SBP) or diastolic pressure (DBP) and 24-h urine excretion of sodium [85]. One small RCT which examined the effect of dietician-supervised dietary sodium restriction (80–100 mmol/ day) for three months (n = 18) demonstrated a significant reduction in urinary sodium excretion (190 ± 75 to 108 ± 48 mEq/d, P < 0.0001), both SBP (146 ± 21 to 116 ± 11 mmHg, P < 0.0001), DBP (89 ± 8 to 72 ± 10 mmHg, P < 0.0001) and use of anti-hypertensive medications. The control group (n = 14) did not show any significant change in urinary sodium, SBP or DBP.

The effect of fish oil on renal hemodynamics and blood pressure was examined in a 12 month randomized double blind study using 6 gram fish oil/day over the study period in cyclosporine–prednisolone treated patients (n = 33) vs. the control group (n = 33) using 6 g/d coconut oil which was ceased at 3 months. Both groups were also advised to restrict salt intake to <3 g/day. At the end of the study period, the intervention group has significantly lower mean arterial pressure (103 vs. 118 mmHg, P = 0.001) and required significantly less antihypertensive medication [86]. Other advantages included a significant higher glomerular filtration rate

(53 vs. 40 mL/min/1.73 m², P = 0.038), effective renal plasma flow (214 vs. 178 mL/min/1.73 m², P = 0.023) and less acute rejection (8 vs. 20, P = 0.029) with a trend toward superior one-year graft survival (97 vs. 84 %, P = 0.097). However, other dietary and lifestyle factors known to have blood pressure lowering effects were not monitored.

It has been postulated that hypertensive kidney transplant recipients may have low levels of nitric oxide (NO) and abnormal NO-mediated vasodilatation; therefore administering of L-arginine (ARG), a precursor of NO, may increase NO bioavailability and may restore the NO-mediated vasodilatory response thus lowering blood pressure. In a randomized crossover study, the blood pressure lowering effects of twice daily of 4.5 g L-arginine over 2 months was examined in 20 hypertensive kidney transplant recipients [87]. After the first 2 months, there was a significant reduction in SBP from baseline (from 155.9 ± 5.0 to 143.2 ± 3.2 mmHg, P = 0.03), DBP was also reduced after supplementation. Once the supplementation was ceased, both SBP and DBP increased significantly. Again confounders such as dietary and lifestyle factors were not monitored.

Effects of weight loss, dietary pattern and structure care programs on blood pressure control in this population have seldom been investigated. However, there is strong evidence of these nutrition interventions in the general or non-kidney transplant populations to lower blood pressure. The Dietary Approaches to Stop Hypertension (DASH) [88] and DASH-sodium [83] trials were controlled feeding dietary trials which examined the effect of dietary pattern to lower blood pressure in the absence of weight loss in the non-renal population. While the sodium intake remained as usual, the combination diet studied in the DASH trial was low in saturated fat (≤7%) and total fat, rich in plant-based foods consisting of wholegrains, nuts, fruit and vegetables and low fat dairy products. Therefore the study diet was high in nutrients and food components that are known to benefit cardiovascular health, e.g. potassium, magnesium, calcium, mono- and poly- and unsaturated fats, vitamin E, dietary fiber and antioxidants. This eight week feeding trial reduced SBP and DBP by 11.4 and 5.5 mmHg (P < 0.001) respectively in the study group compared to the control group that continued with a typical American eating habit which is high in fat and sodium. In the DASH-sodium trial, the additional reduction of sodium levels from the usual diet of ~150 mmol/d to ~100 mmol/d or to ~60 mmol/d reduced SBP by 1.3 mmHg (P = 0.03) and further 1.7 mmHg (P < 0.01) respectively. These landmark trials showed the dose response of sodium restriction to blood pressure control and supported dietary management of hypertension with effects comparable to those of antihypertensive medications. The added benefits of exercise to the DASH diet were demonstrated in the Diet, Exercise, and Weight Loss Intervention Trial (DEW-IT) trial [89] and a 12-week supervised aerobic exercises program [90]. Furthermore, other dietary intervention studies engaging sodium reduction [84,91,92], weight loss [91,93] and limiting of alcohol consumption [94] also demonstrated beneficial effects. In the PREMIER trial [95] the study group received structured dietetic care and intensive behavioral intervention has better changes to diet and physical activity level, thus significant reduction in weight and blood pressure over the control in free living individuals.

In summary, there have been no large scale studies conducted to determine whether nutrition intervention alone is effective in managing hypertension in KTRs. However, a number of small studies with KTRs and in significant clinical trials in the nonrenal transplant population demonstrated the efficacy of nutrition intervention to lower blood pressure. Patients are encouraged to control sodium intake to 80–100 mmol/day or a no added salt diet, together with a healthy balanced diet with optimal energy (calories), rich in wholegrain and plant-based foods, include calcium rich low fat dairy products, limit to no more than two standard drinks of alcohol (20 g) on any day and with at least two alcohol free days per week, and to take up moderate intensity physical activity as per the dietary guidelines recommendation for healthy adults [58,96]. Overweight or obese individuals are encouraged and be supported to lose weight.

FOOD SAFETY

Food-borne illness, such as listeria, may impose a serious infection risk for a person who is immunocompromised. Solid-organ transplant (SOT) recipients, including the KTRs are at increased risk of listeriosis. However, there is little data in the literature on the incidence of listeriosis in KTRs. In a sample of 177 kidney transplant recipients studied, listeria carriage rate was approximately 5.6% and no subjects developed listeria infection [97]. Listeriosis in SOT recipients was found to be uncommon in a matched case-control study of the risk factors, clinical features and outcomes of listeriosis. [98], Over a 12-year study period, among 25,997 SOT recipients in 15 Spanish transplant centers, 30 cases (0.12%) of listeriosis was identified including eight cases in KTRs. Although the incidence was low, 30-day mortality rate was very high. Diabetes mellitus, cytomegalovirus (CMV) infection, and high-dose steroids were identified to be independent risk factors for listeriosis. The source of infection was not reported in this study. In another observational study of 102 cases of listeriosis in KTRs, the manifestations included

meningitis, bacteremia, and pneumonia and a mortality rate of 26% was reported. Neither the incidence rate nor the sources of the infection were reported [99].

In summary, although listeriosis is uncommon, the morbidity and mortality risks are high. There is no study to investigate the role of food hygiene practice to prevent food-borne infection in KTRs. While there is no evidence to support the use of a strict low bacteria diet, it is prudent to observe general food safety measures recommended by the local food safety authorities [100–102]. Listeria is mainly found in certain types of foods, in particular, the ready-to-eat or preprepared foods that have not been handled or stored correctly after processing. Therefore, it is reasonable to advise KTRs to observe good hygiene practice. Foods that are known to harbor listeria should be avoided, e.g. soft cheeses, sandwich meats, sashimi, sushi, paté, cold foods served in buffets, chilled seafood such as raw oysters and smoked fish, especially during the first 3 months posttransplant or any time when high doses of immunosuppressants are used.

HYPOPHOSPHATEMIA

Hypophosphatemia is common in KTRs affecting about 90% of patients in both acute and chronic phases of transplantation. Onset is typically within days to weeks after transplant function is established, severity is maximal during the first weeks–months after transplant when immunosuppressant exposure is highest and in most cases serum phosphate spontaneously returns toward the normal range over the next year [103]. Hypophosphatemia has negative effects on muscular systems causing muscle weakness; in the case of severe hypophosphatemia, rhabdomyolysis, respiratory failure, hemolysis and left ventricular dysfunction may occur. Factors contributing to posttransplant hypophosphatemia include reduced intestinal phosphate absorption, high urinary phosphate losses caused by immunosuppressants and tubular damage, and rapid disposal of phosphate into bone and soft tissues caused by persistent hyperparathyroidism and increased levels of FGF-23 [104–106]. In a 12-week pseudo-randomized controlled study [107] involving early-KTRs with a mean transplant vintage of one month and serum phosphate within the range 0.3–0.75 mmol/L, administration of oral neutral sodium phosphate significantly corrected hypophosphatemia compared to controls who received sodium chloride. All patients were also encouraged to consume a diet rich in phosphorus, e.g. meat and dairy products, during the study period. Those patients receiving the phosphate supplement were also found to have increased muscular adenosine triphosphate (ATP) and phosphodiester content without affecting mineral metabolism. In a prospective intervention study [108] in KTRs with transplant vintage of 41 ± 18 months, supplementation of 1.5 g oral neutral phosphate to usual diet for 15 days led to a significant reduction of serum calcium and 1,25-dihydroxycholecalciferol concentrations ($P < 0.0003$ and $P < 0.0006$, respectively) and these were accompanied by a significant reduction in urinary calcium excretion ($P < 00001$). However, there was a significant increase in serum phosphorus, PTH levels and urinary phosphorus excretion ($P < 0.0001$, $P < 0.0001$ and $P < 0.0001$ respectively). There has been no study to examine if adequate dietary phosphate intake alone could prevent or reverse hypophosphatemia. In managing KTRs with hypophosphatemia, careful clinical judgment and monitoring are required as phosphate supplementation may also have undesired effects including nausea and diarrhea, and as reported in a case of early post-kidney transplant hypercalcemia (2.59 mmol/L) and hypophosphatemia (<0.32 mmol/L), phosphate supplementation ($\sim$1500 mg/d) led to acute phosphate nephropathy [109]. Phosphate supplementation also has the potential to exacerbate hyperparathyroidism in the late posttransplantation period [108]. Our recommendation is to attempt dietary replacement before resorting to supplementation, and only doing so in severe cases (<0.40 mmol/L despite a high phosphate diet).

In summary, KRTs should be encouraged to consume phosphorous-rich foods as part of a healthy diet once the graft is functioning; individalized supplementation of phosphate with careful clinical judgment should be considered if hypophosphatemia persists [110].

OVERWEIGHT/OBESITY

Post-kidney transplant weight gain resulting in overweight (BMI 25–30) and obesity (BMI $\geq$30 kg/m^2) is common, likely due to the combined effects of restoration of kidney function and prednisone in enhancing appetite. A well functioning kidney relieves uremic anorexia, improves sense of well-being and enables removal of previous dietary restrictions required for dialysis. The magnitude of weight gain is typically between 10–35%, it occurs mostly in the first year posttransplant [111–113] and is often associated with an increase in fat mass rather than muscle mass [114,115]. While desirable weight gain may be necessary to correct undernutrition if present, the development and degree of obesity posttransplant are associated with poor early and long term outcomes [116–118]. High BMI at the time of transplant [116,119,120], within one year posttransplant [121,122], high magnitude of weight gain [118] and abdominal obesity [123] are all associated with

inferior outcomes which in the short term include perioperative complications such as wound infection and poor healing [124,125], delayed graft function (DGF), prolonged hospitalization, acute rejection [116]; and long-term chronic allograft nephropathy (CAN) [122] and decreased overall graft and patient survival [116,119,121]. Obesity may act as an independent factor [121] or through the development of co-morbidities e.g. coronary artery disease, hypertension, dyslipidemia and NODAT [117]. Obesity is also known to correlate with other metabolic and hormonal derangements that are associated with poor CV outcomes, these include metabolic syndrome, glucose intolerance, insulin resistance [126–128], inflammation and elevated CRP [129], hypoadiponectinemia [130] and hyperhomocysteinemia [131]. Some studies have shown that with careful management, obesity in KTRs may not be associated with inferior outcomes [132,133].

A number of dietary intervention studies have demonstrated improvements in body weight and other health outcomes in overweight and obese KTRs. In a RCT engaging multidisciplinary lifestyle intervention to modify CV risks in KTRs with abnormal glucose tolerance [134], the study group (n = 56) received supervised care by dietitian while the control group received standard care (n = 46). Dietary intervention consisted of a Mediterranean-style diet with 30% total energy from fat, of low glycemic index with a moderate energy deficit of 500 kcal/day (2000 kJ/day) to aim 0.5 kg of weight loss per week. The mean transplant vintage was approximately 4.3 years. At the 2-year follow-up, the study group had healthier eating habits compared to the control group with significantly lower intake of total fat, 54 g (16–105 g) vs. 65 g (34–118 g), $P = 0.05$ and saturated fat, 10% (5–17%) vs. 13% (4–20%) as a proportion of total energy, $P = 0.05$. There was a trend for the overweight, but not obese patients to lose weight, 4% loss vs. a gain of 0.25% in the study group compared to the control. Weight loss of >5% was correlated with improvement of HDL-cholesterol over time. In addition, patients were given general advice on physical activity to aim 150 minutes of accumulated physical activity per week such as walking and structured activity of daily living as recommended by the National Physical Activity Guidelines for Australians [135]. Despite the individualized goals and plans set for each patient, simple exercise advice did not generate any improvement in reported physical activity or cardio-respiratory fitness measured by peak oxygen uptake (VO$_2$ max) at the end of the study period. In view of the high transplant vintage of ~4.3 years at enrolment, it appears challenging to reverse obesity in these chronic metabolically deranged patients. Perhaps early intervention to prevent undesirable weight gain may be a more effective measure.

In a small nonrandomized prospective intervention study [136], the study group (n = 11) received intensive dietetic intervention weekly for the first four months after transplant then no further input; and weight and BMI data were compared to a historical control group (n = 22) who had received no dietetic intervention. Dietetic intervention included individualized diet prescription for energy and macro- (protein, carbohydrates, fats and alcohol) and micro- (e.g. sodium, calcium and iron) nutrients, dietary fiber, food hygiene and practical advice for weight control such as food choice, behavioral modification and exercise. Both the study and control groups gained weight (BMI) over the study period; at baseline: 67 ± 13 kg (24.1 ± 3.9 kg/m^2) vs. 67 ± 11 kg (23.7 ± 3.4 kg/m^2), NS; at 4 month: 69 ± 12 kg (24.6 ± 3.5 kg/m^2) vs. 74 ± 9 kg (26.3 ± 3.3 kg/m^2), P = 0.01 and 1 year: 73 ± 12 kg (26.1 ± 3.4 kg/m^2) vs. 79 ± 12 kg (27.9 ± 4 kg/m^2), P = 0.01 respectively. The study group had significantly less mean weight gain than the control at 4 months (1.4 vs. 7.1 kg, P = 0.01) and at 1 year (5.5 vs. 11.8 kg, P = 0.01). The results support early intensive dietary advice and follow-up to control weight gain in the first year posttransplant.

As discussed in the dyslipidemia section previously, in a six-month uncontrolled prospective intervention study [74] involving KTRs (n = 23) who were hyperlipidemic and with a BMI >27 kg/m^2, individualized intervention by a dietitian using the American Heart Association (AHA) Step One Diet resulted in a significant decrease in CV risk factors. The significant reductions were intakes of total energy/calories (632 kcal/d, P > 0.001), total fat (9.2%, P > 0.001), cholesterol (131 mg/d P > 0.01); and body weight (3.2 ± 2.9 kg, P < 0.001), body fat measured by triceps skinfold (P < 0.05), bioelectrical impedance (P < 0.001) and infrared interactance (P < 0.01). Serum lipid profile improved in all patients with a decrease in the mean total cholesterol (237 ± 32 vs. 224 ± 36 mg/dL, P < 0.05), and in male only, LDL-cholesterol (156 ± 19 vs. 136 ± 11 mg/dL, P < 0.05).

In summary, although there is limited evidence to suggest nutrition intervention alone is effective in preventing weight gain or reversing obesity, the literature is leaning toward a multifaceted approach to manage obesity, that includes tailoring of immunosuppressants and early structured dietitian intervention [137] engaging healthy eating and exercise as recommended by the local health authorities [58].

MALNUTRITION

In contrast to general thinking, dietary freedom after kidney transplantation does not always associate with better nutrition. Suboptimal nutritional status is often found in KTRs during acute or chronic phases posttransplant due to a number of reasons e.g. pre-existing under-nutrition and co-morbidities, altered protein metabolism, increased metabolic demand and requirements, immunosuppressive medications, in particular corticosteroids which promote muscle catabolism, acute or chronic rejection, infection and inter-current illnesses, inflammation, hospitalization, hormonal and metabolic derangements, suboptimal dietary intake and in cases of severely declining transplant function, uremia.

Protein-energy wasting (PEW) is common in patients with ESKD [138] and is associated with high morbidity and mortality. The prevalence and implications have been well studied in non-transplant ESKD patients [139,140]. However, the prevalence of PEW is often underestimated and data is relatively scarce in the transplant population. In a small cohort of 47 KTRs, the prevalence of malnutrition defined as BMI <21.0 kg/m^2 was 15% [141]. These patients had significantly lower levels of serum protein (66 vs. 77 g/L), albumin (33 vs. 39 g/L) and hemoglobin (102 vs. 121 g/L) compared with patients who had a BMI >21.0 kg/m^2. The key causes of malnutrition were graft failure and co-morbidity. In a cohort of 993 KTRs, malnutrition—inflammation score (MIS) [17,142] was used to assess the relationship between malnutrition—inflammation complex syndrome or PEW and mortality [143]. MIS incorporates the conventional Subjective Global Assessment (SGA) tool and objective parameters including BMI, serum albumin and total iron binding capacity (TIBC) to score the severity of malnutrition and inflammation. Patient's characteristics were mean age 51 ± 13 years, 57% men, 21% diabetes, mean eGFR 51 ± 21 mL/min/1.73 m^2, median transplant vintage 72 months (IQR 39—144), Charlson Comorbidity Index (CCI) 2 [2—4], serum albumin 40 ± 4 g/L and Hb 135 ± 17 g/L. The higher the MIS the more severe the PEW is. MIS categories (% of distribution) were <3 (40%), 3—5 (32%), 6—8 (20%) and ≥8 (8%) suggesting 60% of these patients have some degree of malnutrition. MIS was a significant predictor of all-cause mortality (HR per 1-SD increase, 1.59, 95% CI:1.37—1.85), death with a functioning transplant (HR per 1-SD increase, 1.48, 95% CI:1.23—1.78), and death-censored transplant loss (HR per 1-SD increase, 1.34, 95% CI: 1.04—1.71). Compared with MIS category <3 (well nourished and referent), MIS categories of 3—5, 6—8, and ≥8 have 1.5-, 4- and 7-fold increase in all-cause mortality risk respectively. As previously mentioned, high MIS independently associated with posttransplant anemia and low Hb (P = 0.004) in KTRs with eGFR ≤60 mL/min/1.73 m^2 [18].

In a cohort of 47 KTRs with mean age and transplant vintage of 37.6 ± 10.2 years and 46.4 ± 34.6 years respectively; 44% of patients were rated as malnourished by the SGA score B & C [144]. The well-nourished group

(SGA = A) compared to the malnourished group, has higher serum albumin (44 ± 4 vs. 34 ± 4 g/L, P < 0.0001), BMI (24.6 ± 3.5 vs. 21.9 ± 3.6 kg/m^2, P = 0.02) and mid-arm circumference (P = 0.02), and lower levels of CRP (9.5 ± 5.7 vs. 20.8 ± 9.2 mg/L, P < 0.0001). Twenty-six of 31 (83.4%) patients in the well nourished group had BMI increased from 21.8 ± 3.8 to 24.6 ± 3.6 kg/m^2 after transplantation versus only 3 of 16 patients in the malnourished group (P < 0.0001). In fact the mean BMI in the malnourished group decreased from 23.2 ± 3.6 to 21.9 ± 3.6 kg/m^2. The well nourished group has significantly lower hospitalization rate (P = 0.02) and tended to have a lower frequency of chronic allograft rejection (22.5 vs. 43.7%, P = 0.13).

While obesity is associated with poor outcomes, being underweight (BMI < 18.5 kg/m^2) at transplant has 2-fold (P = 0.02) late or ≥5 years death-censored graft loss compared to patients who have a BMI within normal range (BMI 18.5−24.9 kg/m^2) mainly due to chronic allograft nephropathy [117]. In another analyses performed by the similar researchers [118], weight loss more than 5% was associated with subsequent death (year 1 HR, 1.64, 95% CI: 1.08−2.48, P < 0.019; year 2 HR, 2.09, 95% CI 1.44−3.02, P < 0.013) but not death-censored graft loss. In these studies, nutritional status including SGA, muscle and fat stores, and reasons of weight loss were not known. Therefore it was unsure if the poor outcome was caused by low body weight per se or undesirable factors relating to weight loss e.g. inflammation and intercurrent illnesses.

PEW is known to be associated with poor outcomes in uremic patients [139], these include anemia due to impeded erythropoietin sensitivity [145], muscle wasting leading to impaired cardiac and respiratory muscle function, impaired immune function that compromises wound healing and infection defenses. These similar mechanisms relating to poor outcomes in KTRs are highly plausible. Depressive symptoms were examined in a cross-sectional study of 973 prevalent KTRs [146], MIS was found to correlate moderately and independently associated with the Center for Epidemiologic Studies-Depression Score (CES-D score) r = 0.262; P <0.001 and P < 0.001 respectively after adjusting for important covariables e.g. age, gender and eGFR.

In a cohort of 500 KTRs, a low 1-year serum albumin level of <40 g/L independently predicted patient and graft loss (HR = 1.4, P < 0.0001) [147]. However, effect of serum albumin as marker of inflammation or nutrition in this study was not known. In a French study of 44 KTRs [148], serum albumin was stable in the first year posttransplant, whereas serum prealbumin and retinol binding protein (RBP) decreased from 42.3 ± 10.2 g/L to 30.4 ± 6.3 g/L, P < 0.0001 and from 19.6 ± 6.1 g/L to 6.5 ± 0.2 g/L, P < 0.0001 respectively. Increased total lean body mass was associated with

low steroid doses and the absence of acute rejection and delayed graft function. Other nutritional abnormalities observed in KTRs including low intake and deficiencies of serum vitamins B$_6$ and C, magnesium [149], which appeared primarily relating to the side-effects of immunosuppressive therapy. While diet intake are often appeared adequate in protein and energy intake, deficiencies in folic acid, vitamin D, thiamine, iodine, selenium and iron intake have been reported [150].

In summary, the prevalence and effects of PEW or poor nutritional status in post KTRs cannot be underestimated. Furthermore, suboptimal nutrients intake and the respective low blood status are evident in this population. Therefore, sound clinical practice such as careful monitoring of immunosuppressive medications, prevention and treating infection and inflammation, provision of structured nutritional care including regular assessment, monitoring, education for balanced and adequate nutrition are all important to improve outcomes.

PROTEIN AND ENERGY REQUIREMENTS

The two distinct periods regarding nutritional requirements are the acute and chronic phases posttransplantation. Nutritional demand increases during the acute phase or the first four to six weeks posttransplantation, related to high doses of immunosuppressants, surgical stress and wound healing. Unmet demand may lead to negative nitrogen balance, increased catabolism and decreased anabolism of body protein, resulting in delayed wound healing, loss of muscle mass and a compromised immune system [151−153].

A randomized controlled nitrogen balance study was conducted in 12 consecutive nondiabetic KTRs [154]. From day four after the transplant, these patients were placed on an isocaloric diet of approximately 2100 kcal/day; the control group (n = 6) received a diet providing 70 g protein, 210 g carbohydrate and 109 g fat per day (low protein and high carbohydrate diet) whereas the study group (n = 6) received 210 g protein, 70 g carbohydrate and 109 g fat per day (high protein and low carbohydrate diet). This resulted in final protein intake of 1.0 ± 0.1 (range 0.8−1.1) g/kg/day vs. 2.0 ± 0.3 (range 1.4−3.0) g/kg/day in the control and study groups respectively. During the four-week study period, all patients in the study group maintained positive nitrogen balance and gained an average of 3.2 kg muscle mass whereas patients in the control group remained in negative nitrogen balance and lost an average of 1.3 kg muscle mass (P < 0.005). Cushingoid appearance did not develop in the study group (P = 0.01). A suggestion from this study is that a protein intake of at least

1.4 g/kg/d is required to maintain positive nitrogen balance and limited Cushingoid side effects in KTRs receiving steroids in the immediate transplant phase.

In a prospective intervention study in KTRs with acute tubular necrosis being treated with hemodialysis and prednisone 70 to 120 mg/d, the possible effect of a high-protein, high-energy diet to ameliorate negative nitrogen balance was examined [155]. The high-protein and high energy diet group (n = 8) received protein intake of 1.3 ± 0.06 g/kg/day (energy 33 ± 3 kcal/kg/day) versus a low protein and low energy diet of 0.73 ± 0.03 g/kg/d (energy 20 ± 4 kcal/kg/day) in the control group (P < 0.025). The high-protein and high energy diet group was able to achieve neutral nitrogen balance whereas the controls were in marked negative nitrogen balance or a state of protein wasting throughout the study.

Once graft function is stabilized and immunosuppressive medications are adjusted to maintenance doses, the KRTs enter the chronic posttransplant phase. The optimal levels of protein and energy intake to preserve long-term graft function have yet to be established. In the literature, evidence to support the use of a low protein diet ~0.6g/kg IBW/d to retard deterioration of renal function in CKD patients is still inconclusive and controversial [156,157]. In a prospective cohort study over 11 years with 1624 women enrolled in the Nurses' Health Study [158], high protein intake was not significantly associated with change in estimated GFR in subjects with normal renal function. However, in subjects with early CKD, high protein intake was significantly associated with a change in estimated GFR of −1.69 mL/min/1.73 m^2 (CI, −2.93 to −0.45 mL/min/1.73 m^2) per 10-g increase in protein intake. In usual clinical practice, to strike the balance of preserving renal function, prevention of obesity and malnutrition, KTRs are advised optimal protein near the RDI levels (~0.75 g/kg/d) and energy intakes in line with dietary guidelines for healthy adults of their respective regions.

Inevitably, a significant proportion of KTRs develop chronic allograft dysfunction. In a number of short term studies, KTRs with chronic allograft dysfunction were put on a low-protein diet (0.55 g/kg/day) versus a high-protein diet (2 g/kg/day), whilst both received 35 kcal/kg/day. The low-protein diet was associated with a significant reduction in plasma renin activity and proteinuria without compromising BP, GFR or renal blood flow [159,160]. In long term studies [161,162], 48 patients were advised a normocaloric diet moderate in protein (0.8 g/kg), in sodium (3 g/d), and lipids (<30% of total energy). Data from 30 compliant patients (0.73 ± 0.11 g/kg/day) were compared to the non-compliant group (n = 18) in which patients consumed approximately 1.4 g/kg/day of protein and 5 g/day of sodium. Over a twelve year study period, renal function remained unchanged in the compliant group compared to a 40% progressive decline in the non-compliant group (P < 0.0001).

As anticipated, dialysis will eventually be re-initiated in a significant number of patients. However, re-initiation of dialysis in failing transplant patients imposes tremendous clinical and social burdens, including loss of residual function, hemodynamic instability, PEW, anxiety and significant personal and societal economic cost [163] and every effort should be made to avoid premature commencement. Nutritional and related factors may impact on timing of commencement of dialysis through nutritional status, presence of uremic symptoms and related parameters including acidosis, hyperkalemia and volume overload. All may be helped with timely nutritional intervention. Most patients returning to dialysis will also benefit from advice and re-education about what will be required once dialysis has been commenced.

In summary, in the immediate transplant phase when high dose prednisone is required, a protein intake of at least 1.4 g/kg/d and an adequate energy intake of 30—35 kcal/kg/day are required to maintain positive nitrogen balance. In later stages, when immunosuppressive medications have reached maintenance dose, patients with stable renal function or with declining allograft function should be advised to consume protein intake near the RDI levels (~0.75 g/kg/d) with appropriate energy intake to attain and maintain healthy weight, BMI 20.0—25.0 kg/m^2 [164] and nutritional status.

TABLE 34.1 Principal of Nutritional Management in Post Kidney Transplantation

GENERAL
To maintain optimal nutritional status
To minimize side effects associated with immunosuppression therapy
To correct electrolyte and metabolic abnormalities
To prevent complication and promote good health
ACUTE/EARLY POSTTRANSPLANT PERIOD
To minimize protein catabolism and malnutrition
To promote wound healing
To prevention infection, including practice of food safety
To correct clinically significant electrolyte and metabolic abnormalities caused by restoration of kidney function and immunosuppressive medications
CHRONIC/LONG TERM POSTTRANSPLANT PERIOD
To stabilize and prevent deterioration of renal function
To prevent or minimize (or manage) anemia, obesity, dyslipidemia, diabetes/hyperglycemia, hypertension and bone disease
To prevent or manage malnutrition and nutrient deficiency

NUTRITIONAL MANAGEMENT

In light of the complex metabolic and nutritional changes post kidney transplantation (Figure 34.1), stringent nutrition management for KTRs is recommended with set goals for both acute and chronic phases periods (Table 34.1). There has been little research to examine how such guidelines should be translated into practice. Through a national consultative process for the development of transplant nutrition guidelines in Australia, the

TABLE 34.2A Nutrition Assessment

Nutrition Assessment Parameters and Methods	Targets for Optimal Nutrition
(A) ANTHROPOMETRY	
Weight and weight history	Monitor change
Body mass index (BMI) = Weight ÷ Height^2	21−25 g/m^2
Waist circumference	≤90 cm males; ≤80 cm females
Mid-arm muscle circumference	Compare to standard and monitor change
(B) BIOCHEMISTRY AND LABORATORY RESULTS	
Plasma glucose (fasting)	4.4−6.7 mmol/L (with diabetes)
HbA1c (fasting)	<7% (with diabetes)
Total cholesterol (fasting)	<4.0 mmol/L
LDL-cholesterol (fasting)	<2.5 mmol/L or <2.0 mmol/L (with CHD)
HDL-cholesterol (fasting)	>1.0 mmol/L
Triglycerides(fasting)	<1.5 mmol/L
Serum electrolytes (Na, K, Ca, PO$_4$)	
Serum creatinine, eGFR	Within normal range for unit
Urinary electrolytes	Monitor change
Hemoglobin	Within normal range for unit
Serum albumin	Within normal range for unit
Inflammatory markers (e.g. CRP)	Within normal range for unit Within normal range for unit
(C) CLINICAL SIGNS AND SYMPTOMS	
Blood pressure	<130/85 mmHg <125/75 mmHg (if proteinuria >1 g/d)
Urine output	Monitor input and output
Appetite, nutrition impact symptoms*	Monitor change

TABLE 34.2A Nutrition Assessment—cont'd

Nutrition Assessment Parameters and Methods	Targets for Optimal Nutrition
(D) DIETARY INTAKE	
Diet history (food diary or 24 hour recall)	Compare to recommended intake
Drug/medication review	
Drug-nutrient interactions Side-effects and symptoms*	Manage symptoms, dietary modifications to attain optimal blood parameters and nutrition state
(E) EXERCISE CAPACITY/PHYSICAL ACTIVITY LEVEL	
Subjective Global Assessment (SGA) OR Malnutrition−Inflammation Score (MIS)	Adequate level to attain optimal exercise capacity and body composition A (no sign of malnutrition) <3 (no sign of inflammation− malnutrition)

Others: social history, smoking cessation

* See Table 34.2B.
Modified from the summary of nutrition assessment, The Nutritional Management of Adult Kidney Transplant Recipients Guidelines [3].

combination of scientific evidence, expert opinion and patient experience has led to a general consensus for the need to implement timely structured nutrition care in KTRs [3]. This process follows the frame work of medical nutrition therapy (MNT) [165], which includes (a) referral; (b) nutrition assessment; (c) nutrition diagnosis, intervention and monitoring; and (d) evaluation and follow up. In summary, nutritional assessment and management by a dietitian, as part of a multi-disciplinary renal team, should be offered to all KTRs. Nutritional assessment should be performed soon after transplant and monthly for the first three months and annually thereafter. More frequent consultation may be beneficial when more intensive review is needed or new clinical conditions arise e.g. undesirable change of weight or NODAT. A practical and comprehensive list of nutritional assessment parameters and methods are presented in Table 34.2A, and supplemented by a list of possible side effects of immunosuppressive medications and nutrition related impact symptoms (Table 34.2B). These help formulate individual dietary prescription (Table 34.3) and strategies such as appropriate food choices (Table 34.4) to prevent and manage the key nutrition related health issues that may arise posttransplant. Apart from the specific protein and energy requirements at critical stages posttransplantation, the general nutrition recommendations are in line with those for the general

TABLE 34.2B Possible Side Effects of Immunosuppressants and Nutrition Related Symptoms

Possible Side Effects of Immunosuppressants	Immunosuppressants
Anemia	Azathioprine, everolimus, mycophenolates, sirolimus
Anorexia	Azathioprine, mycophenolates
Diarrhea	Everolimus, mycophenolate, tacrolimus
Delayed wound healing	Everolimus, mycophenolates, prednisone, sirolimus
Gastrointestinal discomfort	Mycophenolates
Hyperglycemia	Cyclosporine, everolimus, prednisone, sirolimus, tacrolimus
Hyperkalemia	Cyclosporine, tacrolimus
Hyperlipidemia	Cyclosporine, everolimus, prednisone, sirolimus, tacrolimus
Hyperphagia	Prednisone
Hypertension	Cyclosporin, tacrolimus
Hyperuricemia	Cyclosporin
Hypomagnesemia	Cyclosporin, everolimus, sirolimus, tacrolimus
Increased catabolism	Prednisone
Nausea	Azathioprine, cyclosporine, mycophenolates, tacrolimus
Vomiting	Cyclosporine, mycophenolates

Modified from the summary of nutrition assessment, The Nutritional Management of Adult Kidney Transplant Recipients Guidelines [3].

population, seeking to avoid deficiency and over-nutrition, and to prevent development of diet related disease such as cancer, hypertension, dyslipidemia, diabetes and obesity.

PRETRANSPLANT STATUS AND POSTTRANSPLANT OUTCOME

Pretransplant nutritional status is known to affect outcomes after transplantation. Direct effects of nutritional status are suggested by the "J-curve" relationship between adverse events posttransplant and BMI. Thus, kidney transplant recipients with BMI <18 (consistent with protein-energy malnutrition) and those with BMI >35 (obesity) incur an excess of morbidity and mortality as compared to those within the normal BMI range. There is much debate among the renal community as to whether transplantation should be offered to morbidly obese patients. It has been observed in some studies

TABLE 34.3 Nutrition Requirements Post Kidney Transplantation

Energy and Nutrients	Requirements*
Energy	Acute phase: 30—35 kcal/kg IBW/d Chronic phase: 30—35 kcal/kg IBW/d Or adequate energy to attain or maintain body weight
Protein	Acute phase: ~1.4 g/kg IBW/d Chronic phase: 0.75—1.0 g/kg IBW/d
Fat	<30% total energy, with 8—10% total energy from n-6 polyunsaturated fat Include n-3 polyunsaturated fat from both plant and marine sources 20% monounsaturated fat <10% saturated and trans fatty acids fats
Carbohydrates	~50% total energy Include a variety of carbohydrates High dietary fiber Low Glycemic Index Limit simple sugars
Calcium	1000 to 1300 mg/d (RDI**)
Phosphorous	1000 to 1300 mg/d (RDI**)
Sodium	80—100 mmol/d (no added salt)
Potassium	Restricted if persistent hyperkalemia present
Iron	10—15 mg/d
Vitamin D	5—15 µg/d (RDI**) + individualized supplementation
Fiber	25—30 g/d
All other nutrients including vitamins and minerals, in particular B_6, B_{12}, magnesium and zinc	RDI** levels
Fluid	Depending on balance and fluid status Approximately 2.0—2.5 liter/d
Alcohol	Limit to <20 g/d, <5days/week

* Supplementation if oral intake alone is unable to meet requirements.
** RDI — Recommended Daily Intake for the general population or age and gender, taking into consideration of body size, nutritional status and physical activity level.

that the presence of obesity pretransplant [166] and at time of transplant was "not" associated with poor patient or graft survival but a greater risk of delayed graft function and surgical wound complications [133,167,168]. However, pretransplant low body weight (BMI <20 kg/m2), low muscle mass measured by serum creatinine [166], and low serum albumin [169] were associated with poor graft and patient survival. Indirect effects of abnormal nutritional status are also evident, mediated through nutrition-related disorders including diabetes,

TABLE 34.4 Healthy Food Choices Post Kidney Transplantation

Food Groups	Main nutrients	Daily Choices* (Serving)	Serving Size	Comments
CORE FOOD GROUPS				
Bread, cereals and grain products	Whole grain carbohydrates, dietary fiber, vitamin E and B vitamins	4–8	1 slice bread ½ cup cooked rice, pasta, noodles, oat porridge, breakfast cereal	Choose wholemeal and wholegrain products
Fruit	Vitamins A and C, potassium and dietary fiber	2–3	1 cup chopped fruit or equivalent in whole fruit	Avoidance of grapefruit in all forms as they interfere with the actions of immunosuppressive medications
Vegetables	Vitamins A and C, folate, iron, potassium magnesium and dietary fiber	5+	½ cup cooked vegetables 1 cup salad vegetables	Choose a variety of colored vegetables in season; traffic light color: red, yellow and green
Meat and meat alternatives (dried beans and legumes)	Protein, phosphorous, iron, zinc and B$_{12}$ and other B vitamins Omega 3 fatty acids and vitamin D (in oily fish)	2	100 g cooked lean meat or chicken 120 g fish 1 cup legumes (beans, lentils etc)	Choose lean cuts of animal protein, remove skin of poultry Eat fish, especially varieties rich in omega-3 fatty acids at least twice per week Eat legumes a few time a week
Nuts and seeds	+ Vitamin E and dietary fiber	1	30g (small handful)	Choose a variety of nuts or seeds (unsalted)
Dairy	Calcium, phosphorous, vitamins B$_2$, A and D	3	1 serve = 250 mL milk or 30 g cheese or 200 g yoghurt	Choose fat reduced options if need to control weight
Fat	Essential fatty acids	1	1 serve = 1 tablespoon	Choose mono- or polyunsaturated fats (e.g. olive, canola or corn oil etc) Limit saturated fats and trans-fats

Notes:
- Limit foods with high fat, especially saturated fat, sugar and sodium (salt) content.
- Observe food hygiene to avoid food–bone infection, e.g. avoid prepared or prepackaged cold or raw salad, cold meat/fish/chicken/seafood/eggs/pate, soft serve ice cream etc.

* *Quantity depending on posttransplant phase, medical condition, nutrition state, body size and physical activity level.*
Adapted from the Dietary Guidelines for Australian adults – a guide to healthy eating, NHMRC 2003 and Food choices after your transplant, patient education material based on the Evidence-Based Practice Guidelines for the Nutritional Management of Kidney Transplant Recipients, CARI and DAA, 2010.

osteoporosis and cardiovascular disease. Therefore, optimal nutritional status including body composition should be maintained in all dialysis patients especially those on the transplant waitlist.

CONCLUSION

This chapter presents the various aspects of nutritional managements and recommendations for the management of KTRs both early and late after transplantation. At present, there is a substantial lack of high level evidence to guide clinical practice. Therefore, large scale randomized control trials to examine the efficacy and safety of nutrition intervention to improve specific health outcomes for KTRs are needed. Until then, audit and evaluation of the implementation of these nutrition guidelines may help to direct and improve clinical practice and patient outcomes.

Acknowledgements

We would like to thank all members of the kidney transplant nutrition guidelines working party for their dedication and enthusiasm for the development of the original guidelines: Karen Fry (guideline project dietitian), Aditi Patwardhan (senior renal dietitian, Royal Prince Alfred Hospital, Sydney), Catherine Ryan (senior renal dietitian, John hunter Hospital, Newcastle), Dr. Paul Trevillian (nephrologist and transplant physician, John Hunter Hospital, Newcastle), Fidye Westgarth (service manager, renal services network, New South Wales, Agency for Clinical Innovation) and Evan Eggins (NSW chair, consumer participation committee, Kidney Health Australia). It was a memorable journey for all of us. Project fund for project dietitian was initially granted by the Greater Metropolitan Clinical Taskforce (GMCT), now Agency for Clinical Innovation (ACI), New South Wales Health in 2006.

References

[1] Fry K, Patwardhan A, Ryan C, et al. Development of evidence-based guidelines for the nutritional management of adult kidney transplant recipients. J Ren Nutr 2009;19(1):101—4.

[2] Nutrition in Kidney Transplant Recipients. Caring for Australasians with Renal Impairment (CARI) Guidelines. Available from: http://www.cari.org.au/trans_nutrition_published.php; 2010.

[3] Evidence based practice guidelines for the nutritional management of adult kidney transplant recipients. Dietitians Association of Australia. Available from: http://daa.collaborative.net.au/files/DINER/TransplantNutrition_Guidelines_FINAL_090628.pdf; 2009.

[4] KDOQI Clinical Practice Guideline and Clinical Practice Recommendations for Anemia in Chronic Kidney Disease. Update of Hemoglobin Target. Available from: http://www.kidney.org/professionals/kdoqi/guidelines_anemia/cpr21.htm; 2007.

[5] Kessler M. Erythropoietin and erythropoiesis in renal transplantation. Nephrol Dial Transplant 1995;10(Suppl. 6):114—6.

[6] Vanrenterghem Y, Ponticelli C, Morales JM, et al. Prevalence and management of anemia in renal transplant recipients: a European survey. Am J Transplant 2003;3(7):835—45.

[7] Shah N, Al-Khoury S, Afzali B, et al. Posttransplantation anemia in adult renal allograft recipients: prevalence and predictors. Transplantation 2006;81(8):1112—8.

[8] Mix TC, Kazmi W, Khan S, et al. Anemia: a continuing problem following kidney transplantation. Am J Transplant 2003;3(11):1426—33.

[9] Einollahi B, Lessan-Pezeshki M, Rostami Z, et al. Anemia after kidney transplantation in adult recipients: prevalence and risk factors. Transplant Proc 2011;43(2):578—80.

[10] Rigatto C, Parfrey P, Foley R, et al. Congestive heart failure in renal transplant recipients: risk factors, outcomes, and relationship with ischemic heart disease. J Am Soc Nephrol 2002;13(4):1084—90.

[11] Molnar MZ, Czira M, Ambrus C, et al. Anemia is associated with mortality in kidney-transplanted patients — a prospective cohort study. Am J Transplant 2007;7(4):818—24.

[12] Chadban SJ, Baines L, Polkinghorne K, et al. Anemia after kidney transplantation is not completely explained by reduced kidney function. Am J Kidney Dis 2007;49(2):301—9.

[13] Sancho A, Pastor MC, Canas L, et al. Posttransplantation anemia: relationship with inflammatory markers, oxidation, and prohepcidin levels. Transplant Proc 2011;43(6):2196—8.

[14] Ghafari A, Noori-Majelan N. Anemia among long-term renal transplant recipients. Transplant Proc 2008;40(1):186—8.

[15] Gossmann J, Thurmann P, Bachmann T, et al. Mechanism of angiotensin converting enzyme inhibitor-related anemia in renal transplant recipients. Kidney Int 1996;50(3):973—8.

[16] Julian BA, Brantley Jr RR, Barker CV, et al. Losartan, an angiotensin II type 1 receptor antagonist, lowers hematocrit in posttransplant erythrocytosis. J Am Soc Nephrol 1998;9(6):1104—8.

[17] Molnar MZ, Keszei A, Czira ME, et al. Evaluation of the malnutrition-inflammation score in kidney transplant recipients. Am J Kidney Dis 2010;56(1):102—11.

[18] Molnar MZ, Czira ME, Rudas A, et al. Association between the malnutrition-inflammation score and posttransplant anaemia. Nephrol Dial Transplant 2011;26(6):2000—6.

[19] Molnar MZ, Mucsi I, Macdougall IC, et al. Prevalence and management of anaemia in renal transplant recipients: data from ten European centres. Nephron Clin Pract 2011;117(2):c127—34.

[20] Poesen R, Bammens B, Claes K, et al. Prevalence and determinants of anemia in the immediate postkidney transplant period. Transpl Int 2011;24:1208.

[21] Karakus S, Kanbay M, Koseoglu HK, et al. Causes of anemia in renal transplant recipients. Transplant Proc 2004;36(1):164—5.

[22] Lorenz M, Winkelmayer WC, Horl WH, et al. Anaemia after renal transplantation. Eur J Clin Invest 2005;35(Suppl. 3):89—94.

[23] Yabu JM, Winkelmayer WC. Posttransplantation anemia: mechanisms and management. Clin J Am Soc Nephrol 2011;6(7):1794—801.

[24] Zadrazil J, Horak P, Horcicka V, et al. Endogenous erythropoietin levels and anemia in long-term renal transplant recipients. Kidney Blood Press Res 2007;30(2):108—16.

[25] Gentil MA, Perez-Valdivia MA, Lopez-Mendoza M, et al. Factor deficiency in the anemia of renal transplant patients with grade III-IV chronic kidney disease: baseline results of the ARES Study. Transplant Proc 2008;40(9):2922—4.

[26] Chadban S, Chan M, Fry K, et al. Nutritional management of anaemia in adult kidney transplant recipients. Nephrology 2010;15:S40—2.

[27] Nutrient reference values. National Health and Research (NH & MRC), Australian Government. Available from: http://www.nrv.gov.au/introduction.htm.

[28] Kidney Disease: Improving Global Outcomes (KDIGO) - Guidelines for Anemia Management. Available from: http://www.kdigo.org/guidelines/topicsummarized/CPG%20Summary%20by%20Topic_Anemia%20Management.html; 2008.

[29] Grotz WH, Mundinger FA, Rasenack J, et al. Bone loss after kidney transplantation: a longitudinal study in 115 graft recipients. Nephrol Dial Transplant 1995;10(11):2096—100.

[30] Almond MK, Kwan JT, Evans K, et al. Loss of regional bone mineral density in the first 12 months following renal transplantation. Nephron 1994;66(1):52—7.

[31] Grotz WH, Mundinger FA, Gugel B, et al. Bone mineral density after kidney transplantation. A cross-sectional study in 190 graft recipients up to 20 years after transplantation. Transplantation 1995;59(7):982—6.

[32] Horber FF, Casez JP, Steiger U, et al. Changes in bone mass early after kidney transplantation. J Bone Miner Res 1994;9(1):1—9.

[33] Lim WH, Coates PS, Russ GR, et al. Hyperparathyroidism and vitamin D deficiency predispose to bone loss in renal transplant recipients. Transplantation 2009;88(5):678—83.

[34] Gallego R, Oliva E, Vega N, et al. Steroids and bone density in patients with functioning kidney allografts. Transplant Proc 2006;38(8):2434—7.

[35] Unal A, Kocyigit I, Sipahioglu MH, et al. Loss of bone mineral density in renal transplantation recipients. Transplant Proc 2010;42(9):3550—3.

[36] Veenstra DL, Best JH, Hornberger J, et al. Incidence and long-term cost of steroid-related side effects after renal transplantation. Am J Kidney Dis 1999;33(5):829—39.

[37] Nikkel LE, Hollenbeak CS, Fox EJ, et al. Risk of fractures after renal transplantation in the United States. Transplantation 2009;87(12):1846—51.

[38] Malluche HH, Monier-Faugere MC, Herberth J. Bone disease after renal transplantation. Nat Rev Nephrol 2010;6(1):32—40.

[39] El-Agroudy AE, El-Husseini AA, El-Sayed M, et al. A prospective randomized study for prevention of postrenal transplantation bone loss. Kidney Int 2005;67(5):2039—45.

[40] El-Agroudy AE, El-Husseini AA, El-Sayed M, et al. Preventing bone loss in renal transplant recipients with vitamin D. J Am Soc Nephrol 2003;14(11):2975—9.

[41] De Sevaux RG, Hoitsma AJ, Corstens FH, et al. Treatment with vitamin D and calcium reduces bone loss after renal transplantation: a randomized study. J Am Soc Nephrol 2002;13(6):1608—14.

[42] Torres A, Garcia S, Gomez A, et al. Treatment with intermittent calcitriol and calcium reduces bone loss after renal transplantation. Kidney Int 2004;65(2):705—12.

[43] Nowacka-Cieciura E, Cieciura T, Baczkowska T, et al. Bisphosphonates are effective prophylactic of early bone loss after renal transplantation. Transplant Proc 2006;38(1):165—7.

[44] Palmer SC, McGregor DO, Strippoli GF. Interventions for preventing bone disease in kidney transplant recipients. Cochrane Database Syst Rev 2007 (3):CD005015.

[45] Yu RW, Faull RJ, Coates PT, et al. Calcium supplements lower bone resorption after renal transplant. Clin Transplant 2011.

[46] Chadban S, Chan M, Fry K, et al. Nutritional interventions for the prevention of bone disease in kidney transplant recipients. Nephrology 2010;15:S43—7.

[47] Chapter 5: Evaluation and treatment of kidney transplant bone disease. Kidney Int 2009;76(S113):S100—10.

[48] Bone disease in the kidney transplant recipient, KDOQI Clinical Practice Guidelines for Bone Metabolism and Disease in Chronic Kidney Disease. Available from: http://www.kidney.org/professionals/kdoqi/guidelines_bone/Guide16.htm.

[49] Dietary Reference Intakes (DRIs), Estimated Average Requirements, Food and Nutrition Board. Available from: http://www.iom.edu/Activities/Nutrition/SummaryDRIs/~/media/Files/Activity%20Files/Nutrition/DRIs/5_Summary%20Table%20Tables%201-4.pdf.

[50] Guitard J, Rostaing L, Kamar N. New-onset diabetes and nephropathy after renal transplantation. Contrib Nephrol 2011;170:247—55.

[51] Bayer ND, Cochetti PT, Anil Kumar MS, et al. Association of metabolic syndrome with development of new-onset diabetes after transplantation. Transplantation 2010;90(8):861—6.

[52] Bee YM, Tan HC, Tay TL, et al. Incidence and risk factors for development of new-onset diabetes after kidney transplantation. Ann Acad Med Singapore 2011;40(4):160—8.

[53] Vincenti F, Friman S, Scheuermann E, et al. Results of an international, randomized trial comparing glucose metabolism disorders and outcome with cyclosporine versus tacrolimus. Am J Transplant 2007;7(6):1506—14.

[54] Luan FL, Stuckey LJ, Ojo AO. Abnormal glucose metabolism and metabolic syndrome in non-diabetic kidney transplant recipients early after transplantation. Transplantation 2010;89(8):1034—9.

[55] Cole EH, Johnston O, Rose CL, et al. Impact of acute rejection and new-onset diabetes on long-term transplant graft and patient survival. Clin J Am Soc Nephrol 2008;3(3):814—21.

[56] Valderhaug TG, Hjelmesaeth J, Hartmann A, et al. The association of early posttransplant glucose levels with long-term mortality. Diabetologia 2011;54(6):1341—9.

[57] Chadban S, Chan M, Fry K, et al. Nutritional management of diabetes mellitus in adult kidney transplant recipients. Nephrology 2010;15:S37—9.

[58] Dietary guidelines for Australian Adults. National Health and Research Council (NH&MRC), Australian Government. Available from: http://www.nhmrc.gov.au/_files_nhmrc/publications/attachments/n33.pdf.

[59] Bantle JP, Wylie-Rosett J, Albright AL, et al. Nutrition recommendations and interventions for diabetes: a position statement of the American Diabetes Association. Diabetes Care 2008;31(Suppl. 1):S61—78.

[60] National Evidence Based Guidelines for the Management of Type 2 Diabetes Mellitus. National Health and Medical Research Council, Australian Government. Available from: http://www.nhmrc.gov.au/guidelines/publications/di16; 2009.

[61] Kasiske B, Cosio FG, Beto J, et al. Clinical practice guidelines for managing dyslipidemias in kidney transplant patients: a report from the Managing Dyslipidemias in Chronic Kidney Disease Work Group of the National Kidney Foundation Kidney Disease Outcomes Quality Initiative. Am J Transplant 2004;4(Suppl. 7):13—53.

[62] Third Report of the Expert Panel on Detection, Evaluation, and Treatment of High Blood Cholesterol in Adults (Adult Treatment Panel III). Available from: http://www.nhlbi.nih.gov/guidelines/cholesterol/.

[63] Kasiske BL, Umen AJ. Persistent hyperlipidemia in renal transplant patients. Medicine (Baltimore) 1987;66(4):309—16.

[64] Segoloni GP, Triolo G, Cassader M, et al. Dyslipidemia in renal transplantation: a 3-year follow-up. Transplant Proc 1993;25(3):2178—9.

[65] Aakhus S, Dahl K, Wideroe TE. Hyperlipidaemia in renal transplant patients. J Intern Med 1996;239(5):407—15.

[66] Ostovan MA, Fazelzadeh A, Mehdizadeh AR, et al. How to decrease cardiovascular mortality in renal transplant recipients. Transplant Proc 2006;38(9):2887—92.

[67] Fazelzadeh A, Mehdizadeh AR, Ostovan MA, et al. Predictors of cardiovascular events and associated mortality of kidney transplant recipients. Transplant Proc 2006;38(2):509—11.

[68] Stachowska E, Wesolowska T, Safranow K, et al. Simple dietary interventions reduce the risk factors of atherosclerosis in renal graft recipients. J Ren Nutr 2005;15(3):291—7.

[69] Stachowska E, Wesolowska T, Olszewska M, et al. Elements of Mediterranean diet improve oxidative status in blood of kidney graft recipients. Br J Nutr 2005;93(3):345—52.

[70] Guida B, Trio R, Laccetti R, et al. Role of dietary intervention on metabolic abnormalities and nutritional status after renal transplantation. Nephrol Dial Transplant 2007;22(11): 3304—10.

[71] The expert Panel. Report of the National Cholesterol Education Program Expert Panel on detection. evaluation and treatment of high blood cholesterol in adults Arch Intern Med 1988;148: 136.

[72] Shen SY, Lukens CW, Alongi SV, et al. Patient profile and effect of dietary therapy on posttransplant hyperlipidemia. Kidney Int Suppl 1983;16:S147—52.

[73] Barbagallo CM, Cefalu AB, Gallo S, et al. Effects of Mediterranean diet on lipid levels and cardiovascular risk in renal transplant recipients. Nephron 1999;82(3):199—204.

[74] Lopes IM, Martin M, Errasti P, et al. Benefits of a dietary intervention on weight loss, body composition, and lipid profile after renal transplantation. Nutrition 1999;15(1):7—10.

[75] Zaffari D, Losekann A, Santos AF, et al. Effectiveness of diet in hyperlipidemia in renal transplant patients. Transplant Proc 2004;36(4):889—90.

[76] Yu-Poth S, Zhao G, Etherton T, et al. Effects of the National Cholesterol Education Program's Step I and Step II dietary intervention programs on cardiovascular disease risk factors: a meta-analysis. Am J Clin Nutr 1999;69(4):632—46.

[77] Cupisti A, D'Alessandro C, Ghiadoni L, et al. Effect of a soy protein diet on serum lipids of renal transplant patients. J Ren Nutr 2004;14(1):31—5.

[78] Chadban S, Chan M, Fry K, et al. Nutritional management of dyslipidaemia in adult kidney transplant recipients. Nephrology 2010;15:S62—7.

[79] Rubin MF. Hypertension following kidney transplantation. Adv Chronic Kidney Dis 2011;18(1):17—22.

[80] Opelz G, Wujciak T, Ritz E. Association of chronic kidney graft failure with recipient blood pressure. Collaborative Transplant Study. Kidney Int 1998;53(1):217—22.

[81] Kasiske BL, Anjum S, Shah R, et al. Hypertension after kidney transplantation. Am J Kidney Dis 2004;43(6):1071—81.

[82] KDIGO clinical practice guideline for the care of kidney transplant recipients. Am J Transplant 2009;9(Suppl. 3):S1—155.

[83] Sacks FM, Svetkey LP, Vollmer WM, et al. Effects on blood pressure of reduced dietary sodium and the Dietary Approaches to Stop Hypertension (DASH) diet. DASH-Sodium Collaborative Research Group. N Engl J Med 2001;344(1):3—10.

[84] Matyas E, Jeitler K, Horvath K, et al. Benefit assessment of salt reduction in patients with hypertension: systematic overview. J Hypertens 2011;29(5):821—8.

[85] Ramesh Prasad GV, Huang M, Nash MM, et al. The role of dietary cations in the blood pressure of renal transplant recipients. Clin Transplant 2006;20(1):37—42.

[86] van der Heide JJ, Bilo HJ, Donker JM, et al. Effect of dietary fish oil on renal function and rejection in cyclosporine-treated recipients of renal transplants. N Engl J Med 1993;329(11): 769—73.

[87] Kelly BS, Alexander JW, Dreyer D, et al. Oral arginine improves blood pressure in renal transplant and hemodialysis patients. JPEN J Parenter Enteral Nutr 2001;25(4):194—202.

[88] Appel LJ, Moore TJ, Obarzanek E, et al. A clinical trial of the effects of dietary patterns on blood pressure. DASH Collaborative Research Group. N Engl J Med 1997;336(16): 1117—24.

[89] Miller 3rd ER, Erlinger TP, Young DR, et al. Results of the Diet, Exercise, and Weight Loss Intervention Trial (DEW-IT). Hypertension 2002;40(5):612—8.

[90] Edwards KM, Wilson KL, Sadja J, et al. Effects on blood pressure and autonomic nervous system function of a 12-week exercise or exercise plus DASH-diet intervention in individuals with elevated blood pressure. Acta Physiol (Oxf) 2011;203(3): 343—50.

[91] Effects of weight loss and sodium reduction intervention on blood pressure and hypertension incidence in overweight people with high-normal blood pressure. The Trials of Hypertension Prevention, phase II. The Trials of Hypertension Prevention Collaborative Research Group. Arch Intern Med 1997;157(6):657—67.

[92] Huggins CE, Margerison C, Worsley A, et al. Influence of dietary modifications on the blood pressure response to antihypertensive medication. Br J Nutr 2011;105(2):248—55.

[93] Mulrow CD, Chiquette E, Angel L, et al. Dieting to reduce body weight for controlling hypertension in adults. Cochrane Database Syst Rev 2000;(2):CD000484.

[94] Xin X, He J, Frontini MG, et al. Effects of alcohol reduction on blood pressure: a meta-analysis of randomized controlled trials. Hypertension 2001;38(5):1112—7.

[95] Elmer PJ, Obarzanek E, Vollmer WM, et al. Effects of comprehensive lifestyle modification on diet, weight, physical fitness, and blood pressure control: 18-month results of a randomized trial. Ann Intern Med 2006;144(7):485—95.

[96] Chadban S, Chan M, Fry K, et al. Nutritional management of hypertension in adult kidney transplant recipients. Nephrology 2010;15:S56—61.

[97] MacGowan AP, Marshall RJ, MacKay IM, et al. Listeria faecal carriage by renal transplant recipients, haemodialysis patients and patients in general practice: its relation to season, drug therapy, foreign travel, animal exposure and diet. Epidemiol Infect 1991;106(1):157—66.

[98] Fernandez-Sabe N, Cervera C, Lopez-Medrano F, et al. Risk factors, clinical features, and outcomes of listeriosis in solid-organ transplant recipients: a matched case-control study. Clin Infect Dis 2009;49(8):1153—9.

[99] Stamm AM, Dismukes WE, Simmons BP, et al. Listeriosis in renal transplant recipients: report of an outbreak and review of 102 cases. Rev Infect Dis 1982;4(3):665—82.

[100] Chadban S, Chan M, Fry K, et al. The CARI guidelines. Food safety recommendations for adult kidney transplant recipients. Nephrology (Carlton) 2010;15(Suppl. 1):S35—6.

[101] Food Standards Australia New Zealand (FSANZ). Listeria and food — the risk to people with weakened immune systems. Available from: http://www.foodstandards.gov.au/_srcfiles/listeria1.pdf.

[102] Food Standards Australia New Zealand (FSANZ). Listeria and Food — commonly asked questions. Available from: http://www.foodstandards.gov.au/_srcfiles/Listeria_Q_%20A_Version_FINAL.pdf#search=%22listeria%20and%20food%22 [Cited June 2008.].

[103] Evenepoel P, Meijers BK, de Jonge H, et al. Recovery of hyperphosphatoninism and renal phosphorus wasting one year after successful renal transplantation. Clin J Am Soc Nephrol 2008;3(6):1829—36.

[104] Torres A, Lorenzo V, Salido E. Calcium metabolism and skeletal problems after transplantation. J Am Soc Nephrol 2002;13(2): 551—8.

[105] Ghanekar H, Welch BJ, Moe OW, et al. Post-renal transplantation hypophosphatemia: a review and novel insights. Curr Opin Nephrol Hypertens 2006;15(2):97—104.

[106] Trombetti A, Richert L, Hadaya K, et al. Early posttransplantation hypophosphatemia is associated with elevated FGF-23 levels. Eur J Endocrinol 2011;164(5):839—47.

[107] Ambuhl PM, Meier D, Wolf B, et al. Metabolic aspects of phosphate replacement therapy for hypophosphatemia after renal transplantation: impact on muscular phosphate content, mineral metabolism, and acid/base homeostasis. Am J Kidney Dis 1999;34(5):875—83.

[108] Caravaca F, Fernandez MA, Ruiz-Calero R, et al. Effects of oral phosphorus supplementation on mineral metabolism of renal transplant recipients. Nephrol Dial Transplant 1998;13(10):2605—11.

[109] Riella LV, Rennke HG, Grafals M, et al. Hypophosphatemia in kidney transplant recipients: report of acute phosphate nephropathy as a complication of therapy. Am J Kidney Dis 2011;57(4):641—5.

[110] Chadban S, Chan M, Fry K, et al. Nutritional management of hypophosphataemia in adult kidney transplant recipients. Nephrology 2010;15:S48—51.

[111] Johnson CP, Gallagher-Lepak S, Zhu YR, et al. Factors influencing weight gain after renal transplantation. Transplantation 1993;56(4):822—7.

[112] Jaggers HJ, Allman MA, Chan M. Changes in clinical profile and dietary considerations after renal transplantation. J Ren Nutr 1996;1996(6):2—20.

[113] Teplan V, Poledne R, Schuck O, et al. Hyperlipidemia and obesity after renal transplantation. Ann Transplant 2001;6(2):21—3.

[114] Qureshi AR, Lindholm B, Alvestrand A, et al. Nutritional status, muscle composition and plasma and muscle free amino acids in renal transplant patients. Clin Nephrol 1994;42(4):237—45.

[115] Dolgos S, Hartmann A, Jenssen T, et al. Determinants of short-term changes in body composition following renal transplantation. Scand J Urol Nephrol 2009;43(1):76—83.

[116] Gore JL, Pham PT, Danovitch GM, et al. Obesity and outcome following renal transplantation. Am J Transplant 2006;6(2):357—63.

[117] Chang SH, Coates PT, McDonald SP. Effects of body mass index at transplant on outcomes of kidney transplantation. Transplantation 2007;84(8):981—7.

[118] Chang SH, McDonald SP. Post-kidney transplant weight change as marker of poor survival outcomes. Transplantation 2008;85(10):1443—8.

[119] Meier-Kriesche HU, Vaghela M, Thambuganipalle R, et al. The effect of body mass index on long-term renal allograft survival. Transplantation 1999;68(9):1294—7.

[120] Cacciola RA, Pujar K, Ilham MA, et al. Effect of degree of obesity on renal transplant outcome. Transplant Proc 2008;40(10):3408—12.

[121] el-Agroudy AE, Wafa EW, Gheith OE, et al. Weight gain after renal transplantation is a risk factor for patient and graft outcome. Transplantation 2004;77(9):1381—5.

[122] Wang K, Liu QZ. Effect analysis of 1-year posttransplant body mass index on chronic allograft nephropathy in renal recipients. Transplant Proc 2011;43(7):2592—5.

[123] Steiger U, Lippuner K, Jensen EX, et al. Body composition and fuel metabolism after kidney grafting. Eur J Clin Invest 1995;25(11):809—16.

[124] Roine E, Bjork IT, Oyen O. Targeting risk factors for impaired wound healing and wound complications after kidney transplantation. Transplant Proc 2010;42(7):2542—6.

[125] Johnson DW, Isbel NM, Brown AM, et al. The effect of obesity on renal transplant outcomes. Transplantation 2002;74(5):675—81.

[126] Teplan V, Schuck O, Stollova M, et al. Metabolic syndrome after renal transplantation. Med Pregl 2007;60(Suppl. 2):28—32.

[127] Armstrong KA, Campbell SB, Hawley CM, et al. Impact of obesity on renal transplant outcomes. Nephrology (Carlton) 2005;10(4):405—13.

[128] Souza GC, Costa C, Scalco R, et al. Serum Leptin, Insulin Resistance, and Body Fat After Renal Transplantation. Journal of Renal Nutrition: the official Journal of the Council on Renal Nutrition of the National Kidney Foundation 2008;18(6):479—88.

[129] Ewers B, Gasbjerg A, Zerahn B, et al. Impact of Vitamin D Status and Obesity on C-Reactive Protein in Kidney-Transplant Patients. Journal of Renal Nutrition: the official journal of the Council on Renal Nutrition of the National Kidney Foundation 2008;18(3):294—300.

[130] Lee MC, Lee CJ, Chou KC, et al. Hypoadiponectinemia correlates with metabolic syndrome in kidney transplantation patients. Transplant Proc 2011;43(7):2601—5.

[131] Teplan V, Schuck O, Stollova M, et al. Obesity and hyperhomocysteinaemia after kidney transplantation. Nephrol Dial Transplant 2003;18(Suppl. 5):v71—3.

[132] Massarweh NN, Clayton JL, Mangum CA, et al. High body mass index and short- and long-term renal allograft survival in adults. Transplantation 2005;80(10):1430—4.

[133] Marcen R, Fernandez A, Pascual J, et al. High body mass index and posttransplant weight gain are not risk factors for kidney graft and patient outcome. Transplant Proc 2007;39(7):2205—7.

[134] Orazio LK, Isbel NM, Armstrong KA, et al. Evaluation of Dietetic Advice for Modification of Cardiovascular Disease Risk Factors in Renal Transplant Recipients. J Ren Nutr 2011;21(6):462—71.

[135] National Physical Activity Guidelines for Australians, Department of Health and Aging, Australian Government. Available from: http://www.health.gov.au/internet/main/publishing.nsf/content/health-pubhlth-strateg-phys-act-guidelines#guidelines_adults.

[136] Patel MG. The effect of dietary intervention on weight gains after renal transplantation. J Ren Nutr 1998;8(3):137—41.

[137] Chadban S, Chan M, Fry K, et al. Nutritional management of overweight and obesity in adult kidney transplant recipients. Nephrology 2010;15:S52—5.

[138] Fouque D, Kalantar-Zadeh K, Kopple J, et al. A proposed nomenclature and diagnostic criteria for protein-energy wasting in acute and chronic kidney disease. Kidney Int 2008;73(4):391—8.

[139] Stenvinkel P, Heimburger O, Lindholm B, et al. Are there two types of malnutrition in chronic renal failure? Evidence for relationships between malnutrition, inflammation and atherosclerosis (MIA syndrome). Nephrol Dial Transplant 2000;15(7):953—60.

[140] de Mutsert R, Grootendorst DC, Axelsson J, et al. Excess mortality due to interaction between protein-energy wasting, inflammation and cardiovascular disease in chronic dialysis patients. Nephrol Dial Transplant 2008;23(9):2957—64.

[141] Djukanovic L, Lezaic V, Blagojevic R, et al. Co-morbidity and kidney graft failure-two main causes of malnutrition in kidney transplant patients. Nephrol Dial Transplant 2003;18(Suppl. 5):v68—70.

[142] Kalantar-Zadeh K, Kopple JD, Block G, et al. A malnutrition-inflammation score is correlated with morbidity and mortality in maintenance hemodialysis patients. Am J Kidney Dis 2001;38(6):1251—63.

[143] Molnar MZ, Czira ME, Rudas A, et al. Association of the malnutrition-inflammation score with clinical outcomes in kidney transplant recipients. Am J Kidney Dis 2011;58(1):101—8.

[144] Sezer S, Ozdemir FN, Afsar B, et al. Subjective global assessment is a useful method to detect malnutrition in renal transplant patients. Transplant Proc 2006;38(2):517–20.

[145] Locatelli F, Andrulli S, Memoli B, et al. Nutritional-inflammation status and resistance to erythropoietin therapy in haemodialysis patients. Nephrol Dial Transplant 2006;21(4):991–8.

[146] Czira ME, Lindner AV, Szeifert L, et al. Association between the Malnutrition-Inflammation Score and depressive symptoms in kidney transplanted patients. Gen Hosp Psychiatry 2011;33(2):157–65.

[147] Dahlberg R, Muth B, Samaniego M, et al. One-Year Serum Albumin is an Independent Predictor of Outcomes in Kidney Transplant Recipients. Journal of Renal Nutrition: the official journal of the Council on Renal Nutrition of the National Kidney Foundation 2010;20(6):392–7.

[148] El Haggan W, Vendrely B, Chauveau P, et al. Early evolution of nutritional status and body composition after kidney transplantation. Am J Kidney Dis 2002;40(3):629–37.

[149] du Plessis AS, Randall H, Escreet E, et al. Nutritional status of renal transplant patients. S Afr Med J 2002;92(1):68–74.

[150] Heaf J, Jakobsen U, Tvedegaard E, et al. Dietary habits and nutritional status of renal transplant patients. Journal of Renal Nutrition: the official journal of the Council on Renal Nutrition of the National Kidney Foundation 2004;14(1):20–5.

[151] Hoy WE, Sargent JA, Hall D, et al. Protein catabolism during the postoperative course after renal transplantation. Am J Kidney Dis 1985;5(3):186–90.

[152] Hoy WE, Sargent JA, Freeman RB, et al. The influence of glucocorticoid dose on protein catabolism after renal transplantation. Am J Med Sci 1986;291(4):241–7.

[153] Seagraves A, Moore EE, Moore FA, et al. Net protein catabolic rate after kidney transplantation: impact of corticosteroid immunosuppression. JPEN J Parenter Enteral Nutr 1986;10(5):453–5.

[154] Whittier FC, Evans DH, Dutton S, et al. Nutrition in renal transplantation. Am J Kidney Dis 1985;6(6):405–11.

[155] Cogan MG, Sargent JA, Yarbrough SG, et al. Prevention of prednisone-induced negative nitrogen balance. Effect of dietary modification on urea generation rate in patients on hemodialysis receiving high-dose glucocorticoids. Ann Intern Med 1981;95(2):158–61.

[156] Johnson DW. Dietary protein restriction as a treatment for slowing chronic kidney disease progression: the case against. Nephrology (Carlton) 2006;11(1):58–62.

[157] Fouque D, Laville M, Boissel JP. Low protein diets for chronic kidney disease in non diabetic adults. Cochrane Database Syst Rev 2006 (2):CD001892.

[158] Knight EL, Stampfer MJ, Hankinson SE, et al. The impact of protein intake on renal function decline in women with normal renal function or mild renal insufficiency. Ann Intern Med 2003;138(6):460–7.

[159] Salahudeen AK, Hostetter TH, Raatz SK, et al. Effects of dietary protein in patients with chronic renal transplant rejection. Kidney Int 1992;41(1):183–90.

[160] Rosenberg ME, Salahudeen AK, Hostetter TH. Dietary protein and the renin-angiotensin system in chronic renal allograft rejection. Kidney Int Suppl 1995;52:S102–6.

[161] Bernardi A, Biasia F, Piva M, et al. Dietary protein intake and nutritional status in patients with renal transplant. Clin Nephrol 2000;53(suppl. 4):3–5.

[162] Bernardi A, Biasia F, Pati T, et al. Long-term protein intake control in kidney transplant recipients: effect in kidney graft function and in nutritional status. Am J Kidney Dis 2003;41(3 Suppl. 1):S146–52.

[163] Molnar MZ, Ojo AO, Bunnapradist S, et al. Timing of dialysis initiation in transplant-naive and failed transplant patients. Nat Rev Nephrol 2012;8(5):284–92.

[164] Chadban S, Chan M, Fry K, et al. Protein requirement in adult kidney transplant recipients. Nephrology 2010;15:S68–71.

[165] Nutrition Care Process, Medical Nutrition Therapy, American Dietetic Association, Evidence Analysis Library. Available from: www.adaevidencelibrary.com/category.cfm?cid=2&;cat=0.

[166] Streja E, Molnar MZ, Kovesdy CP, et al. Associations of pre-transplant weight and muscle mass with mortality in renal transplant recipients. Clin J Am Soc Nephrol 2011;6(6):1463–73.

[167] Bennett WM, McEvoy KM, Henell KR, et al. Morbid obesity does not preclude successful renal transplantation. Clin Transplant 2004;18(1):89–93.

[168] Bennett WM, McEvoy KM, Henell KR, et al. Kidney transplantation in the morbidly obese: complicated but still better than dialysis. Clin Transplant 2011;25(3):401–5.

[169] Molnar MZ, Kovesdy CP, Bunnapradist S, et al. Associations of pretransplant serum albumin with posttransplant outcomes in kidney transplant recipients. Am J Transplant 2011;11(5):1006–15.

Nutritional Management of the Child with Kidney Disease

Vimal Chadha, Bradley A. Warady

Department of Pediatrics, University of Missouri-Kansas City School of Medicine, Kansas City, MO, USA

INTRODUCTION

Protein energy malnutrition (PEM) is a common problem in children with chronic kidney disease (CKD). While the exact prevalence of PEM in children with CKD is not known, an indirect estimate can be gauged from the prevalence of growth failure in these patients, especially during the first few years of life. While several factors such as metabolic acidosis, calcitriol deficiency, renal osteodystrophy, and most importantly tissue resistance to the actions of growth hormone (GH) and insulin-like growth factor-I (IGF-I) contribute to the impaired skeletal growth of children with CKD, malnutrition plays a critical role. Clinical experience suggests that inadequate nutrition may also contribute to an impaired neurodevelopmental outcome in the youngest patients with renal insufficiency [1–4]. Most importantly, physical manifestations of poor growth, such as short stature and low body mass index (BMI), have been associated with an increased risk of mortality in children with CKD [5].

On the other hand, the growing epidemic of obesity has raised concern about over-nutrition and its long-term implications in patients with CKD. Recent data from the International Pediatric Peritoneal Dialysis Network (IPPN) has revealed that being overweight is emerging as a greater problem than under-nutrition among children receiving peritoneal dialysis (PD) in developed countries [6]. In addition, the North American Pediatric Renal Trials and Collaborative Studies (NAPRTCS) database and other reports have shown an increasing prevalence of obesity in pediatric CKD patients awaiting transplantation, as well as in those with earlier stages of CKD [7,8]. Multivariate analysis of BMI Standard Deviation Score (SDS) has shown a U-shaped association between BMI and the risk of death, with extremes in BMI associated with increased

risk of mortality in children with stage 5 CKD [5,9]. Interestingly, this finding contrasts with the data from adults on maintenance dialysis, in whom increased weight seems to be associated with an improved outcome [10].

The goal of this chapter is to provide a comprehensive review of the many factors that impact the nutritional status of infants, children and adolescents with CKD or receiving maintenance dialysis and to provide treatment recommendations. Since the last publication of this chapter in 2004, the National Kidney Foundation — Kidney Disease Outcome Quality Initiative (KDOQI) Clinical Practice Guidelines for Nutrition in Children with CKD: 2008 Update was published in 2009 and included a comprehensive review of the literature and the input of experts in the field [11]. Where appropriate, information derived from those guidelines will be incorporated into this text.

ETIOLOGY OF PROTEIN-ENERGY WASTING

The accumulation of new evidence and novel thinking in the field of nutrition in CKD has resulted in a recent redefinition of the commonly used term "malnutrition". The new term, protein-energy wasting (PEW), has been proposed by The International Society of Renal Nutrition and Metabolism (ISRNM) to describe a "state of decreased body stores of protein and energy". In contrast to simple "malnutrition" that is caused by decreased intake alone, PEW is defined as a complex metabolic syndrome associated with an underlying chronic illness and characterized by a loss of muscle, with or without the loss of fat. While inadequate intake may contribute to PEW, recent evidence indicates that other factors such as systemic inflammation, endocrine perturbations, and abnormal neuropeptide signaling

TABLE 35.1   Causes of Protein-Energy Wasting (PEW) in Children with Chronic Kidney Disease

- Inadequate food intake secondary to:
  - anorexia
  - altered taste sensation
  - nausea/vomiting
  - emotional distress
  - intercurrent illness
  - unpalatable prescribed diets
  - imposed dietary restriction
  - impaired ability to procure food because of socioeconomic situation
- Chronic inflammatory state
- Catabolic response to superimposed illnesses
- Possible accumulation of endogenously formed uremic toxins and/or the ingestion of exogenous toxins
- Removal of nutrients during dialysis procedure
- Endocrine causes such as:
  - resistance to the actions of insulin and IGF-I
  - hyperglucagonemia
  - hyperparathyroidism

play important roles in wasting in the context of CKD. This topic is discussed in detail in Chapters 5, 11 and 12. A good perspective of PEW in children with CKD is provided in a recent review article by Mak et al. [12]. This section provides a brief overview of the causes of PEW as it pertains to children with CKD. The origin of PEW in children with CKD is multifactorial (Table 35.1); however, an inadequate dietary intake is considered a major contributing factor, especially in infants [13]. Nausea and vomiting are common in infants and children with CKD, with delayed gastric emptying and gastroesophageal reflux being detected in as many as 73% of patients with renal insufficiency [14]. Whereas the etiology of these gastrointestinal abnormalities is unclear, factors such as autonomic dysfunction and the actions of uremic toxins on gastric smooth muscle activity have been implicated [15].

The taste sensation of patients with CKD is frequently altered and likely also influences the voluntary nutrient intake. Although zinc depletion has been linked to anorexia, and a low dietary intake of zinc and low serum zinc concentrations have been reported in children with decreased taste acuity undergoing maintenance dialysis [16,17], a benefit of supplementation with zinc in terms of improving taste acuity and appetite has not been clearly demonstrated. Serum levels of a small peptide hormone "leptin" have been shown to be elevated in patients with CKD and those undergoing maintenance dialysis. Produced mainly in adipose tissue and primarily cleared by the kidney, it is speculated that hyperleptinemia might also contribute to uremic anorexia and malnutrition [18–20]. Finally, patients with CKD usually receive multiple medications, and drugs such as angiotensin converting enzyme (ACE)

inhibitors or antihistamines may adversely influence taste perception and, in turn, nutrient intake [21,22].

Adolescents are a unique patient group who appear to be particularly vulnerable to malnutrition due to their poor eating habits. They skip meals, favor fast foods, and in the presence of imposed dietary restrictions, find it difficult to meet the nutritional requirements of normal pubertal growth and development. Finally, the diagnosis/presence of advanced CKD may result in substantial emotional distress in many patients and their families, which may adversely affect nutritional intake. The socioeconomic status of the family might also, on occasion, prevent the patient and family from procuring appropriate food items.

ASSESSMENT OF NUTRITIONAL STATUS

Assessment of the nutritional status of children with CKD requires the evaluation of multiple indices, as there is no single measure that by itself can accurately reflect a patient's nutritional status. A variety of physical measurements and anthropometric data plotted on appropriate growth charts, along with an evaluation of the dietary intake, are required to provide a complete picture. The recommended frequency of the nutritional evaluation depends on both the age of the child and the severity of CKD (Table 35.2).

Evaluation of Nutrient Intake

Dietary recall and food intake records kept in a diary are the two most common methods used for estimating nutrient intake [23,24]. The dietary recall (usually obtained for the previous 24 hours) is a simple, rapid method of obtaining a crude assessment of dietary intake. Since it relies on the patient's (or their parents) memory, the responses may not always be valid. However, the advantages to the recall method are that respondents usually will not be able to modify their eating behavior in anticipation of this dietary evaluation, and they do not have to be literate to provide the information. The most important limitation of the 24-hour recall method is its poor ability to capture the day-to-day variability in dietary intake. Children may be even more susceptible to this limitation than adults because they tend to exhibit more day-to-day variability [25]. Therefore, it may be useful to obtain three 24-hour recalls (preferably including one weekend day) to more completely evaluate the food-intake pattern. A trained dietitian can obtain useful information from patients by using various models of foods and measuring devices to estimate food portion sizes.

Dietary diaries are prospective written reports of foods eaten during a specified length of time,

TABLE 35.2 Recommended Parameters and Frequency of Nutritional Assessment for Children with CKD Stages 2 to 5 and 5D [Ref. 11]

	Minimum Interval in Months									
	Age up to <1 Year			Age 1–3 Years			Age >3 Years			
Measure	CKD 2-3	CKD 4-5	CKD 5D	CKD 2-3	CKD 4-5	CKD 5D	CKD 2	CKD 3	CKD 4-5	CKD 5D
Dietary intake	0.5–3	0.5–3	0.5–2	1–3	1–3	1–3	6–12	6	3–4	3–4
Height or length-for-age percentile or SDS	0.5–1.5	0.5–1.5	0.5–1	1–3	1–2	1	3–6	3–6	1–3	1–3
Height or length velocity-for-age percentile or SDS	0.5–2	0.5–2	0.5–1	1–6	1–3	1–2	6	6	6	6
Estimated dry weight and weight-for-age percentile or SDS	0.5–1.5	0.5–1.5	0.25–1	1–3	1–2	0.5–1	3–6	3–6	1–3	1–3
BMI-for-height-age percentile or SDS	0.5–1.5	0.5–1.5	0.5–1	1–3	1–2	1	3–6	3–6	1–3	1–3
Head circumference-for-age percentile or SDS	0.5–1.5	0.5–1.5	0.5–1	1–3	1–2	1–2	N/A	N/A	N/A	N/A
nPCR	N/A	N/A	N/A	N/A	N/A	N/A	N/A	N/A	N/A	1*

*Only applies to adolescents receiving HD.
N/A, not applicable.

characteristically 3 to 4 days, including a weekend day. A food intake diary provides a more reliable estimate of an individual's nutrient intake than do single day records. The actual number of days chosen to collect food records should depend upon the degree of accuracy needed, the day-to-day variability in the intake of the nutrient being measured, and the cooperation of the patient. Records kept for more than 3 days increase the likelihood of inaccurate reporting because an individual's motivation will typically decrease with an increasing number of days of dietary data collection, especially if the days are consecutive [26].

Food records must be maintained meticulously to maximize the accuracy of the diary. Food intake should be recorded at the time the food is eaten to minimize any reliance on memory. Recording errors can be minimized if proper directions on how to approximate portion sizes and servings of fluid are provided. The dietitian should carefully review the food record with the patient for accuracy and completeness shortly after it is completed. While dietary diaries have been shown to give unbiased estimates of energy intake in normal-weight children younger than 10 years, underreporting is common in adolescents [27,28]. Accordingly, 24-hour recalls may be better suited to adolescents. The intake of calories, macronutrients (carbohydrate, protein and fat), vitamins and minerals derived from interviews or diaries is typically calculated using computer-based programs.

Physical Measurements (Anthropometry)

The evaluation of anthropometric parameters is a fundamental component of the nutritional assessment in pediatrics, and must be accurately measured using calibrated equipment according to standardized techniques, and ideally, by the same person on each occasion [11,29,30]. Recumbent length, height, weight, and head circumference are measured directly, and BMI is calculated as weight (in kg) divided by height (in meters) squared; reference values are available for children older than 2 years of age [31,32]. It is important to note that serial measurements are necessary for the assessment of growth.

Once measured, weight, length/height, head circumference, and BMI should be plotted on the appropriate growth chart, specific for the patient's age and sex. For premature infants, the growth parameters should be plotted after correcting for their gestational age until they are 2 years old. In 2000, the Center for Disease Control (CDC) published revised North American growth reference charts for infants and children up to 20 years of age [33] and in 2006, the World Health Organization (WHO) released new growth standards for children from birth to 5 years of age [34]. The WHO growth *standards* are distinguished from the CDC *reference* charts in two important ways. First, the children contributing to the WHO Growth Standards were specifically selected to represent children growing under ideal conditions, i.e., they had nonsmoking mothers, were from areas of high socioeconomic status, and received regular pediatric health care, including immunizations. In addition, a subset of 882 infants, all breastfed for at least 4 months, provided longitudinal data for 24 months. Second, the study population was of broad ethnic diversity. In turn, an important observation made was that ethnicity had very little impact on growth, indicating that the growth standards reflect a reasonable expectation for growth regardless of ethnicity; only 3% of the variability in growth within the population could be attributed to country of origin [34].

Because the WHO Growth Standards represent ideal growth and ideal growth should be the goal for children with CKD as well, the WHO Growth Standards should be used as the reference for children from birth to 2 years. Thereafter, the differences between the CDC reference curves and the WHO Growth Standards are minimal. For this reason and because the switch is made from length to height measurement at 2 years, this appears to be a reasonable age to make the transition from the WHO Growth Standards to the CDC reference curves [11].

In the general population, undernutrition is defined as weight-for-age, height-for-age, and weight-for-height more negative than −2.0 SD from the reference median [35]. It is important to recognize that the weight-for-age SDS is not particularly useful in isolation as weight-for-age will be low in growth retarded children. Therefore, it should be interpreted in the context of the height-for-age SDS. Accordingly, BMI is an accepted and standard method of assessing weight relative to height [36]. However, BMI is not completely independent of either age or height because of age related changes in body proportions. For this reason, BMI is expressed relative to age in developing children [37], where age functions as a surrogate for both height and maturation. In children with CKD, in whom growth retardation and delayed maturation are common, this approach has limitations. Expressing BMI relative to chronological age in a child with growth and/or maturational delay will result in inappropriate underestimation of his or her BMI compared with peers of similar height and developmental age. To avoid this problem, it may be preferable to express BMI relative to height-age (the age at which the child's height would be on the 50th percentile) in children with CKD [38]. This approach ensures that children with CKD are compared with the most appropriate reference group: those of similar height and maturation. However, caution must be used in applying this approach to children outside the pubertal or peripubertal period, for whom the correlation between height-age and maturation is less clear. BMI relative to chronological age may be more logical in some cases, particularly when sexual maturation is complete.

In addition to absolute values, all anthropometric measurements should be expressed in terms of SDS, (also known as z score) which can be calculated by using data from tables of L, M and S values [39] for each measure and entering them into the following equation:

$$SDS = [(\text{observed measure} \div M) - 1] \div (L \times S)$$

The 2000 Growth Charts LMS tables from the US National Center for Health Statistics, and WHO Growth Standards LMS tables are available on-line [34,40−42]. An SDS within two standard deviations of the mean encompasses 95% of healthy children; an SDS greater than +2.0 or more negative than −2.0 is abnormal and mandates further evaluation.

Recumbent length is measured in children up to approximately 2 years of age or in older children who are unable to stand without assistance. Height is measured when the child is able to stand unassisted. The timing of when the length measurement is changed to height measurement should be noted on the growth chart because of the discrepancy between the two measurements that commonly exist [43].

Weight should be measured while the child is nude (young infants) or with very light clothing. Special attention should be devoted to patients with edema or who are undergoing maintenance dialysis, since changes in weight are more reflective of shifts in fluid balance than true weight gain or loss. It is important to determine the patient's "dry weight," which can be challenging as growing children are expected to gain weight. Five parameters are helpful for this estimate: measured weight, presence of edema, blood pressure, laboratory data, and the dietary interview. The mid-week, post-dialysis weight is used for evaluation purposes in the hemodialysis (HD) patient, and the weight at a monthly visit (minus dialysis fluid in the peritoneal cavity) is used for the child receiving PD. A careful physical examination should be conducted to look for edema in the periorbital, pedal, and other regions of the body. Hypertension that resolves with dialysis is generally indicative of excess fluid weight. Decreased serum sodium and albumin levels may be markers of over-hydration. Likewise, a rapid weight gain in the absence of a significant increase in reported energy intake or decrease in physical activity must be critically evaluated before it is assumed to be dry weight gain.

The head circumference is measured in children up to 36 months of age with a firm, non-stretchable tape. The tape is placed just above the supra-orbital ridges and over the most prominent point on the occiput as the maximum head circumference to the nearest 0.1 cm is recorded.

Some of the previously recommended anthropometric measurements such as triceps skinfold thickness (TSF) and mid-arm circumference (MAC) used to calculate mid-arm muscle circumference and mid-arm muscle area are not recommended by the current K/DOQI Pediatric Nutrition Guidelines [11] as skinfold thickness measurement is extremely operator dependent and lacks precision [44] and in the presence of fluid overload, both MAC and TSF are also likely to be overestimated [38].

Special Studies of Protein Catabolism

Protein equivalent of total nitrogen appearance (PNA), which is sometimes inappropriately referred to as protein catabolic rate (PCR), is a useful tool for the indirect estimation of dietary protein intake. It is based on the simple principle that during steady-state conditions, total nitrogen losses are equal to or slightly less than the total nitrogen intake [45]. The majority of nitrogen losses (approximately 65%) occur as urea excretion in urine and/or dialysate [46]. Nitrogen is also lost as non-urea nitrogen in creatinine, uric acid, feces, skin and hair. Protein loss in urine and/or dialysate is an additional source of nitrogen loss. The total nitrogen losses from the body are represented as total nitrogen appearance (TNA). The PNA can, in turn, be estimated by multiplying the TNA by 6.25 based on the fact that the nitrogen content of protein is relatively constant at 16%. Recognizing the practical difficulties associated with the measurement of all sources of nitrogen loss, in addition to the fact that a portion of these losses (e.g., hair and skin) are small and fixed, several researchers have attempted to derive quantitative relationships between TNA and the easily measurable and most abundant source of nitrogen loss, urea nitrogen [46–50].

The most commonly used formula to estimate dietary protein intake by urinary urea-nitrogen excretion in adults, and published by Maroni et al. [47] is as follows:

$$\text{Protein intake (g/kg/day)} = [\text{urea-N excretion (g/kg/day)} + 0.031] \times 6.25$$

Maroni et al. proposed that the non-urea-N excretion (0.031 g/kg/day) was constant. In contrast, Wingen et al. [48] documented that in children (2 to 18 years of age) the non-urea-N excretion was higher (0.085 ± 0.061 g/kg/day) and was highly correlated to dietary protein intake (r = 0.839). This relationship did not appear to be influenced by the age of the patient. They derived the formula:

$$\text{Protein intake (g/kg/day)} = [\text{urea-N excretion (g/kg/day)} \times 15.39] - 0.8$$

Mendley and Majkowski [46] initially defined the relationship between urea-N and TNA in children undergoing PD as: TNA (g/day) = 1.26 (urea-N appearance) + 0.83. Their data suggested that the non-urea nitrogen appearance in children was greater than that reported by Maroni et al. [47], and supported the observations of Wingen et al. [48]. However, in contrast to Wingen et al.'s observation in children with CKD, the non-urea nitrogen excretion in patients undergoing PD varied by age, being significantly greater in the youngest patients. This is likely due to the relatively greater dialysate protein losses that occur in younger patients. Their formula was subsequently revised to reflect the impact of age as follows:

$$\begin{aligned} \text{TNA} = &\ 1.03\,(\text{urea-N appearance}) + 0.02\,(\text{weight in kg}) \\ &+ 0.56\,(\text{for subjects age 0 to 5 yrs) or} \\ &\ 0.98\,(\text{for subjects age 6 to 15 yrs}) \end{aligned}$$

Edefonti et al. [50] later reported that incorporating the dialysate protein-nitrogen and BSA in the formula yielded the best prediction of TNA in children undergoing PD. He recommended that the TNA be calculated in the following manner:

$$\begin{aligned} \text{TNA(g/day)} = &\ 0.03 + 1.138\,\text{Urea-N}_{\text{urine}} \\ &+ 0.99\,\text{Urea-N}_{\text{dialysate}} + 1.18\,\text{BSA} \\ &+ 0.965\,\text{Protein-N}_{\text{dialysate}} \end{aligned}$$

As protein requirements are primarily determined from fat-free, edema-free body mass, PNA is usually normalized (nPNA) to some function of body weight. The usual weight used to normalize PNA is derived from the urea distribution space ($V_{\text{urea}}/0.58$), as this idealized weight does not include the body fat weight.

Several important limitations of PNA should be recognized with respect to its usage in pediatrics. PNA is known to approximate protein intake only when the patient is in nitrogen equilibrium. However, because of growth, children are in an anabolic state and the PNA will therefore typically underestimate the actual dietary protein intake. It has also been demonstrated that children treated with recombinant human growth (rhGH) hormone may have a significantly increased DPI without exhibiting greater nitrogen excretion, reflective of an anabolic state [46]. On the other hand, in the catabolic patient, child or adult, PNA will exceed protein intake to the extent that there is net degradation and metabolism of endogenous protein pools to form urea. Therefore, PNA can fluctuate from day-to-day and a single measurement of PNA may not reflect the usual protein intake. Additionally, PNA estimates have been found to be inaccurate at extremes of protein intake [51,52].

In patients undergoing maintenance HD, the normalized protein catabolic rate (nPCR), which is equivalent to nPNA, is measured and it is dependent upon the urea generation rate (G) during the inter-dialytic period [53]. While the nPCR can be calculated simultaneously during formal Kt/V estimations by urea kinetic modeling, a simple algebraic formula used in pediatric HD patients [54] has been shown to yield nearly identical nPCR results:

$$\text{nPCR} = 5.43 \times {}_{\text{est}}G/V_1 + 0.17$$

where V_1 is total body water (in L $= 0.58 \times$ post-dialysis weight in kg), and $_{est}G$ is calculated as:

$$_{est}G(mg/min) = [(C_2 \times V_2) - (C_1 \times V_1)]/t$$

where C_1 and V_1 are post-dialysis BUN (mg/dL) and total body water (in dL $= 5.8 \times$ post-dialysis weight in kg), respectively, from the previous HD treatment; C_2 and V_2 are pre-dialysis BUN (mg/dL) and total body water (in dL $= 5.8 \times$ pre-dialysis weight in kg), respectively, from the current HD treatment, and t is time (minutes) from the end of one dialysis treatment to the beginning of the next treatment.

Recent pediatric data demonstrated that nPCR <1 g/kg/d of protein predicted a sustained weight loss of at least 2% per month for three consecutive months in adolescent and young adult-aged patients [55], whereas serum albumin levels could not. However, in younger pediatric HD patients, neither nPCR nor serum albumin level was effective in predicting weight loss.

Other Measures

Serum albumin: Serum albumin was recommended in the 2000 K/DOQI Nutrition Guidelines [56] as a marker of nutritional status because PEM may lead to hypoalbuminemia. Many studies have shown that hypoalbuminemia present at the time of dialysis initiation, as well as during the course of chronic dialysis is a strong independent predictor of patient morbidity and mortality [57–64]. However, despite its clinical utility, serum albumin levels may be insensitive to short-term changes in nutritional status, do not necessarily correlate with changes in other nutritional parameters, and can be influenced by non-nutritional factors such as infection/inflammation, hydration status, peritoneal or urinary albumin losses, and acidemia [65–69]. Therefore, while hypoalbuminemia remains an important component of the general evaluation of patients with CKD, its value as an exclusive marker of nutritional status is questionable.

Bioelectrical impedance analysis (BIA): BIA is an attractive tool for the nutritional assessment of individuals undergoing dialysis because it is noninvasive, painless, relatively inexpensive to perform, and requires minimal operator training. Whereas BIA allows for an accurate assessment of fat free mass in healthy children [70], the estimate of fat free mass of dialysis patients may be confounded by variations in hydration.

Dual energy X-ray absorptiometry (DEXA): Whole body dual energy X-ray absorptiometry (DEXA) is a reliable, noninvasive method to assess the three main components of body composition: fat mass, fat-free mass, and bone mineral mass/density. The accuracy of DEXA is minimally influenced by the variations in

hydration that commonly occur in patients on dialysis. Studies of DEXA in this patient population have demonstrated its superior precision and accuracy when compared to anthropometry, total body potassium counting, creatinine index, and bioelectrical impedance [71–74]. The main limitations to DEXA in pediatrics are its substantial cost and the lack of reliable normal values in children on dialysis.

Subjective Global Assessment (SGA): The Subjective Global Assessment (SGA), a method of nutritional assessment using clinical judgment rather than objective measures, has been widely used to assess the nutritional status of adults with CKD. An SGA specific for the pediatric population has recently been developed and validated in children undergoing major surgery [75], and its applicability in children with CKD is currently being studied. In 2001, the malnutrition–inflammation score (MIS) was introduced as one of the CKD-specific nutritional scoring systems which incorporates seven components of the original SGA plus body-mass index (BMI), serum albumin level, and total iron binding capacity (TIBC) or transferrin level. In adult patients receiving HD, the MIS is strongly associated with inflammation, nutritional status, quality of life, and 5-year prospective mortality [76].

Nutritional physical examination: Finally, the so-called nutritional physical examination can be used as an adjunct to other nutritional assessment and monitoring techniques. The nutritional physical examination involves the assessment of a patient for the presence or absence of physical signs suggestive of nutrient deficiency or excess. A careful examination of the tongue, skin, teeth, breath, and hair may provide important clues to the nutritional status [77].

NUTRITIONAL REQUIREMENTS

The nutritional requirements for children with CKD and those undergoing maintenance dialysis are generally based on the published recommended dietary allowances (RDA) for healthy children [78]. However, it is important to recognize that the RDAs are estimates of the average needs of the normal population, are meant to be applied to children as a group and do not take into account the specific requirements of an individual patient. The American Academy of Pediatrics' Committee on Nutrition states that RDAs cannot be used as a measure of nutritional adequacy in children [79].

The basis for the RDA values vary for different nutrients. While the RDA for energy reflects the average energy intake needed to maintain body weight and activity of well-nourished normal-sized individuals (with an additional provision for infants and children to ensure normal growth), the RDAs for protein are based on protein nitrogen loss (mean + 2SD), and are further adjusted to account for poor protein quality and individual variability [80].

The RDAs for a number of nutrients have been replaced by Dietary Reference Intakes (DRIs) [81]. The new DRIs are comprised of a set of four reference values: *Estimated Average Requirement* (EAR), *Recommended Daily Allowance* (RDA), *Adequate Intake* (AI), *and Tolerable Upper Intake Level* (UL). The EAR is the median usual intake value that is estimated to meet the requirements of half of the healthy individuals in a specific age and gender group, while the other half of individuals are at risk for nutritional deficiency and/or chronic disease. EARs are used to assess the prevalence of nutrient inadequacy in a group of individuals. RDAs are intake levels that, according to the available scientific evidence, meet the nutrient requirement of almost all (>97%) healthy individuals in a specific age and gender group. Adequate Intake values are used when the scientific

evidence is lacking to establish an EAR or an RDA. Adequate Intakes are derived either from experimental data or are approximated from the observed mean nutrient intakes of apparently healthy people. The Tolerable Upper Intake Level is the highest level of daily nutrient intake that is likely to pose no risk of adverse health effects in almost all individuals in a specified group. The UL is not intended to be a recommended intake level and the potential risk for adverse effects increases if the intake exceeds the UL.

Energy Requirements

A variety of studies have shown that the majority of pediatric patients with CKD exhibit an inadequate dietary energy intake [82–86]. Furthermore, the energy intake progressively decreases with worsening renal failure [86]. A number of studies in infants and children on PD have documented mean energy intakes of less than 75% of RDA [87–89], which corresponds to approximately 100% of the estimated energy requirement (EER or EAR) in children older than 3 months. In a large, prospective study of growth failure in children with CKD, caloric intakes were <80% of the RDA for age in more than one-half of food records obtained [90]. While inadequate voluntary energy intake has been clearly demonstrated in infants with CKD [91,92], energy intakes for older children are generally normal relative to their body size [90]. Since energy intake is the principle determinate of growth during infancy, malnutrition has the most marked negative effect on growth in children with congenital disorders leading to CKD [93]. More than half (58.3%) of infants with CKD in the 2008 NAPRTCS report had a height SDS worse than −1.88 (mean for all infants: −2.34) [94].

Energy requirements for children with CKD should be considered to be 100% of the EER for chronological age, that is individually adjusted for the Physical Activity Level (PAL) and BMI [11,95] (Tables 35.3 and 35.4). It is

TABLE 35.3 Equations to Estimate Energy Requirements for Children at Healthy Weights

Age	Estimated Energy Requirement (EER) (kcal/d) = Total Energy Expenditure + Energy Deposition
0–3 mo	EER = [89 × weight (kg) − 100] + 175
4–6 mo	EER = [89 × weight (kg) − 100] + 56
7–12 mo	EER = [89 × weight (kg) − 100] + 22
13–35 mo	EER = [89 × weight (kg) − 100] + 20
3–8 y Boys:	EER = 88.5 − 61.9 × age (y) + PA × [26.7 × weight (kg) + 903 × height (m)] + 20
Girls:	EER = 135.3 − 30.8 × age (y) + PA × [10 × weight (kg) + 934 × height (m)] + 20
9–18 y Boys:	EER = 88.5 − 61.9 × age (y) + PA × [26.7 × weight (kg) + 903 × height (m)] + 25
Girls:	EER = 135.3 − 30.8 × age (y) + PA × [10 × weight (kg) + 934 × height (m)] + 25

Reproduced with permission from Ref: [95].

TABLE 35.4 Physical Activity Coefficients for Determination of Energy Requirements in Children Ages 3–18 Years

	Level of Physical Activity			
Gender	Sedentary	Low Active	Active	Very Active
	Typical activities of daily living (ADL) only	ADL + 30–60 min of daily moderate activity (e.g., walking at 5–7 km/h)	ADL + ≥ 60 min of daily moderate activity	ADL + ≥ 60 min of daily moderate activity + an additional 60 min of vigorous activity or 120 min of moderate activity
Boys	1.0	1.13	1.26	1.42
Girls	1.0	1.16	1.31	1.56

Health Canada: www.hc-sc.gc.ca/fn-an/alt_formats/hpfb-dgpsa/pdf/nutrition/dri_tables-eng.pdf. Reproduced with permission of the Minister of Public Works and Government Services Canada 2008.

important to note that calculated energy requirements are estimates, and some children will require more or less for normal growth; therefore, all dietary prescriptions should be individualized. Energy requirements for patients treated with maintenance HD or PD are similar to those of pre-dialysis patients. In children receiving maintenance PD therapy, variable glucose absorption takes place from the dialysis fluid depending on the PD modality, dialysate glucose concentration, and peritoneal membrane solute transport capacity. In a study of 31 children older than 3 years on ambulatory PD therapy, the mean energy intake derived from peritoneal glucose absorption was 9 kcal/kg/day [96]. Since many children who receive chronic PD are underweight, the prescribed energy intake in them should exclude the estimated calorie absorption from the dialysate as failure to do so may compromise the nutritional quality of the diet. However, some children — and particularly infants receiving PD therapy — gain weight at a faster rate than normal despite oral and/or enteral energy intakes that are lower than the average requirements. Reduced physical activity and increased exposure to high dialysate glucose concentrations for fluid removal may be explanations; in these cases, the calorie contribution from dialysate should be taken into account when estimating energy requirements.

Maximizing caloric intake has been noted to be particularly effective in improving height velocity only in infants with CKD or receiving dialysis [91–93,97,98]. As children older than 2 years of age with CKD do not generally experience catch-up growth [99], the provision of adequate energy intake early in life is crucial. Rizzoni et al. [13] demonstrated that the growth of infants with CKD receiving ≤100% of the RDA averaged 53% (range 10 to 72%) of expected, whereas it averaged 97% (range 61% to 130%) of expected during periods when the energy intake was ≥100% of the RDA. In a study of 35 children younger than 5 years with CKD stages 4 to 5, significant weight gain and accelerated linear growth was demonstrated in those starting enteral feeding at <2 years of age, while improved weight gain and maintenance of growth velocity was observed in those starting enteral feeds at age 2 to 5 years, in each case without exceeding normal energy requirements [91]. If children younger than 3 years with a length (or height) for age < −1.88 SDS fail to achieve expected weight gain and growth when receiving an intake based on chronological age, estimated requirements may be increased by using height-age related recommendations. Finally, while energy supplementation resulting in a total energy intake exceeding the RDA for age has been administered to children treated with long-term dialysis, there are no data that demonstrate a resultant and consistent improvement in growth velocity [100–102]. On the other hand, prevention and treatment of obesity in patients with CKD is important and energy requirements for overweight or obese children are lower and can be estimated by using equations specific for children heavier than a healthy weight [95].

Protein Requirements

Low-protein diets reduce the generation of nitrogenous wastes and inorganic ions, both of which might be responsible for many of the clinical and metabolic disturbances characteristic of uremia. In addition, there is a nearly linear relationship between protein and phosphorus intake [103] which results in the frequent association between hyperphosphatemia and a high protein diet [104]. Accordingly, low-protein diets decrease the development of hyperphosphatemia, metabolic acidosis, hyperkalemia, and other electrolyte disorders. Pediatricians, on the other hand, are rightly concerned about the potential for harmful effects of severe dietary protein restriction, particularly as it pertains to the growth of infants and young children with CKD. Experimental studies in young animals have shown that a decrease in dietary protein intake during the normally rapid period of growth to a level that is sufficient to slow the deterioration of kidney function, does adversely affect growth [105]. As a result, very few studies of dietary protein restriction have been conducted in children with CKD [106,107]. In the largest and most significant pediatric trial, 191 children with CKD stages 3 to 4 were randomized to a reduced dietary protein intake of 100% RDA (0.8 to 1.1 g/kg ideal body weight) or to continue ad libitum intake (mean intake 181% RDA). This modest reduction in protein intake, with maintenance of energy intake greater than 80% RDA in both groups, did not adversely affect growth, serum albumin or the rate of CKD progression within the observation period of 2–3 years [107]. Hence, although there is no evidence for a nephroprotective effect of dietary protein restriction, this study did provide evidence that dietary protein intake can be safely restricted to 0.8 to 1.1 g/kg/d in children with CKD. As in adults, the "restriction" of protein intake is recommended as a means of decreasing the dietary phosphorus intake and the risk for hyperphosphatemia because of its frequent association with cardiovascular disease (CVD) in patients with CKD.

While the spontaneous DPI is reduced in progressive CKD in a manner similar to that of energy intake, the DPI typically remains far in excess of the average requirements, ranging from 150% to 200% of the RDA [84,90,107]. Current K/DOQI Pediatric Nutrition guidelines recommend maintaining the DPI at 100% to 140% of the DRI for ideal body weight in children with CKD stage 3 and at 100% to 120% of the DRI in children with CKD stages 4 to 5 (Table 35.5) [11]. It is

TABLE 35.5 Recommended Dietary Protein Intake in Children with CKD Stages 3—5 and 5D

Age	DRI (g/kg/d)	Recommended for CKD Stage 3(g/kg/d) (100—140% DRI)	Recommended for CKD Stages 4—5 (g/kg/d) (100—120% DRI)	Recommended for HD (g/kg/d)	Recommended for PD (g/kg/d)
0—6 months	1.5	1.5—2.1	1.5—1.8	1.6	1.8
7—12 months	1.2	1.2—1.7	1.2—1.5	1.3	1.5
1—3 years	1.05	1.05—1.5	1.05—1.25	1.15	1.3
4—13 years	0.95	0.95—1.35	0.95—1.15	1.05	1.1
14—18 years	0.85	0.85—1.2	0.85—1.05	0.95	1.0

DRI + 0.1 g/kg/d to compensate for dialysis losses.
DRI + 0.15—0.3 g/kg/d depending on patient age to compensate for peritoneal losses.

important to note that the protein DRI values are lower than the RDA across all age groups [95]. These dietary protein recommendations refer to the needs for a stable child and assume that energy intake is adequate (i.e., it meets 100% of EER). Inadequate caloric intake results in the inefficient use of dietary protein as a calorie source, with a resultant increased generation of urea. Ensuring that caloric needs are met is an important step in assessing protein requirements and modifying protein intake. It is advised that at least 50% of the total protein intake consist of protein of high biologic value such as the protein from milk, eggs, meat, fish, and poultry.

Protein requirements may be increased in patients with proteinuria and during recovery from intercurrent illness and may be adjusted to height age instead of chronological age if evidence of protein deficiency exists. Modification of protein recommendations may also be necessary in obese children. Obese individuals have a greater percentage of body fat, which is much less metabolically active than lean body mass. Therefore, it is believed that basing protein (and energy) requirements of obese individuals on their actual weight may overestimate requirements. Conversely, using ideal body weight for an obese person does not take into account the increase in body protein needed for structural support of extra fat tissue. Therefore, a common practice is to estimate protein requirements of obese individuals based on an "adjusted" weight (i.e., adjusted weight = ideal weight for height + 25% × [actual weight − ideal weight], where 25% represents the percentage of body fat tissue that is metabolically active) rather than their actual body weight [108].

The optimal protein intake for pediatric patients on maintenance dialysis has not yet been well defined. Reviews of nitrogen-balance studies performed in adult dialysis patients with different protein intakes [109—114] conclude that HD patients are in neutral nitrogen balance with a protein intake as low as 0.75 to 0.87 g/kg/d, and PD patients, with 0.9 to 1.0 g/kg/d.

A single nitrogen-balance study has been performed in dialyzed children [96]. In 31 pediatric patients receiving automated PD, the investigators observed a positive correlation between nitrogen balance and DPI and concluded that the DPI should be at least 144% of RDA. However, nitrogen balance also positively correlated with total energy intake, and no multivariate analysis was performed to address whether energy intake, protein intake, or both were independent effectors of nitrogen balance.

A single randomized prospective study in adults [115] and several trials in children have addressed the effect of selectively increasing the amino acid supply in patients on PD therapy. Despite increases in amino acid and dietary protein intake, no significant beneficial effects on nutritional status and longitudinal growth were achieved by this intervention in children, whereas the urea concentration frequently increased [116—120]. These results are compatible with the interpretation that it is not possible to induce tissue anabolism by selectively increasing protein and amino acid ingestion, except in subjects with subnormal baseline protein intake. If more protein is ingested than needed for metabolic purposes, all the excess is oxidized and results in accumulation of nitrogenous-containing end products.

There is some concern that a high DPI may even be harmful to dialyzed children. In a DXA study of body composition in 20 children on long-term PD therapy and with a mean DPI of 144% RDA, protein intake inversely correlated with bone mineral density, bone mineral content, fat-free mass, and plasma bicarbonate level, suggesting that a high protein intake may cause tissue catabolism and bone loss by worsening metabolic acidosis [121]. Finally, the most convincing argument for limiting DPI in dialyzed children is derived from the solid evidence for a key etiologic role of dietary phosphorus load in the pathogenesis of dialysis-associated calcifying arteriopathy. There is a nearly linear relationship between protein and phosphorus intake [103], which results in the frequent association between high quantities of protein in the diet and hyperphosphatemia [122]. Hence, it appears most appropriate to limit protein intake in children on dialysis to the safe levels known to ensure adequate growth and nutrition in healthy children.

Although dialyzed children require larger amounts of protein per unit of body weight compared to adults in order to grow in size and lean body mass, this demand is fully accounted for by the age-adjusted pediatric DRI. Hence, the only additional dietary protein requirement justified by evidence is the replacement of dialytic nitrogen losses. In those on long-term PD therapy, daily peritoneal protein losses decrease with age across childhood from an average of 0.28 g/kg in the first year of life to less than 0.1 g/kg in adolescents [123]. Peritoneal amino acid losses add approximately one-third to the nitrogen lost with protein, resulting in a total additional dietary protein requirement ranging from 0.15 to 0.35 g/kg, depending on patient age (Table 35.5). Patients with high-peritoneal transport characteristics tend to have low serum albumin levels likely due to increased peritoneal protein losses; these patients may have slightly greater protein requirements. Because dialytic protein concentrations can be measured easily, consideration should be given to regular monitoring of peritoneal protein excretion and individual adaptation of the dietary protein prescription according to actual peritoneal losses.

Amino acid and protein losses during HD vary according to dialyzer membrane characteristics and reuse. Whereas losses have not been quantified in children, an average of 8 to 10 g of amino acids and less than 1 to 3 g of protein are lost per HD session in adults [124–127]. On the basis of three HD sessions per week for a 70 kg adult, this equates to 0.08 g/kg/day. Assuming that dialytic amino acid losses are linearly related to urea kinetics, children can be expected to have similar or slightly higher amino acid losses than adults and an added DPI of 0.1 g/kg/d should be appropriate to compensate for pediatric HD losses. Under all conditions, at least 50% of dietary protein intake should be of high biological value to protect body protein and minimize urea generation.

Lipid Requirements

Dyslipidemia is a frequently recognized complication of CKD in children [128], occurs relatively early in the course of CKD (i.e., Stage 3 CKD) and increases in prevalence with decreasing kidney function [129]. Hypercholesterolemia and hypertriglyceridemia have been reported in 69% and 90% of children with CKD stage 5, respectively [130]. Recent data from the CKiD study reported the presence of dyslipidemia in 44% of 250 children with mild to moderate CKD; the most common

abnormality was hypertriglyceridemia in 75% [131]. The dyslipidemia seen in children with CKD has complex underlying metabolic alterations and is characterized by increased levels of serum triglycerides in combination with high levels of VLDL and intermediate-density lipoproteins (IDLs), low levels of HDL particles, and normal or modestly increased levels of total and low density lipoprotein (LDL) cholesterol [128,132,133]. This pattern of dyslipidemia has been labeled "atherogenic". In addition, hypertriglyceridemia has been shown to be an independent contributor to the development of CVD [134,135] and may also accelerate the progression of CKD [136].

The optimal management of dyslipidemia in children with CKD is not clearly defined. Treatment of malnutrition related to impaired kidney function is essential and should supersede any potential rise in lipid levels that might result from it. On the contrary, prevention and treatment of obesity in patients with CKD is an important strategy to reduce the risk of hyperlipidemia [137]. Correction of metabolic acidosis, vitamin D therapy, and correction of anemia with erythropoietin each also seem to have some normalizing effect on dyslipidemia in children with CKD [138–140]. The K/DOQI Dyslipidemia Guidelines' recommendations [141], endorsed by the KDOQI Cardiovascular Guidelines [142], recommend that the dietary and lifestyle recommendations made for adults are also appropriate for post-pubertal children and adolescents with CKD. In 1992, the National Cholesterol Education Program (NCEP) Pediatric Panel Report [143] provided dietary recommendations for all children. These guidelines were recently endorsed by the Expert Panel on Integrated Guidelines for Cardiovascular Health and Risk Reduction in Children and Adolescents [144]. The latter publication recommends that in children with identified hypercholesterolemia, less than 25% to 30% of calories should come from dietary fat, of which ≤7% should be from saturated fatty acids; the daily cholesterol intake should be <200 mg. For serum triglyceride >150 mg/dL, therapeutic lifestyle changes (TLC) are recommended along with a low fat diet and a low intake of simple carbohydrates. The child should be encouraged to ingest complex carbohydrates in lieu of simple sugars and concentrated sweets and to use unsaturated fats such as oils and margarines from corn, safflower, and soy. Plant stanol esters in the form of dietary supplements reduce intestinal cholesterol absorption and may provide a safe and effective means of reducing serum cholesterol.

High intakes of n-3 polyunsaturated fatty acids (omega-3 fatty acids [n-3 FA], docosahexanoic acid [DHA], and eicosapentanoic acid [EPA]) are associated with decreasing TG levels and a decreased risk of heart disease [145,146]. Therefore, EPA and DHA, found almost exclusively in fish and marine sources, must be provided in the diet; the highest sources are fatty fish (e.g., tuna, mackerel, trout, salmon, herring, sardines, and anchovies) [147]. Although n-3 FAs have been found to be extremely safe by both Health Canada and the US Food and Drug Administration, there is insufficient evidence at this time to recommend routine use of n-3 FAs to treat hypertriglyceridemia in children with CKD.

Dietary fiber, particularly naturally occurring viscous fiber, reduces total and LDL cholesterol levels and high intakes have been associated with reduced rates of CVD. The AI for total fiber is based on daily caloric intake, and for all children 1 year and older is 14 g/1000 kcal/d. Dietary fiber is found in most fruits, vegetables, legumes, and whole grains, which are foods restricted in low-potassium and low-phosphorus diets; therefore, meeting normal daily fiber recommendations is challenging for children with CKD. Tasteless mineral- and electrolyte-free powdered forms of fiber (e.g., Unifiber®, Benefiber®) are available to add to meals or drinks if children are unable to meet their fiber intake by diet. High-fiber diets require additional fluid intake, which may not be possible for oliguric or anuric patients with strict fluid restriction.

BONE MINERAL METABOLISM

Calcium

Adequate dietary calcium intake during childhood is necessary for skeletal development and acquisition of optimal peak bone mass [148]. The current recommendation is that patients with CKD should achieve a calcium intake of 100% of the DRI [149] (Table 35.6). Infants and young children usually meet the DRI for calcium with the consumption of adequate volumes of breast milk/formula. Unfortunately, the largest sources

of dietary calcium for most persons are dairy products which are also rich in phosphorus; in turn, phosphorus restriction universally leads to a decreased calcium intake. In these situations, calcium supplementation may be required as low phosphorus, high calcium containing foods such as collards, dandelion greens, kale, rhubarb, and spinach usually do not make up a substantial part of a child's diet. Several products fortified with calcium such as fruit juices and breakfast foods are commercially available and limited studies have suggested that the bioavailability of calcium from these products is at least comparable to that of milk [150]. Calcium can also be supplemented in medicinal forms such as carbonate (40% elemental calcium), acetate (25% elemental calcium), and gluconate (9% elemental calcium) salts of calcium that are commonly used as phosphate binders. When used for calcium supplementation alone, ingesting these products between meals maximizes calcium absorption. Chloride and citrate salts of calcium should be avoided as the former may lead to acidosis in patients with CKD and the latter may enhance aluminum absorption.

On the other hand, excessive calcium intake in conjunction with activated vitamin D analogs can lead to (i) hypercalcemia; (ii) adynamic bone disease; and (iii) systemic calcification. Accordingly, the K/DOQI guidelines recommend that the combined elemental calcium intake from nutritional sources and phosphate binders should not exceed two times the DRI for age, except for ages 9–18 years (both genders) where two times the DRI (2600 mg) exceeds the Tolerable Upper Intake Level (UL) of 2500 mg [149] (Table 35.6). The serum level of total corrected calcium should be maintained within the normal range (8.8–9.5 mg/dL), preferably towards the lower end and definitely not more than 10.2 mg/dL, while the serum calcium and phosphorus product should be kept below 55 mg/dL in adolescents >12 years, and <65 mg/dL in younger children [151].

The calcium balance in patients undergoing maintenance dialysis is also affected by the dialysate calcium concentration. The calcium balance during PD is usually negative with use of a 2.5 mEq/L calcium dialysate and positive with a dialysate calcium concentration of 3.0–3.5 mEq/L [152]. As a result, it may be wise to use a low calcium dialysate (2.5 mEq/L) in children undergoing dialysis who are receiving calcium-containing phosphate binders along with activated vitamin D sterols. On the contrary, a 3.0–3.5 mEq/L calcium dialysate should be used if hypocalcemia is present in a child with elevated PTH (>300 pg/mL) as part of the treatment of secondary hyperparathyroidism (SHPT) and may be needed in children restricted to non-calcium containing phosphate binders only.

TABLE 35.6 Recommended Calcium Intake for Children with CKD Stages 2–5 and 5D

Age	DRI	Upper Limit (for Healthy Children)	Upper Limit for CKD Stages 2–5, 5D (Dietary + Phosphate Binders)
0–6 months	210	ND	≤420
7–12 months	270	ND	≤540
1–3 years	500	2500	≤1000
4–8 years	800	2500	≤1600
9–18 years	1300	2500	≤2500

ND, not determined.
Determined as 200% of the DRI, to a maximum of 2500 mg elemental calcium.

Phosphorus

In an effort to prevent/control CKD-associated bone disease and CVD, serum phosphorus concentrations above the normal reference range for age (Table 35.7), should be avoided in patients with advanced CKD. However, even during the earlier stages of CKD when the serum phosphorus levels are typically within normal range, the dietary phosphorus load is an important determinant of the severity of hyperparathyroidism. Dietary phosphorus restriction decreases PTH levels and increases $1,25(OH)_2D$, whereas dietary phosphorus intakes approximately twice the DRI for age aggravate hyperparathyroidism despite little or no change in serum phosphorus levels (likely the result of elevated FGF-23 levels and enhanced phosphorus excretion) [153]. It is important to note that the higher physiological serum concentrations of calcium and phosphorus that are observed in healthy infants and young children, presumably reflect the increased requirements for these minerals by the rapidly growing skeleton. Rickets due to phosphorus deficiency can occur in preterm infants whose diet provides insufficient quantities of phosphorus, as well as in infants and children with hypophosphatemia due to inherited disorders of renal phosphate transport. Hence, when dietary phosphorus is restricted to control hyperphosphatemia and SHPT in children with CKD, subnormal serum phosphorus values are equally important to avoid. Recently published recommendations suggest that in children with CKD whose serum PTH concentration exceeds the target range (Table 35.7) but whose serum phosphorus concentration remains normal, the dietary phosphorus intake should be restricted to 100% of the DRI; in contrast, the intake should be restricted to 80% of the DRI when the serum phosphorus concentration exceeds the normal reference range for age (Table 35.8) [11].

Despite the need to restrict dietary phosphorus, most clinicians recognize that an overly strict dietary phosphorus restriction is not only often impractical, but it

TABLE 35.7 Age-Specific Normal Ranges of Blood Ionized Calcium, Total Calcium and Phosphorus

Age	Ionized Calcium (mmol/L)	Calcium (mg/dL)	Phosphorus (mg/dL)
0−5 months	1.22−1.40	8.7−11.3	5.2−8.4
6−12 months	1.20−1.40	8.7−11.0	5.0−7.8
1−5 years	1.22−1.32	9.4−10.8	4.5−6.5
6−12 years	1.15−1.32	9.4−10.3	3.6−5.8
13−20 years	1.12−1.30	8.8−10.2	2.3−4.5

Conversion factor for calcium and ionized calcium: mg/dL × 0.25 = mmol/L.
Conversion factor for phosphorus: mg/dL × 0.323 = mmol/L.

TABLE 35.8 Recommended Maximum Oral and/or Enteral Phosphorus (mg/d) Intake for Children with CKD

Age	DRI (mg/d)	High PTH and Normal Phosphorus	High PTH and High Phosphorus
0−6 months	100	≤100	≤80
7−12 months	275	≤275	≤220
1−3 years	460	≤460	≤370
4−8 years	500	≤500	≤400
9−18 years	1250	≤1250	≤1000

Health Canada: www.hc-sc.gc.ca/fn-an/alt_formats/hpfb-dgpsa/pdf/nutrition/dri_tables-eng.pdg. Reproduced with the Permission of the Minister of Public Works and Government Services Canada, 2008. ≤100% of the DRI; ≤80% of the DRI.

can be ill advised as it may lead to an inadvertent poor dietary protein intake with a possible increase in mortality [53]. In addition, extremely low phosphorus diets are typically unpalatable. While young infants are characteristically managed with a low-phosphorus containing milk formula such as Similac PM 60/40 (Abbott Nutrition), or Renastart (Vitaflo Nutrition), or by pretreatment of breast milk, infant formula and cow's milk with sevelamer carbonate (Renvela®) which can effectively reduce the phosphorus content in the supernatant by 80−90% [154,155], it is important to note that some infants may require phosphorus supplementation in the form of sodium phosphate (Neutra Phos) because of their higher physiological needs, as mentioned previously. Most other patients with CKD require oral intestinal phosphate binders to control hyperphosphatemia. Phosphorus control is particularly difficult in vegetarians since for the same total quantity of dietary protein delivered, the phosphorus content is greater in protein derived from vegetable sources (average 20 mg of phosphorus per gm of protein) vs. animal protein (average 11 mg of phosphorus per gram of protein). However, the bioavailability of phosphorus from plant-derived food is very low; therefore, despite their higher specific phosphorus content, some plant sources of protein may actually result in a lower rate of phosphorus uptake per mass of protein than meat based foods [11]. Whereas food labels rarely state the phosphorus content, chocolates, nuts, dried beans, and cola soft drinks are rich in phosphorus and should be avoided; nondairy creamers and certain frozen nondairy desserts may be used in place of milk and ice cream.

Vitamin D

Recent clinical evidence suggests a high prevalence (typically 80% to 90%) of nutritional vitamin D insufficiency in both children and adults with CKD [156]. In

TABLE 35.9 Recommended Supplementation for Vitamin D Deficiency/Insufficiency in Children with CKD

Serum 25(OH)D (ng/mL)	Definition	Ergocaliferol (Vitamin D$_2$) or Cholecalciferol (Vitamin D$_3$) Dosing	Duration (months)
<5	Severe vitamin D deficiency	8000 IU/d orally or enterally × 4 wk or (50,000 IU/wk × 4 wk); then 4000 IU/d or (50,000 IU twice per mo for 2 mo) × 2 mo	3
5−15	Mild vitamin D deficiency	4000 IU/d orally or enterally × 12 wk or (50,000 IU every other wk, for 12 wk)	3
16−30	Vitamin D insufficiency	2000 IU daily or (50,000 IU every 4 wk)	3

a recent publication, Ali et al reported a 20−75% prevalence of vitamin D deficiency (25(OH)D <15 ng/mL) in children with CKD stages 1−5, with higher prevalence rates in Hispanics and African-Americans, likely due to increased melanin content in their skin [156]. This insufficiency may aggravate SHPT in patients with CKD as the availability of 25(OH)$_2$ D becomes a rate limiting step for the synthesis of 1,25(OH)$_2$ D. Accordingly, the latest KDOQI Pediatric Nutrition Guidelines suggest checking serum 25(OH)$_2$ D levels once per year in children with CKD stages 2−5 [11]. If the serum level of 25(OH)$_2$ D is <30 ng/mL, supplementation with vitamin D$_2$ (ergocalciferol) or vitamin D$_3$ (cholecalciferol) is suggested, with the specific dosing regimen dependent on the severity of the deficiency (Table 35.9). Cholecalciferol appears to have higher bioefficacy than ergocalciferol, although long-term comparative trials are lacking in humans [157,158]. During the repletion phase, serum levels of calcium and phosphorus should be measured 1 month following the initiation or a change in the dose of vitamin D and at least every 3 months thereafter. Once patients are replete with vitamin D, supplemental vitamin D should be continued and 25(OH)$_2$ D levels checked yearly [11,151].

ACID−BASE AND ELECTROLYTES

Acid−Base Status

Infants and children normally have a relatively larger endogenous hydrogen ion load (2−3 mEq/kg) than do adults (1 mEq/kg); in turn, metabolic acidosis is a common manifestation of CKD in children and an important negative influence on growth through a number of growth factor specific mechanisms, including reduction in thyroid hormone levels and blunting of IGF response to growth

hormone [159]. Furthermore, studies performed in adults and children have shown that chronic acidosis is associated with increased oxidation of branched-chain amino acids, increased protein degradation [160], and decreased albumin synthesis [161]. Persistent acidosis also has detrimental effects on bone because it alters the normal accretion of hydroxyapatite into bone matrix and causes bone demineralization as bone buffers are increasingly used for neutralizing the excess acid load. Thus, it is recommended that the serum bicarbonate level should be maintained at or above 22 mEq/L in children with CKD by supplementing with oral bicarbonate as needed [11].

Sodium

Sodium requirements in children with CKD are dependent on the underlying kidney disease and the degree of renal insufficiency. Children who have CKD as a result of obstructive uropathy or renal dysplasia are most often polyuric and may experience substantial urinary sodium losses despite advanced degrees of CKD. Sodium depletion adversely affects growth and nitrogen retention [162], and its intake supports normal expansion of the ECF volume needed for muscle development and mineralization of bone [163]. Fine et al. demonstrated poor weight gain in animals deprived of salt with a resultant decreased extracellular volume, bone mass and fat mass [164]. Parekh et al. reported the beneficial effect of a dilute, sodium supplemented (2−4 mEq sodium per 100 mL formula), high-volume (180 to 240 mL/kg per 24 hours, depending on urine output) feeding regimen on the linear growth of 24 young children with severe polyuric CKD. The treated group of patients was able to maintain a nearly normal height SDS despite the presence of significant renal insufficiency [165]. Therefore, infants and children with polyuric salt-wasting forms of CKD who do not have their sodium and water losses corrected may experience vomiting, constipation, and significant growth retardation associated with chronic intravascular volume depletion and a negative sodium balance [165]. It is important to note that normal serum sodium levels do not rule out sodium depletion and the need for supplementation. Sodium supplementation can be given as chloride or bicarbonate, depending upon the patient's acid−base status.

In contrast, children with CKD resulting from a primary glomerular disease, or those who are oliguric or anuric, typically require a sodium and fluid restriction to minimize fluid gain, edema formation, and hypertension. The prescribed fluid intake is usually a fraction of the calculated maintenance volume adjusted for the degree of oliguria. According to the most recent 2005 Dietary Guidelines, the sodium intake for children older than 2 years should be restricted to <1500 mg (65 mmol) [166], which corresponds to sodium intake of 1 to 2 mmol/kg/day for those younger than 2 years. These patients should be advised to avoid processed foods and snacks from fast-food restaurants as the majority (75%) of sodium in the diet comes from salt added during food processing.

Infants receiving PD are predisposed to substantial sodium losses, even when anuric. High ultrafiltration requirements per kilogram of body weight result in removal of significant amounts of sodium chloride. These losses are not adequately replaced through the low sodium content of breast milk (160 mg/L or 7 mmol/L) or standard commercial infant formulas (160 to 185 mg/L or 7 to 8 mmol/L) [167]. Therefore, infants on PD are at risk of developing hyponatremia that can result in cerebral edema and blindness and must be maintained in neutral sodium balance. Sodium supplementation should be individualized based on clinical symptoms, including hypotension, hyponatremia, and/or abnormal serum chloride levels.

Potassium

Potassium homeostasis in children with CKD is usually unaffected until the glomerular filtration rate (GFR) falls to <10% of normal. However, children with renal dysplasia, post-obstructive kidney damage, severe reflux nephropathy, and renal insufficiency secondary to interstitial nephritis often demonstrate renal tubular resistance to aldosterone and may manifest hyperkalemia, even when their GFR is relatively well preserved. The hyperkalemia experienced by these children is exacerbated by volume contraction (and can be particularly common in salt losers) and the majority of the patients respond to salt and water repletion. In patients who are persistently hyperkalemic, dietary potassium intake should be limited. As potassium content is infrequently listed on food labels and cannot be tasted, a list of foods rich in potassium such as chocolates, French fries, potato chips, bananas, green leafy vegetables, dried fruits, and orange juice should be provided to patients and their families. Altering the methods of food preparation, such as soaking vegetables before cooking, helps decrease potassium content. Moderate to severe hyperkalemia may require treatment with a potassium binder such as sodium polystyrene sulfonate (Kayexalate); in hypertensive children, calcium polystyrene sulfonate can be used instead to decrease the sodium load. In the case of infants and young children being fed milk formula, the potassium content of the formula can be reduced by pretreating it with a potassium binder [168]. If constipated, the patient should be treated aggressively as significant quantities of potassium are eliminated through the gastrointestinal route in patients with CKD.

In children undergoing HD, dietary potassium intake should be distributed throughout the day, as high serum concentrations of potassium can develop when a large quantity of potassium is ingested at one time, regardless of the total daily dietary content. On the other hand, some patients receiving PD may become hypokalemic due to potassium losses in the dialysate and will require potassium supplementation.

VITAMINS AND MICRONUTRIENTS

Vitamins and minerals are essential for normal growth and development and either a deficiency or an excess can prove harmful. Unfortunately, the vitamin and mineral needs of pediatric patients with CKD are not clearly defined (other than for Vitamin D), and the limited data that is available is derived from patients undergoing maintenance dialysis. Children with CKD are prone to develop vitamin deficiencies because of anorexia and dietary restrictions, while they are also at risk to develop toxic levels of vitamins when the renal clearance is significantly impaired.

All of the water-soluble vitamins except pyridoxine are eliminated by the kidneys and their clearance in patients with CKD is not known. However, most water-soluble vitamins are lost during maintenance dialysis and, in turn, are routinely supplemented by special vitamin formulations that do not contain vitamin A and D, such as Nephronex (L Lorens Pharmaceuticals), and Nephro-Vite (R & D Laboratories, Inc., Marina Del Rey, CA). Studies conducted in the adult dialysis population have provided evidence of low blood concentrations of water-soluble vitamins and minerals because of inadequate intake, increased losses, and increased needs [169,170]. Deficiency of vitamin B_6 can result from poor dietary intake as well as impaired formation and/or increased clearance of pyridoxal phosphate in the dialysis fluid [171]. Vitamin B_{12} and folic acid, both of which are important for effective erythropoiesis, differ in their peritoneal clearance; while there can be significant losses of folic acid, only small quantities of vitamin B_{12} are lost by this route [172]. Accordingly, supplementation with 0.8 to 1.0 mg folic acid is routinely recommended, while the necessity of vitamin B_{12} supplementation remains unsettled. A higher dose of folic acid (2.5 mg per day) has been suggested for children with CKD as supplemental folic acid has been shown to decrease the elevated homocysteine level that is commonly seen in patients with renal failure and is a potential risk factor for cardiovascular morbidity and mortality [173,174]. In contrast, serum thiamine and riboflavin levels have been reported to be normal in PD patients, with or without supplementation, in association with negligible losses during dialysis [175].

Supplementation with vitamin C is occasionally recommended because of the significant quantity that can be lost during PD [176]. It is important to recognize however, that while adequate levels of vitamin C are necessary for the formation of collagen, an excessive intake of vitamin C in the dialysis population may result in elevated oxalate levels as an end-product of vitamin C metabolism and lead to the development of significant vascular complications [177]. Accordingly, vitamin C intake should not exceed 100 mg/day. Vitamin K deficiency is likely in patients who receive frequent antibiotics and has been reported in a small number of adults [178]. Vitamin A levels are usually elevated in patients undergoing PD despite the lack of vitamin A in the vitamin supplement formulation. The elevated levels are a result of the loss of the kidneys normal ability to excrete vitamin A metabolites [179]. Since elevated levels of vitamin A can be associated with the development of hypercalcemia and complications related to a high calcium-phosphorus product, it is critically important to avoid the use of vitamin supplements that include vitamin A.

In children older than 6 years of age undergoing PD, vitamin supplementation has been associated with normal or greater than normal serum levels of the water-soluble vitamins [176]. However, no published studies have assessed the blood vitamin levels of children undergoing maintenance dialysis in the absence of the use of a vitamin supplement. As most infant milk formulas including Similac PM 60/40 are fortified with both water-soluble and fat-soluble vitamins, most infants with CKD/ESRD receive the DRI/RDA for all vitamins (including vitamin A) by dietary intake alone. Warady et al. [180] reported on the vitamin status of a group of seven infants undergoing PD; their main nutrient intake was infant milk formula (Similac PM 60/40) and they received a water-soluble vitamin supplement (Iberet; Abbott Laboratories, Abbott Park, IL). The combined dietary and supplement intake exceeded the RDA for the water-soluble vitamins in all but one patient who received only 79% of the RDA for vitamin B_6 because of inadequate formula intake. In all cases, the patient's serum concentrations of the water-soluble vitamins were comparable to or greater than the values reported in normal infants. In addition, the serum vitamin A levels were significantly greater than normal values, despite the lack of supplemental vitamin A.

Aluminum, copper, chromium, lead, strontium, tin, and silicon levels have all been noted to be elevated in patients with CKD, reflecting the fact that their clearance is dependent on an adequate GFR [181,182]. Other trace elements have not been well studied in children; however, zinc levels have been shown to be low in malnourished children and should be monitored and supplemented as necessary [181].

Based on the limited data referred to above, the current KDOQI Pediatric Nutrition Guidelines [11] recommend the intake of at least 100% of the DRI for thiamin (B_1), riboflavin (B_2), niacin (B_3), pantothenic acid (B_5), pyridoxine (B_6), biotin (B_8), cobalamin (B_{12}), ascorbic acid (C), retinol (A), α-tocopherol (E), vitamin K, folic acid, copper, and zinc for children with CKD stages 2 to 5, and those receiving maintenance dialysis. They suggest supplementation of vitamins and trace elements if dietary intake alone does not meet 100% of the DRI or if clinical evidence of a deficiency, possibly confirmed by low blood levels of the vitamin or trace element, is present [11]. As most infant milk formulas including Similac PM 60/40 are fortified with both water-soluble and fat-soluble vitamins, the majority of infants with CKD (and not yet on dialysis) receive the dietary reference intakes (DRI) for all vitamins (including vitamin A) by dietary intake alone and do not require vitamin supplementation.

Carnitine

Carnitine is an essential compound in the oxidative process of fatty acids and adenosine triphosphate formation [183], and the kidney is the major site for its synthesis in humans. While there is evidence of carnitine deficiency in patients undergoing HD [184], and far less information regarding its status in those receiving PD, there is little information on the carnitine status of children with CKD. Carnitine deficiency can result in the development of anemia, cardiomyopathy, and muscle weakness [184]. However, most, but not all of the few pediatric studies that have been conducted on the subject of carnitine deficiency in dialysis patients have provided evidence for an increase in the plasma carnitine level after carnitine supplementation with no associated change in any symptoms [185]. As such, there currently is insufficient evidence to support the routine use of carnitine in either the pediatric CKD or dialysis patient populations. However, a trial of carnitine may be indicated when all other causes for the symptoms in question have been excluded, carnitine deficiency has been confirmed, and the patient has been unresponsive to standard therapies [186]. Carnitine deficiency is confirmed by measurements of plasma free and total carnitine with an acyl:free carnitine ratio greater than 0.4 (i.e., [total − free carnitine] ÷ free carnitine) or a total serum carnitine value less than 40 µmol/L [184].

NUTRITION MANAGEMENT

A registered dietitian with experience in pediatric renal diseases should play the central role in the dietary management of children with CKD/ESRD. In addition to possessing knowledge related to nutritional requirements, this person should also be skilled in the evaluation of physical growth, developmental assessment, and the educational and social needs of this special population. The dietitian must be able to establish a positive rapport with both the child and the primary caretakers in order to enhance compliance with the recommended nutritional regimen. The focus of the dietitian's treatment plan is determined by the patient's age. In the case of infants, the parents or primary caretaker who is responsible for feeding the child has the greatest interaction with the dietician; in contrast, adolescents must receive the majority of information directly, as they often eat independently. For children between these two extremes, both the parents and the child are typically involved in different aspects of the dietary management. It is noteworthy that the two most vulnerable groups of patients in terms of the risk for malnutrition are infants and adolescents. While infants are at special risk because of the frequent occurrence of anorexia and emesis, many adolescents have poor eating habits, as mentioned previously.

An individualized nutrition plan taking into account a variety of factors should be developed for each patient by the dietician in consultation with the physician, patient (when appropriate) and family, with clearly defined short and long-term objectives. As cultural food preferences play an important role in the family's ability to adhere to dietary changes, dietary instructions should be tailored to help families modify, but not eliminate cultural food preferences. Background information on cultural diets and translated versions of renal diets and food lists are available for reference [187]. The plan should be modified as necessary according to changes in the child's nutritional status, renal function, dialytic therapy, medication regimen, and psychosocial situation.

Dietary restrictions should be limited as much as possible with a goal of enhancing nutrient intake. Restrictions of nutrients should ideally be imposed only when there is a clear indication, rather than an anticipated need. It is also important to find substitutes for restricted foods so as to maintain an adequate caloric intake. A simple explanation of the role of the nutrient in the body, the rationale for the diet modification, and the desired outcomes to be achieved (e.g. normalization of biochemical parameter, specific amount of weight gain) is helpful in obtaining cooperation of the patient and caretakers, thereby increasing the likelihood of success. Adopting and maintaining changes in eating habits is also easier for a child if family members make similar changes, or at least avoid eating restricted foods in the child's presence. In addition, caregivers outside of the immediate family (e.g. grandparents, school staff, babysitters) should be aware of the diet restrictions and be asked to provide consistency of care in helping the child follow his/her diet. While the ideal goal is full compliance with the prescribed regimen, it is not always a realistic expectation and "partial compliance" is often acceptable. Being very rigid with the dietary prescription adds to parental stress and increases the risk for behavioral eating problems in the young child such as food refusal, gagging, and vomiting.

Oral Supplementation

Infants with CKD requiring fluid restriction or those who have a poor oral intake may require a greater caloric density of their milk formula than the standard 20 kcal/oz. The increase in caloric density should not be achieved by concentrating the milk formula, as this approach will also increase the protein and mineral content. The provision of extra calories can be achieved by adding carbohydrate and/or fat modules to the formula. A glucose polymer such as Polycose (Abbott Nutrition) has a low osmolality and is generally the initial supplement added to infant formulas. Additional calories can be added in the form of corn oil. Oils containing medium chain triglyceride (MCT) are generally not necessary unless there is coexistent malabsorption. However, usage of corn and other oils as additives is not common as they do not mix well with formula and cause problems with tube-feedings. Microlipid (Nestle Nutrition), a 50% fat emulsion from safflower oil with 4.5 kcal/mL and Duocal® (Nutrica North America), a fat and carbohydrate combo modular with 5 kcal per gram of powder (59% calories from carbohydrate and 41% from fat), are common commercially available products for energy supplementation. The latter is not approved for infants younger than 1 year. Older infants may tolerate the addition of corn syrup or sugar, which are readily available and inexpensive. The quantity of both carbohydrate and fat modules can gradually be increased to raise the caloric density to as much as 60 kcal/oz [188]. It is important to wait at least 24 hours following each 2- to 4-kcal/oz incremental increase in concentration to enhance patient tolerance of the formula.

Nutritional therapy, irrespective of the route of administration or caloric density of the formula, should provide a balance of calories from carbohydrate and unsaturated fats within the physiological ranges recommended as the Acceptable Macronutrient Distribution Ranges (AMDR) of the DRI. Recommended AMDR for children older than 4 years are 45–65% from carbohydrate, 25–35% from fat (polyunsaturated/saturated ratio of 1), and 10–30% from protein; children younger than 3 years need a somewhat greater proportion of fat (30–40%) in their diets to meet energy needs. An adequate amount of non-protein calories should be provided for protein-sparing effects. It should, however, be noted that during the advanced stages of uremia, the protein-sparing effect of added fat calories may be inferior to the effect of added concentrated carbohydrate calories [29]. Children beyond infancy characteristically refuse the high-calorie carbohydrate supplements. For them, it is often easier to encourage common foods that have a high caloric content, but a relatively low mineral and protein content. Powdered fruit drinks, frozen fruit flavored desserts, candy, jelly, honey, and other concentrated sweets can be used for this purpose. However, the altered taste acuity associated with uremia may limit the acceptability of these foods. In addition, one may need to avoid high carbohydrate foods in the presence of hypertriglyceridemia. Under these circumstances, unsaturated fats may be the preferred choice of high calorie food sources. Children and adolescents should also be encouraged to use margarine on popcorn, bread, vegetables, rice, and noodles for added calories.

A variety of calorie-dense (1.8 kcal/mL) preparations such as Nepro and Suplena (Abbott Nutrition) have been formulated specifically for renal patients and are commercially available. Suplena has a lower protein content than Nepro (30g/L vs. 70 g/L), and is preferable for pre-dialysis patients. These preparations are characterized by a low renal osmolar load and a low vitamin A and D content. Although initially produced for patients older than 10 years, they have been successfully used in children as young as 3 years; however, it is advisable to dilute them to half to two-thirds strength when used in young children. Recently, Hobbs et al. reported the successful use of these adult renal formulas in seven hyperkalemic infants with improved growth and normalization of the serum potassium level [189].

In contrast to energy intake, the protein requirements of children with CKD are usually met by voluntary, unsupplemented consumption. If the protein intake is insufficient due to concomitant phosphorus restriction in the patient with severely impaired renal function, the protein module, Beneprotein (Nestle Nutrition), a whey protein concentrate, can be added to the formula to increase the protein content. As much as 1 g of Beneprotein , which is equivalent to 0.86 g protein, can be added to each ounce of formula. Semi-synthetic diets supplemented with either amino or keto forms of essential amino acid (EAA) have also been tried to ensure an adequate protein intake. However, the lack of sufficient data in children precludes making any firm recommendation regarding their possible clinical application.

Enteral Nutritional Support

Aggressive enteral feeding should be considered if the nutritional intake by the oral route is sub optimal despite all attempts at oral supplementation. The use of enteral support has resulted in maintenance or improvement of SD scores for weight and/or height in infants and young children with moderate to severe CKD and those undergoing maintenance dialysis [4,13,23,190–193]. In fact, several investigators, including Kari et al. [92] have advocated early enteral feeding at the first sign of growth failure during infancy.

Nasogastric (NG) tubes [191,193–195], gastrostomy catheters [196], gastrostomy buttons [197,198], and gastrojejunostomy tubes [199], have been used to provide supplemental enteral feeding to children with renal disease with encouraging results. The feeding can be given as an intermittent bolus, or more commonly by continuous infusion during the night. Continuous overnight feeds are generally preferred to allow time during the day for regular oral intake. Historically, the NG tube has been used most frequently in infants and young children, as it is easily inserted and is generally well tolerated [193,200]. Ellis et al. reported usage of NG tube by 78% and 68% of children who initiated dialysis at <3 months and 3–20 months of age, respectively [201]. However, this route of therapy is often complicated by recurrent emesis and the need for frequent tube replacement, in addition to the risk of pulmonary aspiration, nasoseptal erosion, and psychological distress of the caretaker because of the cosmetic appearance. Persistent emesis can be addressed by slowing the rate of formula delivery and by the addition of antiemetic agents such as metoclopramide or domperidol. Additionally, whey predominant formulas can be used as they have been shown to stimulate gastric emptying [202,203].

The gastrostomy tube or button has been used as the enteral route of choice by many clinicians, and has the cosmetic advantage of being hidden beneath clothing. Once placed, it can be used within several days. Many, but not all clinicians recommend that the patient should be investigated for gastroesophageal reflux prior to undertaking gastrostomy placement so that a Nissen fundoplication can be created at the same sitting, if required. The reported complications of gastrostomy tubes/buttons include exit-site infection, leakage, obstruction, gastrocutaneous fistula, and peritonitis [204,205]. Peritonitis is potentially the most serious complication and is a likely factor inhibiting the more widespread adoption of gastrostomy as opposed to NG feeding in the PD population [206]. Warady et al. reported that 11 (24%) of 45 episodes of fungal peritonitis were associated with the presence of a gastrostomy tube or button, but there was no statistically significant correlation between the presence of a gastrostomy and the development of fungal peritonitis [207]. To decrease the risk of peritonitis, the gastrostomy should be placed either before or simultaneously during PD catheter placement. In addition, it may be better to avoid combining gastrostomy placement and peritoneal dialysis catheter placement in a severely malnourished patient until the nutritional status and general immunity of the patient can be improved by other means, such as NG tube feeds [205].

A recent report by Rees et al. [208], demonstrated the effectiveness of NG tube and gastrostomy feeding in improving the nutritional status of young (<2 years) children receiving chronic PD. However, the report also revealed marked global variation in feeding strategies and the complex relationship between enteral feeding and growth.

A common and serious complication of using any form of enteral tube feeding is a prolonged and potentially difficult transition from tube to oral feeding [209,210]. Regular non-nutritive sucking and repetitive oral stimulation are recommended for all tube-fed infants. A multidisciplinary feeding team consisting of a dietitian, occupational therapist, and behavioral psychologist can help facilitate the transition from tube to oral feeding.

Alternative Routes of Nutritional Support

The substitution of amino acids for dextrose in the peritoneal dialysis fluid and the provision of parenteral nutrition during hemodialysis sessions (intradialytic parenteral nutrition; IDPN) are two additional aggressive approaches to nutritional supplementation that have had limited pediatric application. Intraperitoneal nutrition has been evaluated in only a small number of children receiving PD and for a limited period of time [211–214]. The quantity of amino acids absorbed from the dialysate routinely exceeded the protein lost in the dialysate. Very little experience with IDPN has been reported in the pediatric population. A short-term study of 10 chronic hemodialysis patients, ages 10 to 18 years, conducted in the Netherlands documented weight gain in nine patients with no significant change in plasma amino acid profile [215]. Similarly, Goldstein et al. [216], demonstrated reversal of weight loss and initiation of weight gain within 6 weeks of IDPN initiation in three malnourished adolescents undergoing hemodialysis. Future studies may prove these routes of nutritional supplementation to be valuable adjuncts to the oral and enteral routes of therapy.

References

[1] Warady BA, Kriley M, Lovell H, et al. Growth and development of infants with end-stage renal disease receiving long-term peritoneal dialysis. J Pediatr 1988;112:714–9.

[2] Geary DF, Haka Ikse K. Neurodevelopmental progress in young children with chronic renal disease. Pediatrics 1989;84:68–72.

[3] Geary DF, Haka Ikse K, Coulter P, et al. The role of nutrition in neurology health and development of infants with chronic renal failure. Adv Perit Dial 1990;6:252–4.

[4] Claris-Appiani A, Arissino GL, Dacco V, et al. Catch-up growth in children with chronic renal failure treated with long-term enteral nutrition. JPEN 1995;19:175–8.

[5] Wong CS, Gipson DS, Gillen DL, et al. Anthropometric measures and risk of death in children with end-stage renal disease. Am J Kidney Dis 2000;36:811–9.

[6] International Pediatric Peritoneal Dialysis Network. About IPPN (online), www.pedpd.org/index.php?id=98; 2011.

[7] Hanevold CD, Ho PL, Talley L, Mitsnefes MM. Obesity and renal transplant outcome: A report of the North American Pediatric Renal Transplant Cooperative Study. Pediatrics 2005;115:352–6.

[8] Filler G, Payne RP, Orrbine E, Clifford T, Drukker A, McLaine PN. Changing trends in the referral patterns of pediatric nephrology patients. Pediatr Nephrol 2005;20:603–8.

[9] Srivaths PR, Wong C, Goldstein SL. Nutrition aspects in children receiving maintenance hemodialysis: impact on outcome. Pediatr Nephrol 2009;25:951–7.

[10] Kopple JD, Zhu X, Lew NL, Lowrie EG. Body weight-for-height relationships predict mortality in maintenance hemodialysis patients. Kidney Int 1999;56:1136–48.

[11] National Kidney Foundation: KDOQI clinical practice guideline for nutrition in children with CKD: 2008 update. Am J Kidney Dis 2009;53(Suppl. 2):S1–S124.

[12] Mak RH, Cheung WW, Zhan JY, Shen Q, Foster BJ. Cachexia and protein-energy wasting in children with chronic kidney disease. Pediatr Nephrol 2012;27:173–81.

[13] Rizzoni G, Basso T, Setari M. Growth in children with chronic renal failure on conservative treatment. Kidney Int 1984;26:52–8.

[14] Ruley EJ, Bock GH, Kerzner B, et al. Feeding disorders and gastroesophageal reflux in infants with chronic renal failure. Pediatr Nephrol 1989;3:424–9.

[15] Bird NJ, Strather CP, O'Doherty MJ, et al. Gastric emptying in patients with chronic renal failure on continuous ambulatory peritoneal dialysis. Nephrol Dial Transplant 1993;9:287–90.

[16] Tamaru T, Vaughn WH, Waldo FB, et al. Zinc and copper balance in children on continuous ambulatory peritoneal dialysis. Pediatr Nephrol 1989;3:309–13.

[17] Coleman JE, Watson AR. Micronutrient supplementation in children on continuous cycling peritoneal dialysis (CCPD). Adv Perit Dial 1992;8:396–401.

[18] Daschner M, Tonshoff B, Blum WF, et al. Inappropriate elevation of serum leptin levels in children with chronic renal failure. European Study Group for Nutritional treatment of Chronic Renal Failure in Childhood. J Am Soc Nephrol 1998;9:1074–9.

[19] Stenvinkel P. Leptin and its clinical implications in chronic renal failure. Miner Electrolyte Metab 1999;25:298–302.

[20] Wolf G, Chen S, Han DC, et al. Leptin and renal disease. Am J Kidney Dis 2002;39:1–11.

[21] Shiffman S. Changes in taste and smell: drug interactions and food preferences. Nutr Rev 1994;52:S11–4.

[22] van der Ejik I, Allman Farinelli MA. Taste testing in renal patients. J Renal Nutr 1997;7:3–9.

[23] Buzzard M. 24-hour dietary recall and food record methods. In: Willett W, editor. New York, NY, Oxford: Nutritional epidemiology; 1998. p. 50–73.

[24] Bross R, Noori N, Kovesdy CP, Murali SB, Benner D, Block G, et al. Dietary assessment of individual with chronic kidney disease. Semin Dial 2010;23:359–64.

[25] Livingstone MB, Robson PJ. Measurement of dietary intake in children. Proc Nutr Soc 2000;59:279–93.

[26] Gersovitz M, Madden JP, Smiciklas-Wright H. Validity of the 24 hr dietary recall and seven-day record for group comparisons. J Am Diet Assoc 1978;73:48–55.

[27] Bandini LG, Cyr H, Must A, Dietz WH. Validity of reported energy intake in preadolescent girls. Am J Clin Nutr 1997;65(Suppl. 4):S1138—41.

[28] Champagne CM, Baker NB, DeLany JP, Harsha DW, Bray GA. Assessment of energy intake underreporting by doubly labeled water and observations on reported nutrient intakes in children. J Am Diet Assoc 1998;98:426—33.

[29] Nelson P, Stover J. Nutrition recommendations for infants, children, and adolescents with end-stage renal disease. In: Gillit D, Stover J, editors. A Clinical Guide to Nutrition Care in End-Stage Renal Disease. Chicago, IL: American Dietetic Association; 1994. p. 79—97.

[30] Centers for Disease Control and Prevention. Using the CDC growth charts: Accurately Weighing and Measuring. Technique, Equipment, Training Modules 2001.

[31] Must A, Dallal GE, Dietz WH. Reference data for obesity: 85 and 95 percentiles of body mass index (wt/ht) and triceps skin fold thickness. Am J Clin Nutr 1991;53:839—46.

[32] Hammer LD, Kraemer HC, Wilson DM, et al. Standardized percentile curves of body-mass index for children and adolescents. AJDC 1991;145:259—63.

[33] Kuczmarski RJ, Ogden CL, Grummer-Strawn LM, et al. CDC growth charts: United States. Adv Data Report no. 2000;314: 1—27.

[34] World Health Organization: WHO Child Growth Standards: Length/Height-for-Age, Weight-for-Age, Weight-for-Length, Weight-for-Height and Body Mass Index-for-Age. Methods and Development. Geneva, Switzerland: World Health Organization; 2006. p. 332.

[35] Peterson KE, Chen LC. Defining undernutrition for public health purposes in the United States. J Nutr 1990;120:933—42.

[36] Cole TJ, Flegal KM, Nicholls D, Jackson AA. Body mass index cut offs to define thinness in children and adolescents: International survey. BMJ 2007;335:194.

[37] Kuczmarski RJ, Ogden CL, Guo SS, et al. 2000 CDC Growth Charts for the United States: Methods and development. Vital Health Stat 2002;11:1—190.

[38] Foster BJ, Leonard MB. Measuring nutritional status in children with chronic kidney disease. Am J Clin Nutr 2004;80:801—14.

[39] Cole TJ. The LMS method for constructing normalized growth standards. Eur J Clin Nutr 1990;44:45—60.

[40] www.cdc.gov/nchs/about/major/nhanes/growthcharts/data files.htm.

[41] www.who.int/childgrowth/standards/technical_report/en/index. html.

[42] World Health Organization. WHO Child Growth Standards: Head Circumference-for-Age, Arm Circumference-for-Age, Triceps Skinfold-for-Age and Subscapular Skinfold-for-Age. Methods and Development. Geneva, Switzerland: World Health Organization; 2007. 234.

[43] WHO Child Growth Standards based on length/height, weight and age. Acta Pediatrica 2006;450(Suppl.):76—85.

[44] Wang J, Thornton JC, Kolesnisk S, et al. Anthropometry in body composition. An overview. Ann N Y Acad Sci 2000;94:317—26.

[45] Kopple JD, Jones MR, Keshaviah PR, et al. A proposed glossary for dialysis kinetics. Am J Kidney Dis 1995;26:963—81.

[46] Mendley SR, Majkowski NL. Urea and nitrogen excretion in pediatric peritoneal dialysis patients. Kidney Int 2000;58: 2564—70.

[47] Maroni BJ, Steinman TI, Mitch WE. A method for estimating nitrogen intake of patients with chronic renal failure. Kidney Int 1985;27:58—65.

[48] Wingen AM, Fabian-Bach C, Mehls O. European Study Group for Nutritional Treatment of Chronic Renal Failure in Childhood. Evaluation of protein intake by dietary diaries and urea-N excretion in children with chronic renal failure. Clin Nephrol 1993;40:208—15.

[49] Kopple JD, Gao XL, Qing DP. Dietary protein, urea nitrogen appearance and total nitrogen appearance in chronic renal failure and CAPD patients. Kidney Int 1997;52:486—94.

[50] Edefonti A, Picca M, Damiani B, et al. Models to assess nitrogen losses in pediatric patients on chronic peritoneal dialysis. Pediatr Nephrol 2000;15:25—30.

[51] Kopple JD. Uses and limitations of the balance technique. J Parenter Enteral Nutr 1987;11:S79—85.

[52] Panzetta G, Tessitore N, Faccini G, et al. The protein catabolic rate as a measure of protein intake in dialysis patients: Usefulness and limits. Nephrol Dial Transplant 1990;5:S125—7.

[53] Shinaberger CS, Kilpatrick RD, Regidor DL, McAllister CJ, Greenland S, Kopple JD, et al. Longitudinal associations between dietary protein intake and survival in hemodialysis patients. Am J Kidney Dis 2006;48:37—49.

[54] Goldstein SL. Hemodialysis in the pediatric patient: State of the art. Adv Renal Rep Ther 2001;8:173—9.

[55] Juarez-Congelosi M, Orellana P, Goldstein SL. Normalized protein catabolic rate versus serum albumin as a nutrition status marker in pediatric patients receiving hemodialysis. J Ren Nutr 2007;17:269—74.

[56] National Kidney Foundation — Kidney Disease Outcomes Quality Initiative. Clinical Practice Guidelines for Nutrition in Chronic Renal Failure. Am J Kidney Dis 2000;35:S1—S140.

[57] Owen Jr WF, Lew NL, Liu Y, et al. The urea reduction ratio and serum albumin concentration as predictors of mortality in patients undergoing hemodialysis. N Eng J Med 1993;329: 1001—6.

[58] Spiegel DM, Breyer JA. Serum albumin: A predictor of long-term outcome in peritoneal dialysis patients. Am J Kidney Dis 1994;23:283—5.

[59] Avram MM, Mittman N, Bonomini L, et al. Markers for survival in dialysis: A seven year prospective study. Am J Kidney Dis 1995;26:209—19.

[60] Churchill DN, Taylor DW, Keshaviah PR. Adequacy of dialysis and nutrition in continuous peritoneal dialysis: association with clinical outcomes. Canada-USA Peritoneal Dialysis Study Group. J Am Soc Nephrol 1996;7:198—207.

[61] Foley RN, Pafrey PS, Harnett JD, et al. Hypoalbuminemia, cardiac morbidity, and mortality in end-stage renal disease. J Am Soc Nephrol 1996;7:728—36.

[62] Fung L, Pollock CA, Caterson RJ, et al. Dialysis adequacy and nutrition determine prognosis in continuous ambulatory peritoneal dialysis patients. J Am Soc Nephrol 1996;7:737—44.

[63] Marcen R, Teruel JL, de la Cal MA, et al. The impact of malnutrition in morbidity and mortality in stable hemodialysis patients. Spanish Cooperative Study of Nutrition in Hemodialysis. Nephrol Dial Transplant 1997;12:2324—31.

[64] Wong CS, Hingorani S, Gillen DL, et al. Hypoalbuminemia and risk of death in pediatric patients with end-stage renal disease. Kidney Int 2002;61:630—7.

[65] Jones CH, Newstead CG, Will EJ, et al. Assessment of nutritional status in CAPD patients: Serum albumin is not a useful measure. Nephrol Dial Transplant 1997;12:1406—13.

[66] Yeun JY, Kaysen JA. Factors influencing serum albumin in dialysis patients. Am J Kidney Dis 1998;32:S118—25.

[67] Ballmer PE, McNurlan MA, Hulter HN, et al. Chronic metabolic acidosis decreases albumin synthesis and induces negative nitrogen balance in humans. J Clin Invest 1995;95:39—45.

[68] Kaysen GA, Rathore V, Shearer GC, et al. Mechanisms of hypoalbuminemia in hemodialysis patients. Kidney Int 1995;48:510—6.

[69] Han DS, Lee SW, Kang SW, et al. Factors affecting low values of serum albumin in CAPD patients. Adv Perit Dial 1996;12: 288–92.

[70] Schaefer F, Georgi M, Zieger A, et al. Usefulness of bioelectric impedance and skinfold measurements in predicting fat-free mass derived from total body potassium in children. Pediatr Res 1994;35:617–24.

[71] Formica C, Atkinson MG, Nyulasi I, et al. Body composition following hemodialysis: Studies using dual-energy X-ray absorptiometry and bioelectrical impedance analysis. Osteoporosis Int 1993;3:192–7.

[72] Stenver DI, Gotfredsen A, Hilsted J, et al. Body composition in hemodialysis patients measured by dual-energy X-ray absorptiometry. Am J Nephrol 1995;15:105–10.

[73] Borovnicar DJ, Wong KC, Kerr PG, et al. Total body protein status assessed by different estimates of fat-free mass in adult peritoneal dialysis patients. Eur J Clin Nutr 1996;50: 607–16.

[74] Woodrow G, Oldroyd B, Smith MA, et al. Measurement of body composition in chronic renal failure: Comparison of skinfold anthropometry and bioelectrical impedance with dual energy X-ray absorptiometry. Eur J Clin Nutr 1996;50: 295–301.

[75] Secker DJ, Jeejeebhoy KN. Subjective Global Nutritional Assessment for children. Am J Clin Nutr 2007;85:1083–9.

[76] Rambod M, Bross R, Zitterkoph J, Benner D, Pithia J, Colman S, et al. Association of malnutrition-inflammation score with quality of life and mortality in hemodialysis patients: a 5-year prospective cohort study. Am J Kidney Dis 2009;53:298–309.

[77] Kight MA, Kelly MP. Conducting physical examination round for manifestations of nutrient deficiency or excess: an essential component of JCAHO assessment performance. Diagn Nutr Network 1995;4:2–6.

[78] Food and Nutrition Board. In: Commission on Life Sciences, National Research Council: Recommended Dietary Allowances. 10th ed. Washington DC: National Academies Press; 1989.

[79] Committee on Nutrition. American Academy of Pediatrics: Pediatric Nutrition Handbook. 4th ed. 1998;489:648–649. p. 126.

[80] Holliday MA. Nutrition therapy in renal disease. Kidney Int 1986;30:S3–6.

[81] Food and Nutrition Boards. Institute of Medicine: Dietary Reference Intakes: Applications in Dietary Assessment. A report of the subcommittees on interpretation and uses of Dietary reference Intakes and Upper Reference Levels of Nutrients, and the Standing Committee on the Scientific Evaluation of Dietary Reference Intakes. Washington DC: National Academies Press; 2001.

[82] Salusky IB, Fine RN, Nelson P, et al. Nutritional status of children undergoing continuous ambulatory peritoneal dialysis. Am J Clin Nutr 1983;38:599–611.

[83] Holliday MA. Calorie deficiency in children with uremia: Effect upon growth. Pediatrics 1972;50:590–7.

[84] Ratsch IM, Catassi C, Verrina E, et al. Energy and nutrient intake of patients with mild to moderate chronic renal failure compared with healthy children: An Italian multicenter study. Eur J Pediatr 1992;151:701–5.

[85] Kuizon BD, Salusky IB. Growth retardation in children with chronic renal failure. J Bone Miner Res 1999;14:1680–90.

[86] Norman LJ, Coleman JE, Macdonald IA, et al. Nutrition and growth in relation to severity of renal disease in children. Pediatr Nephrol 2000;15:259–65.

[87] Broyer M, Niaudet P, Champion G, et al. Nutritional and metabolic studies in children on continuous ambulatory peritoneal dialysis. Kidney Int Suppl 1983;15/24:S106–10.

[88] Macdonald A. The practical problems of nutritional support for children on continuous ambulatory peritoneal dialysis. Human Nutrition: Applied Nutrition 1986;40A:253–61.

[89] Canepa A, Divino Filho JC, Forsberg AM, et al. Children on continuous ambulatory peritoneal dialysis: muscle and plasma proteins, amino acids and nutritional status. Clin Nephrol 1996;46:125–31.

[90] Foreman JW, Abitol CL, Trachtman H, et al. Nutritional intake in children with renal insufficiency: A report of the Growth Failure in Children with Renal Diseases Study. J Am Coll Nutr 1996;15:579–85.

[91] Ledermann SE, Shaw V, Trompeter RS. Long-term enteral nutrition in infants and young children with chronic renal failure. Pediatr Nephrol 1999;13:870–5.

[92] Kari JA, Gonzalez C, Ledermann SE, et al. Outcome and growth of infants with severe chronic renal failure. Kidney Int 2000;57:1681–7.

[93] Betts PR, Magrath G, White RH. Role of dietary energy supplementation in growth of children with chronic renal insufficiency. Br Med J 1977;1:416–8.

[94] North American Pediatric Renal Trials and Collaborative Studies (NAPRTCS) 2008 Annual Report.

[95] Food and Nutrition Board. Dietary reference intakes for energy, carbohydrate, fiber, fat, fatty acids, cholesterol, protein, and amino acids (macronutrients). Food and Nutrition Board. Washington, DC: National Academies; 2002.

[96] Edefonti A, Picca M, Damiani B, et al. Dietary prescription based on estimated nitrogen balance during peritoneal dialysis. Pediatr Nephrol 1999;13:253–8.

[97] Mehls O, Blum WF, Schaefer F, et al. Growth failure in renal disease. Baillieres Clin Endocrinol Metab 1992;6:665–85.

[98] Sedman A, Friedman A, Boineau F, et al. Nutritional management of the child with mild to moderate chronic renal failure. J Pediatr 1996;129:S13–8.

[99] Foreman JW, Chan JCM. Chronic renal failure in infants and children. J Pediatr 1988;113:793–800.

[100] Arnold WC, Danford D, Holliday MA. Effects of caloric supplementation on growth in children with uremia. Kidney Int 1983;24:205–9.

[101] Betts PR, Magrath G. Growth pattern and dietary intake of children with chronic renal insufficiency. Br Med J 1974;2: 189–93.

[102] Simmons JM, Wilson CJ, Potter DE, Holliday MA. Relation of calorie deficiency to growth failure in children on hemodialysis and the growth response to calorie supplementation. N Engl J Med 1971;285:653–6.

[103] Boaz M, Smetana S. Regression equation predicts dietary phosphorus intake from estimate of dietary protein intake. J Am Diet Assoc 1996;96:1268–70.

[104] Shinaberger CS, Greenland S, Kopple JD, et al. Is controlling phosphorus by decreasing dietary protein intake beneficial or harmful in persons with chronic kidney disease? Am J Clin Nutr 2008;88(6):1511–8.

[105] Friedman AL, Pityer R. Benefit of moderate dietary protein restriction on growth in the young animal with experimental chronic renal insufficiency: importance of early growth. Pediatr Res 1989;25:509–13.

[106] Uauy RD, Hogg RJ, Brewer ED, et al. Dietary protein and growth in infants with chronic renal insufficiency: a report from the Southwest Pediatric Nephrology Study Group and the University of California, San Francisco. Pediatr Nephrol 1994;8:45–50.

[107] Wingen AM, Fabian-Bach C, Schaefer F, et al. for the European Study Group for Nutritional Treatment of Chronic Renal Failure in Childhood. Randomized multicenter study of a low-protein

diet on the progression of chronic renal failure in children. Lancet 1997;349:1117—23.

[108] Krenitsky J. Adjusted body weight, pro: Evidence to support the use of adjusted body weight in calculating calorie requirements. Nutr Clin Pract 2005;20:468—73.

[109] Borah MF, Schoenfeld PY, Gotch FA, Sargent JA, Wolfsen M, Humphreys MH. Nitrogen balance during intermittent dialysis therapy of uremia. Kidney Int 1978;14:491—500.

[110] Kopple JD, Shinaberger JH, Coburn JW, Sorensen MK, Rubini ME. Optimal dietary protein treatment during chronic hemodialysis. Trans Am Soc Artif Intern Organs 1969;15: 302—8.

[111] Giordano C, De Santo NG, Pluvio M, et al. Protein requirement of patients on CAPD: A study on nitrogen balance. Int J Artif Organs 1980;3:11—4.

[112] Blumenkrantz MJ, Kopple JD, Moran JK, Coburn JW. Metabolic balance studies and dietary protein requirements in patients undergoing continuous ambulatory peritoneal dialysis. Kidney Int 1982;21:849—61.

[113] Buchwald R, Pena JC. Evaluation of nutritional status in patients on continuous ambulatory peritoneal dialysis (CAPD). Perit Dial Int 1989;9:295—301.

[114] Bergstrom J, Furst P, Alvestrand A, Lindholm B. Protein and energy intake, nitrogen balance and nitrogen losses in patients treated with continuous ambulatory peritoneal dialysis. Kidney Int 1993;44:1048—57.

[115] Misra M, Ashworth J, Reaveley DA, Muller B, Brown EA. Nutritional effects of amino acid dialysate (Nutrineal) in CAPD patients. Adv Perit Dial 1996;12:311—4.

[116] Canepa A, Perfumo F, Carrea A, et al. Long-term effect of amino-acid dialysis solution in children on continuous ambulatory peritoneal dialysis. Pediatr Nephrol 1991;5:215—9.

[117] Canepa A, Perfumo F, Carrea A, et al. Continuous ambulatory peritoneal dialysis (CAPD) of children with amino acid solutions: Technical and metabolic aspects. Perit Dial Int 1990;10:215—20.

[118] Hanning RM, Balfe JW, Zlotkin SH. Effectiveness and nutritional consequences of amino acid-based vs. glucose-based dialysis solutions in infants and children receiving CAPD. Am J Clin Nutr 1987;46:22—30.

[119] Qamar IU, Levin L, Balfe JW, Balfe JA, Secker D, Zlotkin S. Effects of 3-month amino acid dialysis compared to dextrose dialysis in children on continuous ambulatory peritoneal dialysis. Perit Dial Int 1994;14:34—41.

[120] Qamar IU, Secker D, Levin L, Balfe JA, Zlotkin S, Balfe JW. Effects of amino acid dialysis compared to dextrose dialysis in children on continuous cycling peritoneal dialysis. Perit Dial Int 1999;19:237—47.

[121] Azocar MA, Cano FJ, Marin V, Delucchi MA, Rodriguez EE. Body composition in children on peritoneal dialysis. Adv Perit Dial 2004;20:231—6.

[122] Sedlacek M, Dimaano F, Uribarri J. Relationship between phosphorus and creatinine clearance in peritoneal dialysis: Clinical implications. Am J Kidney Dis 2000;36:1020—4.

[123] Quan A, Baum M. Protein losses in children on continuous cycler peritoneal dialysis. Pediatr Nephrol 1996;10:728—31.

[124] Uribarri J. The obsession with high dietary protein intake in ESRD patients on dialysis: Is it justified? Nephron 2000;86:105—8.

[125] Wolfson M, Jones MR, Kopple JD. Amino acid losses during hemodialysis with infusion of amino acids and glucose. Kidney Int 1982;21:500—6.

[126] Chazot C, Shahmir E, Matias B, Laidlaw S, Kopple J. Dialytic nutrition: provision of amino acids in dialysate during hemodialysis. Kidney Int 1997;52:1663—70.

[127] Ikizler T, Flakoll P, Parker R, Hakim R. Amino acid and albumin losses during hemodialysis. Kidney Int 1994;46:830—7.

[128] Querfeld U. Disturbances of lipid metabolism in children with chronic renal failure. Pediatr Nephrol 1993;7:749—57.

[129] National Kidney Foundation. K/DOQI Clinical practice guidelines for chronic kidney disease: evaluation, classification and stratification. Am J Kidney Dis 2002;39(Suppl. 1):S1—S266.

[130] Querfeld U, Salusky IB, Nelson P, Foley J, Fine RN. Hyperlipidemia in pediatric patients undergoing peritoneal dialysis. Pediatr Nephrol 1988;2:447—52.

[131] Wilson AC, Schneider MF, Cox C, et al. Prevalence and correlates of multiple cardiovascular risk factors in children with chronic kidney disease. Clin J Am Soc Nephrol 2011;6:2759—65.

[132] Saland JM, Ginsberg H, Fisher EA. Dyslipidemia in pediatric renal disease: epidemiology, pathophysiology, and management. Curr Opin Pediatr 2002;14:197—204.

[133] Saland JM, Ginsberg HN. Lipoprotein metabolism in chronic renal insufficiency. Pediatr Nephrol 2007;22:1095—112.

[134] Austin MA, Hokanson JE, Edwards KL. Hypertriglyceridemia as a cardiovascular risk factor. Am J Cardiol 1998;81:7B—12B.

[135] Tirosh A, Rudich A, Shochat T, et al. Changes in triglyceride levels and risk for coronary heart disease in young men. Ann Intern Med 2007;147:377—85.

[136] Crook ED, Thallapureddy A, Migdal S, et al. Lipid abnormalities and renal disease: Is dyslipidemia a predictor of progression of renal disease? Am J Med Sci 2003;325:340—8.

[137] Skinner AC, Mayer ML, Flower K, et al. Health status and health care expenditures in a nationally representative sample: How do overweight and healthy-weight children compare? Pediatrics 2008;121:e269—77.

[138] Mak RH. Metabolic effects of erythropoietin in patients on peritoneal dialysis. Pediatr Nephrol 1998;12:660—5.

[139] Mak RH. 1,25-Dihydroxyvitamin D3 corrects insulin and lipid abnormalities in uremia. Kidney Int 1998;53:1353—7.

[140] Mak RH. Effect of metabolic acidosis on hyperlipidemia in uremia. Pediatr Nephrol 1999;13:891—3.

[141] National Kidney Foundation. K/DOQI Clinical practice guidelines for managing dyslipidemias in chronic kidney disease. Am J Kidney Dis 2003;41(Suppl. 3):S1—S91.

[142] National Kidney Foundation. K/DOQI Clinical practice guidelines on cardiovascular disease in dialysis patients. Am J Kidney Dis 2005;45(Suppl. 3):S1—S154.

[143] American Academy of Pediatrics National Cholesterol Education Program. Report of the Expert Panel on Blood Cholesterol Levels in Children and Adolescents. Pediatrics 1992;89:525—84.

[144] Expert Panel on Integrated Guidelines for Cardiovascular Health and Risk Reduction in Children and Adolescents. Summary Report. Pediatrics 2011;s5:S213—256.

[145] Wang C, Harris WS, Chung M, et al. n-3 Fatty acids from fish or fish-oil supplements, but not alpha-linolenic acid, benefit cardiovascular disease outcomes in primary- and secondary-prevention studies: A systematic review. Am J Clin Nutr 2006;84:5—17.

[146] Balk E, Chung M, Lichtenstein A, et al. Effects of omega-3 fatty acids on cardiovascular risk factors and intermediate markers of cardiovascular disease. Evid Rep Technol Assess (Summ) Report no 2004;93:1—6.

[147] Oomen CM, Feskens EJM, Räsänen L, et al. Fish consumption and coronary heart disease mortality in Finland, Italy, and The Netherlands. Am J Epidemiol 2000;151:999—1006.

[148] Baker SS, Cochran WJ, Flores CA, et al. Committee on Nutrition; American Academy of Pediatrics, Policy Statement: Calcium requirements of infants, children and adolescents (RE 9904). Pediatrics 1999;104:1152—7.

[149] Food and Nutrition Board, Institute of Medicine: Dietary Reference Intakes for Calcium, Phosphorus, Magnesium, Vitamin D, and Fluoride. Washington, DC: National Academies Press; 1997.

[150] Andon MB, Peacock M, Kanerva RL, et al. Calcium absorption from apple and orange juice fortified with calcium citrate malate (CCM). J Am Coll Nutr 1996;15:313−6.

[151] National Kidney Foundation. K/DOQI Clinical practice guidelines for bone metabolism and disease in children with chronic kidney disease. Am J Kidney Dis 2005;46(Suppl. 1):S1−S122.

[152] Sieniawska M, Roszkowska-Blaim M, Wojciechowska B. The influence of dialysate calcium concentration on the PTH level in children undergoing CAPD. Perit Dial Int 1996;16:S567−9.

[153] Portale AA, Booth BE, Halloran BP, et al. Effect of dietary phosphorus on circulating concentrations of 1,25-dihydroxyvitamin D and immunoreactive parathyroid hormone in children with moderate renal insufficiency. J Clin Invest 1984;73:1580−9.

[154] Ferrara E, Lemire J, Reznik VM, Grimm PC. Dietary phosphorus reduction by pretreatment of human breast milk with sevelamer. Pediatr Nephrol 2004;19:775−9.

[155] Raaijmakers R, Willems J, Houkes B, Heuvel CS, Monnens LA. Pretreatment of various dairy products with sevelamer: Effective P reduction but also a rise in pH. Perit Dial Int 2008;29(Suppl. 4; abstr):S15A.

[156] Ali FN, Arquelles LM, Langman CB, et al. Vitamin D deficiency in children with chronic kidney disease: uncovering an epidemic. Pediatrics 2009;123:791−6.

[157] Trang HM, Cole DE, Rubin LA, Pierratos A, Siu S, Vieth R. Evidence that vitamin D3 increases serum 25-hydroxyvitamin D more efficiently than does vitamin D2. Am J Clin Nutr 1998;68:854−8.

[158] Houghton LA, Vieth R. The case against ergocalciferol (vitamin D2) as a vitamin supplement. Am J Clin Nutr 2006;84:694−7.

[159] Brungger M, Hulter HN, Krapf R. Effect of chronic metabolic acidosis on the growth hormone/IGF-1 endocrine axis: New cause of growth hormone insensitivity in humans. Kidney Int 1997;51:216−21.

[160] Movilli E, Bossini N, Viola BF, et al. Evidence for an independent role of metabolic acidosis on nutritional status in hemodialysis patients. Nephrol Dial Transplant 1998;13:674−8.

[161] Boirie Y, Broyer M, Gagnadoux MF, et al. Alterations of protein metabolism by metabolic acidosis in children with chronic renal failure. Kidney Int 2000;58:236−41.

[162] Wassner SJ, Kulin HE. Diminished linear growth associated with chronic salt depletion. Clin Pediatr (Phila) 1990;29:719−21.

[163] Ray PE, Lyon RC, Ruley EJ, Holliday MA. Sodium or chloride deficiency lowers muscle intracellular pH in growing rats. Pediatr Nephrol 1996;10:33−7.

[164] Fine BP, Antonia TY, Lestrange N, et al. Sodium deprivation growth failure in the rat: Alterations in tissue composition and fluid spaces. J Nutr 1987;117:1623−8.

[165] Parekh RS, Flynn JT, Smoyer WE, et al. Improved growth in young children with severe chronic renal insufficiency who use specified nutritional therapy. J Am Soc Nephrol 2001;12:2418−26.

[166] US Department of Health and Human Services and US Department of Agriculture: Dietary Guidelines for Americans. Washington, DC: US Government Printing Office; 2005. p 70.

[167] Paulson WD, Bock GH, Nelson AP, Moxey-Mims MM, Crim LM. Hyponatremia in the very young chronic peritoneal dialysis patient. Am J Kidney Dis 1989;14:196−9.

[168] Bunchman TE, Wood EG, Schenck MH, et al. Pretreatment of formula with sodium polystyrene sulfonate to reduce dietary potassium intake. Pediatr Nephrol 1991;5:29−32.

[169] Makoff R. Water-soluble vitamin status in patients with renal disease treated with hemodialysis or peritoneal dialysis. J Renal Nutr 1991;1:56−73.

[170] Makoff R, Dwyer J, Rocco MV. Folic acid, pyridoxine, cobalamin, and homocysteine and their relationship to cardiovascular disease in end-stage renal disease. J Renal Nutr 1996;6:2−11.

[171] Stockberger RA, Parott KA, Lexander SR, et al. Vitamin B6 status of children undergoing continuous ambulatory peritoneal dialysis. Nutr Res 1987;7:1021−30.

[172] Blumberg A, Hanck A, Sander G. Vitamin nutrition in patients on continuous ambulatory peritoneal dialysis (CAPD). Clin Nephrol 1983;20:244−50.

[173] Schroder CH, de Boer AW, Giesen AM, et al. Treatment of hyperhomocysteinemia in children on dialysis by folic acid. Pediatr Nephrol 1999;13:583−5.

[174] Merouani A, Lambert M, Delvin EE, et al. Plasma homocysteine concentration in children with chronic renal failure. Pediatr Nephrol 2001;16:805−11.

[175] Makoff R. Vitamin replacement therapy in renal failure patients. Miner Electrolyte Metab 1999;25:349−51.

[176] Kriley M, Warady BA. Vitamin status of pediatric patients receiving long-term peritoneal dialysis. Am J Clin Nutr 1991;53:1476−9.

[177] Shah GM, Ross EA, Sabo A, et al. Effects of ascorbic acid and pyridoxine supplementation on oxalate metabolism in peritoneal dialysis patients. Am J Kidney Dis 1992;20:42−9.

[178] Reddy J, Bailey RR. Vitamin K deficiency developing in patients with renal failure treated with cephalosporin antibiotics. New Zealand Med J 1980;92:378−9.

[179] Werb R, Clark WF, Lindsay RM, et al. Serum vitamin A levels and associated abnormalities in patients on regular dialysis treatment. Clin Nephrol 1979;12:63−8.

[180] Warady BA, Kriley M, Alon U, et al. Vitamin status of infants receiving long-term peritoneal dialysis. Pediatr Nephrol 1994;8:354−6.

[181] Smythe WR, Alfrey AC, Craswell PW, et al. Trace element abnormalities in chronic uremia. Ann Intern Med 1982;96:302−10.

[182] Thomson NM, Stevens BJ, Humphrey TJ, et al. Comparison of trace elements in peritoneal dialysis, hemodialysis, and uremia. Kidney Int 1983;23:9−14.

[183] Fritz IB. Action of carnitine on long-chain fatty acid oxidation by liver. Am J Physiol 1959;197:297−304.

[184] Belay B, Esteban-Cruciani N, Walsh CA, et al. The use of levocarnitine in children with renal disease: A review and a call for future studies. Pediatr Nephrol 2006;21:308−17.

[185] Lilien MR, Duran M, Quak JM, et al. Oral L-carnitine does not decrease erythropoietin requirement in pediatric dialysis. Pediatr Nephrol 2000;15:17−20.

[186] Eknoyan G, Latos DL, Lindberg J. Practice recommendations for the use of L-carnitine in dialysis related carnitine disorder. National Kidney Foundation Carnitine Consensus Conference. Am J Kidney Dis 2003;41:868−76.

[187] Patel C, Denny M. Cultural Foods and Renal Diets. A Multilingual Guide for Renal Patients. Sections I & II.: CRN Northern California/Northern Nevada.

[188] Yiu VW, Harmon WE, Spinozzi NS, et al. High calorie nutrition for infants with chronic renal disease. J Renal Nutr 1996;6:203−6.

[189] Hobbs JD, Gast TR, Ferguson KB, Bunchman TE, Barletta GM. Nutritional management of hyperkalemic infants with chronic kidney disease, using adult renal formulas. J Renal Nutr 2010;20:121−6.

[190] Balfe JW, Secker DJ, Coulter PE, et al. Tube feeding in children on chronic peritoneal dialysis. Adv Perit Dial 1990;6:257−61.

[191] Brewer ED. Growth of small children managed with chronic peritoneal dialysis and nasogastric tube feedings: 203-month experience in 14 patients. Adv Perit Dial 1990;6:269–72.

[192] Fine RN. Growth in children undergoing continuous ambulatory peritoneal dialysis/continuing cycling peritoneal dialysis/automated peritoneal dialysis. Perit Dial Int 1992;13:S247–50.

[193] Warady BA, Weis L, Johnson L. Nasogastric tube feeding in infants on peritoneal dialysis. Perit Dial Int 1996;16:S521–5.

[194] Warren S, Conley SB. Nutritional considerations in infants on peritoneal dialysis (CPD). Dial Transplant 1983;12:263–6.

[195] Conley SB. Supplemental (NG) feedings of infants undergoing continuous peritoneal dialysis. In: Fine RN, editor. Chronic Ambulatory Peritoneal Dialysis (CAPD) and Chronic Cycling Peritoneal Dialysis (CCPD) in Children, Boston; 1987. p. 263–9.

[196] Watson AR, Taylor J, Balfe JW, et al. Growth in children on CAPD; a reappraisal. In: Khanna R, editor. Advances in Peritoneal Dialysis. Conference; 1985. p. 171–7.

[197] Watson AR, Coleman JE, Taylor EA, et al. Gastrostomy Buttons for Feeding Children on Continuous Cycling Peritoneal Dialysis. In: Khanna R, editor. Advances in Peritoneal Dialysis; 1992. p. 391–5.

[198] Coleman JE, Watson AR, Rance CH, et al. Gastrostomy buttons for nutritional support on chronic dialysis. Nephrol Dial Transplant 1998;13:2041–6.

[199] O'Regan S, Garel L, et al. Percutaneous Gastrojejunostomy for Caloric Supplementation in Children on Peritoneal Dialysis. In: Khanna R, editor. Advances in Peritoneal Dialysis; 1990. p. 273–5.

[200] Kohaut ED, Whelchel J, Waldo FB, et al. Aggressive therapy of infants with renal failure. Pediatr Nephrol 1987;1:150–3.

[201] Ellis EN, Yiu V, Harley F, et al. The impact of supplemental feeding in young children on dialysis: a report of the North American Pediatric Renal Transplant Cooperative Study (NAPRTCS). Pediatr Nephrol 2001;16:404–8.

[202] Fried MD, Khoshoo V, Secker DJ, et al. Decrease in gastric emptying time and episodes of regurgitation in children with spastic quadriplegia fed a whey-based formula. J Pediatr 1992;120:569–72.

[203] Tolia V, Lin CH, Kuhns LP. Gastric emptying using three different formulas in infants with gastroesophageal reflux. J Pediatr Gastrenterol Nutr 1992;15:297–301.

[204] Wood EG, Bunchman TE, Khurana R, et al. Complications of nasogastric and gastrostomy tube feedings in children with end-stage renal disease. Adv Perit Dial 1990;6:262–4.

[205] Watson AR, Coleman JE, Warady BA. When and how to use nasogastric and gastrostomy feeding for nutritional support in infants and children on CAPD/CCPD. In: Fine RN, Alexander SR, Warady BA, editors. CAPD/CCPD in Children. Boston, MA: Kluwer Academic; 1998. p. 281–300.

[206] Murugaru B, Conley SB, Lemire JM, Portman RJ. Fungal peritonitis in children treated with peritoneal dialysis and gastrostomy feeding. Pediatr Nephrol 1991;5:620–1.

[207] Warady BA, Bashir M, Donaldson LA. Fungal peritonitis in children receiving peritoneal dialysis: a report of the NAPRTCS. Kidney Int 2000;58:384–9.

[208] Lesley Rees, Marta Azocar, Dagmara Borzych, et al. Growth in very young children undergoing chronic peritoneal dialysis. J Am Soc Nephrol 2011;22:2303–12.

[209] Kamen RS. Impaired development of oral-motor functions required for normal oral feeding as a consequence of tube feeding during infancy. Adv Perit Dial 1990;6:276–8.

[210] Strologo LD, Principato F, Sinibaldi D, et al. Feeding dysfunction in infants with severe chronic renal failure after long-term nasogastric tube feeding. Pediatr Nephrol 1997;11:84–6.

[211] Hanning RM, Balfe JW, Zlotkin SH. Effect of amino acid containing dialysis solutions on plasma amino acid profiles in children with chronic renal failure. J Pediatr Gastroenterol Nutr 1987;6:942–7.

[212] Hanning RM, Balfe JW, Zlotkin SH. Effectiveness and nutritional consequences of amino acid based vs. glucose based dialysis solutions in infants and children receiving CAPD. Am J Clin Nutr 1987;46:22–30.

[213] Canepa A, Perfumo F, Carrea A, et al. Long-term effect of amino-acid dialysis solution in children on continuous ambulatory peritoneal dialysis. Pediatr Nephrol 1991;5:215–9.

[214] Qamar IU, Levin N, Balfe JW, et al. Effects of 3-month amino-acid dialysis compared to dextrose dialysis in children on continuous ambulatory peritoneal dialysis. Perit Dial Int 1994;14:34–41.

[215] Zachwieja J, Duran M, Joles JA, et al. Amino acid and carnitine supplementation in hemodialysed children. Pediatr Nephrol 1994;8:739–43.

[216] Goldstein SL, Baronette S, Gambrell V, et al. nPCR assessment and IDPN treatment of malnutrition in pediatric hemodialysis patients. Pediatr Nephrol 2002;17:531–4.

36

Nutritional Management of Acute Kidney Injury

Wilfred Druml

Vienna, Austria

INTRODUCTION

Acute kidney injury (AKI) is "more than a kidney disease"; it is a systemic disease process and in many patients, a proxidative, proinflammatory and hypermetabolic clinical syndrome which continues to present one of the most challenging problems in clinical nutrition [1,2]. Patients with AKI from a metabolic point of view represent a heterogenous group of subjects. In designing a nutritional program for a patient with AKI, one must consider not only the metabolic consequences of acute renal dysfunction and the profound alterations in nutrient balances induced by replacement therapy (RRT) but also the metabolic disorders of the underlying disease process and/or associated complications. Usually AKI is a dynamic process, and nutrient requirements may not only differ widely between individual patients but also during the course of disease. Nutritional therapy must also be coordinated with RRT.

Nutrition must present a cornerstone in the management of patients with AKI. The objectives of nutritional therapy exceed conventional goals, and such objectives as amelioration of negative nitrogen balance, limiting loss of lean body mass, stimulation of wound healing, and improvement of immunocompetence, enhance recovery. In addition, metabolic support − in part by using specific substrates ("immunonutrients", "pharmaconutrients") − must be aimed at mitigating the inflammatory state, improving oxygen radical scavenging system, promoting optimal endothelial functions and protecting against tissue injury.

The objectives of nutrition therapy in AKI may differ fundamentally from those for patients with chronic kidney failure (CKD) because diets or infusions that satisfy requirements in stable CKD patients will not necessarily be sufficient for acutely ill, catabolic patients with AKI. Patients with AKI are extremely prone to develop metabolic complications during nutritional support. The tolerance to administering volume and electrolytes is impaired, and metabolic processing of various nutrients is altered. Nutritional therapy for AKI patients requires a more individualized approach and must be more closely monitored than in most other disease states.

For many years, for critically ill patients with AKI requiring nutrition support, parenteral nutrition was the preferred route. However, *enteral* nutrition has become the principal route of nutritional support for all acutely ill patients and also for those with AKI. Nevertheless, enteral and parenteral nutrition should not be viewed as opposing therapies but rather as complementary methods of nutritional support. Often it is impossible to meet requirements by the oral/enteral route alone so supplementary/total parenteral nutrition may become necessary in selected patients.

It is important to note that very few systematic investigations of nutritional therapy in patients with AKI have been conducted, and most of these are older studies and do not reflect current knowledge and practice of nutrition support. But even in acutely ill patients without AKI, recommendations for nutritional support are rarely based on high quality randomized, prospective trials. Thus, statements in this chapter reflect international recommendations which are mostly based only on expert opinion.

METABOLIC ENVIRONMENT OF THE PATIENT WITH AKI

Acute loss of excretory renal function does not affect only water, electrolyte and acid-base balance, but it has a profound effect on the "milieu interieur" with specific and distinct alterations in protein and amino acid,

TABLE 36.1   Important Metabolic Abnormalities Induced by AKI

- Activation of net protein catabolism
- Peripheral glucose intolerance/increase in gluconeogenesis
- Inhibition of lipolysis and reduced plasma fat clearance
- Metabolic acidosis
- Depletion of the antioxidant system
- Reduced vitamin D activation/hyperparathyroidism
- Impaired potassium tolerance
- Other endocrine abnormalities: erythropoietin resistance, resistance to growth factors etc.
- Induction/augmentation of an inflammatory state
- Impairment of immunocompetence

carbohydrate and lipid metabolism and the handling of micronutrients (Table 36.1). The broad pattern of disturbances of physiological functions in AKI exert a pronounced impact on morbidity and mortality [1]. Certainly, in the stable patient with AKI as a mono-organ dysfunction there are some similarities with metabolic findings in CKD.

In many instances however, AKI is not an isolated event but a complication of sepsis, trauma or multiple-organ failure. Thus, the pattern of metabolic disturbances will be determined by the acute uremic state plus the underlying disease processes and/or by such complications as severe infections and additional organ dysfunction and, last but not least, by the type and intensity of renal replacement therapy (RRT) (Table 36.2). Within this clinical context, AKI augments any infectious/inflammatory reaction and induces a pro-oxidative, proinflammatory and hypermetabolic clinical syndrome.

To summarize the metabolic environment in patients with AKI:

- The metabolic environment in a patient with AKI is complex and not only determined by the uremic state but also by the underlying disease processes, associated complications and organ dysfunctions, and also the type and intensity of RRT.
- AKI often represents a systemic inflammatory, pro-oxidative and catabolic syndrome with a profound attributable impact on mortality.

TABLE 36.2   The Metabolic Environment of a Patient with AKI

- Renal failure ("acutely uremic state")
- SIRS*/acute phase reaction — the acute disease state
- Underlying illnesses (type, severity, duration)
- Associated complications (infections, other organ dysfunctions)
- General effects of extracorporal circulation (bioincompatibility etc.)
- Specific effects of RRT (nutrient losses, etc.)

SIRS = systemic inflammatory response syndrome.

- AKI comprises a very heterogenous group of patients with widely differing nutrient requirements among individual patients and also within the same patient during the course of the disease. Thus, AKI requires an individualized approach when designing a nutritional program.
- Patients with AKI are extremely prone to metabolic complications during nutritional support and thus, they must be more closely monitored than patients with most other disease states.

METABOLIC ALTERATIONS SPECIFICALLY ATTRIBUTABLE TO AKI

Energy Metabolism

In experimental animals, AKI decreases oxygen consumption, even when hypothermia and acidosis are corrected ("uremic hypometabolism") [3]. Remarkably, in the multiple organ failure syndrome, oxygen consumption is significantly lower in patients with AKI than in those without impairment of renal function [4]. In patients with uncomplicated AKI, however, oxygen consumption is within the range of healthy subjects. In patients with sepsis and associated AKI, oxygen consumption is increased by approximately 20% to 30% as compared to subjects with uncomplicated AKI [5]. These data indicate that when uremia is well controlled by renal replacement therapy there is little if any change in energy metabolism in patients from the AKI per se, and energy needs (as determined by oxygen consumption) are mainly determined by the underlying disease and associated complications. In contrast to several other acute disease processes, there is rather a tendency to decrease than to increase energy expenditure.

Energy Requirements in Patients with AKI

In acutely ill patients, intake of energy substrates during nutritional support should never exceed actual energy expenditure. Complications, if any, from slightly underfeeding are less deleterious than from overfeeding [6,7]. Increasing energy intake from 30 kcal/kg BW/day to 40 kcal/kg BW/day in patients with AKI increased the rate of metabolic complications, such as hyperglycemia and hypertriglyceridemia, but had no beneficial effects [8].

Patients with AKI should receive 20 to 25 (maximum: 30) kcal/kg BW/day [9]. Even in hypermetabolic conditions such as sepsis or multiple organ dysfunction syndrome, energy expenditure rarely is higher than 130% of calculated basic energy expenditure, and energy intake should not exceed 30 kcal/kg BW/day. During continuous renal replacement therapy (CRRT) the use of lactate or citrate containing substitution fluids can be associated with roughly an additional energy intake of up to 400 kcal/day; the precise amount of this increment in energy intake is difficult to quantify. Other non-traditional sources of energy intake or treatments that reduce in energy expenditure, such as additional glucose infusions or propofol sedation, must be considered when calculating energy intake in nutrition support [7].

Protein- and Amino Acid Metabolism in AKI

A leading feature of metabolic alterations in AKI is the activation of protein catabolism with excessive release of amino acids from skeletal muscle and a sustained negative nitrogen balance [10]. Amino acids are redistributed from muscle tissue to the liver. Hepatic extraction of amino acids from the circulation, hepatic gluconeogenesis and ureagenesis are increased [11]. In the liver, protein synthesis and secretion of acute phase reactants are also stimulated.

Amino acid transport into skeletal muscle is impaired in AKI [12]. This abnormality can be linked both to insulin resistance and to a generalized defect in ion transport in uremia; both the activity and receptor density of the sodium pump are abnormal in adipose cells and muscle tissue [13]. Moreover, there are specific alterations in amino acid metabolism, such as impairment in the conversion of phenylalanine to tyrosine and reduced extrahepatic synthesis of arginine. The elimination of amino acids from the intravascular space is altered. As expected from the stimulation of hepatic extraction of amino acids, overall amino acid clearance and clearance of most glucogenic amino acids is enhanced, and the plasma clearance of phenylalanine, proline and valine is decreased in AKI [14].

As a consequence of these metabolic alterations, imbalances in amino acid pools in plasma and in the intracellular compartments occur, and a characteristic plasma amino acid pattern may be seen in AKI [15]. Plasma concentrations are elevated for cystine, taurine, methionine and phenylalanine and are decreased for valine and leucine.

Metabolic Functions of the Kidney and Protein and Amino Acid Metabolism in AKI

Protein and amino acid metabolism in AKI is also affected by impairment of multiple metabolic functions of the kidney itself. Various amino acids are synthesized or converted by the kidneys and released into the circulation. These include arginine, cysteine, methionine (from homocysteine) and tyrosine [16]. Moreover, the kidney contributes to the elimination of asymmetric dimethylarginine (ADMA), the role of which in the context of AKI remains to be defined [17]. Thus, the impairment of metabolic functions of the kidney can contribute to altered amino acid pools, and amino acids which usually are considered to be non-essential, such as arginine or tyrosine, may become conditionally indispensable in AKI [18].

In addition, the kidney is an important organ for peptide and protein degradation. Many peptides and small proteins are filtered and catabolized at the tubular brush border, and the constituent amino acids are reabsorbed and recycled into the metabolic pool. In AKI, the catabolism of peptides and small proteins, such as inflammatory mediators, are decreased, and inflammation is enhanced. Also catabolism of peptide hormones such as insulin is reduced and insulin requirements can decrease in diabetic patients after development of AKI.

With the increased use of dipeptides in parenteral nutrition support as a source of such amino acids as glutamine and tyrosine, which are not stable or soluble in aqueous solutions, this metabolic function of the kidney may also gain importance for the utilization of these compounds. However, dipeptides currently used as nutritional substrates as sources of glutamine or tyrosine for parenteral nutrition contain alanine or glycine in the N-terminal position and are also rapidly hydrolyzed in the presence of renal dysfunction [19].

Mechanisms of Protein Catabolism in AKI

The causes of hypercatabolism in AKI are complex and manifold and present a combination of nonspecific mechanisms induced by the acute disease process, by the systemic inflammatory syndrome (SIRS), by acidosis, the underlying illness/associated complications, specific effects induced by the acute loss of renal function and finally, the type and intensity of RRT (Table 36.3).

A dominating mechanism of accelerated protein breakdown is the stimulation of hepatic gluconeogenesis from amino acids. In healthy subjects but also in

TABLE 36.3 Protein Catabolism in Acute Renal Failure

CONTRIBUTING FACTORS

- Impairment of metabolic functions by uremic toxins
- Acute phase reaction — systemic inflammatory response syndrome (activation of cytokine network)
- Endocrine factors
  Insulin resistance
  Increased secretion of catabolic hormones (catecholamines, glucagon, glucocorticoids)
  Hyperparathyroidism
  Suppression of release/resistance to growth factors
- Acidosis
- Release of proteases
- Inadequate intake of nutritional substrates
- Renal replacement therapy
  Loss of nutritional substrates
  Activation of protein catabolism

patients with chronic kidney disease (CKD), hepatic gluconeogenesis is suppressed by exogenous glucose infusion. In contrast, in AKI hepatic glucose formation is only decreased but may not be halted by exogenous substrate supply, and gluconeogenesis from amino acids persists even during glucose infusion [20].

These findings have important implications for nutritional support in severely ill patients with AKI, because it is impossible to achieve a positive nitrogen balance during the acute phase of disease. Protein catabolism cannot be suppressed merely by provision of conventional nutritional substrates alone, and thus, for effectively suppressing protein catabolism alternative means for preserving lean body mass must be identified. An important stimulus of muscle protein catabolism in AKI is insulin resistance [21]. In muscle, the maximal rate of insulin-stimulated protein synthesis is depressed by AKI, and protein degradation is increased [11]. An inefficient intracellular energy metabolism stimulates protein breakdown and interrupts the normal control of muscle protein turnover.

Several additional catabolic factors are operative in AKI. The secretion of catabolic hormones (catecholamines, glucagon, glucocorticoids), hyperparathyroidism (which is also frequently present in AKI), suppression and/or decreased sensitivity of growth factors and the release of proteases from activated leucocytes can all stimulate protein breakdown. A central role - as in other acute disease processes – is played by inflammatory mediators such as tumour necrosis factor-α (TNF-α) and interleukins. However, in comparison to other acute disease states this inflammatory reaction is augmented in AKI, both because the kidneys play an important role in the catabolism of cytokines and because the cytokine release is stimulated during tubular injury [22].

Metabolic acidosis has been identified as a major factor in muscle protein breakdown in CKD by stimulating catabolism of protein and oxidation of amino acids by activation of the glucocorticoid dependent ubiquitin-proteasome pathway, independently of azotemia [23,24]. The role of acidosis on metabolism in the context of AKI remains to be demonstrated, and the optimal serum bicarbonate concentration for AKI patients still needs to be defined. In the acute situation (mild) acidosis may even exert some protective actions on organ functions. In patients receiving RRTs, usually acid–base balance is well controlled and can be therapeutically adjusted as desired. In addition to its effects on protein balance, acidosis may be associated with a broad pattern of additional untoward side effects, such as altered bone and mineral metabolism, impaired glucose tolerance, lipolysis and hormone secretion and actions.

Finally, in the patient with AKI, the type and frequency of RRT can profoundly affect protein

metabolism and nutrient balances [25]. Aggravation of protein catabolism, in part, is mediated by the loss of nutritional substrates. In addition, both an activation of protein breakdown and inhibition of muscular protein synthesis can be induced by RRT (see below).

METABOLIC INTERVENTIONS OF CONTROLLING CATABOLISM

Excessive mortality in AKI is tightly correlated with the extent of hypercatabolism but is also associated with the severity of inflammation [26]. No effective methods have been identified to reduce or stop hypercatabolism in the clinical situation. It must be stressed that inhibiting protein catabolism may not present the proper target of therapy, but more "upstream" therapeutic interventions aimed at mitigating the underlying inflammatory process may be required. Principally, hypercatabolism can be modified at four levels of metabolic interventions:

1. Nutrition: Unfortunately, it is impossible to halt hypercatabolism and persisting hepatic gluconeogenesis in severely ill patients with AKI simply by providing conventional nutritional substrates (see above). Novel substrates (e.g., glutamine, leucine or its ketoacid, or structured triglycerides) might exert a more pronounced anti-catabolic response.
2. Endocrine: Experimentally, therapy with hormones [insulin, insulin-like growth factor-I (IGF-I), human growth hormone (rHGH)] or hormone antagonists (antiglucocorticoids) is at least partially effective. Available clinical trial however, with IGF-I and rHGH (described later) have been disappointing.
3. Mediators of inflammation: AKI is a systemic inflammatory state. Therapies to limit inflammatory processes are being experimentally evaluated but have not been tested clinically. Specific nutritional factors such as certain amino acids (glutamine, glycine, arginine), omega-3 fatty acids, or antioxidants may be able to modify the inflammatory response (see below).
4. Interventions to block catabolic pathways: Correction of acidosis is anti-catabolic by blocking the ubiquitin–proteasome proteolytic system. Other experimental interventions that could directly inhibit catabolic pathways are under evaluation.

Certainly, the mystery of accelerated protein and amino acid breakdown in AKI has not been elucidated. It is highly improbable that a single factor is responsible for hypercatabolism in AKI and/or a single agent will reverse accelerated protein degradation.

CLINICAL STUDIES ON PROTEIN CATABOLISM IN AKI

Several studies have tried to quantify protein catabolism in critically ill patients with AKI in order to define the optimal intake of amino acids/protein in these patients. Kierdorf et al. measured a net protein catabolism of about 1.5 g/kg/BW/day and found that provision of 1.5 g amino acids/kg/BW/day was more effective in reducing nitrogen loss than infusion of 0.7 g/kg/day (−3.4 versus −8.1 g N/day). However, a further increase in amino acid intake to 1.74 g/kg/BW/day had no additional effect on nitrogen balance (−3.2 g N/day) [27].

Chima et al. evaluated the protein catabolic rate (PCR, nPNA), urea nitrogen appearance and total nitrogen appearance in 19 critically ill patients undergoing CRRT. A mean PCR of 1.7 +/− 0.6 g/kg BW/day was observed and it was concluded that protein needs in these patients range between 1.6 g and 1.8 g/kg BW/day [28]. In a similar patient group, Macias and coworkers have measured a PCR of 1.4 ± 0.5 g/kg BW/day. There was an inverse relationship between protein and energy provision, and the PCR and nitrogen deficit was less in those patients receiving nutritional support; again a protein-intake of 1.5 to 1.8 g/kg BW/day was recommended [29].

In agreement with these results, newer studies have measured a comparable rate of PCR in patients with AKI on RRT [30]. Leblanc et al. have found a PCR of 1.75 ± 0.82 g/kg BW/d T [31], Fiaccadori et al. a PCR of 1.47 (0.97 to 1.8) g/kg BW/day [8], Marshall MR et al. a PCR of 1.4 ± 0.63 (0.43 to 2.3) g/kg BW/day [32], and finally Ganesan et al. a PCR of 1.57 ± 0.4 g/kg BW/day [33].

Taken together in all these studies a PCR of about 1.5 g/kg BW/day was measured in patients with AKI requiring RRT. But there were wide variations between individual patients and also in the same patient during the course of the disease [28].

AMINO ACID/PROTEIN REQUIREMENTS IN PATIENTS WITH AKI

The most controversial question in nutritional support in patients with AKI concerns the optimal intake of amino acids or protein and few studies only have attempted to define requirements. In non-catabolic patients and during the polyuric recovery phase of AKI, a protein intake of 1.0−1.3 g/kg BW/day was required to achieve a positive nitrogen balance. Thus, the protein intake should be in the same range [34].

As detailed above, in the critically ill patient with AKI undergoing RRT, a PCR of about 1.5 g/kg BW/day was measured. If 0.2 g protein/kg BW/day is added to compensate for amino acid and protein losses associated with RRT a maximum of 1.7 g/kg BW/day is recommended in catabolic patients [9]. In less severely ill patients with a lower degree of net catabolism, 1.2 to 1.5 g/kg BW/day of protein/amino acids may be adequate. It should be noted that 1.5 g kg BW/day of protein/amino acids present the recommendation for acutely ill patients without AKI in general [35,36].

More recently, Australian working groups have assessed higher protein intakes on nitrogen balance in patients with AKI treated with CRRT (see also Chapter 37). Bellomo et al. in a non-randomized study compared a protein intake of 1.2 g/kg BW/day with an intake of 2.5 g/kgBW/day in critically ill patients with ARF on CRRT. Using this high protein intake there was some improvement in nitrogen balance (−5.5g/day vs. −1.92 g/day) but at the cost of an augmented urea generation rate and the need of more aggressive RRT [37]. Similarly, Scheinkestel et al., in a not adequately randomized study, evaluated the impact of three levels of protein and amino acid intake (1.5; 2.0 and 2.5 g/kg BW/day) on nitrogen balance and outcome [38]. In most patients a sequential protocol was employed. Nitrogen balance was inversely related to energy expenditure and was positively related to protein intake. Not surprisingly, nitrogen balance was positively associated with critical care unit/hospital survival, but a causal relationship with the amount of protein/amino acids cannot be concluded from this investigation.

It must be stressed that hypercatabolism cannot be overcome by simply increasing protein or amino acid intake. Even in patients with normal kidney function suffering from sepsis or burns, the provision of more than 1.5 g protein/amino acids/kg BW/day does not abolish net catabolism. There are no proven benefits of more excessive intakes from controlled studies. Any excess protein intake will increase the accumulation of waste products with the potential of aggravating uremic complications, of inducing a hyperammonemic state and leading to an increased need for RRT which, in turn, stimulates muscle protein degradation and increases nutrient losses. Moreover, modulating nitrogen balance may not necessarily accomplish the main goal for nutritional interventions (see above).

CARBOHYDRATE METABOLISM

Glucose metabolism in AKI again is affected both by unspecific mechanisms mediated by the acute disease state and specific effects of acute uremia. A major finding is insulin resistance [39]. Plasma insulin concentrations are elevated, maximal insulin-stimulated glucose uptake by skeletal muscle is decreased and muscular glycogen synthesis is impaired [40].

A second feature of glucose metabolism in AKI is accelerated hepatic gluconeogenesis mainly from conversion of amino acids released during protein catabolism [20]. Hepatic extraction of amino acids and their conversion to glucose and urea production are all increased in AKI. As discussed earlier, in contrast to the non-uremic state and CKD, hepatic gluconeogenesis cannot be suppressed completely by exogenous glucose infusions in AKI. Metabolic acidosis also affects glucose metabolism in AKI by further deteriorating glucose tolerance [41]. Alterations in glucose and protein metabolism in AKI are interrelated, and several factors activating protein catabolism contribute to impaired glucose metabolism. As a consequence of these metabolic alterations hyperglycemia often is present in AKI, and insulin infusions may become necessary in many patients.

Finally, metabolism of insulin is altered in AKI; endogenous insulin secretion is reduced in the basal state and during glucose infusion [42]. Because the kidney is a main organ of insulin disposal, insulin degradation is decreased but surprisingly, insulin catabolism by the liver is also consistently reduced in AKI. The resulting elevations in plasma insulin concentrations may explain the normal blood glucose levels in some patients with AKI.

LIPID METABOLISM

AKI is associated also with specific alterations in lipid metabolism. Total plasma triglyceride concentrations and the triglyceride content of plasma lipoproteins, especially VLDL and LDL, are increased, while total cholesterol and in particular HDL-cholesterol are decreased [43,44]. Additionally, plasma concentrations of apoproteins A I, A II and, B become abnormal. The major cause of lipid abnormalities in AKI is an impairment of lipolysis. The activities of both lipolytic systems, peripheral lipoprotein lipase and hepatic triglyceride lipase, are decreased to less than 50% of normal [45]. Metabolic acidosis may contribute to the impairment of lipolysis in AKI by further inhibiting lipoprotein lipase. This impairment of lipolysis in AKI is in contrast to most other acute disease states where lipolysis usually is accelerated. Increased hepatic triglyceride secretion may contribute to the hypertriglyceridemia of AKI since plasma triglyceride levels do not correlate with triglyceride clearance or postheparin lipolytic activity.

Changes in lipid metabolism develop rapidly; an impairment of fat elimination (as an indicator of lipolysis) becomes apparent within 48 to 96 hours after renal shutdown. A GFR of 30–50 mL/min appears to present the critical threshold for the development of these metabolic alterations.

Particles of artificial fat emulsions used in parenteral nutrition are degraded similarly to endogenous VLDL. Thus, the nutritional consequence of the impaired lipolysis in AKI is a delayed elimination of intravenously infused lipid emulsions (vide infra) [44]. The clearance of fat emulsions is reduced by more than 50% in patients with AKI. Moreover, and relevant for enteral nutrition, intestinal fat absorption is retarded, at least in experimental uremia [46].

Abnormal carnitine levels or metabolism does not contribute to the development of lipid abnormalities in AKI. In contrast to CKD, plasma carnitine levels are increased in AKI [47]. This might be mediated both by an increased release from muscle tissues during catabolism but also by activation of hepatic carnitine synthesis [48].

To summarize the metabolic alterations of macronutrients in critically ill patients with AKI:

- AKI is associated with a distinct pattern of specific metabolic alterations.
- During clinically well controlled acute uremia, energy metabolism is not profoundly affected by AKI. Depending on the severity of the underlying disease process an energy intake of 20–25 (max. 30) kcal/kg BW/day is recommended.
- AKI is often a profoundly catabolic state to which nonspecific (acute phase reactions), mechanisms specific to uremia and also the impact of RRT may contribute.
- Mean protein catabolism in patients is about 1.5 g/kg BW/day. If 0.2 g/kg BW/day are added to compensate for RRT associated losses, a maximum of 1.7 g/kg BW/day is recommended for the protein and amino acid intake.
- In AKI, glucose homeostasis is affected both by induction of an insulin resistant state but also by stimulation of hepatic gluconeogenesis which cannot completely be suppressed by nutritional substrates. Insulin often is required to avoid hyperglycemia, and blood glucose levels should be kept <150 mg/dL (vide infra).
- In contrast to most other acute disease states, AKI is associated with an impairment of lipolysis and of reduction of plasma fat clearing capacity.

MICRONUTRIENTS AND THE ANTIOXIDANT SYSTEM IN AKI

By definition, micronutrients (water soluble and lipid soluble vitamins, trace elements) are essential components of nutrition and any nutrition regimen for patients with AKI must be complete and therefore must contain these substances. Micronutrient requirements in patients with AKI are not well defined, and concise, evidence based recommendations are not available. A further problem with micronutrient treatment for patients with AKI is that currently available diets for enteral nutrition and combinations products of vitamins and trace elements for the addition to parenteral nutrition solutions usually contain micronutrients in amounts that are recommended for healthy adults (RDA; i.e., the recommended daily allowances). These quantities however, do not meet the altered and mostly increased requirements of patients with AKI. Thus, extra supplementation of several vitamins and trace elements may become necessary in addition to the amounts provided in oral, enteral or parenteral nutrition preparations (see below).

One should differentiate "substitution", i.e. covering the (altered) daily requirement of a nutrient, from "supplementation" where higher, even pharmacologic amounts are provided to induce defined effects ("pharmaconutrition") of "key nutrients" such as combinations of various antioxidants [49].

Several micronutrients are components of the antioxidative defence system of the body. In patients with AKI, a severe depression of the antioxidative system and an increase in oxidative stress have been reported which are more pronounced then in other acute disease states [50,51]. Reactive oxygen species are involved in tissue (and kidney) injury in various clinical contexts, and an adequate substitution or even supplementation of micronutrients deserves a much closer attention than previously observed.

Water Soluble Vitamins

Water soluble vitamins are eliminated at a high clearance rate by RRTs. Thus, together with the increased metabolic requirements in acute disease states higher amounts of water soluble vitamin should be given to patients with AKI. An example is thiamine where more than the recommended daily intake for healthy subjects may be removed by RRTs [52]. Severe deficiency states of thiamine associated with symptoms such as lactic acidosis, cardiac failure and variable neuropsychiatric symptoms have been observed in patients with kidney disease [53]. The recommended amount of 3 mg/day of thiamine for healthy subjects is inadequate both to replete the deficiency state and to cover ongoing increased requirements in patients with AKI.

Care should be observed with vitamin C supplementation. The requirements for this vitamin are also higher in patients with AKI than the recommended intake in healthy adults of 75 (women) and 90 (men) mg/day. Potentially, vitamin C may exert renoprotective actions as reported for prevention of contrast induced nephropathy [54]. However, since vitamin C is a precursor of oxalic acid, any excess supplementation can cause secondary oxalosis and should be avoided. Many cases of vitamin C induced AKI have been reported, so the intake should not exceed 250 mg/d [55,56].

Lipid Soluble Vitamins

With the exception of vitamin K, the plasma concentrations of which vary in a broad range, plasma levels of lipid soluble vitamins A, E and D are reduced in patients with AKI [57]. Much interest has been elicited by vitamin D recently. Also in patients with AKI hyperparathyroidism is often present, and the plasma concentrations of 25- and 1, 25-hydroxy-vitamin D_3 are severely depressed [57]. Beyond its effect on mineral metabolism, the steroid hormone vitamin D exerts several pleiotrophic effects involving healthy immune function, intestinal mucosal integrity and glucose metabolism [58]. There currently are no clinical trials in which vitamin D has been administered to AKI patients. In critically ill patients without AKI, even an ultra-high single oral dose of 540,000 U of vitamin D_3 did not cause any side effects or complications [59]. A vitamin D_3 intake of about 1000 U/day may represent a reasonable approach to cover the increased demand. Whether cholecalciferol will be as effective or whether it is necessary to give more active forms of vitamin D_3 (calcitriol or its analogues) is not clear.

Vitamin E is an essential component of the antioxidative defence system. In various experimental situations, vitamin E can prevent the development of renal injury. In combination with vitamin C, vitamin E supplementation reduced the risk of developing organ dysfunction in critically ill patients [60]. In these studies, between 500 IU to 1000 IU were given per day. During long-term vitamin E supplementation of 800 U/day to patients undergoing regular hemodialysis therapy, no side effects were observed.

Some precaution should be taken with vitamin A supplementation in patients with AKI and especially in infants. In experimental AKI, the release of retinol and retinol binding protein from the liver is increased [61]. In a study of 19 pediatric patients developing AKI after hematopoetic stem cell transplantation who required RRT, 17 patients had elevated plasma vitamin A levels during a standard intake, and they showed possible (albeit poorly defined) symptoms of hypervitaminosis A [62].

Trace Elements

A broad range of alterations in trace element homeostasis has been described in patients with kidney disease. However, it is difficult to differentiate whether disorders in trace element metabolism are caused by renal dysfunction or are rather due to the acute disease state and/or inflammation. Decreased plasma concentrations of several trace elements (e.g., selenium, zinc or iron) in patients with AKI may also be an expression of the acute phase reaction. They may not necessarily reflect a deficiency state but rather an altered internal (tissue) distribution. Because of the high degree of protein binding, losses of trace elements during RRT usually are low [52,63].

Caution should be observed with parenteral trace element supplementation in patients with AKI. Parenteral infusion of trace elements circumvents two physiological regulatory elements of trace element homeostasis, intestinal absorption and renal excretion. Thus, the risk of inducing an overdose and toxic effects may be higher than in other patient groups.

Plasma selenium levels are severely depressed in patients with AKI [50]. There are no important losses during intermittent HD, but during CRRT selenium losses can be greater than the RDA [52]. In patients undergoing maintenance HD therapy, selenium supplementation, 300 μg after each HD session, improved the antioxidative defence system [64]. Several intervention studies have been performed in which selenium was administered to critically ill patients [65,66]. The selenium dose in many studies was clearly pharmacologic (up to 2000 μg/day) which can not necessarily be regarded as safe in renal failure patients. Even when the results were conflicting, there is some indication that selenium supplementation can reduce the risk of nosocomial infections and the development of organ failure, and it can potentially also improve survival, an effect especially seen in the most severely ill patients [67].

Zinc is also considered to be a potential phamaconutrient in critically ill patients [68]. Zinc is involved in immune functions, the acute-phase reaction, antioxidative defence mechanisms, glucose homeostasis and wound healing. There is no important loss of zinc during RRTs [52]. Supplementation in patients with AKI higher then 5 mg/day is recommended for healthy adults. In intervention studies in critically ill patients, up to 30 mg/day have been provided.

To summarize micronutrient supplementation in AKI:

- Multiple alterations of micronutrient metabolism occur in AKI, and there is a profound impairment of the antioxidative defense system.
- Micronutrients by definition are essential nutrients and, thus, must be given to patients with AKI, but requirements remain to be defined.
- Water soluble vitamins should be given in higher amounts (possibly double the RDA?), vitamin C intake should not exceed a maximum dose of 250 mg/day.
- Requirements for lipid soluble vitamin K and probably for vitamin A are not increased. Excess vitamin A intake can induce toxic effects.
- With the exception of selenium and zinc, trace elements should be provided according to the recommended daily requirements.
- Selenium and zinc requirements may be higher than the RDA, but excessive quantities should be avoided.
- Whether pharmacologic doses of some micronutrients ("key nutrients") ("pharmaconutrition"), such as selenium or combinations of various antioxidants are beneficial and safe in patients with AKI remains to be shown.

ELECTROLYTES

Derangements in electrolyte balance in patients with AKI are affected by a broad spectrum of factors. These include, but are not limited to, the type and degree of kidney dysfunction, the residual urinary output, the type and intensity of RRT, the underlying disease and extent of hypercatabolism, drug therapy and also the timing, type and composition of nutritional support.

Electrolyte requirements do not only vary considerably between patients but can fundamentally change during the course of the disease. In non-oliguric patients, in subjects undergoing CRRT, and during the polyuric recovery phase of AKI, electrolyte requirements can be considerably increased. Thus, even more than with other nutrient intakes, electrolyte requirements must be evaluated in patients with AKI on a day to day basis, and intakes may need to be adjusted frequently. It should be noted that electrolyte derangements per se, and especially hypokalemia, hypophosphatemia and hypomagnesaemia, increase the risk of developing organ dysfunction and also AKI itself [69,70]. Thus, avoidance of electrolyte derangements must present a primary focus in the metabolic care of patient with AKI.

Potassium

AKI can be complicated by hyperkalemia because of impaired excretion, increased potassium release during accelerated protein catabolism and an altered distribution between intra- and extracellular spaces caused by the uremic state per se, by acidosis, by drugs such as digitalis glycosides, or by beta-antagonists. Actually many patients with AKI may present with decreased potassium levels. When correcting hypokalemia in a patient with AKI, potassium repletion must be performed at a lower rate than in non-renal patients to avoid inducing overshoot hyperkalemia.

Phosphorus

In contrast to chronic kidney disease, hyperphosphatemia usually is of minor relevance in patients with AKI. Nevertheless, hyperphosphatemia per se can cause AKI by precipitation of calcium phosphate crystals within the kidneys ("acute phosphate nephropathy"). This can be due either to release of phosphate from cells (such as in tumor lysis syndrome) or by excess intake of phosphate (such as by using phosphate rich enemas) [71,72].

Both in patients on CRRT, and also on intermittent HD therapy, hypophosphatemia is much more relevant and more common than hyperphosphatemia. Inadequate intake, internal redistribution due to inflammation and increased losses, mainly through RRT (and especially during phosphate-free continuous RRT) can contribute to decreased plasma concentrations [73].

Because of the multiple, well defined side effects of hypophosphatemia, such as respiratory failure, difficulties in weaning from mechanical ventilation, decrease in cardiac contractility, increased risk of infections and decreased survival, attention must be paid to adequate phosphate supplementation and the use of phosphate-containing replacement fluids [73,74]. Hypophosphatemia can also be the consequence of a refeeding syndrome. Since a phosphate-free nutrition is often erroneously provided to patients with AKI, a critical fall in plasma phosphate can occur after initiation of nutrition therapy in subjects with severe malnutrition [75].

Calcium

The majority of patients with AKI are hypocalcemic with a reduction of both protein-bound and ionized calcium fractions [76]. The causes of hypocalcemia are manifold and can include hypoalbuminemia, hyperphosphatemia, citrate anticoagulation, a reduced formation of 1-25(OH)$_2$ vitamin D$_3$ with decreased intestinal calcium adsorption, and potentially, skeletal resistance to the calcemic effect of parathyroid hormone. In most critically ill patients hypocalcemia is present, the magnitude of which correlates with the severity of illness [77].

Hypercalcemia may develop with high dialysate calcium concentrations, immobilisation, acidosis and/or hyperparathyroidism [78]. In AKI caused by rhabdomyolysis, persistent elevations of serum calcitriol may result in a rebound hypercalcemia during the diuretic phase [79]. Acute hypercalcemia per se can cause AKI by inducing acute nephrocalcinosis, arterial calcifications and, interstitial nephritis [80].

Magnesium

Clinically relevant elevations of serum magnesium are rare in patients with AKI. Symptomatic hypermagnesemia can develop during increased oral, enteral or parenteral infusion of magnesium. Hypomagnesemia, on the other hand, is seen more frequently. It can be caused by the acute illness per se, but also by the use of magnesium free replacement fluids for hemofiltration, during citrate anticoagulation, in the diuretic phase of AKI, and after renal transplantation because of increased urinary losses [81,82]. Moreover, several drugs such as cisplatin, aminoglycosides, amphotericin B may cause renal magnesium wasting. Magnesium deficiency may aggravate renal tissue injury, and in patients receiving radiocontrast media, magnesium therapy may be protective especially after nephrotoxic events [83]. In the presence of hypomagnesemia, low serum potassium levels sometimes can only be corrected when magnesium is also provided [84].

To summarize electrolyte supplementation in AKI:

- Electrolyte derangements are frequent in patients with AKI. Avoidance of electrolyte derangements must present a cornerstone in the metabolic care of these patients.
- In patients with AKI not only may excess plasma electrolyte concentrations occur, but frequently deficiency states are present. This is especially true for phosphate depletion during RRT (i.e., CRRT and HD).
- Some electrolyte deficiencies may promote renal tissue injury.
- After initiation of nutrition support, deficiency states, especially for phosphate and potassium, can be induced (i.e., the "refeeding syndrome").
- Electrolyte requirements may vary fundamentally between patients and also in the same patient during the course of the disease. Thus these requirements must be assessed individually on a day-to-day basis.

METABOLIC AND NUTRITIONAL FACTORS AND THE PREVENTION AND THERAPY OF AKI

The potential interactions of nutritional and metabolic factors and interventions with renal function are manifold and can affect renal perfusion, prevention and therapy of tissue injury, and augmentation of celluar regeneration.

Both the oral intake of protein and intravenously infused amino acids increase renal blood flow and glomerular filtration (GFR). Whether this "renal reserve capacity" can be taken into advantage for the prevention or therapy of AKI remains to be shown. In patients with cirrhosis of the liver and functional renal failure, intravenous infusion of amino acids improved renal plasma flow and GFR by approximately 25% [85]. In patients with AKI, a high amino acid infusion (1.5 g/kg BW/day as compared to 0.8 g kg BW/day) increased creatinine clearance and reduced the requirements for diuretics [86].

Studies in experimental animals suggest that certain amino acids may be protective for the kidney. Glutamine, glycine and, to a lesser degree, alanine and taurine, can limit tubular injury in ischemic and nephrotoxic models of AKI [87]. Arginine − possibly by producing nitric oxide − can preserve renal perfusion and tubular function during both nephrotoxic and ischemic injury, whereas inhibitors of nitric oxide synthase exert an opposite effect [88]. Again, evidence from clinical studies using these approaches is scarce and controversial [89].

Intuitively, nutrition in general should accelerate tissue regeneration and possibly also renal tubular repair. In the experimental animal with AKI, provision of amino acids or total parenteral nutrition accelerates recovery of renal function [90]. In patients, however, this has been much more difficult to demonstrate, and only one old study has reported a positive effect of nutrition support on the resolution of AKI [91]. Enteral nutrition seems to exert a specific effect on renal function. Compared to no nutrition or to parenteral nutrition, enteral nutrition accelerated the resolution of experimental AKI [92,93]. Whether this effect is simply mediated by a physiological increase in renal perfusion rather than by anatomical healing remains to be shown.

Various endocrine interventions to hasten renal regeneration after an acute renal injury have been evaluated. In experimental models of AKI, interventions such as thyroxine, rHGH, epidermal growth factor (EGF), IGF-1 and hepatocyte growth factor (HGF)) have been shown to accelerate tubular regeneration. In clinical studies, however, these beneficial effects have not been confirmed. In a small pilot study, infusion of rHGH reduced protein catabolism and improved nitrogen balance [94]. However, administration of rHGH increased the mortality of critically ill patients, many of whom had AKI [95]. A multi-center study of administering IGF-I to AKI patients was terminated early because of the lack of benefit [96]. Administration of triiodothyronine which could potentially upregulate the EGF receptor expression was not only ineffective in patients with AKI but actually increased mortality [97].

It is a remarkable fact that most if not all pharmacologic interventions to prevent or enhance recovery from AKI have failed in the clinical situation [98]. In this context it is interesting to note that several nutritional interventions, such as infusions of glutamine, selenium, combinations of various antioxidants were quite promising at least in some of the available clinical studies (see above).

Hyperglycemia presents a risk factor for the evolution of complications, mainly infections, organ dysfunction and especially AKI (and also of contrast-induced nephropathy [99]). On the other hand glucose control by continuous insulin infusion to prevent hyperglycemia has been shown to avoid evolution of AKI [100].

To summarize the impact of metabolic and nutritional interventions on renal function:

- Metabolic (hyperglycemia) or electrolyte imbalances (hypophosphatemia, hypokalemia, hypomagnesemia) can augment organ dysfunction and also renal injury and increase the risk of additional complications, such as infections.
- Malnutrition per se is a risk factor for renal dysfunction and injury, and nutrition in general may exert a protective and regenerative potential.
- Protein and amino acid intake affect renal perfusion and function.
- Enteral nutrition may exert a specific beneficial effect by improving renal perfusion.
- Various nutrients and especially antioxidative nutrients, i.e. selenium, vitamins C, vitamins E and D may have potential nephroprotective effects.
- Growth factors (such as rHGH, IGF-I) have not been shown to improve the course of disease in patients with AKI.

IMPACT OF RENAL REPLACEMENT THERAPY (RRT) ON METABOLISM AND NUTRIENT BALANCES

The impact of renal replacements therapies (RRT) on metabolism and nutrient balances are manifold and are not only mediated by treatment associated nutrient losses, but also by the obligatory phenomena of bioincompatibility, by the activations of various cascade systems and stimulation of cytokine release, ultimately by the induction of an inflammatory reaction (Table 36.4) [25].

Intermittent Hemodialysis (HD)

During intermittent HD, several water soluble molecules, such as amino acids, vitamins and carnitine are lost. Amino acid losses account for approximately 2 g per hour dialysis session (see also Chapter 11). In many patients with AKI, HD induced phosphate losses are sufficiently great that phosphate replacement is necessary [74].

Protein catabolism is stimulated not only by the amino acid losses but also by activation of protein

TABLE 36.4 Metabolic Effects of Renal Replacement Therapy in ARF

INTERMITTENT HEMODIALYSIS (HD)

Loss of water soluble molecules:
    amino acids
    water soluble vitamins
        other bioactive compounds, such as L-carnitine
        electrolytes (e.g., phosphate!)
Activation of protein catabolism:
    degradation of amino acids
    degradation of proteins and blood cells
Inhibition of protein synthesis
Increase in ROS-production
Consequences of bioincompatiblity:
    (induction and activation of mediator-cascades, of an inflammatory reaction, stimulation of protein catabolism)

CONTINUOUS RENAL REPLACEMENT THERAPY (CRRT)

Heat loss
Excessive load of substrates
    (lactate, citrate, glucose etc.)
Loss of nutrients:
    (amino acids, vitamins, selenium etc.)
Loss of electrolytes (phosphate, magnesium)
Elimination of bioactive peptides and proteins
    (hormones, mediators?, albumin)
Consequences of bioincompatiblity:
    (induction and activation of mediator-cascades, of an inflammatory reaction, stimulation of protein catabolism)

breakdown mediated by induction of inflammatory cytokines. Various inflammatory markers rise during HD and the elevation — and also the stimulation of protein catabolism — persists until several hours after the end of HD. Moreover, it has been suggested that generation of reactive oxygen species is augmented during HD [101,102].

Continuous RRT (CRRT)

In many critical care units CRRT is the preferred modality of RRT for the treatment of patients with AKI. Because of the continuous mode of therapy and associated high fluid turnover of up to 60 L/day or greater, these treatment modalities are associated with a broad pattern of metabolic consequences (Table 36.4). A potentially important side effect of CRRT is the elimination of small and medium sized molecules. In the case of most amino acids, the sieving coefficient approaches 1.0, so the loss of amino acids can be estimated from the volume of the filtrate and the average plasma concentrations. However, because of the electric charges of several amino acids, the sieving coefficient can also exceed 1.0. This is the case for glutamine and arginine, which display the highest losses for amino acids during CRRT [103,104].

Usually, the amino acid losses amount to approximately 0.2 g/L filtrate. Depending on the filtered volume, this means that a total of 5 to 15 g of amino acids are lost per day, which represents about 10% to 15% of the usual amino acid intake. Amino acid losses during continuous hemofiltration (CVVH) and continuous hemodialysis (CVVHD) are of a comparable magnitude [105]. What often is neglected is that depending on the type of RRT, the membrane material used and the effective transmembrane pressure, there may be additional losses of protein of up to 20 g/day [106].

Water soluble vitamins, such as thiamine, folic acid, vitamin B_6 and vitamin C are also eliminated during CRRT, and an intake above the RDA is required to maintain plasma concentrations of these vitamins in patients with AKI [107]. Because of the high protein binding, losses of trace elements during RRT usually are low but can become important with the use of modern high-flux membranes, with RRT using high transmembrane pressure, and if there is an associated leak of albumin or other proteins [52,63,64]. During CRRT, selenium losses by convective transport can exceed the RDA (see above) [52].

Glucose balance during CRRT is dependent on the glucose concentration of the replacement fluid. Solutions designed for peritoneal dialysis should not be used for CRRT, because they promote excessive glucose uptake. Dialysate glucose concentrations should range between 1 g to 2 g/dL to maintain a zero glucose balance.

Uptake of lactate, the organic anion present in replacement fluids, can be considerable during CRRT and within the magnitude of endogenous lactate turnover. During disease states associated with increased lactate formation (such as cardiogenic shock) or decreased lactate clearance (liver insufficiency), bicarbonate based replacement fluids should be used to prevent excessive rises in plasma lactate concentrations.

Recently in several countries, citrate anticoagulation has become a standard procedure during RRT for patients with AKI. Since citrate is predominantly catabolized in the liver, liver dysfunction can result in decreased citrate clearance, and citrate utilization should be monitored using the ratio of total:ionized serum calcium [108]. Moreover, citrate serves as an energy source, and an additional energy intake of up to 400 kcal/day will be associated with citrate anticoagulation.

When phosphate free replacement solutions or dialysate fluids are used for CRRT, phosphate must be supplemented to avoid evolution of hypophosphatemia. An increasing number of commercially available solutions contain phosphate (1.0 to 1.4 mmol/L) [109].

In patients with AKI treated by RRT, nutrition therapy should be given during extracorporal therapy. The endogenous clearance of amino acids is in the range of 80 to 1800 mL/min and thus exceeds the dialytic clearance by 10 to 100 times. Infusion during RRT results in minimal increases in plasma amino acid concentrations, and a small fraction of about 10% of the amino acids infused will be removed in addition to the basal amino acid elimination [14].

To summarize the effects of renal replacement therapy on metabolism and nutrient balances:

- All types of RRTs exert a profound impact on metabolism and nutrient balances.
- Mainly mediated by effects of bioincompatibility, all types of RRTs induce a (low grade) inflammatory syndrome which contributes to protein catabolism.
- Nutrient losses during RRT are important, especially for amino acids and water soluble vitamins and must be considered when designing a nutrition regimen.
- Depending on the type of membrane and additional factors, such as transmembrane pressure, protein losses can also become biologically important.
- Losses of small proteins such as insulin, catecholamines and cytokines are clinically of no importance.
- The use of phosphate-free dialysis fluids or replacement fluids for hemofiltration can result in hypophosphatemia.
- CRRTs may be associated with a substantial intake of metabolic substrates (such as lactate or citrate) which must be taken into consideration when designing nutritional support.

THE EFFECT OF NUTRITION STATUS AND NUTRIENT SUPPLY ON PROGNOSIS

As in other acute and chronic diseases, in patients with AKI a poor nutrition state is associated with an increased risk of complications and a poor prognosis. Fiaccadori and coworkers found that a pre-existing severe malnutrition is present in 42% of patients with AKI and is associated with such complications as sepsis and septic shock, hemorrhage, cardiac arrythmias, cardiogenic shock and respiratory failure. Hospital stay is prolonged, and there is an increase in the hospital-mortality rates [110].

Obesity on the other hand raises the risk of developing AKI [111]. However, a high body mass index (BMI) confers a protective role and improves prognosis in patients with AKI ("reverse epidemiology") [111]. Since obesity is often associated with deficiency states of various nutrients ("sarcopenic obesity") nutrition support should not be withheld in overweight patients.

Last, but not least, of major clinical relevance is the fact that inadequate nutrition may contribute to net protein catabolism and the loss of lean body mass. In experimental animals, starvation potentiates the catabolic response in AKI [112].

PRACTICE OF CLINICAL NUTRITION IN PATIENTS WITH AKI

General Considerations

Nutrition support in critically ill patients with AKI is not fundamentally different from that in patients without renal dysfunction. However, as detailed above, the nutritional regimen must be adapted to the altered metabolism and nutrient requirements and must be coordinated with RRT. The optimal intake of nutrients in patients with AKI is influenced more by the nature of the illness causing AKI, the extent of catabolism, and the type and frequency of RRT rather than renal dysfunction per se. In most clinical situations, daily requirements will exceed the minimal intake recommended for stable CKD patients or the recommended daily allowances (RDA) for normal subjects.

Again, it must be stressed that patients with AKI constitute an extremely heterogeneous group of subjects with widely differing nutrient requirements. Nutritional needs may differ considerably not only between individual patients but, since AKI is a dynamic process, may also vary fundamentally during the course of disease. An individualized approach based on daily assessments of nutrient requirements is mandatory. Nutrient requirements in patients with AKI are summarized in Table 36.5.

At What Degree of Renal Dysfunction should the Nutritional Regimen be Modified for Renal Failure?

Specific metabolic derangements of renal dysfunction occur when renal function falls below about 30% of normal. Thus, at a serum creatinine above ~3 mg/dL, a creatinine clearance below about 40 mL/min or the patients requires RRT (usually RIFLE Stage F or AKIN stage III [113]) the nutrition regimen should consider the metabolic abnormalities of AKI and the altered nutrient requirements induced by RRT.

RIFLE Stage R and I or AKIN Stage I and II

In these early stages of AKI preventive measures to avoid progression to a more severe stage of AKI are of outmost importance. These measures must include metabolic and nutritional interventions to attain such

TABLE 36.5 Nutrient Requirements in ARF*

Energy intake	20—25 (max. 30—35)	kcal/kg/day
Glucose	2—4 (max. 5)	g/kg/day
Lipids	0.8—1.2 (max. 1.5)	g/kg/day
AMINO ACIDS/PROTEIN		
Conservative therapy	0.8—1.2	g/kg/day
+ RRT	1.3—1.5	g/kg/day
+ hypercatabolism	1.5—1.7	g/kg/day
Vitamins	(Mixed vitamin preparations providing the RDAs)	
Water-soluble vitamins		2 × RDA/ day
	(Caution: Vitamin C should be <250 mg/day)	
Lipid-soluble soluble vitamins		1—2 × RDA/day
	(Possibly higher doses for vitamin D)	
Trace elements	(Mixed trace element preparations providing the RDAs)	
		1 × RDA/day
	(Exception possibly selenium at 300 μg/day)	
Electrolytes	(Requirements must be assessed individually)	
	(Caution: Beware of hypokalemia and hypophosphatemia)	

* Please note: Requirements differ between individual patients and may vary considerably in the same patient during the course of the disease!
RDA, recommended dietary allowance.

goals as the maintenance of electrolyte balance, avoidance of hyperglycemia and prevention of malnutrition.

RIFLE Stage F or AKIN Stage III

In this more advanced stage of AKI, RRT is usually employed early in order to minimize the systemic consequences of acute renal dysfunction, to maintain optimal fluid volume and electrolyte balance, and to support hemodynamic and respiratory function. In this stage of AKI, the metabolic consequences of renal dysfunction plus the effects of RRT must be considered.

ORAL NUTRITION IN PATIENTS WITH AKI

Oral nutrition should be encouraged whenever possible. However, this is feasible often only in non-critically ill, non-catabolic patients who present with AKI as an isolated organ dysfunction. These individuals are mostly cared for on open wards. In many situations, AKI is a dynamic process, and nutrition requirements may frequently vary depending on residual renal function, urinary flow, the requirement for RRT, and associated illnesses. Care should be taken to avoid overhydration and induction of electrolyte disorders.

In patients not requiring RRT, the diet should start with about 0.5 g (primarily high-quality) protein/kg BW/day and be gradually increased to about 1.0 g/kg BW/day as long as the SUN remains below 80 mg/dL. By controlling fluid, electrolyte and protein intake the need for RRT may be reduced. Dietary goals in these stable patients are similar to those in CKD patients (see Chapters 14 and 39). In patients requiring RRT, protein intake should be increased to 1.2 to 1.4 g/kg BW/day. An adequate intake of water soluble vitamins and vitamin D should be maintained. The primary goal must be to avoid malnutrition. Diets are similar to those for acutely ill patients on chronic HD therapy (see Chapters 32 and 39).

Anorexia unfortunately, is often a leading symptom. In those patients who do not spontaneously eat adequately, the provision of liquid formula diets or supplements may improve total nutrient intake. Commercially available diets designed for the treatment of patients with CKD can be used for this purpose (see below). For patients with CKD stages 3 and 4, protein and electrolyte restricted diets are available. Patients requiring RRT, may be supplemented with diets containing a moderate amount of protein but with limited amounts of electrolytes (e.g., potassium, magnesium, phosphate). Some of these liquid formula diets have various other nutrients such as carnitine or histidine and are enriched with various flavours to improve the taste. During the dialysis session patients should be encouraged to eat or to drink such nutritious liquid diets (i.e., "intradialytic enteral nutrition").

To summarize oral nutrition in patients with AKI:

- Patients with AKI should receive oral nutrition whenever feasible.
- Care should be taken to avoid overhydration and electrolyte imbalances.
- AKI mostly is a dynamic process and nutritional needs can vary in the same patient, and therefore diets must be adapted frequently to the patient's clinical condition.
- In non-catabolic patients with AKI (as in isolated kidney failure), diets are similar to those for CKD patients.
- Because profound anorexia often is present liquid formula diets can be used to improve oral nutrient intake.
- Intradialytic enteral or parenteral nutrition may be considered to prevent the development of malnutrition.

NUTRITIONAL SUPPORT IN PATIENTS WITH AKI

Who Needs (a Specific Type of) Nutritional Support?

The Decision to Initiate Nutritional Support is Influenced by:

1. The patient's ability to meet his/her nutritional requirements by eating. If a patient is well-nourished and can resume a normal diet within five days, no specific nutritional support is necessary.
2. The nutritional state of the patient. In any patient with evidence of malnourishment, nutritional therapy should be initiated regardless whether the patient will be likely to eat.
3. The severity of disease and degree of accompanying catabolism. In patients with underlying diseases associated with excess protein catabolism, nutritional support should be initiated early.
4. Specific risk constellations (such as immunosuppression, chemotherapy or, agranulocytosis) may require early nutritional interventions.

When Should Nutritional Therapy be Started?

The timing of nutritional support will again be determined by the nutrition state and the severity of disease. The greater the degree of malnutrition and the more pronounced the severity of disease or degree of catabolism, the earlier nutritional therapy should be initiated ("early (enteral) nutrition"). The decision should be made early in the course of disease to avoid the development of deficiencies.

Is Enteral or Parenteral Nutrition the Most Appropriate Means of Providing Nutritional Support for Patients with AKI?

If oral nutrition is not feasible, enteral feeding is the preferred type of nutritional support for all critically ill patients including those with AKI. Nevertheless, a substantial portion of patients with AKI may be intolerant to full enteral feeding, and parenteral nutrition, total or supplementary may become necessary to meet nutritional requirements (see below).

How should Nutritional Support be Started?

Because of the broad spectrum of derangements in substrate utilization and intolerance to various nutrients, both enteral and also parenteral nutrition should be started at a low rate. The rate of administration should be gradually increased over several days until nutritional requirements are met in order to avoid the development of complications.

ENTERAL NUTRITION IN AKI

Without doubt enteral nutrition has become the first and preferred route of nutritional support for patients with AKI. The advantages of enteral nutrition are manifold and include the support of intestinal defense functions against translocation of bacteria and the maintenance of the enteric immune system and thus ultimately, the reduction in infectious complications.

Regarding renal function, enteral nutrition might confer an additional advantage. In experimental AKI it has been reported that enteral as compared to parenteral nutrition can accelerate recovery of renal function [93]. In clinical studies on outcome in patients with AKI requiring RRT, enteral nutrition was a factor associated with an improved survival [114,115].

Regarding the practice of EN in patients with AKI, the impact of acute kidney dysfunction on the intestinal system and especially on gastrointestinal motility is of crucial importance. In uremia a broad spectrum of gastrointestinal alterations has been described, but unfortunately, few studies have investigated these disorders in AKI [116]. Gastric emptying is also retarded and the intestinal transit time is prolonged in AKI [117]. Moreover, any severely catabolic acute disease state, including postoperative and postraumatic conditions are associated with an impairment in the motility of various segments of the gastrointestinal tract. In the critical care setting, this can be augmented by various drugs. Sedation therapy, analgesia with opiates, catecholamines, and other medications may contribute to impairment in intestinal motility.

Thus, in many patients with AKI, the combination of acute kidney dysfunction with various other disorders leads to a profound impairment in gastrointestinal motility which can hamper the achievement of dietary goals during enteral nutrition.

Many patients with AKI will require motility-stimulating drugs, both at the level of the stomach as well as small intestines and the colon. Again, this therapeutic approach has not been specifically investigated in this patient group. In critically ill patients, erythromycin at a low dose (1—2 mg/kg BW up to thrice daily) has been shown to effectively stimulate motility both at the gastric and intestinal level. Alternatives are the combination of metoclopramide (promotion of gastric emptying) and parasympathomimetic drugs such as neostigmine (for stimulation of intestinal motility). Several other medicines currently are under investigation. Prokinetic drugs should be given early, if not prophylactically, to facilitate an early increase in enteral nutrition support to optimal levels. If it is not possible to adequately stimulate motility by these drugs, the placement of a postpyloric jejunal tube should be considered. By this approach often it is possible to achieve the nutritional goals.

However, there still remain a considerable number of patients who cannot be nourished by the enteral route alone and who will require supplemental or total parenteral nutrition (see below).

Enteral Diets for Patients with AKI

No commercial diets are available that have been specifically developed for patients with AKI. Three types of diets have been used in this patient group:

1. Amino acid restricted elemental (mostly powder) diets: These diets originally designed for stable CKD patients should not be used in catabolic patients with AKI because these diets are incomplete and inadequate for acutely ill patient with increased nutrient requirements.
2. Standard formula (liquid) diets as used in non-uremic patients.
3. Formula (liquid) diets adapted either to the needs of patients CKD 3 to 5 not requiring RRT with reduced protein and electrolyte contents or for patients receiving HD. These diets contain a moderately increased protein content and reduced electrolyte (potassium, phosphate, magnesium) concentrations and various other nutrients such as histidine or carnitine.

Worldwide, most healthcare teams use standard diets for patients with AKI as for other (critically ill) patients [9]. It should be noted that in acutely ill patients receiving RRT, hyperkalemia or hyperphosphatemia are rarely clinically important problems. Thus, the use of electrolyte restricted diets usually is not mandatory. The standard diets contain the RDA for micronutrients only for healthy subjects, and one must ensure that water soluble vitamins, vitamin D and possibly also selenium and zinc are adequately supplemented.

"Immunonutrition"

Whether there are advantages to providing a modified standard formula diet, that contains various immuno-modulating substrates, such as fish-oil, antioxidants, nucleotides, or glutamine for patients with AKI remains unclear. The main indications for these modified diets are perioperative situations. But they are not recommended for critically ill patients with severe illnesses (i.e., APACHE II Score >25) [36].

Enteral diets should also contain dietary fiber (water soluble and insoluble). The indication is not as much to reduce uremic toxicity and the inflammatory state, as has been suggested for CKD patients, but rather for the metabolic effects, the protective actions of short chain fatty acids on the colon, and the promotion of motility [118].

Feeding Tubes

Fine pore nasogastric feeding tubes are the standard for enteral feeding. Because feeding tubes often undergo prolonged use, the tubes should be made of biocompatible material, such as silicone or polyurethane. Polyvinylchloride should not be used because it can engender ulcerations in the upper digestive tract. As discussed above, postpyloric feeding tubes should be considered for patients with severe gastrointestinal intolerance and high gastric residual volumes. The tube tip should be positioned well after the ligament of Treitz; a duodenal position should be avoided. Postpyloric tubes should have a second lumen for gastric decompression and gastric administration of medications. Self-advancing (in part electromagnetically visualized) tubes are available which can be positioned within an acceptable time frame (with some experience within less than 20 minutes) without the need for endoscopy [119].

Enteral nutrition should be started early (i.e. within 24 hours of admission) at a low rate and gradually increased during 5 to 7 days [120].

Stress Ulcer Prophylaxis

Enteral nutrition confers some protection against the development of stress ulcers and gastric bleeding. Patients with AKI are usually at high risk for gastric ulcers. Thus for many patients, ulcer prophylaxis, preferably with proton pump inhibitors, will become necessary.

Clinical Studies with Enteral Nutrition in Patients with AKI

In sharp contrast to the worldwide daily routine practice of using enteral nutrition for patients with AKI, only very few systematic studies have been performed. There is only one major study evaluating EN in AKI, and this study is actually more or less a feasibility study comparing patients without AKI (control group) and patients with AKI without and with RRT [121]. A standard formula diet was given; in a subgroup of patients a formula adapted from treatment of CKD patients was used. As compared to patients without renal dysfunction, patients with AKI had higher gastric residual volumes, and there was a trend for more frequent withdrawal of enteral nutrition due to complications. However, in general, enteral nutrition was well tolerated, and nutrient delivery was comparable between all groups. Specific formulas resulted in a higher rate of hypocalcemia and hyperkalemia, but because of lack of randomization no conclusions can be drawn concerning the advantages of such formula diets.

To summarize the use of enteral nutrition (EN) in AKI:

- In patients with AKI who are unable to meet their nutritional needs with oral intake and who require nutritional support, enteral nutrition should be provided whenever possible.
- Even when a quantitatively sufficient amount of enteral nutrition is not possible, one should try to supply at least small amounts of nutrition by the enteral route ("trophic nutrition").
- Enteral nutrition should be started early, i.e. within 24 hours after admission.
- Enteral nutrition should be started slowly (about 25% of requirements) to observe gastrointestinal tolerance, to assure appropriate utilization of nutrients, and to prevent metabolic derangements.
- Prokinetics that stimulate gastrointestinal motility should be started early to improve gastrointestinal tolerance. Placement of a postpyloric feeding tube should be considered when gastrointestinal stasis persists.
- Usually, standard (liquid, formula) diets can be used.
- For many patients with AKI in whom sufficient quantities of nutrients cannot be given by EN, a combination of EN and parenteral nutrition or total parenteral nutrition should be considered (see below).

PARENTERAL NUTRITION IN AKI

Historically, most studies on nutrition support in patients with AKI have been performed using parenteral nutrition (PN). However, because of its well defined advantages, EN should be preferred whenever possible. Nevertheless, for the reasons discussed above, sufficient amounts of enteral nutrition may not be indicated or may not be possible in a considerable proportion of patients with AKI, and supplemental or total parenteral nutrition may become necessary.

Combination of enteral and parenteral nutrition and initiation and progressive increase in the magnitude of parenteral nutrition: Even when parenteral nutrition becomes mandatory, a minimal degree of enteral nutrition ("trophic nutrition") should be attempted whenever possible in order to support the integrity and functions of the intestinal tract (see above).

In general, initiation of parenteral nutrition is recommended not earlier than seven days after admission [35,122]. However, in patients with AKI and severe malnutrition and in subjects requiring RRT with its associated nutrient losses, this delay may be inappropriate, and parenteral nutrition should be started earlier. The increase in parenteral nutrition with AKI should be slower than previously recommended [122]. The goal for the final infusion volume and nutritional intake should not be achieved before four to seven days after initiation.

If parenteral nutrition becomes mandatory, it should be noted that parenteral nutrient infusions are not toxic per se. Many of the negative side affects associated with the parenteral nutrition are due to inadequate planning (excessive energy intake, incomplete solutions), poor practice (too rapid an increase in nutrient intake, too high infusion rates) and insufficient monitoring (hyperglycemia) rather than to the parenteral route of nutrient supply per se.

Components of the Parenteral Nutrition Solution

Amino Acid Solutions

In the early days of nutrition support of patients with AKI amino acid solutions containing essential amino acids only have been used in patients with AKI. This practice was based on a concept of low-protein diet supplemented with essential amino acids in the oral nutrition of patients with CKD. These amino acid solutions are incomplete, have an unbalanced composition, and in large amounts (i.e., >40 g or essential amino acids per day without non-essential amino acids) may cause life threatening complications (such as hyperammonemic coma). They have been abandoned in favor of solutions containing essential and non-essential amino acids.

Complete standard amino acid solutions such as are used for patients without renal dysfunction are recommended for patients with AKI. However, in several countries specific amino acid solutions adapted to the metabolic alterations of AKI are available. These "nephro" solutions contain essential and non-essential amino acids in modified amounts and higher concentrations of conditionally essential amino acids. Some of these solutions are supplemented with a tyrosine containing dipeptide (such as glycyl-tyrosine) as a source for this conditionally essential amino acid in uremia (tyrosine has a low water solubility and cannot be added to an amino acids solution in adequate amounts as a free amino acid) [18,123]. Whether the use of these adapted solutions - beyond normalization of the plasma amino acid pattern and improving nitrogen balance − can in fact alter the course of the disease remains to be shown [124].

Recently, in animal experiments it has been shown that amino acid imbalances not only exert negative effects on protein metabolism but also on more complex cellular functions such as signalling pathways and gene activation [125]. These new insights potentially may also stimulate a renewed interest in disease adapted amino acid solutions.

For the hypercatabolic critically ill patient, glutamine is regarded as a conditionally essential amino acid (recommended intake, 0.3 g kg BW/day) [35]. For glutamine supplementation in patients with AKI only limited evidence is available. In a study comparing a standard parenteral nutrition with a solution enriched with glutamine, the long term survival of critically ill patients was improved [126]. In a post hoc analysis of this study, the improvement in prognosis was most pronounced in patients with AKI (4/24 survivors without glutamine, 14/23 with glutamine, p < 0.02). Glutamine may also exert a nephroprotective potential [87]. Since free glutamine is not stable in aqueous solutions, glutamine containing dipeptides (such as alanyl-glutamine) are used as a glutamine source in parenteral nutrition [122].

Glucose

Glucose should be used as the main energy substrate. In contrast to earlier recommendations, glucose intake must be restricted to <3 to a maximum of 5 g/kg BW/day. A higher glucose intake is not used for energy but will promote lipogenesis with fatty infiltration of the liver, excessive carbon dioxide production, impaired immunocompetence and increase the risk of infectious complications [7].

Glucose tolerance is decreased in AKI, and infusion of insulin is frequently necessary to prevent the development of hyperglycemia. Elevated plasma glucose presents a risk factor not only for infections, but also for renal injury and complications in other organs. The therapeutic target for glucose control during nutritional support in the critically ill is no longer normoglycemia, as had been previously proposed. However, plasma glucose levels should not exceed 150 mg/dL [35]. It should be noted that during parenteral nutrition, insulin requirements are approximately 25% higher than during enteral nutrition [127]. By limiting energy intake and providing a portion of the energy by lipid emulsions in order to decrease glucose infusions, the risk of developing hyperglycemia can be reduced.

Lipid Emulsions

The changes in lipid metabolism associated with AKI should not prevent the use of lipid emulsions during parenteral nutrition. However, the amount of lipids infused must be adjusted to the patient's capacity to clear and utilize lipids. Plasma triglyceride concentrations must be monitored regularly. Usually, 1 g fat/kg BW/day will not substantially increase plasma triglycerides.

Conventional lipid emulsions mostly contain plant oils (soy oil, safflower oil) with a high content of polyunsaturated fatty acids (PUFA). PUFA derived eicosanoids may promote inflammation, vasoconstriction and platelet aggregation. There is an ongoing discussion as to whether lipid emulsions with a lower content of PUFA (replacing soybean oil in part by olive oil, fish oil and/or medium chain triglycerides) should be preferred for parenteral nutrition in critically ill patients.

Alternative oils, and especially fish oil containing omega-3 fatty acids, can serve as precursors for potentially more beneficial eicosanoids. Importantly, these oils may also serve as substrates for a novel class of lipid mediators, protectins and resolvins, which are essential for the resolution of an inflammatory process [128]. In the experimental situation fish oil can exert nephroprotective actions and prolong survival [129]. Unfortunately, systematic clinical studies again are not available in patients with AKI. Nevertheless, in several countries such modified lipid emulsions containing different mixtures of various oils (soy oil, coconut oil, olive oil, fish oil) have recently become available, and various international nutrition societies recommend the use of these modified lipids for parenteral nutrition [36].

Micronutrients

Parenteral nutrition solutions must be complete and thus must also contain all essential micronutrients. Multi-vitamin and multi-trace element preparations are available which can be added directly to the nutrition solution. As discussed above, double the RDA of water soluble vitamins should be provided. If higher selenium supplements are given, the additional selenium should be provided in an additional solution in order to avoid potential adverse interactions (example: between vitamin C and selenium). The increased requirements for vitamin D or analogues should be provided separately, too.

Electrolytes

Electrolyte requirements must be carefully assessed on a day-to-day basis and must be adapted individually. Basic electrolyte requirements can be added to the nutrition solution. More pronounced electrolyte deficits should be provided by separate infusions.

All-in-One Solutions

The use of total nutritional admixtures ("all-in-one" solutions) has become standard worldwide. These solutions either can be obtained as standard products provided by the pharmaceutical industry (usually as multi-chamber-bags (MCB) with a long shelf life) or can be custom-made by the hospital pharmacy or compounding companies. Use of MCBs helps to reduce costs and also the risk of infectious complications [130]. Usually, these MCBs are basic solutions containing the three macronutrients (glucose, amino acids and a lipid emulsion), and also variable amounts of electrolytes. Water and lipid soluble vitamins, trace elements and electrolytes must be added as required before use.

Recent evidence suggests that parenteral nutrition should not be started before 4 to 7 days after admission [122]. Again, many patients with AKI are severely malnourished, and in subjects requiring RRT therapy associated nutrient losses are high. Thus, parenteral nutrition should be started earlier. To ensure maximal nutrient utilisation and avoid metabolic derangements the infusion should be started at a low rate (see above, providing about 25–30% of requirements) and gradually increased over several days. The nutrition solution should be infused continuously over 24 hours to ensure optimal substrate utilization and to avoid marked changes in substrate concentrations in a state of impaired utilization.

Clinical Studies of Parenteral Nutrition in Patients with AKI

As with enteral nutrition, there is a distressingly low number of systematic studies evaluating parenteral nutrition in patients with AKI. Several older studies have assessed isolated aspects of nutritional support, such as the optimal amino acid solution, the severity of protein catabolism, the optimal intake of amino acids or protein. However, prospective, controlled outcome studies have not been performed during the last 25 years.

It should be noted that the nutritional regimens employed in most of these older studies do not meet current standards and practice of nutrition therapy in acutely ill patients with respect to the type and quantity of amino acid solutions, the energy intake, or the nutrient composition of the nutrition solutions. All studies were massively underpowered to assess such hard end points as survival or recovery of renal function. Moreover, in some of these studies, the control group received no nutrition at all or glucose alone. Some of these prospective randomized studies are briefly summarized as follows.

Abel et al. randomly assigned 53 patients with AKI to receive either a mean of 16 g/day of essential amino acids with hypertonic glucose or hypertonic glucose alone [91]. Survival rate was greater in patients receiving essential amino acids and this was especially seen in the sicker patients with serious complications and requiring dialysis therapy. Similarly, Feinstein et al. randomly assigned 30 patients with AKI to three groups, to receive glucose alone, glucose and 21 g/day of essential amino acids or glucose and 21 g/day essential plus 21 g/day nonessential amino acids [131]. In general, results were inconclusive, but there was a trend for a better nitrogen balance and also prognosis in patients receiving more amino acids. In a further prospective trial Feinstein et al. compared in an even smaller group of 13 patients with AKI parenteral nutrition containing 21 g/day of essential amino acids with a solution with a higher amino acid intake (essential plus nonessential amino acids to meet the urea nitrogen appearance rate) [132]. Nitrogen balance was not different and – as was to be expected in such a small trial – recovery of renal function and mortality were comparable. Some of the newer studies have mainly tried to assess the severity of protein catabolism and to define protein requirements in patients with AKI. These studies have been detailed above.

In conclusion, no recent systematic studies on parenteral nutrition using current standards of nutrition support are available for this specific patient group with AKI. No evidence-based statements can be given. Only opinion based recommendations can be offered which are based, in general, on experience with acutely ill patients with some modifications for the patients with AKI [9].

Intradialytic Parenteral Nutrition (IDPN) in Patients with AKI

IDPN has been shown to revert the catabolic effects of hemodialysis into an anabolic condition in clinically stable patients [133]. Moreover, several nutritional indices can be improved by using IDPN [123]. For patients with AKI who are cared for on noncritical care wards and who do not have adequate oral intake, IDPN may offer the possibility to improve total nutrient intake. IDPN may not so much improve the nutrition state as it may prevent the loss of lean body mass. This is the practice in many institutions, but it must be noted that again no systematic studies are available in this specific acutely ill patient group to confirm these benefits.

To summarize parenteral nutrition:

- In patients with AKI who are unable to meet their nutritional needs with oral nutrient intake, who require nutritional support, and who cannot be adequately nourished by enteral nutrition, supplemental or total parenteral nutrition should be considered.
- Even when parenteral nutrition is given, a minimal oral or enteral nutritional intake ("trophic nutrition") should be encouraged to improve gastrointestinal (defense) functions whenever possible.
- Parenteral nutrition solutions must be complete, must contain essential and various non-essential amino acids, glucose, lipids, water- and lipid-soluble vitamins, trace elements and electrolytes.
- If adequate enteral nutrition is impossible or not desired, parenteral nutrition should be initiated earlier than in other patients groups because of the high risk of malnutrition and the high RRT associated nutrient losses in AKI patients (after three to five days).
- Parenteral nutrition should be started slowly (about 30% of calculated requirements) to assure appropriate utilization and to prevent the development of metabolic derangements.
- Any exaggerated energy intake ("hyperalimentation") must be strictly avoided. Glucose control by insulin infusion should maintain plasma glucose levels <150 mg/dL.

COMPLICATIONS OF NUTRITIONAL SUPPORT

Side effects and complications of nutrition support in patients with AKI are not fundamentally different from those in other patients groups. However, for the reasons discussed above, the risk for essentially all nutrition associated complications is increased in the patient with AKI. Gastrointestinal side effects are more frequent, gastric residual volumes are increased, the general tolerance to enteral nutrition is decreased, and thus, close monitoring of enteral nutrition therapy and institution of measures to improve GI motility and tolerance to enteral feedings are mandatory.

Because of the compromised immune functions in AKI, infectious complications originating from the central venous catheter are more frequent [134]. RRT per se presents an additional risk factor for infection in patients with AKI. Tolerance to the administration of excessive volumes is impaired. Careful fluid balance must be observed, and any excess infusion of volume should avoided. Overhydration has been recognized recently as an important factor associated with poor outcome [135]. In contrast to common belief, overhydration also impairs renal function.

Obviously, electrolyte imbalances occur frequently in patients with AKI. It should be noted however, that not only an excesses but also deficiencies of electrolytes, especially for phosphate and potassium, frequently are seen in these patients [73].

Metabolic complications frequently occur in patients with AKI because utilisation of essentially all nutrients is altered or impaired. One reason for gradually increasing the infusion rate of nutritional solutions is to avoid many of the side effects and complications that are associated with nutrition support.

MONITORING OF NUTRITION SUPPORT IN PATIENT WITH AKI

Because of the limited tolerance to various nutrients and the high risk of inducing metabolic derangements in patients with AKI, nutritional therapy requires a tighter schedule of monitoring than in other patient groups. Table 36.6 summarizes laboratory tests used to monitor nutrition support to avoid developing

TABLE 36.6 A Minimal Suggested Schedule for Clinical Monitoring During Nutritional Support

Variables	For the Patient Who is Metabolically:	
	Unstable	Stable
BLOOD OR SERUM:		
Glucose, potassium	1–6 × daily	daily
Electrolytes (sodium, chloride)	daily	3 × weekly
Calcium, phosphate, magnesium	daily	3 × weekly
Osmolality	daily	1 × weekly
Urea N/daily rise in BUN	daily	daily
Triglycerides	daily	2 × weekly
Arterial blood gas analysis/pH	daily	1 × weekly
Urea nitrogen appearance:		
(estimate of protein catabolism)	2 × weekly	1 × weekly
Ammonia	2 × weekly	1 × weekly
Transaminases and bilirubin	2 × weekly	1 × weekly

metabolic complications. The frequency of testing will depend on the metabolic stability of the patient. Plasma concentrations of glucose, potassium, and phosphate should be monitored repeatedly after initiating nutrition therapy.

Glucose Control

As discussed earlier, hyperglycemia presents a risk factor for kidney dysfunction in acute disease states. On the other hand, AKI per se is associated with insulin resistance. Thus, glucose control by insulin infusions is mandatory in most patients with AKI. In contrast to earlier recommendations, however, glucose control should not be too tight and should not aim for normoglycemia, but rather should maintain plasma glucose concentrations below 150 mg/dL. Optimally, an algorithm for glucose control should be followed.

Triglycerides

Due to the impairment of lipolysis and retarded plasma clearing capacity for triglycerides, adjustments in lipid infusions may become necessary. Simultaneous infusion of propofol (a drug which is dissolved in a 10% lipid emulsion), which frequently is used for sedation therapy can be associated with a substantial intake of lipids. This potential source of lipids must be taken into consideration when designing a nutrition regimen.

Electrolyte Balance

It is a commonplace that AKI is associated with various electrolyte imbalances, and a tight schedule of monitoring is mandatory. Nevertheless, it again should be stressed that the risk of electrolyte deficiency states is increased.

References

[1] Druml W. Acute renal failure is not a "cute" renal failure!. Intensive Care Med 2004;30:1886–90.

[2] Kelly KJ. Acute renal failure: much more than a kidney disease. Semin Nephrol 2006;26:105–13.

[3] Om P, Hohenegger M. Energy metabolism in acute uremic rats. Nephron 1980;25:249–53.

[4] Soop M, Forsberg E, Thorne A, Alvestrand A. Energy expenditure in postoperative multiple organ failure with acute renal failure. Clin Nephrol 1989;31:139–45.

[5] Schneeweiss B, Graninger W, Stockenhuber F, et al. Energy metabolism in acute and chronic renal failure. Am J Clin Nutr 1990;52:596–601.

[6] Arabi YM, Tamim HM, Dhar GS, et al. Permissive underfeeding and intensive insulin therapy in critically ill patients: a randomized controlled trial. Am J Clin Nutr 2011;93:569–77.

[7] Dissanaike S, Shelton M, Warner K, O'Keefe GE. The risk for bloodstream infections is associated with increased parenteral caloric intake in patients receiving parenteral nutrition. Crit Care 2007;11:R114.

[8] Fiaccadori E, Maggiore U, Rotelli C, et al. Effects of different energy intakes on nitrogen balance in patients with acute renal failure: a pilot study. Nephrol Dial Transplant 2005;20:1976–80.

[9] Cano N, Fiaccadori E, Tesinsky P, et al. ESPEN Guidelines on Enteral Nutrition: Adult renal failure. Clin Nutr 2006;25:295–310.

[10] Flugel-Link RM, Salusky IB, Jones MR, Kopple JD. Protein and amino acid metabolism in posterior hemicorpus of acutely uremic rats. Am J Physiol 1983;244:E615–23.

[11] Clark AS, Mitch WE. Muscle protein turnover and glucose uptake in acutely uremic rats. Effects of insulin and the duration of renal insufficiency. J Clin Invest 1983;72:836–45.

[12] Maroni BJ, Haesemeyer RW, Kutner MH, Mitch WE. Kinetics of system A amino acid uptake by muscle: effects of insulin and acute uremia. Am J Physiol 1990;258:F1304–10.

[13] Druml W, Kelly RA, May RC, Mitch WE. Abnormal cation transport in uremia. Mechanisms in adipocytes and skeletal muscle from uremic rats. J Clin Invest 1988;81:1197–203.

[14] Druml W, Fischer M, Liebisch B, Lenz K, Roth E. Elimination of amino acids in renal failure. Am J Clin Nutr 1994;60:418–23.

[15] Druml W, Burger U, Kleinberger G, Lenz K, Laggner A. Elimination of amino acids in acute renal failure. Nephron 1986;42:62–7.

[16] Garibotto G, Sofia A, Saffioti S, Bonanni A, Mannucci I, Verzola D. Amino acid and protein metabolism in the human kidney and in patients with chronic kidney disease. Clin Nutr;29:424–433.

[17] Nijveldt RJ, Siroen MP, Teerlink T, van Leeuwen PA. Elimination of asymmetric dimethylarginine by the kidney and the liver: a link to the development of multiple organ failure? J Nutr 2004;134:2848S–52S. discussion 2853S.

[18] Druml W, Roth E, Lenz K, Lochs H, Kopsa H. Phenylalanine and tyrosine metabolism in renal failure: dipeptides as tyrosine source. Kidney Int Suppl 1989;27:S282–6.

[19] Druml W, Lochs H, Roth E, Hubl W, Balcke P, Lenz K. Utilization of tyrosine dipeptides and acetyltyrosine in normal and uremic humans. Am J Physiol 1991;260:E280–5.

[20] Cianciaruso B, Bellizzi V, Napoli R, Sacca L, Kopple JD. Hepatic uptake and release of glucose, lactate, and amino acids in acutely uremic dogs. Metabolism 1991;40:261–9.

[21] Hu Z, Wang H, Lee IH, Du J, Mitch WE. Endogenous glucocorticoids and impaired insulin signaling are both required to stimulate muscle wasting under pathophysiological conditions in mice. J Clin Invest 2009;119:3059–69.

[22] Zager RA, Johnson AC, Hanson SY, Lund S. Ischemic proximal tubular injury primes mice to endotoxin-induced TNF-alpha generation and systemic release. Am J Physiol Renal Physiol 2005;289:F289–97.

[23] Lecker SH, Mitch WE. Proteolysis by the ubiquitin-proteasome system and kidney disease. J Am Soc Nephrol 2011;22:821–4.

[24] Bailey JL, Mitch WE. Twice-told tales of metabolic acidosis, glucocorticoids, and protein wasting: what do results from rats tell us about patients with kidney disease? Semin Dial 2000;13:227–31.

[25] Druml W. Metabolic aspects of continuous renal replacement therapies. Kidney Int Suppl 1999:S56–61.

[26] Simmons EM, Himmelfarb J, Sezer MT, et al. Plasma cytokine levels predict mortality in patients with acute renal failure. Kidney Int 2004;65:1357–65.

[27] Kierdorf H. Continuous versus intermittent treatment: clinical results in acute renal failure. Contrib Nephrol 1991;93:1–12.

[28] Chima CS, Meyer L, Hummell AC, et al. Protein catabolic rate in patients with acute renal failure on continuous arteriovenous hemofiltration and total parenteral nutrition. J Am Soc Nephrol 1993;3:1516−21.

[29] Macias WL, Alaka KJ, Murphy MH, Miller ME, Clark WR, Mueller BA. Impact of the nutritional regimen on protein catabolism and nitrogen balance in patients with acute renal failure. JPEN J Parenter Enteral Nutr 1996;20:56−62.

[30] Fiaccadori E, Cremaschi E, Regolisti G. Nutritional assessment and delivery in renal replacement therapy patients. Semin Dial 2011;24:169−75.

[31] Leblanc M, Garred LJ, Cardinal J, et al. Catabolism in critical illness: estimation from urea nitrogen appearance and creatinine production during continuous renal replacement therapy. Am J Kidney Dis 1998;32:444−53.

[32] Marshall MR, Golper TA, Shaver MJ, Alam MG, Chatoth DK. Urea kinetics during sustained low-efficiency dialysis in critically ill patients requiring renal replacement therapy. Am J Kidney Dis 2002;39:556−70.

[33] Ganesan MV, Annigeri RA, Shankar B, et al. The protein equivalent of nitrogen appearance in critically ill acute renal failure patients undergoing continuous renal replacement therapy. J Ren Nutr 2009;19:161−6.

[34] Hasik J, Hryniewiecki L, Baczyk K, Grala T. [Minimal protein requirements in patients with acute kidney failure]. Pol Arch Med Wewn 1979;61:29−36.

[35] Martindale RG, McClave SA, Vanek VW, et al. Guidelines for the provision and assessment of nutrition support therapy in the adult critically ill patient: Society of Critical Care Medicine and American Society for Parenteral and Enteral Nutrition: Executive Summary. Crit Care Med 2009;37:1757−61.

[36] Singer P, Berger MM, Van den Berghe G, et al. ESPEN Guidelines on Parenteral Nutrition: intensive care. Clin Nutr 2009;28:387−400.

[37] Bellomo R, Seacombe J, Daskalakis M, et al. A prospective comparative study of moderate versus high protein intake for critically ill patients with acute renal failure. Ren Fail 1997;19:111−20.

[38] Scheinkestel CD, Adams F, Mahony L, et al. Impact of increasing parenteral protein loads on amino acid levels and balance in critically ill anuric patients on continuous renal replacement therapy. Nutrition 2003;19:733−40.

[39] Basi S, Pupim LB, Simmons EM, et al. Insulin resistance in critically ill patients with acute renal failure. Am J Physiol Renal Physiol 2005;289:F259−64.

[40] May RC, Clark AS, Goheer MA, Mitch WE. Specific defects in insulin-mediated muscle metabolism in acute uremia. Kidney Int 1985;28:490−7.

[41] Weisinger J, Swenson RS, Greene W, Taylor JB, Reaven GM. Comparison of the effects of metabolic acidosis and acute uremia on carbohydrate tolerance. Diabetes 1972;21:1109−15.

[42] Cianciaruso B, Sacca L, Terracciano V, et al. Insulin metabolism in acute renal failure. Kidney Int Suppl 1987;22:S109−12.

[43] Druml W, Laggner A, Widhalm K, Kleinberger G, Lenz K. Lipid metabolism in acute renal failure. Kidney Int Suppl 1983;16:S139−42.

[44] Druml W, Fischer M, Sertl S, Schneeweiss B, Lenz K, Widhalm K. Fat elimination in acute renal failure: long-chain vs. medium-chain triglycerides. Am J Clin Nutr 1992;55:468−72.

[45] Druml W, Zechner R, Magometschnigg D, et al. Post-heparin lipolytic activity in acute renal failure. Clin Nephrol 1985;23:289−93.

[46] Schurr D, Levy E, Goldstein R, Stankiewicz H, Pomeranz A, Drukker A. Intestinal fat malabsorption in the uremic rat. Int J Pediatr Nephrol 1987;8:129−34.

[47] Druml W. Nutritional management of acute renal failure. J Ren Nutr 2005;15:63−70.

[48] Wanner C, Riegel W, Schaefer RM, Horl WH. Carnitine and carnitine esters in acute renal failure. Nephrol Dial Transplant 1989;4:951−6.

[49] Jones NE, Heyland DK. Pharmaconutrition: a new emerging paradigm. Curr Opin Gastroenterol 2008;24:215−22.

[50] Metnitz GH, Fischer M, Bartens C, Steltzer H, Lang T, Druml W. Impact of acute renal failure on antioxidant status in multiple organ failure. Acta Anaesthesiol Scand 2000;44:236−40.

[51] Himmelfarb J, McMonagle E, Freedman S, et al. Oxidative stress is increased in critically ill patients with acute renal failure. J Am Soc Nephrol 2004;15:2449−56.

[52] Berger MM, Shenkin A, Revelly JP, et al. Copper, selenium, zinc, and thiamine balances during continuous venovenous hemodiafiltration in critically ill patients. Am J Clin Nutr 2004;80:410−6.

[53] Madl C, Kranz A, Liebisch B, Traindl O, Lenz K, Druml W. Lactic acidosis in thiamine deficiency. Clin Nutr 1993;12:108−11.

[54] Spargias K, Alexopoulos E, Kyrzopoulos S, et al. Ascorbic acid prevents contrast-mediated nephropathy in patients with renal dysfunction undergoing coronary angiography or intervention. Circulation 2004;110:2837−42.

[55] Stepien KM, Prinsloo P, Hitch T, McCulloch TA, Sims R. Acute renal failure, microangiopathic haemolytic anemia, and secondary oxalosis in a young female patient. Int J Nephrol 2011;2011:679160.

[56] Canavese C, Petrarulo M, Massarenti P, et al. Long-term, low-dose, intravenous vitamin C leads to plasma calcium oxalate supersaturation in hemodialysis patients. Am J Kidney Dis 2005;45:540−9.

[57] Druml W, Schwarzenhofer M, Apsner R, Horl WH. Fat-soluble vitamins in patients with acute renal failure. Miner Electrolyte Metab 1998;24:220−6.

[58] Lee P, Nair P, Eisman JA, Center JR. Vitamin D deficiency in the intensive care unit: an invisible accomplice to morbidity and mortality? Intensive Care Med 2009;35:2028−32.

[59] Amrein K, Sourij H, Wagner G, et al. Short-term effects of high-dose oral vitamin D3 in critically ill vitamin D deficient patients: a randomized, double-blind, placebo-controlled pilot study. Crit Care 2011;15:R104.

[60] Nathens AB, Neff MJ, Jurkovich GJ, et al. Randomized, prospective trial of antioxidant supplementation in critically ill surgical patients. Ann Surg 2002;236:814−22.

[61] Gerlach TH, Zile MH. Upregulation of serum retinol in experimental acute renal failure. Faseb J 1990;4:2511−7.

[62] Lipkin AC, Lenssen P. Hypervitaminosis in pediatric hematopoietic stem cell patients requiring renal replacement therapy. Nutr Clin Pract 2008;23:621−9.

[63] Pasko DA, Churchwell MD, Btaiche IF, Jain JC, Mueller BA. Continuous venovenous hemodiafiltration trace element clearance in pediatric patients: a case series. Pediatr Nephrol 2009;24:807−13.

[64] Koenig JS, Fischer M, Bulant E, Tiran B, Elmadfa I, Druml W. Antioxidant status in patients on chronic hemodialysis therapy: impact of parenteral selenium supplementation. Wien Klin Wochenschr 1997;109:13−9.

[65] Angstwurm MW, Engelmann L, Zimmermann T, et al. Selenium in Intensive Care (SIC): results of a prospective randomized, placebo-controlled, multiple-center study in patients with severe systemic inflammatory response syndrome, sepsis, and septic shock. Crit Care Med 2007;35:118−26.

[66] Andrews PJ, Avenell A, Noble DW, et al. Randomised trial of glutamine, selenium, or both, to supplement parenteral nutrition for critically ill patients. Bmj 2011;342:d1542.

[67] Heyland DK, Dhaliwal R, Suchner U, Berger MM. Antioxidant nutrients: a systematic review of trace elements and vitamins in the critically ill patient. Intensive Care Med 2005;31:327—37.

[68] Heyland DK, Jones N, Cvijanovich NZ, Wong H. Zinc supplementation in critically ill patients: a key pharmaconutrient? JPEN J Parenter Enteral Nutr 2008;32:509—19.

[69] Santos MS, Seguro AC, Andrade L. Hypomagnesemia is a risk factor for nonrecovery of renal function and mortality in AIDS patients with acute kidney injury. Braz J Med Biol Res 2011;43:316—23.

[70] Seguro AC, de Araujo M, Seguro FS, Rienzo M, Magaldi AJ, Campos SB. Effects of hypokalemia and hypomagnesemia on zidovudine (AZT) and didanosine (ddI) nephrotoxicity in rats. Clin Nephrol 2003;59:267—72.

[71] Markowitz GS, Perazella MA. Acute phosphate nephropathy. Kidney Int 2009;76:1027—34.

[72] Haas M, Ohler L, Watzke H, Bohmig G, Prokesch R, Druml W. The spectrum of acute renal failure in tumour lysis syndrome. Nephrol Dial Transplant 1999;14:776—9.

[73] Demirjian S, Teo BW, Guzman JA, et al. Hypophosphatemia during continuous hemodialysis is associated with prolonged respiratory failure in patients with acute kidney injury. Nephrol Dial Transplant 2011;26:3508—14.

[74] Schiffl H, Lang SM. Severe acute hypophosphatemia during renal replacement therapy adversely affects outcome of critically ill patients with acute kidney injury. Int Urol Nephrol 2012.

[75] Gariballa S. Refeeding syndrome: a potentially fatal condition but remains underdiagnosed and undertreated. Nutrition 2008;24:604—6.

[76] Tan HK, Bellomo R, M'Pisi DA, Ronco C. Ionized serum calcium levels during acute renal failure: intermittent hemodialysis vs. Continuous hemodiafiltration. Ren Fail 2002;24:19—27.

[77] Hastbacka J, Pettila V. Prevalence and predictive value of ionized hypocalcemia among critically ill patients. Acta Anaesthesiol Scand 2003;47:1264—9.

[78] Pietrek J, Kokot F, Kuska J. Serum 25-hydroxyvitamin D and parathyroid hormone in patients with acute renal failure. Kidney Int 1978;13:178—85.

[79] Graziani G, Calvetta A, Cucchiari D, Valaperta S, Montanelli A. Life-threatening hypercalcemia in patients with rhabdomyolysis-induced oliguric acute renal failure. J Nephrol;24:128—131.

[80] Moyses-Neto M, Guimaraes FM, Ayoub FH, Vieira-Neto OM, Costa JA, Dantas M. Acute renal failure and hypercalcemia. Ren Fail 2006;28:153—9.

[81] Satish R, Gokulnath G. Serum magnesium in recovering acute renal failure. Indian J Nephrol 2008;18:101—4.

[82] Soliman HM, Mercan D, Lobo SS, Melot C, Vincent JL. Development of ionized hypomagnesemia is associated with higher mortality rates. Crit Care Med 2003;31:1082—7.

[83] de Araujo M, Andrade L, Coimbra TM, Rodrigues Jr AC, Seguro AC. Magnesium supplementation combined with N-acetylcysteine protects against postischemic acute renal failure. J Am Soc Nephrol 2005;16:3339—49.

[84] Hamill-Ruth RJ, McGory R. Magnesium repletion and its effect on potassium homeostasis in critically ill adults: results of a double-blind, randomized, controlled trial. Crit Care Med 1996;24:38—45.

[85] Badalamenti S, Gines P, Arroyo V. Renal effects of amino acid administration in cirrhosis. Gastroenterology 1993;104:1886.

[86] Singer P. High-dose amino acid infusion preserves diuresis and improves nitrogen balance in non-oliguric acute renal failure. Wien Klin Wochenschr 2007;119:218—22.

[87] Kim YS, Jung MH, Choi MY, et al. Glutamine attenuates tubular cell apoptosis in acute kidney injury via inhibition of the c-Jun N-terminal kinase phosphorylation of 14-3-3. Crit Care Med 2009;37:2033—44.

[88] Schramm L, Seibold A, Schneider R, Zimmermann J, Netzer KO, Wanner C. Ischemic acute renal failure in the rat: effects of L-arginine and superoxide dismutase on renal function. J Nephrol 2008;21:229—35.

[89] Miller HI, Dascalu A, Rassin TA, Wollman Y, Chernichowsky T, Iaina A. Effects of an acute dose of L-arginine during coronary angiography in patients with chronic renal failure: a randomized, parallel, double-blind clinical trial. Am J Nephrol 2003;23: 91—5.

[90] Toback FG. Regeneration after acute tubular necrosis. Kidney Int 1992;41:226—46.

[91] Abel RM, Beck Jr CH, Abbott WM, Ryan Jr JA, Barnett GO, Fischer JE. Improved survival from acute renal failure after treatment with intravenous essential L-amino acids and glucose. Results of a prospective, double-blind study. N Engl J Med 1973;288:695—9.

[92] Roberts PR, Black KW, Zaloga GP. Enteral feeding improves outcome and protects against glycerol-induced acute renal failure in the rat. Am J Respir Crit Care Med 1997;156:1265—9.

[93] Mouser JF, Hak EB, Kuhl DA, Dickerson RN, Gaber LW, Hak LJ. Recovery from ischemic acute renal failure is improved with enteral compared with parenteral nutrition. Crit Care Med 1997; 25:1748—54.

[94] Saadeh E, Ikizler TA, Shyr Y, Hakim RM, Himmelfarb J. Recombinant human growth hormone in patients with acute renal failure. J Ren Nutr 2001;11:212—9.

[95] Takala J, Ruokonen E, Webster NR, et al. Increased mortality associated with growth hormone treatment in critically ill adults. N Engl J Med 1999;341:785—92.

[96] Hirschberg R, Kopple J, Lipsett P, et al. Multicenter clinical trial of recombinant human insulin-like growth factor I in patients with acute renal failure. Kidney Int 1999;55:2423—32.

[97] Acker CG, Singh AR, Flick RP, Bernardini J, Greenberg A, Johnson JP. A trial of thyroxine in acute renal failure. Kidney Int 2000;57:293—8.

[98] Joannidis M, Druml W, Forni LG, et al. Prevention of acute kidney injury and protection of renal function in the intensive care unit. Expert opinion of the Working Group for Nephrology. ESICM. Intensive Care Med 2010;36:392—411.

[99] Marenzi G, De Metrio M, Rubino M, et al. Acute hyperglycemia and contrast-induced nephropathy in primary percutaneous coronary intervention. Am Heart J 2011;160:1170—7.

[100] Schetz M, Vanhorebeek I, Wouters PJ, Wilmer A, Van den Berghe G. Tight blood glucose control is renoprotective in critically ill patients. J Am Soc Nephrol 2008;19:571—8.

[101] Bitla AR, Reddy PE, Manohar SM, Vishnubhotla SV. Pemmaraju Venkata Lakshmi Narasimha SR. Effect of a single hemodialysis session on inflammatory markers. Hemodial Int 2011;14:411—7.

[102] Caglar K, Peng Y, Pupim LB, et al. Inflammatory signals associated with hemodialysis. Kidney Int 2002;62:1408—16.

[103] Berg A, Norberg A, Martling CR, Gamrin L, Rooyackers O, Wernerman J. Glutamine kinetics during intravenous glutamine supplementation in ICU patients on continuous renal replacement therapy. Intensive Care Med 2007;33:660—6.

[104] Frankenfield DC, Reynolds HN. Nutritional effect of continuous hemodiafiltration. Nutrition 1995;11:388—93.

[105] Maxvold NJ, Smoyer WE, Custer JR, Bunchman TE. Amino acid loss and nitrogen balance in critically ill children with acute renal failure: a prospective comparison between classic hemofiltration and hemofiltration with dialysis. Crit Care Med 2000;28:1161—5.

[106] Tang XY, Ren JA, Gu GS, Chen J, Fan YP, Li JS. [Protein loss in critically ill patients during continuous veno-venous hemofiltration]. Zhonghua Wai Ke Za Zhi 2011;48:830–3.

[107] Morena M, Cristol JP, Bosc JY, et al. Convective and diffusive losses of vitamin C during haemodiafiltration session: a contributive factor to oxidative stress in haemodialysis patients. Nephrol Dial Transplant 2002;17:422–7.

[108] Meier-Kriesche HU, Gitomer J, Finkel K, DuBose T. Increased total to ionized calcium ratio during continuous venovenous hemodialysis with regional citrate anticoagulation. Crit Care Med 2001;29:748–52.

[109] Broman M, Carlsson O, Friberg H, Wieslander A, Godaly G. Phosphate-containing dialysis solution prevents hypophosphatemia during continuous renal replacement therapy. Acta Anaesthesiol Scand 2011;55:39–45.

[110] Fiaccadori E, Lombardi M, Leonardi S, Rotelli CF, Tortorella G, Borghetti A. Prevalence and clinical outcome associated with preexisting malnutrition in acute renal failure: a prospective cohort study. J Am Soc Nephrol 1999;10:581–93.

[111] Druml W, Metnitz B, Schaden E, Bauer P, Metnitz PG. Impact of body mass on incidence and prognosis of acute kidney injury requiring renal replacement therapy. Intensive Care Med 2010;36:1221–8.

[112] Baliga R, George VT, Ray PE, Holliday MA. Effects of reduced renal function and dietary protein on muscle protein synthesis. Kidney Int 1991;39:831–5.

[113] KDIGO Clinical Practice Guideline for Acute Kidney Injury. Kidney Int Suppl 2012;2:1–138.

[114] Metnitz PG, Krenn CG, Steltzer H, et al. Effect of acute renal failure requiring renal replacement therapy on outcome in critically ill patients. Crit Care Med 2002;30:2051–8.

[115] Scheinkestel CD, Kar L, Marshall K, et al. Prospective randomized trial to assess caloric and protein needs of critically ill, anuric, ventilated patients requiring continuous renal replacement therapy. Nutrition 2003;19:909–16.

[116] Druml W, Mitch WE. Enteral nutrition in renal disease. In: Rolandelli, Bankhead, Boullata, Campher, editors. Clinical Nutrition: Enteral and Tube Feeding. 4th ed. Philadelphia: WB Saunders; 2005. p. 471–85.

[117] Silva AP, Freire CC, Gondim FA, et al. Bilateral nephrectomy delays gastric emptying of a liquid meal in awake rats. Ren Fail 2002;24:275–84.

[118] Krishnamurthy VM, Wei G, Baird BC, et al. High dietary fiber intake is associated with decreased inflammation and all-cause mortality in patients with chronic kidney disease. Kidney Int 2011.

[119] Holzinger U, Brunner R, Miehsler W, et al. Jejunal tube placement in critically ill patients: A prospective, randomized trial comparing the endoscopic technique with the electromagnetically visualized method. Crit Care Med 2011;39:73–7.

[120] Doig GS, Heighes PT, Simpson F, Sweetman EA, Davies AR. Early enteral nutrition, provided within 24 h of injury or intensive care unit admission, significantly reduces mortality in critically ill patients: a meta-analysis of randomised controlled trials. Intensive Care Med 2009;35:2018–27.

[121] Fiaccadori E, Maggiore U, Giacosa R, et al. Enteral nutrition in patients with acute renal failure. Kidney Int 2004;65:999–1008.

[122] Casaer MP, Mesotten D, Hermans G, et al. Early versus late parenteral nutrition in critically ill adults. N Engl J Med 2011;365:506–17.

[123] Smolle KH, Kaufmann P, Holzer H, Druml W. Intradialytic parenteral nutrition in malnourished patients on chronic haemodialysis therapy. Nephrol Dial Transplant 1995;10:1411–6.

[124] Smolle KH, Kaufmann P, Fleck S, et al. Influence of a novel amino acid solution (enriched with the dipeptide glycyltyrosine) on plasma amino acid concentration of patients with acute renal failure. Clin Nutr 1997;16:239–46.

[125] Roth E, Druml W. Plasma amino acid imbalance: dangerous in chronic diseases? Curr Opin Clin Nutr Metab Care;14:67–74.

[126] Griffiths RD, Jones C, Palmer TE. Six-month outcome of critically ill patients given glutamine-supplemented parenteral nutrition. Nutrition 1997;13:295–302.

[127] van den Berghe G, Wouters P, Weekers F, et al. Intensive insulin therapy in the critically ill patients. N Engl J Med 2001;345:1359–67.

[128] Mayer K, Seeger W. Fish oil in critical illness. Curr Opin Clin Nutr Metab Care 2008;11:121–7.

[129] Hassan IR, Gronert K. Acute changes in dietary omega-3 and omega-6 polyunsaturated fatty acids have a pronounced impact on survival following ischemic renal injury and formation of renoprotective docosahexaenoic acid-derived protectin D1. J Immunol 2009;182:3223–32.

[130] Turpin RS, Canada T, Liu FX, Mercaldi CJ, Pontes-Arruda A, Wischmeyer P. Nutrition therapy cost analysis in the US: premixed multi-chamber bag vs. compounded parenteral nutrition. Appl Health Econ Health Policy 2011;9:281–92.

[131] Feinstein EI, Blumenkrantz MJ, Healy M, et al. Clinical and metabolic responses to parenteral nutrition in acute renal failure. A controlled double-blind study. Medicine (Baltimore) 1981;60:124–37.

[132] Feinstein EI, Kopple JD, Silberman H, Massry SG. Total parenteral nutrition with high or low nitrogen intakes in patients with acute renal failure. Kidney Int Suppl 1983;16:S319–23.

[133] Pupim LB, Flakoll PJ, Brouillette JR, Levenhagen DK, Hakim RM, Ikizler TA. Intradialytic parenteral nutrition improves protein and energy homeostasis in chronic hemodialysis patients. J Clin Invest 2002;110:483–92.

[134] Parienti JJ, Dugue AE, Daurel C, et al. Continuous renal replacement therapy may increase the risk of catheter infection. Clin J Am Soc Nephrol 5:1489–1496.

[135] Prowle JR, Echeverri JE, Ligabo EV, Ronco C, Bellomo R. Fluid balance and acute kidney injury. Nat Rev Nephrol 6:107–115.

37

Nutritional Management of Patients Treated with Continuous Renal Replacement Therapy

Horng-Ruey Chua[1,2], Rinaldo Bellomo[2]

[1]Division of Nephrology, University Medicine Cluster, National University Hospital, National University Health System, Singapore [2]Department of Intensive Care, Austin Hospital, Melbourne, Australia

INTRODUCTION

Continuous renal replacement therapy (CRRT) is a technique to dialyze patients in a gradual and more physiologic way. By lowering the dialysate or replacement fluid flow to near one tenth of that in intermittent therapy, and extending treatment in a continuous manner to often more than 24 hours; rates of solute clearance, osmolality shift and ultrafiltration are significantly reduced, resulting in better hemodynamic tolerability and stability. As such, CRRT is the preferred option in critically ill patients who suffer from acute kidney injury (AKI), with or without baseline chronic renal impairment [1]; and also in those with end-stage renal disease (ESRD) on maintenance hemodialysis who are critically ill [2]. It accounts for 82% of all dialysis modalities used in intensive care units [3,4].

Critical illness confers derangements to body metabolism, with increased hepatic gluconeogenesis, protein catabolism, lipolysis, and loss of lean body mass [5,6]. Though CRRT facilitates nutritional support by efficient azotemic and volume control, it can lead to loss of water-soluble nutrients of low molecular weight with extended therapy. Prolonged extracorporeal circulation possibly increases inflammation and exacerbates the catabolic state of patients. As such, the impact of CRRT on nutrition is significant.

In this chapter, we shall review the nutritional implications of CRRT, with emphasis on nutrient balance, and discuss recommendations on nutritional support to date.

MODES OF CRRT

Solute clearance in CRRT is achieved by diffusion, convection, and membrane adsorption. These processes occur on and across a membrane with variable pore selectivity, usually from 20–30 kDa, which in turn affects solute permeability and water movement (flux). The adjustable trans-membrane pressure allows volume removal (ultrafiltration) to be finely titrated. Blood circulation can be arteriovenous, or venovenous via a single dual lumen catheter, the latter being adopted by most modern machines [7,8].

Continuous venovenous hemodialysis (CVVHD) involves a counter-current dialysate flow to blood across the hemodialyzer membrane, and allows mainly solute diffusion, with small degree of convection from ultrafiltration (Figure 37.1A). In contrast, continuous venovenous hemofiltration (CVVH) generates a much higher volume removal (effluent) across the hemofilter membrane, in excess of the desired ultrafiltration, to induce convective solute removal. The excess plasma lost needs to be substituted with a replacement fluid, which is infused before or after the hemofilter (pre- or post-filter respectively), or both in variable proportions (Figure 37.1B). Continuous venovenous hemodiafiltration (CVVHDF) is a combination of the above (Figure 37.1C). Blood-membrane contact and membrane adsorption facilitates solute removal in all modes. Dialysates and replacement fluids contain electrolytes at physiological concentrations with various buffers for alkalization.

In CVVH, solute removal depends on its sieving coefficient (SC = effluent/plasma concentration) and its

Nutritional Management of Renal Disease
http://dx.doi.org/10.1016/B978-0-12-391934-2.00037-0

(A) **CVVHD**

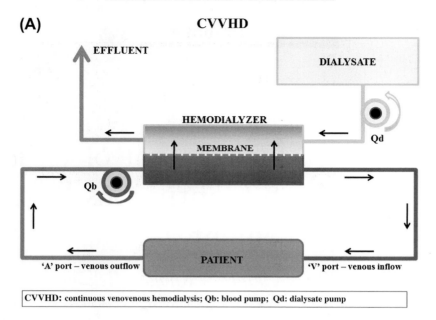

CVVHD: continuous venovenous hemodialysis; Qb: blood pump; Qd: dialysate pump

(B) **CVVH**

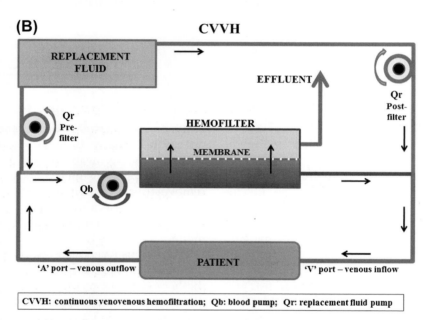

CVVH: continuous venovenous hemofiltration; Qb: blood pump; Qr: replacement fluid pump

FIGURE 37.1 Modes of continuous renal replacement therapy. This figure is reproduced in color in the color plate section.

clearance (SC × effluent rate). Most nutritional substrates are small and their SC approximates 1.0, and clearances are affected chiefly by effluent rate. Pre-filter replacement dilutes the actual plasma concentration entering the hemofilter and reduces the effective clearance, but compensates by prolonging filter life through hemodilution and prevention of clotting [9]. With conventional intensity in CVVH, the differences in small solute clearance with pre- or post-filter replacements are negligible [10]. For that matter, the current optimal dose of CRRT is around 20–25 mL/kg/h of effluent rate, with no difference in clinical outcomes compared to 35 mL/kg/h [11,12]. This is estimated at 2 L/hr based on 25 ml/kg/hr in an 80 kg adult. In practice,

there is also no appreciable difference in small solute clearance between CVVHD and CVVH at prescribed dose of 35 mL/kg/h [13]. As such, the difference in nutrient losses between various modes of CRRT is small.

GENERIC EFFECTS OF CRRT ON ENERGY METABOLISM

Measurement of Energy Expenditure (EE)

A stable bicarbonate pool is essential for gas exchange measurement. Extracorporeal removal or gain of CO_2 affects VCO_2 (rate of CO_2 production), and confounds

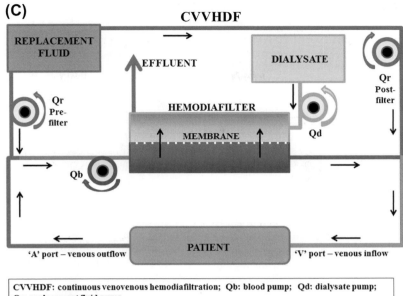

FIGURE 37.1 *(Continued).*

EE quantification with indirect calorimetry (IC) [14,15]. The impact of CRRT on IC is probably minimal, since solute clearance is gradual. In addition, effluent nitrogen loss during CRRT is used in place of (if anuric), or in combination with urinary nitrogen loss, for calculation of EE using proprietary formulas incorporating results of IC. Amino acid nitrogen loss in the effluent (see below) likely confounds the results. Furthermore, actual EE obtained using IC in these patients, exceeds predicted EE using the Schofield equation (adjusted for stress factors) by 19% (if predicted EE is less than 2500 kcal/day); while actual EE is 6% less than predicted (if predicted EE is more than 2500 kcal/day) [16]. Clinicians are reminded to note these limitations.

Hypothermia

Extracorporeal blood circulation induces heat loss, and higher dialysate or replacement fluid flow administered at room temperature leads to a lower core body temperature [17,18]. Short interval (up to 120 minutes) of such heat loss does not affect hepatosplanchnic or gastric mucosal energy consumption and balance significantly. EE is instead reduced with drop in core temperature, provided shivering is prevented with adequate sedation [19]. The effect of heat dissipation with more prolonged therapy is unknown, and may add to negative energy balance. The heating module in modern CRRT machines may attenuate this effect.

Membrane Biocompatibility

Early generation regenerated cellulose (cuprophan) natural membranes are less biocompatible than modern synthetic membranes (e.g. polyamide, polysulfone, polyacrylonitrile), and the former invokes more complement activation with blood-membrane contact [20,21], which may aggravate protein catabolism [22–24]. A systematic review however found no differences in protein catabolic rate between these different membranes in patients on maintenance hemodialysis [25]. Similar studies are limited in CRRT, and most centers today routinely use high flux synthetic membranes. Though there are no apparent differences in small solute SC or clearance and complement activation between high flux modified cellulose and synthetic membranes in CRRT [26], the impact with more prolonged therapy is unknown.

Membrane Adsorption

High flux synthetic membranes have adsorptive properties, which are influenced by electrostatic interactions, hydrophilicity and hydrophobicity. This is an important clearance mechanism for plasma proteins or peptides of higher molecular weight range which restricts routine convection or diffusion, such as cytokines, inflammatory mediators [27,28], and albumin (66 kDa). Adsorption on polymethylmethacrylate membranes results in in-vitro albumin loss of 2.5 g over 12 hours, but less so (less than 0.5 g) with polysulfone or polyacrylonitrile membranes [29]. Adsorptive losses can be easily neglected as these are not measurable in the effluent.

Buffers

The various buffers utilized in CRRT fluids include bicarbonate, or bicarbonate yielding substrates such as acetate, lactate, and citrate. Citrate, and metabolites of acetate and lactate, undergo oxidation in the Krebs cycle and generate calories. Complete oxidation of 1 mmol of acetate and 1 mmol of lactate release about 0.21 kcal and 0.33 kcal of energy respectively, of which 16% to 23% could be expended when the process is diverted into gluconeogenesis or lipogenesis [30]. In addition, 6% of lactate infused will be eliminated during CRRT [31]. Assuming a buffer solution containing 40 mmol/L of lactate running at 2 L/h, this alone accounts for 500 kcal/day of calories. Use of lactate-based solutions for CRRT also worsens glycemia compared to bicarbonate-based solutions [31].

Regional citrate anticoagulation (RCA) has been increasingly used in CRRT. Citrate binds to plasma calcium to inhibit anticoagulation, and has a SC near 1.0. While energy metabolism of citrate is less studied, loss of citrate in CRRT is shown to be proportional to effluent volume, up to 40–60% with an effluent flow rate of 2–3.5 L/h respectively [32]. Citrate's contribution to calorie intake should be less than lactate.

SPECIFIC EFFECTS ON NUTRIENT BALANCE

Glucose and Insulin

Glucose and insulin have molecular weights of 180 Da and 6000 Da respectively. Glucose homeostasis depends on the balance between plasma and CRRT fluid glucose. Results of relevant studies are summarized in Table 37.1.

Historically, glucose-rich peritoneal dialysates were used in CRRT. 51–360 g/day of glucose can be absorbed, depending on the concentration of glucose in these fluids, with corresponding calorie gain of 205–1436 kcal/day [33–36]. For example, 1.5% Dianeal (Baxter) contains 1.5 g/dL (83 mmol/L) of glucose, which at 1 L/h flow rate, contributed 5.8 g/h of glucose and 550 kcal/day [33]. This increases proportionally with higher fluid flow rates and higher fluid glucose concentration [33,35], but tends to plateau at a flow rate of 2 L/h [35]. Consequentially, this can worsen the hyperglycemic and hyperosmolar states encountered

in critical illness and renal impairment [34,36]. Such fluids are now rarely used worldwide.

On the other hand, 40–80 g/day of glucose can be lost, if glucose free CRRT fluids are used [37,38]. The use of glucose-containing fluids result in more glucose loss, but this is offset by the higher net glucose absorbed [36,37]. Higher loss is associated with higher effluent volume and higher plasma glucose concentrations, and can reduce the effective calorie delivered with nutrition therapy [37]. Reduced calorie intake may be compensated by the catabolic diversion of amino acids into endogenous gluconeogenesis. This led to suggestions for physiologic fluid glucose concentrations to establish glucose homeostasis [38,39].

CRRT fluids used today are either glucose free or have low glucose content. The ideal fluid glucose level is unknown. In critical illness, intensive plasma glucose control (80–110 mg/dL or 4.4–6.1 mmol/L) with insulin leads to increased hypoglycemic events [40–43] and increased patient mortality [43], compared to conventional control (up to 200 mg/dL or 11.1 mmol/L). The target plasma glucose range in such scenario is recommended at 144–180 mg/dL (8–10 mmol/L) [44,45]. In addition, CRRT has an independent risk association with hypoglycemia [46], and in particular, use of bicarbonate-based replacement fluids with glucose concentration of 100 mg/dL (5.5 mmol/L), compared to lactate-based replacement fluids of higher glucose composition [47]. Using a fluid with a similar glucose content to optimal plasma level may help to prevent hypoglycemia and glucose variability, which are otherwise associated with increased mortality [48,49].

Insulin loss during CRRT is trivial (1%), compared to endogenous secretion or exogenous administration rates, and is unlikely to be clinically relevant [34].

Lipids

Effluent samples in CRRT are mostly lipid free, with trace amounts of cholesterol and triglycerides detectable, and there is no arteriovenous gradient for lipids across the hemodiafilter to suggest membrane adsorption [33]. Lipid homeostasis is not significantly affected by CRRT.

Amino Acids (AA)

The molecular weights of proteins range from 55–220 kDa, well above the cut-off of standard CRRT membranes; while that of AA is only 110 Da (75–204 Da). AA loss during CRRT has been studied mostly in the context of total parenteral nutrition (PN). The relevant findings are summarized in Table 37.2A,B.

TABLE 37.1 Summary of Studies on Glucose Balance in CRRT

Study	Bellomo 1991 [33]	Bellomo 1992 [34]	Bonnardeaux 1992 [35]	Monaghan 1993 [36]	Frankenfield 1995 [37]
PATIENTS	($n = 9$) PROSPECTIVE	($n = 16$) PROSPECTIVE	($n = 10$) PROSPECTIVE	($n = 20$) PROSPECTIVE	($n = 17$) PROSPECTIVE
Intake	TPN	TPN/EN	—	TPN	TPN
RRT	CAVHDF	CAVHDF/CVVHDF	CAVHDF	CAVH	CAVHDF
RF	NaCl/NaHCO₃, *Post-filter* —	— —	0.5% Dianeal, *Post-filter* —	1.5% Dianeal, *Pre-filter* mean 1.4 L/h	NaCl ± D5%*, *Post-filter* ≈ 0.5 L/h
Dialysate	1.5–4.25% Dianeal 1–2 L/h	1.5% Dianeal 1 L/h	0.5–4.25% Dianeal 0–4 L/h	none	NaCl + HCO₃ ≈ 1.2 L/hr
Plasma glucose	<180 mg/dL	178 mg/dL pre-HDF 207 mg/dL at 24 h	— —	133 mg/dL pre HF 276 mg/dL during HF	162 mg/dL (D5%) 169 mg/dL (no D5%)
Glucose gain and	139–360 g/day	134 g/day	51 g/day	286 g/day	234 g/day
Energy gain	553–1436 kcal/day	536 kcal/day	205 kcal/day (0.5% Dianeal at 2 L/h)	1142 kcal/day	936 kcal/day (with D5% in RF)
Glucose loss	—	—	—	≈ 181 g/day	57 g/day (no D5% given) 82 g/day (D5% given)
Insulin loss	—	689 mU/day	—	—	—
Others	↑ glucose uptake a/w ↑ dialysate glucose & ↑ dialysate flow	trivial loss of insulin (≈ 1% of secretion/administration)	Glucose gain with 0.5% Dianeal plateaued at dialysate flow of 2 L/h	Glucose gain ↑ linearly with ↑ RF up to 2.5 L/h	Plasma glucose and effluent volume predicted glucose loss

Dextrose 5% solution added in variable proportions to replacement fluid.

Note: 1.5% Dianeal contains 1.5 g/dL of glucose.

RRT: renal replacement therapy; CAVH: continuous arteriovenous hemofiltration; CAVHDF: continuous arteriovenous hemodiafiltration; RF: replacement fluid; CVVHDF: continuous venovenous hemodiafiltration; TPN: total parenteral nutrition; EN: enteral nutrition; HDF: hemodiafiltration; HF: hemofiltration; ≈: approximately; D5%: dextrose 5% solution: information not available; ↑: increase; a/w: associated with.

TABLE 37.2A   Summary of Studies on Amino Acid Balance in CRRT

Study	Davenport 1989 [59]	Davies 1991 [53]	Frankenfield 1993 [50]	Kihara 1997 [57]
Patients	*(n = 8)*	*(n = 6)*	*(n = 19)*	*(n = 6)*
NUTRITION	TPN	TPN	TPN	TPN
Protein/AA intake	0.7 g/kg/day*	0.7–1.4 g//kg/day*	2.2 g/kg/day	0.5 g/kg/day*
CRRT	CVVH	CAVHDF	CAVHDF/CVVHDF	Slow HD‡ × 10 h
Bld AA levels	Most within normal range but Gln/Gla low	12 of 19 AA levels low e.g. Ser, Gln, Tau, Try, Iso	All equal or higher than those in control†, except Tau	Ser, Asg lower than normal range
AA clearance (mL/min)	—	3-methyl-His (33.7) Gly (27.6)	—	Cys (36.5) Leu (25.4)
AA loss (g)	3.8–7.4 g/day (*Highest: Ala, Pro, Gln/Gla*)	—	10–16 g/day vs. 5 g/day in control† (*Gln 2 g/day*)	6.2 g (per session) (*Highest: Gln/Gla, Ala*)
Total Nitro loss (g)	—	—	—	8.4 g/day
AA Nitro loss	*(0.6 g–1.1 g/day)*	—	—	*(≈ 1.0 g/day)*
% of intake lost	up to 11% of daily Nitro intake	up to 12.1% of daily protein intake *Highest for Tyr, Lys, Val*	6–9% of daily AA intake vs. 3% in control†	16% of daily AA intake

* Values adjusted as for presumed body weight of 80 kg;
† controls are patients with no AKI at initiation of study;
‡ intensity close to that of CRRT

RRT: renal replacement therapy; AA: amino acid; Nitro: nitrogen; AKI: acute kidney injury; TPN: total parenteral nutrition; —: not reported; CVVH: continuous veno-venous hemofiltration; CAVHDF: continuous arterio-venous hemodiafiltration; CVVHDF: continuous veno-venous hemodiafiltration; HD: hemodialysis; h: hour; CVVHD: continuous veno-venous hemodialysis; HF: hemofiltration; ESRD: end-stage renal disease; EN: enteral nutrition; PN: parenteral nutrition; Gln: glutamine; Gla: glutamic acid; Ala: alanine; Pro: proline; Ser: serine; Cys: cysteine; Leu: leucine; Arg: arginine; Tau: taurine; Try: tyrosine; Iso: isoleucine; ≈: approximately; His: histidine; Gly: glycine; Lys: lysine; Val: valine; Phe: phenylalanine; Asg: asparagine.

TABLE 37.2B Summary of Studies on Amino Acid Balance in CRRT

Study	Novak 1997 [54]	Maxvold 2000 [55]	Bellomo 2002 [51]	Scheinkestel 2003 [52]
Patients	*(n = 6)*	*(n = 6) (peds)*	*(n = 7)*	*(n = 11)*
NUTRITION	TPN	TPN	TPN	TPN
Protein/AA intake	1.2 g/kg/day	1.5 g/kg/day	2.5 g/kg/day	incremental up to 2.5 g/kg/day
CRRT	CVVHDF	CVVH/CVVHD	CVVHDF	CVVHD
Bld AA levels	Most lower than normal eg: Gln, Val, Leu, Iso, Tyr	—	All higher or normal except Asg, His, Tau	AA levels significantly higher at 2.5 g/kg/day intake
AA clearance (mL/min)	Only Gln reported (18.6)	HF: Cys (75.4), Arg (46.1)[#], HD: Cys (53.1), Gln (31.0)[#]	Tyr (45.5), Asg (24.4)	—
AA loss (g)	—	12.5 g (HF), 11.6 g (HD) (per day/1.73 m^2) (*Highest Gln, Lys, Pro*)	12 g/day (*Highest Ala, Val, Lys*)	—
Total Nitro loss (g) *AA Nitro loss*	≈ 27.4 g/day *(0.6 g/day)*	≈ 22 g/day/1.73 m^2 *(≈ 2.0 g/day/1.73 m^2)*	24.3 g/day —	— —
% of intake lost	4.5% of daily AA intake	11–12% of daily AA intake	5–21% of daily AA intake *highest % loss for Tyr*	17% of total AA intake *(87% loss for Tyr)*

[#]*clearance expressed in mL/min/1.73 m^2*

RRT: renal replacement therapy; AA: amino acid; Nitro: nitrogen; AKI: acute kidney injury; CVVH: continuous veno-venous hemofiltration; CAVHDF: continuous arterio-venous hemodiafiltration; CVVHDF: continuous veno-venous hemodiafiltration; HD: hemodialysis; h: hour; CVVHD: continuous veno-venous hemodialysis; HF: hemofiltration; ESRD: end-stage renal disease; EN: enteral nutrition; ≈: approximately; Gln: glutamine; Gla: glutamic acid; Ala: alanine; Pro: proline; Ser: serine; Cys: cysteine; Leu: leucine; Arg: arginine; Tau: taurine; Try: tyrosine; Iso: isoleucine; His: histidine; Gly: glycine; Lys: lysine; Val: valine; Phe: phenylalanine; Asg: asparagine; peds: pediatrics.

BLOOD LEVELS Blood AA levels tend to be higher than or normal compared to reference range or control, in patients on CRRT with protein intake of more than 2 g/kg/day [50–52], while levels are lower than normal range when protein intake is less [53,54]; the significance of which is unknown.

SC OF AA Majority of individual AA has a high SC near 1.0, such as cysteine, arginine, alanine, and glutamine; except for glutamic acid (0.25–0.5) [53,55]. Glutamic acid has a low isoelectric pH, and it assumes a negative surface charge at physiological pH [56]. It is postulated that AAs with similarly low isoelectric pH can be repelled by the negative surface charge on most synthetic membranes, and thus reduce their SC [55], but this trend has not been consistently observed.

AA CLEARANCES AA clearances range from 20–45 mL/min in patients on CRRT [51,53,54,57], as compared to about 200 ml/min in patients on intermittent hemodialysis [58]. AA clearances increase with higher dialysate flow rate [53], and can be 30–40% higher in CVVH compared to CVVHD, and this difference is more apparent with individual AA of higher clearance [55]. However, there is no consistent trend in the differential clearance of any particular AA.

AA LOSSES Protein intake of more than 1.5 g/kg/day is associated with AA loss of about 12 g/day [50,51,55], and AA loss seems less with lower protein intake [57,59]. AA losses account for 5% to a substantial 20% of daily AA intake [50–55,57,59]. Importantly, fractional AA loss (with respect to intake) reduces instead with increased protein intake [52]. Individual blood AA levels correlate well to corresponding losses in CRRT [50,52,57,59], and there is weak evidence that overall AA loss is marginally higher in CVVH than CVVHDF, and with higher intensity of treatment [53,60]. In addition, there is selectivity in individual AA losses, with glutamine and alanine being lost in greater absolute amounts [51,55,57,59], and tyrosine having the highest fractional loss per intake [51-53]. All three are non-essential AA under normal physiological states.

NITROGEN BALANCE Total nitrogen loss in CRRT is about 25 g/day [51,54,55], of which 10% is contributed by AA nitrogen loss [54,55,57], while the rest is likely from protein catabolism; and these result in a negative nitrogen balance. Nitrogen balance in these patients can be improved with increased protein intake, with highest blood AA levels and nitrogen balance achieved at protein intake of 2.5 g/kg/day [51,52].

Vitamins and Trace Elements

These micronutrients have important wound healing, immunomodulatory and antioxidant effects in critical illness [61,62]. Relevant studies in CRRT are summarized in Table 37.3.

BLOOD LEVELS In patients on CRRT, blood levels of vitamins C and E, zinc and selenium are lower, while that of chromium is higher, than healthy controls and normal reference ranges. Low vitamin levels might be associated with increased oxidative utilization in critical illness, and higher chromium might reflect its dependence on renal excretion [63,64]. Hours to days of CRRT can reduce blood levels of folate, pyridoxine-5'-phosphate (P-5'-P, an important moiety of vitamin B_6), zinc and selenium significantly [64,65].

EFFLUENT LOSSES Losses of micronutrients enough to cause significant decrease in blood levels or large fractional losses of usual intake include vitamins C, B_1, B_6 (P-5'-P), folate, chromium and selenium. Specifically, about 68 mg/day of vitamin C, 0.3 mg/day of folate, and 4 mg/day of vitamin B_1 (thiamine) are lost [63–65]. More than twice the daily supplementation of vitamin B_1 and selenium can be lost. Zinc, however, is present in some citrate preparations and replacement fluids, which may instead result in a net gain [64,66,67]. The effect of intensity and mode of CRRT on these losses are unclear.

Electrolytes

Effective treatment of severe hyperkalemia by CRRT may take hours, due to its slow clearance; in which intermittent hemodialysis may be preferred [68]. On the other hand, prolonged CRRT with potassium poor or free fluids will cause hypokalemia, unless potassium is replaced centrally, or incorporated into CRRT fluids with nursing protocols [69].

Hypocalcemia and hypermagnesemia are frequently observed in AKI and ESRD, and the subsequent balances are affected by corresponding levels in CRRT fluids [70]. Calcium can be lost at 60–76 mg/L (1.5–1.9 mmol/L) of effluent or up to 2.7 g/day, while magnesium loss is about 0.6 g/day [66,71]. Frequent hypocalcemia can develop despite 6.4 mg/dL of calcium in replacement fluids [70], whereas fluid magnesium levels up to 3.65 mg/dL may help to minimize CRRT loss [66]. There are no known optimal fluid levels, and frequent monitoring is necessary.

In RCA, citrate chelates calcium and magnesium, and since CRRT fluids that accompany RCA do not contain calcium, algorithms are required for systemic calcium infusion with regular monitoring of ionized calcium levels. Severe hypomagnesemia is rare as CRRT fluids still contain magnesium, though higher loss is anticipated and may require increased replacement [72,73].

Prolonged CRRT with RCA together with immobilization over weeks is associated with bone resorption

TABLE 37.3   Summary of Studies on Vitamin and Trace Element Balance in CRRT

Study	Story 1999 [63]	Fortin 1999 [65]	Klein 2002 [66]	Berger 2004 [64]	Churchwell 2007 [115]
Patients	*(n = 8)*	*(n = 10)*	*(n = 6)*	*(n = 11)*	*(n = 10)*
RRT	CVVH	CVVH/CVVHDF	CVVH/CVVHDF	CVVHDF	CVVHDF
Control	9 ICU pts, 9 healthy pts	none	6 ICU pts with no AKI	none	none
Intensity†	2L/hr	1.8 L/h	1.4–2.2 L/h	1.7 L/h	2.5 L/h
Bld levels	Lower vC, vE, Sel, Zn, higher Chrom (than healthy controls)	marked ↓ folate and P5P over 5d of CRRT	—	Lower Zn, Sel (than reference range) ↓ levels after CRRT × 8 h	Huge interpatient variability
Effluent losses	vC: 68 mg/d Cu: 0.5 mg/d Chrom: 0.02 mg/d	Folate 0.29 mg/d P5P: 0.02 mg/d	Zn: 0.5 mg/d	vB1: 4 mg/d* Cu: 0.4 mg/d* Sel: 0.08 mg/d*	Zn: 0.07 mg/d Cu: 0.01 mg/d Sel: 0.004 mg/d Chrom: 0.004 mg/d Manga: 0.0002 mg/d
Comments	No Zn in effluent; Fat soluble vA, vD, vE are not lost	P5P (active moiety of vB6)	Excessive Zn lost as Zn present in TCA	Sel lost at 2× of daily supplementation; (Net Zn gained from RF)	Fractional loss (per intake): Chrom: 42% Sel: 6.7%

* Net loss after factoring in baseline quantity in replacement fluid;
†inferred from details on effluent/dialysate flow/replacement fluid rates;
RRT: renal replacement therapy; Bld: blood; CVVH: continuous venovenous hemofiltration; CVVHDF: continuous venovenous hemodiafiltration; ICU: intensive care unit; pts: patients; d: day; AKI: acute kidney injury; TCA: trisodium citrate anticoagulant; CRRT: continuous renal replacement therapy; RF: replacement fluid; vA: vitamin A; vB1: vitamin B1/thiamine; vC: vitamin C; vD: vitamin D; vE: vitamin E; P5P: pyridoxal-5′-phosphate; Chrom: chromium; Cu: copper; Manga: manganese; Sel: selenium; Zn: zinc.

and relative hypercalcemia, which mask the hypocalcemia accompanying RCA, leading to gradual reduction in systemic calcium requirement. This can result in severe bone loss and spontaneous fracture [74].

Hypophosphatemia in CRRT occurs in 11–65% of cases, depending on the intensity and duration of treatment [75,76]. Hypophosphatemia is associated with prolonged respiratory failure, cardiac arrhythmias, prolonged hospitalization, and increased mortality [77–81]. Ad hoc phosphate replacement during CRRT results in variability of serum phosphate levels, and necessitates frequent monitoring. The off-label addition of phosphate directly into CRRT fluids has apparently good clinical efficacy and safety profile [82,83]. However, spiking of the solution adds to nursing and pharmacy work-time, with potential for breach in sterility and medical errors. The use of pre-prepared phosphate containing solutions for CRRT is a new attractive and convenient option [84]. The time of initiation of such fluids and the effects on electrolyte balance have not been well reported.

RECOMMENDATIONS ON NUTRITIONAL THERAPY

General Principles

1. AKI by itself does not affect resting EE [85], and nitrogen catabolism in critical illness overwhelms any catabolic effect of AKI or CRRT per se [86]. The overall nutritional requirement during CRRT is primarily determined by the underlying condition.
2. The optimal timing, delivery and intensity of nutritional therapy in critical care remain uncertain.
3. CRRT facilitates unrestricted nutritional support by efficient volume and azotemic control [51,87]. Protein intake should not be limited to avoid uremia.
4. The supplementation of nutritional losses during CRRT to minimize negative body balance is believed to be beneficial, but has not been tested in adequately powered RCTs.

An overview of the recommendations is shown in Figure 37.2.

Timing and Delivery of Nutritional Therapy

The preferred mode of nutritional support in critical illness is early enteral nutrition (EN) [88,89]. Possible benefits include the maintenance of gut integrity, decreased bacterial translocation and less systemic inflammation [90]; and stress ulcer prophylaxis. EN compared to PN is associated with reduced infectious complications, cost, and length of stay [91,92].

Early feeding is assumed to be essential to avert malnutrition, which is otherwise associated with worse outcomes [93,94]. Early EN in acute medical/surgical/trauma/burns patients is associated with reduced infectious complications and length of hospitalization [95]. However, early full dose compared to delayed full dose EN in critical illness is associated with opposite outcomes to the above [96]. In the absence of more definite evidence, all patients (who often cannot tolerate a full oral intake) should receive EN within 24 to 48 hours following admission titrated to gut tolerance [88,89].

Permissive Underfeeding and Supplemental PN

The target goal of nutrition remains ill defined. Interestingly, short term hypocaloric feeding (up to two weeks) is associated with benefits such as reduced metabolic burden, endogenous lipid mobilization, improved glycemic control and reduced infectious events, compared to normo- or hypercaloric feeding; but at the expense of possible negative nitrogen balance [97]. A recent RCT in critically ill patients on EN (12–19% received RRT) further demonstrated that permissive underfeeding (60–70% of predicted calorie requirement) versus full feeding was associated with reduced mortality [98]. Even trophic feeding for initial six days at 15.8% compared to 74.8% of goal calories results in similar clinical outcomes including mortality [99]. In addition, early supplemental PN does not lead to improved clinical outcomes [100], and a multi-center RCT showed that late (after day 8) compared to early (within 48 hours) supplemental PN for insufficient EN was associated with reduced duration of ICU stay and hospitalization, infections, healthcare cost, duration of mechanical ventilation and RRT days [101]. The latest evidence thus suggests that early PN supplementation for insufficient EN due to gut intolerance is not necessary. This does not equate to total or prolonged avoidance of nutritional therapy beyond two weeks, which remain physiologically unsound [102,103].

Macronutrients

Calorie requirements can be measured using IC to calculate EE, or estimated using predictive equations or empirically by weight [88,89]. There are limitations to these and no evidence to suggest the benefit of any method over the other. Providing 25–35 kcal/kg/day of calories with 1.5–1.8 g/kg/day of protein in patients with AKI on CRRT appears to allow the optimal balance between protein catabolism and nitrogen balance [104]. This empirical calorie amount seems consistent with predicted or calculated requirement using IC [16]. Increasing calorie intake to 40 kcal/kg/day does not improve protein balance, but instead leads to worsened

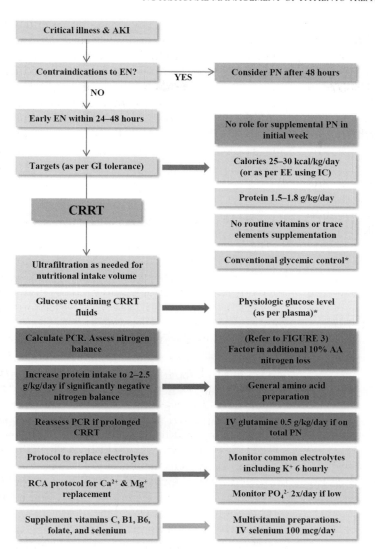

FIGURE 37.2 Algorithm for nutritional therapy. This figure is reproduced in color in the color plate section.

AKI: acute kidney injury; EN: enteral nutrition; PN: parenteral nutrition; GI: gastro-intestinal; EE: energy expenditure; IC: indirect calorimetry; CRRT: continuous renal replacement therapy; PCR: protein catabolic rate; RCA: regional citrate anticoagulation.
*: target plasma glycemia of 144–180 mg/dL.

glycemic control, increased triglycerides and volume administered [105].

CRRT fluids should contain glucose comparable to desired plasma level of 144 to 180 mg/dL to avoid hypoglycemia or glucose variability.

The optimal protein intake is unclear, and the flexibility of adjusting intake is limited by the composition in standard enteral formulas. For example, Isosource® 1.5 cal (Nestle) contains 1.5 kcal/mL of calories and 16.9 g of protein per 250 mL. Intake of 30 kcal/kg/day only delivers 1.4 g/kg/day of protein.

Higher protein intake of 2.5 g/kg/day results in a near positive or positive nitrogen balance, and offers the only active measure to reduce the tendency for

protein catabolism, apart from treating the underlying disease [51,52]. A positive nitrogen balance is associated with improved patient survival in critical illness, but improved survival is not a direct effect of increased protein intake [16]. However, there is a progressive, dose related association between increased protein intake and clinically significant improvement in renal function in critically ill patients [106]. Supplementing protein to a target of 2.0–2.5 g/kg/day may be desirable, in patients on prolonged CRRT with excessively negative nitrogen balance. Therefore, we recommend infrequent monitoring of protein catabolic rate and nitrogen balance in such patients. Equations to guide clinical estimations are shown in Figure 37.3.

1. **TNA = UNA + other nitrogen appearance**
   - TNA: total nitrogen appearance over 24 hours
   - UNA: urea nitrogen appearance over 24 hours

2. **UNA = ([UN]$_{urine}$ x UV) + ([UN]$_{effluen}$ x EV) + change in body UN content**
   - [UN]$_{urine}$: urea nitrogen concentration in urine
   - [UN]$_{effluent}$: urea nitrogen concentration in CRRT effuent
   - UV: urine volume over 24 hours
   - EV: CRRT effluent volume over 24 hours

3. **Change in body UN content over 24 hours = ([BUN] x total body water)$_{current\ day}$ minus ([BUN] x total body water)$_{day\ before}$**
   - [BUN]: blood urea nitrogen concentration
   - total body water $\approx$ 0.6 x body weight (males) or 0.5 x body weight (females)

4. Other nitrogen appearance includes:
   - Amino acid nitrogen loss in CRRT (estimated 10% of TNA)
   - Creatinine nitrogen, other protein losses, skin losses, and gastrointestinal losses (not routinely measured)
   - UNA is thus estimated at 65–75% of TNA
   - $\rightarrow$ **Therefore TNA $\approx$ UNA $\div$ 0.7**

5. **Nitrogen balance = nitrogen intake – TNA**
   - Nitrogen intake = 0.16 x daily protein intake (nitrogen content of protein is about 16%)

6. Conversely to the above, **PCR = TNA x 6.25**
   - PCR: protein catabolic rate

The above equations are limited by the various assumptions, and serve only to provide a clinically useful approximation of nitrogen balance and protein catabolic rate.

FIGURE 37.3　Estimation of nitrogen balance and protein catabolic rate for clinical use

There is no evidence that specific administration of essential AA in preference to general AA preparations lead to any improved clinical outcomes [107]. It is inferred from the general ICU setting, that IV glutamine supplementation of 0.3–0.5 g/kg/day might improve outcome and reduce ICU mortality for patients on total PN [108,109], and it is opinion-based that in CRRT a higher supplementation may be needed [110], but with caution exercised in patients with co-existing fulminant hepatic failure, whose supranormal plasma glutamine levels is linked to hyperammonemia [111]. Role of glutamine supplementation in EN is not defined.

Micronutrients

Micronutrients lost in CRRT should be replaced [112, 113]. That includes increased supplementation of vitamin C, folate, thiamine, and pyridoxine. The desired dose is unknown. In our center, we routinely prescribe Cernevit™ (multivitamin for infusion) for patients on CRRT, which contains all the above.

Selenium can be supplemented intravenously at 100 mcg/day in view of loss [114]. Zinc need not be supplemented as it may have instead a positive balance in CRRT.

Strict nursing protocols to monitor and replace serum potassium; and if RCA is used, serum calcium and magnesium, are essential. It is our opinion that physiologic potassium levels in CRRT fluids of 4 mmol/L (if severe hyperkalemia is absent) helps to prevent iatrogenic hypokalemia and minimize risk of arrhythmias.

The role of correcting hypophosphatemia more aggressively is unclear, and the threshold serum phosphate level to trigger replacement is undefined. We believe that the use of phosphate containing replacement fluids (at 0.8 mmol/L) beyond day 3 of CRRT will help to prevent hypophosphatemia effectively, reduce variability in body phosphate levels, and should translate into an improved outcome.

CONCLUSION

CRRT has provided unparalleled precise extracellular volume and uremic control in critical illness, and has greatly facilitated nutritional support in patients, which is otherwise impeded by AKI or ESRD. The negative impact on nutritional management is primarily due to critical illness itself and less so the iatrogenic nutrient losses during CRRT. The adequacy and appropriateness of nutrition supplementation, especially protein intake, and the effect on protein energy wasting, safety profile, and clinical outcomes, should be the target for future research in this field.

Acknowledgements

Dr Horng-Ruey Chua was a recipient of the Singapore Health Manpower Development Programme (HMDP) award in 2010, which was co-funded by the Ministry of Health (MOH) Singapore, and National University Health System (NUHS) Singapore. The funds were used for his training in Austin Hospital, Melbourne, Australia.

References

[1] Uchino S, Kellum JA, Bellomo R, Doig GS, Morimatsu H, Morgera S, et al. Acute renal failure in critically ill patients:

a multinational, multicenter study. JAMA: the Journal of the American Medical Association 2005;294(7):813−8.

[2] Bell M, Granath F, Schon S, Lofberg E, Ekbom A, Martling CR. End-stage renal disease patients on renal replacement therapy in the intensive care unit: short- and long-term outcome. Crit Care Med 2008;36(10):2773−8.

[3] Gatward JJ, Gibbon GJ, Wrathall G, Padkin A. Renal replacement therapy for acute renal failure: a survey of practice in adult intensive care units in the United Kingdom. Anaesthesia 2008;63(9):959−66.

[4] Bagshaw SM, Uchino S, Bellomo R, Morimatsu H, Morgera S, Schetz M, et al. Timing of renal replacement therapy and clinical outcomes in critically ill patients with severe acute kidney injury. J Crit Care 2009;24(1):129−40.

[5] Brealey D, Singer M. Hyperglycemia in critical illness: a review. J Diabetes Sci Technol 2009;3(6):1250−60.

[6] Rennie MJ. Anabolic resistance in critically ill patients. Crit Care Med 2009;37(Suppl. 10):S398−9.

[7] Cerda J, Ronco C. Modalities of continuous renal replacement therapy: technical and clinical considerations. Seminars in dialysis 2009;22(2):114−22.

[8] Abi Antoun T, Palevsky PM. Selection of modality of renal replacement therapy. Seminars in dialysis 2009;22(2):108−13.

[9] Uchino S, Fealy N, Baldwin I, Morimatsu H, Bellomo R. Predilution vs. post-dilution during continuous veno-venous hemofiltration: impact on filter life and azotemic control. Nephron Clin Pract 2003;94(4):c94−8.

[10] Nurmohamed SA, Jallah BP, Vervloet MG, Beishuizen A, Groeneveld AB. Predilution versus postdilution continuous venovenous hemofiltration: no effect on filter life and azotemic control in critically ill patients on heparin. ASAIO Journal 2011;57(1):48−52.

[11] Palevsky PM, Zhang JH, O'Connor TZ, Chertow GM, Crowley ST, Choudhury D, et al. Intensity of renal support in critically ill patients with acute kidney injury. The New England journal of medicine 2008;359(1):7−20.

[12] Bellomo R, Cass A, Cole L, Finfer S, Gallagher M, Lo S, et al. Intensity of continuous renal-replacement therapy in critically ill patients. New Engl J Med 2009;361(17):1627−38.

[13] Ricci Z, Ronco C, Bachetoni A, D'Amico G, Rossi S, Alessandri E, et al. Solute removal during continuous renal replacement therapy in critically ill patients: convection versus diffusion. Crit Care 2006;10(2):R67.

[14] Brandi LS, Bertolini R, Calafa M. Indirect calorimetry in critically ill patients: clinical applications and practical advice. Nutrition 1997;13(4):349−58.

[15] Lev S, Cohen J, Singer P. Indirect calorimetry measurements in the ventilated critically ill patient: facts and controversies − the heat is on. Critical Care Clin 2010;26(4):e1−9.

[16] Scheinkestel CD, Kar L, Marshall K, Bailey M, Davies A, Nyulasi I, et al. Prospective randomized trial to assess caloric and protein needs of critically Ill, anuric, ventilated patients requiring continuous renal replacement therapy. Nutrition 2003;19(11-12):909−16.

[17] Matamis D, Tsagourias M, Koletsos K, Riggos D, Mavromatidis K, Sombolos K, et al. Influence of continuous haemofiltration-related hypothermia on haemodynamic variables and gas exchange in septic patients. Intensive Care Med 1994;20(6):431−6.

[18] Yagi N, Leblanc M, Sakai K, Wright EJ, Paganini EP. Cooling effect of continuous renal replacement therapy in critically ill patients. Am J Kidney Dis 1998;32(6):1023−30.

[19] Rokyta Jr R, Matejovic M, Krouzecky A, Opatrny Jr K, Ruzicka J, Novak I. Effects of continuous venovenous haemofiltration-induced cooling on global haemodynamics, splanchnic oxygen

and energy balance in critically ill patients. Nephrology, Dialysis, Transplantation: official publication of the European Dialysis and Transplant Association − European Renal Association 2004;19(3):623−30.

[20] Ivanovich P, Chenoweth DE, Schmidt R, Klinkmann H, Boxer LA, Jacob HS, et al. Symptoms and activation of granulocytes and complement with two dialysis membranes. Kidney Internat 1983;24(6):758−63.

[21] Woffindin C, Hoenich NA. Blood-membrane interactions during haemodialysis with cellulose and synthetic membranes. Biomaterials 1988;9(1):53−7.

[22] Gutierrez A. Protein catabolism in maintenance haemodialysis: the influence of the dialysis membrane. Nephrology, Dialysis, Transplantation: official publication of the European Dialysis and Transplant Association − European Renal Association; 1996; 11(Suppl. 2):2108−11.

[23] Gutierrez A, Alvestrand A, Wahren J, Bergstrom J. Effect of in vivo contact between blood and dialysis membranes on protein catabolism in humans. Kidney Internat 1990;38(3):487−94.

[24] Hakim RM. Clinical implications of hemodialysis membrane biocompatibility. Kidney Internat 1993;44(3):484−94.

[25] Macleod AM, Campbell M, Cody JD, Daly C, Donaldson C, Grant A, et al. Cellulose, modified cellulose and synthetic membranes in the haemodialysis of patients with end-stage renal disease. Cochrane database of systematic reviews 2005;(3):CD003234.

[26] Pichaiwong W, Leelahavanichkul A, Eiam-ong S. Efficacy of cellulose triacetate dialyzer and polysulfone synthetic hemofilter for continuous venovenous hemofiltration in acute renal failure. J Med Assoc Thai 2006;89(Suppl. 2):S65−72.

[27] De Vriese AS, Colardyn FA, Philippe JJ, Vanholder RC, De Sutter JH, Lameire NH. Cytokine removal during continuous hemofiltration in septic patients. Journal of the American Society of Nephrology: JASN 1999;10(4):846−53.

[28] Matsuda K, Hirasawa H, Oda S, Shiga H, Nakanishi K. Current topics on cytokine removal technologies. Ther Apher 2001;5(4):306−14.

[29] Yamashita AC, Tomisawa N. Which solute removal mechanism dominates over others in dialyzers for continuous renal replacement therapy? Hemodial Int 2010;14(Suppl. 1):S7−13.

[30] Chiolero R, Mavrocordatos P, Burnier P, Cayeux MC, Schindler C, Jequier E, et al. Effects of infused sodium acetate, sodium lactate, and sodium beta-hydroxybutyrate on energy expenditure and substrate oxidation rates in lean humans. Am J Clin Nutr 1993;58(5):608−13.

[31] Bollmann MD, Revelly JP, Tappy L, Berger MM, Schaller MD, Cayeux MC, et al. Effect of bicarbonate and lactate buffer on glucose and lactate metabolism during hemodiafiltration in patients with multiple organ failure. Intens Care Med 2004;30(6):1103−10.

[32] Mariano F, Tedeschi L, Morselli M, Stella M, Triolo G. Normal citratemia and metabolic tolerance of citrate anticoagulation for hemodiafiltration in severe septic shock burn patients. Intens Care Med 2010;36(10):1735−43.

[33] Bellomo R, Martin H, Parkin G, Love J, Kearley Y, Boyce N. Continuous arteriovenous haemodiafiltration in the critically ill: influence on major nutrient balances. Intens Care Med 1991; 17(7):399−402.

[34] Bellomo R, Colman PG, Caudwell J, Boyce N. Acute continuous hemofiltration with dialysis: effect on insulin concentrations and glycemic control in critically ill patients. Crit Care Med 1992;20(12):1672−6.

[35] Bonnardeaux A, Pichette V, Ouimet D, Geadah D, Habel F, Cardinal J. Solute clearances with high dialysate flow rates and

glucose absorption from the dialysate in continuous arteriovenous hemodialysis. Am J Kidney Dis 1992;19(1):31−8.

[36] Monaghan R, Watters JM, Clancey SM, Moulton SB, Rabin EZ. Uptake of glucose during continuous arteriovenous hemofiltration. Crit Care Med 1993;21(8):1159−63.

[37] Frankenfield DC, Reynolds HN, Badellino MM, Wiles 3rd CE. Glucose dynamics during continuous hemodiafiltration and total parenteral nutrition. Intens Care Med 1995;21(12):1016−22.

[38] Druml W. Metabolic aspects of continuous renal replacement therapies. Kidney Internat Supplement 1999;72:S56−61.

[39] Schetz M, Leblanc M, Murray PT. The Acute Dialysis Quality Initiative−part VII: fluid composition and management in CRRT. Adv Ren Replace Ther 2002;9(4):282−9.

[40] Brunkhorst FM, Engel C, Bloos F, Meier-Hellmann A, Ragaller M, Weiler N, et al. Intensive insulin therapy and pentastarch resuscitation in severe sepsis. New Engl J Med 2008;358(2):125−39.

[41] Wiener RS, Wiener DC, Larson RJ. Benefits and risks of tight glucose control in critically ill adults: a meta-analysis. JAMA: the journal of the American Medical Association 2008;300(8):933−44.

[42] Preiser JC, Devos P, Ruiz-Santana S, Melot C, Annane D, Groeneveld J, et al. A prospective randomised multi-centre controlled trial on tight glucose control by intensive insulin therapy in adult intensive care units: the Glucontrol study. Intensive Care Med 2009;35(10):1738−48.

[43] Finfer S, Chittock DR, Su SY, Blair D, Foster D, Dhingra V, et al. Intensive versus conventional glucose control in critically ill patients. New England J Med 2009;360(13):1283−97.

[44] Standards of medical care in diabetes − 2010. Diabetes Care 2010;33(Suppl. 1):S11−61.

[45] Egi M, Finfer S, Bellomo R. Glycemic control in the ICU. Chest 2011;140(1):212−20.

[46] Arabi YM, Tamim HM, Rishu AH. Hypoglycemia with intensive insulin therapy in critically ill patients: predisposing factors and association with mortality. Crit Care Med 2009;37(9):2536−44.

[47] Vriesendorp TM, van Santen S, DeVries JH, de Jonge E, Rosendaal FR, Schultz MJ, et al. Predisposing factors for hypoglycemia in the intensive care unit. Crit Care Med 2006;34(1):96−101.

[48] Egi M, Bellomo R, Stachowski E, French CJ, Hart G. Variability of blood glucose concentration and short-term mortality in critically ill patients. Anesthesiology 2006;105(2):244−52.

[49] Egi M, Bellomo R, Stachowski E, French CJ, Hart GK, Taori G, et al. Hypoglycemia and outcome in critically ill patients. Mayo Clin Proc. 2010;85(3):217−24.

[50] Frankenfield DC, Badellino MM, Reynolds HN, Wiles 3rd CE, Siegel JH, Goodarzi S. Amino acid loss and plasma concentration during continuous hemodiafiltration. JPEN J Parenter Enteral Nutr 1993;17(6):551−61.

[51] Bellomo R, Tan HK, Bhonagiri S, Gopal I, Seacombe J, Daskalakis M, et al. High protein intake during continuous hemodiafiltration: impact on amino acids and nitrogen balance. Int J Artif Organs 2002;25(4):261−8.

[52] Scheinkestel CD, Adams F, Mahony L, Bailey M, Davies AR, Nyulasi I, et al. Impact of increasing parenteral protein loads on amino acid levels and balance in critically ill anuric patients on continuous renal replacement therapy. Nutrition 2003;19(9):733−40.

[53] Davies SP, Reaveley DA, Brown EA, Kox WJ. Amino acid clearances and daily losses in patients with acute renal failure treated by continuous arteriovenous hemodialysis. Crit Care Med 1991;19(12):1510−5.

[54] Novak I, Sramek V, Pittrova H, Rusavy P, Lacigova S, Eiselt M, et al. Glutamine and other amino acid losses during continuous venovenous hemodiafiltration. Artif Organs 1997;21(5):359−63.

[55] Maxvold NJ, Smoyer WE, Custer JR, Bunchman TE. Amino acid loss and nitrogen balance in critically ill children with acute renal failure: a prospective comparison between classic hemofiltration and hemofiltration with dialysis. Crit Care Med 2000;28(4):1161−5.

[56] Schultz RM, Liebman MN, Proteins I. Composition and structure. In: Devlin TM, editor. Textbook of biochemistry with clinical correlations. 3rd ed. New York: Wiley-Liss, Inc; 1992. p. 25−90.

[57] Kihara M, Ikeda Y, Fujita H, Miura M, Masumori S, Tamura K, et al. Amino acid losses and nitrogen balance during slow diurnal hemodialysis in critically ill patients with renal failure. Intens Care Med 1997;23(1):110−3.

[58] Hynote ED, McCamish MA, Depner TA, Davis PA. Amino acid losses during hemodialysis: effects of high-solute flux and parenteral nutrition in acute renal failure. JPEN J Parenter Enteral Nutr 1995;19(1):15−21.

[59] Davenport A, Roberts NB. Amino acid losses during continuous high-flux hemofiltration in the critically ill patient. Crit Care Med 1989;17(10):1010−4.

[60] Mokrzycki MH, Kaplan AA. Protein losses in continuous renal replacement therapies. Journal of the American Society of Nephrology: JASN 1996;7(10):2259−63.

[61] Prelack K, Sheridan RL. Micronutrient supplementation in the critically ill patient: strategies for clinical practice. J Trauma 2001;51(3):601−20.

[62] Berger MM, Shenkin A. Update on clinical micronutrient supplementation studies in the critically ill. Curr Opin Clin Nutr Metab care 2006;9(6):711−6.

[63] Story DA, Ronco C, Bellomo R. Trace element and vitamin concentrations and losses in critically ill patients treated with continuous venovenous hemofiltration. Critical Care Med 1999;27(1):220−3.

[64] Berger MM, Shenkin A, Revelly JP, Roberts E, Cayeux MC, Baines M, et al. Copper, selenium, zinc, and thiamine balances during continuous venovenous hemodiafiltration in critically ill patients. Am J Clin Nutr 2004;80(2):410−6.

[65] Fortin MC, Amyot SL, Geadah D, Leblanc M. Serum concentrations and clearances of folic acid and pyridoxal-5-phosphate during venovenous continuous renal replacement therapy. Intens Care Med 1999;25(6):594−8.

[66] Klein CJ, Moser-Veillon PB, Schweitzer A, Douglass LW, Reynolds HN, Patterson KY, et al. Magnesium, calcium, zinc, and nitrogen loss in trauma patients during continuous renal replacement therapy. JPEN J Parent Enteral Nutr 2002;26(2):77−92. discussion -3.

[67] Zappitelli M, Juarez M, Castillo L, Coss-Bu J, Goldstein SL. Continuous renal replacement therapy amino acid, trace metal and folate clearance in critically ill children. Intensive Care Med 2009;35(4):698−706.

[68] Kraus MA. Selection of dialysate and replacement fluids and management of electrolyte and Acid-base disturbances. Seminars in Dialysis 2009;22(2):137−40.

[69] Brooks G. Potassium additive algorithm for use in continuous renal replacement therapy. Nurs Crit Care 2006;11(6):273−80.

[70] Morimatsu H, Uchino S, Bellomo R, Ronco C. Continuous venovenous hemodiafiltration or hemofiltration: impact on calcium, phosphate and magnesium concentrations. Internat J Artif Organs 2002;25(6):512−9.

[71] Locatelli F, Pontoriero G, Di Filippo S. Electrolyte disorders and substitution fluid in continuous renal replacement therapy. Kidney Internat Suppl 1998;66:S151−5.

[72] Davenport A, Tolwani A. Citrate anticoagulation for continuous renal replacement therapy (CRRT) in patients with acute kidney injury admitted to the intensive care unit. Nephrol Dial Transplant Plus 2009;2(6):439—47.

[73] Mariano F, Bergamo D, Gangemi EN, Hollo Z, Stella M, Triolo G. Citrate anticoagulation for continuous renal replacement therapy in critically ill patients: success and limits. Int J Nephrol 2011;2011:748320.

[74] Wang PL, Meyer MM, Orloff SL, Anderson S. Bone resorption and "relative" immobilization hypercalcemia with prolonged continuous renal replacement therapy and citrate anticoagulation. Am J Kidney Dis United States 2004. p. 1110—1114.

[75] Palevsky PM, Zhang JH, O'Connor TZ, Chertow GM, Crowley ST, Choudhury D, et al. Intensity of renal support in critically ill patients with acute kidney injury. N Engl J Med United States: 2008 Massachusetts Medical Society 2008; p. 7—20.

[76] Bellomo R, Cass A, Cole L, Finfer S, Gallagher M, Lo S, et al. Intensity of continuous renal-replacement therapy in critically ill patients. N Engl J Med United States: 2009 Massachusetts Medical Society 2009; p. 1627—1638.

[77] Geerse DA, Bindels AJ, Kuiper MA, Roos AN, Spronk PE, Schultz MJ. Treatment of hypophosphatemia in the intensive care unit: a review. Crit Care 2010;14(4). R147.

[78] Demirjian S, Teo BW, Guzman JA, Heyka RJ, Paganini EP, Fissell WH, et al. Hypophosphatemia during continuous hemodialysis is associated with prolonged respiratory failure in patients with acute kidney injury. Nephrol Dial Transplant 2011.

[79] Cohen J, Kogan A, Sahar G, Lev S, Vidne B, Singer P. Hypophosphatemia following open heart surgery: incidence and consequences. Eur J Cardiothorac Surg 2004;26(2):306—10.

[80] Schwartz A, Gurman G, Cohen G, Gilutz H, Brill S, Schily M, et al. Association between hypophosphatemia and cardiac arrhythmias in the early stages of sepsis. Eur J Intern Med 2002;13(7): 434.

[81] Shor R, Halabe A, Rishver S, Tilis Y, Matas Z, Fux A, et al. Severe hypophosphatemia in sepsis as a mortality predictor. Ann Clin Lab Sci. 2006;36(1):67—72.

[82] Troyanov S, Geadah D, Ghannoum M, Cardinal J, Leblanc M. Phosphate addition to hemodiafiltration solutions during continuous renal replacement therapy. Intens Care Med 2004; 30(8):1662—5.

[83] Santiago MJ, Lopez-Herce J, Urbano J, Bellon JM, del Castillo J, Carrillo A. Hypophosphatemia and phosphate supplementation during continuous renal replacement therapy in children. Kidney Int 2009;75(3):312—6.

[84] Broman M, Carlsson O, Friberg H, Wieslander A, Godaly G. Phosphate-containing dialysis solution prevents hypophosphatemia during continuous renal replacement therapy. Acta Anaesthesiol Scand 2011;55(1):39—45.

[85] Schneeweiss B, Graninger W, Stockenhuber F, Druml W, Ferenci P, Eichinger S, et al. Energy metabolism in acute and chronic renal failure. Am J Clin Nutr 1990;52(4):596—601.

[86] Bellomo R, Ronco C. How to feed patients with renal dysfunction. Curr Opin Crit Care 2000;6(4):239—46.

[87] Bellomo R, Seacombe J, Daskalakis M, Farmer M, Wright C, Parkin G, et al. A prospective comparative study of moderate versus high protein intake for critically ill patients with acute renal failure. Renal Failure 1997;19(1):111—20.

[88] McClave SA, Martindale RG, Vanek VW, McCarthy M, Roberts P, Taylor B, et al. Guidelines for the Provision and Assessment of Nutrition Support Therapy in the Adult Critically Ill Patient: Society of Critical Care Medicine (SCCM) and American Society for Parenteral and Enteral Nutrition (A.S.P.E.N.). J Parent Enteral Nutr 2009;33(3):277—316.

[89] Kreymann KG, Berger MM, Deutz NE, Hiesmayr M, Jolliet P, Kazandjiev G, et al. ESPEN Guidelines on Enteral Nutrition: Intensive care. Clin Nutr 2006;25(2):210—23.

[90] Jabbar A, Chang WK, Dryden GW, McClave SA. Gut immunology and the differential response to feeding and starvation. Nutr Clin Pract 2003;18(6):461—82.

[91] Heyland DK, Dhaliwal R, Drover JW, Gramlich L, Dodek P. Canadian clinical practice guidelines for nutrition support in mechanically ventilated, critically ill adult patients. JPEN J Parent Enteral Nutr 2003;27(5):355—73.

[92] Simpson F, Doig GS. Parenteral vs. enteral nutrition in the critically ill patient: a meta-analysis of trials using the intention to treat principle. Intens Care Med 2005;31(1):12—23.

[93] Giner M, Laviano A, Meguid MM, Gleason JR. In 1995 a correlation between malnutrition and poor outcome in critically ill patients still exists. Nutrition 1996;12(1):23—9.

[94] Fiaccadori E, Lombardi M, Leonardi S, Rotelli CF, Tortorella G, Borghetti A. Prevalence and clinical outcome associated with preexisting malnutrition in acute renal failure: a prospective cohort study. J Am Soc Nephrol 1999; 10(3):581—93.

[95] Marik PE, Zaloga GP. Early enteral nutrition in acutely ill patients: a systematic review. Critical Care Med 2001;29(12): 2264—70.

[96] Ibrahim EH, Mehringer L, Prentice D, Sherman G, Schaiff R, Fraser V, et al. Early versus late enteral feeding of mechanically ventilated patients: results of a clinical trial. JPEN J Parent Enteral Nutr 2002;26(3):174—81.

[97] Owais AE, Bumby RF, MacFie J. Review article: permissive underfeeding in short-term nutritional support. Aliment Pharmacol Ther 2010;32(5):628—36.

[98] Arabi YM, Tamim HM, Dhar GS, Al-Dawood A, Al-Sultan M, Sakkijha MH, et al. Permissive underfeeding and intensive insulin therapy in critically ill patients: a randomized controlled trial. Am J Clinical Nutr 2011;93(3):569—77.

[99] Rice TW, Mogan S, Hays MA, Bernard GR, Jensen GL, Wheeler AP. Randomized trial of initial trophic versus full-energy enteral nutrition in mechanically ventilated patients with acute respiratory failure. Critical Care Med 2011;39(5): 967—74.

[100] Kutsogiannis J, Alberda C, Gramlich L, Cahill NE, Wang M, Day AG, et al. Early use of supplemental parenteral nutrition in critically ill patients: Results of an international multicenter observational study. Critical Care Med 2011.

[101] Casaer MP, Mesotten D, Hermans G, Wouters PJ, Schetz M, Meyfroidt G, et al. Early versus Late Parenteral Nutrition in Critically Ill Adults. New Engl J Med 2011.

[102] Sandstrom R, Drott C, Hyltander A, Arfvidsson B, Schersten T, Wickstrom I, et al. The effect of postoperative intravenous feeding (TPN) on outcome following major surgery evaluated in a randomized study. Ann Surg 1993;217(2):185—95.

[103] Heyland DK, MacDonald S, Keefe L, Drover JW. Total parenteral nutrition in the critically ill patient: a meta-analysis. JAMA: the journal of the American Medical Association 1998;280(23): 2013-9.

[104] Macias WL, Alaka KJ, Murphy MH, Miller ME, Clark WR, Mueller BA. Impact of the nutritional regimen on protein catabolism and nitrogen balance in patients with acute renal failure. J Parent Enteral Nutr 1996;20(1):56—62.

[105] Fiaccadori E, Maggiore U, Rotelli C, Giacosa R, Picetti E, Parenti E, et al. Effects of different energy intakes on nitrogen balance in patients with acute renal failure: a pilot study. Nephrology, Dialysis, Transplantation: official publication of the European Dialysis and Transplant Association — European Renal Association 2005;20(9):1976—80.

[106] Doig GS, Simpson F, Finfer S, Delaney A, Davies AR, Mitchell I, et al. Effect of evidence-based feeding guidelines on mortality of critically ill adults: a cluster randomized controlled trial. JAMA 2008;300(23):2731—41.

[107] Li Y, Tang X, Zhang J, Wu T. Nutritional support for acute kidney injury. Cochrane database of systematic reviews (Online) 2010;(1):CD005426.

[108] Novak F, Heyland DK, Avenell A, Drover JW, Su X. Glutamine supplementation in serious illness: a systematic review of the evidence. Critical Care Med 2002;30(9):2022—9.

[109] Wernerman J, Kirketeig T, Andersson B, Berthelson H, Ersson A, Friberg H, et al. Scandinavian glutamine trial: a pragmatic multi-centre randomised clinical trial of intensive care unit patients. Acta Anaesthesiol Scand 2011;55(7):812—8.

[110] Wernerman J. Glutamine supplementation. Ann Intens Care 2011;1:25.

[111] Clemmesen JO, Kondrup J, Ott P. Splanchnic and leg exchange of amino acids and ammonia in acute liver failure. Gastroenterology 2000;118(6):1131—9.

[112] Casaer MP, Mesotten D, Schetz MR. Bench-to-bedside review: metabolism and nutrition. Crit Care 2008;12(4):222.

[113] Wiesen P, Van Overmeire L, Delanaye P, Dubois B, Preiser JC. Nutrition disorders during acute renal failure and renal replacement therapy. JPEN J Parent Enteral Nutr 2011;35(2):217—22.

[114] Chiolero R, Berger MM. Nutritional support during renal replacement therapy. Contrib Nephrol 2007;156:267—74.

[115] Churchwell MD, Pasko DA, Btaiche IF, Jain JC, Mueller BA. Trace element removal during in vitro and in vivo continuous haemodialysis. Nephrology, Dialysis, Transplantation: official publication of the European Dialysis and Transplant Association — European Renal Association 2007;22(10):2970—7.

Anorexia and Appetite Stimulants in Chronic Kidney Disease

Juan Jesús Carrero, Peter Stenvinkel

Division of Renal Medicine, Karolinska Institutet, Stockholm, Sweden

GENERAL CONSIDERATIONS

Diminished appetite in patients with chronic kidney disease (CKD) is an important contributor to inadequate nutrient intake that leads together with other concurrent risk factors to the uremic protein-energy wasting (PEW) syndrome. The drive to eat is a primal drive of all species, and without ingestion of food to provide energy to fuel all functions, survival is not possible. The problem arises when diminished appetite becomes chronically present, profoundly affecting body homeostasis by altering the equilibrium between energy intake and energy expenditure and mobilizing the use of body stores for this purpose. Anorexia (from mild to severe forms) is a common detrimental condition in many chronic diseases with an inflammatory, malnutrition or cachectic component, such as CKD. Anorexia, however, is a complex term that involves not only metabolic signals but also anomalies in the system organs involved in nutrient intake as well as psychological and acquired aspects, including a desire for pleasure, social behavior and customs.

Some definitions and a few words about the feeling of hunger are necessary to introduce this chapter. Appetite is the desire to eat food, felt as hunger. Appetite serves to regulate adequate energy intake to maintain metabolic needs. It is regulated by a close interplay between the digestive tract, adipose tissue and the brain. Anorexia is the decreased sensation of appetite. This term is often used interchangeably with anorexia nervosa. However, anorexia ranges from mild to severe, some of which is relatively harmless, while others indicate a serious clinical condition or pose a significant risk. In CKD patients we mainly encounter mild/moderate forms of anorexia, that is, diminished or low appetite, which contribute to reduced nutrient intake.

Humans eat in episodes, i.e., meals. During the meals, people usually eat until they are comfortably full (satiation), after which they do not eat for a certain time (satiety). Immediately after a meal, there is a low drive to eat. This drive builds up again until the moment of the next eating episode. The moment of the next eating episode is not only dependent on internal factors, but to a large extent is also determined by external (conditioned) environmental factors (cues). Many of environmental cues are highly dependent on the time of the day. Cultural cues, habits and traditions apply as well. Humans eat not only to satisfy their appetite but also for many other reasons, e.g., sensory hedonics, sensory stimulation, tension reduction, social pressure and boredom [1,2]. Thus, anorexia is hard to quantify and also, treatment of anorexia is complex and must involve a global multifaceted approach.

PREVALENCE OF ANOREXIA, METHODS OF ASSESSMENT AND CLINICAL IMPLICATIONS

Anorexia is a common finding in CKD patients which typically develops when glomerular filtration rate is less than 10–25% of normal and increases in severity with the progression towards end stage renal disease [3]. Appetite can be measured in two ways. First, it can be measured with the help of subjective ratings. When used appropriately, subjective ratings have been shown to be reproducible, sensitive to exposures of food components and predictive of food intake. However, it should be noted that appetite may not always be accessible to patient introspection and that people do not always eat when they are hungry and do not always refrain when satiated. Second, appetite can be measured by actual food intake. The degree to which food intake reflects appetite is nevertheless debatable, as there are many factors that may intervene: cognitive factors such as dietary restraint and external factors such as availability, hedonic properties of food and social circumstances. Most studies on anorexia in CKD use rating scales to assess appetite, such as the visual analogue scale (VAS) [4]. More inaccurate but perhaps easily implementable in the clinical setting is the use of self-reports of the patient's appetite [5–8], which have shown to validly correlate with both dietary energy and protein intake [6]. The simplicity of this question is as follows: "How would you grade your appetite in the last week?" according to a 4-point scale: (a) good; (b) sometimes bad; (c) often bad; and (d) always bad [5].

While the prevalence of this condition in early CKD stages is, to our knowledge, unknown, it is reported in generally 35–50% of the patients on dialysis [9] as shown in contemporary studies (Figure 38.1), with a higher proportion of self-reported poor appetite on dialysis treatment days [10]. The consequences of anorexia in this setting are important and should not be underestimated. Four medium–large sample size studies consistently show that a worsening in appetite progressively associates with increased mortality risk [5–8,11] (Figure 38.2). In addition, anorexia increases hospitalization rates by up to 22%, with the costs that this implies for healthcare [6,8,12]. Finally, anorexia is perceived by dialysis patients as a significant worsening in their quality of life [7,11].

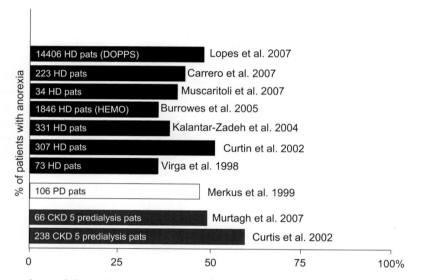

FIGURE 38.1 Reported prevalence of diminished appetite in ESRD, PD and HD patients from recent cohort studies.

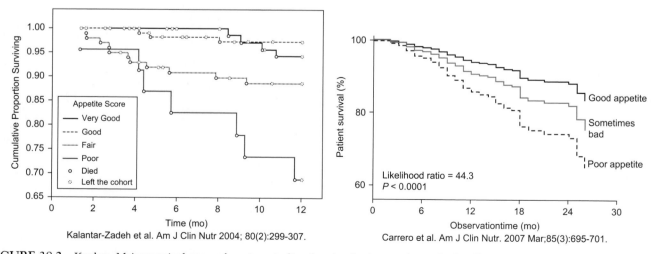

Kalantar-Zadeh et al. Am J Clin Nutr 2004; 80(2):299-307.

Carrero et al. Am J Clin Nutr. 2007 Mar;85(3):695-701.

FIGURE 38.2 Kaplan–Meier survival curves from two studies showing the impact that a single self-report on patient's appetite has on the prediction of 1-year and 2-years mortality. Both studies included prevalent patients undergoing hemodialysis. *Reproduced with permission from Refs [5,7].*

PATHOGENESIS OF ANOREXIA IN CKD

A spontaneous decrease in dietary protein intake and appetite occurs with progressive reduction in renal function [13,14]. Traditionally, diminished appetite has been considered a sign of uremic intoxication [15]. However, anorexia cannot be confined only to appetite regulators, as it links to several other important complications of CKD that need to be put in context. A correct understanding of the multifactorial causes of uremic anorexia is necessary to appropriately tackle this problem. Multiple causes of diminished appetite in the uremic population are discussed below and summarized in Table 38.1. The vast majority of the findings presented in this section pertain to end-stage renal disease (ESRD) or dialysis populations. Very limited information presently exists on the causes of diminished appetite and the extent of this reduction in non-dialyzed populations.

Indirect Contributors to Uremic Anorexia

A number of abnormalities commonly present in CKD may indirectly affect and/or mask the feeling of hunger in these patients, likely influencing and limiting dietary intake. The enjoyment of food depends not only on its taste but also on its odor as it approaches the mouth and the release of volatile organic substances within the mouth. In addition, the temperature and texture of the food, as well as the masticatory sounds, all produce the ultimate sensory experience. All of these

TABLE 38.1 Summary of Potential Mechanisms Contributing to Diminished Appetite and Undernutrition in CKD Patients

Causes of Anorexia in CKD	Comment
DISRUPTED MOLECULAR SIGNALING	
Altered CCK, PYY, ghrelin	Satiety arises earlier in dialysis patients during meal consumption. Ghrelin administration may have potential as therapy
Cytokine and adipokine retention	By both central and peripheral mechanisms. Potential as therapy through antagonism of the melanocortin-4 receptor
Low branched-chain amino acids	Leading to increased serotonin (appetite suppressant) production. Potential as therapy by oral supplementation
FACTORS INHERENT TO THE DIALYSIS PROCEDURE	
Glucose absorption in dialysate	Feeling of fullness, inhibition of appetite by glucose degradation products, delayed gastric emptying by dialysate exchange
Retention of uremic suppressants/toxins	Unknown molecules of middle-size
ALTERATIONS IN THE ORGANS INVOLVED IN NUTRIENT INTAKE	
Oral manifestations: taste abnormalities, dry mouth, tongue coating, mucosal inflammation or oral ulceration	Problems with swallowing and food perception. Possibilities for treatment
Tooth problems: missing/decayed teeth, periodontitis	Problems with chewing, patient may avoid high-fiber foods. Possibilities for treatment.
Impaired olfactory function	Affects taste and food perception. Related to systemic inflammation and malnutrition in CKD
Functional gastrointestinal disturbances: gastric distension, constipation, motility disorders and impaired gastric emptying, diabetic gastroparesis	Will influence patients in their choice of food items that may associate with painful digestion/evacuation. Possibilities for treatment
Infections in the gastrointestinal tract	Possibly contributing also to systemic inflammation. Possibilities for treatment
SOCIAL, PSYCHOSOCIAL CAUSES	
Depression and anxiety, attitude towards disease	
Poor physical activity	
Loneliness and limited ability to do daily living (cooking, buying groceries…etc)	
Economical limitations	
Poor nutritional knowledge on available food choices	

factors and more are altered to some extent with CKD. For instance, a number of characteristic uremic *oral manifestations* such as taste abnormalities (palatability, acuity, metal flavor), dry mouth, tongue coating, mucosal inflammation or oral ulceration (that will altogether ultimately lead to swallowing problems) can contribute to inappetence. Swallowing disorders are *de facto* associated both with aspiration and decreased food intake. Taste loss is common in pediatric CKD, with a recent Australian report showing that children with CKD had a significantly lower taste identification score and of those, about one-third suffered taste loss [16]. The strong association between decreased taste function and loss in eGFR in that study suggests that uremia *per se* is responsible for such abnormalities [16]. Peritoneal dialysis (PD) patients have been reported to have difficulties in detecting salty and bitter tastes in foods as compared to age- and sex-matched controls with normal renal function [17], observations which may be useful when designing

dietary supplements and devising meal plans to help patients consume nutritionally adequate diets. In addition, a relative aversion for sucrose (sweet) taste has been also reported in both animal-models of uremia and pediatric CKD patients [18]. It is plausible that abnormally low preferences for sweet foods can contribute to insufficient caloric intake.

Typical *dental problems* such as higher decayed, missing or filled teeth and the increased prevalence of periodontitis in the CKD population likewise create chewing and/or biting problems, making patients less likely to consume high-fiber foods such as bread, fruits or vegetables and therefore risking their essential nutrient intake [9]. *Depression* (Figure 38.3) and *anxiety* will obviously influence the willingness to eat [8,19], and *olfactory function* is also impaired in hemodialysis patients and related to the severity of protein energy wasting (PEW) [20]. Poor physical activity may also be linked to deprived appetite: in an analysis from the

FIGURE 38.3 Lack of appetite is associated with signs of depression. This figure shows percentage of patients with higher levels of symptoms of depression by degree of being bothered by lack of appetite. Downhearted and blue (n = 14,008); Down in the dumps (n = 8623); Center for Epidemiological Studies Depression Screening Index (CES-D) score (n = 6952). *Reproduced with permission from Ref. [8].*

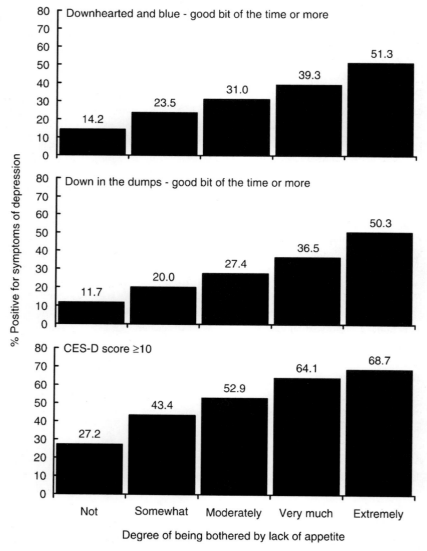

multinational DOPPS, regular exercisers had higher health related quality of life, physical functioning and sleep quality scores, as well as better appetite [21].

Loss of appetite in uremia is related to a number of common *gastrointestinal disturbances*, including gastric distension, constipation, motility disorders and impaired gastric emptying [22,23], all of which will create discomfort associated with nutrient digestion and subsequent food aversion. In line with this, dialysis patients with dyspepsia were reported to be more often malnourished and to have low dietary intake and delayed gastric emptying [24]. Given that diabetes is a frequent comorbidity in dialysis patients, *chronic diabetic gastroparesis* may also be an additional problem resulting in reduced nutrient intake. With prolonged diabetes, the vagus nerve becomes damaged and develops autonomic neuropathy. This disturbance results in prolonged abdominal distension and an exacerbated feeling of satiety, in addition to severely impacting in patient's quality of life. Other indirect causes of anorexia may relate to stomach irritation caused by medicines such as iron compounds or phosphate binders. Enlarging the complexity of this syndrome, gastrointestinal infections are important and underestimated contributors to anorexia in CKD. In the classic study by Aguilera et al. [25], *Helicobacter pylori* infection in patients undergoing PD was associated with a poor nutritional status, increased systemic inflammation and worsened appetite scales (as evaluated by VAS). More recently, bowel bacterial overgrowth syndrome was also proposed as a cause of anorexia and inflammation in PD patients [26]. Most interestingly, general antibiotic treatment of these two infections yielded a significant improvement in both inflammatory markers and VAS appetite scores [25,26].

Drugs can affect food intake, and food intake can also affect, in turn, the efficacy of some drugs and food—drug interactions. Some drugs that may decrease appetite, disturb and disrupt taste the gastrointestinal tract. This is the case, for instance, for many immunosuppressants used in kidney transplant patients, whose reported side effects include nausea, vomiting and diminished appetite. Decreased appetite and nausea were also the more commonly reported adverse events in type-2 diabetic patients with CKD receiving bardoxolone methyl [27]. Most CNS stimulants can also lead to anorexia, and certain antihypertensive drugs (captopril) may result in abnormalities in taste/smell of food. Drugs such as codeine and morphine can decrease peristalsis causing constipation. Drugs can also affect absorption, metabolism and excretion of nutrients. For instance, NSAIDs can alter gastric acidity impacting on intestinal mucosa, and antibiotics can bind to some nutrients such as Fe, Mg and Zn, affecting absorption.

Lastly, we should bear in mind that CKD is eminently a disease of the old, and it is difficult to separate uremia-induced appetite loss from the diminished appetite that naturally develops with age. Additional factors, more difficult to evaluate and to treat, that may promote low nutrient intake are loneliness (living alone, being a widow or divorcee, social isolation), limited ability to do activities of daily living (manage themselves, cook or buy groceries), or economic restraints. Lack of education on adequate dietary needs and uremia-specific dietary restrictions can result in poor dietary intake with an inadequate selection of food choices. Diseases that interfere with the ability of the person to eat or prepare food, e.g., stroke, tremors, or arthritis, can all lead to decreased food intake.

Uremic Anorexia and Early Satiety

The front line in the hunger/satiety cycle is the gastric phase, responsible for the short-term regulation of appetite. Studies on meal termination show that the main reason to stop eating at the end of a meal is fullness or absence of hunger, which refers to a sensation of fullness in the stomach. Another reported reason is a decline in the pleasantness or reward value of the food being eaten. The sensation of fullness is related to peripheral physiologic measures: meal volume and composition induces gastric distension, which stimulates baroreceptors leading to gastric release of appetite regulators responsible for inhibiting gastric motility and inducing central satiety via primary CNS phenomena. The relative contribution of pleasantness and fullness to meal termination depends on the balance between these two factors. Very pleasant-tasting meals may result in a higher food intake and a greater fullness at meal termination.

An initial observation at this level is that dialysis patients with diminished appetite show *slower eating* and *feeling of fullness* before the meals as compared to non-anorectic patients and controls [28] (Figure 38.4). Early satiety and slow gastric emptying in dialysis patients have been linked to dysregulation of short-term appetite modulators from the *gastrointestinal* tract, all of which seem elevated in CKD patients, most likely because of uremic retention. Of these mediators, *cholecystokinin (CCK)*, *glucagon-like peptide 1 (GLP-1)* and *peptide YY (PYY)* release by duodenal cells are perhaps the most important. In PD patients, CCK levels were associated with fullness and hunger perception [29], and PYY levels were significantly elevated in hemodialysis (HD) patients [30], with meal provocation studies disclosing a marked dysregulation of PYY during the postprandial secretion [31], altogether leading to earlier satiety. To the best of our knowledge, only one report assesses GLP-1 circadian variation in uremia and reports no alterations in HD patients as compared to controls [30]. However, based on the common finding of histological evidence of chronic inflammation in the uremic

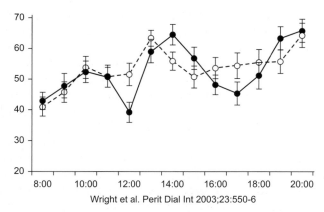

Wright et al. Perit Dial Int 2003;23:550-6

FIGURE 38.4 Mean fullness scores at hourly time points for healthy controls (closed diamonds) and patients undergoing peritoneal dialysis (open circles). While fullness and satiety peaks in healthy controls are marked by each episode meal (i.e., breakfast, lunch and dinner), such peaks are much flattened in peritoneal dialysis patients, meaning that they have a general feeling of fullness along the day and a weaker eating drive. *Reproduced with permission from Ref. [28].*

contradictory given its orexigenic action and that has been interpreted as a sign of resistance to the action of ghrelin. However, it is likely that other concurrent conditions, like pre-existent PEW, may have masked and confounded these observations in cross-sectional analyses [35]. Ghrelin circulates in plasma in two major forms: acyl ghrelin, which promotes food intake, and the abundant desacyl ghrelin (>90%), which on the contrary may induce a negative energy balance by decreasing appetite and delay gastric emptying [36]. Consequently, desacyl ghrelin levels have been found elevated in anorectic HD patients as compared to non-anorectic ones [37], this observation being more prominent in men [38]. Interestingly, the acyl-ghrelin form was reported lower in HD patients and did not exhibit the premeal spike as observed in healthy controls [30]. Counteracting the effects of ghrelin is the recently identified gastric peptide *obestatin*, recently reported low in HD patients [39].

gastrointestinal tract (i.e. esophagitis, gastritis, enteritis and colitis), it can be speculated that impairment of the intestinal barrier function is present. In connection with this, satiety was reported to be more pronounced in PD than in HD patients [28], and associated with abdominal distension due to glucose absorption [15,32].

Ghrelin is another orexigenic peptide released from the stomach, which increases appetite and adjusts both short- and long-term energy balance through the expression of orexigenic neuropeptides and increased growth hormone release. Although the postprandial regulation of ghrelin seems unaffected [33], ghrelin levels are reported elevated in dialysis patients [34], a finding possibly due to uremic retention. This seems

Uremic Anorexia, a Matter of Retention and Disrupted Signaling

The decline of glomerular filtration rate in CKD patients is associated with a significant reduction in food intake and progressive anorectic signs [13,14]. A plausible explanation for this is that inhibition of appetite is caused by retention in body fluids of one or more appetite suppressant. This was suggested in early animal studies where rats given an intraperitoneal injection of plasma ultrafiltrate from uremic patients decreased food intake, as opposed to rats injected with plasma ultrafiltrate from healthy volunteers [40] (Figure 38.5). Such a finding is consistent with the observation that, after commencement of dialysis, food intake and

FIGURE 38.5 Anorexia as a sign of uremic intoxication. Rats given an i.p. injection of plasma ultrafiltrate from uremic patients with decreased food intake, as opposed to rats injected with plasma ultrafiltrate from healthy volunteers (A). This inhibition of food intake seemed to be dose dependent (B). *Reproduced with permission from Ref. [40].*

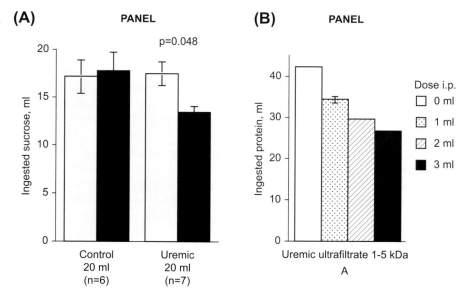

nutritional markers usually improve, at least temporarily. Similarly, it can be hypothesized that the accumulation of these appetite suppressers may reach maximum peak before each dialysis treatment, and indeed there seems to be lower food intake during dialysis days [10].

Factors inherent to the dialysis procedure may further aggravate these symptoms, as animal studies demonstrated that PD solutions with increasing glucose concentration gradually inhibit ingestive behavior [41] (Figure 38.6). Glucose uptake and use have long been central features of many hypotheses about meal initiation because of the central role of glucose in the regulation of energy metabolism, which is due to its exclusivity as an energy source for the central nervous system, its limited storage, its high turnover rate, and its tight regulation. This is the basis for the glucostatic theory for short-term appetite regulation, which postulates that glucoreceptors in the brain detect changes in the rate of glucose utilization. A decrease in glucose utilization represented the stimulus for meal initiation, and an increase in glucose utilization represented the onset of satiety. Peritoneal absorption of large glucose amounts may contribute to this effect. Although there is no strong evidence suggesting that PD patients are more often malnourished than HD patients, it seems however that PD patients are more often bothered by diminished appetite than HD patients [42]. PD fluid exchange has been shown to delay gastric emptying and thus lead to fullness interfering with appetite sensations [43]. Interestingly, a 3.86% glucose-based dialysate infusion decreased total and acyl-ghrelin in a similar way as normal postprandial feeding in 10 PD patients, which would imply that the satiety induced by a PD glucose-exchange equals that of a single lunch or dinner [33]. Glucose degradation products (GDP) have also been suggested as mediators of uremic anorexia, as heat sterilization of glucose PD solutions (thus increasing GDP production) inhibited intraoral intake of mice in a dose-dependent manner as compared to filter

sterilization [44]. Lactate and bicarbonate/lactate buffered PD solutions have been associated with better oral intake than glucose solutions in nephrectomized rats [45]. In a randomized controlled trial, 5 weeks of bicarbonate/lactate solutions in PD patients was associated with a better anorectic profile (depicted as elevated acyl-ghrelin, growth hormone (GH) and adiponectin) compared with traditional lactate solutions [46].

Research in the last decade has focused on identifying the molecules that are dysregulated in uremic anorexia. The best studied of these pathways pertain to proinflammatory cytokines and distorted secretion of adipokines. *Leptin* is the product of the *ob* gene as produced by adipocytes and provides information on the availability of body fat stores to the hypothalamus. Hyperleptinemia is present in uremia, and although *leptin* is an important central mediator of uremic anorexia in animal models acting primarily on hypothalamic neurons [47], clinical studies have yet not been able to demonstrate a role of leptin in this process [48,49]. A state of leptin resistance due to systemic inflammation has been proposed. Leptin actions may be difficult to assess in uremic patients, where rapid changes in body composition occur. For instance, because poor appetite is accompanied with increased fat mass loss [5], declining leptin levels may reflect such loss. The one study showing that low leptin levels predicted poor outcome in dialysis patients probably reflects the detrimental effects of a state of PEW and loss of fat mass on outcome [50]. Growing evidence in the general population suggests a pathophysiological role for leptin in hypertension, CVD, osteoporosis and endothelial dysfunction [51]. Since leptin is produced by abdominal fat and because central obesity is associated with increased inflammation, malnutrition and poor outcome in HD patients [52], it was demonstrated that the effects of hyperleptinemia on CKD outcome are a consequence of abdominal obesity [53]. Supporting this concept, a recent study [54] assessed longitudinal determinants of leptin change in HD patients. In that study, leptin, dietary energy and protein intake and biochemical markers of nutrition and body composition (both anthropometry and bioimpedance analysis) were measured at baseline and at 6, 12, 18 and 24 months following enrollment in 101 prevalent HD patients. The study observed a general decrease in leptin values, but no significant associations were noted between leptin levels and changes in dietary protein or energy intake, or laboratory nutritional markers [54]. Thus, it is likely that leptin levels reflect fat mass depots, rather than independently contributing to uremic anorexia or modifying nutritional status in chronic hemodialysis patients. Although leptin levels may be a consequence of other concurrent risk factors, antagonizing leptin receptors at the hypothalamus may represent a future therapeutic target discussed below.

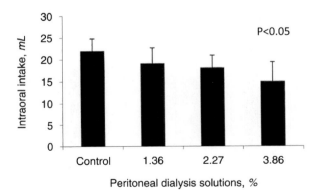

FIGURE 38.6 Peritoneal dialysis solutions with increasing glucose concentration gradually inhibited ingestive behavior in animal models with partial nephrectomy. *Reproduced with permission from Ref. [44].*

Visfatin, recently revisited as a novel adipokine, was previously known as nicotinamide phosphoribosyltransferase (NAMPT), a ubiquitously expressed intracellular protein linked to cellular energy homeostasis, and the rate-limiting step for cell synthesis of nicotinamide adenine dinucleotide [55]. Intracellular visfatin is upregulated in times of low-nutrient availability and promotes cell survival during starvation [55]. Interestingly, and as opposed to serum visfatin levels, visfatin concentrations in human cerebrospinal fluid (CSF) decrease with rising body fat, leading to the hypothesis that centrally acting visfatin is linked to the development of obesity, and reduced CSF visfatin or the development of resistance to its effects may play a role in altered body weight regulation [56]. In ESRD patients the reported hypervisfatinemia [57] may be a counterregulatory response to central visfatin resistance, as elevated visfatin levels were associated with uremic anorexia and low fasting serum amino acids (AAs), glucose and blood lipids, altogether suggesting reduced plasma nutrient availability [58].

Uremic serum amino acid imbalances may contribute to a "brain hyperserotoninergic-like syndrome" that favors anorexia. The altered uremic AA pattern includes reduced essential/non-essential AAs ratio and lower branched-chain AAs [59]. A low plasma level of branched-chain AAs theoretically favors high levels of free tryptophan in the CSF. Tryptophan is the precursor of serotonin, a mediator of appetite suppression. In addition, the nitric oxide (NO) system is altered in uremia, with the accumulation of NO synthase inhibitors that interfere with tryptophan metabolism and enhance serotonin production [15]. This hypothesis has not been, to my knowledge, confirmed in CKD [59]. However, agreeing with this, oral branched-chain AA supplementation was shown to improve appetite in a placebo-controlled double-blind small study on malnourished dialysis patients [60].

Some appetite related nervous-system derived hormones seem also altered in uremia: increased neuropeptide Y has been reported in HD patients [30,61] and did not display any circadian variation [30]. This sustained elevation in NPY may suggest increased tonic hypersecretion in uremia [62]. Norepinephrine levels have been reported marginally elevated in HD patients but did not exhibit the normal nocturnal dip either [30]. Finally, it has been proposed that the commonly observed suppressed parasympathetic activity in CKD patients may directly or indirectly contribute to anorexia [30]. Indeed, the vagus nerve is the central mediator of adipokines, cytokines, PYY and ghrelin in reaching their hypothalamic receptors. Some basic studies support this concept: abdominal vagotomy abolished the PYY-induced decline in feeding [63]. While intravenous PYY administration to control rats resulted in a significant reduction in food consumption compared with saline, PYY given to vagotomized rats did not reduce food intake [63]. In rats, vagotomy abolishes ghrelin-stimulated feeding [64]; in humans, ghrelin does not stimulate appetite in those who had surgical procedures involving vagotomy [65].

Last but not least, the interaction between sex hormones and peptide release disorders may also contribute to appetite loss, as suggested by the observations of sex differences in the severity of uremic anorexia [5]. In animal models, inflammation-induced anorexia was shown more severe in male rats [66], while estradiol and progesterone have inhibitory effects on anorexia [67]. Also, the existence of sex-specific orexigenic and anorexigenic mechanisms in response to inflammation has been suggested in rats, implying sex differences in the upregulation of leptin and ghrelin [68]. This observation links to clinical studies using megestrol acetate as a mean to improve caloric intake in dialysis patients (discussed below).

Uremic Anorexia and Inflammation, an Integrative Factor

An increased loss of appetite is consistently accompanied by higher *inflammation* (Figure 38.7). Levels of CRP, IL-6 or TNF-α have been associated with uremic anorexia [5,7,69,70], in connection with the capacity of cytokines to inhibit feeding through both peripheral

FIGURE 38.7 Markers of systemic inflammation increase across worsening appetite categories in a cohort of patients undergoing maintenance hemodialysis. *Adapted from Ref. [5].*

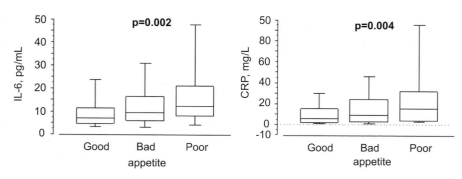

and brain mechanisms [71]. Cytokines are capable of inducing anorexia by influencing on meal size, duration and frequency differentially. Specific cytokines access the brain acting directly on hypothalamic neurons and/or generate mediators targeting both peripheral and/or brain target sites [15,71]. However, the pleiotropic nature of proinflammatory cytokines clearly impinges upon the development of common complications in CKD [72], some of them reinforcing, through a vicious circle, its links to anorexia. For instance, in dialysis patients, depressive symptoms seemed to worsen in the presence of increased IL-6 levels [73]. Chronic inflammatory processes in the periodontium are associated with an elevation of inflammatory markers in HD patients [74]. Impaired olfactory function associates with inflammation [20], and CRP directly blocks the effects of leptin upon satiety and weight reduction [75], making it possible that systemic uremic inflammation further contributes to leptin resistance. Alterations in the gastrointestinal tract, such as dyspepsia and nausea were associated with an increased variability of the inflammatory response in dialysis patients [76]. IL-1 and TNF-α interfere with tryptophan and serotonin turnover [77]. TNF-α decreases NO levels and increases sympathetic activity [78], and low serum amino acids are, in part, a consequence of systemic inflammation [79]. Altogether, interactions at this level emphasize the importance of the inflammation—PEW interplay and its role in exacerbating poor outcomes [80].

Central effects of both adipokines and cytokines on anorexia are mediated by the hypothalamic melanocortin-4 receptor (MC4-R) system. Both the activated macrophage and the activated adipocyte secrete these molecules to plasma and, via the vagus afferent nerve, activate the melanocortin receptor system altering the balance food intake/energy expenditure. Pharmacologic manipulation has shown that agonizing the MC4-R causes weight loss and antagonizing the MC4-R produces weight gain. Interestingly, Cheung et al. [81] reported that intraperitoneal administration of MC4-R antagonists stimulated food intake and weight gain in uremic mice. Most interesting in this study is the secondary observation that neuropeptide signaling pathways also affected expression of key proteins involved in muscle mass maintenance [81], linking uremic anorexia and muscle catabolism by common pathways. Interestingly, numerous classes of MC4-R antagonists have been reported and patented, but it is still too early to be able to apply these therapies in the clinical setting.

TREATMENT OF ANOREXIA IN CKD

To date, no official guidelines exist with regards to the treatment of anorexia in CKD and therefore, the following statements reflect the authors' opinion, this topic is also being reviewed excellently elsewhere [82]. Given the multifactorial nature of anorexia in uremia, it seems reasonable to state that the correct treatment should likely be multifaceted.

As a first step one should screen and if possible treat the underlying causes of anorexia discussed earlier, including gastrointestinal infections and disorders, poor oral and dental health, the presence of periodontitis or diabetic gastroparesis. A comprehensive nutritional, dietary, and appetite assessment to identify whether nutritional stores are too low is recommended. A detailed personal interview with the patients may help us to detect other psychological or social situations that further enhance low food intake, such as problems related to self-feeding, access to food, and eventually, identification of active psychic, social, medical, dialytic, or medicinal related issues that could affect food intake. In the case of diabetic gastroparesis, several nutritional recommendations can be given, including (1) to eat small frequent meals, since high volumes can slow gastric emptying; (2) to consider mechanically altered foods (pureed, ground); (3) not to limit fat, which can provide additional calories; and (4) to stand up for at least one to two hours after eating.

Nutritional counseling to correct reduced or unhealthy nutrient intake should be given to all patients on a regular basis as a means of promoting food intake and to improve the patient's knowledge on food options with respect to their disease. The importance of adequate nutritional support is backed up by an intervention study where the rate of change in serum albumin level was significantly greater among dialysis patients randomized to dietary counseling alone than among those who received oral supplements [83]. Nutritional support in the form of oral supplements or intradialytic parenteral nutrition is nevertheless a valid alternative to ensure adequate nutrition. The usefulness of nutritional support in CKD patients has been largely demonstrated in many studies and will not be discussed in this chapter. However, and connecting to the hypothesized role of branched-chain AA deficiencies in promoting anorexia, it is worth stressing the results from a randomized controlled cross-over trial with 28 malnourished PD patients where daily branched-chain AAs supplementation (12 g/day) for 6 months resulted in improved nutritional status and increased spontaneous oral food intake as compared to the group receiving placebo [60]. A more recent study also observed improvements in albumin and protein catabolic rate together with a decrease in systemic CRP after supplementation of oral amino acids versus placebo [84]. Lastly, promotion of physical exercise and salutary lifestyle modifications may indirectly impact on the patient's energy and calorie intake through improved general well-being [21].

After underlying causes have been treated and adequate nutritional counsel been given, the appetite issue could be tackled by optimizing dialysis regimes. In fact, the increase in the number of dialysis sessions through short daily HD or nocturnal HD has been shown to improve appetite and food intake [85–88]. Although difficult to quantify, this may be due to elimination of certain toxins and appetite suppressants, but likely also to a general feeling of well-being, increased physical activity, fewer dietetic restrictions and the decreased dose of medications linked to the modification in dialysis frequency/dose. In PD, one study also reported an improvement in appetite scales through applying increased daily dialysate volume [89]. Alternation with non-glucose based solutions has also been associated with increased nutrient intake or a more anorexigenic profile in animal and clinical studies [44–46].

Finally, the use of appetite stimulants should be considered. Among the various available medications available for this purpose, megestrol acetate is the only one studied in clinical studies of CKD. Megestrol acetate is a synthetic hormone (progestogen) whose effects on appetite stimulation have mainly been studied in cancer cachexia. Table 38.2 summarizes available studies and main results with megestrol acetate in CKD. All studies, including two with a randomized controlled design, report improvements in appetite and dietary intake, weight gain and albumin increase [77,79,81–84,90–97]. A limitation of these studies is nevertheless the relatively small sample size. Although in principle megestrol acetate could be a valid option for treating uremic anorexia, caution is needed in the close monitoring and follow-up of patients for possible side-effects. A few of these studies report sporadic cases of overhydration, hyperglycemia and ACTH secretion [86,96,97]. The only study performed in pediatric CKD patients observed a case of cushingoid features [95]. Initial evidence suggests that subcutaneous acyl-ghrelin administration improves short-term (single dose and one-week treatment) energy intake and energy balance in mildly to moderately malnourished dialysis patients [98,99]. These results, although highly promising, should still be interpreted with caution until further research evaluates the safety and tolerance of long-term ghrelin administration in dialysis patients [100].

TABLE 38.2 Summary of Reported Studies using Megestrol Acetate as a Mean to Improve Anorexia and Nutritional Status in Patients with Chronic Kidney Disease

Study, Year	Number of Patients (Dialysis Modality)	Dose	Study Design	Outcomes
Boccanfuso et al. 2000 [90]	17 (HD)	400 mg/day for 6 mo.	Prospective observational	↑appetite and weight
Costero et al. 2004 [91]	32 (PD)	160 mg/day for 6 mo.	Uncontrolled	↑appetite and weight
Rammohan et al. 2005 [92]	10 (HD)	400 mg/day for 4 mo.	Uncontrolled	↑weight, albumin, energy intake, quality of life
Monfared et al. 2009 [93]	22 (HD) hypoalbuminemic	80 mg/day for 2 mo.	Randomized controlled	↑albumin and protein catabolic rate
Yeh et al. 2010 [94]	9 (HD) wasted male patients	800/day for 5 mo.	Randomized controlled	↑ weight (both fat and fat-free mass) and exercise capacity. ↑appetite and wellbeing (trends).
Hobbs et al. 2010 [95]	25 pediatric CKD patients	Tapered doses 14.4 mg/kg/d for 5.4 mo.	Retrospective observational	↑weight Side effects: cushingoid features (n=1)
Gołebiewska et al. 2011 [96]	12 (HD) hypoalbuminemic	160 mg/day for 6 mo.	Uncontrolled	↑weight, albumin, subjective global assessment. **Side effects:** overhydration, excessive weight gain, hyperglycemia.
Fernández-Lucas et al. 2011 [97]	16 (HD)	160 mg/day for 3 mo.	Uncontrolled	↑weight, albumin, creatinine, protein catabolic rate **Side effects:** hyperglycemia and ACTH secretion.

HD, hemodialysis; PD, peritoneal dialysis.

References

[1] Morley JE. Anorexia of aging: Physiologic and pathologic. Am J Clin Nutr 1997;66:760−73.

[2] de Graaf C, Blom WA, Smeets PA, Stafleu A, Hendriks HF. Biomarkers of satiation and satiety. Am J Clin Nutr 2004;79:946−61.

[3] Carrero JJ. Mechanisms of altered regulation of food intake in chronic kidney disease. J Ren Nutr 2011;21:7−11.

[4] Hylander B, Barkeling B, Rossner S. Changes in patients' eating behavior: In the uremic state, on continuous ambulatory peritoneal dialysis treatment, and after transplantation. Am J Kidney Dis 1997;29:691−8.

[5] Carrero JJ, Qureshi AR, Axelsson J, Avesani CM, Suliman ME, Kato S, et al. Comparison of nutritional and inflammatory markers in dialysis patients with reduced appetite. Am J Clin Nutr 2007;85:695−701.

[6] Burrowes JD, Larive B, Chertow GM, Cockram DB, Dwyer JT, Greene T, et al. Self-reported appetite, hospitalization and death in haemodialysis patients: Findings from the hemodialysis (hemo) study. Nephrol Dial Transplant 2005;20:2765−74.

[7] Kalantar-Zadeh K, Block G, McAllister CJ, Humphreys MH, Kopple JD. Appetite and inflammation, nutrition, anemia, and clinical outcome in hemodialysis patients. Am J Clin Nutr 2004;80:299−307.

[8] Lopes AA, Elder SJ, Ginsberg N, Andreucci VE, Cruz JM, Fukuhara S, et al. Lack of appetite in haemodialysis patients − associations with patient characteristics, indicators of nutritional status and outcomes in the international DOPPS. Nephrol Dial Transplant 2007;22:3538−46.

[9] Carrero JJ. Identification of patients with eating disorders: Clinical and biochemical signs of appetite loss in dialysis patients. J Ren Nutr 2009;19:10−5.

[10] Burrowes JD, Larive B, Cockram DB, Dwyer J, Kusek JW, McLeroy S, et al. Effects of dietary intake, appetite, and eating habits on dialysis and non-dialysis treatment days in hemodialysis patients: Cross-sectional results from the hemo study. J Ren Nutr 2003;13:191−8.

[11] Kanamori H, Nagai K, Matsubara T, Mima A, Yanagita M, Iehara N, et al. Comparison of the psychosocial quality of life in hemodialysis patients between the elderly and non-elderly using a visual analogue scale: The importance of appetite and depressive mood. Geriatr Gerontol Int 2012 Jan;12(1):65−71.

[12] Bossola M, Giungi S, Luciani G, Tazza L. Appetite in chronic hemodialysis patients: A longitudinal study. J Ren Nutr 2009;19:372−9.

[13] Ikizler TA, Greene JH, Wingard RL, Parker RA, Hakim RM. Spontaneous dietary protein intake during progression of chronic renal failure. J Am Soc Nephrol 1995;6:1386−91.

[14] Bossola M, Muscaritoli M, Tazza L, Panocchia N, Liberatori M, Giungi S, et al. Variables associated with reduced dietary intake in hemodialysis patients. J Ren Nutr 2005;15:244−52.

[15] Carrero JJ, Aguilera A, Stenvinkel P, Gil F, Selgas R, Lindholm B. Appetite disorders in uremia. J Ren Nutr 2008;18:107−13.

[16] Armstrong JE, Laing DG, Wilkes FJ, Kainer G. Smell and taste function in children with chronic kidney disease. Pediatr Nephrol 2010;25:1497−504.

[17] Middleton RA, Allman-Farinelli MA. Taste sensitivity is altered in patients with chronic renal failure receiving continuous ambulatory peritoneal dialysis. J Nutr 1999;129:122−5.

[18] Bellisle F, Dartois AM, Kleinknecht C, Broyer M. Perceptions of and preferences for sweet taste in uremic children. J Am Diet Assoc 1990;90:951−4.

[19] Bossola M, Ciciarelli C, Di Stasio E, Panocchia N, Conte GL, Rosa F, et al. Relationship between appetite and symptoms of depression and anxiety in patients on chronic hemodialysis. J Ren Nutr 2012 Jan;22(1):27−33.

[20] Raff AC, Lieu S, Melamed ML, Quan Z, Ponda M, Meyer TW, et al. Relationship of impaired olfactory function in ESRD to malnutrition and retained uremic molecules. Am J Kidney Dis 2008;52:102−10.

[21] Tentori F, Elder SJ, Thumma J, Pisoni RL, Bommer J, Fissell RB, et al. Physical exercise among participants in the dialysis outcomes and practice patterns study (DOPPS): Correlates and associated outcomes. Nephrol Dial Transplant 2010;25:3050−62.

[22] Aguilera A, Bajo MA, Espinoza M, Olveira A, Paiva AM, Codoceo R, et al. Gastrointestinal and pancreatic function in peritoneal dialysis patients: Their relationship with malnutrition and peritoneal membrane abnormalities. Am J Kidney Dis 2003;42:787−96.

[23] Bossola M, Luciani G, Rosa F, Tazza L. Appetite and gastrointestinal symptoms in chronic hemodialysis patients. J Ren Nutr 2011 Nov;21(6):448−54.

[24] Van Vlem B, Schoonjans R, Vanholder R, De Vos M, Vandamme W, Van Laecke S, et al. Delayed gastric emptying in dyspeptic chronic hemodialysis patients. Am J Kidney Dis 2000;36:962−8.

[25] Aguilera A, Codoceo R, Bajo MA, Diez JJ, del Peso G, Pavone M, et al. Helicobacter pylori infection: A new cause of anorexia in peritoneal dialysis patients. Perit Dial Int 2001;21(Suppl. 3):S152−6.

[26] Aguilera A, Gonzalez-Espinoza L, Codoceo R, Jara Mdel C, Pavone M, Bajo MA, et al. Bowel bacterial overgrowth as another cause of malnutrition, inflammation, and atherosclerosis syndrome in peritoneal dialysis patients. Adv Peritoneal Dialysis 2010;26:130−6.

[27] Pergola PE, Raskin P, Toto RD, Meyer CJ, Huff JW, Grossman EB, et al. Bardoxolone methyl and kidney function in CKD with type 2 diabetes. New Engl J Med 2011;365:327−36.

[28] Wright M, Woodrow G, O'Brien S, King N, Dye L, Blundell J, et al. Disturbed appetite patterns and nutrient intake in peritoneal dialysis patients. Perit Dial Int 2003;23:550−6.

[29] Wright M, Woodrow G, O'Brien S, Armstrong E, King N, Dye L, et al. Cholecystokinin and leptin: Their influence upon the eating behaviour and nutrient intake of dialysis patients. Nephrol Dial Transplant 2004;19:133−40.

[30] Suneja M, Murry DJ, Stokes JB, Lim VS. Hormonal regulation of energy-protein homeostasis in hemodialysis patients: An anorexigenic profile that may predispose to adverse cardiovascular outcomes. Am J Physiol 2011;300:E55−64.

[31] Perez-Fontan M, Cordido F, Rodriguez-Carmona A, Penin M, Diaz-Cambre H, Lopez-Muniz A, et al. Short-term regulation of peptide YY secretion by a mixed meal or peritoneal glucose-based dialysate in patients with chronic renal failure. Nephrol Dial Transplant 2008;23:3696−703.

[32] Chung SH, Carrero JJ, Lindholm B. Causes of poor appetite in patients on peritoneal dialysis. J Ren Nutr 2011;21:12−5.

[33] Perez-Fontan M, Cordido F, Rodriguez-Carmona A, Garcia-Naveiro R, Isidro ML, Villaverde P, et al. Acute plasma ghrelin and leptin responses to oral feeding or intraperitoneal hypertonic glucose-based dialysate in patients with chronic renal failure. Kidney Int 2005;68:2877−85.

[34] Rodriguez Ayala E, Pecoits-Filho R, Heimburger O, Lindholm B, Nordfors L, Stenvinkel P. Associations between plasma ghrelin levels and body composition in end-stage renal disease: A longitudinal study. Nephrol Dial Transplant 2004;19:421−6.

[35] Carrero JJ, Nakashima A, Qureshi AR, Lindholm B, Heimburger O, Barany P, et al. Protein-energy wasting modifies

the association of ghrelin with inflammation, leptin, and mortality in hemodialysis patients. Kidney Int 2011;79:749—56.

[36] Asakawa A, Inui A, Fujimiya M, Sakamaki R, Shinfuku N, Ueta Y, et al. Stomach regulates energy balance via acylated ghrelin and desacyl ghrelin. Gut 2005;54:18—24.

[37] Muscaritoli M, Molfino A, Chiappini MG, Laviano A, Ammann T, Spinsanti P, et al. Rossi Fanelli F. Anorexia in hemodialysis patients: The possible role of des-acyl ghrelin. Am J Nephrol 2007;27:360—5.

[38] Carrero JJ, Heimburger O, Lindholm B, Stenvinkel P, et al. In reply to mofino. Am J Clin Nutr 2007;86:1551—3.

[39] Mafra D, Guebre-Egziabher F, Cleaud C, Arkouche W, Mialon A, Drai J, et al. Obestatin and ghrelin interplay in hemodialysis patients. Nutrition 2010 Nov-Dec;26(11—12):1100—4.

[40] Anderstam B, Mamoun AH, Sodersten P, Bergstrom J. Middle-sized molecule fractions isolated from uremic ultrafiltrate and normal urine inhibit ingestive behavior in the rat. J Am Soc Nephrol 1996;7:2453—60.

[41] Zheng ZH, Anderstam B, Qureshi AR, Heimburger O, Wang T, Sodersten P, et al. Heat sterilization of peritoneal dialysis solutions influences ingestive behavior in non-uremic rats. Kidney Int 2002;62:1447—53.

[42] Strid H, Simren M, Johansson AC, Svedlund J, Samuelsson O, Bjornsson ES. The prevalence of gastrointestinal symptoms in patients with chronic renal failure is increased and associated with impaired psychological general well-being. Nephrol Dial Transplant 2002;17:1434—9.

[43] Schoonjans R, Van Vlem B, Vandamme W, Van Vlierberghe H, Van Heddeghem N, Van Biesen W, et al. Gastric emptying of solids in cirrhotic and peritoneal dialysis patients: Influence of peritoneal volume load. Eur J Gastroenterol Hepatol 2002;14: 395—8.

[44] Zheng ZH, Sederholm F, Anderstam B, Qureshi AR, Wang T, Sodersten P, et al. Acute effects of peritoneal dialysis solutions on appetite in non-uremic rats. Kidney Int 2001;60:2392—8.

[45] Zheng ZH, Anderstam B, Yu X, Qureshi AR, Heimburger O, Lindholm B. Bicarbonate-based peritoneal dialysis solution has less effect on ingestive behavior than lactate-based peritoneal dialysis solution. Perit Dial Int 2009;29:656—63.

[46] Rodriguez-Carmona A, Perez-Fontan M, Guitian A, Peteiro J, Garcia-Falcon T, Lopez-Muniz A, et al. Effect of low-gdp bicarbonate-lactate-buffered peritoneal dialysis solutions on plasma levels of adipokines and gut appetite-regulatory peptides. A randomized crossover study. Nephrol Dial Transplant 2012 Jan;27(1):369—74.

[47] Cheung W, Yu PX, Little BM, Cone RD, Marks DL, Mak RH. Role of leptin and melanocortin signaling in uremia-associated cachexia. J Clin Invest 2005;115:1659—65.

[48] Bossola M, Muscaritoli M, Valenza V, Panocchia N, Tazza L, Cascino A, et al. Anorexia and serum leptin levels in hemodialysis patients. Nephron Clin Pract 2004;97:c76—82.

[49] Rodriguez-Carmona A, Perez Fontan M, Cordido F, Garcia Falcon T, Garcia-Buela J. Hyperleptinemia is not correlated with markers of protein malnutrition in chronic renal failure. A cross-sectional study in predialysis, peritoneal dialysis and hemodialysis patients. Nephron 2000;86:274—80.

[50] Scholze A, Rattensperger D, Zidek W, Tepel M. Low serum leptin predicts mortality in patients with chronic kidney disease stage 5. Obesity (Silver Spring Md.) 2007;15:1617—22.

[51] Carrero JJ, Cordeiro AC, Lindholm B, Stenvinkel P. The emerging pleiotrophic role of adipokines in the uremic phenotype. Current Opinion in Nephrology and Hypertension 2010;19:37—42.

[52] Cordeiro AC, Qureshi AR, Stenvinkel P, Heimburger O, Axelsson J, Barany P, et al. Abdominal fat deposition is associated with increased inflammation, protein-energy wasting and worse outcome in patients undergoing haemodialysis. Nephrol Dial Transplant 2010;25:562—8.

[53] Zoccali C, Postorino M, Marino C, Pizzini P, Cutrupi S, Tripepi G. Waist circumference modifies the relationship between the adipose tissue cytokines leptin and adiponectin and all-cause and cardiovascular mortality in haemodialysis patients. J Intern Med 2011;269:172—81.

[54] Beberashvili I, Sinuani I, Azar A, Yasur H, Feldman L, Averbukh Z, et al. Longitudinal study of leptin levels in chronic hemodialysis patients. Nutr J 2011;10:68.

[55] Yang H, Yang T, Baur JA, Perez E, Matsui T, Carmona JJ, et al. Nutrient-sensitive mitochondrial NAD+ levels dictate cell survival. Cell 2007;130:1095—107.

[56] Hallschmid M, Randeva H, Tan BK, Kern W, Lehnert H. Relationship between cerebrospinal fluid visfatin (PBEF/NAMPT) levels and adiposity in humans. Diabetes 2009;58:637—40.

[57] Yilmaz MI, Saglam M, Carrero JJ, Qureshi AR, Caglar K, Eyileten T, et al. Serum visfatin concentration and endothelial dysfunction in chronic kidney disease. Nephrol Dial Transplant 2008;23:959—65.

[58] Carrero JJ, Witasp A, Stenvinkel P, Qureshi AR, Heimburger O, Barany P, et al. Visfatin is increased in chronic kidney disease patients with poor appetite and correlates negatively with fasting serum amino acids and triglyceride levels. Nephrol Dial Transplant 2010;25:901—6.

[59] Bossola M, Scribano D, Colacicco L, Tavazzi B, Giungi S, Zuppi C, et al. Anorexia and plasma levels of free tryptophan, branched chain amino acids, and ghrelin in hemodialysis patients. J Ren Nutr 2009;19:248—55.

[60] Hiroshige K, Sonta T, Suda T, Kanegae K, Ohtani A. Oral supplementation of branched-chain amino acid improves nutritional status in elderly patients on chronic haemodialysis. Nephrol Dial Transplant 2001;16:1856—62.

[61] Zoccali C, Mallamaci F, Tripepi G, Benedetto FA, Parlongo S, Cutrupi S, et al. Prospective study of neuropeptide Y as an adverse cardiovascular risk factor in end-stage renal disease. J Am Soc Nephrol 2003;14:2611—7.

[62] Deshmukh S, Phillips BG, O'Dorisio T, Flanigan MJ, Lim VS. Hormonal responses to fasting and refeeding in chronic renal failure patients. Am J Physiol 2005;288:E47—55.

[63] Koda S, Date Y, Murakami N, Shimbara T, Hanada T, Toshinai K, et al. The role of the vagal nerve in peripheral PYY3-36-induced feeding reduction in rats. Endocrinology 2005;146:2369—75.

[64] Date Y, Murakami N, Toshinai K, Matsukura S, Niijima A, Matsuo H, et al. The role of the gastric afferent vagal nerve in ghrelin-induced feeding and growth hormone secretion in rats. Gastroenterology 2002;123:1120—8.

[65] le Roux CW, Neary NM, Halsey TJ, Small CJ, Martinez-Isla AM, Ghatei MA, et al. Ghrelin does not stimulate food intake in patients with surgical procedures involving vagotomy. J Clin Endocrinol Metab 2005;90:4521—4.

[66] Lennie TA. Sex differences in severity of inflammation-induced anorexia and weight loss. Biol Res Nurs 2004;5:255—64.

[67] Eckel LA. Estradiol: A rhythmic, inhibitory, indirect control of meal size. Physiol Behav 2004;82:35—41.

[68] Gayle DA, Desai M, Casillas E, Beloosesky R, Ross MG. Gender-specific orexigenic and anorexigenic mechanisms in rats. Life Sci 2006 Sep;13;79(16):1531—6.

[69] Bossola M, Luciani G, Giungi S, Tazza L. Anorexia, fatigue, and plasma interleukin-6 levels in chronic hemodialysis patients. Ren Fail 2010;32:1049—54.

[70] Aguilera A, Codoceo R, Selgas R, Garcia P, Picornell M, Diaz C, et al. Anorexigen (TNF-alpha, cholecystokinin) and orexigen

(neuropeptide Y) plasma levels in peritoneal dialysis (PD) patients: Their relationship with nutritional parameters. Nephrol Dial Transplant 1998;13:1476—83.

[71] Plata-Salaman CR. Cytokines and feeding. Int J Obes Relat Metab Disord 2001;25(Suppl. 5):S48—52.

[72] Carrero JJ, Yilmaz MI, Lindholm B, Stenvinkel P. Cytokine dysregulation in chronic kidney disease: How can we treat it? Blood Purif 2008;26:291—9.

[73] Sonikian M, Metaxaki P, Papavasileiou D, Boufidou F, Nikolaou C, Vlassopoulos D, et al. Effects of interleukin-6 on depression risk in dialysis patients. Am J Nephrol 2010;31: 303—8.

[74] Chen LP, Chiang CK, Chan CP, Hung KY, Huang CS. Does periodontitis reflect inflammation and malnutrition status in hemodialysis patients? Am J Kidney Dis 2006;47:815—22.

[75] Chen K, Li F, Li J, Cai H, Strom S, Bisello A, et al. Induction of leptin resistance through direct interaction of c-reactive protein with leptin. Nature Med 2006;12:425—32.

[76] Snaedal S, Heimburger O, Qureshi AR, Danielsson A, Wikstrom B, Fellstrom B, et al. Comorbidity and acute clinical events as determinants of c-reactive protein variation in hemodialysis patients: Implications for patient survival. Am J Kidney Dis 2009;53:1024—33.

[77] Cangiano C, Laviano A, Muscaritoli M, Meguid MM, Cascino A. Rossi Fanelli F. Cancer anorexia: New pathogenic and therapeutic insights. Nutrition 1996;12:S48—51.

[78] Ando T, Dunn AJ. Mouse tumor necrosis factor-alpha increases brain tryptophan concentrations and norepinephrine metabolism while activating the HPA axis in mice. Neuroimmunomodulation 1999;6:319—29.

[79] Suliman ME, Qureshi AR, Stenvinkel P, Pecoits-Filho R, Barany P, Heimburger O, et al. Inflammation contributes to low plasma amino acid concentrations in patients with chronic kidney disease. Am J Clin Nutr 2005;82:342—9.

[80] Carrero JJ, Stenvinkel P. Persistent inflammation as a catalyst for other risk factors in chronic kidney disease: A hypothesis proposal. Clin J Am Soc Nephrol 2009;4(Suppl. 1):S49—55.

[81] Cheung WW, Rosengren S, Boyle DL, Mak RH. Modulation of melanocortin signaling ameliorates uremic cachexia. Kidney Int 2008;74:180—6.

[82] Bossola M, Giungi S, Luciani G, Tazza L. Interventions to counteract anorexia in dialysis patients. J Ren Nutr 2011;21:16—9.

[83] Akpele L, Bailey JL. Nutrition counseling impacts serum albumin levels. J Ren Nutr 2004;14:143—8.

[84] Bolasco P, Caria S, Cupisti A, Secci R, Saverio Dioguardi F. A novel amino acids oral supplementation in hemodialysis patients: A pilot study. Ren Fail 2011;33:1—5.

[85] O'Sullivan DA, McCarthy JT, Kumar R, Williams AW. Improved biochemical variables, nutrient intake, and hormonal factors in slow nocturnal hemodialysis: A pilot study. Mayo Clin Proc 1998;73:1035—45.

[86] Galland R, Traeger J, Arkouche W, Cleaud C, Delawari E, Fouque D. Short daily hemodialysis rapidly improves

nutritional status in hemodialysis patients. Kidney Int 2001;60: 1555—60.

[87] Spanner E, Suri R, Heidenheim AP, Lindsay RM. The impact of quotidian hemodialysis on nutrition. Am J Kidney Dis 2003;42:30—5.

[88] Galland R, Traeger J, Arkouche W, Delawari E, Fouque D. Short daily hemodialysis and nutritional status. Am J Kidney Dis 2001;37:S95—8.

[89] Liakopoulos V, Krishnan M, Stefanidis I, Savaj S, Ghareeb S, Musso C, et al. Improvement in uremic symptoms after increasing daily dialysate volume in patients on chronic peritoneal dialysis with declining renal function. Int Urol Nephrol 2004;36:437—43.

[90] Boccanfuso JA, Hutton M, McAllister B. The effects of megestrol acetate on nutritional parameters in a dialysis population. J Ren Nutr 2000;10:36—43.

[91] Costero O, Bajo MA, del Peso G, Gil F, Aguilera A, Ros S, et al. Treatment of anorexia and malnutrition in peritoneal dialysis patients with megestrol acetate. Adv Peritoneal Dialysis 2004;20:209—12.

[92] Rammohan M, Kalantar-Zadeh K, Liang A, Ghossein C. Megestrol acetate in a moderate dose for the treatment of malnutrition-inflammation complex in maintenance dialysis patients. J Ren Nutr 2005;15:345—55.

[93] Monfared A, Heidarzadeh A, Ghaffari M, Akbarpour M. Effect of megestrol acetate on serum albumin level in malnourished dialysis patients. J Ren Nutr 2009;19:167—71.

[94] Yeh SS, Marandi M, Thode Jr HC, Levine DM, Parker T, Dixon T, et al. Report of a pilot, double-blind, placebo-controlled study of megestrol acetate in elderly dialysis patients with cachexia. J Ren Nutr 2010;20:52—62.

[95] Hobbs DJ, Bunchman TE, Weismantel DP, Cole MR, Ferguson KB, Gast TR, et al. Megestrol acetate improves weight gain in pediatric patients with chronic kidney disease. J Ren Nutr 2010;20:408—13.

[96] Golebiewska JE, Lichodziejewska-Niemierko M, Aleksandrowicz-Wrona E, Majkowicz M, Lysiak-Szydlowska W, Rutkowski B. Influence of megestrol acetate on nutrition, inflammation and quality of life in dialysis patients. Int Urol Nephrol 2012 Aug;44(4):1211—22.

[97] Fernandez Lucas M, Teruel JL, Burguera V, Sosa H, Rivera M, Rodriguez Palomares JR, et al. [treatment of uraemic anorexia with megestrol acetate]. Nefrologia 2010;30:646—52.

[98] Ashby DR, Ford HE, Wynne KJ, Wren AM, Murphy KG, Busbridge M, et al. Sustained appetite improvement in malnourished dialysis patients by daily ghrelin treatment. Kidney Int 2009;76:199—206.

[99] Wynne K, Giannitsopoulou K, Small CJ, Patterson M, Frost G, Ghatei MA, et al. Subcutaneous ghrelin enhances acute food intake in malnourished patients who receive maintenance peritoneal dialysis: A randomized, placebo-controlled trial. J Am Soc Nephrol 2005;16:2111—8.

[100] Carrero JJ, Stenvinkel P. Nutrition: Can ghrelin improve appetite in uremic wasting? Nat Rev Nephrol 2009;5:672—3.

Oral and Enteral Supplements in Kidney Disease and Kidney Failure

Noel J. Cano

Centre Hospitalier Universitaire de Clermont-Ferrand, Université d'Auvergne, Unité de Nutrition Humaine,
INRA, CRNH Auvergne, Clermont-Ferrand, France

INTRODUCTION

The term "protein-energy wasting" (PEW) has been recommended to designate the loss of body protein mass and fuel reserves in individuals with chronic kidney disease (CKD) or acute kidney injury (AKI) [1]. Kidney diseases include a wide range of pathological states which can both influence nutritional intakes and nutrient metabolism. In fact, CKD, end-stage renal disease (ESRD) treated by maintenance hemodialysis (MHD) or chronic peritoneal dialysis (CPD), and AKI, exhibit very different nutritional and metabolic conditions that require specific nutritional management. The pathophysiology of PEW and its prevalence, as well as the rationale for the use of oral nutritional supplements (ONS) and enteral nutrition (tube feeding, EN) differs according to the type and stage of kidney disease.

In patients with conservatively treated CKD, PEW is the consequence of several factors which usually appear in association with a reduction in the glomerular filtration rate. These factors include a decrease in spontaneous food intake, metabolic derangements and endocrine disturbances (Table 39.1) (see Chapter 11) [1−3]. It is noteworthy that a number of these factors, which also engender losses of muscle mass and fat stores, are similarly found in other chronic diseases such as chronic respiratory diseases, chronic heart failure, chronic infections and cancers. These factors include anorexia, physical inactivity, anemia, inflammation, insulin resistance, hypogonadism [4]. These causes of PEW (see Chapter 11) constitute the nutritional phenotype of these chronic diseases. The prevalence of PEW in conservatively treated CKD increases together with the degree of reduction in renal function and can be close to 50 per cent of people with stage 4 CKD [1].

In MHD and CPD patients, additional causes of nutritional depletion, including dialysis-associated factors and acidemia, are responsible for an increase in the prevalence of PEW, which can reach up to 75% according to some measurements of PEW (Table 39.1). In MHD patients, the independent impact of PEW on the survival was demonstrated in the 1980s [5−7]. The beneficial effects of ONS are now recognized in MHD but remain poorly documented in CPD patients [8,9]. PEW is found in 50% of AKI patients hospitalized in intensive care units [10]. These patients are characterized by a very high catabolic rate leading to major losses of body proteins. During AKI, PEW is associated with an increase in mortality rate [10]. EN, given alone or in association with parenteral nutrition, is a key component of the management of these patients [8,11−14].

Because of the high prevalence of PEW in renal diseases and of its deleterious effect on patients' quality of life, hospitalization rate and mortality, nutritional guidelines to address the prevention and treatment of PEW have been developed by professional and scientific kidney and nutrition organizations. These guidelines address nutritional evaluation and monitoring, nutrient requirements and the management of PEW in patients with kidney disorders. ONS and EN are now considered as the routes of choice for nutritional support in these conditions [8,9,14−16]. Parenteral nutrition is only recommended when ONS or tube feeding cannot ensure adequate nutritional intakes. These guidelines regarding ONS and EN in CKD should take into account two important issues: (1) Due to the lack of large randomized controlled trials assessing the effects of nutritional support on nutritional status, body functioning, morbidity and mortality in patients with kidney diseases, guidelines often rely primarily on expert

Nutritional Management of Renal Disease
http://dx.doi.org/10.1016/B978-0-12-391934-2.00039-4

TABLE 39.1   Causes of Protein-Energy Wasting in Chronic Kidney Disease

Chronic organ disease-related causes of PEW	Anorexia Inflammation Insulin resistance Hypogonadism Anemia Poor physical activity	Co-morbidities Multiple hospitalizations Multiple drug therapies Depression Loneliness Poor economic status
Causes of decreased food intake in CKD	Dietary restrictions: water, protein, phosphorus, sodium, potassium Dysgueusia	Abnormal plasma amino acids Uremic toxins Digestive symptoms, gastroparesis
Other causes of PEW in CKD	Abnormal splanchnic metabolism of nutrients Metabolic acidemia Abnormal growth factor metabolism	Decreased 1,25-dihydroxyvitamin D synthesis Increased serum levels of cortisol, glucagon, adrenaline Hyperparathyroidism
MHD associated factors	Glucose, amino acids and hydrosoluble losses Decreased protein synthesis	Increased protein catabolism Blood-membrane interaction-induced inflammation and protein degradation
CPD associated factors	Protein and micronutrient losses Abdominal discomfort	Anorexia due to glucose absorption from dialysis fluid Peritonitis

opinion [8,14–17]; (2) At present, few oral or enteral formulas specifically adapted to the metabolic needs of patients with kidney disease have been designed and evaluated for their efficacy with regard to both nutritional benefits and prognostic effects. The kidney disorders addressed in this chapter include conservatively treated CKD including CKD 1–5, nephrotic syndrome, ESRD with MHD or CPD, and AKI.

ORAL AND ENTERAL (TUBE FEEDING) NUTRITION IN CKD PATIENTS

The nutritional challenge in patients with conservatively treated CKD is to simultaneously ensure, on the one hand, the preservation of renal function using low protein diets (if such diets do slow progression) and, on the other hand, the prevention or treatment of PEW. Indeed, PEW in patients commencing MHD is associated with higher mortality rates during the first year of MHD. Such a challenge requires a close monitoring of dietary intakes and nutritional status of CKD patients in order to detect PEW (Table 39.2). This condition is generally identified by insufficient nutrient intake, decreased body mass, loss of muscle mass, often reduced fat mass, and low serum albumin or transthyretin [1] (see Chapter 10). In patients with advanced CKD and no obvious severe, superimposed catabolic illness, the occurrence of PEW in spite of nutritional management is an indication to initiate dialysis treatment [16]. Although ONS and EN may be useful in CKD patients with PEW, these treatments have been poorly investigated. Because systematic trials are not available, present guidelines are considered as expert-opinion based [8,9,14–17].

Nutritional and Metabolic Setting

Causes of PEW in CKD are given in Table 39.1. Spontaneous oral intakes progressively decline during the progression of CKD: it has been reported that, for each 10 mL/min decrease in creatinine clearance, dietary protein intakes decrease by 0.064 g/kg per day [18]. Patients with CKD frequently present with digestive symptoms. Impaired gastrointestinal motility can be a limit for the tolerance of EN. Gastroparesis, which is most pronounced in diabetic patients, may be improved by prokinetic agents and by the management of diabetes and diabetic neuropathy. The following are among the metabolic disturbances associated with CKD that should be taken into account when determining strategies for nutritional support in CKD: insulin resistance and disturbed blood glucose control, abnormal plasma lipid clearances, increased protein degradation, inflammation, metabolic acidemia, hyperparathyroidism, altered vitamin D metabolism and hyperkalemia. Correction of acidemia in CKD patients is shown to improve serum albumin and transthyretin levels [19].

Indications for Oral Nutritional Supplements and Enteral Nutrition in Conservatively Treated CKD

Essential amino acid and ketoacid preparations that are given with very low protein diets and prescribed as part of the regular diet for such patients are not addressed in this chapter (see Chapter 14) [20]. Guidelines for protein, energy intakes and for some mineral and vitamin needs are given in other chapters in this book [8,14,17]. An energy intake of at least

TABLE 39.2 Criteria for Protein-Energy Wasting According to the International Society for Renal Nutrition and Metabolism (Ref. [1])

Serum chemistry	• Albumin <38 g/L (by bromocresol method, approximately 35 g/L by immunonephelemetry) • Transthyretin (prealbumin) <300 mg/L • Cholesterol <1 g /L
Body mass	• Body mass index <23 kg/m^2 • Unintentional body weight loss >5% over 3 months or 10% over 6 months • Total body fat percentage <10%
Muscle mass	• Muscle wasting >5% over 3 months or 10% over 6 months • Reduced arm muscle mass area >10% in relation to 50th percentile • Creatinine appearance
Dietary intake	• Unintentional dietary protein intake <0.80 g/kg/d for at least 2 months • Unintentional dietary energy intake <25 kcal/kg/d for at least 2 months

30–35 kcal/kg BW/day is associated with a better nitrogen balance and is recommended in conservatively treated CKD patients. When spontaneous feeding cannot meet these requirements, ONS may be useful to ensure that the recommended intakes are met, to prevent the occurrence of PEW, or to treat this condition. ONS and EN with specialized formulas have been recommended for protein-energy wasted CKD patients [8]. Polymeric nutritive mixtures which are protein and electrolyte-restricted and which have high energy density are available. A number of these diets are shown to be well tolerated and able to improve protein and calorie intakes [21]. However, their effects on nutritional parameters, morbidity and survival have not been studied. Because such formulas are not available in every country, standard ONS and EN that are used for people without kidney disease are often employed for CKD patients with PEW. The prescription of such supplements should take into account their protein, phosphorus, sodium and potassium content.

In addition to its use for patients with PEW, EN is indicated in CKD patients who are unable to eat adequately, cannot take sufficient ONS for their needs, who have acute stress conditions or who have certain neurological diseases, dementia, or pharyngeal or esophageal obstruction [8,22]. EN is first administered through a nasogastric tube. When EN is planned to last more than one month, a perendoscopic or radiologic gastrostomy should be considered.

ORAL AND ENTERAL NUTRITION FOR PATIENTS WITH NEPHROTIC SYNDROME

Nutritional and Metabolic Particularities of Nephrotic Syndrome

Patients with nephrotic syndrome exhibit specific metabolic disorders that should be taken into account when designing their nutritional management. Insulin resistance is frequent and can be worsened by corticosteroid and other immunosuppressive treatments [23]. Metabolic studies showed similar rates of whole body protein metabolism in patients with the nephrotic syndrome as compared to controls. However, tissue-specific studies show that liver protein synthesis is increased whereas muscle protein synthesis reduced [24]. Patients with the nephrotic syndrome also exhibit abnormalities in lipid metabolism that mainly consist of increased plasma concentrations of LDL-cholesterol, lipoprotein (a), and VLDL [25]. These patients are also characterized renal by sodium retention [26], hypocalcemia and low serum vitamin D levels due to the urinary losses of vitamin D and vitamin D transport protein [27].

Nutritional Requirements, Oral Nutritional Supplements and Enteral Nutrition in Patients with the Nephrotic Syndrome

A personalized dietetic evaluation is needed in patients with nephrotic syndrome. High protein diets, which had been proposed to prevent PEW, were shown to increase proteinuria and reduce renal function [24,28]. On the other hand, modestly restricted low protein diets have been shown to decrease proteinuria, to increase serum albumin levels and to maintain nitrogen (protein) balance [28]. It should be emphasized that such regimens have only been investigated in clinically stable patients and during short-term studies (e.g., one month). Therefore, the long-term effects of modestly reduced protein diets on nutritional status, as well as their tolerance by clinically unstable patients, are unknown [24,27,28]. The risk of PEW during long-term treatment with low protein diets has not been evaluated in nephrotic patients. A protein supply of 1 g/kg BW/day or 0.8 g protein/kg BW/day plus the compensation of urinary protein losses appears to be a good approach (see Chapter 26). Monitoring nephrotic patients by urinary urea excretion and urinary protein losses makes it possible to assess adherence to the prescribed regimen [28,29]. Other dietary recommendations include an energy intake of 30 to 35 kcal/kg BW/day, the exclusion of sugars that have rapid gastrointestinal absorption, and a limited fat intake [27]. Therapies which reduce protein-uria contribute to an improved serum lipid profile [25]. Regular exercise, vitamin D and calcium supplementation have been proposed to prevented osteoporosis [27]. Because of water and sodium retention, sodium chloride intake should not exceed 4 g/day in adults [26,29]. The effects of ONS and EN have not been evaluated for the treatment of nephrotic patients with PEW. Because such patients may need a nutritive assistance, ONS as well as EN should be prescribed as in other conservatively treated CKD patients.

ORAL AND ENTERAL NUTRITION IN CHRONIC DIALYSIS PATIENTS

Most of the clinical research that has addressed the pathophysiology, prevalence and treatment of PEW in CKD has been performed in MHD or CPD patients [8,9]. In MHD and CPD patients, the reported incidence and prevalence of PEW varies from 25 to 70% according to the nutritional parameters that are assessed [30]. An increased mortality risk associated with PEW has been described since the 1980s [5,6]. Numerous clinical trials, including seven randomized studies in MHD patients with documented nutritional wasting, showed the ability of ONS to improve nutritional parameters in these individuals (Table 39.3) [9,31]. One prospective study showed, during a two-year follow-up, that the improvement in nutritional status with ONS administration, as assessed by an increase in serum transthyretin, was associated with a two-fold increase in survival, an improvement of the Karnofsky activity score and a reduction of hospitalization rates [32]. The clinical response to ONS of CPD patients with PEW is still poorly studied.

Specific Issues Related to Protein-Energy Wasting (PEW) in Maintenance Dialysis Patients

In addition to the causes of PEW that are commonly found in non-dialyzed CKD patients, MHD and CPD are associated with many additional nutritional and metabolic alterations that further increase the risk of PEW (Table 39.1). Anorexia is a major cause of protein-energy depletion in MHD [33,34]. Because MHD patients eat less than their needs, nutritional supplementation is a key component of their management. The contribution of unfavorable economic status and psychological disorders to the genesis of PEW has

been emphasized. The negative role of these factors on the prognosis of MHD patients has been recently described in a DOPPS report: poorer social support and other adverse psychosocial conditions are associated with higher mortality risk, lower adherence to medical care, and poorer physical quality of life [35].

Most studies of resting energy expenditure in MHD patients reported rates of energy consumption similar to healthy, age-matched normal subjects (for review see [31]). Severe hyperparathyroidism [36], high serum IL-6 concentrations [37] and possibly hemodialysis sessions [38] have been associated with an increase in energy expenditure. A hemodialysis treatment transiently decreases plasma amino acid concentrations by dialytic removal of these compounds, and there is a subsequent decrease in protein synthesis [39]. Moreover, the hemodialysis procedure engenders an increase in protein catabolism [40], which is enhanced if non-biocompatible membranes are used [41]. Both the uremic syndrome and the hemodialysis procedure lead to inflammatory conditions that may enhance protein catabolism. Interventional studies indicate that MHD patients with PEW may undergo an anabolic response to nutritional support even when systemic inflammation, as evidenced by elevated serum C-reactive protein, is present [32,42,43]. Associated disease processes such as infections enhance protein catabolism and must be treated. Similarly, the correction of metabolic acidemia can reduce protein catabolism [44]. Another factor engendering protein-energy depletion can be an insufficient dialysis prescription. An inadequate dialysis dose is associated with increased risk of PEW [30]. Conversely, the use of high permeability membranes is associated with improvement in serum albumin levels and survival [45]. Such positive effects of high permeability membranes on survival may only be observed in patients with low serum albumin [46].

CPD-related causes of PEW are shown in Table 39.1. Usually protein losses during CPD range from 5 to 15 g/day and can reach 100 g/day during peritonitis. Amino acid losses are usually close to 3—4 g/day. Protein losses are accompanied by losses of protein bound substances, such as trace elements. Elimination of water-soluble substances is lower than in MHD. Because peritoneal solutions with high glucose content are used, CPD is associated with a glucose uptake that can reach 100 g/day. Consequently, total energy intake usually is higher in CPD than in MHD patients. Such a high glucose intake should be considered for the calculation of calorie supply. Indeed, glucose absorption from the dialysate can cause obesity [47,48], hyperglycemia, induction or aggravation of diabetes, increased LDL-cholesterol and hypertriglyceridemia. As compared with MHD, CPD is usually associated with a better renal residual function for about the first two years of chronic dialysis therapy [49].

TABLE 39.3 Controlled Randomized and Crossover Studies that Evaluated Oral Nutritional Supplements vs. Control in HD and PD Patients with Symptoms of Undernutrition

Authors (Reference)	Nutritional Entry Criteria, Number of Patients	Dialysis Modality	Type Study	ONS Content	Length (Days)	Parameters Significantly Improved by ONS
Acchiardo 1982 [5]	Low SA, transferrin, n = 15	MHD	Randomized	EAA + His	105	SA, transferrin, bone density
Tietze 1991 [97]	Low transferrin, BW, n = 43	MHD	Randomized, CO	Fish protein	1280	BW, LBM, plasma amino acid profile
Eustace 2000 [98]	SA <38 g/L, n = 47	MHD CPD	Randomized	EAA + His +Tyr, 10.8 g/day EAA	90	SA, Muscle strength
Hiroshige 2001 [70]	Elderly, SA <35g/L, n = 19	MHD	Randomized, CO	BCAA, 12 g/day	180	BW, Lean body mass, fat mass, SA, Muscle strength
Sharma 2002 [99]	BMI <20, SA<40g/L, n = 47	MHD	Randomized	15 g Protein/HD	30	SA, functional score
Gonzalez-Espinoza 2005 [100]	BMI <20, low SA, n = 28	CPD	Randomized	Egg albumin	180	Dietary energy and protein intake SA, nPNA
Teixidó-Planas 2005 [101]	PEW/SGA, n = 65	CPD	Randomized	Standard protein 20 g	180	BW, TTR, AMC, LBM (noncompliance, intolerance)
Fouque 2008 [43]	nPNA <1 g/kg/day, n = 86	MHD	Randomized	CKD specific ONS (Renilon®, Nutricia, Schiphol, The Netherlands)	90	Dietary energy and protein intake, quality of life
Moretti 2009 [102]	Low SA, n = 49	MHD CPD	Randomized, CO	Standard ONS	365	SA, nPNA

PEW: protein-energy wasting; MHD: maintenance hemodialysis; CPD: chronic peritoneal dialysis; BMI: body mass index; BW: body weight; TTR: serum transthyretin; ONS: oral nutritional supplements; AA: amino acids; EAA: essential amino acids; CO: crossover; SA: serum albumin; BCAA: branched chain amino acids; TSF: triceps skinfold thickness; AMC: arm muscle circumference; nPNA: normalized protein nitrogen appearance, n: number of patients.

Nutritional Management of MHD and CPD with Oral Nutritional Supplements (ONS) and Enteral Nutrition (EN)

Guidelines for Nutritional Management of Dialysis Patients

Recommendations for routine nutritional monitoring in MHD and CPD patients are given in Table 39.4. Such monitoring is necessary to detect and treat MHD patients with PEW. Unstable and wasted patients may require monitoring at shorter intervals. Nutritional assessment should particularly include evaluation for the criteria of PEW which are given in Table 39.2 [1]. Severe PEW requiring nutritional intervention can be diagnosed by a decrease in BMI <20 kg/m^2, body weight loss $>10\%$ within 6 months, serum albumin <35 g/L and transthyretin <300 mg/L [32]. The assessment of appetite is a simple and useful clinical tool for identifying dialysis patients at higher risk for mortality [34]. Measurements of triceps skinfold thickness (TSF) enables one to estimate body fat mass, and arm muscle circumference (AMC = arm circumference $-$ 3.14 $\times$ TSF) allows for estimation of muscle mass [50]. Body composition can be evaluated by bioelectrical impedance analysis (BIA) and DEXA, taking into account changes in body water compartments [51]. Handgrip strength is correlated with muscle mass and prognosis in MHD and CPD patients [52,53].

Recommendations for dietary intake of macronutrients, minerals and micronutrients for conservatively treated CKD, MHD and CPD patients are discussed in other chapters. MHD patients with PEW commonly ingest energy intakes of 20–24 kcal/kg/day. Thus, nutritional supplements must provide about 10 kcal/kg/day to attain the recommended intake [14]. Abnormalities of glucose metabolism and fat clearance should be considered. Fat should account for 30 to 40% of total energy supply. The value of adding carnitine (0.5 to 1 g daily) remains debatable, and most workers in the field do not consider it necessary to provide supplemental carnitine to CKD or ESRD patients [54]. Due to the glucose absorption from peritoneal dialysate, calorie intakes in CPD patients are often close to 30 kcal/kg/day. Given the usual spontaneous protein intakes reported in most protein-energy wasted chronic dialysis patients (0.8 to 1.0 g/kg/day), approximately 0.3 g protein/kg/day should be provided by nutritional supplementation to these individuals [14]. Standard protein mixtures are commonly used. Total phosphorus intake should not exceed 10–15 mg/kg/day. Since most proteins in normal foods contain 10–13 mg phosphorus/g, most chronic dialysis patients who have an adequate dietary protein intake will need phosphate binders. A renal dietitian is needed to counsel patients on the foods that are low in phosphorus.

Due to dialysis-induced losses, water-soluble vitamins should be supplied to MHD patients. Management of vitamin D is discussed in Chapter 19 and also Chapter 21. European Best Practice Guidelines (EBPG) also recommend providing MHD patients with supplements of thiamin, riboflavin, cobalamin, niacin, biotin, pantothenic acid and tocopherol should be supplemented (expert opinion) [15]. When large loads of glucose are given, the usual dietary intake of thiamin

TABLE 39.4   Routine Nutritional Assessment in MHD and CPD Patients. These Guidelines give, for Each Parameter, Intervals for Measurements and Recommended Values

NKF K/DOQI, NKF [17] (hemodialysis and peritoneal dialysis)	• Predialysis (MHD) or stabilized (CPD) serum albumin: monthly. Serum albumin should be $\geq$40 g/L by bromocresol green method* • Percentage of usual post-dialysis (hemodialysis) or post-drain (peritoneal dialysis) body weight, monthly • Percentage of standard (NHANES II) body weight, every 4 months • Subjective global assessment (SGA) every 6 months • Dietary interview and/or diary nPNA, every 6 months
EBPG guidelines on nutrition [15] (hemodialysis)	• Dietary interviews: every 6–12 months or every 3 months in patients over 50 years of age or on hemodialysis for more than 5 years. • Body weight and body mass index. Average post-dialysis body weight over the month and percentage change in the average BW. Body mass index should be BMI $>$23.0 • nPNA: 1 month after beginning of hemodialysis and three-monthly thereafter. Normalized PNA should be above 1.0 g/kg • Serum albumin: 1 month after beginning of hemodialysis and three monthly thereafter. Serum albumin should be $>$40 g/L by bromocresol green method* • Serum transthyretin should be $>$300 mg/L • Serum cholesterol should be $>$ minimal laboratory threshold value

*Bromocresol green method is a poorly specific method to measure serum albumin concentrations. The value of 40 g/L obtained by this method is approximately equivalent to 37 g/L by the reference method, immunonephelometry. Predialysis: obtaining the measurement immediately before an individual hemodialysis treatment; Stabilized CPD: obtaining the measurement after it is no longer changing during the CPD treatment.

(0.5–1.5 mg/day) should be supplemented (thiamin hydrochloride, 1–5 mg/day) [55]. In CPD patients, supplemental vitamin E may be considered to reduce cardiovascular risk [56] (please also see Chapters 24, 33 and 40). Although routine hemodialysis does not induce significant losses of most trace elements, serum zinc and selenium levels should be assessed in patients with PEW, and, if needed, supplements of these elements should be given (please also see Chapter 23).

Other Nutritional Management Issues for Dialysis Patients

The management of anorexia in MHD patients is best served by an integrated therapeutic strategy that includes optimal dialysis dose and frequency, nutritional supplements, physical exercise, anti-inflammatory strategies, correction of plasma low branched chain amino acid concentrations and attention to associated psychological and economic issues [57]. With regard to appetite stimulating drugs, although megestrol acetate and ghrelin administration show encouraging results on appetite and body composition [58–62], large randomized, controlled trials are needed before guidelines can be proposed [57]. Dietary counseling is reported to improve nutritional status in MHD patients [42]. These data argue for holding regular (twice-yearly) sessions with a dietician during which the patient's nutrient intake is assessed and adjusted and oral supplements are prescribed as needed (Table 39.4).

Nutritional support for MHD patients includes ONS, intradialytic parenteral nutrition (IDPN), and EN (tube feeding). The following practical rules may improve the efficiency of ONS [8,31]: (1) In order to perform true nutritional supplementation and not simply a nutritional substitution, ONS should be given separately from regular meals, usually one to two hours after the main meals. (2) ONS should be given during hemodialysis sessions to prevent dialysis procedure-associated alterations of protein metabolism. (3) A late evening meal or ONS feeding may be useful to reduce the length of nocturnal nutrient deprivation and the associated increased consumption of endogenous protein and fat mass. Few specific ONS for dialysis patients are commercially available [43]. Among the standard ONS that have been developed for the general population of sick people, it is preferable to use ones that are protein and energy dense. Care must be taken to ensure that the potassium and phosphorus content of these ONS are not excessive for the dialysis patient. Table 39.3 summarizes the results of randomized trials of ONS administration versus no nutritional support for MHD and CPD patients who had evidence of PEW. Although these clinical trials were heterogeneous with regard to study design, the measured nutritional outcomes improved in the seven controlled trials conducted in MHD patients. ONS, similarly to IDPN, can provide approximately 10 kcal/kg/day. Such a calorie supply makes it possible to attain the recommended levels of protein and energy intakes only when the patient's spontaneous oral intake provides more than 20 kcal/kg/day. The French Intradialytic Nutrition Evaluation Study (FINES) showed that, independent of serum C-reactive protein, ONS induced a sustained improvement of body mass index and serum albumin and transthyretin. No advantage was observed when IDPN was added to ONS [32]. Interestingly, multivariate Cox model analyses indicated that an early response to nutritional support, as assessed by an increase in serum transthyretin concentrations by more than 30 mg/L within three months, independently predicted a 54% decrease in mortality, an improvement of the Karnofsky score, and a decrease in hospitalization rates during the two-year follow-up. In diabetic patients, no survival benefit was observed with the nutritional supplements. This observation is consistent with previous data showing that survival of diabetic MHD patients is not independently predicted by nutritional status [63]. The FINES data showed that ONS is able to improve nutritional and clinical outcome endpoints, and that IDPN should be proposed only in patients with poor compliance to ONS or who do not tolerate it. Although the FINES yielded much information of clinical value, a limitation of this study was the lack of a comparison control group for ONS that did not receive any nutritional support.

In CPD patients with PEW, intraperitoneal parenteral nutrition (IPPN) consists of the intraperitoneal administration usually of a 1.1% amino acid-based solution [64]. IPPN is shown to improve nutritional parameters [65,66] but not survival [67]. IPPN, which can be associated with hypokalemia, hypophosphatemia and acidemia, requires close monitoring [65]. Modification of the composition of IPPN solutions should reduce the likelihood that patients who will develop these metabolic complications. IPPN cannot provide for the full nutritional needs of the patient. IPPN may be useful in stable CPD patients who are eating but whose food intakes are insufficient to satisfy their nutritional needs [56].

Tube feeding is indicated in chronic dialysis patients when PEW is associated with spontaneous intakes less than 0.8 g protein and 20 kcal/kg/day, and dietary intake does not improve sufficiently with nutritional counseling or ONS. In these patients, EN is preferable to parenteral nutrition because EN helps to maintain normal digestive tract structure and function [8]. A few cohort studies have addressed the effects of EN in MHD patients; their nutritional parameters improved

[21,68,69]. Enteral nutrition is most often used when ONS and/or IDPN are not able to satisfy nutritional requirements, in conditions such as severe anorexia, swallowing troubles secondary to neurologic or head and neck diseases, the perioperative period and superimposed systemic illnesses. In these situations EN should provide all of the required macro- and micronutrients. Protein and energy dense nutritive mixtures are preferably used. When prescribing EN for CKD, ESRD or AKI patients, the water, sodium, potassium and phosphorus content of the preparation should be taken into account. Because the duration of EN feeding usually exceeds one month, a gastrostomy, most often an endoscopic placed gastrostomy, is often needed to ensure a reliable long-term route for nutritional support.

The following algorithm for nutritional support of chronic dialysis patients with PEW has been proposed by the European Society of Clinical Nutrition and Metabolism [14] (Figure 39.1):

A. In patients presenting with mild nutritional depletion, as defined by insufficient spontaneous intakes, dietary counseling, and, if necessary, ONS should be prescribed.
B. In patients exhibiting PEW and spontaneous intakes ≥20 kcal/kg BW/day, dietary counseling and ONS should be prescribed. IDPN in MHD and IPPN in CPD may be considered in patients unable to comply with ONS. EN can be necessary when ONS, IDPN or IPPN cannot meet nutritional requirements.
C. In patients with PEW and spontaneous intakes <20 kcal/kg BW/day, or in stress conditions, a daily nutritional support is necessary. EN should be preferred to total parenteral nutrition.

Some protein-energy wasted MHD patients do not respond to nutritional support. In these patients, therapeutic approaches, including treatments aiming to improve appetite, to decrease protein breakdown and/or to promote protein synthesis, have been proposed in the EBPG [15]:

• Exercise training, which is demonstrated to improve protein synthesis and to increase muscle performance and possibly muscle mass, should be proposed after cardiovascular assessment establishes its safety.
• Similarly, in the case of severe malnutrition resistant to optimal nutritional intervention, a three to six-month course of androgenic compounds may be given to MHD patients in the absence of contraindications; such patients should be monitored at regular intervals for side effects (hirsutism, voice change, priapism, alteration in plasma lipids, liver tests and blood tests for prostate cancer).
• EBPG also suggest consideration of a six to 12-month trial of daily dialysis (either short daily or long nocturnal) as therapy for MHD patients who are frail, exhibit a failure to thrive and/or have PEW that is resistant to nutritional support and other therapies.

In order to improve protein nutrition, such other therapies as the administration of essential or branched-chain amino acid supplements [70] and the modulation of inflammation, for example by pentoxifylline, have been proposed [71,72]. These data suggest that an integrated multimodal management, combining nutritional support, exercise and, in selected patients, anabolic and anti-catabolic agents may be the optimal treatment for PEW in chronic dialysis patients [73].

FIGURE 39.1 Decisional tree for nutritional intervention in chronic dialysis patients (adapted from Ref. [14]). BMI, body mass index; IDPN, intradialytic parenteral nutrition; IPPN, intraperitoneal parenteral nutrition; EN, enteral nutrition; PN, parenteral nutrition.

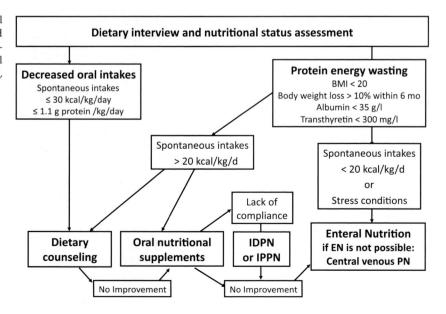

ORAL AND ENTERAL NUTRITION IN ACUTE KIDNEY INJURY

Depending on the cause of renal failure and its clinical presentation, two types of AKI patients must be considered: those with isolated renal disease, characterized by a high rate of recovery, and those with AKI complicating a severe disease, as is found in intensive care units. In intensive care patients, AKI is most often associated with other organ dysfunctions and a systemic inflammatory response syndrome which are responsible for the poor prognosis. The overall mortality rate in oligo-anuric AKI patients, which has not decreased during the last three decades, is about 40% to 60%. The nutritional management now appears as one of the main goals of the treatment of AKI patients, together with renal replacement therapies and the treatment of the underlying disease. AKI requires a close integration between nutritional support and renal replacement therapy (RRT), particularly in patients treated by highly efficient RRT, such as continuous veno-venous hemofiltration (CVVH), or prolonged intermittent hemodialysis such as sustained low-efficiency dialysis (SLED). There have been several recently published reviews and guideline papers on this subject [8,14,74]. From a metabolic point of view, chronic dialysis patients with acute inflammatory stress conditions are similar to patients with AKI and should receive similar nutritional therapy. Statements made for AKI therefore apply also to these former patient groups as well.

Nutrition and Nutrient Metabolism During Acute Kidney Injury

A prospective cohort study in 309 patients showed that severe PEW, as evaluated at admission by subjective global assessment, was present in 42% of patients with AKI [10]. In this study, the length of stay and the in-hospital mortality were increased in protein-energy wasted patients. PEW is now recognized as a predictor of in-hospital mortality independently of complications and comorbidities. In AKI, both protein and energy metabolism are greatly altered.

Animal studies of muscle protein metabolism published in the seventies showed that, during the early course of AKI, muscle protein degradation was increased and that, in the later course of AKI, both protein degradation and synthesis became abnormal [75]. The nitrogen balance of AKI patients varies according to the severity of renal failure, underlying disease and co-morbidities. Metabolic acidemia is a key element of abnormal protein metabolism during AKI. The association of AKI with severe sepsis, trauma or multi-organ failure is responsible for the systemic inflammatory response syndrome. The severity of protein catabolism can be evaluated for a urea nitrogen appearance (UNA) or, more precisely, a total nitrogen appearance that is greater than daily nitrogen intake, which indicates negative protein balance [76].

In intensive care patients with AKI, mean energy expenditure is similar to that of non-AKI patients with similar degrees of catabolic stress; i.e., close to 27 kcal/kg BW/day [77]. Glucose oxidation is decreased during AKI [78]. In contrast, fat oxidation is increased, as shown by the low respiratory quotient exhibited by these patients [78]. Increased oxidation of fat is found in spite of the abnormalities in plasma lipid patterns reported in these patients; namely, hypertriglyceridemia, an increase in triglyceride-rich particles, and a decrease in plasma lipolytic activities [79]. In AKI patients as compared with healthy controls, the clearance of triglycerides with long and medium-chain fatty acids were shown to be reduced by 66 and 69%, respectively [80].

The main modalities for dialysis treatment of critically ill patients with AKI are continuous renal replacement therapies (CRRT), and particularly CVVH and veno-venous hemodiafiltration (CVVHD-F) and sustained low-efficiency dialysis (SLED). However, standard intermittent hemodialysis is still frequently employed. These therapies can induce significant losses of electrolytes and water soluble nutrients [81]. CVVH and CVVHDF induce a loss of about 0.2 g amino acids/l of ultra filtrate (up to 10—15 g amino acids per day) (for review, [14,74]). Protein losses vary according to the hemofiltration filters and techniques used and range from 0.5 to 5—10 g/day; losses appear to be lower with polysulfone membrane and tubing [82—86]. Similar to lipids, substantial quantities of lipid-soluble vitamins are not lost during renal replacement therapies.

In AKI patients, micronutrient disturbances include reduced plasma concentrations of water-soluble vitamins, altered activation of vitamin D_3 contributing to secondary hyperparathyroidism, low serum levels of vitamin A, vitamin E, zinc and selenium. These reduced serum levels may lead to a profound depression of the antioxidant system. Micronutrient losses into dialysate have been reported: the largest losses of water soluble vitamins are observed for vitamins B_1, B_6, C (600 µmol/d), and folate (600 nmol/d) [87,88]; regarding trace elements, significant losses of selenium and copper in the dialysate, but not of zinc, have been reported [88]. Zinc deficiency in AKI patients has been attributed to the dilution of the circulating compartment by large quantities of infused fluids and to inadequate intakes [88].

The administration of large amounts of lactate in the substitution fluid, or of citrate as anticoagulant, can cause such complications as increased serum lactate or citrate and lead to metabolic alkalosis [14]. During CRRT, hypokalemia, hypophosphatemia, hypomagnesemia and hypocalcemia may occur, and the electrolyte composition of dialysate and replacement solutions should be designed to prevent such alterations. The nutritional management should also be designed to prevent the occurrence of a refeeding syndrome [8,89].

Nutritional Support in Acute Kidney Injury

Due to the lack of large randomized trials, present guidelines are mainly based on expert opinions. According to both the American (and European) Society of Parenteral and Enteral Nutrition (ASPEN and ESPEN) guidelines, the primary goals of nutritional support should be the same as those in other catabolic conditions in the ICU. They should aim at providing an optimal amount of energy, protein and micronutrients, in order to maintain nutritional status, avoid further metabolic derangements, enhance wound healing and kidney repair, support immune function, and reduce mortality. Nutritional goals may also include the attenuation of their inflammatory status and improvement of the oxygen radical scavenging system and endothelial function [90].

Routes for nutritional support are given in Table 39.5 and Figure 39.2. The following is according to ESPEN guidelines [8,14]: (1) In uncomplicated AKI, when spontaneous alimentation is insufficient, ONS may be useful to meet estimated requirements; (2) In ICU patients, nasogastric tube is considered as the standard access for the administration of EN (jejunal tube placement may be indicated in the presence of severe impairment of gastrointestinal motility); (3) In some cases where requirements cannot be met via the enteral route, supplementary parenteral nutrition may be needed [12].

Energy requirements in AKI patients, as determined from indirect calorimetry data, are not different from that of other ICU patients [77]. Nitrogen balance studies did not show an advantage of increasing non-protein energy above 30 kcal/kg BW/day, i.e. approximately 35 kcal/kg BW/day of total calories [91,92]. Carbohydrate and fat supplies should be provided taking into account the metabolic disturbances of these two substrates.

Protein requirements depend on the metabolic status of the patients, the use of replacement therapies and their modalities [8,11,14] (Table 39.5). Protein nitrogen appearance (PNA) studies in ICU patients with AKI showed values close to 1.5 g protein/kg/day [91,92–94]. In these patients, their nitrogen requirement has been estimated to be equivalent to the sum of the daily PNA and the amino acid losses into dialysate. There are no data demonstrating advantages of a specific protein composition or amino acid formulation in AKI patients. Therefore, standard sources for the protein or amino acid intake are recommended.

Serum phosphorus, magnesium and calcium should be closely monitored in severely ill patients with AKI in order to compensate losses. It is assumed that an EN mixture satisfying protein energy needs covers most of micronutrient needs. However, some specific micronutrient requirements should be considered. Due to the decrease in the renal degradation of retinol-binding protein, plasma retinol is increased during renal failure [95]. Although retinol intoxication is not reported in AKI patients, such patients should be monitored for signs of potential vitamin A toxicity during supplementation (see Chapter 24). Inappropriate vitamin C administration may result in secondary oxalosis. However, an intake of vitamin C greater than 50 mg/day may be necessary in ICU patients given a report of losses during CRRT of 600 μmol/day (i.e. 100 mg/day) of vitamin C. Thus a vitamin C intake up to 100 mg per day may be needed. Trace elements, which mainly circulate in a protein-bound form, appeared to be less affected by CRRT [87]. However, selenium losses do occur, and selenium supplements should be given [88]. These data demonstrate the need for monitoring the micronutrient status of AKI patients, both because possible deficiencies may occur and because excessive supplementation may result in toxicity.

A decision tree for nutritional support in AKI patients with PEW has been suggested [14,96] (Figure 39.2).

TABLE 39.5 Route for Nutritional Supply and Nutritional Requirements in Patients with AKI

Metabolic Status, Conservative or Renal Replacement Therapy	Typical Route for Nutritional Intake	Protein (or Essential and Non-Essential Amino Acids)[a]	Total Energy (Kcal), Carbohydrates (CHO) Lipids (fat)
Mild catabolism, conservative therapy	Food, ONS	0.6–0.8 (max. 1.0) g/kg/day	20–30 kcal/kg/day[a] 3–5 (max. 7) g CHO/kg/day
Moderate catabolism, extracorporeal therapy	EN and/or parenteral nutrition	1.0–1.5 g/kg/day	0.8–1.2 (max. 1.5) g fat/kg/day
Severe catabolism, CRRT	EN and/or parenteral nutrition	Up to 1.7–2.5 g/kg/day	

[a]Adapted for the degree of hypercatabolism and for individual needs in patients who are underweight or obese. CRRT: Continuous renal replacement therapy; ONS: oral nutritional supplements; EN: enteral nutrition (tube feeding).
(from Refs [14,89,96])

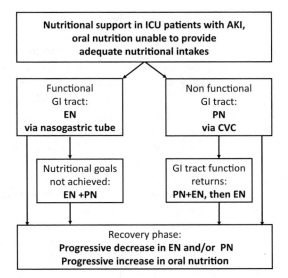

FIGURE 39.2 Decisional tree for nutritional intervention in patients with acute kidney insufficiency (adapted from Ref. [14]). ICU, intensive care unit; CVC, central venous catheter.

According to these guidelines, the route for nutritional support depends on the digestive tract status: (1) when the gastrointestinal tract functions normally, nutrition should be given orally and/or by enteral nutrition; (2) when nutritional goals cannot achieved solely through the gastrointestinal tract, parenteral nutrition should be initiated, either in addition to EN, or given exclusively if the digestive tract is not at all functional; (3) In the recovery phase, when gastrointestinal function returns, oral nutrition should be progressively reintroduced, together with a decrease in EN or parenteral nutrition.

CONCLUSIONS

Kidney diseases include very different nutritional and metabolic conditions that require specific nutritional management. Patients with CKD generally share with patients who have other chronic diseases a common phenotype which is responsible for similar losses of muscle mass, visceral proteins, and fat stores. The causes for PEW in these individuals include anorexia, reduced elective nutrient intake, physical inactivity, anemia, inflammation, insulin resistance and hypogonadism. Although data concerning the treatment of PEW in conservatively treated CKD patients are scarce, ONS or EN can be indicated when PEW or superimposed acute diseases occur. MHD and CPD contribute additional causes for PEW. The independent adverse effect of PEW on the survival of chronic dialysis patients has been known for over 30 years. In MHD patients, the beneficial effects of ONS on improving protein-energy status have been demonstrated. In non-diabetic patients, improvement in nutritional status during nutritional

support has been associated with increased survival. EN via tube feeding, given alone or in association with parenteral nutrition, is a key element in the treatment of hypercatabolic patients with AKI who either have or are at risk for developing PEW.

References

[1] Fouque D, Kalantar-Zadeh K, Kopple J, et al. A proposed nomenclature and diagnostic criteria for protein-energy wasting in acute and chronic kidney disease. Kidney Int 2008;73:391–8.

[2] Kopple JD, Chumlea WC, Gasman JJ, et al. Relationship between GFR and nutritional status of patients with chronic renal failure. J Am Soc Nephrol 1994;5:335 (abstr).

[3] Ikizler TA, Hakim RM. Nutrition in end-stage renal disease. Kidney Int 1996;50:343–57.

[4] Evans WJ, Morley JE, Argiles J, et al. Cachexia: a new definition. Clin Nutr 2008;27:793–9.

[5] Acchiardo SR, Moore LW, Latour PA. Malnutrition as the main factor of morbidity and mortality in hemodialysis patients. Kidney Int 1983;24(Suppl. 16):S199–203.

[6] Cano N, Fernandez JP, Lacombe P, et al. Statistical selection of nutritional parameters in hemodialyzed patients. Kidney Int Suppl 1987;22:S178–80.

[7] Owen Jr WF, Lew NL, Liu Y, Lowrie EG, Lazarus JM. The urea reduction ratio and serum albumin concentration as predictors of mortality in patients undergoing hemodialysis. N Engl J Med 1993;329:1001–6.

[8] Cano N, Fiaccadori E, Tesinsky P, et al. ESPEN Guidelines on Enteral Nutrition: Adult renal failure. Clin Nutr 2006;25:295–310.

[9] Kalantar-Zadeh K, Cano NJ, Budde K, et al. Diets and enteral supplements for improving outcomes in chronic kidney disease. Nat Rev Nephrol 2011;7:369–84.

[10] Fiaccadori E, Lombardi M, Leonardi S, Rotelli CF, Tortorella G, Borghetti A. Prevalence and clinical outcome associated with preexisting malnutrition in acute renal failure: a prospective cohort study. J Am Soc Nephrol 1999;10:581–93.

[11] Kopple JD. The nutritional management of the patient with acute renal failure. JPEN 1996;20:3–12.

[12] Fiaccadori E, Maggiore U, Giacosa R, et al. Enteral nutrition in patients with acute renal failure. Kidney Int 2004;65:999–1008.

[13] Druml W. Nutritional management of acute renal failure. J Ren Nutr 2005;15:63–70.

[14] Cano NJ, Aparicio M, Brunori G, et al. ESPEN Guidelines on Parenteral Nutrition: adult renal failure. Clin Nutr 2009;28:401–14.

[15] Fouque D, Vennegoor M, ter Wee P, et al. EBPG guideline on nutrition. Nephrol Dial Transplant 2007;22(Suppl. 2):ii45–87.

[16] Brown RO, Compher C. ASPEN clinical guidelines: nutrition support in adult acute and chronic renal failure. JPEN J Parenter Enteral Nutr 2010;34:366–77.

[17] Clinical practice guidelines for nutrition in chronic renal failure. K/DOQI, National Kidney Foundation. Am J Kidney Dis 2000;35:S1–140.

[18] Ikizler TA, Greene JH, Wingard RL, Parker RA, Hakim RM. Spontaneous dietary protein intake during progression of chronic renal failure. J Am Soc Nephrol 1995;6:1386–91.

[19] Verove C, Maisonneuve N, El Azouzi A, Boldron A, Azar R. Effect of the correction of metabolic acidosis on nutritional status in elderly patients with chronic renal failure. J Ren Nutr 2002;12:224–8.

[20] Fouque D, Aparicio M. Eleven reasons to control the protein intake of patients with chronic kidney disease. Nat Clin Pract Nephrol 2007;3:383–92.

[21] Cockram DB, Hensley MK, Rodriguez M, et al. Safety and tolerance of medical nutritional products as sole sources of nutrition in people on hemodialysis. J Ren Nutr 1998;8:25–33.

[22] Druml W, Mitch WE. Enteral nutrition in renal disease. In: Rombeau JL, Rolandelli RH, editors. Enteral and tube feeding. Philadelphia: Saunders, WB; 1997. p. 439–61.

[23] Roth KS, Amaker BH, Chan JC. Nephrotic syndrome: pathogenesis and management. Pediatr Rev 2002;23:237–48.

[24] Maroni BJ, Staffeld C, Young VR, Manatunga A, Tom K. Mechanisms permitting nephrotic patients to achieve nitrogen equilibrium with a protein-restricted diet. J Clin Invest 1997;99:2479–87.

[25] Kronenberg F. Dyslipidemia and nephrotic syndrome: recent advances. J Ren Nutr 2005;15:195–203.

[26] Doucet A, Favre G, Deschenes G. Molecular mechanism of edema formation in nephrotic syndrome: therapeutic implications. Pediatr Nephrol 2007;22:1983–90.

[27] Orth SR, Ritz E. The nephrotic syndrome. N Engl J Med 1998;338:1202–11.

[28] Castellino P, Cataliotti A. Changes of protein kinetics in nephrotic patients. Curr Opin Clin Nutr Metab Care 2002;5:51–4.

[29] Haute autorité de santé. Syndrome néphrotique idiopatique de l'adulte. Protocole national de diagnostic et de soins pour une maladie rare, www.has-sante.fr/portail/upload/docs/application/pdf/2008-06/pnds_sni_adulte_2008-06-24_15-35-43_506.pdf; 2008.

[30] Aparicio M, Cano N, Chauveau P, et al. Nutritional status of haemodialysis patients: a French national cooperative study. French Study Group for Nutrition in Dialysis. Nephrol Dial Transplant 1999;14:1679–86.

[31] Heng AE, Cano NJ. Nutritional problems in adult patients with stage 5 chronic kidney disease on dialysis (both haemodialysis and peritoneal dialysis). NDT Plus 2010;3:109–17.

[32] Cano NJ, Fouque D, Roth H, et al. Intradialytic parenteral nutrition does not improve survival in malnourished hemodialysis patients: a 2-year multicenter, prospective, randomized study. J Am Soc Nephrol 2007;18:2583–91.

[33] Kalantar-Zadeh K, Block G, McAllister CJ, Humphreys MH, Kopple JD. Appetite and inflammation, nutrition, anemia, and clinical outcome in hemodialysis patients. Am J Clin Nutr 2004;80:299–307.

[34] Carrero JJ, Qureshi AR, Axelsson J, et al. Comparison of nutritional and inflammatory markers in dialysis patients with reduced appetite. Am J Clin Nutr 2007;85:695–701.

[35] Untas A, Thumma J, Rascle N, et al. The associations of social support and other psychosocial factors with mortality and quality of life in the dialysis outcomes and practice patterns study. Clin J Am Soc Nephrol 2011;6:142–52.

[36] Cuppari L, de Carvalho AB, Avesani CM, Kamimura MA, Dos Santos Lobao RR, Draibe SA. Increased resting energy expenditure in hemodialysis patients with severe hyperparathyroidism. J Am Soc Nephrol 2004;15:2933–9.

[37] Horacek J, Sulkova SD, Fortova M, et al. Resting energy expenditure and thermal balance during isothermic and thermoneutral haemodialysis heat production does not explain increased body temperature during haemodialysis. Nephrol Dial Transplant 2007;22:3553–60.

[38] Ikizler TA, Wingard RL, Sun M, Harvell J, Parker RA, Hakim RM. Increased energy expenditure in hemodialysis patients. J Am Soc Nephrol 1996;7:2646–53.

[39] Kobayashi H, Borsheim E, Anthony TG, et al. Reduced amino acid availability inhibits muscle protein synthesis and decreases activity of initiation factor eIF2B. Am J Physiol Endocrinol Metab 2003;284:E488–98.

[40] Ikizler TA, Pupim LB, Brouillette JR, et al. Hemodialysis stimulates muscle and whole body protein loss and alters substrate oxidation. Am J Physiol Endocrinol Metab 2002;282:E107–16.

[41] Gutierrez A, Alverstrand A, Wahren J, Bergström J. Effect of in vivo contact between blood and dialysis membranes on protein catabolism in humans. Kidney Int 1990;38:487–94.

[42] Leon JB, Majerle AD, Soinski JA, Kushner I, Ohri-Vachaspati P, Sehgal AR. Can a nutrition intervention improve albumin levels among hemodialysis patients? A pilot study. J Ren Nutr 2001;11:9–15.

[43] Fouque D, McKenzie J, de Mutsert R, et al. Use of a renal-specific oral supplement by haemodialysis patients with low protein intake does not increase the need for phosphate binders and may prevent a decline in nutritional status and quality of life. Nephrol Dial Transplant 2008;23:2902–10.

[44] Movilli E, Viola BF, Camerini C, Mazzola G, Cancarini GC. Correction of metabolic acidosis on serum albumin and protein catabolism in hemodialysis patients. J Ren Nutr 2009;19:172–7.

[45] Chauveau P, Nguyen H, Combe C, et al. Dialyzer membrane permeability and survival in hemodialysis patients. Am J Kidney Dis 2005;45:565–71.

[46] Locatelli F, Martin-Malo A, Hannedouche T, et al. Effect of membrane permeability on survival of hemodialysis patients. J Am Soc Nephrol 2009;20:645–54.

[47] Choi SJ, Kim NR, Hong SA, et al. Changes in body fat mass in patients after starting peritoneal dialysis. Perit Dial Int 2011;31:67–73.

[48] Pellicano R, Strauss BJ, Polkinghorne KR, Kerr PG. Longitudinal body composition changes due to dialysis. Clin J Am Soc Nephrol 2011;6:1668–75.

[49] McKane W, Chandna SM, Tattersall JE, Greenwood RN, Farrington K. Identical decline of residual renal function in high-flux biocompatible hemodialysis and CAPD. Kidney Int 2002;61:256–65.

[50] Frisancho AR. New norms of upper limb fat and muscle areas for assessment of nutritional status. Am J Clin Nutr 1981;34:2540–5.

[51] Cano NJ, Miolane-Debouit M, Leger J, Heng AE. Assessment of body protein: energy status in chronic kidney disease. Semin Nephrol 2009;29:59–66.

[52] Qureshi AR, Alvestrand A, Danielsson A, et al. Factors predicting malnutrition in hemodialysis patients: a cross-sectional study. Kidney Int 1998;53:773–82.

[53] Wang AY, Sea MM, Ho ZS, Lui SF, Li PK, Woo J. Evaluation of handgrip strength as a nutritional marker and prognostic indicator in peritoneal dialysis patients. Am J Clin Nutr 2005;81:79–86.

[54] Hurot JM, Cucherat M, Haugh M, Fouque D. Effects of L-carnitine supplementation in maintenance hemodialysis patients: a systematic review. J Am Soc Nephrol 2002;13:708–14.

[55] Locatelli F, Fouque D, Heimburger O, et al. Nutritional status in dialysis patients: a European consensus. Nephrol Dial Transplant 2002;17:563–72.

[56] Dombros N, Dratwa M, Feriani M, et al. European best practice guidelines for peritoneal dialysis. 8. Nutrition in peritoneal dialysis. Nephrol Dial Transplant 2005;20(Suppl. 9):ix28–33.

[57] Bossola M, Giungi S, Luciani G, Tazza L. Interventions to counteract anorexia in dialysis patients. J Ren Nutr 2011;21:16–9.

[58] Yeh SS, Marandi M, Thode Jr HC, et al. Report of a pilot, double-blind, placebo-controlled study of megestrol acetate in elderly dialysis patients with cachexia. J Ren Nutr 2010;20: 52–62.

[59] Costero O, Bajo MA, del Peso G, et al. Treatment of anorexia and malnutrition in peritoneal dialysis patients with megestrol acetate. Adv Perit Dial 2004;20:209–12.

[60] Rammohan M, Kalantar-Zadeh K, Liang A, Ghossein C. Megestrol acetate in a moderate dose for the treatment of malnutrition-inflammation complex in maintenance dialysis patients. J Ren Nutr 2005;15:345–55.

[61] Monfared A, Heidarzadeh A, Ghaffari M, Akbarpour M. Effect of megestrol acetate on serum albumin level in malnourished dialysis patients. J Ren Nutr 2009;19:167–71.

[62] Ashby DR, Ford HE, Wynne KJ, et al. Sustained appetite improvement in malnourished dialysis patients by daily ghrelin treatment. Kidney Int 2009;76:199–206.

[63] Cano NJ, Roth H, Aparicio M, et al. Malnutrition in hemodialysis diabetic patients: evaluation and prognostic influence. Kidney Int 2002;62:593–601.

[64] Wang T, Lindholm B. Peritoneal dialysis solutions. Perit Dial Int 2001;21(Suppl. 3):S89–95.

[65] Mehrotra R, Kopple JD. Protein and energy nutrition among adult patients treated with chronic peritoneal dialysis. Adv Ren Replace Ther 2003;10:194–212.

[66] Kopple JD, Bernard D, Messana J, et al. Treatment of malnourished CAPD patients with an amino acid based dialysate. Kidney Int 1995;47:1148–57.

[67] Li FK, Chan LY, Woo JC, et al. A 3-year, prospective, randomized, controlled study on amino acid dialysate in patients on CAPD. Am J Kidney Dis 2003;42:173–83.

[68] Douglas E, Lomas L, Prygrodzka F, Woolfson AMJ, Knapp MS. Nutrition and malnutrition in renal patients: the role of nasogastric nutrition. Proc EDTA 1982;11:17–20.

[69] Holley JL, Kirk J. Enteral tube feeding in a cohort of chronic hemodialysis patients. J Ren Nutr 2002;12:177–82.

[70] Hiroshige K, Sonta T, Suda T, Kanegae K, Ohtani A. Oral supplementation of branched-chain amino acid improves nutritional status in elderly patients on chronic haemodialysis. Nephrol Dial Transplant 2001;16:1856–62.

[71] Biolo G, Ciocchi B, Bosutti A, Situlin R, Toigo G, Guarnieri G. Pentoxifylline acutely reduces protein catabolism in chronically uremic patients. Am J Kidney Dis 2002; 40:1162–72.

[72] Gonzalez-Espinoza L, Rojas-Campos E, Medina-Perez M, Pena-Quintero P, Gomez-Navarro B, Cueto-Manzano AM. Pentoxifylline decreases serum levels of tumor necrosis factor alpha, interleukin 6 and C-reactive protein in hemodialysis patients: results of a randomized double-blind, controlled clinical trial. Nephrol Dial Transplant 2012;27:2023–8.

[73] Cano NJ, Heng AE, Pison C. Multimodal approach to malnutrition in malnourished maintenance hemodialysis patients. J Ren Nutr 2011;21:23–6.

[74] Fiaccadori E, Cremaschi E. Nutritional assessment and support in acute kidney injury. Curr Opin Crit Care 2009;15:474–80.

[75] Mitch WE, Clark AS. Muscle protein turnover in uremia. Kidney Int 1983;24(Suppl. 16):S2–8.

[76] Druml W. Nutritional management of acute renal failure. Am J Kidney Dis 2001;37:S89–94.

[77] Faisy C, Guerot E, Diehl JL, Labrousse J, Fagon JY. Assessment of resting energy expenditure in mechanically ventilated patients. Am J Clin Nutr 2003;78:241–9.

[78] Schneeweiss B, Graninger W, Stockenhuber F, et al. Energy metabolism in acute and chronic renal failure. Am J Clin Nutr 1990;52:596–601.

[79] Druml W, Laggner A, Widhalm K, Kleinberger G, Lenz K. Lipid metabolism in acute renal failure. Kidney Int 1983; 24(Suppl. 16):S139–42.

[80] Druml W, Fischer M, Sertl S, Schneeweiss B, Lenz K, Widhalm K. Fat elimination in acute renal failure: long-chain vs. medium-chain triglycerides. Am J Clin Nutr 1992;55:468–72.

[81] Druml W. Metabolic aspects of continuous renal replacement therapies. Kidney Int Suppl 1999;72:S56–61.

[82] Morgera S, Slowinski T, Melzer C, et al. Renal replacement therapy with high-cutoff hemofilters: Impact of convection and diffusion on cytokine clearances and protein status. Am J Kidney Dis 2004;43:444–53.

[83] Krieter DH, Lemke HD, Wanner C. A new synthetic dialyzer with advanced permselectivity for enhanced low-molecular weight protein removal. Artif Organs 2008;32:547–54.

[84] Yamashita AC, Tomisawa N. Importance of membrane materials for blood purification devices in critical care. Transfus Apher Sci 2009;40:23–31.

[85] Kawanishi H. Preferred performance of the high-performance membrane in the case of online hemodiafiltration. Contrib Nephrol 2011;173:36–43.

[86] Yumoto M, Nishida O, Moriyama K, et al. In vitro evaluation of high mobility group box 1 protein removal with various membranes for continuous hemofiltration. Ther Apher Dial 2011;15:385–93.

[87] Bellomo R, Boyce N. Acute continuous hemodiafiltration: a prospective study of 110 patients and a review of the literature. Am J Kidney Dis 1993;21:508–18.

[88] Berger MM, Shenkin A, Revelly JP, et al. Copper, selenium, zinc, and thiamine balances during continuous venovenous hemodiafiltration in critically ill patients. Am J Clin Nutr 2004;80: 410–6.

[89] Wooley JA, Btaiche IF, Good KL. Metabolic and nutritional aspects of acute renal failure in critically ill patients requiring continuous renal replacement therapy. Nutr Clin Pract 2005;20:176–91.

[90] Lameire N, Van Biesen W, Vanholder R. Acute renal failure. Lancet 2005;365:417–30.

[91] Macias WL, Alaka KJ, Murphy MH, Miller ME, Clark WR, Mueller BA. Impact of the nutritional regimen on protein catabolism and nitrogen balance in patients with acute renal failure. JPEN J Parenter Enteral Nutr 1996;20:56–62.

[92] Fiaccadori E, Maggiore U, Rotelli C, et al. Effects of different energy intakes on nitrogen balance in patients with acute renal failure: a pilot study. Nephrol Dial Transplant 2005;20: 1976–80.

[93] Chima CS, Meyer L, Hummell AC, et al. Protein catabolic rate in patients with acute renal failure on continuous arteriovenous hemofiltration and total parenteral nutrition. J Am Soc Nephrol 1993;3:1516–21.

[94] Leblanc M, Garred LJ, Cardinal J, et al. Catabolism in critical illness: estimation from urea nitrogen appearance and creatinine production during continuous renal replacement therapy. Am J Kidney Dis 1998;32:444–53.

[95] Cano N, Di Costanzo-Dufetel J, Calaf R, et al. Prealbumin-retinol-binding-protein-retinol complex in hemodialysis patients. Am J Clin Nutr 1988;47:664–7.

[96] Fiaccadori E, Parenti E, Maggiore U. Nutritional support in acute kidney injury. J Nephrol 2008;21:645–56.

[97] Tietze IN, Pedersen EB. Effect of fish protein supplementation on aminoacid profile and nutritional status in haemodialysis patients. Nephrol Dial Transplant 1991;6:948–54.

[98] Eustace JA, Coresh J, Kutchey C, et al. Randomized double-blind trial of oral essential amino acids for dialysis-associated hypoalbuminemia. Kidney Int 2000;57:2527–38.

[99] Sharma M, Rao M, Jacob S, Jacob CK. A controlled trial of intermittent enteral nutrient supplementation in maintenance hemodialysis patients. J Ren Nutr 2002;12:229—37.

[100] Gonzalez-Espinoza L, Gutierrez-Chavez J, del Campo FM, et al. Randomized, open label, controlled clinical trial of oral administration of an egg albumin-based protein supplement to patients on continuous ambulatory peritoneal dialysis. Perit Dial Int 2005;25:173—80.

[101] Teixido-Planas J, Ortiz A, Coronel F, et al. Oral protein-energy supplements in peritoneal dialysis: a multicenter study. Perit Dial Int 2005;25:163—72.

[102] Moretti HD, Johnson AM, Keeling-Hathaway TJ. Effects of protein supplementation in chronic hemodialysis and peritoneal dialysis patients. J Ren Nutr 2009;19:298—303.

40

Intradialytic Parenteral Nutrition, Intraperitoneal Nutrition and Nutritional Hemodialysis

Ramanath Dukkipati

Division of Nephrology and Hypertension, Harbor-UCLA Medical Center, Torrance, CA, USA

INTRODUCTION

Protein-energy wasting (PEW) is one of the strongest risk factors for adverse outcomes and death in chronic dialysis patients. Nonrandomized studies, some of which are retrospective, indicate that improving protein-energy status by nutritional interventions may improve outcomes in these patients, although this has not been tested in large-scale, prospective, randomized clinical trials. Indicators of PEW include decreased body mass index, and muscle mass, low serum levels of albumin and transthyretin, decreased appetite and food intake, and measures indicating inflammation. There is a consensus that dietary counseling and oral nutritional supplements should be the first step in the management of patients with PEW who have low nutrient intakes, once disease states that prevent digestion and absorption of nutrients are ruled out as a cause of PEW. Enteral tube feeding is a physiological method to provide nutrients as this method uses the patient's gastrointestinal tract for absorption of nutrients. However many patients are reluctant to accept enteral tube as a method of feeding or cannot receive sufficient nutrients to satisfy their daily requirements by enteral nutrition.

INTRADIALYTIC PARENTERAL NUTRITION (IDPN)

For these latter individuals, intradialytic parenteral nutrition (IDPN) offers an alternative method for providing additional nutrients to a patient undergoing maintenance hemodialysis (MHD). When IDPN is given, it is normally administered with each hemodialysis. It is generally started at the beginning of a hemodialysis session, where it is infused into the venous line distal to the hemodialyzer, and is continued until the end or near the end of the dialysis treatment. It should be emphasized that since most MHD patients undergo hemodialysis only three times weekly, IDPN must be viewed as only an adjuvant for nutritional therapy, and it cannot be used as the sole source of nutritional support unless patients receive hemodialysis more frequently.

The nutritional components of a typical IDPN solution are listed in Table 40.1 and the components of commonly prescribed oral nutritional supplements are listed in Table 40.2. IDPN solutions are commonly prepared from base solution components. Base solutions for amino acids, carbohydrates and lipids from which IDPN solutions are prepared can vary in concentration; up to 10% of essential and nonessential amino acids, 50 or 70% d-glucose, and 10 or 20% lipids or no lipids. Additional components commonly include macro-electrolytes and often trace elements and multivitamin formulations. The mineral content of the amino acid, carbohydrate and lipid solutions must be taken into consideration when prescribing additional minerals to be added to the IDPN solution. The composition of the final IDPN solution can be altered depending on the patient's nutritional needs and metabolic characteristics and the length of their dialysis treatment time, although the modifying the IDPN content often increases the cost of formulating the solution.

Studies of the Nutritional and Metabolic Effects of IDPN

Many patients receive hemodialysis treatments at a time when they haven't ingested food for many hours.

Nutritional Management of Renal Disease
http://dx.doi.org/10.1016/B978-0-12-391934-2.00040-0

TABLE 40.1 Current Recommended IDPN Formulations

Dextrose (Infusion Rates)	Lipids (Infusion Rates)	Protein
Moderate to high dextrose Carbohydrate controlled 4–6 mg d-glucose/ kg/minute Noncarbohydrate controlled 6–8 mg d-glucose/ kg/minute	Lipids 4 mg/kg/minute or 12–12.5 g/hour	Amino acids 0.6 to 0.8 g/kg per hemodialysis treatment or per one IDPN bag
Low dextrose ≤3 mg/kg/minute	Lipids 4 mg/kg/minute or 12–12.5 g/hour	Amino acids 0.6 to 0.8 g/kg per hemodialysis treatment or per one IDPN bag
Low dextrose, no lipids ≤3 mg/kg/minute	No lipids	Amino acids 0.6 to 0.8 g/kg per hemodialysis treatment or per one IDPN bag

Dextrose and lipids are calculated based on variable infusion rate. Amino acids are calculated based on daily protein requirements or allowances for nonpregnant nonlactating, normal adults or nondialyzed patients with chronic kidney disease which is 1.2 to 1.6 g/kg/day.
These solutions are designed to be infused in four hours but some nephrologists may infuse over three hours in MHD patients who have substantial renal function.

It is therefore relevant that Ikizler et al. and Pupim et al. (Figure 40.1) investigated the acute effects of hemodialysis on protein turnover in MHD patients who were in the postabsorptive state [1]. In 11 clinically stable MHD patients who were fasted for at least 10 hours prior to the initiation of the study, total body protein, forearm protein synthesis and degradation were measured. These were measured before, during and 2 hours after hemodialysis was completed. The patients

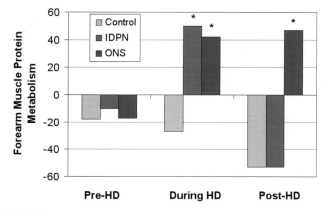

FIGURE 40.1 Effect of IDPN and Oral nutritional therapy on Forearm muscle homeostasis. *(Adapted from Pupim and coworkers [3]). HD, hemodialysis; ONS, oral nutritional supplement; IDPN, intradialytic parenteral nutrition. This figure is reproduced in color in the color plate section.*

received a constant infusion of L-(1-^{13}C) leucine and L-(ring-^{2}H$_5$) phenylalanine starting two hours before hemodialysis and lasting two hours into the post dialysis session. Degradation of total body protein and forearm muscle protein increased significantly during dialysis and remained increased at two hours after dialysis. Increase in protein synthesis was observed in forearm but not in the total body during hemodialysis and protein synthesis increased in the post-dialysis period. Net protein loss in the forearm increased significantly during dialysis but decreased to baseline levels after dialysis. Protein synthesis in the forearm but not the total body also increased during hemodialysis, and protein synthesis in both compartments was increased post-dialysis as compared with baseline levels. During hemodialysis, total-body net protein balance became significantly more negative. In the post-dialysis period

TABLE 40.2 Content of Selected Nutrients in Some Currently Available Oral Nutritional Formulations

	Total Carbohydrates (g)	Total Protein (g)	Total Fat (g)	Total Calories (Kcal)	Kcal/mL
Nepro (240 mL)	39.4	19.1	22.7	425	1.8
Nepro (1000 mL)	166.8	81	96	1800	1.8
Boost glucose control (237 mL)	20	14	12	250	1.06
Boost glucose control (1000 mL)	84	58.2	49.4	1060	1.06
Boost (240 mL)	41	10	4	240	1.0

These nutrients indicate the total amount present in the volume of the solution indicated in the first column.
These nutritional supplements also contain other macroelectrolytes, trace elements and multiple vitamins.

total-body protein balance decreased significantly, and compared to baseline was significantly more negative.

There is reason to believe that IDPN may improve nutritional status of patients with PEW that is at least partly due to inadequate protein or energy intake. First, data clearly indicate that the great preponderance of amino acids infused during IDPN are retained in the body and not removed by the dialyzer [2]. Also, in clinically stable MHD patients, there is at least a transient increase in protein anabolism during IDPN.

Pupim et al. also studied seven MHD patients who were clinically stable with no evidence of PEW while they received IDPN during a 4-hour hemodialysis [1]. Patients were fasted for 10 hours, and they received the same amino acid isotope infusion as described above. Each IDPN provided solutions of 300 mL of 15% essential and nonessential amino acids, 150 mL of 50% glucose and 150 mL of 20% lipids. When the fasting patients received IDPN, total body protein and forearm protein synthesis were more positive and total body protein degradation decreased as compared to when the patients did not receive IDPN (see above). During IDPN, the patients also had significantly more positive forearm protein balance and net total-body protein balance as compared to when they did not receive IDPN. The enhanced anabolic state observed during IDPN abated after the 2-hour post-dialysis period. It is unclear if the anabolic response observed during the hemodialysis session with IDPN would have reoccurred in subsequent hemodialysis sessions if the use of IDPN had been continued.

This same team of researchers subsequently compared intradialytic oral nutrition (IDON) to IDPN and also to no nutritional support in a separate study of eight clinically stable MHD patients [3]. The IDON provided 57 g of amino acids, 48 g of lipids, 109 g of carbohydrates and a total of 1090 kcal. This solution was given in three equal feedings at 30, 90 and 150 minutes after the onset of the 4-hour hemodialysis. The IDPN solution contained 59 g of amino acids, 26 g of lipids, 197 g of carbohydrates and 752 kcal. This IDPN solution was given starting 30 minutes after the initiation of hemodialysis and continued until the end of the hemodialysis session. Compared with no nutritional supplementation, both IDPN and oral nutrition displayed a significant increase in total body protein synthesis and decrease in total body protein degradation. Net total body protein balance was significantly positive. At two hours after the completion of the hemodialysis session total body protein synthesis was still elevated only when the patients received IDON. Protein degradation did not differ significantly between the IDON and IDPN groups, but net total-body protein balance was significantly more negative with IDON as compared to IDPN or no nutritional treatment. In the two hours after dialysis, forearm protein balance was also significantly more positive when patients were given oral nutrition as compared to IDPN or no nutritional treatment. Although forearm protein degradation was similar among these three different treatments and during the 2-hour post-dialysis session, the net forearm protein balance was significantly more positive during both IDON and IDPN as compared to no nutritional support. Thus, these short-term studies suggest that IDON may provide as safe and at least as effective a way as IDPN for providing nutritional supplements to MHD patients.

Limitations of the Clinical Trials of IDPN

Virtually all of the studies that have examined the effectiveness of IDPN are limited by one or more aspects of the experimental design, such as small sample size and, hence, inadequate statistical power, absence of a control group, poorly described inclusion criteria or the fact that not all of patients receiving IDPN treatment met the criteria for a diagnosis of PEW. Commonly, studies did not describe the dose of dialysis received. The duration of the treatment and follow-up periods were often short. Many studies did not control the intake of food or oral nutritional supplements. Occasionally, studies also offered defined amounts of food or oral nutritional supplements to the IDPN treated or control patients. Due to these limitations, definitive conclusions regarding the effectiveness in IDPN in different patient populations cannot be drawn from the nonrandomized and the randomized studies. Some of the more seminal and influential of the nonrandomized IDPN studies, summarized in Table 40.3, and the randomized trials of IDPN, summarized in Table 40.4, will be reviewed.

Nonrandomized Studies of IDPN

The first report of the use of IDPN in MHD patients was by Heidland and Kult [4]. They administered IDPN to 18 patients undergoing hemodialysis thrice weekly during a 60-week period of study. For the last 90 minutes of each hemodialysis session, patients were given 16.7 g of essential amino acids, including histidine and 250 mL of a mixture of D/L − malic acid, xylitol and sorbitol. Some nonessential amino acids were added to the above mixture during the first three months. In 13 of the 18 patients, therapy was discontinued after 16 weeks. During each dialysis session, close to 100 grams of protein in food was also prescribed. However, there was a variable intake of food. Serum albumin and total protein levels were reported to increase significantly after 30 weeks of IDPN. Discontinuation of IDPN after 30 weeks, resulted in significant fall in serum transferrin

TABLE 40.3 Selected Nonrandomized Trials of IDPN

Study	Design	Treatment Duration	No. w/ PEW	Parameters Measured	Outcome
Heidland & Kult, 1975 [14]	18 pts; 16.75 g EAA, 100 kcal; no control	60 wks	Most did not	Alb, total protein, complement levels, transferrin	Increase in serum Alb, total protein, transferrin, complement levels after 16 wks therapy in 13 pts. When therapy was discontinued for 6 wks, decrease in serum complement and transferrin.
Piriano 1981 [5]	16 pts: 16.5 g EAA + 1 NEAA, 200 g glucose 5 pts: 10.2 g glucose/ EAA only	20 wks	5 (in EAA group lost >15% of usual BW)	BW	In EAA + NEAA group, 8 pts gained >10% BW, other 8 lost weight. Pts in EAA group gained weight if did not have acute illness.
Powers 1989 [15]	18 pts; 250 mL 50% glucose, 250 mL RenAmin[a]	46–165 infusions	All	Weight gain, Alb, TSF, MAMC	Weight gain (12.6 ± 4.9 lb) in 11 of 18 pts. No change in serum Alb.
Bilbrey 1989 [16]	20 pts; 50 g EAA + NEAA, 50 g lipids, 125 g glucose	90 days minimum	All	BW, MAMC	Only MAMC improved.
Matthys 1991 [17]	10 pts; 16.75 g EAA	3 mos	All	Quality of life, Hct, BW, degree of edema	BW increased starting from first month of therapy (p < 0.01). Scoring index of general condition increased (p < 0.01).
Bilbrey 1993 [18]	47 pts; 400 mL 15% AA, 150 mL 70% glucose, 250 mL 20% lipids	90 days minimum	All	Alb, transferrin, mortality	29 survived, 18 died. Survivors had increase in Alb, transferrin. No data on cause of death.
Chertow 1994 [7]	1679 pts: 1.2 g protein/ kg, 15 kcal/kg 22,517 pts: no IDPN	12 mos or until death		Alb, URR, odds of death	Decrease in mortality in IDPN-treated pts who had serum Alb ≤3.3 g/dL.
Capelli 1994 [19]	50 pts: 50 g EAA, 50 g lipids, 125 g glucose, dietary suppl	9 mos	All had Alb <3.5 g/dL, BW < 90% of desirable	Alb, BW, mortality	32 of 50 treated pts & 16 of 31 untreated pts survived. Weight gain in treated survivors, no

Study	Treatment	Duration	Inclusion	Outcome measures	Results
Foulks 1994 [20]	72 pts; 0.64 g N/kg, 3.78 kcal/kg as lipids, glucose (discontinued once IDPN started) 31 pts: dietary suppl	mean of 159 days in responders, 222 days in nonresponders	BW or BW loss >10% over 2 mos	Mortality, hosp. rate	weight gain in survivors who were untreated. No weight gain in nonsurvivors in either group. 6 mo of IDPN before change in weight or serum Alb. Decreased mortality and hosp rate in responders.
Smolle 1995 [21]	16 pts; 0.8 g/kg EAA + NEAA	16 wks		Alb, skin test reactivity, WBC, SCr	NA[b]
Cranford 1998 [22]	43 pts; 63 g EAA + NEAA, 18.4 g lipids, 92.5 g carbohydrates	6 mos		Alb, BUN, hospitalizations	NA[b]
Hiroshige 1998 [8]	10 pts: 200 mL 50% glucose, 200 mL 7% EAA, 200 mL 20% lipids; 18 pts: dietary counseling	12 mos	All	BW, BMI, TSF, MAMC, Alb, transferrin, plasma AA profile, mortality	All IDPN-treated pts survived, 5 pts without IDPN therapy died (3 due to sepsis, 1 due to GI bleeding) during study period.
Mortelmans 1999 [23]	26 pts (16 pts completed study, 10 pts withdrew); 250 mL 50% glucose, 250 mL 20% lipids, 250 mL 7% AA	9 mos	All	BW, MAMC, lean body mass, transferrin, serum pre Alb levels	BW increased (p < 0.05); serum transferrin, transthyretin increased. TSF increased (p < 0.05). No such change in pts who withdrew.
Blondin 1999 [24]	45 pts[c]	6 mos	All had mean Alb <3.2 g/dL ± 0.4	Alb, BUN, morbidity, URR, hosp. rate	Decrease in hosp rate (p < 0.05), increase in serum Alb (p < 0.05).
Cherry 2002 [25]	24 pts; 250 or 500 mL 10% AA, 250 mL 50% glucose, 250 mL 20% fat emulsion	4.3 mos (mean)	All	Alb, dry BW	Increase in dry BW, serum Alb.
Dezfuli 2009 [26]	196 pts. IDPN No control group	3–12 months	All	Serum albumin	72% of patients had increase in serum Alb. with a mean increase of 0.4 g/dL.

Abbreviations: NA, not available; BUN, blood, urea, nitrogen; IDPN, intradialytic parenteral nutrition; HD, hemodialysis; PEW, Protein-energy wasting; EAA, essential amino acids; NEAA, nonessential amino acids; Alb, albumin; MAMC, mid-arm muscle circumference; TSF, triceps skinfold; URR, urea reduction ratio; BMI, body mass index; PNA, protein equivalent of total nitrogen appearance; IV, intravenous.

TABLE 40.4   Randomized Prospective Trials of IDPN

First Author of Study	Design	Treatment Duration	No. w/ PEW	Parameters Measured	Outcome
Wolfson 1982 [2]	8 pts. EAA + NEAA + glucose solution versus normal saline	NA	NA	Plasma amino acid levels	Unclear if plasma amino acid levels increased
Toigo 1989 [27]	11 pts: 26.5 g modified EAA 10 pts 24 g EAA + NEAA	6 mos	None	Nerve conduction velocity, Alb	Decrease in Alb in EAA + NEAA group
Cano 1990 [9]	12 pts: 0.08 g N/kg (per HD session) from EAA + NEAA, 1.6 g/kg (per HD session) lipids 14 pts: no intervention	3 mos	All	BW, appetite, MAMC	Increase in calorie (9 kcal/kg/d) and protein intake (0.25 g/kg/d) in IDPN-treated pts
McCann 1999 [28]	19 pts; 70% glucose, 15% amino acids, 20% lipids	11 wks	NA	Delivered Kt/v, URR	Reduction in delivered Kt/v in pts who received amino acid-containing IDPN
Navarro 2000 [29]	17 pts	3 mos	NA	NA	Positive net balance of amino acids. Increase in PNA, Alb, transferrin
Cano 2006 [30]	17 pts: olive oil-based IV lipid emulsion 18 pts: soybean oil-based IV lipid emulsion	5 wks	NA	NA	Both groups showed similar improvement in nutritional status, plasma lipid, oxidative and inflammatory parameters
Cano 2007 [11]	89 pts: IDPN 93 pts: control	12 mos	All	Primary end point, all-cause mortality; secondary endpoints, hosp rate, BW, Karnofsky score, BMI	No difference in hospitalization rate or mortality between two groups

Note: Only clinical trials with eight patients or more are listed.
Abbreviations: NA, not available; IDPN, intradialytic parenteral nutrition; HD, hemodialysis; PEW, Protein-energy wasting; EAA, essential amino acids; NEAA, nonessential amino acids; Alb, albumin; MAMC, mid-arm muscle circumference; URR, urea reduction ratio; BMI, body mass index; PNA, protein equivalent of total nitrogen appearance; IV, intravenous.

levels along with a decrease in several complement proteins and hemoglobin levels.

Piriano reported on 21 MHD patients who had lost at least 10% of their dry weight and then were treated with IDPN for 20 weeks [5]. Sixteen of these patients were treated with IDPN, which provided an average of 400 mL of 8.5% essential amino acids and nonessential amino acids with 400 mL of 50% glucose at each dialysis session. The other patients (five out of 21 patients) were given a solution containing essential amino acids and 50% glucose. These five patients had lost at least 15% of their dry weight. The volume of IDPN provided, the dialysis dose and the co-morbid conditions are not clear. In both of these groups there was no increase in serum albumin levels and neither group experienced weight gain. However, in patients who received the essential and nonessential amino acids and who did not have hyperparathyroidism there was gain in their body weight.

In 47 MHD patients with severe PEW who received IDPN for 3 months, Bilbrey et al. reported that survivors had a significant increase in serum albumin levels (from 3.30 ± 0.38 (SD) to 3.71 ± 0.30 g/dL; $p < 0.001$) and transferrin levels (165 ± 37 to 200 ± 62 mg/dL; $p < 0.001$) [16]. In the nonsurvivors, there was no increase in serum albumin or serum transferrin levels. Duration of IDPN therapy, dialysis dose and co-morbid conditions were not reported.

In a retrospective study, Capelli et al., compared survival of 50 patients who received IDPN to 31 patients who did not [6]. The body weights of patients treated with IDPN were 10% less than their desirable weight and/or had at least a 10% weight loss. All 81 patients in the study had low serum albumin levels. In the control group, low body weights or a history of recent weight loss were not consistently present. At the beginning of the study, oral nutritional supplements and/or nutritional counseling were given for two months for all the patients in the study. Patients who did not respond to this nutritional treatment, were then given IDPN. The IDPN given provided a 10% or 20% lipid emulsion (20–500 kcal/dialysis session), 50 g of essential amino acids per dialysis session and a variable amount of D-glucose based on the diabetic status of the patient. Mortality was 48% in controls versus 36% in the IDPN-treated patients ($p > 0.05$), but time to death in the nonsurvivors was significantly greater in the IDPN treated patients: 16.9 ± 7.9 (SD) versus 7.5 ± 4.2 months ($p < 0.01$).

Foulks et al. reported the results of a nonrandomized study of 72 patients with PEW who failed to respond to dietary counseling and who received IDPN (20). Responders were classified as those who manifested at least a 10% increase in dry body weight or an increase in serum albumin of ≥ 0.5 g/dL while they received IDPN. Mortality was significantly lower in the patients who responded to IDPN. The serum albumin before IDPN was inaugurated and was significantly lower in the responders as compared to the nonresponders (2.2 ± 0.7 (SD) versus 3.0 ± 0.8 g/dL; ($p < 0.0001$). The body weights were similar in the responders and nonresponders both before and after treatment with IDPN. During the six months prior to initiation of IDPN, responders had higher hospitalization rates ($p < 0.0001$). However during IDPN therapy, only 52% of responders were hospitalized as compared with 76% of nonresponders ($p < 0.0001$). The hospitalization rate decreased significantly only in the responders. It is possible that the improved clinical course of the responders was due to the IDPN and the patients' enhanced nutritional status. However, it is also likely that the increased morbidity of the nonresponders impaired their ability to respond to the IDPN or to demonstrate the rise in serum albumin of ≥ 0.5 g/dL.

The largest study of IDPN retrospectively compared 1679 MHD patients who received IDPN to 22,517 control MHD patients who did not receive IDPN [7]. The IDPN prescriptions were not uniform in the 1679 patients. After adjustment for case mix and predialysis serum creatinine levels, those patients who had baseline serum albumin concentrations ≤ 3.3 g/dL and were treated with IDPN, as compared to those who had similar serum albumin levels but who did not receive IDPN, displayed a significant reduction in the odds ratio for death at 1 year. The IDPN treated patients who had serum albumin levels ≥ 3.5 g/dL showed a significant increase in 1-year mortality. The survival effect of IDPN was greater in those MHD patients who had predialysis serum creatinine levels of 8.0 mg/dL or lower.

In another nonrandomized study, Hiroshige et al. reported results of IDPN therapy in 10 MHD patients who had PEW and were greater than 70 years of age [8]. Eighteen other MHD patients with PEW who refused IDPN were treated with dietary counseling and serve as controls. The IDPN treated group received therapy for one year. The IDPN solutions that they received contained 200 mL of 50% glucose, 200 mL of a 20% lipid emulsion and 200 mL of 7.1% essential amino acids per dialysis session. There were no major differences in baseline nutritional measures between the two groups. During the IDPN treatment, there was a significant increase in serum albumin and transferrin, body weight, triceps skinfold thickness and mid-arm muscle circumference in the IDPN treated group. All of the patients in the control group showed a significant decrease in all these parameters. The control group also displayed a decrease in plasma essential amino acid concentrations during the course of the study. In the IDPN treated group, plasma levels of essential amino acids and some nonessential amino acids increased and 3-methylhistidine levels fell. There were no deaths in the IDPN treated group as compared to five deaths in the control group. (p < 0.02).

RANDOMIZED PROSPECTIVE CONTROLLED TRIALS OF IDPN

Randomized studies of IDPN are summarized in Table 40.3. Twenty-six MHD patients with PEW were studied by Cano et al. for 12 weeks [9]. Twelve patients received IDPN, and 14 patients with a similar degree of PEW did not. The patients receiving IDPN demonstrated a significant increase in body weight, serum albumin and transthyretin (prealbumin) levels, mid-arm muscle circumference, skin test reactivity, plasma leucine concentrations and apolipoprotein A-1 levels. The control patients did not manifest an increase in any of these measures. For many of these markers, the IDPN group had statistically nonsignificant lower baseline values which could have predisposed to the increase in these values during IDPN. The IDPN solution provided 1.6 g/kg body weight of fat and 0.08 g/kg of nitrogen from essential and nonessential amino acids. Although plasma apolipoprotein A-1 levels increased, plasma lipid levels did not change. The authors concluded that the high fat content of the IDPN solutions is effective and safe.

Guarnieri et al. studied 18 MHD patients, most but not all of whom had PEW [10]. Patients were randomly assigned to one of three IDPN treatment regimens according to the amino acid content of the solutions. Patients received either (1) only essential amino acids; (2) a combination of essential and nonessential amino acids; (3) no amino acids with an isocaloric infusion of 5% glucose. Minerals, vitamins and trace elements were given with each of the three IDPN treatments. These infusions were given thrice weekly for two months. There was a significant increase in body weight (p < 0.05) only in the patients who received essential amino acids alone. This was the only change in any of the three groups.

In a subsequent study, 21 MHD patients were randomly assigned to receive IDPN for six months. 11 patients received only essential amino acids as the nitrogen source, and 10 patients received a mixture of essential and nonessential amino acids. The mean serum albumin level was normal at baseline, and the average baseline energy intake prior to IDPN initiation was low. The mean baseline body weight and protein intake were marginally decreased. During IDPN with the essential and nonessential amino acids, but not with the essential amino acids alone, there was a significant

decrease in serum albumin levels and an increase in normalized protein nitrogen appearance (nPNA).

The largest prospective randomized study was the French Interdialytic Nutrition Evaluation Study (FineS) [11]. One hundred and eighty six patients, aged 18–80 years, undergoing MHD for more than six months were randomly assigned to receive IDPN (n = 93) or to not receive IDPN (n = 93). IDPN was given during dialysis sessions for one year. Both the IDPN treated group and the control group receive oral nutritional supplementation. Patients included in the study had at least two of the following indicators of PEW: (1) edema free weight loss of greater than 10% over the previous 6 months; (2) serum albumin <3.5 g/dL; (3) body mass index <20 kg/m^2; (4) serum transthyretin <30 mg/dL. The exclusion criteria were (1) single pool Kt/V <1.2; (2) total parenteral nutrition received within the three months preceding the study; (3) severe comorbid conditions that adversely affect 1-year survival (4) less than 12 hours of dialysis treatment per week; (5) fasting serum triglyceride levels >300 mg/dL; (6) hospitalization at the time of randomization. The nutritional intake, including energy intake, from all sources was monitored at baseline and at 3, 6, 12, 18 and 24 months after the onset of IDPN. The follow-up period was up to 2 years.

At months 3, 6 and 12, IDPN provided with each hemodialysis the equivalent of 6.6 ± 2.6 (SD), 6.4 ± 2.1 and 6.1 ± 2.2 kcal/kg and 0.26 ± 0.08, 0.25 ± 0.09 and 0.24 ± 0.10 g/kg of amino acids. To estimate the time-averaged daily dose, these estimates should be multiplied by 3 (3 hemodialysis per week) and divided by 7 (the number of days in the week). At months 3, 6 and 12, oral supplements provided 5.9 ± 2.6, 5.8 ± 2.5 and 5.6 ± 2.7 kcal/kg/d and 0.39 ± 0.18, 0.38 ± 0.18 and 0.37 ± 0.18 g protein/kg/d. There was patient to patient variability as well as variability among hemodialysis centers with regard to the intake of nutrients from the IDPN and from spontaneous eating.

The results indicated no statistical difference in mortality, hospitalization rates and indicators of PEW between the patients assigned to IDPN and the control patients. Both treatment groups showed no change from baseline in Karnofsky scores, nor was there any difference between the two groups in the change in these scores from baseline. The authors noted that although this was the largest prospective randomized trial to date, it was still underpowered. Since both groups receive oral nutritional supplementation, it is not unlikely that the failure to demonstrate any differences in outcome between the IDPN and control groups may have been due to the substantial intake of oral nutritional supplements that both groups received. Those patients in both treatment arms who had an increase in serum transthyretin to greater than 30 mg/L within the first three months of the trial displayed an approximately 50% decrease in mortality at two years.

ADVANTAGES AND DISADVANTAGES OF IDPN

Advantages to IDPN include the nutritional support that it provides to patients with each dialysis session independent of their appetite, anorexia or gastrointestinal function. Since the nutrition is given intravenously, the compliance of the patients or the willingness or the ability of the patient to cooperate does not materially affect this aspect of their nutritional intake. There is no need for an additional vascular access, because IDPN is given through the patient's pre-existing access. The nutrient composition and the quantity of IDPN can be controlled and modified as needed. The excess fluid administered with intravenous infusions can be removed as it is infused during hemodialysis and will not add to the water load of the patient.

Disadvantages of IDPN therapy given in the current format are that the nutrition supplementation can be given only for about 9 to 12 hours weekly as it is given only during dialysis. Therefore, IDPN, as it is usually provided three times weekly, cannot be the sole source for adequate nutrition. Since IDPN is given intravenously, it presents a nonphysiological circumvention of the gut-nutrient interactions. Hence, it does contribute to the direct trophic effects of oral or enteral nutrition on the gastrointestinal tract. There is rapid clearance of nutrients from the blood with IDPN — much faster than is found with oral or enteral feeding into the stomach. Usually IDPN adds significantly to the costs to dialysis therapy.

INDICATIONS FOR IDPN

In patients who can eat there is a consensus that nourishment should be provided using the oral route. Tube feeding should be considered in patients who are unable to maintain adequate protein—energy status solely by eating. Tube feeding is more physiologic than intravenous feeding and can have valuable trophic effects on the gastrointestinal tract. Tube feeding is also safe and is inexpensive. For MHD patients who cannot be adequately nourished by oral intake and tube feeding or for whom these routes of nourishment are not safe, IDPN should be considered. IDPN cannot be used as the sole source of nutrition for patients who undergo MHD only thrice weekly. Some MHD patients whose nutritional needs cannot be met by a combination of oral intake or tube feeding, and IDPN may require total parenteral nutrition. Definitive indications for IDPN are difficult to identify, because benefits regarding morbidity and mortality have not been shown conclusively in randomized trials of IDPN. The lack of trials that demonstrate improved morbidity, mortality or quality of life with IDPN may reflect the fact that there are no randomized prospective clinical trials of IDPN that have the combination of adequate sample sizes, sufficiently long duration of study, appropriate key outcome measures and an experimental protocol with the necessary rigorous design.

BOX 40.1

MEDICARE PART D CRITERIA FOR APPROVAL TO INITIATE IDPN (INTERVENTION FOR MALNUTRITION: PATIENT QUALIFICATION CRITERIA)

1. Patient given intensive dietary counseling, emphasizing need for increased protein and/or calorie intake, for a minimum of one month with no evidence of clinical improvement (i.e. rise in serum albumin and/or weight)
2. Initiation of oral supplementation attempted with no improvement in and/or weight gain after one to two months
3. Evidence of continued protein malnutrition as documented by:
   A) Three month average serum albumin <3.5 g/dL
   B) Progressive decline in serum albumin over three months to <3.5 g/dL
   C) nPNA (nPCR) <0.8 or documentation of inadequate protein intake

   or

   Evidence of continued calorie malnutrition as documented by:
   A) Current weight <90% of ideal body weight
   B) BMI <18 or
   C) Weight loss greater than 5% over three months.
4. Recommendation by physician for prescribing IDPN therapy

IDPN IN THE UNITED STATES

Currently, approval for the initiation of IDPN for a MHD patient is based on the insurance coverage of the particular patient. Patients with Medicare may have their IDPN covered by the Part D program of Medicare if they are outpatients. For hospitalized patients IDPN is covered under Medicare Part A. The criteria that Medicare uses to approve initiation of IDPN coverage are summarized in Box 40.1. The coverage of IDPN by Medicaid (insurance coverage by the state for qualified individuals) is not uniform. Many state Medicaid programs in the United States do cover IDPN. The private insurance carriers loosely follow Medicare criteria for approval of IDPN, but coverage for IDPN is uneven and some costs may be transferred to the patient. Most Health Maintenance Organizations (HMOs) do not provide coverage for IDPN. Medicare, Medicaid and most commercial private insurance carriers recommend that IDPN is to be discontinued if serum albumin is >3.8 g/dL for more than three consecutive months.

NUTRITIONAL HEMODIALYSIS AND INTRAPERITONEAL NUTRITION

Nutritional Hemodialysis

Adding essential and nonessential amino acids to hemodialysate will result in an uptake of amino acids into blood, which can be substantial [12]. When 139 g of amino acid mixture is added to the dialysate there is a net transfer of 39 g of amino acids from dialysate into the patient [12]. When 46 g of a mixture of 20 amino acids are added to the dialysate the amino acid concentrations remain similar to those in the plasma of fasting patients. A limitation of this treatment is that in order to not excessively increase the osmolality of hemodialysate containing amino acids, the amount of glucose in the hemodialysate must be substantially reduced or eradicated altogether. Therefore, the total energy intake from the hemodialysate will be grossly inadequate for the patient's daily needs. Of course, the needed glucose and lipids can be either ingested or infused intravenously during dialysis. At the least, providing amino acids during hemodialysis should eradicate the catabolic effects of amino acid losses during hemodialysis that patients will sustain when they fast during this procedure. Theoretically, this should be a less expensive treatment than IDPN for providing adequate nutrition during hemodialysis. Lowering the hemodialysate flow rate has been done by some investigators to increase fractional extraction of amino acids and glucose from the dialysate into blood [12]. The advantage of this approach is the reduced cost, but the disadvantage is the decreased efficiency of dialysis.

Intraperitoneal Nutrition

Addition of amino acids to the peritoneal dialysate appears to increase protein synthesis and the concentrations of several serum proteins and amino acids [13]. It also allows a reduction in the dialysate glucose concentration which is often of metabolic benefit to the patient. Generally, a mixture of essential and nonessential amino acids is added to a typical dialysate solution, except for the possible reduction in glucose concentration, to attain a final concentration of 1.1% amino acids. This solution is used for one or two peritoneal dialysate exchanges each day. To ensure uptake of about 80% of the amino acid content dwell times of four to six hours are recommended.

Again, in order to prevent excessive osmolality of the dialysate solutions, the energy that can be provided from these solutions is not substantial. Patients should be encouraged to consume a nutrient intake or undertake tube feeding that provides at least most of their needs for energy and most other nutrients when they receive intraperitoneal nutrition. However, care must be taken to prevent an excessive load of amino acids and protein from the combined intakes of intraperitoneal and oral or enteral nutrition. High serum urea nitrogen levels, metabolic acidosis and even some uremic symptoms can develop from such intakes.

FIGURE 40.2 Decision pathway in managing patients with protein-energy wasting.

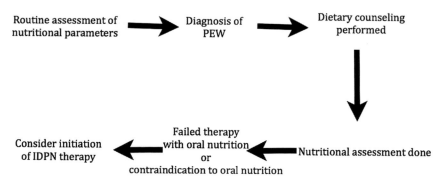

References

[1] Pupim LB, Flakoll PJ, Brouillette JR, Levenhagen DK, Hakim RM, Ikizler TA. Intradialytic parenteral nutrition improves protein and energy homeostasis in chronic hemodialysis patients. The Journal of clinical investigation Aug 2002;110(4):483–92.

[2] Wolfson M, Jones MR, Kopple JD. Amino acid losses during hemodialysis with infusion of amino acids and glucose. Kidney Int Mar 1982;21(3):500–6.

[3] Pupim LB, Majchrzak KM, Flakoll PJ, Ikizler TA. Intradialytic oral nutrition improves protein homeostasis in chronic hemodialysis patients with deranged nutritional status. J Am Soc Nephrol: JASN Nov 2006;17(11):3149–57.

[4] Heidland A, Kult J. Long-term effects of essential amino acids supplementation in patients on regular dialysis treatment. Clin Nephrol Jun 1975;3(6):234–9.

[5] Piraino AJ, Firpo JJ, Powers DV. Prolonged hyperalimentation in catabolic chronic dialysis therapy patients. JPEN. J Parenteral Enteral Nutr Nov-Dec 1981;5(6):463–77.

[6] Capelli JP, Kushner H, Camiscioli TC, Chen SM, Torres MA. Effect of intradialytic parenteral nutrition on mortality rates in end-stage renal disease care. Am J Kidney Dis: The Official Journal of the National Kidney Foundation Jun 1994;23(6):808–16.

[7] Chertow GM, Ling J, Lew NL, Lazarus JM, Lowrie EG. The association of intradialytic parenteral nutrition administration with survival in hemodialysis patients. Am J Kidney Dis: The Official Journal of the National Kidney Foundation Dec 1994;24(6):912–20.

[8] Hiroshige K, Iwamoto M, Kabashima N, Mutoh Y, Yuu K, Ohtani A. Prolonged use of intradialysis parenteral nutrition in elderly malnourished chronic haemodialysis patients. Nephrology, Dialysis, Transplantation: official publication of the European Dialysis and Transplant Association – European Renal Association Aug 1998;13(8):2081–7.

[9] Cano N, Labastie-Coeyrehourq J, Lacombe P, et al. Perdialytic parenteral nutrition with lipids and amino acids in malnourished hemodialysis patients. Am J Clin Nutr Oct 1990;52(4): 726–30.

[10] Guarnieri G, Faccini L, Lipartiti T, et al. Simple methods for nutritional assessment in hemodialyzed patients. Am J Clin Nutr Jul 1980;33(7):1598–607.

[11] Cano NJ, Fouque D, Roth H, et al. Intradialytic parenteral nutrition does not improve survival in malnourished hemodialysis patients: a 2-year multicenter, prospective, randomized study. J Am Soc Nephrol: JASN Sep 2007;18(9):2583–91.

[12] Chazot C, Shahmir E, Matias B, Laidlaw S, Kopple JD. Dialytic nutrition: provision of amino acids in dialysate during hemodialysis. Kidney Int Dec 1997;52(6):1663–70.

[13] Kopple JD, Bernard D, Messana J, et al. Treatment of malnourished CAPD patients with an amino acid based dialysate. Kidney Int Apr 1995;47(4):1148–57.

[14] Heidland A, Kult J. Long-term effects of essential amino acids supplementation in patients on regular dialysis treatment. Clin Nephrol 1975;3(6):234–9.

[15] Powers DV, Piriano AJ. Prolonged intradialysis hyperalimentation in chronic hemodialysis patients with an amino acid solution RenAmin formulated for renal failure. Kinny JM, Brown PR; Perspect Clin Nutr 1989:191–205.

[16] Bilbrey GL, Cohen TL. Identification and treatment of protein calorie malnutrition in chronic hemodialysis patients. Dialysis Transplant 1989;18:669–77.

[17] Matthys DAVR, Ringoir SM. Benefit of intravenous essential amino acids in catabolic patients on chronic hemodialysis. Acta Clin Belg 1991;46:150–8.

[18] GL B. Is intradialtic parenteral nutrition of benefit in hemodialysis patients? IDPN is benefecial for selected dialysis patients. Semin Dial 1993;6:168–70.

[19] Capelli JP, Kushner H, Camiscioli TC, Chen SM, Torres MA. Effect of intradialytic parenteral nutrition on mortality rates in end-stage renal disease care. Am J Kidney Dis 1994;23(6): 808–16.

[20] Foulks CJ. The effect of intradialytic parenteral nutrition on hospitalization rate and mortality in malnourished hemodialysis patients. J Renal Nutr 1994;4:5–10.

[21] Smolle KH, Kaufmann P, Holzer H, Druml W. Intradialytic parenteral nutrition in malnourished patients on chronic haemodialysis therapy. Nephrol Dial Transplant 1995;10(8):1411–6.

[22] Cranford W. Cost effectiveness of IDPN therapy measured by hospitalizations and length of stay. Nephrol News Issues 1998;12(9):33–5. 37–39.

[23] Mortelmans AK, Duym P, Vandenbroucke J, et al. Intradialytic parenteral nutrition in malnourished hemodialysis patients: a prospective long-term study. JPEN J Parenter Enteral Nutr 1999;23(2):90–5.

[24] Blondin J, Ryan C. Nutritional status: a continuous quality improvement approach. Am J Kidney Dis 1999;33(1):198–202.

[25] Cherry NSK. Efficacy of intradialytic parenteral nutrition in malnourished hemodialysis patients. Am J Health Syst Pharm 2002;59:1736–41.

[26] Dezfuli A, Scholl D, Lindenfeld SM, Kovesdy CP, Kalantar-Zadeh K. Severity of hypoalbuminemia predicts response to intradialytic parenteral nutrition in hemodialysis patients. J Renal Nutr: the official journal of the Council on Renal Nutrition of the National Kidney Foundation Jul 2009;19(4):291–7.

[27] ToigoG SR, Tamaro G, Bianco A, Giuliani V, Dardi F, Vianello S, et al. Effect of intraveous supplementation of a new essential amino acid formulation in hemodialysis patients. Kidney Int 1989;36(Suppl. 27):278–81.

[28] McCann L, Feldman C, Hornberger J, et al. Effect of intradialytic parenteral nutrition on delivered Kt/V. Am J Kidney Dis 1999;33(6):1131–5.

[29] Navarro JF, Mora C, Leon C, et al. Amino acid losses during hemodialysis with polyacrylonitrile membranes: effect of intradialytic amino acid supplementation on plasma amino acid concentrations and nutritional variables in nondiabetic patients. Am J Clin Nutr Mar 2000;71(3):765–73.

[30] Cano NJ, Saingra Y, Dupuy AM, et al. Intradialytic parenteral nutrition: comparison of olive oil versus soybean oil-based lipid emulsions. Br J Nutr Jan 2006;95(1):152–9.

41

Therapeutic Use of Growth Factors in Renal Disease

Bo Feldt-Rasmussen[1], Ralph Rabkin[2]

[1]Department of Nephrology, Rigshospitalet, University of Copenhagen, Denmark
[2]Stanford University Medical Center, Stanford, California, USA

INTRODUCTION

Despite conventional dialysis treatment for end-stage renal disease (ESRD), the mortality and morbidity in adult patients undergoing chronic maintenance dialysis (CMD) is high [1,2]. Many interventions have been tested but it has so far been difficult to document clinical significant effects on morbidity and mortality. However, recently it was shown in the SHARP study that lowering of LDL cholesterol using a combination of simvastatin and ezetimibe has some beneficial clinical effect. Even in the SHARP study, the morbidity and mortality of ESRD patients who received these medicines remain high. This may, at least in part, be related to another important cardiovascular risk factor, protein-energy wasting (PEW), which is closely associated with a high risk of death and hospitalization in this patient population [3,4]. There is still an unmet medical need to develop more effective treatments to enhance the protein-energy status of these patients in order to improve their poor prognosis [5,6].

Before considering the therapeutic use of growth factors for the management of malnourished patients with renal disease, it should be kept in mind that some basic steps often are sufficient to prevent or correct PEW in many patients, and it is important to institute these measures before considering more complicated regimens [6]. First, it is essential to provide the appropriate amounts of calories and proteins to meet the patient's daily needs. Although this may appear straightforward, it is not always easily carried out in anorexic, seriously ill patients. Next, providing oral bicarbonate supplements — or for patients receiving renal replacement therapy, increasing the dialysate bicarbonate concentration — may suppress protein breakdown in acidemic subjects. Acidemia

stimulates muscle proteolysis [7]. Any coexistent or superimposed diseases, such as diabetes or infection, need to be effectively treated; increasing dialysis to provide a Kt/V above 1.2 is another essential step in preventing and correcting PEW [8]. This general approach may need to be modified for the individual patient according to the etiology of the malnourished state. This falls into two major categories: inadequate food intake, usually resulting from a loss of appetite, and increased catabolism, often with impaired net protein synthesis [2,7]. These categories usually overlap.

It is important that the clinician recognize that several of the common parameters used to evaluate the nutritional state of patients with ESRD, such as the serum transferrin, prealbumin (transthyretin), and albumin levels, are severely affected by chronic inflammation, a common event in patients receiving renal replacement therapy [2,9]. It has been shown that prolonged subclinical inflammation, detectable by measurements that include serum C-reactive protein and amyloid A levels, is a frequent cause of low serum albumin levels in patients undergoing dialysis, and these low levels are the result of a decrease in protein synthesis [10]. This effect is induced by proinflammatory cytokines, such as tumor necrosis factor alpha and certain interleukins, and in some patients these cytokines may be the cause of refractory PEW. Although it is established that protein-energy malnutrition and chronic inflammation adversely affect the patient's long-term outcome, it is now evident that both conditions are separately predictive of an increase in morbidity, and treatment should be directed accordingly [6,11].

Aggravating the negative effects of PEW in patients with renal failure are the endocrine changes that occur as renal function declines [12]; these may be worsened further by anorexia, acidemia and chronic inflammation.

Cytokines, as mentioned above, are elevated in chronic kidney disease (CKD) and correlate with the degree of cachexia in these patients [13,14]. Animal studies have shown that the complex hypothalamic neuropeptide signaling system may be disturbed by these cytokines and consequently alter appetite and energy expenditure and play an important role in the development of PEW in uremia [15,16]. One major orexigenic hormone affected in CKD is ghrelin which is largely produced in the upper gastrointestinal tract [17]. Its actions are mediated through the growth hormone secretagogue receptor (GHSR) in the hypothalamus, and despite elevated serum levels of ghrelin in CKD, its salutary effects on food intake are suppressed. Early clinical studies suggest that ghrelin may be an effective treatment for anorexia in CKD patients.

In addition to the alterations in the production, secretion, and metabolism of hormones that occur in uremia, an especially important endocrine change is insensitivity to the action of hormones such as insulin, growth hormone (GH), and insulin-like growth factor-I (IGF-I) [12]. Although the mechanisms of resistance are not fully understood, in the case of insulin it appears to be the result of a defect in postreceptor signal transduction [18]. With respect to GH, resistance largely has been attributed to insensitivity to IGF-I [12]. Expression of this growth factor is regulated by GH and mediates many of the actions of GH. However, the situation may be more complex because, as discussed later, GH-mediated receptor signal transduction via the JAK/STAT (Janus kinase/signal transducer and activator of transcription) pathway also is impaired in uremia [19]. Hence, there appears to be resistance to the actions of GH independently of IGF-I resistance. In contrast to insulin and GH, resistance to IGF-I is mainly caused by increased sequestration of IGF-I by circulating high-affinity IGF-binding proteins (IGFBPs) that increase in concentration in renal failure [20], although post-IGF-I receptor signaling defect also may be present [21]. Compounding the adverse effects of uremia on the GH-IGF-I axis are the suppressive effects of protein-calorie malnutrition and chronic inflammation. Malnutrition, even in the absence of uremia, causes a depression of IGF-I production, and serum IGF-I levels decrease [22,23]. The GH-IGF-I axis also is depressed by acidemia and potassium depletion [22,24]. Thus, when managing severely malnourished patients with renal failure, these endocrine changes must be taken into account, and any underlying causes should be corrected whenever possible. Also, given that GH therapy is effective in promoting body growth in children with renal failure [22,25–28], it would seem reasonable to administer GH or IGF-I to patients with renal failure and PEW who are unresponsive to standard therapy, so as to promote anabolism.

TREATMENT OF PROTEIN-ENERGY WASTING (PEW) IN ESRD PATIENTS

PEW and high mortality remain a challenge in the treatment of maintenance hemodialysis (MHD) patients. Several interventions are available including dietary intervention, intradialytic parenteral nutrition and treatment with anabolic steroids (e.g., nandrolone) [29,30], but they are often of limited efficacy and not without compliance problems and adverse effects. There is a need to develop more effective treatments to enhance the protein-energy status of MHD patients. One such approach is the use of recombinant growth factors and anabolic steroids for patients with PEW who are refractory to standard nutritional therapy [31]. In this chapter the role of growth factors is of particular relevance; our main focus will be the role of growth hormone and insulin-like-growth factor-I (IGF-I) in the treatment and prevention of PEW in patients with CKD.

THERAPEUTIC USE OF GROWTH FACTORS IN RENAL DISEASE

Several recent clinical studies have begun to address the potential use of growth hormone and IGF-I, ghrelin and a super agonist of GH-releasing hormone in the management of wasting in uremia. But to date there are no adequately powered placebo-controlled randomized clinical trials that have assessed whether such interventions prolong survival and/or reduce morbidity in MHD patients. Although not generally thought of as growth factors, anabolic steroids also have shown promise in the management of uremic wasting. Insulin, essential for normal growth, is also anabolic, but because of its hypoglycemic action, it generally is reserved for the management of the patient with diabetes or for catabolic intensive care unit patients. The following discussion reviews the use of growth factors in the management of wasting in renal failure and to a minor extent the potential use of growth factors to augment renal function in advanced CRF and to enhance recovery from acute tubular necrosis.

GROWTH FACTORS IN THE MANAGEMENT OF WASTING IN RENAL DISEASE

Growth Hormone (GH)

One of the most successful therapeutic applications of a recombinant growth factor in clinical nephrology has been in the treatments of growth failure in children with chronic renal failure (CRF) [32]. The other is treatment of anemia with erythropoietin. Encouraging results also have been obtained in several small studies examining the use of GH in the management of PEW in adults with ESRD [22,28,33–39]. Before going into details regarding the therapeutic usage of GH in renal disease, however, a brief description of the physiology of the GH-IGF-I system and the changes that occur in renal failure will be provided.

Growth Hormone Physiology and Perturbations in Renal Failure

Growth hormone is a 22-kD, 191-amino acid protein synthesized in the pituitary gland and released into the circulation in pulsatile manner (Figure 41.1). These processes are regulated largely by two hypothalamic hormones: somatostatin, which is inhibitory, and growth hormone-releasing hormone, which is stimulatory [40–43]. In addition, other factors that influence GH production and secretion include the peptide hormones ghrelin, leptin and neuropeptide Y, and fatty acids and other nutrients [44]. Together these factors appear to coordinate GH secretion and metabolism. Nutrient intake regulates GH secretion in a manner that tends to preserve lean body mass during energy restriction. Fasting increases pulsatile GH secretion in humans [40,41]. Oral or intravenous glucose loads acutely decrease serum GH levels by increasing the release of somatostatin. Insulin-induced acute hypoglycemia increases GH secretion by decreasing somatostatin release. Arginine, and certain other amino acids, intravenously infused or taken as a high-protein meal, strongly increases GH secretion. Free fatty acids also reduce GH secretion by a direct suppressive effect on the pituitary gland.

Apart from its action to promote longitudinal bone growth, GH induces amino acid uptake and protein synthesis in muscle, resulting in a positive nitrogen balance [45]. GH also has lipolytic effects on fat and muscle that leads to increased fat mobilization and a decrease in body fat. This, together with its action on protein synthesis, leads to an increase in the absolute and percentage lean body mass. It also modulates carbohydrate, fluid, and electrolyte balance and influences the immune system. In addition, GH regulates the expression of IGF-I, IGF binding proteins (IGFBPs), and the acid-labile subunit that binds with IGF-I and IGFBP-3. Many, but not all, of the effects of GH are mediated through the actions of IGF-I, including essentially all of the anabolic effects of IGF-I [40,42].

In patients with CRF, fasting plasma GH levels usually are normal or even elevated, especially in those with more severe renal failure [28,43]. Generally, GH production is decreased, although in some prepubertal children it actually may be increased [43,46,47], and

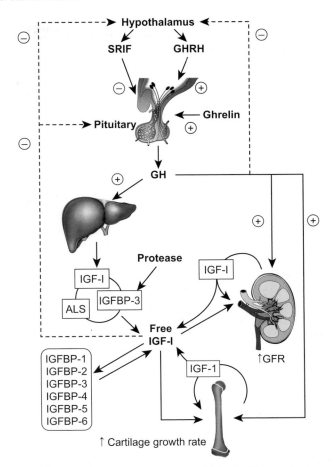

FIGURE 41.1 The growth hormone-IGF-I axis. The synthesis and release of growth hormone (GH) from the pituitary are controlled by the hypothalamic hormones GH-releasing hormone (GHRH) and somatostatin (SRIF), which in turn are regulated by feedback (dashed lines) from blood GH and insulin-like growth factor-I (IGF-I) concentrations. The endogenous GH-releasing peptide, called ghrelin also stimulates GH release. Circulating GH acts directly on many organs to stimulate IGF-I production, with IGF-I production in the liver providing the main source of blood IGF-I. Most of the IGF-I in the circulation is bound to IGF-binding protein-3 (IGFBP-3) in a ternary complex with acid-labile subunit (ALS); a smaller fraction is bound to the five other IGFBP. A small fraction of the total IGF-I in blood is in a bioactive-free fraction. In the kidney, IGF-I increases renal plasma flow and GFR, whereas on bone it acts on the epiphysial plate, which leads to longitudinal bone growth. As illustrated, GH also has direct effects on many organs, including kidney and cartilage, which can be independent of IGF-I action. *(This figure is republished with permission of the American Society of Nephrology; Roelfsema V, Clark RG. J Am Soc Nephrol, 2001;12:1297-1306.)*

adults with ESRD have an exaggerated release of GH in response to GH-releasing hormone [48]. Because GH is largely cleared from the circulation through the kidney, its metabolic clearance rate is reduced in CRF [49], and this accounts for the normal or elevated plasma GH levels in CRF, even in the presence of reduced GH production [50]. Despite these normal or elevated GH levels, children with CRF have retarded body growth and require large doses of GH to promote body growth [50,51]. Resistance to GH also has been demonstrated in the uremic rat [52–54]. Although the mechanism of GH resistance is not fully understood, there is evidence of resistance to IGF-I action [21,55] and possibly a defect in GH-receptor expression [52,53] which has, however, more recently been questioned [56,57].

The growth hormone receptor, a transmembrane glycoprotein, is distributed in tissues throughout the body including the liver, heart, kidney, intestine, lung, muscle, pancreas, brain, and testes [40,58]. Each GH molecule binds two receptors, inducing receptor dimerization. This is followed by receptor signal transduction that is mediated through the receptor intracellular domain [59]. A truncated variant of GH known as the growth hormone-binding protein (GHBP) is present in the circulation and also binds GH with relatively high affinity [60]. In humans GHBP is generated largely by proteolytic cleavage of the GH receptor. The expression of the intact GH receptor appears to be regulated by GH; chronically elevated serum GH levels increase GH binding in liver, whereas acute increases in GH tend to down regulate GH receptor expression [23]. Nutrients also influence the GH receptor and GHBP abundance. In humans the GHBPs bind approximately 50% of the circulating GH, slowing its clearance and reducing its bioavailability. Circulating GHBPs in humans are believed to reflect tissue GH receptor abundance and are used as an indirect measurement of GH number, although the validity of this assumption has not been tested rigorously [60].

There are several reports of low GHBP levels in patients with CRF [61–63], and this has been taken to indicate that cellular GH levels are reduced in renal failure, although there is no direct evidence to support this conclusion. In contrast to these reports, a study of 69 children with CRF failed to show low GHBP levels [64]. However, this interpretation requires caution, because the controls used for comparison were obtained from an older study. Some support for a defect at the level of the GH receptor is provided from studies with uremic rats that show reduced hepatic GH receptor messenger RNA (mRNA) levels and reduced growth plate GH receptor protein levels [52,53]. However, there are studies that indicate that hepatic GH receptor protein levels are unaltered by uremia [19,65] and that reduced food intake is the main cause of reduced GH receptor expression [52,65].

Another potential cause of GH resistance is a defect in the post GH receptor signaling pathway at one or more sites [57]. Studies of uremic rats demonstrated a convincing defect in the pathway that involves the tyrosine kinase janus kinase 2 (JAK2). Along this GH activated pathway, Jak2 phosphorylates and thus activates members of a protein family that serve as both signal transducers and activators of transcription (STAT) [19,66,67]. This signaling pathway is illustrated in Figure 41.2. Although GH receptor binding and the levels of the downstream proteins — namely, JAK2, STAT5, 3, and 1 — were unaffected by uremia, tyrosine phosphorylation and nuclear translocation of these proteins were depressed. Because activation of STAT5, in particular STAT5b, is required for stimulating IGF-I expression and normal growth, it was concluded that this defect in JAK-STAT phosphorylation contributes to the GH-resistant state and, hence, the stunted body growth and wasting seen in uremia.

The GH/JAK2 pathways are regulated by several factors. These include tyrosine phosphatases that deactivate the signaling proteins and suppressors of cytokine signaling (SOCS) proteins that are induced by GH and that serve as negative feedback regulators of GH signaling. These proteins are also induced by proinflammatory cytokines [68]. Both of these groups of regulators appear to play a role in uremic GH resistance. The SOCS proteins play an especially important role when there is underlying inflammation [66,69,70]. It also should be recognized that malnutrition alone impairs GH-stimulated IGF-I gene transcription and translation [23]; thus, malnutrition in uremia may worsen the resistance to GH. Finally, there is evidence that in uremia, resistance to GH is to a large part caused by insensitivity to the action of IGF-I, its major mediator [21,28,71].

Important Clinical Studies of the Effects of Treatment with Growth Hormone in ESRD Patients

Treatment with GH has been demonstrated to increase both short-term and adult height in pediatric patients with a variety of different growth disorders including chronic renal failure [25–28]. An important question is whether this anabolic effect on growth can translate into improving the nutritional status of MHD patients with protein-energy wasting. This seems to be the case. Short-term studies in MHD patients given repetitive doses of GH, IGF-I, or carnitine have shown an anabolic effect with each of these agents [72,73]. Results from studies in animals suggest that low dose GH is cardioprotective in uremia [74]. There have been several longer-term controlled, trials of growth hormone administration in patients with ESRD with different doses and durations of treatment for each study [34,75,76]. The design and results of four of these clinical trials are summarized in Table 41.1 [76–79]. The study of Kotzman et al. [79] had a duration of 3 months. The GH-treated patients displayed a significant increase in procollagen I, carboxy terminal peptide, an indicator of bone formation and bone mineral density, and a decrease

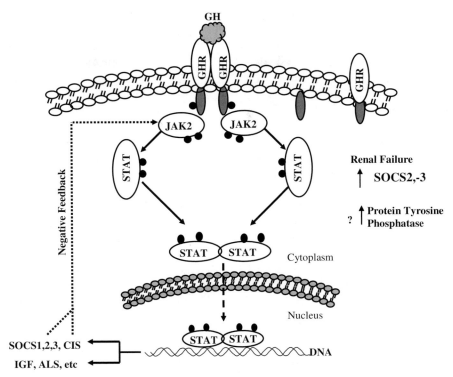

FIGURE 41.2 Growth hormone mediated JAK2/STAT signal transduction. GH activates several signaling pathways via Janus kinase2 (JAK2) including the JAK/STAT (signal transducer and activator of transcription) pathway [19,20]. Binding of GH binding to its receptor, activates JAK2 which then self-phosphorylates followed by phosphorylation of the GHR and subsequently STAT 1a, 3, 5a and 5b, members of a larger family of cytoplasmic transcription factors. These phosphorylated STATs form dimers that enter the nucleus where they bind to specific DNA sequences and activate their target genes including IGF-1 and some suppressors of cytokine signaling (SOCS). Deletion of STAT5 expression leads to retarded body growth and STAT5b is required for GH mediated IGF-1 gene expression. In renal failure phosphorylation of JAK2 and the downstream signaling molecules STAT5, STAT3 and STAT1 are impaired as is the nuclear levels of phosphorylated STAT proteins. This important cause of uremic GH resistance may result in part from upregulation of SOCS2 and SOCS3 expression with suppressed GH signaling and increased protein-tyrosine phosphatase activity with enhanced dephosphorylation and deactivation of the signaling proteins. *(Reprinted with permission from Rabkin R et al. Pediatr Nephrol. 2005;20(3):313-318.)*

in the phagocytic activity of polymorphonuclear leukocytes. No changes in body composition measures or in serum nutritional markers were observed. The next three studies had a duration of six months each, and they all showed improvements in markers of nutrition as indicated by lean body mass or serum albumin (Table 41.1). In the study of Johannsson et al. [76], an improvement of muscle strength was also shown (P < 0.01; Table 41.1). Jensen et al. [78] studied MHD patients who were given subcutaneous injections of GH, 4 IE/m²/day (n = 9), or placebo (n = 10), for six months each, in a randomized, double-blind, prospective clinical trial (Table 41.1). After six months of therapy, the GH-treated group showed an increase in lean body mass and in serum type III collagen N-terminal propeptide and a decrease in fat mass. The placebo-treated group displayed no significant changes with treatment. The results also raised questions about one of the most important safety issues with GH treatment; the left ventricular muscle mass increased [78].

Based on these findings, we planned a proof-of-concept study. This fourth trial was also designed as a dose-finding study in order to identify an effective dose that minimized such side effects as the observed increase in left ventricular mass [78]. The effect of three different doses of GH, 20, 35 and 50 μg/kg/day (Norditropin; Novo Nordisk, Bagsværd, Denmark), were studied in 139 adult CHD patients [77]. The effects of these three doses on serum albumin and lean body mass were the primary study end points. The main results are shown in Table 41.1 [76—79] and Figure 41.3 [77]. Treatment with GH led to statistically significant gains in serum albumin and lean body mass as compared with placebo (P < 0.001). Statistically significant beneficial changes in other (cardiovascular) biomarkers of mortality (homocysteine, transferrin, high-density lipoprotein) as well as health-related quality of life were also observed [77].

The risk of death and hospitalization rates in ESRD patients correlate strongly with indicators of low protein mass, as indicated by low serum albumin and decreased edema-free, fat-free body mass (i.e., lean body mass LBM) as well as with chronic inflammation. Hence, the beneficial effects suggested by these small randomized

TABLE 41.1 Clinical, Prospective Randomized Trials on the Effects of Growth Hormone Treatment in Adult Hemodialysis Patients

Study	Johansson et al. [76]	Jensen et al. [78]	Kotzman et al. [79]	Feldt-Rasmussen et al. [77]
Number of patients	20	31	19	139
Mean age (SD) of patients	73 [9]	49 (no SD) range 18–70	59 [13]	60 [14]
Study duration (months)	6	6	3	6
GH dose per injection (µg/kg)	67	32	35	Low 20, medium 35, high 50
Dosing interval	Three times a week	Daily	Three times a week	Daily
Cumulated GH dose per week (µg/kg/week)	200	225	243	Low 140, medium 245, high 350
Significance of S-albumin increase	$P < 0.001$	ND	NS	$P = 0.08$
Lean body mass increase (kg) and p-value	ND	3.2, $P < 0.001$	NS	2.5, $P < 0.001$
Fat mass reduction (kg)	ND	3.3, $P < 0.01$	NS	2.9, $P < 0.001$
Significance of muscle strength increase	$P < 0.01$	ND	ND	NS
Significance of quality of life improvement	ND	ND	$P < 0.05$	$P < 0.04$

GH, growth hormone; SD, standard deviation; ND, not done; NS, nonsignificant.

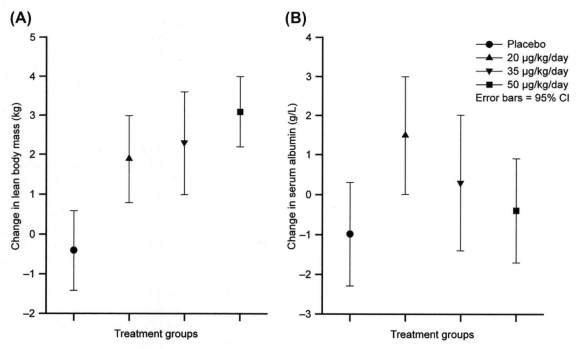

FIGURE 41.3 Mean change in lean body mass (A) and serum albumin (B) from baseline to the end of study for patients taking growth hormone (GH) (at three different doses) compared with placebo. Changes in lean body mass were significantly greater for all the GH treatment groups compared with placebo ($P < 0.001$). An overall increase in serum albumin levels of 1.49 g/L approached significance as compared with placebo in the 20 µg/kg group ($P = 0.063$). A drop in serum albumin levels was seen in all groups initially, but was more pronounced at the higher doses of GH. The initial drop was followed by a steady increase in serum albumin in GH-treated groups as compared with a steady-state level in the placebo group. *(This figure is republished with permission of the American Society of Nephrology from Feldt-Rasmussen et al., 2007 [89].)*

studies would seem to be of major importance. The association may be even more important because PEW occurs in approximately 40% of ESRD patients [80]. The possibility that improved measures of PEW may lead to decreased mortality and/or morbidity was recently underscored by several cross-sectional and longitudinal evaluation of cohorts containing up to 58,000 ESRD patients who were followed for up to two years. These studies showed that both higher serum-albumin and body weight, as well as an increase in these measures are strongly associated with greater survival [81,82].

Therefore a decision was made to conduct a more definitive prospective, randomized clinical trial in hypoalbuminemic patients undergoing MHD. This study, called the OPPORTUNITY Trial®, was planned to involve 2500 MHD patients, up to 50% of whom had diabetes mellitus. Patients were recruited from 22 countries. The clinical endpoints were mortality, morbidity and markers of body protein mass, inflammation, exercise capacity and health related quality of life [83]. The study was terminated by decision of the sponsor in 2009 after inclusion of 800 patients (due to recruitment problems). At the time of closure, the majority of the patients had only participated in the trial for a few weeks. The study, therefore, was considered inconclusive and could not add further information with respect to whether GH treatment improves mortality and morbidity in hypoalbuminemic MHD patients [84]. However, as noted in the dose finding study [85], several biomarkers of (cardiovascular) mortality and morbidity did improve in this incomplete trial [84]. Thus, according to our present knowledge, treatment with GH leads to statistically significant gains in lean body mass and significant beneficial changes in other (cardiovascular) biomarkers of mortality, but it is not known whether there are long-term benefits on morbidity and mortality. More recently a super-agonist of GH-releasing hormone has been tested in a clinical trial in patients with CKD stages 4 and 5. It showed very promising results with rapid improvement of nutritional status in these patients [86]. Longer termed studies are needed.

Safety Aspects of Growth Hormone Therapy

Despite its evidently beneficial effects, it is uncertain whether the long-term use of pharmacological doses of GH may induce undesirable effects. GH treatment of MHD patients is associated with an initial increase in serum glucose in one study [75] but not in another [76]. In our phase 2 study of GH treatment in MHD patients, serum glucose rose transiently but hyperglycemia was not induced [77]. This transient effect on serum glucose may be mediated through effects on insulin sensitivity [87]. An initial decrease in insulin

sensitivity with GH therapy followed by increased sensitivity may be related to a rise in LBM and a decrease in fat mass as was observed in our phase 2 study [77]. Such a bi-phasic response may explain the initial rise in fasting plasma glucose that was observed.

Several studies have reported that GH deficient adults without kidney failure develop increased left ventricular hypertrophy after GH treatment [88,89]. In our phase 2 study, no changes in left ventricular mass was however observed and echocardiography showed no differences between the placebo and the GH treatment groups [83,90]. Sodium and water retention can be observed when giving GH to individuals with normal kidney function. This effect is most likely the result of stimulation of sodium reabsorption in the kidneys [91]. This may be a problem for patients with preserved kidney function, but would hardly affect MHD patients who have little or no renal function.

GH may stimulate differentiation of beta-cell lymphoid precursors [92], and IGF-I may promote cancer growth in vitro [93]. There is, therefore, a concern that GH might induce cancer or promote cancer proliferation. This is particularly relevant because there is an increased risk of cancer in ESRD patients. In a recent retrospective, observational study, children who began to receive GH treatment when they had chronic renal insufficiency and who then received a kidney transplant, had a borderline significantly higher incidence of lympho-proliferative disease than did children with a kidney transplant who had not received GH [94]. The odds ratio, adjusted for age and time when manifestations of the lympho-proliferative disease occurred, was 1.88 (95% confidence interval 1.00−3.55, p = 0.05). Moreover, a large proportion of the GH treatment treated transplant recipients who developed lympho-proliferative disease were Epstein−Barr virus positive, which is a risk factor for this semi-malignant disease. Other studies in children with advanced CKD who were treated with GH to increase stature report GH treatment to be safe [95]. A recent consensus statement of several endocrine societies state, "There is no evidence that GH replacement in adults increases risk of de-novo malignancies or recurrence" [96]. Taking together there is no support for a role for GH in inducing cancer, although GH possibly might stimulate the growth of pre-existing cancer.

Therefore, the foregoing information, taken together, indicate that GH might prove to be of value in reducing mortality and morbidity of patients on long-term hemodialysis.

Insulin-Like Growth Factor I (IGF-I)

Whereas GH is a major promoter of growth in children and exerts anabolic actions even in adults such as enhanced protein synthesis, reduced protein degradation, increased fat mobilization and increased gluconeogenesis, IGF-I is the major mediator of these actions [8]. IGF-I and IGF-II function principally through their activation of the IGF-I receptor (IGF-IR), a transmembrane tyrosine kinase structurally related to the insulin receptor [97]. IGF-IR is widely expressed. Through its coupling to signaling cascades, such as the PI3K and MAPK (ERK) pathways, IGF-I controls cellular proliferation, survival and differentiation. Normally, IGF-I is produced in tissues throughout the body, including kidney, muscle and bone, through the influence of GH and nutrients (Figure 41.1) [12,23,40,71,98]. IGF-I has general growth-promoting and anabolic properties [40]. IGF-I is also locally produced, which is important for promoting body growth [40]. Circulating IGF-I is bound to high-affinity IGFBPs of which seven have been described [98]. Serum IGF-I levels are normal in well-nourished adults receiving chronic dialysis and are reduced in protein-energy wasted adults receiving chronic dialysis. IGF-I has been used as a marker of malnutrition or PEW. Due to their low molecular mass (7.6 kDa) the glomerular filtration of IGF-I and IGF-II should occur at a relatively high rate. However, since 95% or more of the circulating IGFs are sequestered in complexes with IGFBPs, principally a 150-kDa ternary complex of IGF-I or IGF-II, IGFBP-3 and the acid labile subunit (about 150 and 45 kDa), glomerular filtration of these protein complexes occur at very low rates [98]. As discussed earlier, resistance to IGF-I develops in the uremic state and appears to be caused by a reduction in bioavailable IGF-I due to increased trapping by circulating high-affinity IGF-binding proteins (IGFBPs) that increase in concentration in renal failure [20], although a post-IGF-I receptor signaling defect also may be present [21].

Studies of Insulin-Like Growth Factor-I Treatment

Despite the development of resistance in uremia to IGF-I, administration of pharmacological doses of recombinant human IGF-I induces an anabolic response [55]. Combining treatment with GH and IGF-I may induce an even stronger anabolic action than that attained with GH alone [42,99]. In conclusion, more studies are required to evaluate whether long-term IGF-I treatment, either alone or together with GH, can improve the nutritional status, body composition, quality of life, morbidity and mortality of protein-energy wasted patients with ESRD. But first we need a better understanding of the pathophysiology of GH/IGF in CKD, for this may well lead to the development of more effective strategies for the use of IGF-I in the management of PEW.

Ghrelin

Ghrelin is a 28-amino orexigenic peptide secreted largely from the stomach and small intestine in response to a decrease in gastrointestinal contents. Ghrelin secretion is suppressed by eating. This peptide stimulates appetite and promotes food intake [17,100]. Three products arise from the ghrelin gene, namely acyl ghrelin which is converted to des-acyl ghrelin, and obestatin. Acyl ghrelin binds to the GH secretagogue receptor (GHS-R) type 1a which is expressed in hypothalamic arcuate nuclei, heart, lung, pancreas, intestine and adipose tissue. Activation of the hypothalamic GHS-R receptor by acyl ghrelin stimulates GH secretion, appetite and weight gain (adiposity). Indeed some of the anabolic actions of ghrelin may be mediated by GH. Acyl ghrelin also has positive effects on the cardiovascular system and inhibits inflammation [17,101,102]. It appears that ghrelin stimulates appetite after binding to the GHS-R receptor by sending out a signal to neurons containing neuropeptide Y and agouti-related peptide that promote their release. These latter peptides, in turn, inhibit the release of melanocortin, an appetite suppressor. In contrast to acyl-ghrelin, des-acyl ghrelin and obestatin inhibit food intake and gastro-intestinal motility and decrease body weight. Several studies in both CKD patients who do not require dialysis treatment and those undergoing MHD [17,44] have shown that serum total ghrelin levels are elevated and that this elevation is due to an increase in des-acyl-ghrelin levels which comprise 90% of the circulating hormone. Peritoneal dialysis patients have lower ghrelin levels. Of note, Carrero et al. 2011 [101] studying 217 hemodialysis patients reported that in patients with PEW, low serum total ghrelin and elevated serum leptin, the risk for cardiovascular mortality was markedly increased. Since these patients were more anorectic, the investigators suggested that this might be a clinical condition where ghrelin therapy may be particularly useful.

Studies of Ghrelin Treatment

There have been few clinical or preclinical studies of ghrelin therapy in CKD. In rats with CKD, treatment with either ghrelin or ghrelin analogues for two weeks significantly increased food intake, suppressed muscle proteolysis, increased lean body mass and tended to lower serum proinflammatory cytokine levels as compared to saline treated controls [102]. Another animal study showed that treatment with ghrelin increased food intake and induced muscle mitochondrial changes and lowered tissue triglycerides, favoring insulin action and muscle anabolism [103]. In a clinical randomized, double-blind, placebo-controlled crossover study, in which peritoneal dialysis patients were treated with a single subcutaneous injection of ghrelin, ghrelin increased immediate food intake by 57% versus placebo treated controls [104]. A comparable effect on food intake was observed in a double-blinded randomized crossover study, where protein-energy wasted dialysis patients were treated for seven days with ghrelin; a sustained positive change in energy balance was observed [105]. Treatment caused a modest but temporary lowering of blood pressure and no significant adverse effects. Clinical studies in other wasting diseases including anorexia nervosa, chronic obstructive lung disease and congestive heart failure, indicate that ghrelin therapy may be of value in these conditions [106]. There is therefore a clear need for long term clinical trials evaluating the efficacy of this peptide hormone in the management of PEW in CKD.

Androgenic Steroids

Testosterone, the male steroid hormone, is essential for normal sexual differentiation, growth and development and maintenance of secondary sexual characteristics [107]. In addition to its androgenic actions, testosterone and its active metabolites have important anabolic effects such as promoting nitrogen (protein) retention and increasing muscle mass and body weight [29,108]. These compounds have therefore been misused in strength-intensive sports [109]. Anabolic androgenic steroids have also been used in clinical practice since the 1940s for the treatment of chronic debilitating illnesses, trauma, burns, surgery and radiation therapy [88,110]. Testosterone circulates in plasma largely bound to proteins, and in advanced renal failure testosterone levels fall. Indeed in about two-thirds of the males with ESRD, testosterone levels are low, and it has been suggested that this decline in plasma testosterone contributes to uremic muscle wasting [111].

In view of its anabolic properties and its value in such other wasting conditions as aging and chronic illnesses [108], there has been interest in using androgens for the management of the protein-energy wasted renal failure patient [107]. This seems reasonable, especially in males with low testosterone levels where replacement therapy simply to correct these low levels may be sufficient [111]. However, when considering the long term use of androgens especially in high doses, it is essential to take into account not only its potential benefits, but also its potential adverse effects [107,109]. The latter include stimulation of growth of sub-clinical prostatic carcinoma or benign prostatic hypertrophy, thrombotic episodes, hypertension, peripheral edema, gynecomastia, disturbed liver function, sleep apnea and, in females, virilization. However, several small studies suggest that the non-17 alpha-alkylated androgen, nandrolone, may be safer to use, and that it is effective at increasing weight gain and serum protein levels in ESRD patients [29,112]. Furthermore concerns about the potential adverse effects of testosterone on the prostate have encouraged the development of selective androgen receptor modulators that increase muscle mass without affecting the prostate [110]. Interestingly earlier small short term studies suggested that androgens also may be of value by enhancing the responsiveness to erythropoietin in CKD patients [112]. However given the ready availability of effective erythropoiesis stimulating agents, the potential adverse effects of androgens, and the lack of strong evidence of a long term ability of testosterone or its congeners to maintain hemoglobin levels of ESRD patients at the target range, their use for this purpose is not recommended [113].

Anabolic-androgenic steroid therapy appears to be an exciting alternative to improve the protein-muscle status of patients with chronic renal disease. In a double-blind placebo controlled trial, 29 patients were randomized to either placebo or nandrolone decanoate for six months [114]. Serum creatinine and lean body mass were significantly greater in the nandrolone group. The results of functional tests, such as timed walking and stair climbing, also significantly improved in the nandrolone group, whereas they worsened in the placebo group. In addition to the increase in lean body mass, there is also the potential for increasing bone mineral density [111]. Based on these data the role of androgens should be further evaluated in long term, large scale, prospective controlled trials of patients with renal failure and PEW in which, lean body mass, functional status, quality of life, morbidity and mortality are monitored.

Use of Growth Factors in Chronic Kidney Disease with Preserved Renal Function

Growth hormone and IGF-I induce glomerular hyperfiltration when injected in normal adults [115,116]. The GH effect is likely to be mediated through the release of IGF-I [117]. When administered to patients with CKD stage 4, who had an eGFR of 20 mL/min or lower, there was no change in GFR in response to GH [118]. In contrast, administration of IGF-I to patient groups with similar eGFR levels augments renal function [119,120] but the effect seems to be time-limited [119]. Others have, however, shown a sustained increase in GFR for up to 45 days [121]. It is therefore possible that IGF-I can produce a sustained increase in renal function in patients with advanced renal failure without troubling side effects.

Insulin

Insulin is a universal anabolic hormone. Its potential role as a growth factor in renal disease is discussed elsewhere. In this chapter, we will briefly mention its potential role in improving hyperglycemia in hospitalized individuals, and particularly in intensive care unit (ICU) patients, since elevated blood glucose has been related to higher mortality rates and other adverse outcomes [122–125]. Postoperative hyperglycemia is a significant predictor of postoperative infection and longer hospitalization in patients who had undergone surgery [122,124].

Studies in patients with acute myocardial infarction [126] or who are admitted to the ICU have demonstrated a beneficial effect of intensive insulin treatment with regard to the time spent on mechanical ventilation, length of stay and mortality [126,127]. A recent randomized controlled trial in the ICU-environment [128] and a meta-analysis [129], however, have not confirmed these findings. This is probably due to episodes of hypoglycemia in vulnerable patients [128,130]. Therefore, it is of utmost importance to ensure that intensive glycemic control does not induce hypoglycemia. More frequent monitoring of the blood glucose level in insulin treated in-patients than has tended to be performed in these previous studies is therefore mandatory in order to detect and prevent episodes of severe hypoglycemia.

CONCLUSION

Although growth factors and anabolic steroids offer the potential for improving protein-energy status, body composition, quality of life and even the muscle strength and physical performance of protein-energy wasted patients with renal failure, further large scale and prolonged interventional studies are required before these agents can be used in clinical practice. The research should include an assessment of the impact of growth factors on body composition, functional ability, quality of life and morbidity and mortality with careful monitoring for potential side effects including progression of CKD. Since PEW in CKD is a complex process, it can be anticipated that a successful study may require a broad approach applying several therapeutic modalities concurrently. For example, the use of a potent anabolic agent such as an androgenic steroid, plus an agent such as ghrelin which acts largely by improving appetite and perhaps suppressing inflammation, together with nutrient supplements and a physical exercise regimen may be one such approach. In the meantime, much can be done to improve the nutritional status of the patient with kidney failure. This includes ensuring that the patient is receiving and is ingesting needed nutrients in sufficient amounts to improve lean body mass, even if this requires tube feeding or parenteral nutrition; the elimination of any source of chronic inflammation, ensuring that the MHD patient receives optimal dialysis therapy, and finally encouraging increased mobility and participation in an exercise regimen. The latter should not be overlooked, since muscle disuse alone leads to muscle atrophy. Finally, with regard to the pre-ESRD patient and the potential for improving renal function by administering recombinant IGF-I, although the preliminary results are encouraging, far more extensive evaluation are required before such treatment can be considered appropriate for clinical use.

References

[1] U.S.Renal Data System. USRDS 2007 Annual Data Report: Atlas of chronic kidney disease and end-stage renal disease in the United States. Bethesda, MD: National Institutes of Health, National Institute of Diabetes and Digestive and Kidney Diseases; 2007. H207 Reference tables. 2011.

[2] Riella MC. Malnutrition in dialysis: malnourishment or uremic inflammatory response? Kidney Int 2000 March;57(3):1211–32.

[3] Kalantar-Zadeh K, Block G, McAllister CJ, Humphreys MH, Kopple JD. Appetite and inflammation, nutrition, anemia, and clinical outcome in hemodialysis patients. Am J Clin Nutr 2004 August;80(2):299–307.

[4] Kalantar-Zadeh K, Kopple JD, Block G, Humphreys MH. A malnutrition-inflammation score is correlated with morbidity and mortality in maintenance hemodialysis patients. Am J Kidney Dis 2001 December;38(6):1251–63.

[5] Ikizler TA, Hakim RM. Nutrition in end-stage renal disease. Kidney Int 1996 August;50(2):343–57.

[6] Kopple JD. Therapeutic approaches to malnutrition in chronic dialysis patients: the different modalities of nutritional support. Am J Kidney Dis 1999 January;33(1):180–5.

[7] Mitch WE, Maroni BJ. Factors causing malnutrition in patients with chronic uremia. Am J Kidney Dis 1999 January;33(1): 176–9.

[8] Ikizler TA, Wingard RL, Hakim RM. Interventions to treat malnutrition in dialysis patients: the role of the dose of dialysis, intradialytic parenteral nutrition, and growth hormone. Am J Kidney Dis 1995 July;26(1):256–65.

[9] Stenvinkel P, Heimburger O, Lindholm B, Kaysen GA, Bergstrom J. Are there two types of malnutrition in chronic renal failure? Evidence for relationships between malnutrition, inflammation and atherosclerosis (MIA syndrome). Nephrol Dial Transplant 2000 July;15(7):953–60.

[10] Kaysen GA. Inflammation nutritional state and outcome in end stage renal disease. Miner Electrolyte Metab 1999 July;25(4-6): 242–50.

[11] Ikizler TA, Wingard RL, Harvell J, Shyr Y, Hakim RM. Association of morbidity with markers of nutrition and inflammation in chronic hemodialysis patients: a prospective study. Kidney Int 1999 May;55(5):1945–51.

[12] Rabkin R. Growth factor insensitivity in renal failure. Ren Fail 2001 May;23(3-4):291–300.

[13] Cheung WW, Paik KH, Mak RH. Inflammation and cachexia in chronic kidney disease. Pediatr Nephrol 2010 April;25(4):711–24.

[14] Kalantar-Zadeh K, Balakrishnan VS. The kidney disease wasting: inflammation, oxidative stress, and diet-gene interaction. Hemodial Int 2006 October;10(4):315–25.

[15] Mak RH, Cheung W, Cone RD, Marks DL. Orexigenic and anorexigenic mechanisms in the control of nutrition in chronic kidney disease. Pediatr Nephrol 2005 March;20(3):427–31.

[16] Mak RH, Cheung WW, Zhan JY, Shen Q, Foster BJ. Cachexia and protein-energy wasting in children with chronic kidney disease. Pediatr Nephrol 2011 February 6.

[17] Cheung WW, Mak RH. Ghrelin in chronic kidney disease. Int J Pept 2010;2010:7. Article ID 567343.

[18] Mak RH. Insulin and its role in chronic kidney disease. Pediatr Nephrol 2008 March;23(3):355—62.

[19] Schaefer F, Chen Y, Tsao T, Nouri P, Rabkin R. Impaired JAK-STAT signal transduction contributes to growth hormone resistance in chronic uremia. J Clin Invest 2001 August;108(3):467—75.

[20] Rabkin R, Schaefer F. New concepts: growth hormone, insulin-like growth factor-I and the kidney. Growth Horm IGF Res 2004 August;14(4):270—6.

[21] Ding H, Gao XL, Hirschberg R, Vadgama JV, Kopple JD. Impaired actions of insulin-like growth factor 1 on protein Synthesis and degradation in skeletal muscle of rats with chronic renal failure. Evidence for a postreceptor defect. J Clin Invest 1996 February 15;97(4):1064—75.

[22] Rabkin R. Nutrient regulation of insulin-like growth factor-I. Miner Electrolyte Metab 1997;23(3-6):157—60.

[23] Thissen JP, Ketelslegers JM, Underwood LE. Nutritional regulation of the insulin-like growth factors. Endocr Rev 1994 February;15(1):80—101.

[24] Kuemmerle N, Krieg Jr RJ, Latta K, Challa A, Hanna JD, Chan JC. Growth hormone and insulin-like growth factor in non-uremic acidosis and uremic acidosis. Kidney Int Suppl 1997 March;58:S102—5.

[25] Fine RN. Growth hormone treatment of children with chronic renal insufficiency, end-stage renal disease and following renal transplantation — update 1997. J Pediatr Endocrinol Metab 1997 July;10(4):361—70.

[26] Haffner D, Schaefer F, Nissel R, Wuhl E, Tonshoff B, Mehls O. Effect of growth hormone treatment on the adult height of children with chronic renal failure. German Study Group for Growth Hormone Treatment in Chronic Renal Failure. N Engl J Med 2000 September 28;343(13):923—30.

[27] Hokken-Koelega AC, Stijnen T, de Muinck Keizer-Schrama SM, Wit JM, Wolff ED, de Jong MC, et al. Placebo-controlled, double-blind, cross-over trial of growth hormone treatment in prepubertal children with chronic renal failure. Lancet 1991 September 7;338(8767):585—90.

[28] Tonshoff B, Blum WF, Mehls O. Derangements of the somatotropic hormone axis in chronic renal failure. Kidney Int Suppl 1997 March;58:S106—13.

[29] Navarro JF, Mora C. In-depth review effect of androgens on anemia and malnutrition in renal failure: implications for patients on peritoneal dialysis. Perit Dial Int 2001 January;21(1):14—24.

[30] Kopple JD. National kidney foundation K/DOQI clinical practice guidelines for nutrition in chronic renal failure. Am J Kidney Dis 2001 January;37(1 Suppl. 2):S66—70.

[31] Chen Y, Fervenza FC, Rabkin R. Growth factors in the treatment of wasting in kidney failure. J Ren Nutr 2001 April;11(2):62—6.

[32] Santos F, Moreno ML, Neto A, Ariceta G, Vara J, Alonso A, et al. Improvement in growth after 1 year of growth hormone therapy in well-nourished infants with growth retardation secondary to chronic renal failure: results of a multicenter, controlled, randomized, open clinical trial. Clin J Am Soc Nephrol 2010 July;5(7):1190—7.

[33] Garibotto G, Barreca A, Russo R, Sofia A, Araghi P, Cesarone A, et al. Effects of recombinant human growth hormone on muscle protein turnover in malnourished hemodialysis patients. J Clin Invest 1997 January 1;99(1):97—105.

[34] Hansen TB, Gram J, Jensen PB, Kristiansen JH, Ekelund B, Christiansen JS, et al. Influence of growth hormone on whole body and regional soft tissue composition in adult patients on hemodialysis. A double-blind, randomized, placebo-controlled study. Clin Nephrol 2000 February;53(2):99—107.

[35] Iglesias P, Diez JJ. Recombinant human growth hormone therapy in adult dialysis patients. Int J Artif Organs 2000 December;23(12):802—4.

[36] Ikizler TA, Wingard RL, Breyer JA, Schulman G, Parker RA, Hakim RM. Short-term effects of recombinant human growth hormone in CAPD patients. Kidney Int 1994 October;46(4):1178—83.

[37] Ikizler TA, Wingard RL, Flakoll PJ, Schulman G, Parker RA, Hakim RM. Effects of recombinant human growth hormone on plasma and dialysate amino acid profiles in CAPD patients. Kidney Int 1996 July;50(1):229—34.

[38] Schulman G, Wingard RL, Hutchison RL, Lawrence P, Hakim RM. The effects of recombinant human growth hormone and intradialytic parenteral nutrition in malnourished hemodialysis patients. Am J Kidney Dis 1993 May;21(5):527—34.

[39] Ziegler TR, Lazarus JM, Young LS, Hakim R, Wilmore DW. Effects of recombinant human growth hormone in adults receiving maintenance hemodialysis. J Am Soc Nephrol 1991 December;2(6):1130—7.

[40] Butler AA, Le RD. Control of growth by the somatropic axis: growth hormone and the insulin-like growth factors have related and independent roles. Annu Rev Physiol 2001;63:141—64.

[41] Pombo M, Pombo CM, Garcia A, Caminos E, Gualillo O, Alvarez CV, et al. Hormonal control of growth hormone secretion. Horm Res 2001;55(Suppl. 1):11—6.

[42] Roelfsema V, Clark RG. The growth hormone and insulin-like growth factor axis: its manipulation for the benefit of growth disorders in renal failure. J Am Soc Nephrol 2001 June;12(6):1297—306.

[43] Schaefer F, Veldhuis JD, Stanhope R, Jones J, Scharer K. Alterations in growth hormone secretion and clearance in peripubertal boys with chronic renal failure and after renal transplantation. Cooperative Study Group of Pubertal development in Chronic Renal Failure. J Clin Endocrinol Metab 1994 June;78(6):1298—306.

[44] Mafra D, Guebre-Egziabher F, Fouque D. Endocrine role of stomach in appetite regulation in chronic kidney disease: about ghrelin and obestatin. J Ren Nutr 2010 March;20(2):68—73.

[45] Jorgensen JO, Rubeck KZ, Nielsen TS, Clasen BF, Vendelboe M, Hafstrom TK, et al. Effects of GH in human muscle and fat. Pediatr Nephrol 2010 April;25(4):705—9.

[46] Schaefer F, Hamill G, Stanhope R, Preece MA, Scharer K. Pulsatile growth hormone secretion in peripubertal patients with chronic renal failure. Cooperative Study Group on Pubertal Development in Chronic Renal Failure. J Pediatr 1991 October;119(4):568—77.

[47] Tonshoff B, Veldhuis JD, Heinrich U, Mehls O. Deconvolution analysis of spontaneous nocturnal growth hormone secretion in prepubertal children with preterminal chronic renal failure and with end-stage renal disease. Pediatr Res 1995 January;37(1):86—93.

[48] Ramirez G, Bercu BB, Bittle PA, Ayers CW, Ganguly A. Response to growth hormone-releasing hormone in adult renal failure patients on hemodialysis. Metabolism 1990 July;39(7):764—8.

[49] Haffner D, Schaefer F, Girard J, Ritz E, Mehls O. Metabolic clearance of recombinant human growth hormone in health and chronic renal failure. J Clin Invest 1994 March;93(3):1163—71.

[50] Blum WF, Ranke MB, Kietzmann K, Tonshoff B, Mehls O. Growth hormone resistance and inhibition of somatomedin activity by excess of insulin-like growth factor binding protein in uraemia. Pediatr Nephrol 1991 July;5(4):539–44.

[51] Zadik Z, Frishberg Y, Drukker A, Blachar Y, Lotan D, Levi S, et al. Excessive dietary protein and suboptimal caloric intake have a negative effect on the growth of children with chronic renal disease before and during growth hormone therapy. Metabolism 1998 March;47(3):264–8.

[52] Chan W, Valerie KC, Chan JC. Expression of insulin-like growth factor-1 in uremic rats: growth hormone resistance and nutritional intake. Kidney Int 1993 April;43(4):790–5.

[53] Edmondson SR, Baker NL, Oh J, Kovacs G, Werther GA, Mehls O. Growth hormone receptor abundance in tibial growth plates of uremic rats: GH/IGF-I treatment. Kidney Int 2000 July;58(1):62–70.

[54] Mak RH, Pak YK. End-organ resistance to growth hormone and IGF-I in epiphyseal chondrocytes of rats with chronic renal failure. Kidney Int 1996 August;50(2):400–6.

[55] Fouque D, Peng SC, Kopple JD. Impaired metabolic response to recombinant insulin-like growth factor-1 in dialysis patients. Kidney Int 1995 March;47(3):876–83.

[56] Greenstein J, Guest S, Tan JC, Tummala P, Busque S, Rabkin R. Circulating growth hormone binding protein levels and mononuclear cell growth hormone receptor expression in uremia. J Ren Nutr 2006 April;16(2):141–9.

[57] Rabkin R, Sun DF, Chen Y, Tan J, Schaefer F. Growth hormone resistance in uremia, a role for impaired JAK/STAT signaling. Pediatr Nephrol 2005 March;20(3):313–8.

[58] Carter-Su C, Smit LS. Signaling via JAK tyrosine kinases: growth hormone receptor as a model system. Recent Prog Horm Res 1998;53:61–82.

[59] Lanning NJ, Carter-Su C. Recent advances in growth hormone signaling. Rev Endocr Metab Disord 2006 December;7(4):225–35.

[60] Baumann G. Growth hormone binding protein 2001. J Pediatr Endocrinol Metab 2001 April;14(4):355–75.

[61] Baumann G. Growth hormone binding protein and free growth hormone in chronic renal failure. Pediatr Nephrol 1996 June;10(3):328–30.

[62] Postel-Vinay MC, Tar A, Crosnier H, Broyer M, Rappaport R, Tonshoff B, et al. Plasma growth hormone-binding activity is low in uraemic children. Pediatr Nephrol 1991 July;5(4):545–7.

[63] Tonshoff B, Cronin MJ, Reichert M, Haffner D, Wingen AM, Blum WF, et al. Reduced concentration of serum growth hormone (GH)-binding protein in children with chronic renal failure: correlation with GH insensitivity. The European Study Group for Nutritional Treatment of Chronic Renal Failure in Childhood. The German Study Group for Growth Hormone Treatment in Chronic Renal Failure. J Clin Endocrinol Metab 1997 April;82(4):1007–13.

[64] Powell DR, Liu F, Baker BK, Hintz RL, Lee PD, Durham SK, et al. Modulation of growth factors by growth hormone in children with chronic renal failure. The Southwest Pediatric Nephrology Study Group. Kidney Int 1997 June;51(6):1970–9.

[65] Villares SM, Goujon L, Maniar S, ehaye-Zervas MC, Martini JF, Kleincknecht C, et al. Reduced food intake is the main cause of low growth hormone receptor expression in uremic rats. Mol Cell Endocrinol 1994 December;106(1-2):51–6.

[66] Sun DF, Zheng Z, Tummala P, Oh J, Schaefer F, Rabkin R. Chronic uremia attenuates growth hormone-induced signal transduction in skeletal muscle. J Am Soc Nephrol 2004 October;15(10):2630–6.

[67] Zheng Z, Sun DF, Tummala P, Rabkin R. Cardiac resistance to growth hormone in uremia. Kidney Int 2005 March;67(3):858–66.

[68] Tan JC, Rabkin R. Suppressors of cytokine signaling in health and disease. Pediatr Nephrol 2005 May;20(5):567–75.

[69] Chen Y, Biada J, Sood S, Rabkin R. Uremia attenuates growth hormone-stimulated insulin-like growth factor-1 expression, a process worsened by inflammation. Kidney Int 2010 July;78(1):89–95.

[70] Garibotto G, Russo R, Sofia A, Ferone D, Fiorini F, Cappelli V, et al. Effects of uremia and inflammation on growth hormone resistance in patients with chronic kidney diseases. Kidney Int 2008 October;74(7):937–45.

[71] Hirschberg R, Adler S. Insulin-like growth factor system and the kidney: physiology, pathophysiology, and therapeutic implications. Am J Kidney Dis 1998 June;31(6):901–19.

[72] Fouque D, Peng SC, Shamir E, Kopple JD. Recombinant human insulin-like growth factor-1 induces an anabolic response in malnourished CAPD patients. Kidney Int 2000 February;57(2):646–54.

[73] Kopple JD, Brunori G, Leiserowitz M, Fouque D. Growth hormone induces anabolism in malnourished maintenance haemodialysis patients. Nephrol Dial Transplant 2005 May;20(5):952–8.

[74] Rabkin R, Awwad I, Chen Y, Ashley EA, Sun D, Sood S, et al. Low-dose growth hormone is cardioprotective in uremia. J Am Soc Nephrol 2008 September;19(9):1774–83.

[75] Iglesias P, Diez JJ, Fernandez-Reyes MJ, Aguilera A, Burgues S, Martinez-Ara J, et al. Recombinant human growth hormone therapy in malnourished dialysis patients: a randomized controlled study. Am J Kidney Dis 1998 September;32(3):454–63.

[76] Johannsson G, Bengtsson BA, Ahlmen J. Double-blind, placebo-controlled study of growth hormone treatment in elderly patients undergoing chronic hemodialysis: anabolic effect and functional improvement. Am J Kidney Dis 1999 April;33(4):709–17.

[77] Feldt-Rasmussen B, Lange M, Sulowicz W, Gafter U, Lai KN, Wiedemann J, et al. Growth hormone treatment during hemodialysis in a randomized trial improves nutrition, quality of life, and cardiovascular risk. J Am Soc Nephrol 2007 July;18(7):2161–71.

[78] Jensen PB, Hansen TB, Frystyk J, Ladefoged SD, Pedersen FB, Christiansen JS. Growth hormone, insulin-like growth factors and their binding proteins in adult hemodialysis patients treated with recombinant human growth hormone. Clin Nephrol 1999 August;52(2):103–9.

[79] Kotzmann H, Yilmaz N, Lercher P, Riedl M, Schmidt A, Schuster E, et al. Differential effects of growth hormone therapy in malnourished hemodialysis patients. Kidney Int 2001 October;60(4):1578–85.

[80] Mehrota R, Kopple JD. Causes of protein-energy malnutrtion in chronic renal failure. In: Kopple JD, Massry SG, editors. Nutritional Management of Renal Disease. Baltimore, MD: Lippincott Williams & Wilkins; 2004. p. 167–82. 2011.

[81] Kalantar-Zadeh K, Kilpatrick RD, Kuwae N, McAllister CJ, Alcorn Jr H, Kopple JD, et al. Revisiting mortality predictability of serum albumin in the dialysis population: time dependency, longitudinal changes and population-attributable fraction. Nephrol Dial Transplant 2005 September;20(9):1880–8.

[82] Kalantar-Zadeh K, Kopple JD, Kilpatrick RD, McAllister CJ, Shinaberger CS, Gjertson DW, et al. Association of morbid obesity and weight change over time with cardiovascular survival in hemodialysis population. Am J Kidney Dis 2005 September;46(3):489–500.

[83] Kopple JD, Cheung AK, Christiansen JS, Djurhuus CB, El NM, Feldt-Rasmussen B, et al. OPPORTUNITY: a randomized clinical trial of growth hormone on outcome in hemodialysis patients. Clin J Am Soc Nephrol 2008 November;3(6):1741−51.

[84] Kopple JD, Cheung AK, Christiansen JS, Djurhuus CB, El NM, Feldt-Rasmussen B, et al. OPPORTUNITYTM: a large-scale randomized clinical trial of growth hormone in hemodialysis patients. Nephrol Dial Transplant 2011 July 12.

[85] Feldt-Rasmussen B, Lange M, Sulowicz W, Gafter U, Lai KN, Wiedemann J, et al. Growth hormone treatment during hemodialysis in a randomized trial improves nutrition, quality of life, and cardiovascular risk. J Am Soc Nephrol 2007 July;18(7):2161−71.

[86] Niemczyk S, Sikorska H, Wiecek A, Zukowska-Szczechowska E, Zalecka K, Gorczynska J, et al. A super-agonist of growth hormone-releasing hormone causes rapid improvement of nutritional status in patients with chronic kidney disease. Kidney Int 2010 March;77(5):450−8.

[87] Norrelund H. The metabolic role of growth hormone in humans with particular reference to fasting. Growth Horm IGF Res 2005 April;15(2):95−122.

[88] Amato G, Carella C, Fazio S, La MG, Cittadini A, Sabatini D, et al. Body composition, bone metabolism, and heart structure and function in growth hormone (GH)-deficient adults before and after GH replacement therapy at low doses. J Clin Endocrinol Metab 1993 December;77(6):1671−6.

[89] Cuneo RC, Salomon F, Wilmshurst P, Byrne C, Wiles CM, Hesp R, et al. Cardiovascular effects of growth hormone treatment in growth-hormone-deficient adults: stimulation of the renin-aldosterone system. Clin Sci (Lond) 1991 November;81(5):587−92.

[90] Kober L, Rustom R, Wiedmann J, Kappelgaard AM, El NM, Feldt-Rasmussen B. Cardiovascular effects of growth hormone in adult hemodialysis patients: results from a randomized controlled trial. Nephron Clin Pract 2010;115(3):c213−26.

[91] Moller J, Nielsen S, Hansen TK. Growth hormone and fluid retention. Horm Res 1999;51(Suppl. 3):116−20.

[92] Sumita K, Hattori N, Inagaki C. Effects of growth hormone on the differentiation of mouse B-lymphoid precursors. J Pharmacol Sci 2005 March;97(3):408−16.

[93] Grimberg A, Cohen P. Role of insulin-like growth factors and their binding proteins in growth control and carcinogenesis. J Cell Physiol 2000 April;183(1):1−9.

[94] Dharnidharka VR, Talley LI, Martz KL, Stablein DM, Fine RN. Recombinant growth hormone use pretransplant and risk for post-transplant lymphoproliferative disease − a report of the NAPRTCS. Pediatr Transplant 2008 September;12(6):689−95.

[95] Banerjee I, Clayton PE. Growth hormone treatment and cancer risk. Endocrinol Metab Clin North Am 2007 March;36(1):247−63.

[96] Ho KK. Consensus guidelines for the diagnosis and treatment of adults with GH deficiency II: a statement of the GH Research Society in association with the European Society for Pediatric Endocrinology, Lawson Wilkins Society, European Society of Endocrinology, Japan Endocrine Society, and Endocrine Society of Australia. Eur J Endocrinol 2007 December;157(6):695−700.

[97] LeRoith D, Werner H, Beitner-Johnson D, Roberts Jr CT. Molecular and cellular aspects of the insulin-like growth factor I receptor. Endocr Rev 1995 April;16(2):143−63.

[98] Feld S, Hirschberg R. Growth hormone, the insulin-like growth factor system, and the kidney. Endocr Rev 1996 October;17(5):423−80.

[99] Kupfer SR, Underwood LE, Baxter RC, Clemmons DR. Enhancement of the anabolic effects of growth hormone and insulin-like growth factor I by use of both agents simultaneously. J Clin Invest 1993 February;91(2):391−6.

[100] Hillman JB, Tong J, Tschop M. Ghrelin biology and its role in weight-related disorders. Discov Med 2011 June;11(61):521−8.

[101] Carrero JJ, Nakashima A, Qureshi AR, Lindholm B, Heimburger O, Barany P, et al. Protein-energy wasting modifies the association of ghrelin with inflammation, leptin, and mortality in hemodialysis patients. Kidney Int 2011 April;79(7):749−56.

[102] Deboer MD, Zhu X, Levasseur PR, Inui A, Hu Z, Han G, et al. Ghrelin treatment of chronic kidney disease: improvements in lean body mass and cytokine profile. Endocrinology 2008 February;149(2):827−35.

[103] Barazzoni R, Zhu X, Deboer M, Datta R, Culler MD, Zanetti M, et al. Combined effects of ghrelin and higher food intake enhance skeletal muscle mitochondrial oxidative capacity and AKT phosphorylation in rats with chronic kidney disease. Kidney Int 2010 January;77(1):23−8.

[104] Wynne K, Giannitsopoulou K, Small CJ, Patterson M, Frost G, Ghatei MA, et al. Subcutaneous ghrelin enhances acute food intake in malnourished patients who receive maintenance peritoneal dialysis: a randomized, placebo-controlled trial. J Am Soc Nephrol 2005 July;16(7):2111−8.

[105] Ashby DR, Ford HE, Wynne KJ, Wren AM, Murphy KG, Busbridge M, et al. Sustained appetite improvement in malnourished dialysis patients by daily ghrelin treatment. Kidney Int 2009 July;76(2):199−206.

[106] Muller TD, Perez-Tilve D, Tong J, Pfluger PT, Tschop MH. Ghrelin and its potential in the treatment of eating/wasting disorders and cachexia. J Cachexia Sarcopenia Muscle 2010 December;1(2):159−67.

[107] Iglesias P, Carrero JJ, Diez JJ. Gonadal dysfunction in men with chronic kidney disease: clinical features, prognostic implications and therapeutic options. J Nephrol 2012 January;25(1):31−42.

[108] Bhasin S, Woodhouse L, Storer TW. Androgen effects on body composition. Growth Horm IGF Res 2003 August;13(Suppl. A):S63−71.

[109] Handelsman DJ. Androgen misuse and abuse. Best Pract Res Clin Endocrinol Metab 2011 April;25(2):377−89.

[110] Bhasin S, Storer TW. Anabolic applications of androgens for functional limitations associated with aging and chronic illness. Front Horm Res 2009;37:163−82.

[111] Johansen KL. Testosterone metabolism and replacement therapy in patients with end-stage renal disease. Semin Dial 2004 May;17(3):202−8.

[112] Johnson CA. Use of androgens in patients with renal failure. Semin Dial 2000 January;13(1):36−9.

[113] II. Clinical practice guidelines and clinical practice recommendations for anemia in chronic kidney disease in adults. Am J Kidney Dis 2006 May;47(5 Suppl. 3):S16−85.

[114] Johansen KL, Mulligan K, Schambelan M. Anabolic effects of nandrolone decanoate in patients receiving dialysis: a randomized controlled trial. JAMA 1999 April 14;281(14):1275−81.

[115] Hirschberg R, Rabb H, Bergamo R, Kopple JD. The delayed effect of growth hormone on renal function in humans. Kidney Int 1989 March;35(3):865−70.

[116] Hirschberg R, Brunori G, Kopple JD, Guler HP. Effects of insulin-like growth factor I on renal function in normal men. Kidney Int 1993 February;43(2):387−97.

[117] Hirschberg R, Kopple JD, Blantz RC, Tucker BJ. Effects of recombinant human insulin-like growth factor I on glomerular dynamics in the rat. J Clin Invest 1991 April;87(4):1200−6.

[118] Haffner D, Zacharewicz S, Mehls O, Heinrich U, Ritz E. The acute effect of growth hormone on GFR is obliterated in chronic renal failure. Clin Nephrol 1989 December;32(6):266−9.

[119] Vijayan A, Behrend T, Miller SB. Clinical use of growth factors in chronic renal failure. Curr Opin Nephrol Hypertens 2000 January;9(1):5—10.

[120] O'Shea MH, Miller SB, Hammerman MR. Effects of IGF-I on renal function in patients with chronic renal failure. Am J Physiol 1993 May;264(5 Pt 2):F917—22.

[121] Vijayan A, Franklin SC, Behrend T, Hammerman MR, Miller SB. Insulin-like growth factor I improves renal function in patients with end-stage chronic renal failure. Am J Physiol 1999 April;276(4 Pt 2):R929—34.

[122] Ainla T, Baburin A, Teesalu R, Rahu M. The association between hyperglycaemia on admission and 180-day mortality in acute myocardial infarction patients with and without diabetes. Diabet Med 2005 October;22(10):1321—5.

[123] Jones KW, Cain AS, Mitchell JH, Millar RC, Rimmasch HL, French TK, et al. Hyperglycemia predicts mortality after CABG: postoperative hyperglycemia predicts dramatic increases in mortality after coronary artery bypass graft surgery. J Diabetes Complications 2008 November;22(6):365—70.

[124] McAlister FA, Majumdar SR, Blitz S, Rowe BH, Romney J, Marrie TJ. The relation between hyperglycemia and outcomes in 2,471 patients admitted to the hospital with community-acquired pneumonia. Diabetes Care 2005 April; 28(4):810—5.

[125] Monteiro S, Monteiro P, Goncalves F, Freitas M, Providencia LA. Hyperglycaemia at admission in acute coronary syndrome patients: prognostic value in diabetics and non-diabetics. Eur J Cardiovasc Prev Rehabil 2010 April;17(2):155—9.

[126] van den BG, Wouters P, Weekers F, Verwaest C, Bruyninckx F, Schetz M, et al. Intensive insulin therapy in the critically ill patients. N Engl J Med 2001 November 8;345(19):1359—67.

[127] van den BG, Wilmer A, Hermans G, Meersseman W, Wouters PJ, Milants I, et al. Intensive insulin therapy in the medical ICU. N Engl J Med 2006 February 2;354(5):449—61.

[128] Finfer S, Chittock DR, Su SY, Blair D, Foster D, Dhingra V, et al. Intensive versus conventional glucose control in critically ill patients. N Engl J Med 2009 March 26;360(13):1283—97.

[129] Griesdale DE, de Souza RJ, van Dam RM, Heyland DK, Cook DJ, Malhotra A, et al. Intensive insulin therapy and mortality among critically ill patients: a meta-analysis including NICE-SUGAR study data. CMAJ 2009 April 14;180(8):821—7.

[130] Wiener RS, Wiener DC, Larson RJ. Benefits and risks of tight glucose control in critically ill adults: a meta-analysis. JAMA 2008 August 27;300(8):933—44.

42

Nutritional Prevention and Treatment of Kidney Stones

Marvin Grieff, David A. Bushinsky

University of Rochester School of Medicine, Rochester, NY, USA

INTRODUCTION

Diet is a key determinant of urinary composition, which governs urinary saturation and the propensity for stone formation. The prevalence of kidney stones is increasing in the United States and kidney stones now appear to affect 5.2% of the total population [9]. It is likely that this increase in stone formation is attributable to dietary and lifestyle changes and the increase is far too rapid to be explained by mutations in the genome. For example, the increased incidence of stones in women has been attributed to an increase in female body mass index [1,2].

Though there are pharmacological treatments for recurrent kidney stones, alterations in diet will significantly reduce rates of stone formation [10]. There are many mechanisms by which alterations in diet will influence the rate of kidney stone formation. There are general dietary effects on kidney stones formation and specific dietary recommendations based on stone type. In this chapter we will discuss how various dietary components alter urine saturation and stone formation. We will also discuss the relationship between diet, obesity and how bariatric surgery effects stone formation; as well as recent data on how dietary melamine can lead to stone formation.

PATHOPHYSIOLOGY OF KIDNEY STONE FORMATION

Urinary tract stones result from a phase change in which dissolved substances form into a solid. This phase change is driven by increasing urinary saturation of the substances forming the stone [11]. Saturation is defined as the ratio of the concentration of a substance in the urine to its solubility. Saturation is calculated from measured components in the urine by a complex computer algorithm generally either the EQUIL II or JESS programs. Stones cannot form in urine that is undersaturated and increasing saturation, leading to supersaturation with respect to a solid phase correlates strongly with the rate of stone formation.

Supersaturation can be altered by many factors, and most obviously by changing urine volume [12]. More dilute urine will lead to a decrease in the concentration of dissolved substances and thus decrease the degree of supersaturation and the likelihood of stone formation. Urine calcium and oxalate are the determinants of calcium oxalate supersaturation, urine calcium, phosphate, and pH are the main effectors of calcium phosphate supersaturation while uric acid supersaturation is governed principally by urate excretion and urine pH.

Urine volume is affected primarily by fluid intake and extrarenal fluid loss. Urine calcium is determined by intestinal calcium absorption, renal tubule calcium reabsorption and bone resorption [13]. Approximately 20–25% of dietary calcium is absorbed by the intestine, which is governed, to a large extent, by the level of 1,25-dihydroxyvitamin D_3. Circulating calcium is about 40% bound to plasma protein, mostly albumin. Non protein bound calcium, either as free ionized calcium or calcium complexed to anions, is ultrafiltered at the glomerulus. Approximately, 50–60% is reabsorbed in the proximal convoluted tubule and then lesser amounts in the thick ascending limb of the loop of Henle as well as the distal convoluted tubule. Calcium reabsorption in the nephron is influenced by sodium balance with calcium reabsorption increasing with volume depletion and by parathyroid hormone which increases tubular calcium reabsorption. Increasing calcium reabsorption in the renal tubules will decrease urine calcium excretion and

Nutritional Management of Renal Disease
http://dx.doi.org/10.1016/B978-0-12-391934-2.00042-4

supersaturation with respect to the calcium oxalate and calcium phosphate solid phases. Increased dietary sodium, a fixture of many American diets, will increase urine calcium excretion.

Urine oxalate excretion is derived from the sum of intestinal absorption and endogenous production. Dietary approaches to prevent kidney stones have focused on limiting intestinal oxalate absorption which is influenced by dietary oxalate content and by dietary calcium which binds oxalate and prevents its absorption (see Enteric hyperoxaluria below).

GENERAL DIETARY EFFECTS ON KIDNEY STONES

Fluid Intake

One of the most effective dietary recommendations to prevent kidney stones is for a patient to increase their fluid intake. The resultant increase in urine volume leads to a decrease in urine supersaturation and would be expected to decrease the incidence of stones. Pak et al. demonstrated that increasing the urine volume led to a decrease in saturation with respect to calcium oxalate, calcium phosphate and monosodium urate [14]. Epidemiological studies have demonstrated that stone formers have lower urine volumes compared to controls [15–17]. A randomized study by Borghi et al. demonstrated that increasing the fluid intake, without any other maneuver to decrease stone risk, to maintain a urine output of more than two liters decreased the 5-year stone recurrence from 27% to 12% [18].

Influence of Fluid Type on Stone Recurrence

The association of various kinds of fluids with stone recurrence has been examined in large populations. In a prospective observational study Curhan et al. examined the effect of various beverages on the risk of recurrent stone formation in men [19]. They found that caffeinated and decaffeinated coffee, tea, beer and wine decreased the risk of recurrent stones, while apple juice increased the risk by 35% per 8 oz. glass ingested daily and grapefruit juice increased the risk by 37% per 8 oz. glass ingested daily. In a similar prospective study of stone-forming women, Curhan et al. demonstrated that ingestion of caffeinated and decaffeinated coffee, tea and wine were associated with a decrease in stone recurrence while grapefruit juice was associated with an increase in stone recurrence [16]. Neither study demonstrated an increase in stone risk with ingestion of colas.

Mineral Water

The influence of mineral water on stone formation is influenced by the calcium and bicarbonate content in the water. Cauderella et al. randomized stone formers to three types of mineral water and found no evidence that hard water, with a higher calcium content, was more lithogenic than soft water [20]. Those subjects who drank water with the highest calcium intake had an increase in urine calcium and parallel decrease in urinary oxalate with no significant change in urinary saturation with respect to calcium oxalate. Kessler et al. demonstrated that bicarbonate-rich mineral water increases urine pH and urine citrate and decreases the supersaturation of both calcium oxalate and uric acid [21]. Karagulle et al. demonstrated that bicarbonate-rich mineral water alkalinized the urine and decreased the supersaturation of uric acid; however it also increased supersaturation with respect to calcium phosphate [22].

Coffee and Tea

The data by Curhan suggests that caffeinated coffee and tea are beneficial in preventing kidney stones [16,19]. However, Massey and Sutton administered caffeine to both stone-formers and non-stone formers and demonstrated an increase in urine calcium excretion [23]. This small study used only a single dose of caffeine and may not reflect the effect of long-term use of caffeinated beverages on stone recurrence.

Various types of tea appear to differ as to whether they are effective in preventing kidney stones. Mackay et al. determined the oxalate content of various teas, and demonstrated that black teas have a much higher oxalate content than herbal teas and thus may be more lithogenic [24]. Though studies by Curhan et al. demonstrated that tea ingestion is associated with a protective effect on kidney stones, since the oxalate content of teas differ, it is not clear that all teas affect stone recurrence rates similarly [16,19].

Grapefruit Juice

Grapefruit juice does not appear to be as beneficial as other beverages in preventing recurrent kidney stones [16,19]. The mechanism by which grapefruit juice increases the risk of kidney stones is unknown. Goldfarb and Asplin administered grapefruit juice to normal volunteers [25] and found an increase in urine oxalate and citrate compared to administration of water. However there was no change in urinary supersaturation with respect to calcium oxalate, calcium phosphate or uric acid.

Alcohol Intake

Hirvonen in a study of Finnish smokers found that beer intake was inversely related to stone risk and each bottle of beer decreased the risk of kidney stones by 40% [26]. Curhan found that wine ingestion was also associated with a lower incidence of stones [16,19].

Lemonade Versus Orange Juice

Lemonade, a source of citrate, has been touted as being beneficial for kidney stones. Citrate decreases urinary supersaturation and thus stone formation by binding with calcium and forming a soluble calcium-citrate complex. However, studies examining the effect of lemonade on nephrolithiasis do not show a consistent benefit beyond the increase in urine volume. Patients with hypocitraturic nephrolithiasis given lemonade made with 120 mL of concentrated lemon juice with 2 liters of water have a significant increase in urinary citrate [27,28]. Penniston has shown that drinking lemonade will increase urine citrate and urine volume [29]. These studies suggest that lemonade could be used as a source of citrate in hypocitraturic stone formers. However, Koff et al. found that lemonade was not as effective as potassium citrate in increasing urine citrate. They compared the administration of potassium citrate to lemonade in stone formers and found that lemonade failed to alkalinize the urine or increase urine citrate [30].

Orange juice may have beneficial effects on preventing kidney stones. Odvina et al. compared the effect of drinking orange juice to lemonade on stone risk. They found that orange juice provided better urinary alkalinization and a higher urine citrate than lemonade [31]. Coe et al. randomized hypercalciuric stone formers to drinking two six ounce glasses of calcium fortified orange juice per day or two eight ounce glasses of milk per day and determined urinary supersaturation in each group [32]. They did not find any difference in urinary calcium oxalate, brushite or urate supersaturation with milk compared to calcium fortified orange juice.

Soft Drinks

The effect of soft drinks on stone prevention is unclear. Shuster et al. demonstrated that stone formers with a decrease in soda intake had a decrease in stone recurrence [33]. Passman et al. compared the effect of Le Bleu bottled water, Fresca and caffeine-free diet Coke on stone risk in non-stone forming adults to a control fluid intake which was self-selected [34]. They found that urine volumes were significantly higher and supersaturation of calcium oxalate lower for any of the fluids compared to the control. However they did not find a significant benefit on stone risk with ingestion of Fresca or caffeine-free diet Coke compared to water.

Calcium Intake

Dietary calcium should not be restricted in an attempt to prevent stone recurrence. Many have assumed that restriction of dietary calcium would decrease the incidence of stone recurrence; however both observational data and controlled trials clearly demonstrate the opposite. Curhan et al. performed an observational cohort study of 45,619 men between the ages of 40 and 75 and demonstrated that dietary calcium was inversely associated with the risk of kidney stones [15]. Curhan et al. found the same result in an observational cohort study of 96,245 women [17]. Borghi et al. performed a randomized study comparing stone formation rates in patients prescribed a normal calcium, low salt, low protein diet to those prescribed a low calcium diet [35]. At 5 years of follow-up, the risk of recurrent nephrolithiasis decreased by approximately 50% in those on the normal calcium, low salt, low protein diet compared to those on the low calcium diet (Figure 42.1). While this latter study did not directly compare a normal calcium to a low calcium diet, in aggregate these studies provide strong evidence that dietary calcium restriction should not be recommended to prevent recurrent kidney stones.

There are conflicting data on the risk of recurrent nephrolithiasis with calcium supplementation in patients

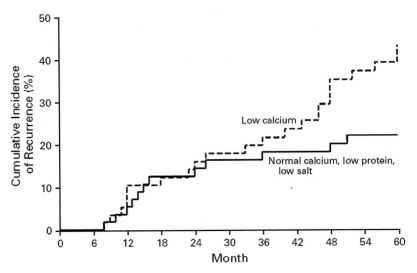

FIGURE 42.1 A normal calcium, low protein, low salt diet decreases stone recurrence when compared to a normal calcium diet. Relative risk was 0.49 (95% confidence interval, 0.24 to 0.98, p = 0.04). Reprinted with permission from Borghi et al. [35].

with kidney stones. In a review by Heaney, stone risk was examined in twelve randomized studies of calcium supplementation and there was no significant increase in kidney stones [36]. It is important to note that these studies did not focus on stone formers. However in a large randomized study of 36,282 postmenopausal women enrolled in the Women's Health Initiative, Jackson et al. found that calcium and vitamin D supplementation increased the risk of kidney stones [37]. In a retrospective analysis, Curhan et al. demonstrated that calcium supplementation increased the risk for stone formation in women [38]. The variability in the risk of calcium supplementation inducing stone formation is not currently understood.

The mechanism by which a low calcium intake increases the predisposition to form recurrent kidney stones appears due to interaction between calcium and oxalate in the intestine. Most patients who form calcium-stones have idiopathic hypercalciuria, a condition in which intestinal absorption of calcium is abnormally high [39]. Taylor et al. examined the influence of various dietary factors on urinary calcium excretion [40]. They confirmed that stone formers had elevated urinary calcium compared to non-stone formers. However, they found that the variation in urinary calcium as a result of changes in dietary calcium was relatively small; about 11 mg more per 24 hours in the quartile with the highest calcium intake as compared to those with the lowest calcium intake. Most calcium stones consist of calcium oxalate and the effect of variations of dietary calcium intake on stone formation appear due to intestinal binding of calcium to oxalate. Lemann found that the higher the dietary calcium intake the lower the urinary oxalate excretion [41].

Hess et al. administered different diets to normal subjects [42] and found that a high oxalate diet resulted in a high urine oxalate, but that adding dietary calcium to a high oxalate diet decreased urine oxalate and led to decreased urinary crystallization. Calcium supplements also decrease the absorption of oxalate and decrease urinary oxalate [43].

Thus patients with kidney stones should not decrease their dietary calcium intake below the age and gender recommended intake as doing so may increase the fraction of dietary oxalate which is absorbed. It is not clear whether calcium supplements have the same protective effect against kidney stones as the increased calcium absorption may outweigh the effect of binding dietary oxalate. Indeed, the study by Curhan et al. and the data from the Women's Health Initiative suggests that calcium supplements may actually increase the risk for kidney stones [37,38]. We recommend that patients obtain about 1 g of elemental calcium per day. We generally recommend that calcium be obtained from dietary sources such as milk or cheese rather than in pill form

as the latter may be more rapidly absorbed and result in peaks of calcium excretion though there is no firm experimental evidence for this recommendation. It is prudent to monitor the effect of any calcium supplementation on urine calcium excretion in a patient who forms kidney stones.

Protein Intake

A diet high in protein appears to be a factor in the increasing prevalence of kidney stones. A high protein intake increases the risk of kidney stones by at least two mechanisms, by increasing urinary calcium excretion and thus calcium oxalate supersaturation and by decreasing urinary pH which would favor uric acid precipitation. In humans metabolic acidosis increases urinary calcium excretion [44]. Lutz et al. demonstrated in healthy women that a high protein intake will increase both renal acid excretion as well as urinary calcium [45]. Administration of sodium bicarbonate reverses the increase in urinary calcium induced by the high protein intake. Subsequently, Sebastian et al. demonstrated that potassium bicarbonate will decrease urine calcium in women who have a high protein intake [46]. Others have found that high protein diets increase both urine calcium and oxalate excretion in those with underlying hyperoxaluria which promotes calcium oxalate precipitation [47].

The increase in stone formation due to high protein diets may also be due to the acidic urine promoting the precipitation of uric acid. The increase in renal acid excretion with high protein intake is due to the sulfur containing amino acids cystine and methionine which generate metabolic acids during metabolism. Breslau compared the effect of three forms of dietary protein; vegetarian protein, vegetable and egg protein, and animal protein on urine acid excretion. They found that high animal protein intake favors uric acid stone formation as it lowers urine pH. The reduction in urinary pH is correlated with an increase in urinary sulfate [48]. The high animal, as opposed to vegetable, protein increased urine calcium excretion; however there was an associated decrease in urinary oxalate excretion. None of the diets appeared to favor either calcium oxalate or calcium phosphate precipitation. Nguyen et al. demonstrated that the effect of a high animal protein diet on urinary oxalate was variable and unpredictable [47]. Thus a high animal protein diet clearly will promote uric acid stone formation.

The clinical effectiveness of low protein diet in prevention of recurrent nephrolithiasis is not clear. In a randomized controlled study Hiatt et al. found that a low animal, high fiber diet was associated with a higher incidence of recurrent stones compared to the control diet [49]. In a randomized study, Dussol et al. could not demonstrate a beneficial effect of low animal protein diets on recurrent stones [50]. However the study by Borghi et al. comparing a low calcium diet to a normal calcium low animal protein low salt diet demonstrated a lower rate of stone recurrence on the latter diet [35]. Thus while low animal protein diets alone have not demonstrated a reduction in kidney stone recurrence combination therapy using a low animal protein diet with a normal calcium low salt diet clearly reduces nephrolithiasis. It is our practice to recommend that animal protein intake not exceed approximately 1.0 g/kg/day [51].

Sodium Intake

High sodium intake appears to increase the incidence and prevalence of kidney stones. In mammals calcium clearance parallels sodium clearance indicating that increasing dietary sodium intake will lead to an increase in urine calcium excretion [52]. In stone formers a reduction of dietary sodium restriction will decrease urine calcium excretion [53,54]. Urinary calcium decreases linearly with urine sodium, so that even small changes in dietary sodium will lead to a decrease in urine calcium excretion. [54]. Nouvenne et al. has shown in calcium oxalate stone formers that after 3 months of dietary sodium restriction urine calcium decreased by 38% in males and 34% in females [55]. The decrease in urine calcium excretion with dietary sodium restriction has been associated with a decrease in stone recurrence. Again, Borghi et al. has shown that the combination of a normal calcium, low animal protein diet decreased stone recurrence [35]. Which components of this diet, alone or in combination, accounted for the reduction in recurrent stone formation is not known.

Thiazide diuretics are used commonly to decrease urine calcium excretion in stone formers. Thiazides are effective in reducing urine calcium excretion only if sodium is restricted as well. Brickman et al. compared males treated with a thiazide diuretic to those treated with a thiazide diuretic who had their urinary sodium losses replaced [56]. The thiazide diuretic decreased urine calcium by an average of 52% by four days of treatment, however this reduction in urine calcium excretion did not occur if urinary sodium losses were replaced (Figure 42.2) [56,57].

A recent study suggests that sodium restriction may not be beneficial in all stone formers. In a group of hypocitraturic calcium oxalate stone formers, Stoller demonstrated that sodium supplementation led to an increase in urine volume and a decrease in supersaturation with respect to calcium oxalate [58]. Urine calcium before sodium supplementation averaged 98 mg/day and after sodium supplementation increased to only 135 mg/day. Though this single study is intriguing, it

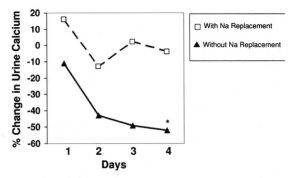

FIGURE 42.2 The decrease in urine calcium with hydrochlorothiazide treatment does not occur with sodium replacement. Data from Brickman et al. [56]. *P < 0.01 versus baseline. Reprinted with permission from Grieff and Bushinsky [57].

is only a single study in non hypercalciuric stone formers and may not be applicable to the vast majority of recurrent stone formers. Salt supplementation has many other negative consequences that argue against recommending this treatment even if further studies find it to be effective in reducing recurrent stone formation.

In patients with nephrolithiasis we generally recommend limiting daily sodium intake to a maximum of 3000 mg (approximately 130 mEq) [51]. Adherence to this dietary recommendation can be monitored when a 24-hour urine collection is collected in the follow-up of the recurrent kidney stone former.

Vitamin C Intake

Vitamin C can be metabolized to oxalate and thus has been examined as a risk factor for kidney stone formation. Curhan et al. did not find an increased risk of stone formation in women taking vitamin C [59]. However, Taylor et al. found that kidney stone formation was associated with a higher vitamin C intake in men when examined at 14 years of follow-up [60]. The reason for this discordance is not clear. In patients with hyperoxaluria, restriction of vitamin C supplements appears prudent.

Sugar Intake

A higher sugar intake has been associated with a predisposition to develop nephrolithiasis. In 1969, Lemann et al. demonstrated an increase in urine calcium excretion after intake of both glucose and sucrose, especially in stone formers and their relatives [61]. Additional fructose has been implicated in increasing the rate of kidney stone formation. Fructose intake has increased greatly over the past decades with the common use of high-fructose corn syrup. Taylor and Curhan prospectively studied women enrolled in the

Nurses Health Studies I and II and found that a higher fructose intake predicted the development of kidney stones [62]. Nguyen et al. infused seven healthy subjects with intravenous fructose and found an increase in urine calcium and oxalate excretion [63]. Though a higher sugar intake has been associated with a higher risk for kidney stones to date there have been no studies to demonstrate that a modification of sugar intake will alter the rate of stone formation.

EFFECT OF DIET BASED ON URINARY FINDINGS

The complete evaluation of the recurrent kidney stone former includes both a dietary history as well as a 24-hour urine collection which includes measurements of volume, calcium, sodium, urate and oxalate [51,64]. Dietary recommendations are based on the goal to optimize 24-hour urine values (Table 42.1). Fluid intake should be increased to achieve optimal urine volume (see under "Fluid intake" above). Urinary ion and fluid excretion are a continuum, there are no absolute values for individual parameters at which point a stone will or will not form. Each contributes to supersaturation which is what ultimately controls whether a stone will or will not form.

Hypercalciuria

Calcium Intake

Most patients with nephrolithiasis have idiopathic hypercalciuria in which there is generally increased intestinal absorption of dietary calcium. However it is clear that low calcium diets are associated with a higher incidence of kidney stones [15,17,35]. Taylor et al. analyzed the relationship between dietary calcium intake and urinary calcium excretion from large population databases including the Health Professional Follow-up Study (men) and the Nurses Health Studies I and II (women). They found that stone formers did absorb and excrete a larger proportion of ingested calcium, but these differences were small in the usual ranges of

TABLE 42.1 Optimal 24-Hour Urine Values

Volume	>2 liters
Calcium	<300 mg or <3.5–4 mg/kg in men; <250 mg or <3.5–4 mg/kg in women.
Sodium	<3000 mg or 130 mEq
Uric acid	<800 mg in men; 750 mg in women.
Oxalate	<40 mg

After Monk and Bushinsky [51].

dietary calcium [40]. They found several other factors influenced urinary calcium as well, including urinary magnesium, sulfate, citrate, phosphorus, and volume.

Calcium intake should not be restricted for a number of reasons in patients with idiopathic hypercalciuria. If patients cannot adequately reabsorb filtered calcium in the renal tubule, a low calcium diet will result in a loss of bone mineral as there is no other source of calcium in the body. Indeed many patients with idiopathic hypercalciuria have decreased bone mineral density and an increased rate of fractures. A reduction in dietary calcium will also allow absorption, and subsequent excretion, of dietary oxalate. Thus patients should not restrict dietary calcium, rather they should eat age and gender appropriate amounts of dietary calcium, generally about a gram of elemental calcium a day.

Sodium Intake

Urinary sodium and calcium excretion are closely linked [52] and dietary sodium should be restricted in hypercalciuric stone formers. Dietary sodium restriction will decrease urine calcium excretion [53,54]. Nouvenne et al. demonstrated that 3 months of dietary sodium restriction in calcium oxalate stone formers decreased urine calcium by 38% in males and 34% in females [55].

Dietary sodium restriction also has a major role in the hypocalciuric effect of thiazides, and sodium restriction should be reinforced in patients treated with thiazides. Brickman et al. studied males treated with a thiazide diuretic and compared them to those treated with a thiazide diuretic with replacement of urinary sodium losses [56]. The thiazide diuretic was only effective in decreasing urine calcium if urinary sodium was not replaced (Figure 42.2) [56,57].

Potassium Intake

Potassium administration decreases urine calcium excretion while potassium deprivation increases urine calcium excretion [65]. Taylor et al. examined the diets in the large populations of: the Health Professionals Follow-up Study, Nurses' Health Studies I and II. In one study he and his colleagues demonstrated that a higher potassium diet was associated with a lower urine calcium [40].

The DASH (Dietary Approaches to Stop Hypertension) diet which is high in fruits and vegetables is associated with a lower risk of kidney stones [3]. The DASH diet results in decreased urine calcium possibly because it is low in sodium and high in potassium. Unfortunately the DASH diet includes fruits and vegetables which are also high in oxalate. Recommending the DASH diet to stone formers should only be done with the caveat that foods high in oxalate not be consumed (Table 42.2).

TABLE 42.2 Foods High in Oxalate

Beans (including foods derived from beans including tofu, soy milk)

Beer

Beets

Berries (including juice containing berries)

Black tea

Celery

Chocolate, cocoa

Eggplant

Figs

Greens: collard greens, dandelion greens, endive, escarole, kale, leeks, mustard greens, parsley, sorrel, spinach, Swiss chard, watercress.

Green peppers

Lemon, lime and orange peel

Nuts

Okra

Rhubarb

Sweet potato

Adapted from Monk RD, Bushinsky DA. Kidney Stones. In: Melmed S, Polonsky KS, Larsen RP, Kronenberg HM, eds. Williams Textbooks of Endocrinology, 12th edn. Philadelphia, PA: Elsevier, 2011: 1350—1367.

Hyperuricosuria

Hyperuricosuria generally defined as a urine uric acid excretion above 800 mg/day in men, and 750 mg/day in women and is a risk factor for the formation of calcium oxalate stones [11]. Uric acid is the end-product of purine metabolism and hyperuricosuria often results from a diet high in purine intake. Animal protein from beef, poultry and fish contain high amounts of purines [66]. Though dietary restriction of these foods decreases urine uric acid, to date there are no studies which show that dietary purine restriction will prevent recurrent calcium oxalate stones.

Hyperoxaluria

Oxalate is present in most plant but not animal tissues [67]. Once ingested, about 30% is degraded by anaerobic intestinal florae. The remaining oxalate is absorbed by active transport in the small intestine and by passive diffusion along the length of the small and large intestine. Intestinal oxalate absorption is quite variable and can range from as low as 10—20% to as high as 100%.

The causes of hyperoxaluria can be divided into: (1) Primary hyperoxaluria due to defects in inborn errors of metabolism causing excess oxalate generation; (2) Enteric hyperoxaluria due to intestinal hyperabsorption usually as a result of fat malabsorption; and (3) Idiopathic hyperoxaluria which may be due to a number of factors including low calcium diet, excess dietary oxalate as well as variations in intestinal oxalate transport [11,67]. The magnitude of the oxalate excretion in enteric hyperoxaluria and idiopathic hyperoxaluria can be altered by manipulation of the patient's diet.

Epidemiological studies have helped determine the role of various dietary factors on urine oxalate excretion. Curhan et al. analyzed the impact of various factors on urinary oxalate in 3348 stone formers and non-stone forming participants from the Nurses Health Studies I and II as well as the Health Professionals Follow-up Study [68]. They found that body mass index, total fructose intake, and 24-h urinary potassium, magnesium, and phosphorus were each directly associated with an increase in urinary oxalate excretion while age and dietary calcium were inversely associated with urinary oxalate. Interestingly, the quartile of participants with the highest oxalate intake excreted only 1.7 mg/day more oxalate than those in the lowest quartile of intake (P trend 0.0001). In addition, participants consuming greater than 1000 mg/day of vitamin C excreted only 6.8 mg/d more urinary oxalate than participants consuming <90 mg/d (P trend <0.001). Thus, the effects of dietary oxalate on urinary oxalate are relatively minor and suggest that dietary oxalate restriction may have limited effectiveness in decreasing urine oxalate excretion and preventing recurrent stone formation.

Neither animal nor human studies have clarified the role for dietary oxalate restriction in stone formation. A rat model of recurrent calcium stones was utilized to determine the effect of varying dietary oxalate on the risk of kidney stone formation. The genetic hypercalciuric stone-forming (GHS) rat has been studied extensively to determine the pathophysiology of kidney stone formation and can be utilized to study therapeutic approaches for the prevention of recurrent stone formation. These rats have been inbred for over 95 generations and now excrete eight to ten times as much urine calcium as control rats and universally form calcium containing kidney stones. Bushinsky et al. administered varying amounts of oxalate to the GHS rats and found that the risk for stone formation based on changes in urinary supersaturation did not vary with dietary oxalate [69]. In this study, the increase in urine oxalate excretion due to increasing dietary oxalate was offset by a decrease in urine calcium excretion. Similarly in a study in humans, administration of an oxalate load led to an increase in urine oxalate, but this was mitigated by administering calcium with the meal [70]. Others have demonstrated that a reduction in dietary oxalate in conjunction with other dietary recommendations to prevent nephrolithiasis led to a reduction in the risk for recurrent stone formation [71,72]. Thus, the effectiveness of a low oxalate diet alone on preventing recurrent kidney stone formation is not clear. However dietary oxalate restriction along with other dietary recommendations to reduce kidney stones, may be a reasonable recommendation for a hyperoxaluric stone former.

Even if a clinician decides to recommend restriction of dietary oxalate in a hyperoxaluric stone former it is often difficult to determine the oxalate content of foods. Measurements of the oxalate content in foods depends on how the food is prepared, when in the preparation process the oxalate is measured as well as the method of measurement [73]. Nonetheless, Massey recommends avoidance of the following foods: spinach, rhubarb, beets (roots and leaves), black teas (not green or herbal), chocolate, some tree nuts, bran concentrates and cereals, and legumes (beans, peanuts, soybeans and some soyfoods). In terms of tea, Mackay et al. determined the oxalate content of various teas, and found that black teas have a much higher oxalate content than herbal teas and thus may be more lithogenic [24]. Patients with hyperoxaluria are generally given a list of high oxalate foods to avoid (Table 42.2) and their oxalae excretion is followed by 24 h urine measurements of not only oxalate but supersaturation with respect to calcium oxalate as well.

Calcium intake is a determinant of oxalate absorption [67]. In the intestinal lumen oxalate is present in the salt form bound to calcium and not as free oxalate. Decreasing calcium intake will lead to more free oxalate and intestinal absorption. Several investigators have demonstrated in humans that increasing dietary calcium, for example by drinking milk, will decrease urine oxalate excretion [42,74—76].

Enteric Hyperoxaluria

Enteric hyperoxaluria is due to excessive oxalate absorption in patients with bowel disease and leads to increased rates of stone formation. In patients with ileal disease, the increase in urine oxalate excretion can be mitigated by a decrease in dietary oxalate. Urine oxalate is also increased after small bowel resection and intestinal bypass and the increase is proportional to the severity of steatorrhea [77]. In these cases excess oxalate absorption occurs in the colon and can be reversed by perfusion with calcium [78]. It is thought that in these cases the luminal calcium complexes with the free fatty acids, rather than with the oxalate, allowing the oxalate to be absorbed. The absorbed oxalate is excreted in the urine resulting in hyperoxaluria. Thus in patients with steatorrhea induced enteric hyperoxaluria it is prudent to not only recommend a low fat and low oxalate diet but that calcium should be taken with meals.

DIETARY RECOMMENDATIONS BASED ON STONE TYPE

Calcium Stones

Dietary recommendations in the presence of idiopathic calcium stones should be based on the urinary abnormalities as described above (see Effect of diet based on urinary findings above) [51,64,79].

Uric Acid Stones

Uric acid precipitates in acid urine, and excessively acid urine, and not excess uric acid excretion is the primary risk factor for the formation of uric acid stones. Pak et al. compared the serum and urine chemistries of uric acid stone formers to controls and found that uric acid stone formers had a higher serum uric acid, a lower 24-hour urine uric acid excretion and a lower urinary pH [80]. The decreased urine pH is felt to be due to an insufficient production of urinary ammonium [81]. Malouf et al. compared subjects with the metabolic syndrome to controls, and found that these patients had a lower urine pH as less of their net acid excretion was less in the form of ammonium and more in the form of titratable acidity [82]. The decreased rate of ammonium excretion was thought to be due to renal tubule insulin resistance. It is not clear whether reversal of the metabolic syndrome will lead to a decrease in the rate of recurrent nephrolithiasis in these patients.

Cystine Stones

Cystine stones result from an excess of urinary cystine, due to a genetic defect in renal reabsorption of dibasic amino acids including cystine [11]. Cystine is relatively insoluble in aqueous solutions such as urine with an upper limit of solubility is 243 mg/L [11]. The urinary excretion of cystine in cystinuria ranges between 350—500 mg/day and can easily exceed the upper limit of solubility unless patients are instructed to drink large amounts of fluid. Sodium restriction has been found to significantly decrease urine cystine excretion [83].

The dietary recommendation to prevent recurrent cystine stones focus on a high fluid intake and salt restriction. Sufficient fluid intake should be ingested so that the measured urinary cystine excretion remains soluble, generally more than 3 liters a day [84]. Higher urine output has been shown to reduce recurrence of cystine stones [85].

OBESITY AND KIDNEY STONES

Obesity and Kidney Stones

The increase in the prevalence of kidney stones is associated with the increasing prevalence of obesity [9]. Several investigators have shown that the risk of kidney stones is directly correlated with an increased body mass index [2,86]. For unclear reasons this association appears greater in females than in males. It is not known if weight loss will reduce the risk of recurrent stone formation. In particular, the Atkins diet, which has a low carbohydrate and high protein content would be expected to increase the risk for kidney stones.

Bariatric Surgery and Kidney Stones

The risk of kidney stone formation is increased after some types of bariatric surgery. Hyperoxaluria as well as hypocitraturia frequently occur after Roux-en-Y gastric bypass surgery leading to increase urinary supersaturation and stone formation despite weight loss [7]. As opposed to Roux-en-Y gastric bypass surgery, restrictive gastric surgery for bariatric indications is not associated with marked hyperoxaluria [5,6].

After Roux-en-Y surgery hyperoxaluria is likely due to fat malabsorption [4]. Current recommendations to prevent stones in patients with hyperoxaluria after this procedure include a high fluid intake, low oxalate and a low fat diet. Calcium with meals may also bind intestinal oxalate and aid in decreasing oxalate absorption and subsequent excretion.

MELAMINE STONES

Melamine is an inedible synthetic compound used in a variety of commercial products [8]. Due to its high nitrogen content it has been used as an adulterant to boost the apparent protein content of products such as milk-based infant formula and pet foods. Melamine forms crystals in the urinary tract and may result in nephrolithiasis and acute kidney injury. Outbreaks of melamine stones in Chinese children were reported and in late September, 2008 the World Health Organization reported 54,000 cases of melamine-induced illness [87].

References

[1] Scales Jr CD, Curtis LH, Norris RD, et al. Changing gender prevalence of stone disease. J Urol 2007;177:979—82.

[2] Nowfar S, Palazzi-Churas K, Chang DC, Sur RL. The relationship of obesity and gender prevalence changes in united states inpatient nephrolithiasis. Urology 2011;78:1029.

[3] Taylor EN, Fung TT, Curhan GC. DASH-style diet associates with reduced risk for kidney stones. J Am Soc Nephrol 2009;20:2253—9.

[4] Kleinman JG. Bariatric surgery, hyperoxaluria, and nephrolithiasis: a plea for close postoperative management of risk factors. Kidney Int 2007;72:8—10.

[5] Penniston KL, Kaplon DM, Gould JC, Nakada SY. Gastric band placement for obesity is not associated with increased urinary risk of urolithiasis compared to bypass. J Urol 2009;182:2340—6.

[6] Semins MJ, Asplin JR, Steele K, et al. The effect of restrictive bariatric surgery on urinary stone risk factors. Urology 2010;76:826—9.

[7] Sinha MK, Collazo-Clavell ML, Rule A, et al. Hyperoxaluric nephrolithiasis is a complication of Roux-en-Y gastric bypass surgery. Kidney Int 2007;72:100—7.

[8] Bhalla V, Grimm PC, Chertow GM, Pao AC. Melamine nephrotoxicity: an emerging epidemic in an era of globalization. Kidney Int 2009;75:774—9.

[9] Stamatelou KK, Francis ME, Jones CA, Nyberg LM, Curhan GC. Time trends in reported prevalence of kidney stones in the United States: 1976-1994. Kidney Int 2003;63:1817—23.

[10] Goldfarb S. Dietary factors in the pathogenesis and prophylaxis of calcium nephrolithiasis. Kidney Int 1988;34:544—55.

[11] Coe FL, Evan A, Worcester E. Kidney stone disease. J Clin Invest 2005;115:2598—608.

[12] Bushinsky DA, Coe FL, Moe O. Nephrolithiasis. In: Brenner and Rector's The Kidney. 8th ed. Philadelphia: Saunders Elsevier; 2007. p. 1299.

[13] Mount AS, Yu ASL. Transport of inorganic solutes: Sodium, chloride, potassium, magnesium, calcium and phosphate. In: Brenner and Rector's The Kidney. 8th ed. Philadelphia: Saunders Elsevier; 2007. p. 156.

[14] Pak CY, Sakhaee K, Crowther C, Brinkley L. Evidence justifying a high fluid intake in treatment of nephrolithiasis. Ann Intern Med 1980;93:36—9.

[15] Curhan GC, Willett WC, Rimm EB, Stampfer MJ. A prospective study of dietary calcium and other nutrients and the risk of symptomatic kidney stones. N Engl J Med 1993;328:833—8.

[16] Curhan GC, Willett WC, Speizer FE, Stampfer MJ. Beverage use and risk for kidney stones in women. Ann Intern Med 1998;128:534—40.

[17] Curhan GC, Willett WC, Knight EL, Stampfer MJ. Dietary factors and the risk of incident kidney stones in younger women: Nurses' Health Study II. Arch Intern Med 2004;164:885—91.

[18] Borghi L, Meschi T, Amato F, Briganti A, Novarini A, Giannini A. Urinary volume, water and recurrences in idiopathic calcium nephrolithiasis: a 5-year randomized prospective study. J Urol 1996;155:839—43.

[19] Curhan GC, Willett WC, Rimm EB, Spiegelman D, Stampfer MJ. Prospective study of beverage use and the risk of kidney stones. Am J Epidemiol 1996;143:240—7.

[20] Caudarella R, Rizzoli E, Buffa A, Bottura A, Stefoni S. Comparative study of the influence of 3 types of mineral water in patients with idiopathic calcium lithiasis. J Urol 1998;159:658—63.

[21] Kessler T, Hesse A. Cross-over study of the influence of bicarbonate-rich mineral water on urinary composition in comparison with sodium potassium citrate in healthy male subjects. Br J Nutr 2000;84:865—71.

[22] Karagulle O, Smorag U, Candir F, et al. Clinical study on the effect of mineral waters containing bicarbonate on the risk of urinary stone formation in patients with multiple episodes of CaOx-urolithiasis. World J Urol 2007;25:315—23.

[23] Massey LK, Sutton RA. Acute caffeine effects on urine composition and calcium kidney stone risk in calcium stone formers. J Urol 2004;172:555—8.

[24] McKay DW, Seviour JP, Comerford A, Vasdev S, Massey LK. Herbal tea: an alternative to regular tea for those who form calcium oxalate stones. J Am Diet Assoc 1995;95:360—1.

[25] Goldfarb DS, Asplin JR. Effect of grapefruit juice on urinary lithogenicity. J Urol 2001;166:263—7.

[26] Hirvonen T, Pietinen P, Virtanen M, Albanes D, Virtamo J. Nutrient intake and use of beverages and the risk of kidney stones among male smokers. Am J Epidemiol 1999;150:187—94.

[27] Kang DE, Sur RL, Haleblian GE, Fitzsimons NJ, Borawski KM, Preminger GM. Long-term lemonade based dietary manipulation

in patients with hypocitraturic nephrolithiasis. J Urol 2007; 177(1358):62. discussion 1362; quiz 1591.

[28] Seltzer MA, Low RK, McDonald M, Shami GS, Stoller ML. Dietary manipulation with lemonade to treat hypocitraturic calcium nephrolithiasis. J Urol 1996;156:907–9.

[29] Penniston KL, Steele TH, Nakada SY. Lemonade therapy increases urinary citrate and urine volumes in patients with recurrent calcium oxalate stone formation. Urology 2007;70: 856–60.

[30] Koff SG, Paquette EL, Cullen J, Gancarczyk KK, Tucciarone PR, Schenkman NS. Comparison between lemonade and potassium citrate and impact on urine pH and 24-hour urine parameters in patients with kidney stone formation. Urology 2007;69:1013–6.

[31] Odvina CV. Comparative value of orange juice versus lemonade in reducing stone-forming risk. Clin J Am Soc Nephrol 2006;1:1269–74.

[32] Coe FL, Parks JH, Webb DR. Stone-forming potential of milk or calcium-fortified orange juice in idiopathic hypercalciuric adults. Kidney Int 1992;41:139–42.

[33] Shuster J, Jenkins A, Logan C, et al. Soft drink consumption and urinary stone recurrence: a randomized prevention trial. J Clin Epidemiol 1992;45:911–6.

[34] Passman CM, Holmes RP, Knight J, Easter L, Pais V, Assimos DG. Effect of soda consumption on urinary stone risk parameters. J Endourol 2009;23:347–50.

[35] Borghi L, Schianchi T, Meschi T, et al. Comparison of two diets for the prevention of recurrent stones in idiopathic hypercalciuria. N Engl J Med 2002;346:77–84.

[36] Heaney RP. Calcium supplementation and incident kidney stone risk: a systematic review. J Am Coll Nutr 2008;27:519–27.

[37] Jackson RD, LaCroix AZ, Gass M, et al. Calcium plus vitamin D supplementation and the risk of fractures. N Engl J Med 2006; 354:669–83.

[38] Curhan GC, Willett WC, Speizer FE, Spiegelman D, Stampfer MJ. Comparison of dietary calcium with supplemental calcium and other nutrients as factors affecting the risk for kidney stones in women. Ann Intern Med 1997;126:497–504.

[39] Coe FL, Parks JH, Favus MJ. Diet and calcium: the end of an era? Ann Intern Med 1997;126:553–5.

[40] Taylor EN, Curhan GC. Demographic, dietary, and urinary factors and 24-h urinary calcium excretion. Clin J Am Soc Nephrol 2009;4:1980–7.

[41] Lemann Jr J, Pleuss JA, Worcester EM, Hornick L, Schrab D, Hoffmann RG. Urinary oxalate excretion increases with body size and decreases with increasing dietary calcium intake among healthy adults. Kidney Int 1996;49:200–8.

[42] Hess B, Jost C, Zipperle L, Takkinen R, Jaeger P. High-calcium intake abolishes hyperoxaluria and reduces urinary crystallization during a 20-fold normal oxalate load in humans. Nephrol Dial Transplant 1998;13:2241–7.

[43] Levine BS, Rodman JS, Wienerman S, Bockman RS, Lane JM, Chapman DS. Effect of calcium citrate supplementation on urinary calcium oxalate saturation in female stone formers: implications for prevention of osteoporosis. Am J Clin Nutr 1994;60:592–6.

[44] Lemann Jr J, Gray RW, Maierhofer WJ, Cheung HS. The importance of renal net acid excretion as a determinant of fasting urinary calcium excretion. Kidney Int 1986;29:743–6.

[45] Lutz J. Calcium balance and acid-base status of women as affected by increased protein intake and by sodium bicarbonate ingestion. Am J Clin Nutr 1984;39:281–8.

[46] Sebastian A, Harris ST, Ottaway JH, Todd KM, Morris Jr RC. Improved mineral balance and skeletal metabolism in postmenopausal women treated with potassium bicarbonate. N Engl J Med 1994;330:1776–81.

[47] Nguyen QV, Kalin A, Drouve U, Casez JP, Jaeger P. Sensitivity to meat protein intake and hyperoxaluria in idiopathic calcium stone formers. Kidney Int 2001;59:2273–81.

[48] Breslau NA, Brinkley L, Hill KD, Pak CY. Relationship of animal protein-rich diet to kidney stone formation and calcium metabolism. J Clin Endocrinol Metab 1988;66:140–6.

[49] Hiatt RA, Ettinger B, Caan B, Quesenberry Jr CP, Duncan D, Citron JT. Randomized controlled trial of a low animal protein, high fiber diet in the prevention of recurrent calcium oxalate kidney stones. Am J Epidemiol 1996;144:25–33.

[50] Dussol B, Iovanna C, Rotily M, et al. A randomized trial of low-animal-protein or high-fiber diets for secondary prevention of calcium nephrolithiasis. Nephron Clin Pract 2008;110: c185–94.

[51] Monk RD, Bushinsky DA. Kidney stones. In: Melmed S, Polonsky KS, Larsen RP, Kronenberg HM, editors. Williams Textbook of Endocrinology. 12th ed. Philadelphia, PA: Elsevier, Inc.; 2011. p. 1350.

[52] Walser M. Calcium clearance as a function of sodium clearance in the dog. Am J Physiol 1961;200:1099–104.

[53] Breslau NA, McGuire JL, Zerwekh JE, Pak CY. The role of dietary sodium on renal excretion and intestinal absorption of calcium and on vitamin D metabolism. J Clin Endocrinol Metab 1982;55:369–73.

[54] Muldowney FP, Freaney R, Moloney MF. Importance of dietary sodium in the hypercalciuria syndrome. Kidney Int 1982; 22:292–6.

[55] Nouvenne A, Meschi T, Prati B, et al. Effects of a low-salt diet on idiopathic hypercalciuria in calcium-oxalate stone formers: a 3-mo randomized controlled trial. Am J Clin Nutr 2010;91: 565–70.

[56] Brickman AS, Massry SG, Coburn JW. Changes in serum and urinary calcium during treatment with hydrochlorothiazide: studies on mechanisms. J Clin Invest 1972;51:945–54.

[57] Grieff M, Bushinsky DA. Diuretics and disorders of calcium homeostasis. Semin Nephrol 2011;31:535–41.

[58] Stoller ML, Chi T, Eisner BH, Shami G, Gentle DL. Changes in urinary stone risk factors in hypocitraturic calcium oxalate stone formers treated with dietary sodium supplementation. J Urol 2009;181:1140–4.

[59] Curhan GC, Willett WC, Speizer FE, Stampfer MJ. Intake of vitamins B6 and C and the risk of kidney stones in women. J Am Soc Nephrol 1999;10:840–5.

[60] Taylor EN, Stampfer MJ, Curhan GC. Dietary factors and the risk of incident kidney stones in men: new insights after 14 years of follow-up. J Am Soc Nephrol 2004;15:3225–32.

[61] Lemann Jr J, Piering WF, Lennon EJ. Possible role of carbohydrate-induced calciuria in calcium oxalate kidney-stone formation. N Engl J Med 1969;280:232–7.

[62] Taylor EN, Curhan GC. Fructose consumption and the risk of kidney stones. Kidney Int 2008;73:207–12.

[63] Nguyen NU, Dumoulin G, Henriet MT, Regnard J. Increase in urinary calcium and oxalate after fructose infusion. Horm Metab Res 1995;27:155–8.

[64] Monk RD, Bushinsky DA. Nephrolithiasis and nephrocalcinosis. In: Floege J, Johnson RJ, Feehally J, editors. Comprehensive Clinical Nephrology. 4th ed. St. Louis, MO: Elsevier, Inc.; 2010. p. 687.

[65] Lemann Jr J, Pleuss JA, Gray RW, Hoffmann RG. Potassium administration reduces and potassium deprivation increases urinary calcium excretion in healthy adults [corrected]. Kidney Int 1991;39:973–83.

[66] Coe FL, Moran E, Kavalich AG. The contribution of dietary purine over-consumption to hyperpuricosuria in calcium oxalate stone formers. J Chronic Dis 1976;29:793–800.

[67] Massey LK, Roman-Smith H, Sutton RA. Effect of dietary oxalate and calcium on urinary oxalate and risk of formation of calcium oxalate kidney stones. J Am Diet Assoc 1993;93: 901–6.

[68] Taylor EN, Curhan GC. Determinants of 24-hour urinary oxalate excretion. Clin J Am Soc Nephrol 2008;3:1453–60.

[69] Bushinsky DA, Bashir MA, Riordon DR, Nakagawa Y, Coe FL, Grynpas MD. Increased dietary oxalate does not increase urinary calcium oxalate saturation in hypercalciuric rats. Kidney Int 1999;55:602–12.

[70] de OG, Mendonca C, Martini LA, Baxmann AC, et al. Effects of an oxalate load on urinary oxalate excretion in calcium stone formers. J Ren Nutr 2003;13:39–46.

[71] Lieske JC, Tremaine WJ, De Simone C, et al. Diet, but not oral probiotics, effectively reduces urinary oxalate excretion and calcium oxalate supersaturation. Kidney Int 2010;78: 1178–85.

[72] Pak CY, Odvina CV, Pearle MS, et al. Effect of dietary modification on urinary stone risk factors. Kidney Int 2005;68: 2264–73.

[73] Massey LK. Food oxalate: factors affecting measurement, biological variation, and bioavailability. J Am Diet Assoc 2007. 107:1191,4; quiz 1195–6.

[74] Smith LH. Diet and hyperoxaluria in the syndrome of idiopathic calcium oxalate urolithiasis. Am J Kidney Dis 1991;17: 370–5.

[75] Savage GP, Charrier MJ, Vanhanen L. Bioavailability of soluble oxalate from tea and the effect of consuming milk with the tea. Eur J Clin Nutr 2003;57:415–9.

[76] Nouvenne A, Meschi T, Guerra A, et al. Diet to reduce mild hyperoxaluria in patients with idiopathic calcium oxalate stone formation: a pilot study. Urology 2009. 73:725,30, 730.e1.

[77] Parks JH, Worcester EM, O'Connor RC, Coe FL. Urine stone risk factors in nephrolithiasis patients with and without bowel disease. Kidney Int 2003;63:255–65.

[78] Modigliani R, Labayle D, Aymes C, Denvil R. Evidence for excessive absorption of oxalate by the colon in enteric hyperoxaluria. Scand J Gastroenterol 1978;13:187–92.

[79] Worcester EM, Coe FL. Clinical practice. Calcium kidney stones. N Engl J Med 2010;363:954–63.

[80] Pak CY, Sakhaee K, Peterson RD, Poindexter JR, Frawley WH. Biochemical profile of idiopathic uric acid nephrolithiasis. Kidney Int 2001;60:757–61.

[81] Sakhaee K, Adams-Huet B, Moe OW, Pak CY. Pathophysiologic basis for normouricosuric uric acid nephrolithiasis. Kidney Int 2002;62:971–9.

[82] Maalouf NM, Cameron MA, Moe OW, Adams-Huet B, Sakhaee K. Low urine pH: a novel feature of the metabolic syndrome. Clin J Am Soc Nephrol 2007;2:883–8.

[83] Jaeger P, Portmann L, Saunders A, Rosenberg LE, Thier SO. Anticystinuric effects of glutamine and of dietary sodium restriction. N Engl J Med 1986;315:1120–3.

[84] Shekarriz B, Stoller ML. Cystinuria and other noncalcareous calculi. Endocrinol Metab Clin North Am 2002;31:951–77.

[85] Barbey F, Joly D, Rieu P, Mejean A, Daudon M, Jungers P. Medical treatment of cystinuria: critical reappraisal of long-term results. J Urol 2000;163:1419–23.

[86] Curhan GC, Willett WC, Rimm EB, Speizer FE, Stampfer MJ. Body size and risk of kidney stones. J Am Soc Nephrol 1998; 9:1645–52.

[87] Langman CB, Alon U, Ingelfinger J, et al. A position statement on kidney disease from powdered infant formula-based melamine exposure in Chinese infants. Pediatr Nephrol 2009; 24:1263–6.

43

Herbal Supplements in Patients with Kidney Disease

Alison l. Steiber

Department of Nutrition, School of Medicine, Case Western Reserve University, Cleveland, OH, USA

INTRODUCTION

The impact of herbal supplements on kidney function as well as the interaction between herbal supplements and commonly used treatments for patients with kidney disease will be reviewed in this chapter. Herbal medicine, as defined by Jonas and Levin in the *Essentials of Complementary and Alternative Medicine*, is "a healing approach that uses medicinal plants singly or in combination to treat disease and as a preventive to promote health and well-being" [1]. Any form of the plant or plant product can be included in this definition, for example the leaves, stem, flowers, roots, seeds or even extract of the plant can be used to enhance health.

It is difficult to pinpoint the exact number of adults who are using herbal medicines; part of the difficulty stems from a variety of terms used in research surveys. However, use of herbal medicine in the general population and specifically in those patients with chronic diseases is thought to be very high. In a 2004 report from the Center on Disease Control, 62% of adults were found to use some form of complementary and alternative medicine (CAM) during the previous year [2]. More recently and more specific to herbals, the 2007 National Health Interview Survey (NHIS) showed that approximately 18% of American adults had used a non-vitamin/non-mineral natural product [3]. Of the adults using natural products, fish oil/omega 3 fatty acids were the most popular at 37.4%.

Herbal medicine is often considered by the general public to be "more natural" and therefore "safe" when compared to conventional medicine. Unfortunately, this way of thinking is flawed. Many of the herbal products on the market today have multiple ingredients and

these ingredients may or may not be at concentrations to be pharmacologically active. An example of a herbal product having multiple chemicals was highlighted by Dr. Stephen Bent in a paper from Grand Rounds at the University of California, San Francisco Medical Center [4]. In this paper, Dr. Bent describes ginkgo biloba as having at least 33 different chemical constituents.

In contrast to drugs, the Dietary Supplement Health and Education Act (DSHEA), passed in 1994, allows herbal medicines to be produced and sold with no evidence of safety or efficacy. In fact, of the most commonly purchased herbal products sold in the USA only 5 out 10 have evidence of efficacy (ginkgo biloba, garlic, St. John's Wort, soy and kava kava) [4]. It should be noted that even the evidence that exists has limitations regarding methodological issues, various product preparations and primary outcomes.

There are three basic ways in which herbal medicines may be unsafe: (i) due to the presence of contaminants [5]; (ii) due to the presence of biologically active compounds; or (iii) due to herbal-to-drug or herbal-to-herbal interactions. A recent example of the risk of contamination was outlined in a case study by Prakash et al. [5] where a patient presented with a significant decline in renal function and abnormal presentation of symptoms. Upon investigation, it was discovered that the patient had been consuming an Ayuvedic herbal product from India. Each tablet of this herbal product had 236.7 mcg of lead which had resulted in lead poisoning and subsequent rapid progression of renal failure in the patient.

A well-documented negative effect of a biologically active compound, aristolochic acid, has been shown to cause Fanconi's syndrome nephropathy characterized by increased low molecular weight proteins in urine,

Nutritional Management of Renal Disease
http://dx.doi.org/10.1016/B978-0-12-391934-2.00043-6

chronic interstitial renal fibrosis, and proximal tubular toxicity [6]. This compound was in Chinese herbals used for weight loss. In a case study describing 105 Belgium women taking the Chinese herbal, 43 developed end-stage renal disease and 39 had prophylactic kidney removal [7].

Finally, with multiple chemical compounds, some of which are biologically active, it is not difficult to understand the risk that herbal medicines may interact with drugs, foods and other supplements. Herbals can interfere with absorption, metabolism, and potentially the excretion of other metabolites found in conventional medicine and nutrients from food [1]. A classic example of a herbal product interacting with the metabolism is St. John's Wort which is metabolized by the cytochrome P450 enzyme system in the liver and thus interferes with the metabolism of other drugs which use the same system.

To more completely understand herbal metabolism, a brief discussion on the cytochrome P450 enzymatic system may be worthwhile, as both St. John's Wort and aristolochic acid are nephrotoxic and are metabolized by this system. Cytochrome P450, a detoxifying system with subclasses that metabolize foreign toxins, is the most important xenobiotic-metabolizing enzyme system, and is found primarily in the liver [8]. However, there are both cytochrome P450 systems and non-P450 enzymes in the kidney as well. This enzyme system is responsible for metabolizing many commonly used medications, such as morphine-derived pain reducing agents, oral contraceptives and chemotherapeutic agents [4].

An overview of herbal supplements and how they relate to the kidney follows with specific emphasis on acute kidney injury, chronic kidney disease, and transplant.

ACUTE KIDNEY INJURY

Publications describing herbal effects on acute kidney function are outlined in Table 43.1. This table demonstrates the use of supplements for a variety of reasons, from weight loss to constipation to diabetes and a wide range of biological chemicals which have potentially negative side effects related to kidney function.

Aristolochic Acid Nephrology

The negative effects of aristolochic acid have been so well documented that it has its own type of nephropathy, aristolochic acid nephropathy (AAN). This type of nephropathy, previously called Chinese herbal nephropathy, usually presents with sub-acute renal failure with severe anemia or as Fanconi's syndrome, and typically results in a rapid progression to end-stage renal disease [20,21]. Histological examination shows that AAN causes an interstitial renal failure due to severe fibrosis complicated by neoplastic transformation in the urothelium. Additionally, aristolochic acid is a risk factor for Balkan endemic nephropathy [8]. The metabolites from aristolochic acid metabolism, by cytochrome P450, are aristolactums primarily found in urine and feces. It is unknown whether these metabolites are the cause of AAN or whether the aristolactums are further metabolized by the kidney and the subsequent products cause the toxicity (see Figure 43.1).

In 2001, a list of products containing aristolochic acid was published by the Federal Drug Administration as a warning to consumers (see Table 43.2).

Herbal Teas

It is important to be aware that herbal teas, as well as herbal pills, can have harmful effects. Vanderperren et al. [9] describe a case study where a 52-year-old woman was using a tea containing senna to self-treat constipation. The women had been using the tea for three years when she developed symptoms such as a loss of appetite, weakness, low blood glucose and elevated serum creatinine. One month after discontinuation of the tea, the kidney function laboratory markers were within normal limits.

CHRONIC KIDNEY DISEASE

Herbal use in the dialysis population is particularly difficult for both patient and healthcare provider in terms of determining safety and efficacy. A paucity of data is available describing herbal excretion, dialytic clearance, and interaction with other drugs. In a 2007 study by Duncan et al. [22], dialysis patients were surveyed on CAM use. A total of 294 patients were given paper surveys and 153 patients completed the survey (52%). Of the responders, 18% said they were currently using some form of CAM, 63% indicated they would be willing to try a type of CAM, and 19% said they would never use CAM. Of those who were currently using CAM, the most commonly consumed herbals were St. John's Wort, ginkgo, vitamin B_{12}, and melatonin. While these findings are interesting the study sample was quite small with only 12 patients in the CAM user group. Thus the data cannot be generalized to the larger hemodialysis population. However, this study does highlight the importance of a thorough assessment to identify use of herbal supplements. Table 43.3 outlines herbs which may impact patients with chronic kidney disease who are receiving dialysis.

TABLE 43.1 Herbal Supplements and Acute Kidney Injury

Active Compound	Herb/plant	Reference	Reason for Use	Symptoms	Other
Anthraquinone glycoside	*Sennae fructus angustifoliae* as tea (1 liter tea, 70 g dry senna)	Vanderperren et al. Ann Pharmacother 2005; 39, 1353–7 [9]	Self-medication for constipation	Weakness, loss of appetite, confusion, cold extremities, blood glucose 40 mg/dL, creatinine 3.2 mg/dL, polyuria developed after admission to ICU, high urine levels of metals, including cadmium	Renal function loss may be due to long-term laxative use, or cytotoxic effect on kidneys by herb or cadmium, although samples of senna from patient's house not found to be adulterated with cadmium or other metal.
Aristolochic acid	*Akebia* species, Boui, Mokutsu, Mu-tong, *Aristolochia* species (*Stephania* species)	Bagnis et al. AJKD. 2004; 44 (1), 1–11 [6]	Ingredient in herbal "slimming pills", Chinese herbals for hepatitis B	Aristolochic acid-nephropathy: Fanconi's syndrome, increased low molecular weight proteins in urine, chronic interstitial renal fibrosis, proximal tubular toxicity	Also a risk factor for carcinomas of the urinary tract in animals and humans
Aloesin (aloeresin A/B)	*Cape aloes*	Luyckx et al. [6,10]	Laxative	Acute ologuric renal failure, interstitial nephritis (IV administration)	
Sciadopitysin	*Taxus celebica*	Lin et al. [6,11]	Diabetes therapy	Acute tubular necrosis, fever, GI upset, hemolysis	
Atractyloside	*Callilepsis laureola*	Seedat and Hitchcock [6,12]	Vermifuge or purgative (Zulu)		
Glycyrrhizic acid/ glycyrrhetinic acid	*Glycyrrhiza glabra*, *G. radix* (licorice), *G. uralensis* (gancao)	Stewart et al. [6,13]	Cough mixtures, teas	Aldosterone-like effect, inhibition of renal steroid dehydrogenase enzyme, proximal tubulopathy	

(Continued)

TABLE 43.1 Herbal Supplements and Acute Kidney Injury—cont'd

Active Compound	Herb/plant	Reference	Reason for Use	Symptoms	Other
Glycyrrhizic acid, aristolochic acid	Boui-ougi-tou (Chinese herbs/drugs mixture)	Stewart et al. and [6,13,14]	Cure for obesity	Fanconi's tubulopathy	
Ephedrine	Ma huang (usually as tea)	Powell et al. [15]	Asthma, cold/flu, fever/chills, aches, edema	Hypertension, kidney stones	
Anticholinergic substances (scopolamine, hyoscyamine, atropine)	*Datura metel*, *Rhododendron molle*	Chan et al. [16]		Acute urine retention	
	Vaccinium macrocarpon (cranberry)	Harkins et al. [17]		Oxalate stones in high risk patients	
Paraphenylenediamine	Takaout Roumia	Bagnis et al. and Sir Hashim [6,18]	Substitute for *Tamaris orientalis* in hair dye	Acute tubular necrosis, rhabdomyolysis	
Sodium or potassium dichromate	Substituted for herbal ingredients	Wood et al. [19]		Acute renal failure, albuminuria, pyuria, hematuria, interstitial nephritis	

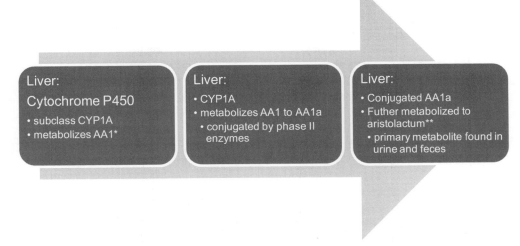

FIGURE 43.1   Metabolism of aristolochic acid as adapted from Xio et al., Kidney Int. 2008 [8]. * = aristolochic acid 1, the most toxic derivative of aristolochic acid. ** = exact location of this action is not known, possibly both the liver and kidney.

TABLE 43.2   Federal Drug Administration List of Herbal Products Containing Aristolochic Acid

Product Name	Manufacturer/Distributor
Rheumixx	PharmaBotanixx, Irvine, CA (Distributor), Sun Ten Laboratories, Inc., Irvine, CA (Manufacturer)
BioSlim	Doctor's Natural Weight Loss System Slim Tone Formula Thane International, LaQuinta, CA (Distributor)
Prostatin	Herbal Doctor Remedies, Monterey Park, CA (Distributor)
Fang Ji Stephania	Lotus Herbs Inc., LaPuente, CA (Distributor)
Mu Tong *Clematis armandi*	Lotus Herbs Inc., LaPuente, CA (Distributor)
Temple of Heaven Chinese Herbs Radix aristolochiae	Mayway Corporation, Oakland, CA (Distributor) and Almira Alchemy, Alachua, FL (Distributor)
Meridian Circulation	East Earth Herb Inc. (Brand name Jade Pharmacy), Eugene, OR
Qualiherb Chinese Herbal Formulas Dianthus Formulas Ba Zheng San	QualiHerb (Division of Finemost), Cerritos, CA (Distributor)
Clematis & Carthamus Formula 21280 (two samples)	QualiHerb (Division of Finemost), Cerritos, CA (Distributor)
Virginia Snake Root, Cut *Aristolochia serpentaria* (two samples)	Penn Herb Co., Philadelphia, PA (Manufacturer)
Green Kingdom Akebia Extract	Green Kingdom Herbs, Bay City, MI (Manufacturer) Ava Health, Grove City, OH (Distributor)
Green Kingdom Stephania Extract	Green Kingdom Herbs, Bay City, MI Ava Health (Distributor)
Neo Concept Aller Relief	BMK International, Inc., Wellesley, MA (Distributor), Sun Ten Labs, Irvine, CA (Manufacturer)
Mu Tong *Clematis armandi*	Botanicum.com, Winnipeg, Canada and Pembina, ND
Fang Ji Stephania	Botanicum.com, Winnipeg, Canada and Pembina, ND
Stephania tetrandra, roots, whole [1]	Ethnobotanical, Racine, WI

Product labeling states "Not for human consumption".
See www.fda.gov/Food/DietarySupplements/Alerts/ucm095297.htm Accessed on 8 October 2011, page last updated on 5 May 2009.

TABLE 43.3 Herbal Supplements with Potential for Impacting Patients on Dialysis

Supplement	Reference	Claimed Benefits	Risks/Side Effects/Drug Interactions	Kidney Effects	Other
Garlic (*Allium sativum*)	ADA Dietary Supplements Natural Medicines Database Banerjee et al. [23]	Reduces cholesterol, reduces blood pressure, treats *H. pylori* infection, treats diarrhea, cancer prevention, treat diabetes, immune system stimulation, reduces blood pressure.	May increase bleeding time, use with caution before surgery because of anti-aggregation effects, especially with warfarin, ginger, ginkgo. Decreases cytochrome P450 enzyme substrates: cyclosporine, some calcium channel blockers. Decreases efficacy of anti-retrovirals especially protease inhibitors: do not combine. In rats, high doses have been shown to be toxic perhaps due to pro-oxidant effects, or inhibition of alkaline phosphatase or alcohol dehydrogenase. High doses of garlic homogenate can change cellular architecture of kidneys in rats. May cause GI distress.	Shown to decrease lipid peroxidation in heart, kidney and liver in rats red garlic homogenate. May lower blood lipids, particularly oxidized LDL through enhanced nitric oxide production. Some animal studies have indicated that garlic is renoprotective when administered before known nephrotoxins.	Many types of garlic preparations, they have different properties and efficacy because of different chemical compositions from processing.
St John's Wort (*Hypericum perforatum*)	ADA Dietary Supplement Shibayama et al. [24] Natural Medicines Database	Reduces depression, increases well-being. Does seem to have positive effects similar in scope to antidepressants in patients with moderate depression. Mixed results in major depression.	GI symptoms, dizziness, headache, hypoglycemia, photosensitivity are side effects. Should not be used by individuals with Alzheimer's. Abrupt discontinuation may cause anxiety, headaches, insomnia. Causes hypotension in anesthesia. Additive effects with antidepressant drugs may	Pre-treatment with St John's Wort has been shown to reduce cisplatin nephrotoxicity in rats with normal baseline kidney function. How this translates to humans/CKD is unclear.	Multiple reports of organ transplant rejection after cyclosporine + St John's Wort

| Ginseng (*Panax ginseng, Panax japonicus, Panax qinquefolius, Eleutherococcus senticosus*) Active compound is Saponins ginsenosides | ADA Dietary Supplements Natural Medicines Database Liao et al. [25] Kim et al. [26] Roemheld-Hamm & Dahl [27] | Improves exercise, QOL, energy, mood, sexual function, helps control blood glucose levels. | be dangerous. Decreases effectiveness of contraceptives, protease inhibitors, digoxin, anti-epileptics, antipsychotics, immunosuppressives, and anti-coagulants. Do not combine with drugs metabolized through the cytochrome P450 pathway including beta blockers, anti-inflammatories, also do not combine with phenobarbitol, phenytoin (speeds metabolism of both, decreases seizure control) and narcotics. Extremely high doses 3 g root per day (or 600 mg extract) may cause hypertension, edema, lower doses are safe for up to 4 weeks. *Eleutherococcus senticosus* (Siberian ginseng) is contraindicated for HTN. Changes blood coagulation, unclear if inhibits or encourages platelet aggregation but do not combine with warfarin. Interacts with corticosteroids, digoxin, furosemide, diabetes medications (due to blood glucose lowering effects). Has mild hormone effects, can interfere with contraceptives, hormone therapy, avoid if history of estrogen related cancers. Some reports of insomnia, perhaps due to stimulant effects. | Study in rats with streptozotocin induced diabetes showed lower blood glucose levels and less diabetic nephropathy (lower creatinine and urinary protein levels compared to controls) when fed heat treated American ginseng. Case report of 83 YO female with renal insufficiency experiencing brachycardia and increased digoxin levels after ingestion of ginseng for approximately 1 mo. Ginseng is known to increase digoxin, perhaps due to their similar structures. The kidneys are the main organ responsible for digoxin removal. | Reports of contaminated ginseng products: 8/20 had high levels of pesticides, 2/20 had lead levels and 7/20 had low levels of ginsenosides (active compounds) |

(Continued)

TABLE 43.3   Herbal Supplements with Potential for Impacting Patients on Dialysis—cont'd

Supplement	Reference	Claimed Benefits	Risks/Side Effects/Drug Interactions	Kidney Effects	Other
Ginkgo biloba	ADA Dietary Supplements Kim et al. [28] Natural Medicines Database	Improves memory, improves circulation.	May cause GI upset including diarrhea, nauseas vomiting at high doses. Interacts with seizure medications, can decrease clotting when on anticoagulant drugs, but may also increase risk of intercranial bleeding. Interacts with certain antidepressants (buspirone, fluoxetine, St John's Wort) to create hypomania. Reduces efficacy of thiazide diuretics, should not be combined with anticonvulsants as the ginkgo toxin can cause seizures, can also change the action of diabetes drugs, can cause spontaneous bleeding when combined with ibuprofen.	Study in 33 PD patients showed that ginkgo biloba extract (150 mg/day for 8 weeks) decreased D-dimer levels compared to the control group. No changes in bleeding time, albumin or CRP were noted, however one patient dropped out due to GI side effects.	Ginkgo seeds are poisonous, leaves are used
Melatonin	ADA Dietary Supplements Herrera et al. [29] Koch et al. [30,31] Natural Medicines Database	Regulates circadian rhythms including in jet lag, helps with migraines, reduces cancer risk, enhances sex drive.	Long-term effects unknown, seems safe short term. Can interfere with immunosuppressive drugs and other sleep medications. Use caution when combining with anti-diabetic drugs, anticoagulant drugs, central nervous system depressants (additive sedative effects).	Nine new HD patients receiving IV iron and ruHEPP had increased oxidative stress compared to matched controls but those who were administered oral melatonin (0.29 mg/kg) 1 h prior to EPO had lower measures of oxidative stress compared to those who received to placebo before EPO (lower plasma malondialdehyde, RBC glutathione, and catalase). In 20 daytime HD patients, crossover design 3 mg melatonin administered at 10 pm for 6 weeks improved subjective and	

CoQ10 (ubiquinone)	ADA dietary supplements Shojaei et al. [32]	Antioxidant effects claimed: improve health in heart disease, HTN, exercise, cancer, prevents migraines.	GI distress including appetite suppression, vomiting, diarrhea, nausea may occur. May reduce efficacy of warfarin and have additive effect with anti-hypertensives.	objective measures of sleep time and quality and nights of dialysis and non-dialysis days. CoQ10 when administered alone or in combination with carnitine for 3 months lowered lipoprotein (a) levels in HD patients on statins compared to those on statins only. No adverse effects were noted.	Smoking, HMG COA reductase drugs may deplete body stores. B-6 is required for endogenous synthesis.
Noni Juice (from *Morinda citrifolia*)	ADA Dietary Supplements Natural Medicines Database	Cancer prevention, increased immunity, reduced BP, reduced cholesterol levels, pain relief, diabetes control.	Potassium content similar to orange juice, risk of hyperkalemia, should not be combined with ACE inhibitors, ARBS and potassium sparing diuretics. May also reduce efficacy of warfarin, reports of hepatoxicity from Noni juice consumption, reversed with termination of consumption.		
Echinacea (*Echinacea angustifolia, E. pallid, E. purpurea*)	ADA Dietary Supplements Natural Medicines Database	Boosts immune function, protects against colds and URI, UTIs, yeast infections.	Can cause fever, GI upset, taste alterations, dry mouth, headache, dizziness, insomnia. Patients with grass allergies should use with caution as anaphylaxis has been reported. Decreases efficacy of immunosuppressants, should be avoided in patients with autoimmune diseases, also not to be combined with hepatoxic medications. Can increase plasma levels of caffeine by 30% due to inhibition of cyt P450, avoid with other cyt P450 substrate drugs.		

(Continued)

TABLE 43.3 Herbal Supplements with Potential for Impacting Patients on Dialysis—cont'd

Supplement	Reference	Claimed Benefits	Risks/Side Effects/Drug Interactions	Kidney Effects	Other
Glucosamine	ADA Dietary Supplements Natural Medicines Database	Reduces pain in joints from osteoarthritis by protecting and producing collagen and other cartilage components. Mixed results: may be safer than but as effective as NSAIDS, other studies show no results.	May impact blood glucose control, should monitor patients with DM. Patients with shellfish allergy should not consume. Additive effect with warfarin, should not be combined.	Anecdotal reports of induced renal toxicity.	
Ginger (Zingiber officinale)	ADA Dietary Supplements Natural Medicines Database Onwuka et al. [33] Shanmugam et al. [34]	Anti-nausea (pregnancy, chemo, post-surgery), loss of appetite, treats migraines.	May increase the effect of anticoagulants and glucose lowering drugs (may increase blood glucose). May have additive effect with calcium channel blockers.	Animal studies indicate it is a protective antioxidant compound against oxidative and nephrotoxic agents including cadmium, with statistically significant decreases in lipid peroxidation and kidney damage (shrinkage) in rats compared to cadmium treated without ginger. It also protects against alcoholic kidney damage including reversing tubule degeneration at a dose of 100 mg/kg ginger extract 1/day for 30 days.	GRAS status
Soy	Roemheld-Hamm et al. [27] and Imani et al. [35] and Siefker and DiSilvestro [36]	Menopause symptoms, hypocholesterolemic, antioxidant, anti-inflammatory properties.	May lower coagulation factor IX. Soy isoflavones may be elevated in patients on dialysis treatment as they are not well cleared.	Studies indicate soy lowers cholesterol and blood pressure.	
Flaxseed	ADA Dietary Supplements Sankaran et al. [37]	Laxative, manage IBS symptoms, improves blood lipids, improves inflammatory symptoms, reduces heart disease risk.	Requires extra fluid consumption (150 mL/10 g flaxseed) or risk of impaction; may interact with warfarin therapy. Flaxseed lignins are a phytoestrogen and it is unclear their effect on hormone sensitive cancers, may compete for uptake with exogenous hormones like contraceptives.	Flaxseed oil based diets in diabetic rats and mice with polycystic kidney disease (PKD) have prevented renal injury when initiated early in the disease state, but when initiated later (2 months in PKD rats, similar to stage 3 CKD) renal injury is not ameliorated but inflammation is reduced.	

			Flaxseed may have anticoagulant effects (through n-3 fatty acid prostaglandin pathway), concerns for surgical bleeding, and additive effects with anticoagulant medications. May increase triglycerides in individuals with hypertriglyceridemia. May have additive effect with glucose lowering drugs, high fiber content may also inhibit absorption of other drugs, including furosemide.	
Black cohosh (*cimicifuga racemosa*)	ADA Dietary Supplements Roemhel-Hamm et al. [27].	Reduces premenstrual and postmenopausal symptoms.	Although not a hormone, it affects hormones so should be avoided in women with breast cancer or who are pregnant. GI upset may occur, may also cause weight gain, cramping. Long-term use discouraged, may be safe for up to six months. Must be avoided in individuals with existing liver disease or who are taking hepatoxic drugs due to its potential hepatoxicity (49 reports of hepatoxicity). May inhibit cyt P450 so avoid with substrate drugs, one case report of negative effects when combined with Lipitor.	Remifemin is brand name of standardized extract
Lutein	ADA Dietary Supplements Sundl et al. [38]	Treats age related macular degeneration and cataracts.	No data on drug interactions. So far proven safe and effective even with long-term use.	PD patients have been found to have lower lutein levels (and other carotenoids) than healthy matched controls and within PD patients lower carotenoid status correlates with higher inflammatory markers. No research on how lutein supplementation affects these parameters.

(Continued)

TABLE 43.3   Herbal Supplements with Potential for Impacting Patients on Dialysis—cont'd

Supplement	Reference	Claimed Benefits	Risks/Side Effects/Drug Interactions	Kidney Effects	Other
Milk thistle (*Silybum marianum*)	ADA Dietary Supplements Vessal [39] Natural Medicines Database	Improves liver health including treating viral hepatitis and alcoholic cirrhosis, improves appetite, used to manage diabetes.	GI upset including nausea, diarrhea, allergic reaction may occur. May interact with antiretrovirals, cytochrome P450 metabolized drugs, may speed clearance of statins, diazepam, digosin, morphine. May chelate iron.	Milk thistle extract, fed for 4 weeks at 1.2 mg/kg to streptozotocin induced diabetic rats lead to lower serum glucose, serum urea, higher eGFR and lower 24-hour urinary protein than streptomycin diabetic rats not receiving the supplement, and did not affect the parameters of control (non-diabetic) rats who received the supplement. The silymarin itself (100 mg/kg) improved parameters in the diabetic rats but was not statistically significant. It is suggested that the mechanism is through ROS scavenging.	
Saw Palmetto (*Serenoa repens*)	ADA Dietary Supplements Natural Medicines Database	Improves enlarged prostate, prevents prostate cancer, prevents male alopecia, diuretic, anti-inflammatory.	Anti-coagulant, should be discontinued before surgery. Should not be mixed with other anticoagulant medications. May interact with hormone medications through anti-estrogenic effects.		

FIVE HERBALS WITH SOME PROVEN EFFICACY

1 St. John's Wort

St. John's Wort is primary used as an anti-depressant and through multiple randomized clinical trials has been shown to be effective in mild to moderate depression. A meta-analysis was conducted by Linde et al. [40], which reviewed the pertinent clinical trials to determine whether the active ingredient in St. John's Wort was effective in reducing mild or moderate depression. To be included in this analysis the study had to meet the following criteria: (a) randomized and double-blind; (b) patients with depressive disorders; (c) compared extracts of St. John's Wort with placebo or standard antidepressants; and finally, (d) clinical outcomes such as scales assessing depressive symptoms. Thirty-seven clinical trials were ultimately contained within the meta-analysis. The effect of St. John's Wort was larger in moderate or mild depression than in severe depression. The relative risk for reduction of depression symptoms by St John's Wort from six larger trials was 1.71 (95% CI, 1.40–2.09) and from five smaller trials was 6.13 (95% CI, 3.63 to 10.38) [40].

The primary active ingredients in St. John's Wort are hypericin and pseudohypericin. The mechanism of both hypericin and pseudohypericin related to improving mild and moderate depression is the inhibition of re-uptake of serotonin into the central nervous system [41]. It may be hypothesized that depression is caused by a reduction in functional activity of monoamines such as the centrally acting neurotransmitters: serotonin, dopamine and norepinephrine. Inhibition of re-uptake of serotonin by St. John's Wort results in increased concentration of serotonin in specific nerve synapse and thus improves functionality of serotonin.

Bioavailability of St. John's Wort is poor; it is estimated at 14% for hypericin and 21% for pseudohypericin [41]. Excretion of the compound in St. John's Wort is through the kidneys and it has a half-life of 25 to 26.5 hours for hypericin and 16 to 36 hours for pseudo-hypericin [42].

In the non-CKD population a concentration of 0.2 to 2.5% of hypericin is suggested for efficacy. However, no data were found on a safe dose for patients with CKD. It is possible that in end-stage renal disease patients, St. John's Wort compounds may accumulate in the body since their typical route of excretion is no longer available, but there are no data to substantiate this possibility.

Side effects in people taking St. John's Wort are rare and may include photosensitivity. However, drug interactions are a concern. St. John's Wort may interfere with the action of monoamine oxidase inhibitors and selective serotonin reuptake inhibitors; it may antagonize reserpine and reduce serum concentrations of cyclosporine, indinavir, and possibly other drugs used to control HIV infection. Additionally the active compounds may reduce estrogen concentrations from oral contraceptives, decrease the efficacy of digoxin, irinotecan and other cancer treatment drugs, seizure control drugs, such as Dilantin and phenobarbital, and finally, warfarin and related anticoagulants may be impacted by St. John's Wort [22]. Due to the effects on cyclosporine, transplant patients must be monitored closely for use of this herb, and doses of either the cyclosporine or St. John's Wort may need to be altered to prevent risk of rejection.

2 Garlic: *Alium sativum*

Reported benefits of garlic are on cardiovascular disease symptoms such as: reduced serum lipid concentrations (total cholesterol, low density lipoprotein (LDL) and triglycerides) and blood pressure, increased fibrinolytic activity, antibiotic properties, enhanced natural killer cells, and lengthened clotting time [22,41]. In the non-CKD population there are randomized clinical trials demonstrating the effectiveness of garlic as a hypocholesterolemic supplement. Kannar et al. [43] conducted a 12-week, double-blind, randomized clinical trial in patients with hypercholesterolemia. All patients received dietary counseling on low fat intake and then the treatment group received an enteric coated garlic powder tablet while the other arm received a placebo. The treatment tablet contained 9.6 mg of allicin. The treatment group (n = 22) had a significant reduction in total cholesterol (−0.36 mmol/L) and LDL (−0.44 mmol/L) while the placebo group did not change significantly.

Alternatively, a meta-analysis was conducted by Jepson et al. [44] to assess the effects of garlic for the treatment of peripheral arterial occlusive disease; unfortunately only one study met the inclusion criteria and it was small without statistically significant results. No clinical trials testing the efficacy or safety of garlic in the dialysis patients were found.

Due to the effects on clotting time, patients who are on blood thinning medications such as heparin, coumadin, or even aspirin may be at risk. Additionally, patients who are scheduled for surgery should be advised to withhold consumption of garlic prior to the procedure [45].

The active ingredient in garlic is allicin, an organic disulfide, which is formed when the substance, alliin, in garlic cloves is crushed or pressed. Crushing the garlic clove releases the enzyme allinase which converts alliin into allicin. When interpreting data on garlic as an intervention, it is important to know the amount of

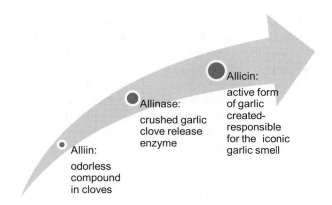

FIGURE 43.2 Formation of active compound, allicin, in garlic cloves.

active allicin in the garlic preparation. Allicin is metabolized in the liver to an inactive compound and eliminated. Since garlic is metabolized and eliminated by the liver, it may be safe for CKD patients to consume garlic for cholesterol and blood pressure as long as increased time for blood clotting is monitored (see Figure 43.2).

The mechanism of garlic as a lipid lowering agent is not well understood; however it is hypothesized that allicin reduces the activity of HMG CoA reductase. HMG CoA reductase is an enzyme in the initial step of cholesterol synthesis; therefore, allicin may reduce endogenously manufactured cholesterol.

3 Ginkgo

Ginkgo biloba has been used to improve or stabilize mental function, improve memory, and to improve cerebral and peripheral disease. Ginkgo biloba was tested in 66 chronic peritoneal dialysis patients by Kim et al. [28] to determine whether the herb improves hemostatic factors and inflammation. The patients were randomized to either a control group or to receive ginkgo biloba at a dose of 160 mg/day for eight weeks. At baseline of the study there were no statistically significant differences between the control and ginkgo biloba groups for age, gender ratio, presence of diabetes and cardiovascular disease, and time on dialysis. At the end of eight weeks, the only parameters which changed significantly were D-dimer which is an index of fibrin turnover and intravascular thrombogenesis. D-dimer decreased from 0.92 ± 0.59 μg/mL to 0.75 ± 0.48 μg/mL ($p < 0.05$) in the ginkgo group but did not change significantly in the control group. It may be that an active component of ginkgo biloba impacts coagulation factors and thus the D-dimer.

The impact on coagulating factors is also the reason that patients undergoing surgical procedures or using anti-coagulating medications, such as heparin, should discontinue use of ginkgo biloba or closely monitor coagulation parameters as ginkgo may cause extended clotting times. Additional potential side effects of ginkgo are: gastrointestinal complaints, headache, and allergic skin reactions [45].

Soy

Soy contains high amounts of isoflavones and phytoestrogens. Women with ESRD may be particularly interested in soy products due to the reported effects on reducing menopausal symptoms, such as hot flashes. The phytoestrogens in soy products are thought to be responsible for reducing the menopausal symptoms in addition to their potentially beneficial effects on osteoporosis and cardiovascular prevention. Furthermore, soy food products have sufficient data demonstrating efficacy for cholesterol reduction to warrant statements indicating this effect on food labels.

Recently, a few small trials have been published on soy supplementation in dialysis patients. An unblinded, randomized trial was conducted [35] on the impact of soy on plasma coagulating factors. This study included 36 peritoneal dialysis patients (18 on soy and 18 as control) who were followed for eight weeks. The soy group received 28-g packets of raw, textured soy flour containing 14 g of soy protein and 233 mg of phosphorus. Patients were not included in the study if their baseline serum phosphorus was greater than 5.5 mg. At baseline there were no significant differences in any demographic characteristics except for B_{12} supplement intake (more patients were taking this supplement in the soy group). At the end of the eight weeks there was no statistically significant difference in serum phosphorus, as might be expected (soy group 3.5 ± 1.0 mg/dL vs. control 3.7 ± 0.9 mg/dL). However, there was a significant decrease in coagulation factor IX (baseline soy group 135 ± 33.5 % activity vs. 8 weeks 112.5 ± 32 % activity). This decrease in coagulation factor IX may be a risk factor for patients on dialysis, especially if they are receiving other anti-coagulating medications or herbal supplements.

Another small trial, this one in hemodialysis patients, used soy verses whey protein and tested the safety and efficacy of these different proteins on oxidized LDL concentrations. The study randomized 17 hemodialysis patients to receive either soy (n = 7, 25 mg protein and 52 mg flavones) or whey (n = 9) for four weeks. There were no statistically significant changes in laboratory values between pre- and post-intervention for either group, except serum creatinine which significantly decreased in the whey group. A significant difference in mean change of oxidized LDL was found between groups with the soy group decreasing by 31.02% and the whey group increasing by 11.12% (p < 0.05) [36].

In a 2008 longitudinal study on 41 patients with type 2 diabetes and nephropathy, the soy treatment arm received 35% animal proteins, 35% textured soy protein, and 30% vegetable proteins while the control arm received 70% animal proteins and 30% vegetable proteins for four years [46]. This small randomized clinical trial resulted in improved cardiovascular risk factors from the consumption of soy, such as: plasma glucose (mean change in the soy protein versus control groups: -18 ± 3 vs. 11 ± 2 mg/dL; P < 0.03), total cholesterol (-23 ± 5 vs. 10 ± 3 mg/dL; p < 0.01), LDL cholesterol (-20 ± 5 vs. 6 ± 2 mg/dL; p < 0.01), serum triglyceride (-24 ± 6 vs. -5 ± 2 mg/dL; p < 0.01) concentrations, serum CRP concentrations (-1.31 ± 0.6 vs. 0.33 ± 0.1 mg/L; p < 0.02), proteinuria (-0.15 ± 0.03 vs. 0.02 ± 0.01 g/day; p < 0.001), and urinary creatinine (-1.5 ± 0.9 vs. 0.6 ± 0.3 mg/dL, p < 0.01).

From these small studies in pre-dialysis and dialysis patients, soy use appears to have some efficacy and from the longitudinal study in pre-dialysis patients, it appears to have a lower risk of side effects. However, similar to the other herbal products, soy may impact coagulation factors thus careful monitoring of clotting parameters would be warranted in patients consuming high amounts of soy.

5 Kava Kava

Kava extracts come from the rhizomes of a perennial shrub in the South Pacific Islands. The term kava comes from both the kava plant and the kava extracts [47] and is typically consumed as either a capsule or table containing either ethanolic or acetonic extracts. The active ingredients in kava are kavapyrones, also known as kavalactones, which have psychoactive properties. In the western populations, kava kava has been used for anxiety. In 2009, a randomized, double-blind crossover study was published on the aqueous extract of kava [48]. The 60 adult subjects had one month of elevated, generalized anxiety (>10 on the Beck Anxiety Inventory) prior to enrolling in the study. During the treatment phase of the study (length = 1 week) the patients received five tablets of kava per day, each containing 50 mg of kavalactones. The pooled analysis across phases (using differences from pretreatment scores) demonstrated a significant effect across phases in favor of kava [F(1.35) = 26.18; p < 0.0001] and a strong effect size [48].

It is important to note that the clinical trial above used the aqueous extract form of kava and the duration of the intervention period was only one week. There have been many reports by Teschke et al. [49] on the hepatic toxicity of the ethanolic or acetonic extract. In an analysis of kava kava [50], when quantitative tools for assessing causality were used, the data strongly supported a cause and effect relationship between kava consumed and hepatotoxicity.

Therefore, although data have demonstrated the effectiveness of aqueous kava extract on anxiety in healthy adults, patients must be cautioned that there are strong data on hepatotoxicity and that there are no clinical trials involving patients with CKD.

TRANSPLANT

Patients who have received a transplant need to be particularly aware of herbal supplements which are metabolized by the cytochrome P450 enzymatic system. The P450 system metabolizes some of the anti-rejection medications prescribed post-transplant such as cyclosporine; therefore, ingestion of herbals which use the same enzymatic system may result in decreased drug concentrations and thus put the patient at an increased risk of rejection. Some examples of herbal supplements which use the cytochrome P450 system are St. John's Wort, echinacea and melatonin.

CLINICAL IMPLICATIONS

As stated in the introduction of this chapter, surveys have been conducted indicating a high use of herbal supplements in both the general and CKD populations. It is not uncommon for patients to withhold information on their herbal supplement use from healthcare providers. Given the potential for contaminants and herb-to-drug or herb-to-herb interactions it is imperative that heath care providers know what patients are consuming so they can educate patients on potential risks. To date, there are no validated, CKD specific questionnaires which include information on herbal or other CAM use. Therefore, clinicians need to conduct thorough, individualized assessments with specific questions regarding herbal use in their CKD patients.

In summary, herbal use is probably high in patients with CKD and many herbs have active components which may interact with other medications or which may have direct negative effects on the health of the patients. There are few studies using herbs as the primary intervention in patients with CKD. However, there are some studies which demonstrate both reasonable safety and some effectiveness in CKD such as soy. More studies need to be conducted with CKD patients to assure safety and determine effectiveness of the most commonly used herbals.

References

[1] Wayne Jonas MaJSL PhD, MPH B, editor. Essentials of Complementary and Alternative Medicine. Philadelphia: Lippincott Williams &Wilkins; 1999.

[2] Barnes PM, Powell-Griner E, McFann K, Nahin RL. Complementary and alternative medicine use among adults: United States, 2002. Adv Data 2004 May;27(343):1–19.

[3] Medicine NCfCaA. What is Complementary and Alternative Medicine, [NCCAM Publication No. D347]. Available from: www.NCCAM.NIH.gov/health/whatiscam/#natural;2010 [updated 01.04.11; cited 15.08.11].

[4] Bent S. Herbal medicine in the United States: review of efficacy, safety, and regulation: grand rounds at University of California, San Francisco Medical Center. J Gen Intern Med 2008 Jun;23(6): 854–9.

[5] Prakash S, Hernandez GT, Dujaili I, Bhalla V. Lead poisoning from an Ayurvedic herbal medicine in a patient with chronic kidney disease. Nat Rev Nephrol 2009 May;5(5):297–300.

[6] Isnard Bagnis C, Deray G, Baumelou A, Le Quintrec M, Vanherweghem JL. Herbs and the kidney. Am J Kidney Dis 2004 Jul;44(1):1–11.

[7] Nortier JL, Martinez MC, Schmeiser HH, Arlt VM, Bieler CA, Petein M, et al. Urothelial carcinoma associated with the use of a Chinese herb (Aristolochia fangchi). N Engl J Med 2000 Jun 8;342(23):1686–92.

[8] Xiao Y, Ge M, Xue X, Wang C, Wang H, Wu X, et al. Hepatic cytochrome P450s metabolize aristolochic acid and reduce its kidney toxicity. Kidney Int 2008 Jun;73(11):1231–9.

[9] Vanderperren B, Rizzo M, Angenot L, Haufroid V, Jadoul M, Hantson P. Acute liver failure with renal impairment related to the abuse of senna anthraquinone glycosides. Ann Pharmacother 2005 Jul-Aug;39(7-8):1353–7.

[10] Luyckx VA, Ballantine R, Claeys M, Cuyckens F, Van den Heuvel H, Cimanga RK, et al. Herbal remedy-associated acute renal failure secondary to Cape aloes. Am J Kidney Dis 2002 Mar;39(3):E13.

[11] Lin JL, Ho YS. Flavonoid-induced acute nephropathy. Am J Kidney Dis 1994 Mar;23(3):433–40.

[12] Seedat YK, Hitchcock PJ. Acute renal failure from Callilepsis laureola. S Afr Med J 1971 Jul 31;45(30):832–3.

[13] Stewart PM, Wallace AM, Valentino R, Burt D, Shackleton CH, Edwards CR. Mineralocorticoid activity of liquorice: 11-beta-hydroxysteroid dehydrogenase deficiency comes of age. Lancet 1987 Oct 10;2(8563):821–4.

[14] Tomlinson B, Chan TY, Chan JC, Critchley JA, But PP. Toxicity of complementary therapies: an eastern perspective. J Clin Pharmacol 2000 May;40(5):451–6.

[15] Powell T, Hsu FF, Turk J, Hruska K. Ma-huang strikes again: ephedrine nephrolithiasis. Am J Kidney Dis 1998 Jul;32(1): 153–9.

[16] Chan JC, Chan TY, Chan KL, Leung NW, Tomlinson B, Critchley JA. Anticholinergic poisoning from Chinese herbal medicines. Aust N Z J Med 1994 Jun;24(3):317–8.

[17] Harkins KJ. What's the use of cranberry juice? Age Ageing 2000 Jan;29(1):9–12.

[18] Sir Hashim M, Hamza YO, Yahia B, Khogali FM, Sulieman GI. Poisoning from henna dye and para-phenylenediamine mixtures in children in Khartoum. Ann Trop Paediatr. 1992; 12(1):3–6.

[19] Wood R, Mills PB, Knobel GJ, Hurlow WE, Stokol JM. Acute dichromate poisoning after use of traditional purgatives. A report of 7 cases. S Afr Med J 1990 Jun 16;77(12):640–2.

[20] Bakhiya N, Arlt VM, Bahn A, Burckhardt G, Phillips DH, Glatt H. Molecular evidence for an involvement of organic anion transporters (OATs) in aristolochic acid nephropathy. Toxicology 2009 Oct 1;264(1-2):74–9.

[21] Kong PI, Chiu YW, Kuo MC, Chen SC, Chang JM, Tsai JC, et al. Aristolochic acid nephropathy due to herbal drug intake manifested differently as Fanconi's syndrome and end-stage renal failure – a 7-year follow-up. Clin Nephrol 2008 Dec;70(6): 537–41.

[22] Duncan HJ, Pittman S, Govil A, Sorn L, Bissler G, Schultz T, et al. Alternative medicine use in dialysis patients: potential for good and bad!. Nephron Clin Pract 2007;105(3):c108–13.

[23] Banerjee SK, Mukherjee PK, Maulik SK. Garlic as an antioxidant: the good, the bad and the ugly. Phytother Res. 2003 Feb;17(2):97–106.

[24] Shibayama Y, Kawachi A, Onimaru S, Tokunaga J, Ikeda R, Nishida K, et al. Effect of pre-treatment with St John's Wort on nephrotoxicity of cisplatin in rats. Life Sci. 2007 Jun 20;81(2): 103–8.

[25] Liao WI, Lin YY, Chu SJ, Hsu CW, Tsai SH. Bradyarrhythmia caused by ginseng in a patient with chronic kidney disease. Am J Emerg Med 2010 May;28(4)(538):e5–6.

[26] Kim HY, Kang KS, Yamabe N, Nagai R, Yokozawa T. Protective effect of heat-processed American ginseng against diabetic renal damage in rats. J Agric Food Chem. 2007 Oct 17;55(21): 8491–7.

[27] Roemheld-Hamm B, Dahl NV. Herbs, menopause, and dialysis. Semin Dial 2002 Jan-Feb;15(1):53–9.

[28] Kim SH, Lee EK, Chang JW, Min WK, Chi HS, Kim SB. Effects of Ginkgo biloba on haemostatic factors and inflammation in chronic peritoneal dialysis patients. Phytother Res. 2005 Jun; 19(6):546–8.

[29] Herrera J, Nava M, Romero F, Rodriguez-Iturbe B. Melatonin prevents oxidative stress resulting from iron and erythropoietin administration. Am J Kidney Dis 2001 Apr;37(4):750–7.

[30] Koch BC, Hagen EC, Nagtegaal JE, Boringa JB, Kerkhof GA, Ter Wee PM. Effects of nocturnal hemodialysis on melatonin rhythm and sleep-wake behavior: an uncontrolled trial. Am J Kidney Dis 2009 Apr;53(4):658–64.

[31] Koch BC, Nagtegaal JE, Hagen EC, van der Westerlaken MM, Boringa JB, Kerkhof GA, et al. The effects of melatonin on sleep-wake rhythm of daytime haemodialysis patients: a randomized, placebo-controlled, cross-over study (EMSCAP study). Br J Clin Pharmacol 2009 Jan;67(1):68–75.

[32] Shojaei M, Djalali M, Khatami M, Siassi F, Eshraghian M. Effects of carnitine and coenzyme Q10 on lipid profile and serum levels of lipoprotein(a) in maintenance hemodialysis patients on statin therapy. Iran J Kidney Dis 2011 Mar;5(2):114–8.

[33] Onwuka FC, Erhabor O, Eteng MU, Umoh IB. Protective effects of ginger toward cadmium-induced testes and kidney lipid peroxidation and hematological impairment in albino rats. J Med Food 2011 Jul-Aug;14(7-8):817–21.

[34] Shanmugam KR, Ramakrishna CH, Mallikarjuna K, Reddy KS. Protective effect of ginger against alcohol-induced renal damage and antioxidant enzymes in male albino rats. Indian J Exp Biol. 2010 Feb;48(2):143–9.

[35] Imani H, Tabibi H, Atabak S, Rahmani L, Ahmadinejad M, Hedayati M. Effects of soy consumption on oxidative stress, blood homocysteine, coagulation factors, and phosphorus in peritoneal dialysis patients. J Ren Nutr 2009 Sep;19(5):389–95.

[36] Siefker K, DiSilvestro RA. Safety and antioxidant effects of a modest soy protein intervention in hemodialysis patients. J Med Food 2006. Fall;9(3):368–72.

[37] Sankaran D, Bankovic-Calic N, Cahill L, Yu-Chen Peng C, Ogborn MR, Aukema HM. Late dietary intervention limits benefits of soy protein or flax oil in experimental polycystic kidney disease. Nephron Exp Nephrol 2007;106(4):e122–8.

[38] Sundl I, Roob JM, Meinitzer A, Tiran B, Khoschsorur G, Haditsch B, et al. Antioxidant status of patients on peritoneal dialysis: associations with inflammation and glycoxidative stress. Perit Dial Int 2009 Jan-Feb;29(1):89—101.

[39] Vessal G, Akmali M, Najafi P, Moein MR, Sagheb MM. Silymarin and milk thistle extract may prevent the progression of diabetic nephropathy in streptozotocin-induced diabetic rats. Ren Fail. 2010 Jul;32(6):733—9.

[40] Linde K, Ramirez G, Mulrow CD, Pauls A, Weidenhammer W, Melchart D. St John's wort for depression — an overview and meta-analysis of randomised clinical trials. BMJ 1996 Aug 3;313(7052):253—8.

[41] Duncan MG. The effects of nutritional supplements on the treatment of depression, diabetes, and hypercholesterolemia in the renal patient. J Ren Nutr 1999 Apr;9(2):58—62.

[42] Kerb R, Brockmoller J, Staffeldt B, Ploch M, Roots I. Single-dose and steady-state pharmacokinetics of hypericin and pseudo-hypericin. Antimicrob Agents Chemother 1996 Sep;40(9): 2087—93.

[43] Kannar D, Wattanapenpaiboon N, Savige GS, Wahlqvist ML. Hypocholesterolemic effect of an enteric-coated garlic supplement. J Am Coll Nutr 2001 Jun;20(3):225—31.

[44] Jepson RGKJ, Leng GC. Garlic for peripheral arterial occlusive disease. Cochrane Database of Systematic Reviews 1997;(2).

[45] Jonas WBL, Jeffrey S, editors. Essentials of Complementary and Alternative Medicine. Lippincott Wiliams and Wilkins; 1999.

[46] Azadbakht L, Atabak S, Esmaillzadeh A. Soy protein intake, cardiorenal indices, and C-reactive protein in type 2 diabetes with nephropathy: a longitudinal randomized clinical trial. Diabetes Care 2008 Apr;31(4):648—54.

[47] Teschke R, Genthner A, Wolff A. Kava hepatotoxicity: comparison of aqueous, ethanolic, acetonic kava extracts and kava-herbs mixtures. J Ethnopharmacol 2009 Jun 25;123(3): 378—84.

[48] Sarris J, Kavanagh DJ, Adams J, Bone K, Byrne G. Kava Anxiety Depression Spectrum Study (KADSS): a mixed methods RCT using an aqueous extract of Piper methysticum. Complement Ther Med 2009 Jun;17(3):176—8.

[49] Teschke R. Kava hepatotoxicity — a clinical review. Ann Hepatol 2010 Jul-Sep;9(3):251—65.

[50] Teschke R, Fuchs J, Bahre R, Genthner A, Wolff A. Kava hepatotoxicity: comparative study of two structured quantitative methods for causality assessment. J Clin Pharm Ther 2010 Oct;35(5):545—63.

Drug—Nutrient Interactions in Renal Failure

Raimund Hirschberg

UCLA, Division of Nephrology and Hypertension, Harbor-UCLA Medical, Torrance, CA, USA

INTRODUCTION

Foods and prescribed or over-the-counter medicines can interact in multiple ways. Such interactions may result in reduced or increased drug effects or in (often subtle) nutritional deficiencies. Drug efficacy may be reduced due to food-induced delayed or decreased absorption from the gastrointestinal tract. Diet or nutrients may induce or inhibit drug-metabolizing enzymes and increase or decrease the rate of metabolism of a given drug. The rate of excretion of the drug or of active or toxic metabolites may also be altered by dietary effects.

The most commonly observed drug—food interaction is altered drug absorption from the gastrointestinal tract, usually a decrease in the rate of absorption. Less commonly, the drug absorption rate may be increased if taken concurrently with foods. Drugs can also induce certain specific nutrient deficiencies particularly for vitamins and minerals.

In patients with chronic kidney disease (CKD) or end-stage renal disease (ESRD), drug—nutrient interactions may lead to overt nutritional deficiencies particularly when the general nutritional status is poor or there are specific, subclinical nutritional deficiencies. This chapter will focus on interactions between drugs typically prescribed to renal patients and foods.

EFFECT OF FOOD INTAKE ON DRUG ABSORPTION

The intestinal absorption of many drugs is slowed when administered concurrently with food, either because of delayed gastric emptying or because of dilution of the drug in the intestinal contents. Some medications, such as central α_2-adrenergic drugs, can reduce gastrointestinal motility and delay the emptying of the stomach and, hence, increase oral—fecal transit time [1]. In contrast, calcium channel blockers do not appear to affect gastrointestinal motility [2]. Table 44.1 lists several drugs that may be prescribed to patients with CKD and which may interfere with the gastric emptying rate. Table 44.2 lists drugs that are absorbed more slowly when given concurrently with meals. To optimize drug absorption, these medicines should be given one hour before or two hours after meals. However, there are a few commonly administered

TABLE 44.1 Drugs Affecting the Gastric Emptying Rate (GER)[1]

Increase GER	Decrease GER
Metoclopamide	Anticholinergics
Reserpine	Atropine
Sodium bicarbonate	Amitriptyline
Ondensetron	Imipramine
Analgesics	
Morphine	
Pentazocine	
Isoniazid	
Chloroquine	
Phenytoin	
Aluminum hydroxide	
Phenothiazines	
Chlorpromazine	
Diphenylhydramine	
Promethazine	
Sympathomimetics	
Levodopa	
Amantadine	

[1]Adapted from [82,83].

TABLE 44.2 Drugs Undergoing Reduced or Delayed Absorption if Administered with Food

Acetaminophen	Ferrous sulfate[2]	Nifedipine
Amoxicillin	Fosinopril	Norfloxacin
Ampicillin	Furosemide	Ofloxacin
Aspirin	Glipizide	Oxacillin
Benazepril	Hydralazine[3]	Oxytetracycline[2]
Captopril	Ibuprofen	Penicillamine
Cephalexin	Indomethacin	Pravastatin
Cephaclor	Isoniazid	Ramipril
Cimetidine[1]	Ketoconazole	Rifampin
Ciprofloxacin[1]	Ketoprofen	Simvastatin
Clindamycin	Levodopa	Spironolactone
Demeclocycline	Levothyroxine[3]	Sulindac
Digoxin	Lisinopril	Tacrolimus
Docycycline	Methotrexate	Tetracycline[2]
Enalapril	Misoprostol	Zidovudine
Erythromycin	Nicardipine	Zink salts

[1]Concurrent administration with caffeine-containing foods may increase caffeine uptake
[2]Mainly dairy products
[3]Particularly enteral formulas.

oral medicines that will undergo more effective absorption when administered with foods (Table 44.3). In most circumstances the food-dependent increase in drug absorption may enhance drug efficacy. However, serious toxic side effects may arise, such as when lithium or cyclosporine is given with foods.

TABLE 44.3 Drugs that are Absorbed More Effectively If Given with Food

Buspirone	Griseofulvin
Carbamazepine	Isradipine
Cefpodoxime	Labetolol
Cefuroxime	Lithium salts
Chlorothiazide	Metoprolol
Cyclosporine	Morphine
Diazepam	Nitrofurantoin
Dicumarol	Propaphenone
Diltiazem	Propranolol
Etretinate	Quinidine
Famotidine	Sertraline
Felodipine	Triclopidine

Dietary contents can also reduce gastrointestinal drug uptake by inhibiting organic acid transport proteins (OATPs). Naringin and flavonoids in fruits, fruit juices and vegetables such as grapefruit and orange juice have been shown to inhibit OATP1A2 [3]. The uptake of drugs that are transported by this protein (fexofenadine, L-thyroxine, atenolol, ciprofloxacin) can be reduced by as much as 50% [3]. Etoposide absorption is also substantially reduced by grapefruit juice [4].

Subclinical or overt iron deficiency is commonly observed in patients with advanced CKD or end-stage renal disease. Low or empty iron stores may be caused by reduced nutrient and, hence, iron intakes as well as subtle iron losses. Iron deficiency is the most common reason for resistance to erythropoietin in patients with renal failure. Experimental studies have shown that administration of the phosphate binder calcium carbonate ($CaCO_3$) with foods reduces the bioavailability of iron from oral iron sulfate [5]. Apparently, in the presence of calcium, iron is taken up normally into the gut mucosa, but the transfer through mucosal cytoplasm and/or basolateral membranes is reduced. This interaction is bypassed by intravenous iron administration.

EFFECTS OF NUTRIENTS ON DRUG METABOLISM

Dietary Protein and Lipids

The hepatic clearance of some drugs is reduced in renal failure [6]. Drugs that are metabolized by oxidation, conjugation or both processes may be predisposed to decreased hepatic clearance in CKD. High protein diets can raise the activity of drugs that are metabolized through cytochrome P-450-dependent mixed function oxidases [7]. High protein diets accelerate the metabolic clearance of some drugs such as theophylline and propranolol by about 30 to 60% compared to low protein diets [8].

Low protein diets also reduce the activity of xanthine oxidase [9] and increase the plasma levels of allopurinol and oxipurinol. Since oxipurinol accounts for some of the adverse effects of allopurinol, the concurrent prescription of low protein diets and allopurinol may increase the likelihood of allopurinol toxicity [9]. The prescription of low protein diets to patients with CKD may reduce also the sulfate conjugation of some drugs, although clinical studies directly examining this question in patients or normal subjects are lacking. Drug sulfation depends on the availability of sulfur-containing amino acids and the possible release of sulfur in the gut by the action of intestinal sulfatases.

Cruciferous Vegetables and Drug Metabolism

Drug metabolism can be affected by other compounds derived from certain foods. For example, various indoles that originate from cruciferous vegetables such as cabbage and Brussels sprouts, enhance oxidation and increase the metabolic clearance rate of medicines. Such foods also may enhance drug glucuronidation in healthy subjects, e.g., for acetaminophen [10]. Diet-derived compounds may affect the activity of the P-450 enzyme species, and such substances can compete as substrates for the P-450-dependent monooxygenase system [11]. Indole-3-carbinol and related compounds that are present in cruciferous vegetables, particularly Brussels sprouts, are potent inducers of the intestinal P-450 IA1 (CYP1A1) and hepatic CYP1A1 and CYP1A2 isoenzymes [12].

Nutrients and Cytochrome P-450-Dependent Drug Metabolism

Increased dietary protein augments hepatic microsomal cytochrome P-450 content probably through tryptophan and sulfur amino acids [13]. In contrast, the activity of this enzyme system is reduced by low protein, high carbohydrate or fat diets, flavonoids (i.e., contained in citrus fruits and some vegetables), large doses of riboflavin and possibly during total parenteral nutrition [12]. The cytochrome P-450IIE1 (CYP2E1) isoenzyme is induced by dietary lipids [14]. This isoenzyme participates in the metabolism of acetaminophen, enflurane and halothane [11]. Moreover, the CYP2E1 isoenzyme is also activated by fasting, as well as by thiamine deficiency [14]. Several other alterations in the micronutrient status can affect the oxidative metabolism of drugs (Table 44.4).

Cytochrome P-450 Isoenzyme Activity and Citrus Juice Compounds

Flavonoids, such as naringin, are present in rather large amounts in citrus fruits, citrus juices and some vegetables. The related aglycone, naringenin, is readily formed in humans from its precursor. This compound, like other flavonoids, inhibits the cytochrome P-450 3A4 isoenzyme. Grapefruit juice which is perhaps the food most potently inhibiting CYP3A4 contains naringenin but also psoralen derivatives which are also thought to inhibit this isoenzyme [15]. In-vitro studies identified several other compounds that were extracted from grapefruit juice and inhibit CYP3A4 [16]. Many different flavonoids can severely inhibit CYP3A4 (as much as 100% in-vitro). These compounds are also found in other citrus juices and fruits, fennel, bell pepper, celery, carrots as well as ginkgo biloba [17]. In clinical studies in

TABLE 44.4 Effects of Vitamin and Trace Element Alterations on Oxidative Drug Metabolism[1]

Vitamin A deficiency	↓ P-450
	↓ Metabolism of aminopyrine, Coumadin
Vitamin A, high dose	↑ Metabolism of Coumadin
Niacin deficiency	↓ Metabolism of anesthetics
Riboflavin deficiency	↓ NADPH:P-450 reductase
	↑ Aminopyrine metabolism
Vitamin C deficiency	↓ P-450
	↓ NADPH:P-450 reductase
	↓ Monooxigenase activities
Folic acid deficiency	↓ Induction of P-450IIB1 by barbiturates
Aluminum, high dose	↓ Hepatic P-450
Selenium deficiency	↓ Induction of P-450 by phenobarbital
Zinc deficiency	↓ Phenobarbital and aminopyrine metabolism

[1]Adapted from [11].

normal subjects naringin inhibits the metabolism of the CYP3A4 substrate nisoldipine only moderately giving rise to the importance of other compounds in grapefruit juice as inhibitors of this cytochrome P-450 isoenzyme [18]. Although the effect of these grapefruit juice compounds on CYP3A4 may be clinically more important, they also tend to inhibit several other cytochrome P-450 isoenzymes such as CYP1A2, CYP2C9, CYP2C19 and CYP2D6 [16,17].

CYP3A4 is present in relatively large concentrations in the wall of the small intestine where it contributes to the first pass metabolism of several drugs limiting the amount of active drug that reaches the blood stream. The inhibition of CYP3A4 by compounds in grapefruit juice and other citrus fruit juices is clinically important since this isoenzyme plays a major role in the metabolism of drugs that are commonly used in patients with CKD or end-stage renal disease. These include cyclosporine A, the dihydropyridine calcium channel blockers nifedipine, nimodipine, felodipine, nitrendipine and nisoldipine; the calcium channel blocker verapamil; saquinavir; diazepam, midazolam, triazolam, terfenadine and lovastatin [15,18,19]. The bioavailability of these drugs is increased by co-administration with grapefruit juice and, perhaps, even more so in subjects consuming large amounts of citrus juices chronically. For example, ingestion of diazepam, 5 mg, with 250 mL of grapefruit juice as compared to water increases the diazepam area-under-the-curve 3.2-fold [20]. The drug—nutrient interaction between compounds in citrus juices and dihydropyridine calcium channel blockers has significant clinical implications. First, the increased plasma levels of the drugs may raise the incidence of adverse effects. Second, in hypertensive patients treated with dihydropyridines, sporadic concomitant ingestion of grapefruit juice may cause symptomatic hypotension. Third, the combination of a dihydropyridine antihypertensive with grapefruit juice can increase the therapeutic efficacy. This has been illustrated in a published case report [21].

Large doses of vitamin C given as nutritional supplements to patients without ascorbic acid deficiency may increase the rate of oxidative drug metabolism [22]. High vitamin C intakes can also reduce the rate of sulfate conjugation of drugs, such as acetaminophen, by competing for the available sulfate. Dietary supplementation with large doses of pyridoxine may increase the metabolism and decrease the therapeutic efficacy of levodopa, since this vitamin is a cofactor for the dopa decarboxylase [23]. In contrast, St. John's Wort induces CYP3A4 and accelerates metabolism of some drugs.

Nutrients and Urinary Excretion of Drugs

The deficiency in some trace elements such as iron, zinc, copper, and selenium has been shown to influence the mixed function oxidase system in experimental animals, but for most such elements, studies in humans are not available. Moreover, even marked iron deficiency in man does not appear to affect oxidative drug metabolism.

In CKD the half-life of drugs that are primarily metabolized by hepatic glucuronidation may be prolonged [24,25]. There is circumstantial evidence that renal insufficiency per-se reduces hepatic drug clearance [26]. Although it is possible that fasting, malnutrition or specific nutrient deficiencies may alter the hepatic glucuronidation of some drugs, the literature at present does not provide clearly supportive data.

The urinary excretion of certain drugs or of bioactive or toxic metabolites does not only depend on the degree of renal failure, i.e. GFR or creatinine clearance, but also on urinary pH [27]. In patients with normal renal function and even in patients with moderate or even advanced CKD, urinary pH depends largely on dietary intakes, at least during the post-absorptive period. A low protein diet produces more alkaline urine, and conversely, a high protein diet results in more acidic urine. Drugs or drug metabolites that are weak bases are more efficiently excreted in acidic urine, whereas more alkaline urine will promote the excretion of drugs or metabolites that are weak acids. Foods that potentially acidify the urine include meats, fish, eggs, cheese,

bread, cranberries, plums and prunes. More alkaline urine can be caused by milk, various fruits and all vegetables except corn and lentils [28].

INTERACTIONS OF FOOD SUPPLEMENTS WITH DRUGS

Patients with advanced CKD and those on maintenance dialysis are often prescribed food supplements, such as vitamins and iron preparations, or phosphate binders. Specific interactions between certain drugs and these food supplements have been described that may not only reduce the blood levels of the drug but may reduce the drug efficacy. Thus, it may be necessary to separate the timing of the intake of the food supplement from that of the drug. In general, the drug should be taken one hour before or two hours after the supplement, but in some circumstances this period of time should be even longer (up to 4 h).

Supplemental folic acid decreases the blood levels of phenobarbital [29] and may lead to break-through seizures. Pyridoxine (vitamin B_6) when given in large dosages (400 mg/day) can also reduce the serum levels of phenobarbital, possibly by increasing the activity of pyridoxal phosphate-dependent enzymes. In animal experiments, large doses of pyridoxine may reduce the activity of isonicotinic acid against tuberculosis. Pyridoxine appears to form a Schiff base with isonicotinic acid which is then excreted in the urine or removed during dialysis [30]. Concomitant therapy with pyridoxine and L-dopa in patients with Parkinson's disease reduces the efficacy of the latter drug and worsens the disease symptoms.

Excess intake of vitamin E can induce a hemorrhagic state in laboratory animals caused by vitamin K deficiency [31]. Patients on Coumadin therapy are at risk for developing hemorrhages that result from unwarranted further suppression of the vitamin K-dependent clotting factors by concomitant intake of vitamin E. It has been suggested that megadoses of vitamin C (>1 g/day) may lead to vitamin B_{12} deficiency apparently by destruction of vitamin B_{12} by vitamin C when they are taken together.

Clinically important interactions occur between iron supplements or phosphate binders and fluoroquinolone antibiotics [32]. Bioavailability of ciprofloxacin is reduced if the drug is co-administered with aluminum hydroxide-containing phosphate binders. Magnesium hydroxide as well as aluminum hydroxide reduce the bioavailability of ciprofloxacin by as much as 90% when given concomitantly or within <0.5 hours, and a lesser but still significant reduction occurs when the drug is given within up to 4 hours after the antacid [33]. Similar reductions in the bioavailability occur for other fluoroquinolone antibiotics, such as norfloxacin, ofloxacin and enoxacin when administered up to four hours after intake of aluminum, magnesium or calcium containing phosphate binders [34]. A significant decrease in the bioavailability of fluoroquinolones was also described by several authors to occur upon co-administration with several oral iron supplement preparations such as ferrous sulfate, fumarate or gluconate. Calcium-containing phosphate binders or antacids have also been shown to reduce the bioavailability of tetracyclines [35]. Sevelamer does not appear to have such effects on drug bioavailability. The reduction of iron absorption from diet or ferrous sulfate due to co-administration of calcium-containing phosphate binders has been discussed earlier in this chapter.

DRUG-INDUCED NUTRITIONAL DEFICIENCIES

Several prescribed or over-the-counter medicines reduce appetite and food intake. In patients with CKD or on maintenance dialysis this may aggravate an already poor nutritional status and may contribute to frank malnutrition. However, of greater concern are more specific interactions of prescribed drugs with micronutrients, mainly with certain vitamins and minerals.

Drug-Induced Vitamin Deficiencies

Vitamin metabolism and requirements in renal disease and renal failure are described in Chapter 24. Thiamine deficiency may be aggravated or caused by chronic alcoholism. The literature, at present, does not suggest that specific short-term or long-term drug therapies may cause vitamin B_1 deficiency. However, thiamine deficiency may occur in severely ill patients who undergo parenteral nutrition [36,37]. Thiamine is a co-enzyme for pyruvate dehydrogenase, and thiamine deficiency may cause the acute onset of unexplained, severe lactic acidosis [36–38]. Riboflavin deficiency can be caused or aggravated by long-term administration of chlorpromazine or amitriptyline. Pyridoxine deficiency may be caused by long-term treatment with isoniazid. It is recommended that vitamin B_6 supplements (10–15 mg/day) should be prescribed for the entire period of time that isoniazid is taken. Vitamin B_6 deficiency may also be caused by hydralazine and penicillamine [23]. High doses of pyridoxine hydrochloride reduce the serum levels of anticonvulsants and may reduce the clinical seizure control. Chronic vitamin B_{12} deficiency may develop during long-term treatment with colchicine or cimetidine [39,40].

Several drugs antagonize folic acid and may cause megaloblastic anemia. These include phenytoin, phenobarbital, sulphasalazine, triamterene, trimethoprim, trimetrexate and methotrexate [41–43]. On the other hand, folate supplementation may interact with these medicines and reduce their clinical efficacy. Daily dosages of folate of more than 5 mg reduces the plasma levels of phenytoin and phenobarbital and may reduce their therapeutic efficacy [44]. A risk for the development of niacin deficiency may exist when treatment with isoniazid is prescribed. During such treatment, concurrent administration of niacin (100 mg/day) may be advisable. Retinoids and possibly retinol increase the blood cyclosporine levels [45]. Vitamin A supplements should be avoided in renal patients. In addition to Coumadin anticoagulants, there are a number of drugs that can cause vitamin K deficiency and that may induce or enhance severe bleeding. This has been described particularly with the administration of moxalactam, cefotetan, cefamandole, cefoperazone and other cephalosporins that contain the methylthiotetrazole side chain. Vitamin K supplements should be administered concurrently with these antibiotics [46,47]. Weaker anti-vitamin K effects have been shown with tetracycline and cholestyramine [48]. Ingestion of megadoses of vitamin E can cause vitamin K deficiency and should be avoided [31].

Drug-induced osteomalacia can be due to chronic intake of anticonvulsants, isoniazid and possibly cimetidine. Anticonvulsant therapy with phenytoin, phenobarbital, or carbamazepine results in reduced levels of 24,25-dihydroxyvitamin D_3, and this may play a role in the anticonvulsant-induced osteomalacia [49]. In patients with CKD this drug-induced risk for osteomalacia may be additive to the increased risk of renal bone disease. Patients undergoing chronic dialysis therapy are often supplemented with 1,25-dihydroxycholecalciferol or analogues. However, in patients with moderate CKD not receiving 1,25-dihydroxycholecalciferol, vitamin D supplements should be given concurrently with the above drug treatments.

Drug-Induced Mineral and Trace Element Deficiencies

As a rule, the intakes of many minerals such as Na, K, Mg, Ca and P correlate with the intake of nitrogen [50]. Mineral and trace element deficiencies may develop due to poor nutritional intakes and elderly patients are at greater risk. Mineral depletion can occur due to poor gastrointestinal absorption and/or enhanced renal excretion, the latter mainly in patients with lesser degrees of CKD. Both, reduced absorption and enhanced excretion of minerals can be caused by drug therapy. Potassium, calcium, magnesium, iron and zinc are the most common minerals that become depleted in patients with CKD. Drug-induced potassium deficiency in patients with chronic renal failure most commonly results from diuretic therapy and can be caused by both thiazide and loop diuretics. With diuretic therapy, magnesium deficiency may also develop.

Concurrent intake of aminoglycosides and cephalosporin antibiotics can be interactive and cause potassium (and magnesium) depletion, particularly when intakes of these minerals are low which may occur with ingestion of low protein diets. Hypokalemia can also occur with gentamycin toxicity and during treatment with amphotericin B. Potassium deficiency may also be caused by laxative abuse with resulting potassium losses through the gastrointestinal tract. Lithium carbonate and levodopa can contribute to potassium deficiency [51]. Hypokalemia and potassium depletion worsen blood pressure levels in hypertensive patients and may contribute to the thiazide-induced carbohydrate intolerance [52].

Calcium deficiency can be caused by poor dietary intake, primary malabsorption or vitamin D-deficiency-induced malabsorption, or drug-induced hypercalciuria. Primary calcium malabsorption can result from enteropathy caused by neomycin, colchicine, methotrexate and corticosteroids [53]. Aluminum and magnesium hydroxide may reduce calcium absorption. Phenytoin and phenobarbital may interfere with vitamin D metabolism as described above. Loop diuretics, such as furosemide and ethacrynic acid can cause hypocalcemia secondary to hypercalciuria [54]. In patients with chronic renal failure combined treatments with drugs that interfere with calcium metabolism are not uncommon.

Hypercalcemia in patients with CKD may result in soft tissue calcification and nephrocalcinosis that may contribute to the progression of renal disease or may itself cause CKD. The long-term combined intakes of large amounts of calcium carbonate and (vitamin D-fortified) milk can lead to severe chronic hypercalcemia and nephrocalcinosis causing CKD, the so-called milk-alkali syndrome [55]. In CKD, hypercalcemia may result from the intake of calcium-containing phosphate binders and/or vitamin D derivatives.

Hyperoxalemia and hyperoxaluria can be caused or aggravated by vitamin C supplementation, even at moderate doses (i.e., 500 mg/day) [56]. Patients who eat relatively large amounts of foods that generate oxalate (e.g., green salads) and take moderate or megadoses of vitamin C have an increased risk to develop hyperoxalemia-associated complications [56].

Zinc deficiency may be caused or worsened by total parenteral nutrition without adequate zinc intake [57]. Administration of penicillamine or corticosteroids have also been associated with zinc deficiency [58]. Zinc depletion causes or contributes to clinical symptoms that are often observed in patients with CKD, such as loss of appetite and altered taste and smell sensation. Loss of taste or smell may lead to reduced food intake and, hence, malnutrition. Aspirin (even at the low dose of 81 mg/day), ibuprofen and other non-steroidal anti-inflammatory drugs may cause occult gastrointestinal bleeding and contribute to iron losses [59]. Iron depletion and anemia may also be caused by poor food intake or reduced bioavailability from non-heme iron in foods such as due to concomitant calcium-containing phosphate binders. This has been discussed above. There are not sufficient data to indicate whether there are important drug interactions with other trace elements, such as selenium, molybdenum, chromium, manganese, rubidium and others.

TAURINE AND ACE-INHIBITOR EFFECTS

The amino acid taurine blocks actions of angiotensin II by inhibiting cellular Ca^{++}-uptake and angiotensin II signaling [60]. In experimental in-vitro and in-vivo studies taurine food supplements were found to have renal antifibrogenic effects comparable to those of ACE-inhibitors [61].

Serum and blood cell taurine levels tend to be lower in diabetics compared to normal subjects and taurine food supplements can normalize taurine levels [62]. Foods rich in taurine include seafood, particularly crustaceans and molluscs, and lesser amounts are present in beef, pork and lamb [63]. Taurine containing food supplements are available over the counter. Whether increased dietary taurine will indeed reduce the progression of renal disease and/or reduce the cardiovascular mortality in chronic dialysis patients is unknown due to the lack of respective clinical trials. Nevertheless, this may be an example of collaborative, beneficial drug—nutrient interaction.

NUTRIENT INTERACTIONS WITH ORAL ANTICOAGULANTS

Until recently, Coumadin was the mainstay of oral anticoagulation therapy in non-renal as well as CKD-patients. This drug is a prime example of the importance of foods that can interfere with drug actions. This is mainly because of the small therapeutic window between under- and overdose as well as its reduced efficacy by dietary vitamin K intakes. Table 44.5 summarizes commonly consumed foods with relatively high vitamin K content. In contrast, the intake of large amounts of vitamin E can cause vitamin K deficiency [31].

TABLE 44.5 Commonly Consumed Foods High in Vitamin K Content

Beef liver	Cheese	Lettuce
Broccoli	Collard greens	Spinach
Brussels sprouts	Green tea	Soybean
Cabbage	Lentils	Turnip greens

Several novel orally effective small molecule factor Xa or thrombin enzyme inhibitor anticoagulants have recently been approved by regulatory agencies (rivaroxaban, dabigatran) or are in various stages of clinical and registrative development in the US and Europe (apicaban, edoxaban, betrixaban). Rivaroxaban and dabigatran are approved for patients with CKD stages 1-3B but not or only with caution in CKD 4 and 5. High fat, high calorie diets tend to reduce the rate of absorption of dabigatran but overall drug availability is not substantially different from fasting [64]. Similar food interactions were shown for rivaroxaban [65]. Other important food interactions have not yet emerged. Since these drugs are in clinical use for only a short period of time, other drug nutrient interactions may come to attention.

Apixaban, edoxaban and rivaroxaban are mainly metabolized through CYP3A4. Thus, nutrients and food supplements that induce CYP3A4 such as St. John's Wort might reduce drug levels and anticoagulant efficacy. Over-anticoagulation could occur with large amounts of citrus juice intake due to CYP3A4 inhibition. Thus far, this has not materialized. Betrixaban and dabigatran are not metabolized by CYP450 enzymes.

INTERACTIONS OF CALCINEURIN INHIBITORS WITH NUTRIENTS

Treatments with cyclosporine A or tacrolimus continue to be part of many immunosuppressive regimens that are used in kidney transplantation. Cyclosporine has several side effects which include nephrotoxicity, hepatotoxicity, hypertrichosis, gingival hyperplasia and hyperuricemia and gout (7% of patients), the latter particularly when used together with loop diuretics [66]. Cyclosporine is incompletely absorbed from the gastrointestinal tract and administration of the drug with foods tends to increase absorption. Oral administration of cyclosporine A together with food and bile salts increases the bioavailability of the drug apparently due to improved absorption. However, co-administration of cyclosporine with bile salts alone does not raise the cyclosporine blood levels [67]. The incomplete absorption of intact cyclosporine is, in part,

caused by metabolism in the small bowel wall [68]. Cyclosporine is metabolized by oxidation in liver microsomes through the cytochrome P-450 3A isoenzyme system [69]. This enzyme system is also expressed in the small bowel wall which explains the first-pass metabolism of cyclosporine A [70].

Cyclosporine A is a highly lipid-soluble drug, and about 40% of cyclosporine in plasma is bound to lipoproteins. Thus, it is reasonable to speculate that dietary fat intakes or the fat content of meals may raise the gastrointestinal absorption and plasma levels of cyclosporine A but this has not been confirmed in clinical trials.

As indicated above, citrus juices, particularly grapefruit juice, reduce the metabolic rate of Cyclosporine and raise its blood levels [71], possibly through the inhibitory effects of flavonoids and other compounds on cytochrome P-450 3A enzymes [15]. The inhibition of CYP3A4 by grapefruit juice and other citrus juices and fruits raises the area-under-the-curve and causes an increase in the 24 hr trough cyclosporine level [72]. St. John's Wort and caspofungin induces CYP3A4 activity. Other drugs that inhibit or reduce cyclosporine A levels due to effects on CYP3A are listed in Tables 44.6 and 44.7.

Both cyclosporine and tacrolimus can cause a number of metabolic complications including phosphorous,

TABLE 44.6 Drugs that Increase Blood Cyclosporine A Levels Due to Inhibition of or Competition with CYP3A Isoenzymes[1]

Ceftazidime	Ketoconazole
Cimetidine	Nicardipine
Diltiazem	Norfloxacin
Erythromycin	Omeprazole
Fluconazole	Ponsinomycin
Imipenem	Ranitidine
Itraconazole	Verapamil

[1]Adapted from [66,84].

TABLE 44.7 Drugs that Decrease Blood Cyclosporine A Levels Due to Induction of CYP3A Isoenzymes[1]

Barbiturates	Nafcillin
Benzodiazepines	Phenytoin
Carbamazepin	Rifampicin
Cephalosporins	Trimethoprim
Isoniazid	Valproic acid

[1]Adapted from [66].

magnesium or potassium depletion, hyperkalemia, glucose intolerance and diabetes mellitus and hyperlipoproteinemia. Tacrolimus is mainly metabolized through CYP3A enzymes. Hence, food/food supplement interactions can affect tacrolimus blood levels: St. John's Wort (as well as caspofungin) induces CYP3A and may decrease tacrolimus blood levels. Grapefruit juice which blocks this enzyme system increases blood levels. Drug inhibitors of CYP3A (calcium channel blockers and azoles) can increase tacrolimus levels.

Absorption of tacrolimus from the gastrointestinal tract is substantially influenced by food: Absorption is greatest with fasting. High fat diets reduce tacrolimus absorption and drug availability more than high carbohydrate diets [73].

ENTERAL TUBE FEEDING AND ORAL DRUG ADMINISTRATION

Enteral tube feeding may be a necessary or desirable mode of nutrient delivery in some patients with CKD or ESRD either transiently during periods of acute, severe illness or for longer periods of time. In such patients, drugs may be administered preferably by intravenous routes, but enteral drug administration sometimes may be necessary, since many medicine preparations are not available for intravenous infusion.

Several considerations should be taken into account when giving oral drug preparations through enteral feeding tubes. First, oral medicines should be delivered into the stomach to ensure proper preparation for subsequent drug absorption in the jejunum. Second, drugs should be used in liquid form rather than as crushed tablets. Third, slow-release or enteric-coated tablets should not be crushed at all. Fourth, drugs may not be compatible with the tube feeding formula and should not be mixed with formula. Thus, tubes should be flushed with water before and after drug administration. Fifth, the osmolality of some liquid drug preparations may be very high and may add to the osmolality of the formula. A complete list of commercially available liquid preparations of commonly used drugs has been published elsewhere [74,75].

Only few studies have examined the bioavailability of drugs when administered with enteral formulas, and this information is not available for most medicines. Phenytoin bioavailability, for example, is much reduced when given with enteral formulas as compared to a similar dose given orally [76,77]. Effervescent potassium tablet preparations causes marked coagulation of the enteral formula, whereas potassium chloride or gluconate solutions are compatible [78]. Administration of aluminum-containing phosphate binders with some enteral formulas can lead to precipitation of formula proteins with the aluminum salts and gastrointestinal plug formation can occur [79]. Case reports have suggested that enteral tube feeding causes resistance to warfarin [79,80]. Apparently, this results from the antagonistic effect of vitamin K that is present in enteral formulas [74]. In patients undergoing treatment with warfarin, a formula with a lesser vitamin K content should be used and will improve the response to warfarin. There is also evidence that warfarin may directly bind to the feeding tube reducing drug availability [81]. Some drug compounds are light sensitive and inactivated by light exposure and preparation and tube administration should be performed in the dark (nifedipine, nicardipine, metronidazole, amiodarone, furosemide) [75].

Little is known about interactions of many other drugs that may be used in patients with renal failure undergoing tube feeding. Hence, close monitoring of the plasma drug levels, treatment response, and compatibility with the formula are necessary.

References

[1] Nagata M, Osumi Y. Central alpha-2-adrenoreceptor-mediated inhibition of grastric motility in rats. Jpn J Pharmacol 1993;62:329—30.

[2] Baba T, Ishizaki T. Recent advances in pharmacological management of hypertension in diabetic patients with nephropathy. Effects of antihypertensive drugs on kidney function and insulin sensitivity. Drugs 1992;43:464—89.

[3] Bailey DG. Fruit juice inhibition of uptake transport: a new type of food-drug interaction. Br J Clin Pharmacol 2010;70:645—55.

[4] Greenblatt DJ. Analysis of drug interactions involving fruit beverages and organic anion-transporting polypeptides. J Clin Pharmacol 2009;49:1403—7.

[5] Wienk KJ, Marx JJ, Lemmens AG, et al. Mechanism underlying the inhibitory effect of high calcium carbonate intake on iron bioavailability from ferrous sulphate in anaemic rats. Br J Nutr 1996;75:109—20.

[6] Touchette M, Slaughter R. The effect of renal failure on hepatic drug clearance. DICP 1991;25:1214—24.

[7] Anderson K, Conney A, Kappas A. Nutrition and oxidative drug metabolism in man: Relative influence of dietary lipids, carbohydrates, and protein. Clin Pharmacol Ther 1979;26:493—501.

[8] Fagan T, Walle T, Oexmann M, et al. Increased clearance of propranolol and theophylline by high-protein compared with high-carbohydrate diet. Clin Pharmacol Ther 1987;41:402—6.

[9] Berlinger W, Park G, Spector R. The effect of dietary protein on the clearance of allopurinol and oxypurinol. N Engl J Med 1985;313:771—6.

[10] Pantuck E, Pantuck C, Anderson K, et al. Effect of brussels sprouts and cabbage on drug conjugation. Clin Pharmacol Ther 1984;35:161—9.

[11] Yang C, Brady J, Hong J. Dietary effects on cytochromes P-450, xenobiotic metabolism, and toxicity. FASEB J 1992;6:737—44.

[12] Vang O, Jensen M, Autrup H. Induction of cytochrome P450 1A1 in rat colon and liver by indole-3-carbinol and 5,6-benzo-flavone. Carcinogenesis 1990;11:1259—63.

[13] Evarts R, Mostafa M. Effects of indole and tryptophane on cytochrome P-450, dimethylnitrosamine demethylase, and arylhydrocarbon hydroxylase activities. Biochem Pharmacol 1981;30:517—22.

[14] Yoo J, Park H, Ning S, et al. Effects of thiamine deficiency on hepatic cytochromes P450 and drug-metabolizing enzyme activities. Biochem Pharmacol 1990;39:519—25.

[15] Fuhr U. Drug interactions with grapefruit juice. Extent, probable mechanism and clinical relevance. Drug Safety 1998;18:251—72.

[16] Tassaneeyakul W, Guo LQ, Fukuda K, et al. Inhibition selectivity of grapefruit juice components on human cytochromes P450. Arch Biochem Biophys 2000;378:356—63.

[17] Kimura Y, Ito H, Ohnishi R, et al. Inhibitory effects of polyphenols on human cytochrome P450 3A4 and 2C9 activity. Food Chem Toxicol 2010;48:429—35.

[18] Bailey DG, Arnold JM, Munoz C, et al. Grapefruit juice—felodipine interaction: mechanism, predictability, and effect of naringin. Clin Pharmacol Therapeut 1993;53:637—42.

[19] Guengerich F, Kim D. In-vitro inhibition of dihydropyridine oxidation and aflatoxin B1 activation in human liver microsomes by naringenin and other flavonoids. Carcinogenesis 1990;11:2275—9.

[20] Ozdemir M, Aktan Y, Boydag BS, et al. Interaction between grapefruit juice and diazepam in humans. Eur J Drug Metab Pharmacokinet 1998;23:55—9.

[21] Pisarik P. Blood pressure-lowering effect of adding grapefruit juice to nifedipine and terazosin in a patient with severe renovascular hypertension. Arch Fam Med 1996;5: 413—6.

[22] Houston J. Effect of vitamin C supplement on antipyrine disposition in man. Br J Clin Pharmacol 1977;4:236—9.

[23] Shigetomi S, Kuchel O. Defective 3,4-dihydroxyphenylalanine decarboxylation to dopamine in hydralazine-treated hypertensive patients may be pyridoxine remedial. Am J Hypertension 1993;6:33—40.

[24] Brater D. Clinical pharmacology of loop diuretics in health and disease. Eur Heart J 1992;13:10—4.

[25] Fillastre J, Montay G, Bruno R, et al. Pharmacokinetics of sparfloxacin in patients with renal impairment. Animicrob Agents Chemother 1994;38:733—7.

[26] Dreisbach AW, Lertora JJ. The effect of chronic renal failure on drug metabolism and transport. Expert Opin Drug Metab Toxicol 2008;4:1065—74.

[27] Lamy P. Effects of diet and nutrition on drug therapy. J Am Geriatr Soc 1982;30:S99—S112.

[28] Roe D. Therapeutic significance of drug—nutrient interactions in the elderly. Pharmacol Rev 1984;36:109S—22S.

[29] Botez M, Botez T, Ross-Chouinard A, et al. Thiamine and folate treatment in chronic epileptic patients: A controlled study with the Wechsler IQ scale. Epilepsy Res 1993;16:157—63.

[30] McCune R, Deuschle K, McDermott W. The delayed appearance of isoniazid antagonism by pyridoxine in-vivo. Ann Rev Tuberc 1957;76:1106—9.

[31] Kappus H, Diplock A. Tolerance and safety of vitamin E: A toxicological position report. Free Radical Biol Med 1992;13:55—74.

[32] Golper T, Hartstein A, Morthland V, et al. Effects of antacids and dialysis dwell times on multiple-dose pharmacokinetics of oral ciprofloxacin in patients on continuous ambulatory peritoneal dialysis. Antimicrob Agents Chemother 1987;31: 1787—90.

[33] Nix D, Watson W, Lerner M, et al. Effects of aluminum and magnesium antacids and ranitidine on the absorption of ciprofloxacin. Clin Pharmacol Therapeut 1989;46:700—5.

[34] Redandt J, Marchbanks C, Dudley M. Interactions of fluoroquinolones with other drugs: Mechanisms, variability, clinical significance and management. Clin Infect Dis 1992;14:272—84.

[35] Deppermann K, Lode H. Fluoroquinolones: Interaction profile during enteral absorption. Drugs 1993;45:65—72.

[36] Naito E, Ito M, Takeda E, et al. Molecular analysis of abnormal pyruvate dehydrogenase in a patient with thiamine-responsive congenital lactic acidosis. Pediatr Res 1994;36:340—6.

[37] Sanz París A, Albero Gamoa R, Acha Pérez FJ, et al. Thiamine deficiency associated with parenteral nutrition: apropos of a new case. Nutricion Hosp 1994;9:110—3.

[38] Hamalatha S, Kerr D, Wexler I, et al. Pyruvate dehydrogenase complex deficiency due to a point mutation (P188L) within the thiamine pyrophosphate binding loop of the E1 alpha subunit. Hum Mol Gen 1995;4:315—8.

[39] Force R, Nahata M. Effect of histamine H2-receptor antagonists on vitamin B12 absorption. Ann Pharmacother 1992;26:1283—6.

[40] Palopoli J, Waxman J. Recurrent aphthous stomatitis and vitamin B12 deficiency. South Med J 1990;83:475—7.

[41] Carl G, Smith M. Phenytoin-folate interaction: Differing effects of the sodium salt and the free acid of phenytoin. Epilepsia 1992;33:372—6.

[42] Casserly C, Stange K, Chren M. Severe megaloblastic anemia in a patient receiving low dose methotrexate for psoriasis. J Am Acad Dermatol 1993;29:477—80.

[43] Elmazar M, Nau H. Trimetoprim potentiates valproic acid-induced neural tube defects in mice. Reprod Toxicol 1993;7:249—54.

[44] Baylis E, Crowley J, Preece J, et al. Influence of folic acid on blood phenytoin levels. Lancet 1971;1:62—4.

[45] Shah I, Whiting P, Omar G, et al. The effects of retinoids and terbinafine on the human microsomal metabolism of cyclosporine. Br J Dermatol 1993;129:395—8.

[46] Kaiser C, McAuliffe J, Barth R, et al. Hypoprothrombinemia and hemorrhage in a surgical patient treated with cefotetan. Arch Surg 1991;126:524—5.

[47] Kikuchi S, Ando A, Minato K. Acquired coagulopathy caused by administration of parenteral broard spectrum antibiotics. Jpn J Clin Pathol 1991;39:83—90.

[48] Westphal J, Vetter D, Brogard J. Hepatic side-effects of antibiotics. J Antimicrob Chemother 1994;33:387—401.

[49] Zerwekh J, Homan R, Tindall R, et al. Decreased serum 24, 25-dihydroxyvitamin D concentration during long-term anticonvulsant therapy in adult epileptics. Ann Neurol 1982;12:184—6.

[50] Kopple J, Hirschberg R. Nutrition and peritoneal dialysis. In: Mitch W, Klahr S, editors. Nutrition and the Kidney. Boston: Little, Brown and Company; 1993. p. 290—313.

[51] Shirley D, Singer D, Sagnella G, et al. Effect of a single test dose of lithium carbonate on sodium and potassium excretion in man. Clin Sci 1991;81:59—63.

[52] Murphy M, Lewis P, Kohner E, et al. Glucose intolerance in hypertensive patients treated with duretics. A 14 year follow-up. Lancet 1982;2:1293—5.

[53] Race T, Paes I, Faloon W. Intestinal malabsorption induced by oral colchicine. comparison with neomycin and cathartic agents. Am Med Sci 1981;259:32—41.

[54] Eknoyan G, Suki W, Martinez-Maldonato M. Effect of diuretics on urinary excretion of phosphate, calcium and magnesium in thyroparathyroidectomized dogs. J Lab Clin Med 1970;76: 257—66.

[55] Newmark K, Nugent P. Milk-alkali syndrome: A consequence of chronic antacid abuse. Postgrad Med 1993;93. 149—150 & 156.

[56] Mitwalli A, Oreopoulos D. Hyperoxaluria and hyperoxalemia: One more concern for the nephrologist. Int J Artific Org 1985;8:71−4.

[57] Chen W, Chiang T, Chen T. Serum zinc and copper during long-term parenteral nutrition. J Formosan Med Assoc 1991;90:1075−80.

[58] Milanino R, Frigo A, Bambara L, et al. Copper and zinc status in rheumatoid arthritis: Studies of plasma, erythrocytes, and urine and their relationship to disease activity markers and pharmacological treatment. Clin Exp Rheumat 1993;11:271−81.

[59] Goldwasser P, Koutelos T, Abraham S, et al. Serum ferritin, hematocrit and mean corpuscular volume in hemodialysis. Nephron 1994;67:30−5.

[60] Schaffer SW, Lombardini JB, Azuma J. Interaction between the actions of taurine and angiotensin II. Amino Acids 2000;18:305−18.

[61] Cruz CI, Ruiz-Torres P, del Moral RG, et al. Age-related progressive renal fibrosis in rats and its prevention with ACE inhibitors and taurine. Am J Physiol Renal Physiol 2000;278: F122−129.

[62] Franconi F, Bennardini F, Mattana A, et al. Plasma and platelet taurine are reduced in subjects with insulin-dependent diabetes mellitus: effects of taurine supplementation. Am J Clin Nutr 1995;61:1115−9.

[63] Zhao X, Jia J, Lin Y. Taurine content in Chinese food and daily intake of Chinese men. Adv Exp Med Biol 1998;442:501−5.

[64] Stangier J, Eriksson BI, Dahl OE, et al. Pharmacokinetic profile of the oral direct thrombin inhibitor dabigatran etexilate in healthy volunteers and patients undergoing total hip replacement. J Clin Pharmacol 2005;45:555−63.

[65] Kubitza D, Becka M, Zuehlsdorf M, et al. Effect of food, an antacid, and the H2 antagonist ranitidine on the absorption of BAY 59-7939 (rivaroxaban), an oral, direct factor Xa inhibitor, in healthy subjects. J Clin Pharmacol 2006;46: 549−58.

[66] Danovitch G. Immunosuppressive medications and protocols for kidney transplantation. In: Danovitch G, editor. Handbook of Kidney Transplantation. Boston: Little, Brown and Company; 1992. p. 67−103.

[67] Lindholm A, Henriccson S, Dahlqvist R. The effect of food and bile acid administration on the relative bioavailability of cyclosporine. Br J Clin Pharmacol 1990;29:541−8.

[68] Kolars J, Awni W, Merion R, et al. First-pass metabolism of cyclosporine by the gut. Lancet 1991;338:1488−90.

[69] Fahr A. Cyclosporine clinical pharmacokinetics. Clin Phamacokinet 1993;24:472−95.

[70] Christians U, Sewing K. Cyclosporine metabolism in transplant patients. Pharmacol Ther 1993;57:291−345.

[71] Herlitz H, Edgar B, Hedner T, et al. Grapefruit juice: A possble source of variability in blood concentrations of cyclosprone A. Nephr Dial Transpl 1993;8:375.

[72] Brunner LJ, Munar MY, Vallian J, et al. Interaction between cyclosporine and grapefruit juice requires long-term ingestion in stable renal transplant recipients. Pharmacotherapy 1998;18:23−9.

[73] Vicari-Christensen M, Repper S, Basile S, et al. Tacrolimus: review of pharmacokinetics, pharmacodynamics, and pharmacogenetics to facilitate practitioners' understanding and offer strategies for educating patients and promoting adherence. Prog Transplant 2009;19:277−84.

[74] Melnik G. Pharmacologic aspects of enteral nutrition. In: Rombeau J, Coldwell M, editors. Clinical Nutrition: Enteral and Tube feeding. Philadelphia: W.B. Sauders Company; 1990. p. 472−509.

[75] Behnken I, Gaschott T, Stein J. [Enteral nutrition: drug administration via feeding tube]. Z Gastroenterol 2005;43:1231−41.

[76] Au Yeung SC, Ensom MH. Phenytoin and enteral feedings: does evidence support an interaction? Ann Pharmacother 2000;34:896−905.

[77] Worden J, Wood C, Workman C. Phenytoin and nasogastric feedings. Neurology 1994;34:132.

[78] Scott D. Addition of potassium supplements to mild-based tube feedings. J Hum Nutr 1980;34:85−90.

[79] Valli C, Schultheiss H, Asper R, et al. Interaction of nutrients with antacids: A complication during enteral tube feeding. Lancet 1986;1:747−8.

[80] Howard P, Hannaman K. Warfarin resistance linked to enteral nutrition products. J Am Diet Assoc 1985;85:713−5.

[81] Klang M, Graham D, McLymont V. Warfarin bioavailability with feeding tubes and enteral formula. JPEN J Parenter Enteral Nutr 2010;34:300−4.

[82] Nimmo W. Drugs, disease and altered gastric emptying. Clin Pharmacokinet 1976;1:189−203.

[83] Prescott L. Gastric emptying and drug absorption. Br J Clin Pharmacol 1974;1:189−90.

[84] Couet W, Istin B, Sinuta P, et al. Effect of ponsinomycin on cyclosporine pharmacokinetics. Eur J Clin Pharmacol 1990;39:165−7.

Exercise Training for Individuals with Advanced Chronic Kidney Disease

Thomas W. Storer

Section of Endocrinology, Diabetes, and Nutrition, Boston University School of Medicine, Boston MA, USA

INTRODUCTION

More than 20 million people in the United States, about 10% of the adult population, have chronic kidney disease (CKD) [1] 571,000 patients receive treatment for end-stage renal disease (ESRD) at a cost of over $42 billion Medicare and non-Medicare dollars annually, and in 2008, 88,620 of those people receiving hemodialysis (HD) died [2]. Primary contributors to ESRD are diabetes mellitus, hypertension, glomerulonephritis, cystic disease of the kidney, urologic disease, and others with death from cardiovascular disease accounting for about 50% of deaths [3]. On average, life expectancy after initiation of dialysis is approximately eight years in patients aged 40−44 and 4.5 years for those 60−64 years of age. This is 4−5 times less than that for age-matched healthy persons [4]. Heart disease is common in persons receiving HD. In a 2004 report, approximately 80% of the 1846 patients receiving HD were noted to have some form of heart disease; nearly 40% had ischemic heart disease and 40% presented with CHF [5]. Chronic renal disease is now considered a coronary heart disease risk equivalent [6−8].

Mortality is significantly related to the optimal dialysis dose [9], age, race, heart failure, physical functioning and comorbidity scores [10]. Of these predictive factors, only physical functioning can be easily and directly improved. As illustrated in Figure 45.1, sedentary behavior, especially prevalent in the ESRD population, is thought to directly impact a number of co-morbidities, inflammation, oxidative stress and survival, although proof of a causal relationship between sedentary behavior and these disorders is lacking. Exercise training has mitigated these negative effects in healthy individuals and possibly in people with CKD. As with the general population, regular

exercise training (planned, structured, repetitive, and purposive in improving or maintaining physical fitness) [11] and increased physical activity (any bodily movement that results in energy expenditure) result in substantial benefit for persons with ESRD.

CHARACTERISTICS OF ADVANCED CKD PATIENTS

Definition

This chapter addresses exercise training for individuals with advanced chronic kidney disease (CKD). For the purposes of this chapter, advanced CKD refers to stage 4 or 5 CKD, including patients undergoing maintenance hemodialysis (HD) or chronic peritoneal dialysis, and renal transplant recipients with stage 4 or 5 CKD. When relevant, advanced CKD may also refer to people, including renal transplant recipients, with stage 3b CKD (i.e., with glomerular filtration rates of 30−44.9 mL/min/1.73 m^2).

Individuals with advanced CKD exhibit malaise and diminished capacity for virtually any form of exercise apart from self-care [12−14]. These patients are severely deconditioned, exhibit significant skeletal muscle weakness [15−19] and have abnormal muscle morphology [20,21]. The cause of weakness is not entirely understood, but muscle atrophy, myopathy, deconditioning, malnutrition and carnitine deficiency have been proposed as contributors [17−19]. Peak oxygen uptake ($\dot{V}O_2$ peak), strength and physical function levels in patients with ESRD are approximately 60% to 70% of age-matched healthy individuals, even with the use of erythropoietin stimulating agents [21−24], and contribute to the malaise, low exercise tolerance [25,26], and poor physical functioning in patients with

Nutritional Management of Renal Disease
http://dx.doi.org/10.1016/B978-0-12-391934-2.00045-X

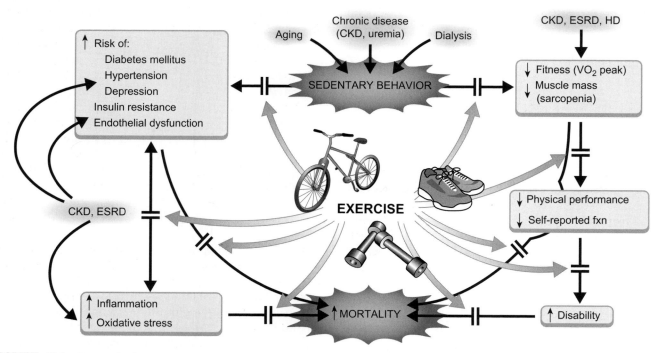

FIGURE 45.1 Potential adverse effects of sedentary behavior and chronic kidney disease and potential beneficial effects of exercise interventions. *fxn = function. From Johansen KL. Exercise in the end-stage renal disease population. J Am Soc Nephrol 2007; 18: 1845–1854.

ESRD as determined by objective measurements and self-reporting. In a national study of over 2400 new dialysis patients, 75% described severe limitations in vigorous activities, and 42% of patients acknowledged severe limitations in moderate activities such as moving a table or vacuuming [27]. Dialysis patients have significantly greater muscle atrophy in contractile areas as compared with healthy controls, even when corrected for habitual activity level [16]. Atrophy is proportional to muscle weakness and reduced physical performance, as determined by gait speed [16]. In addition, the limitation in peak oxygen uptake ($\dot{V}O_2$ peak), the highest oxygen uptake achieved during an incremental exercise test and an indicator of functional capacity, may be due, in part, to impaired skeletal muscle function. However, this impaired skeletal muscle function may be improved with exercise training with consequent improvements in $\dot{V}O_2$ peak.

Excitation-contraction coupling, central activation, and specific tension, when the latter is expressed as the ratio of maximal voluntary strength to contractile cross-sectional area (CSA), are not different between HD patients and controls [17,21]. This suggests that muscle atrophy is a major cause of muscle weakness and the ensuing decrements in physical function. More than 60% of ESRD patients are over age 65 and are sarcopenic [28], and when compared with healthy age matched controls, these patients have significant muscle fiber atrophy and greater contractile area

atrophy even when corrected for habitual activity level [17]. Loss of edema free lean mass in HD patients, whether as a consequence of a chronic catabolic state, uremic myopathy, or decreased levels of androgens, growth hormone, and/or the insulin-like growth factor (IGF) system, is a common observation [29]. In addition to the myriad functional limitations experienced by those with ESRD, the loss of edema free lean body mass (LBM) common to this population may portend increased risk of mortality [30]. The Dialysis Morbidity and Mortality Study reports that mortality risks, expressed as relative risk (RR), were greatest in patients with ESRD who had severe limitations in moderate (RR, 1.72) or vigorous (RR, 1.51) physical activity when compared with those with minimal or no limitations. For HD patients who exercised 2 to 3 vs 4 to 5 times per week, mortality risks were substantially lower; RR = 0.74 and RR = 0.70, respectively [31]. It is eminently clear that individuals receiving HD have an important need for interventions that mitigate the effects of ESRD on physical function and possibly morbidity, and mortality and that may reduce risks due to co-morbidities, especially cardiovascular disease. Interventions that result in improved physical function would be welcome in the ESRD population. Well applied and regularly practiced exercise training and increased physical activity is just such as intervention. Data collected for over 40 years in this area have demonstrated significant physical performance and health-related benefits in those HD patients who reasonably comply with exercise training guidelines. Many of these benefits are presented below.

VALUE OF EXERCISE AND PHYSICAL ACTIVITY IN ADVANCED CKD

In the general population, lifestyle change, including physical activity and exercise training, are listed among the highest priorities for improving health and reducing chronic disease risk [32,33]. The health related benefits gained from participation in regular exercise and physical activity are many (Table 45.1) with positive effects on most organ systems plus psychological benefits. Epidemiological data suggest that the benefits seen in healthy individuals might occur in patients with most chronic diseases including ESRD. Forty-five years ago, Jetty and colleagues reported a case study that investigated the feasibility of administering exercise training to a patient receiving HD [34]. The twice weekly exercise program conducted on non-dialysis days was associated with improved functional capacity, improved mood, and decreased blood phosphorous levels. Patricia Painter, a research pioneer in the application of exercise training with HD patients, investigated the effects of 6 months of thrice weekly cycle exercise with duration progressing up to 30 continuous minutes during the second or third hour of dialysis [25]. After 6-months, a significant 23% improvement in $\dot{V}O_2$ peak was reported with no change in the control group. Compliance in the training group was 91%. This study was the first to show that significant benefit could be achieved by performing regular, simple cycling exercise during the hemodialysis procedure. Thirty-five years later, this seminal work has been confirmed many times, not only showing benefits for aerobic capacity but also for several other health and performance related variables (Table 45.1) as reported in several reviews [35–39].

Aerobic capacity, $\dot{V}O_2$ peak, is recognized as the best non-invasive parameter for assessing the integrated function of the cardiopulmonary and muscular systems [40–42]. Consequently, $\dot{V}O_2$ peak has been studied extensively in HD patients and its positive changes due to exercise training have been well documented [24,35–37]. Table 45.2 summarizes $\dot{V}O_2$ peak before and after training in randomized controlled trials of HD patients and in a few cases, with healthy, age matched controls. These studies have also been the most frequently cited in systematic reviews and meta-analyses [24,35–37,43]. The exercise training design features of these studies are given in Table 45.3. Several results should be noted. First, changes in $\dot{V}O_2$ peak were smaller in the two studies using home exercise [44,45]. This is likely due to issues of poor compliance and lack of supervision. Second, the overall improvement in $\dot{V}O_2$ peak for HD patients undergoing exercise training in these studies is about 23% or 4.3 mL/kg/min/min. This represents a 1.2 MET increase where 1 MET is equivalent to the resting metabolic rate expressed as an oxygen uptake ($\dot{V}O_2$) of 3.5 mL/kg/min. Third, based on the studies reviewed in Table 45.2, $\dot{V}O_2$ peak in HD patients is less than half of age-matched healthy people and after training is still only about 54% of values from healthy controls. Although seemingly small, the 1.2 MET improvement in $\dot{V}O_2$ peak brings about important benefits as discussed below.

Aerobic capacity is an independent predictor of mortality, has high prognostic ability, and outperforms traditional risk factors and other exercise test responses (including markers of ischemia) for predicting outcomes in people with and without CVD, patients with CHF, hypertension, diabetes, or obesity [45–55] even when estimated from treadmill time rather than direct measurement [50]. Several studies have now shown in people without CKD that increasing aerobic capacity, especially in those with very low fitness, e.g., <5–6 METs ($\dot{V}O_2$ peak of 17.5 – 21 mL/kg/min) has a significant impact on reducing cardiovascular and all-cause mortality. In people without CKD, improving from this low fitness category, which is approximately the fitness level of those HD patients who have volunteered for study, every 1 MET increase in $\dot{V}O_2$ peak reduces mortality risk by 10–25% [48,56,57]. In 2011, Aspenes et al. who studied 4631 normal Norwegian men and women reported that each 5 mL/kg/min lower peak $\dot{V}O_2$ was associated with a 56% higher odds of cardiovascular risk clustering [46]. Inasmuch as many HD patients often have some form of intercurrent cardiovascular disease accounting for approximately 30% of their morbidity and mortality [58], improvement of $\dot{V}O_2$ peak might be of major benefit. In addition, increasing one's capacity for work decreases the relative percentage of that capacity required to perform at more common submaximal levels of functioning. Hence, exercise training regimens designed to improve aerobic capacity should be of significant benefit to the HD patient.

Less is known about the prognostic ability of $\dot{V}O_2$ peak in HD patients. Sietsema studied 175 end-stage renal disease (ESRD) subjects who had completed cardiopulmonary exercise testing (CXT) with measurement of $\dot{V}O_2$ peak to determine its value in predicting survival [59]. There were 23 deaths during the 39-month follow-up period with 19 deaths in subjects who were below the median $\dot{V}O_2$ peak of 17.5 mL/kg/min and four deaths in the subjects who were above the median.

TABLE 45.1 Summary of Benefits with Exercise Training in Selected Randomized Clinical Trials of Patients with Advanced CKD*

	Variable	Change with Exercise Training	Type, Intensity, Duration, Frequency, Supervision
Cardiovascular and aerobic performance	$\dot{V}O_2$ peak	Increase	Any
	SBP at rest	Decrease	Any
	DBP at rest	Decrease	Any
	HR at rest	Decrease	Any
	HRmax	Increase	Any
Musculoskeletal	Muscle strength	Increase	PRT
	Type I fiber area	No change	
	Mid-thigh muscle area	Equivocal increase	Any
	Thigh muscle attenuation	Increase	Resistance training
Physical performance	Sit-to-stand	No change	
	Gait speed	Increase	Endurance training >60% capacity
	Stair climb	No change	
Body composition	Fat mass	No change	
	Circumferences	No change	
Physical activity	Various measures	Increase	Any
Lipids and glucose	Triglycerides	No change	
	Total cholesterol	No change	
	HDL-C	Increase	Any
	LDL-C	Equivocal decrease	
	Glucose metabolism	No change	
Inflammation	IL-6	No change	
	Lymphocytes	No change	
	Protein catabolic rate	No change	
	Depression	Equivocal decrease	
	HR-QOL	Equivocal increase	

* Summarized from Heiwe and Jacobson, 2011 [36]

This difference was statistically significant (P = 0.009) and proved to be a better predictor of mortality than other traditional predictor variables. Although this was a retrospective study with a relatively small number of deaths, it gives insight into the possible value of increasing $\dot{V}O_2$ peak and hence the value of regular exercise training in the HD population. More research examining the causal nature of these relationships is needed.

Progressive resistance exercise training (PRT) has the potential to specifically address the well appreciated muscle dysfunction observed in advanced CKD, as it is the most potent exercise stimulus for anabolic adaptations. In healthy individuals, these adaptations include increased LBM, skeletal muscle fiber hypertrophy, increased muscle strength, power, and fatigability, and improved physical performance. These changes have been reported for both men and women of all ages [60,61] including older men in their 90s [62]. Likewise, significant increases in muscle performance and LBM have been reported after PRT in patients with COPD [63] and HIV infection [64]. Based on these observations in healthy individuals and patients with some chronic diseases, PRT applied to patients with ESRD holds promise.

TABLE 45.2 Changes in Aerobic Capacity ($\dot{V}O_2$ peak) from Randomized Clinical Trials in Exercising Hemodialysis Patients, Non-Exercising Controls, and Age-Matched Healthy Individuals

Study[ref]		Test mode	HD Exercise		HD home Exercise		HD CTRL		Healthy CTRL	
			Mean	SD	Mean	SD	Mean	SD	Mean	SD
Akiba 1995 [172]	Pre	CE	19.5				21.1			
	Post		20.0				18.2			
Carmack 1995 [44]	Pre	CE	10.7	4			10.0	3		
	Post		14.4	5			10.9	3		
Carney 1987 [173]	Pre	CE	17.9	4						
	Post		21.0	7						
Deligiannis 1999 [222]	Pre	TM	16.6	6	16.3	5	16.3	5	42.4	10
	Post		23.7	8	19	5	15.8	5		
Deligiannis 1999 [222]	Pre	TM	17.0	6			16.0	4	42.0	9
	Post		24.0	7			16.0	6	43.0	7
Goldberg 1983 [165]	Pre		21.0	7			20.0	7		
	Post		25.0	9			20.0	8		
Konstantindou 2002 [167]	Pre	TM	16.5†	6	16.2	5	16.3	5		
	Post		22.4†	7	19.0	5	15.8	5		
Koufaki 2002 [223]	Pre	CE	17.0	6			19.5	5		
	Post		19.9	6			18.8	5		
Kouidi 1997 [224]	Pre	TM	16.8	6			16.1	4		
	Post		23.2	8			15.9	4		
Kouidi 2009 [168]	Pre	TM	16.4	5			16.7	4		
	Post		21.4	7			16.5	5		
Molstead 2004 [177]	Pre	CE	18.8				23.1			
	Post		20.9				24.0			
Ouzouni 2009 [169]	Pre	TM	20.9	5			20.3	4		
	Post		25.3	5			20.1	3		
Painter 2002 [86]	Pre	TM	18.5	6			18.8	3		
	Post		20.8	9			17.7	4		
Tsuyuki 2003 [178]	Pre	TM	21.5	3			22.2	7		
	Post		27.0	6			21.7	5		
Van Vilsteren 2005 [45]	Pre	CE	25.4	6			26.1	11		
	Post		28.0	9			26.3	11		
Averages	Pre		18.3	5.4	16.3	5.0	18.8	5.2	42.2	9.5
	Post		22.6	7.2	19.0	5.0	18.4	5.3	43.0	7.0
	Δ		4.3		2.7		−0.4			
	% Δ		23%		17%		−2%		2%	

TABLE 45.3 Characteristics of Endurance Exercise Training Program Studies in Randomized Clinical Trials of Hemodialysis Patients

Reference	Akiba, 1995 [172]	Carmack, 1995 [44]	Carney, 1987 [173]	Deligiannis, 1999 [222]	Deligiannis, 1999 [163]	Goldberg, 1983 [165]	Konstantindou, 2002 [167]
Groups	HD-EX HD-NEX	HD-EX HD-NEX	HD-EX HD-NEX	HD-EX HD-NEX Healthy NEX	G1: EX-ND G2: EX-HD G3: NX-C G4: Healthy-C	HD-EX HD-NEX	G1: EX-ND G2: EX-HD G3: Ex Home G4: NX G5: Healthy-C
HD yrs	6	Not reported	2.9	6.3	6.2	2.5	6.1
M/F	9/11	48/21	8	32/28	23/15	15/10	31/17
Age (yr)	39.5	44.1		48	48.9	37.5	48.5
Study wks	12	10	24	24	24	52	24
Timing	Unknown	HD + other	ND	ND	G1: ND G2: ND-Home	HD	G1: ND G2: HD G3: Home
Supervision	Y	N	Y/N	Y	Y/N	Y	Y/Y/N
Type	Cycle	Cycle + other	Walk/jog	Calisthenics: steps, swimming, ball games	Cycle Treadmill Calisthenics: steps, stretching, +RT after 2 months	Walk/jog Cycle	G1: ET + RT G2: ET + RT G3: ET + Flex G4: NEX
Frequency (days/wk)	3	3	3	3/4	3	3	3, 3, 5, 0
Duration (min)	10 to >20	20–30	45–60	50	50	45	60, 60, 30, 0
Intensity	80% WRmax	Not reported	50–80% VO$_2$peak	60–70% HRmax	G1: 60–70% HRmax G2: 50–60% HRmax	50–60% VO$_2$peak	G1: 60–70% HRmax G2: 70% HRmax G3: 50% HRmax
Progression (exercise group only)	Intensity	Not reported	Intensity	Adjusted periodically to increase performance	Basketball, football, swimming	70–75% VO$_2$peak and up to 60 min	Basketball, football, swimming
Compliance (%)	Not Reported	84%	Not reported	Not reported	Not reported	100%	G1 = 76% G2 = 83% G3 = 83% G4 = 100%

Reference	Koufaki, 2002 [223]	Kouidi, 1997 [224]	Kouidi, 2009 [168]	Molstead, 2004 [177]	Ouzouni, 2009 [169]	Painter, 2002 [86]	Tsuyuki, 2003 [178]	van Vilsteren, 2005 [45]
Groups	HD-EX HD-NEX	HD-EX HD-NEX	HD-EX HD-NEX	HD-EX HD-NEX	HD-EX HD-NEX	HD-EX HD-NEX	HD-EX HD-NEX	HD-EX HD-NEX
HD yrs	3.5	6	6.3	1.8	1.8	5.4	2.3	3.9
M/F	24/9	15/16	18/12	22/11	27/6	9/10	14/15	68/34
Age (yr)	54.3	53	54	55.3	50.2	47.8	39.9	54.5
Study wks	12		40	20	40	20		12
Timing	HD	ND	HD	Not reported	HD	HD	ND	Pre-HD PRT HD Cycle
Supervision	Y	Y	Y	Yes	Yes	Yes	Yes	
Type	Cycle		Cycle, walk, jog, aerobics, games	Steps, circuit training, spin cycle, RT	Cycle, RT	Cycle	Cycle; jog	PRT + cycle
Frequency (days/wk)	3	3/4	3	2	3	3	2.5	2.5
Duration (min)	6–40	90	40-ET 30-RT	60	60–90	10/30	30	PRT ~20 CE : 20–30
Intensity	90% VO$_2$@AT	50–60% VO$_2$max	ET-60-70 HRmax	RPE = 14–17/20	RPE= 13–14/20	RPE = 12–13 70% HRpeak	50—60% HRpeak	60% WRpeak
Progression (exercise group only)	WR and Time	Add games last 8–12 weeks	ET = ↑time to 40 min RT = ↑resist	Not reported	ET: ↑time to 60 min RT: ↑reps, sets, resist	Add 2–3 min intervals RPE = 15–17	Not reported	Increase to maintain RPE = 12/20
Compliance (%)	Not reported	83	EX = 88%	74	Not reported	Not reported	Not reported	88%

TABLE 45.4 Characteristics of Resistance Exercise Training Interventions in Randomized Clinical Trials of CKD Patients

	Castaneda, 2001 [67]	Cheema, 2007 [100]	Chen, 2010 [68]	DePaul, 2002 [225]	Johansen, 2006 [65]
Groups	Diet + RT Diet + ShamEx	HD-RT HD-NEX	HD-RT HD-NEX	HD-ET + RT HD-NEX	HD-RT HD-NEX
HD yrs	NA	2.4	3.7	4.2	NR
M/F	17/9	34/15	23/21	23/14	26/14
Age (yr)	65	62.6	69.0	54.5	55.5
Study wks	12	12	24	12	12
Timing	Scheduled at research center	HD	HD	ET: HD RT: before or after HD	HD
Supervision	Yes	Yes	Yes	Yes	Yes
Type	RT: 5 pneumatic resistance exercises	RT: 10 free weight exercises	Ankle weights 8 exercises	ET: CE RT: Leg Pulley weights	Ankle weights 5 lower extremity exercises
Freq (d/wk)	3	3	2	3	3
Duration (sets × reps or min)	3 × 8	2 × 8	2 × 8	ET: 20 min RT: 1−3 × 10	2-3 × 10
Intensity	80% most recent 1-RM	RPE = 15−17/20 ("hard to very hard")	OMNI RPE = 6/10 (60% 1-RM)	ET: RPE = 4/10 RT:50% 5-RM	60% 3-RM
Progression (exercise group only)	Resistance increased to maintain 80% of most recent 1-RM	↑load to maintain RPE = 15−17/20	↑load when OMNI RPE <6	ET: ↑load when RPE <4/10 RT: ↑ load to 125% base 5-RM	↑ to 3 sets; then ↑ load
Variables assessed (selected)	Upper and lower extremity strength* Muscle fiber area* Mid-thigh area	Muscle CSA Muscle attenuation* Total strength* Arm and leg girth* 6-MWD BMI* log CRP* Self-reported PA* Vitality*	Knee extensor strength* Body composition SPPB*	Combined right/left quadriceps and hamstring strength* 6-MWD QOL	Quadriceps CSA* muscle strength* LBM Fat mass* Gait speed Stair climb time Sit-to-stand Objective PA Self-reported PA*
Compliance (%)	90−91	85	89	75	89%

	Kopple, 2007 [66]	Molstead, 2004 [177]	Segura-Orti, 2009 [171]	Yurtkuran, 2007 [69]
Groups	HD-ET; HD-RT, HD-ET + RT; HD-NEX	HD-EX HD-NEX	HD: LI ET HD: HI RT	HD-EX; HD-NEX
HD yrs	3.9	1.8	3.5	1.8
M/F	31/20	22/11	18/7	16/24
Age (yr)	43.9	55.3	55.9	39.8
Study wks	21	20	24	12

TABLE 45.4 Characteristics of Resistance Exercise Training Interventions in Randomized Clinical Trials of CKD Patients—cont'd

	Kopple, 2007 [66]	Molstead, 2004 [177]	Segura-Orti, 2009 [171]	Yurtkuran, 2007 [69]
Timing	HD	Not reported probably NHD	HD:RT	NHD
Supervision	Yes	Yes	Yes	Yes
Type	ET: CE RT: LP, LC; LE; CP ET + RT: Both	Stepping, circuit training, spin cycle, RT	LI-ET: aerobic exercise HI-RT: weights and elastic bands	EX: Modified Yoga
Freq (d/wk)	3	2	3	2
Duration (sets × reps or min)	ET: 20—40 min RT: 1—3 × 12-15 ET + RT: 1/2 ET and RT	60 min	3 × 15 for 4 exercises	15—30 min
Intensity	ET: 50% VO$_2$pk RT: 70% 5-RM ET + RT: same at ET and RRT	RPE = 14—17/20	RPE = 12—15/20	NR
Progression (exercise group only)	ET:↑ D + I as tolerated RT: 3 sets; 6-8 reps; 80% new 5-RM ET + RT: same as ET and RT	increase intensity to maintain RPE = 14—17/20	↑ Intensity to maintain RPE = 14—17/20	↑ Intensity as strength improved
Variables assessed (selected)	mRNA for IGF-1 isoforms IGF1-BP2,3 myostatin body composition	Leg strength* stair climb steps SF-36 PF*	Knee extension strength* sit-to-stand 6-MWD SF-36	Grip strength*
Compliance (%)	NR	74	84	"Good"

* Indicates significant improvement in exercise only groups relative to controls.
RT is resistance training; ET is endurance training; HD is hemodialysis; NEX is no exercise controls; RM is repetitions maximum; RPE is rating of perceived exertion; CSA is cross sectional area; 6-MWD is six-minute walk distance; BMI is body mass index; CRP is C-reactive protein; QOL is quality of life; LI is low intensity and HI is high intensity; NHD is non-dialysis days.

Given the well-appreciated muscle dysfunction known to accompany ESRD, it is somewhat surprising that only a few studies have investigated the anabolic effects of PRT in this population of patients. (Table 45.4) In the first study of resistance exercise training conducted during dialysis, Johansen and colleagues [65] compared changes in LBM and muscle size resulting from resistance exercise training and/or weekly injections of nandrolone decanoate (ND) in a 2 × 2 factorial design. Twelve weeks of PRT alone did not prove to be an adequate stimulus for increasing LBM, but quadriceps muscle cross sectional area (CSA) increased significantly. Conversely, subjects randomized to receive ND experienced greater gains in these measures and the effects were additive in subjects receiving both ND and PRT. Kopple and colleagues [66] compared the anabolic response in ESRD subjects randomized to 21 weeks of endurance training (ET), PRT, combined ET plus PRT, or non-exercising controls. Changes in skeletal muscle transcriptional levels of several growth factors were used to examine the anabolic response to these modes of training. The subjects randomized to PRT alone exhibited no change in fat-free mass (DEXA) as well as no significant changes in several muscle mRNA growth factors other than increased levels of insulin-like growth factor-IEa (IGF-IEa) (Table 45.4). Myostatin mRNA decreased by 23% in this group, but the change was not significant possibly due to the small number of subjects in this group . The authors identified several factors that might have influenced these results including the severe deconditioning and comorbidities of the patients in all groups, an inadequate training stimulus for the RT group, the possibility of myopathies that might have impaired training responses, or a type II statistical error because of the relatively small sample sizes. When all HD patients undergoing exercise training were compared together, there were significant increases with exercise in muscle transcriptional levels for a number of growth factors, and the mRNA for myostatin decreased significantly.

Castaneda et al. examined the effects of a low protein diet with or without PRT in a 12-week RCT of patients with chronic renal insufficiency (Table 45.4). Despite the protein restriction, trained subjects had significantly greater improvement in several measures of muscle strength (average 32% increase) compared to a 13% decrease in non-exercising subjects. In addition, the trained subjects exhibited maintainance of body weight and increased total body potassium and type I and II muscle fiber areas, whereas controls were observed to undergo a decrease in these measures; the differences in the changes were significant [67].

In a 24 week study, Chen et al. demonstrated that HD patients randomized to low intensity PRT (about 60% 1-RM) for the lower extremity conducted during the second hour of dialysis had significantly greater improvements in physical function (short physical performance battery, SPPB), knee extensor strength, and physical activity levels than subjects in the attention control group [68]. Similarly, some, but not all studies of patients with CKD randomized to PRT with or without added endurance training have shown significant improvements in muscle strength, 6-minute walk distance, stair climb performance, sit-to-stand transitions, self-reported physical function, and quality of life. Significant changes in these variables are noted in Table 45.4. Even an interdialytic modified yoga program resulted in significant improvements in handgrip strength relative to controls [69].

Recently, an Australian group described the effects of 12 and 24 weeks of PRT on markers of muscle performance, physical function, body composition and associated variables. (Table 45.4). Initially, 49 HD patients were randomized to 12 weeks of PRT during dialysis or to a non-exercising control group. After interim measurements at 12 weeks, the trained subjects continued training for an additional 12 weeks, whereas the control group crossed over to the same PRT program as the original exercise group. The primary outcome variables were midthigh CSA and thigh muscle attenuation, an indicator of intramuscular lipid accumulation; lower attenuation was reported to reflect better muscle quality. After the first 12-week phase of the study, no significant improvement in thigh CSA was seen in the group receiving PRT, and there was no significant change between groups in this measurement. Thigh muscle attenuation decreased by 1.2% (P > 0.05) in the PRT group, but this change resulted in a significant difference when compared with the 0.34% increase in the control group. At 24 weeks, the change in thigh muscle CSA was significantly greater in the group that had trained for 24 weeks versus the crossover group who had completed 12 weeks of training. There was no difference in attenuation between the groups at 24 weeks. Substantial improvements in variables associated with an anabolic response such as strength and physical function were observed.

There is no evidence in studies with HD patients that exercise training results in increased LBM. Limited and often inconsistent data do suggest anabolic effects in the form of significant increases in muscle CSA, muscle fiber size, muscle growth factors and their transcriptional levels, and decreased levels of myostatin and atrophic fibers from these interventions, particularly with PRT and combined training modes (Tables 45.1–45.3). Importantly, these changes are generally observed with improvements in less proximal measures of anabolism (i.e., muscle function and physical performance) that are of great functional benefit.

Observational data suggest that regular physical activity may be beneficial for improving survival in HD patients. These patients are extraordinarily inactive. One report showed 35% less activity than in sedentary healthy individuals [70] and two studies that analyzed physical activity data reported by over 2200 HD patients in the US Renal Data System Dialysis Morbidity and Mortality Study Wave 2 reported a 62% greater mortality risk in patients who were sedentary (never or almost never exercised) versus non-sedentary (i.e., those with physical activity on < 1 day/week to daily) at the time dialysis was initiated [31,71]. Although a causal relation is not yet proven or tested, the associative data so far available suggest that increasing $\dot{V}O_2$ peak, muscle performance, physical function, and habitual physical activity in patients with CKD should be a high priority in their usual care, and specific exercise training and physical activity guidance should be considered part of routine therapy for the advanced CKD patient. Conspicuously lacking, however, are data on the sustainability of these positive changes, and whether there is sustained improvement in important health outcomes, such as survival, morbidity, and risk factors, especially cardiovascular risk factors [58]. Since most available data are based on studies of less than 6 months duration, longer studies are needed to demonstrate whether sustainability of benefit does occur.

PRINCIPLES OF EXERCISE TRAINING

Basic Principles

Specificity

Exercise guidelines for the general population [32,33,72] as well as for various patient groups [73–76] encourage multi-modal exercise that includes endurance (aerobic) exercise training, progressive resistance exercise training (PRT), and attention to other dimensions of physical fitness including flexibility and balance [77]. These guidelines are based on the recognition that each of these modes of training offers unique benefits with only little crossover between types of training. For example, endurance training is the preferred mode of exercise for developing parameters of aerobic performance and submaximal endurance. These are valuable outcomes and in the HD population, numerous studies have shown endurance exercise training to result in significant physical, psychological, and quality of life benefit without adverse events [35,37,43]. However, in healthy young and older individuals as well as those with muscle atrophy due to sarcopenia or effects of chronic disease, PRT is the preferred training modality [77,78].

Overload

Without increasing effort beyond the usual, little to no improvement will occur. Overload in exercise training is considered to provide positive outcomes when appropriately and progressively applied. Overload requires an increase in exercise frequency, duration, and or intensity for further gains.

Progression

As people exercise regularly with certain intensities, frequencies, and durations, they adapt and reach a plateau in performance. In order for improvements to continue, there must be increases in the intensity, frequency, and/or duration as described below. This process is repeated until targets for risk reduction, physical function, or other clinical or patient important outcomes are achieved. In many older individuals and patient groups, progression may be slow, but in order to improve while combating the effects of disease on deteriorating physical performance, continued progression is important. The notion of progressive exercise training had its origin with DeLorme and Watkins over 60 years ago in their work rehabilitating soldiers [79]. However, legend describes Milo of Crotona, an Olympic wrestler in the 6th century BC, who was said to lift his new-born calf and carry it for a mile every day until Milo was lifting and carrying the fully grown bull; a clear example of the principles of overload and progressive exercise training. In the case of the advanced CKD patient, progression should continue indefinitely, albeit slowly, in order to overcome age and disease related decrements in physical abilities.

Individualization

Each person has unique capabilities and limitations due to age, medical history, exercise training history, comorbidities, years on dialysis, etc. Therefore, each exercise training prescription must be individually developed and monitored for responsiveness. Exercise prescriptions should be considered as dynamic with the dose altered as the individual responds to the training stimulus. For many people with advanced kidney failure, particularly when they are elderly, the prescription for exercise training may need to be quite modest.

Reversibility

While this seems self-evident, failure to maintain a regular training schedule will result in detraining and loss of improvements. Patients should be encouraged to remain as regular as possible with their exercise routines. Even some activity, even if not with the recommended duration and intensity, is better than none.

Warm-Up

The warm-up is designed to increased muscle/tendon suppleness, stimulate blood flow to the periphery, increase body temperature, and enhance free, coordinated movement. Depending on the planned exercise intensity, a general 5–15 min whole body warm-up of gradually increasing intensity to the intensity target should precede the conditioning period. At rest, muscle receives only about 15–20% of the cardiac output; during moderate exercise, this increases to about 70%. Beneficial effects of warm up include increased muscle temperature through increased blood flow; increased myocardial blood flow; rightward shift of the oxyhemoglobin dissociation curve facilitating oxygen delivery; and possible reduction in cardiac dysrhythmias [80]. For resistance exercise, movement through the intended range of motion for the selected exercise with light resistance will provide a muscle-specific increase in blood flow and temperature and improved neuromuscular activation including greater conduction velocities and faster activation of muscle fibers [81].

Cool Down

In upright exercise, a gradual decrease in exercise intensity over a 5–10 minute period prevents blood pooling in the lower extremities by maintaining the action of the peripheral muscle pump. Possible consequences of blood pooling include hypotension, fainting and cardiac dysrhythmias [77]. Cool down also facilitates heat dissipation and more rapid removal of lactic acid and catecholamines from the blood.

PATIENT ASSESSMENT

Prior to the onset of an exercise training program, patients with CKD should undergo a clinical exercise test that at a minimum includes incremental exercise on a treadmill or cycle ergometer to peak work rate with electrocardiographic (ECG) and blood pressure monitoring throughout rest, exercise, and recovery. In many cases, exercise echocardiography or imaging studies may be important additional measures. When resources allow, the exercise test should include complete cardiopulmonary exercise test (CXT) procedures with measurement of respiratory gas exchange and pulmonary minute ventilation. The CXT can add important diagnostic data including parameters of aerobic performance ($\dot{V}O_2$ peak, anaerobic threshold) cardiovascular performance (ECG, blood pressure, chronotropic index, ventilatory efficiency slope, oxygen uptake efficiency slope), as well as insight into ventilatory and/or gas exchange limitations. See references 39–41 for details.

Assessing patients with CKD provides objective insight into physical abilities, quantifies exercise tolerance, aids in developing exercise training guidelines, and provides a baseline for monitoring progress and program efficacy. These assessments may also be used to identify relationships between exercise intensity and symptoms such as cardiac abnormalities or musculoskeletal limitations.

Common assessments associated with physical performance and exercise training include measures of aerobic function (cardiorespiratory endurance), muscle performance, flexibility, and in older individuals and in patients with chronic diseases, physical function, and balance [77]. Table 45.5 summarizes several options for assessing various dimensions of health related fitness and physical performance.

Aerobic Function and Cardiopulmonary Endurance

Assessment instruments for endurance performance include laboratory methods such as cardiopulmonary exercise testing (CXT) using incremental and constant work-rate (CWR) protocols performed on treadmills or cycle ergometers [40,82]. Analysis of gas exchange data collected with metabolic measurement systems adds precision and allows evaluation of the integrated function of the cardiovascular, pulmonary, and muscular systems [40,83] A symptom-limited CXT can be valuable in defining the specific physiologic limitations to exercise, assessing the safety of exercise, formulating the exercise prescription, and providing a baseline for progress monitoring [40]. Key variables to measure during this assessment include $\dot{V}O_2$ peak, $\dot{V}O_2$ at the anaerobic (lactate) threshold, ($\dot{V}O_2$ θ), as well work rates and heart rates at these markers of aerobic performance. Specific guidelines for administering and interpreting cardiopulmonary exercise tests assessments (CXT, CWR, functional tests) have been published [40,83,84].

Because of their profound muscle weakness, most advanced CKD patients terminate an exercise test because of leg fatigue before a plateau in oxygen uptake is achieved, thus not meeting the primary criteria defining maximal oxygen uptake [41]. In addition to oxygen delivery limitations (low hemoglobin, low ventricular performance) there are also both an overall smaller muscle mass and dysfunctional mitochondria that affect oxygen extraction through significantly reduced complex IV activity in CKD/HD patients as compared with healthy controls [85]. Hence, $\dot{V}O_2$ peak is considered as an index of functional capacity in patients with CKD. Painter points out, however, that $\dot{V}O_2$ peak may not reflect the functional impact of exercise training in HD patients [86]. Submaximal CWR tests are particularly appealing in this regard, because unlike maximal incremental exercise testing that investigates the limits of tolerance, CWR tests assesses ability to sustain exercise at levels of work more commonly encountered in everyday life [87]. In one study investigating the effects of 9 weeks of endurance exercise cycling in HD patients, $\dot{V}O_2$ peak increased by 22% in exercising subjects [26]. However, endurance time on a CWR test, using 80% of baseline WRpeak, increased by 144%, from 5.5 min to 13.4 min. This improvement was likely an underestimation, as the CWR test in this study was constrained to 15 min. The improved $\dot{V}O_2$ peak predicts an increased capacity for exercise and reduced risk, but the large increase in CWR time suggests the potential for substantial improvements in the ability to perform every day activities that may lead to improvements in quality of life.

When CXT with gas exchange analysis is not feasible or is inappropriate, incremental and CWT cycle or treadmill tests can still be performed with monitoring of the blood pressure, heart rate, the electrocardiogram and work rate (treadmill speed and grade or power output in watts during cycle ergometry). Time to peak exercise provides an index of functional capacity and peak work rate reflects exercise tolerance. Symptoms of exercise intolerance, including blood pressure and ECG abnormalities, at submaximal work rates may be useful in setting exercise training intensities to avoid these signs and symptoms of intolerance. Functional exercise tests such as 6-minute walk distance tests [88,89] and shuttle walk tests [90–92] are practical, time saving, inexpensive, and can provide helpful information for setting the exercise prescription and for progress monitoring. Specific guidelines for administering the 6-minute walk test and the shuttle walk test are available [88,91,93].

Muscle Performance

Muscle performance includes three specific functional attributes: strength, power, and fatigability (local muscle endurance). *Strength*, the greatest force that can be developed against a resistance one time only, is usually assessed with the one-repetition maximum (1-RM) procedure [94]. This method requires a gradual progression of increasing resistance to muscular movement to the maximum resistance that can be overcome one time only. The 1-RM procedure has been administered safely in the elderly [62], and in many chronic disease states, including patients with COPD [95, 96], lower risk cardiac patients [97—99], and CKD patients [37,100,101] but it may not be routinely appropriate for use in the ESRD population due to the higher risk for fracture and tendon rupture [102—104]. In this case, dynamic muscle strength can be estimated with the 3-RM or 5-RM procedure in which resistance is gradually increased to a level where only three or five repetitions can be performed in good form before

TABLE 45.5 Methods for Assessing Dimensions of Health Related Fitness and Physical Performance in Patients with CKD

Methods of Assessment	Outcome Variable(s)	Equipment	Dimension of Performance	References
CARDIOPULMONARY FUNCTION AND ENDURANCE				
CXT	VO$_2$peak	TM or cycle ergometer Metabolic Measurement System	Aerobic capacity	[40,83]
	WRpeak		Work capacity	
	HRpeak		Chronotropic response	
	Anaerobic threshold		Ability for prolonged work	
	CXT duration		Surrogate for aerobic capacity	
CWR test	CWR duration	TM or cycle ergometer	Submaximal aerobic endurance	
MUSCLE PERFORMANCE				
3-RM/5-RM	Strength	Elastic, free weights, or machine weights	Surrogates for muscle strength	[65,105—107]
Handgrip		Handgrip dynamometer		[226—229]
Repetitions to failure	Fatigability	Elastic, free weights, or machine weights	Local muscle endurance	[26]
at 80% ×-RM value				
PHYSICAL PERFORMANCE — OBJECTIVE MEASURES				
SPPB	0—12 score	Stopwatch, chair, 4-m walk course	PF	[126]
NSRI-PF	Time		Integrated PF	[230]
Chair stands	Time or number of stands	Chair; stopwatch	PF; surrogate for leg power	[131]
Stair Climb	Time and power	Staircase; timing system	PF; surrogate for leg power	[132]
Lift and Lower	Number of shelves	Shelves; weight	Upper extremity PF	[132]
6-MWD	Distance and gait speed	20—30-m straight course; timer	PF; gait speed	[88,231]
Timed walks	Gait speed	Measured course 6-m to 400-m	Gait speed	[129]
Timed-up-and-go (TUG)	Time	Chair, measured course	Integrated PF	[232]
PHYSICAL PERFORMANCE — SUBJECTIVE MEASURES				
PF-10		PF-10 inventory	Self-reported PF	

(Continued)

TABLE 45.5   Methods for Assessing Dimensions of Health Related Fitness and Physical Performance in Patients with CKD—cont'd

Methods of Assessment	Outcome Variable(s)	Equipment	Dimension of Performance	References
FLEXIBILITY				
Forward trunk flexion	Centimeters reached	Sit-and-reach box	Integrated flexibility	[116—118]
Rotational trunk flexion	Centimeters reached	Meter stick	Rotational flexibility	
BALANCE				
Single leg balance	Time in balance	Stopwatch	Balance	[126]
Semi-tandem balance	Time in balance	Stopwatch	Balance	[126]
Berg Balance Test	Berg score	Step stool, mat table, chair with arms, Tape measure, stopwatch, and pen.	Balance	[233]
Timed tandem walk	Time and errors	6-m course; stopwatch	Dynamic balance	[114]
PHYSICAL ACTIVITY OBJECTIVE MEASURES				
Pedometers	Step counts	Pedometer	Spontaneous PA	[234]
Accelerometers	Step counts; time in Different activity levels	Accelerometer (Triaxial)		[235]
PHYSICAL ACTIVITY SUBJECTIVE MEASURES				
Logs	PA Score	Logs	Self-reported PA — PF-10	
Questionnaires	PA Score	Questionnaires		[236]
Quality of Life				
KDQOL				[237,238]
SF-36				[239]

the resistance can no longer be overcome. The 3-RM and 5-RM have been shown to predict 1-RM with reasonable accuracy in healthy individuals [105—107], but no studies have examined this relationship in CKD patients.

Similar in concept to the CWR endurance tests, *local muscle endurance* can be assessed using submaximal resistance. Targeted exercises with 70—90% of the 1-RM, 3-RM, or 5-RM evaluates the ability of a particular group of muscles to make repetitive contractions at submaximal loads before fatigue leads to failure to complete the next repetition.

Muscle power, the rate of muscle contraction, is associated with a variety of physical performance measures including sit-to-stand transitions, stair climb time and power, and gait speed [26,108,109] and may be a better predictor of functional performance than strength [110,111]. Despite its strong association with physical performance, muscle power is difficult to measure without specialized equipment [26,109,112]. However, some studies have used measurements of the time taken to complete a number of sit to stand transitions (e.g., 5—10) as a surrogate for leg power measurements [113]. Musculoskeletal limitations can be further assessed and addressed through referral to a physical therapist or exercise physiologist.

When the results from muscle strength, muscle endurance, or muscle power assessments are used to develop exercise training intensities, for progress monitoring, or to evaluate program efficacy, the type of resistance (Table 45.5) and movement pattern of the specific exercises should be identical.

Balance and Flexibility

Balance

In addition to the three static balance tests described below within the Short Physical Performance Battery (SPPB), dynamic balance can be assessed using a timed tandem walk where subjects walk heel-to-toe, as quickly as possible over a 6-meter course [114]. Test–retest reliability of this procedure is r = 0.94, P = 0.001.

Flexibility

Loss of flexibility contributes to restricted mobility in daily activities in older individuals. Since no single measurement indicates loss of flexibility at all joints [115], multiple or integrated tests of flexibility can be considered. The modified sit-and-reach test [116] primarily assesses hamstring flexibility and to a lesser extent, low back and calf flexibility in the sagittal plane and the standing trunk rotation test assesses the integrated flexibility of the ankles, knees, trunk, shoulder, and neck in the horizontal plane [117,118]. Test-retest reliability for these tests is high, r = 0.83, and interclass reliability is 0.98 and 0.99 in elderly subjects [115,119].

Physical Function

As humans grow older, they experience a decline in physical function that contributes to increased risk of falls, fractures, disability, mortality, and poor quality of life [120–125]. Indeed, physical function has been described as a mirror to an individual's health [120,124,126]. Limitations in physical function are associated with increased risk of disability, mortality, hospitalization, and poor quality of life [127–131]. Objective measures of physical function reflect the ease with which one performs typical activities of daily living (ADL). These include walking, stair climbing, rising from a chair, and lifting and lowering objects. Many of these tests have been developed for the frail elderly [108] and as such often have ceiling effects when applied to other populations [132–134]. That is, when a person's ability reaches a certain level, no further improvement is seen on these measures with increased ability. However, given the extremely low functional ability of people with advanced CKD, many of the common tests of physical function may be entirely appropriate for this population. Several of these measures are summarized in Table 45.5.

Overend and colleagues studied the relative and absolute reliability of the 6-minute walk test and the number of sit-to-stand transitions completed in 30 seconds [135]. Interclass correlations for the two functional measures were good (0.93 for both), suggesting good reliability, but the significant differences between trial 1 and trial two for the 6-minute walk (19-m) and chair stands (one repetition) suggest the use duplicate trials for these tests to ensure baseline stability. The minimal detectable changes determined from these data were 77-meters for the 6-minute walk test and 2.6 repetitions for the chair stands. Since the minimal detectable difference describes the random variability in scores of a truly stable participant, changes greater than these values can give confidence that a true change will have occurred 95% of the time.

Self-reported physical function has also been evaluated in CKD patients. Knight et al. reported hazard ratios for one year mortality in 15,000 dialysis patients using the physical component summary (PCS) from the SF-36 [136]. Compared to patients with a PCS score greater than 50, individuals scoring 20–29 had a mortality hazard ratio of 1.62; those scoring 30–39 had a hazard ratio of 1.32 and patients whose PCS was lower than 20 had a hazard ratio of 1.97. Finally, patients whose PCS declined over 1 year had additional risk of mortality with an increased hazard ratio of 1.25 per 10-point decline in PCS score.

COMPONENTS OF THE EXERCISE TRAINING PRESCRIPTION

Formal guidelines for prescribing exercise in healthy adults have been evolving since at least 1975 [137]. Since then, the American College of Sports Medicine has provided regular updates to these recommendations and most recently, evidence-based guidelines for exercise training in apparently healthy younger [32] and older adults [72]. The 2008 Physical Activity Guidelines for Americans from the U.S. Department of Health and Human Services [33] have contributed to the ease of understanding and more widespread dissemination of these recommendations [77]. These guidelines, with certain modifications, comprise the framework for evidence-based exercise training recommendations in cardiac [82,98,138] and pulmonary rehabilitation programs [73,76] and for recommendations from authorities for exercise for the CKD population [35,37,38,139]. Although at this time, there are no recognized formal guidelines for "renal rehabilitation" programs, the concepts embodied in these other guidelines should be directly applicable for patients with advanced CKD, although with specific modifications. Johansen has suggested [38] that until evidence-based guidelines are available for exercise training in HD patients, the guidelines developed for healthy older persons [72] may be appropriate for use in this patient group. This suggestion is altogether reasonable and in fact does establish the structure for most research studies of exercise training in individuals undergoing HD. This section provides a general description of the defining elements of exercise training including the **Mode** of activity and the **Frequency**, **Duration**, and **Intensity** of training. The basic principles that underlie these components may be used for any mode of exercise and, with appropriate modifications, for people with most chronic diseases. Examples of these elements will be given for endurance and resistance exercise training as well as for flexibility and balance in the next section. Details for prescribing these elements in HD patients will be provided later in the chapter.

Mode

The mode of exercise is defined as the general category of exercise, i.e., endurance (aerobic) exercise training, resistance training, flexibility, and balance. Each of these modes provides a unique contribution to improving physical performance and for risk reduction. Within each mode are various **Types** of exercise. For example, endurance exercise training is best accomplished when large muscle groups are used in continuous, rhythmical patterns of movement [82]. Good examples of endurance training activities are those that require minimal skill or fitness and include walking, cycling, water-aerobics, and slow dancing. More vigorous endurance activities include jogging/running, rowing, elliptical exercise, and faster paced dancing.

Types of resistance exercise training generally consider the nature of resistance used. Good examples, many of which are low cost options, include ankle weights, dumbbell weights, machine weights, and elastic resistance (tubing or bands).

Recommended types of stretching include static (active or passive), dynamic, ballistic and proprioceptive neuromuscular facilitation (PNF) [32,72,82]. Static stretching requires slow movement to a stretched posture that is held for 10−30 seconds (active), or the stretched position is held by a partner and/or by holding onto a limb, towel, stretch band, etc. (passive). Caution is advised with ballistic (bouncing using body momentum to produce the stretch) so as not to invoke a reflexive muscle contraction due to an excessively fast movement or movement through a range of motion that is too far for comfort. Dynamic stretching includes slow, gradual transitions from one body position to another with progressively increasing range of motion. PNF stretching can be performed in a number of ways but usually involves a preliminary 5−10 second isometric contraction of the muscle to be stretched followed immediately by a static stretch of this muscle, usually passively with an experienced partner helping to sustain the stretched posture. Whether stretching is useful for injury prevention, low back pain, or delayed onset muscle soreness is controversial [140]. However, stretching may be helpful for enhancing postural stability and balance, particularly when it is augmented by resistance exercise training [141,142]. These are clearly of value in older individuals, particularly those weakened by chronic disease.

Frequency

Frequency is expressed for all training modes as the number of days per week for exercise. Recommended frequency varies with the medical and exercise history of the individual as well as with acute exacerbations. Training frequency may be different for different modes, although two or more modes of exercise might be performed in a given training session. For example stretching, endurance exercise, and resistance exercise could be performed during the same visit to the dialysis center although this does not necessarily suggest that two or more modes should be performed in EVERY exercise session. Current guidelines for healthy individuals currently recommend 5 days per week of moderate intensity endurance exercise and two or more days per week for resistance exercise [32,33,72].

Duration

Duration defines the amount of time spent during each mode of training on any given training day. For endurance training, this typically means total time spent at an elevated heart rate or perception of effort (see Intensity, below). For resistance training, duration is generally expressed as a volume defined by the product of the number of sets (e.g., 1 to 3), of repetitions (complete cycles) and total number of exercises performed. For example, two sets of 10 repetitions for eight exercises yield a volume of 160 repetitions ($2 \times 10 \times 8$). For healthy older persons one set of 10−15 repetitions for each major muscle group is recommended. Similar recommendations are suggested for patients with COPD and cardiovascular disease. For stretching exercises, duration can be expressed as the product of the length of time a stretch is held, and the number of stretches performed.

Intensity

Intensity refers to the level of exertion during exercise training which is prescribed and measured differently for different modes of exercise. Common among endurance and resistance training intensities is the use of subjective rating of effort known as ratings of perceived exertion or RPE.

Endurance Exercise

Intensity can be measured objectively with heart rate, oxygen uptake, blood lactate, or work rate. Setting a target heart rate based on a percentage of maximal heart rate (%HRmax) or percentage of the heart rate reserve (%HRR, where HRR is HRmax − HRrest) achieved during a CXT (Table 45.6) is appealing because of its ease of use. However, training intensities based on heart rate may be unreliable in HD patients, as described below in **Exercise training program design for patients with advanced CKD.** If a CXT has been performed with measurements of oxygen uptake ($\dot{V}O_2$), a percentage of $\dot{V}O_2$ peak or $\dot{V}O_2$ reserve ($\dot{V}O_2$ R) where $\dot{V}O_2$ R = $\dot{V}O_2$ peak − $\dot{V}O_2$ rest may be used to set the intensity level. Subjectively, intensity can be estimated with ratings of perceived exertion using the Borg 6−20 RPE scale [143], the Borg 0−10 category ratio scale [144], the Omni scale (a pictorial scale with ratings from 0−10) [145,146], or arbitrary 0−10 scales [32,72]. Scherr et al. have recently demonstrated in 2560 Caucasian men and women, aged 13−83 years, that ratings of perceived exertion on the Borg 6-20 RPE scale were strongly correlated with heart rate (r = 0.74, p = 0.001) and blood lactate (r = 0.83, p = 0.001) [147]. Moreover, this study showed that these relationships were independent of sex, age, exercise test modality (treadmill of cycle ergometer), physical activity level, or coronary artery disease status. An RPE of 11 corresponded to the lactate threshold and was suggested as reasonable exercise intensity ("fairly light" to "somewhat hard") for less fit and untrained individuals. Since the lactate threshold is a marker of one's ability to perform prolonged work

without a net lactate accumulation [147], an RPE of 11−13 could serve as an appropriate guideline for low fit individuals while an RPE of 13−15 (vigorous exercise) would be more appropriate for more fit and active people. Prediction equations for both heart rate and blood lactate from RPE are available [147]. Although these recommendations seem reasonable, there are no data to indicate their validity in patients with pathologies other than coronary artery disease.

It is easier to use one of the subjective perceptual scales, and these scales are perhaps the most practical method for assessing exercise intensity once the patient has a good understanding of how one should perceive a given level of effort. Guidelines for this purpose have been published [88,143,148]. Indeed, current recommendations for assessing exercise intensity in both healthy younger and older people have attempted to simplify intensity guidelines by suggesting use of "moderate" (e.g., brisk walking and noticeable increases in heart rate) and "vigorous" (jogging with rapid breathing and substantial increase in heart rate) ranges of effort which correspond to 5−6 and 7−8 on an arbitrary 10 point scale, respectively [32,33,72].

Interval training that uses alternating bouts of higher and lower intensity exercise has been used safely and effectively in patients with COPD [149−152], various types of heart disease [133−136,153−156], and in people with other cardiometabolic diseases [157,158]. Examples include high intensity intervals using 80% to 105% $\dot{V}O_2$ peak alternated with lower intensity intervals (70-70% $\dot{V}O_2$ peak) in various ratios, e.g. 1:1, 1:2, 4:3, 0.5:4 repeated 4−6 times. Burgomaster et al trained eight healthy young men and women using 4−7 30-second maximal efforts on a cycle ergometer interspersed with 4 minute recovery periods [159]. A total of six training

TABLE 45.6 Methods for Calculating Relative Endurance Exercise Training Intensities Including Different Measures that Indicate Roughly Equivalent Degrees of Exercise Intensity

	% HRmax	% $\dot{V}O_2$ max	%HRreserve or %$\dot{V}O_2$ reserve	RPE 6−20 [123]	RPE 0−10 [124]
Very light	<57	<37	<30	<9	0−1
Light	37−45	37−45	30−39	9−11	2-3
Moderate	64−76	46−63	40−59	12−13	3-4
Vigorous	77−95	64−90	60−89	14−17	5−7
Near maximal to maximal	≥96	≥91	≥90	≥18	8−10

%HR rate reserve is HRmax-HRrest; %$\dot{V}O_2$ reserve is $\dot{V}O_2$ max-$\dot{V}O_2$ rest; RPE 6−20 is Borg's Rating of Perceived Exertion Scale; RPE 0−10 is Borg's Category Ratio Scale of perceived effort and pain.
Adapted from Garber et al., 2011 [77].

sessions were evenly distributed over two weeks. A control group did not train. Time to fatigue at work rates equivalent to 80% baseline $\dot{V}O_2$ peak increased by 100% with no change in controls. These impressive improvements in endurance occurred after an average total high intensity exercise time of 14—16 minutes and a total training time including the rest intervals of about 90 minutes over two weeks suggesting the time efficiency of this training method. Hwang et al. summarized findings of six RCT using high intensity interval training compared with continuous endurance training in cohorts of patients with cardiometabolic diseases including overweight or obese patients, individuals diagnosed with the metabolic syndrome, coronary artery disease or heart failure, or post-coronary artery bypass graft surgery (n = 94) [157]. Total energy expenditure between high intensity interval and continuous training groups was held equal. Adherence to high intensity interval training was between 70 and ≥90%. Compared to continuous endurance exercise training, high intensity interval training yielded significantly higher $\dot{V}O_2$ peak, weighted mean difference = 3.6 (95% CI, 2.28—4.91) mL/kg/min. There were no differences between types of training for BMI, body weight, waist circumference, blood pressure, or serum lipids.

Resistance Exercise

In this mode, exercise intensity is usually expressed as a percentage of the maximal load that can be lifted once (1-RM) during an initial assessment. Alternatively, the load that can be lifted for a given range of repetitions, i.e., 10—15 repetitions per set, may be used. The 1-RM test is highly effort dependent [94] and presents some risk of injury. However, the 1-RM test has been safely administered to healthy individuals without musculoskeletal limitations [160] and even to pulmonary disease patients [95,96], and lower risk cardiac patients [97,98]. However, use of alternative forms of resistance, such as elastic bands or tubing or body weight resistance, affects the ability to attain a 1-RM. Limitations of 1-RM testing in ESRD patients will be discussed below.

Many studies have used percentages of the 1-RM (% 1-RM) for training intensity prescriptions. Ideally, 1-RM values are retested after adaptation to training since the 1-RM will have likely increased as training progresses. Without reestablishing the 1-RM, subsequent training loads will no longer represent the originally chosen % 1-RM. There may be some disadvantage, in using % 1-RM as a guide to training intensity. First, the training stimulus at a fixed percentage of 1-RM varies with the muscle mass used and the training state of the subject [161,162]. Thus, 70% of 1-RM for the leg press exercise may result in a different number of repetitions completed per set than for triceps extensions at the same 70% 1-RM load. Second, the number of repetitions

that can be performed at 50% 1-RM versus 85% 1-RM varies considerably. At least in healthy individuals, 50% 1-RM loads correspond to greater than 15 repetitions; similarly, 85% of 1-RM corresponds to about 6 repetitions [94]. These different combinations of loads and repetitions predict different training effects [161]. Third, assigning loads based on % 1-RM requires frequent reassessment of the 1-RM so that the load may be increased proportionally as strength increases over time. This can be tedious, time consuming, and difficult for patients. An alternative approach proposed by Nelson et al. for older, healthy adults makes use of subjective ratings of effort in which moderate exercise is equivalent to 5—6 on a zero to 10 scale (0 = no movement) and high intensity exercise at 7—8 on a 0—10 scale [72]. Another approach uses a given range of repetitions to near failure or inability to complete the next repetition in good form. For example, initial training loads might include sets of 10—15 RM (resistance is selected that can be lifted for at least 10 repetitions but not more than 15 repetitions) which represents about 65—75% 1-RM. As training progresses, prescribed repetitions-maximum often decrease, e.g. to 6—10 RM, which is equivalent to about 75—85% 1-RM [94]. This method of repetitions to near failure is self-adjusting for maintenance of relatively constant training loads. As a general rule, when an individual is able to complete three consecutive training sessions with all prescribed repetitions, the load should be increased enough to maintain the prescription, e.g., at 10—15-RM.

Rest Interval

Especially with resistance exercise training, consideration for rest between efforts, e.g., a set in resistance training, an interval in endurance training, or days between training sessions is important to allow sufficient time for recovery before the next effort. Rest intervals are often overlooked in guidelines for exercise training and left to the practitioner or individual. For endurance exercise interval training, rest between higher intensity efforts may be passive or active with the latter using lower intensity exercise. Often the effort-to-rest ratio is 1:1 or 1:2, but the practitioner may choose any ratio appropriate for a given patient. Rest between days for endurance training depends on the medical condition and training state of the subject as well as on training intensity and objectives. As fitness improves, the need for rest days in the form of no exercise decreases so long as intensity is in the moderate range. Even with vigorous intensity exercise such as interval training, with proper progression, a patient could exercise the next day if the intensity was in the light to moderate range. It is reasonable, even for patients with advanced CKD, to progress to five or more days per week of moderate intensity exercise.

For *resistance exercise*, rest intervals between sets are often guided by the training objective, health and fitness of the participant, and exercise training history. Current evidence-based guidelines for healthy adults suggest 2–3 minutes for rest between sets. This would be appropriate for most patient groups as well. Shorter rest intervals are used by more well conditioned individuals particularly when the primary objective is muscle hypertrophy (45–60 sec) or muscle endurance (15–30 sec) [94]. Since most resistance training for all the major muscle groups is performed 2 to 3 days/wk, at least one rest day should be given before exercising the same body part again.

Progression

A gradual increase in exercise volume through adjustments in frequency, duration, and intensity should occur until the training objective is achieved. For endurance exercise, practitioners should consider the time available to participants, as this will help decide whether frequency or duration should be increased bearing in mind the objective of five or more days per week and 30 minutes or more per day. Since injury risk may be greater with higher intensity exercise, first achieving one's frequency and duration goals is a reasonable approach. Absolute intensity should be increased, i.e., work rate, so that relative intensity remains the same as fitness improves. For example, with training, higher work rates (walking speeds and grades, cycle resistance) will be required to maintain the same target heart rate or RPE. Similar approaches are used in resistance exercise training through increases in sets, resistance, and training days. While one set of an exercise for each major muscle group is effective in low fitness or untrained individuals, particularly for improving muscle endurance, greater benefits to improving muscle strength, hypertrophy, and power are seen with 2–4 sets [77].

EXERCISE TRAINING PROGRAM DESIGN FOR PATIENTS WITH ADVANCED CKD

There are no specific evidence-based guidelines for prescribing exercise to improve physical function and quality of life, or reduce morbidity and mortality in CKD patients. However, guidelines from the National Kidney Foundation Kidney Disease Outcome Quality Initiative (NKF KDOQI) [138], systematic reviews [35–37] and recommendations from experts [38,139] as well as evidence based guidelines for healthy individuals [32,33,72,77,82,98], people with COPD [73,75,76,93] and

cardiovascular disease [74,82,98,163] have provided a framework for general exercise training recommendations. Endurance exercise guidelines are summarized in Table 45.7, and resistance training guidelines are listed in Table 45.8. For comparison, evidence-based guidelines for endurance and resistance exercise training for healthy younger and older individuals as well as for patients with cardiovascular disease and COPD are included.

Objectives of Exercise Training for Advanced CKD Patients

The objectives for an exercise training program include the following:

- Assess individual patients for exercise history and physical functional abilities (see Table 45.5).
- Develop and assist the patient in implementing safe and effective exercise training.
- Provide guidelines for unsupervised exercise, e.g. home exercise, as well as for lifestyle physical activity.
- Provide appropriate supervision and monitoring to detect changes in clinical status and provide ongoing surveillance data to the patients' healthcare providers to enhance medical management.
- Increase exercise capacity, physical function, quality of life, and survival.
- Decrease risk factors associated with CKD and ESRD.
- Provide patient and family education to maximize secondary/tertiary prevention, e.g., risk factor modification.

When to Exercise

Both intradialytic [25,26,45,65,66,68,86,100,164–171] and interdialytic [15,19,166,172–178] exercise training programs have been used successfully and safely in studies with HD patients. In general, supervised programs are preferred when possible. If training is conducted during dialysis, it should be done either before or during the first 90–120 min of treatment to avoid the risk of hypotensive responses. Unsupervised home programs have had mixed success [37]. Three studies have directly compared home versus supervised intra- or interdialytic exercise on various primary outcomes including VO_2 peak, anaerobic threshold, 6-minute walk test, and aortic pulse wave velocity [166,167,176]. Patients randomized to supervised programs on non-dialysis days had the greatest improvement from baseline in aerobic capacity, but incurred the highest dropout rates as compared with intradialytic training. Some improvement in the primary outcomes was demonstrated in all of the three exercise training schedules [166,167,176]. Intradialytic exercise may be the preferred exercise time since it not only provides increased opportunity for supervision

TABLE 45.7　Summary of Evidence-Based and Clinical Practice Guidelines for Cardiovascular Endurance (Aerobic) Exercise Training in Healthy Young and Older Individuals, Cardiac Patients and People with COPD. For Comparison, Existing Recommendations for Endurance Exercise Prescription in CKD are Included

Group	Supervision	Type	Frequency (d/wk)	Intensity	Duration (min)	Notes
Healthy younger [32]	NS	Large muscle group, rhythmical, continuous exercise: T, C, AE, A/LE, R	≥5	Moderate and	30–60	Target volume recommendations: ≥500–1000 MET min/wk Increase pedometer step counts to ≥7000 steps/d
			≥3	Vigorous	20–60	
Healthy older [72]	NS	Large muscle group, rhythmical, continuous exercise: T, C, AE, A/LE, R	≥5	Moderate (5–6/10) and	≥30	Duration should be accumulated in bouts of at least 10 min
			≥3	Vigorous (7–8/10)	≥20	Duration should be continuous for at least 20 min/d
Cardiac rehabilitation (outpatient) [74,82]	Supervised and unsupervised	Large muscle group, sustained exercise: T, C, AE, A/LE, R	4–7	RPE = 11–14; 40–80% HRR/VO$_2$R; THR < angina, ST-depression, BP thresholds; to tolerance*	20–60	Intermittent, short duration exercise may be necessary initially; both continuous and interval training may be used
COPD [73,75,76]	Supervised	Walk; cycle; UB ergometer	≥3	Low and/or High Intervals	Build to >30	Intermittent, short duration exercise may be necessary initially; higher intensity recommended when appropriate
	Supervised	CE, T	3–5	≥50–60% WRpeak or 4–5/10 RPE	20–60	
	Supervised		3–5	Higher intensity 70–80% WRpeak	20–60 in bouts of 30–180 sec	Higher intensity interval training if appropriate. Work:Rest has not been defined but 1:1 or 1:2 may be used if patient cannot sustain recommended intensity

CURRENT RECOMMENDATIONS FOR ENDURANCE EXERCISE PRESCRIPTION IN HD PATIENTS

Group	Supervision	Type	Frequency (d/wk)	Intensity	Duration min)	Notes
NKF K/DOQI [138]	NS	NS	Most to 7	Moderate	30	Guideline 14.4.a.i: Refer severely deconditioned HD patients to cardiac rehabilitation Guideline 14.4.a.ii: start with very low intensity and duration
Johansen [38]	NS	Walking	3	Moderate as tolerated	10–30	
Brenner [35]		Adapted cycle ergometer	3	RPE 12–15/20	30–90 (includes RT)	Exercise during dialysis is preferred particularly to ensure adherence
Meta-analysis exercise in CKD [37]	Supervised	Large muscle group, sustained exercise e.g., cycle walk, jog	3	"high intensity"	30–90 (includes RT)	These summary recommendations were stated as the strategy to "increase aerobic capacity as effectively as possible" and includes the recommendation of a 4–6 mo supervised program
ACSM [82]	Supervised and unsupervised	Walk; cycle	3–5	40–<60% VO2R; RPE = 11–13/20	20–60 min	Duration could be in bouts of at least 10 min with goal of accumulating 20–60 min

NS = Not stated; T= treadmill; CE = cycle ergometer; AE = arm ergometer; A/LE = arm plus leg ergometer; R = rowing; MET min = MET level of exercise × duration of exercise where 1 MET is the resting metabolic rate ($VO_2 = 3.5$ mL/kg/min or ~1.3 Kcal/min for 75 kg/person); HRR is heart rate reserve: HRmax − HRrest; VO_2R is oxygen uptake (VO_2) reserve = VO_2max − VO_2rest. IF HR and VO_2 are determined from a maximal exercise test use the peak values for HRmax and VO_2max.
Healthy younger adults (18–65 yr): Moderate intensity is 40–59% HRR or VO_2R; 64–76% HRmax; 46–63% VO2max; RPE = 12–13/20 (fairly light to somewhat hard). Vigorous intensity is 60–89% HRR or VO_2R; 77–95% HRmax; 64–90% VO2max; RPE = 14–17/20 (to somewhat hard − very hard). More favorable results are seen at higher intensities.
Healthy older adults (≥65 yr): Moderate intensity is 5–6 on a 10 point scale. Vigorous intensity is 7–9 on a 10 point scale.
Moderate and vigorous training may also be mixed when appropriate. More favorable results are seen at higher intensities.
COPD: Low intensity = dyspnea rating 3–5/10 [144] High intensity = 60–80% WRpeak. More favorable results are seen at higher intensities.
CARDIAC: * If maximal exercise test data are not available, THR = HRrest + 20 beats per minute increasing based on RPE signs and symptoms and normal physiologic responses.
CKD − Heiwe & Jacobson [37]: Any exercise regardless of type, intensity or supervision will improve aerobic capacity.

TABLE 45.8 Summary of Evidence-Based and Clinical Practice Guidelines for Progressive Resistance Exercise Training in Healthy Young and Older Individuals and Cardiac Patients

Group	Type	Frequency (d/wk)	Intensity	Duration Sets x Reps)	Exercises (Number)	Notes
Healthy younger [32,77]	A variety of equipment and/or body weight can be used. See text	2—3	60—70% 1-RM (novice) 80% 1-RM (experienced)	1—4 sets 8—12	Each major muscle group	<50% 1-M to improve muscular endurance Rest intervals of 2—3 minutes between sets
Healthy older [72,77]		2—3	40—50% 1-RM (novice) 5—6 on 10 point scale	≥ 1 set 10—15 reps	8—10	Nelson et al. [72] recommend moderate (5—6) intensity exercise with vigorous intensity (7—8/10) as an option for more fit and experienced people, preferably with supervision
Cardiac rehabilitation (outpatient) [98]		2—3	30—40% 1-RM (upper body 50—60% 1-RM (lower body)	1 set 12—15 reps	8—10	See Williams et al. [98] for details and contraindications; training loads might increase to 50—80% 1-RM

and adherence but also makes use of what is otherwise a long bout of sedentary time.

Parsons and King-VanVlack have suggested that an element of the exercise prescription unique to HD patients is the timing of exercise training, specifically for exercise during dialysis or on non-dialysis days [58]. In addition to the attributes noted above, these authors suggest that exercise during dialysis may increase dialysis efficacy. They point out that movement of solutes from tissues to blood and optimizing flow between blood and dialyzer is a rate limiting step for removal of many solutes including uremic toxins. Exercise results in an increased cardiac output and increased distribution of blood flow to the active muscle, thereby enhancing solute removal essentially by increasing the tissue mass exposed to dialysis [23]. Results of studies examining the effect of exercise on urea clearance (Kt/Vurea) are mixed. Two studies found no change in Kt/Vurea after 8—16 weeks of moderate 30—45 minutes cycle exercise during dialysis [170,179]. However, the effectiveness of exercise training on urea clearance may not have been optimized in these studies, since exercise was conducted into the third hour of dialysis. One 8-week study, in which patients performed either aerobic or resistance exercise training for 10—30 minutes during hemodialysis had no effect on Kt/Vurea [180]. It is possible that the 10—30 minute aerobic or resistance training used in this study was of insufficient time or intensity to observe an effect on Kt/Vurea. Conversely, three studies reported 5—19% improvements in Kt/Vurea [45,181,182]. The possibility of improved dialysis efficacy, i.e., reduced uremia and improved overall clinical status, might engender benefits for skeletal muscle and provide another advantage for intradialytic, as opposed to interdialytic exercise training [37].

Barriers to Overcome

It is recognized that maintenance HD patients encounter significant impediments to maintaining a regular exercise program [35,43,183,184]. Commonly reported barriers to participation include fatigue on dialysis and nondialysis days [183], transportation limitations [184,185], lack of encouragement [185], and low motivation [186]. The recently reported Network 11 study of physical activity in 1323 ESRD patients revealed that lack of motivation, fatigue, perception of being too sick, and no place to exercise or lack of exercise equipment were the most frequently cited barriers to participation in physical activity [187]. Lack of motivation, the most frequently reported perceived barrier to participation in exercise [186,188], has also been associated with less physical activity [183]. Barriers to conducting exercise training in the dialysis center have also been reported [189]. Dialysis staff may not recognize some patients who might benefit from exercise because they perceive time limitations due to the complications of dialysis, risks of exercise, or uncertainty regarding benefits from exercise as limiting factors [190]. Dialysis center staff has also been reluctant to encourage exercise among dialysis patients because they believe it is not their responsibility to do so, and usually they do not they have the skills to implement exercise training [185,186]. Possibly of particular importance is that dialysis staffing and healthcare worker to dialysis patient ratios in the United States generally allow little time for dialysis staff to spend time on encouraging, assisting and monitoring exercise training of patients in chronic dialysis units.

Two studies have revealed that nephrologists typically do not counsel their patients regarding exercise, query physical activity or exercise habits, or provide guidelines for implementing exercise training [184,190]. Interestingly, while the vast majority of nephrologists agreed that exercise was potentially beneficial, the physicians surveyed thought that dialysis patients would not be interested in learning about exercise, were concerned about the risks of exercise, and believed their patients would not increase their physical activity even if counseled to do so [190]. In a separate study these physician opinions were counter to those reported by patients; i.e., they would increase activity if recommended by their physician [184]. These two studies, conducted by the same group, reported that despite accumulating evidence for the value of exercise in HD patients, there have been no changes in counseling behavior over the intervening seven years between studies. These problems are compounded by lack of interest and lack of training on the part of dialysis center staff as well as lack of appropriate exercise equipment and space. The latter impediments have been overcome using simple, inexpensive cycle ergometers [25] and resistance exercise equipment [191]. Novel weight machines have also been developed for resistance training while the patient is situated in the dialysis chair [192].

COMPONENTS OF THE EXERCISE TRAINING SESSION

Warm-Up

This should consist of at least 5—10 min of low intensity (e.g., RPE 9-11) general aerobic and muscle specific resistance exercise. Light stretching may be included after the warm-up, interspersed during exercise, or as part of the cool down. At least one 30-60 second stretch for each of the major muscle groups should be included with range of motion extending to the point of feeling tightness or mild discomfort.

Conditioning

Comprehensive exercise training including aerobic, resistance, flexibility, and balance exercise should be performed either together in the same session (60—90 minutes) or dispersed throughout the week. For endurance (aerobic) exercise, bouts of 10 min are acceptable if the individual progresses to the ability to accumulate at least 30 min/day. On some days, endurance exercise and resistance exercise may be performed separately with flexibility and balance training integrated within each session. Cool down: at least 5—10 min of low (RPE <11) intensity activities should be performed at the end of each conditioning session.

Endurance Exercise Training Guidelines

Type

Cycle ergometry performed at the dialysis chair is the most practical type of endurance exercise during HD. Most commercially available cycle ergometers require slight modification or adjustments in positioning to provide effective yet reasonably comfortable training. Ideally, patients undergoing exercise training during the HD session should lie in the chair while exercising so as to reduce the risk of hypotension or of falling. For interdialytic exercise, available and patient-preferred types of aerobic exercise may be used. Whereas walking might be the most readily available and easiest type of exercise, other exercise modes such as cycling, swimming, rowing, or arm ergometry can be used. A meta-analysis of exercise training in HD patients published in 2011 concluded that any mode of exercise training yielded a statistically significant difference in improvement in many health related fitness and physical function measures when compared to non-exercising controls [37].

Frequency

Overall, patients with CKD should attempt to perform endurance exercise of moderate duration 5 or more days/week. Initially, 3 days/week might be an appropriate target in order to gradually adapt to unaccustomed exercise and to contribute to compliance. As fitness improves, achieving the evidence-based guideline of 5 days/week is recommended. For HD patients, intradialytic exercise may be preferred where there is the availability of supervision in facilities that offer exercise training; this may improve compliance. When feasible, additional interdialytic exercise should be recommended, ideally with supervision and guidance, but home exercise, such as walking or stationary cycling and/or modest resistance exercise training should also be recommended. Logs of training sessions will assist practitioners in monitoring compliance and provide rationale for adjusting components of the patient's exercise training program.

Duration

Current evidence based guidelines for endurance exercise duration in healthy individuals [32,72] and patient groups [73-76,82] suggest ≥30 minutes per session with a target of accumulating ≥150 minutes per week of endurance exercise training. Based on these evidence based guidelines for non-CKD patients, as well as expert recommendations for HD patients [35,37,38,82,138], an initial target of 30 minutes of low to moderate intensity exercise is recommended. It is not currently known whether in HD patients further increases in the duration of time that they undergo endurance exercise each day will bring about proportional improvements.

In many cases, especially when HD patients are very deconditioned, it may be necessary to use a lower duration of exercise at the onset of training, such as bouts of 5–10 minutes. Duration of exercise training can then be increased progressively as tolerated. Indeed, protocols for exercise duration for healthy older adults includes the option of accumulating 30 minutes of exercise per day in bouts of 10 minutes or more [72].

Intensity

Endurance exercise training for HD patients should begin with lower intensities and progress to higher intensity as tolerated and safe. Evidence in healthy individuals suggests that intensity as low as 30% $\dot{V}O_2$ peak or RPE of 10–11 would be an appropriate starting point in these patients [193-195]. Although some research studies have used a percentage of HRmax to guide training intensity in HD subjects [86,167,168,174,178], it may be difficult to do so in these patients because of conditions such as autonomic dysregulation due to changes in blood volume [196], medications such as ß-blockers and some calcium channel blockers [82], and non-cardiac related limitations to exercise such as pulmonary disease [40] or myopathy [15,197,198]. The use of prediction equations from submaximal exercise variables, such as peak exercise time or treadmill speed and grade [199] or the commonly used 220 minus age in years, to predict HRmax may be employed to select initial levels of exercise intensity [200,201] but with the caveat that prediction errors may be greater than 10 beats per minute [201]. Performing a clinical exercise test to peak exercise would improve the usefulness of heart rate indices for intensity prescription, because an actual HRpeak would be obtained by this method. When the test is repeated with similar peak efforts, the reproducibility of HRpeak is about ± 2 beats per minute. While this approach might be most useful in nondialyzed CKD patients, even objectively determined HR indices for training intensity in HD may not be as reliable as other objective measures such as $\dot{V}O_2$ or WR, if these data are available and are feasible to use. If objective data are not available to set the training intensity, use of one of the perceptual scales [143-145,202] or the 0-10 point scale advocated for healthy older individuals [72] could be used. Table

45.6 summarizes several approaches to objectively and subjectively determine exercise intensity. Light to moderate levels of exertion would be the most appropriate choices for most HD patients, at least until exercise becomes regular and fitness improves. At this point, higher intensity work might be introduced.

Only one study has specifically examined high intensity interval training in HD patients [203]. This small, uncontrolled pilot study provided 12 weeks of thrice weekly, semi-recumbent cycle exercise using high intensity intervals during the first hour of dialysis. Two minutes of high intensity exercise was interspersed with two minutes of active, low intensity exercise. Because of the unreliability of heart rate as an index of exercise intensity, Borg's rating of perceived exertion scale (RPE) [143] was used. High intensity was defined as >17 on the 6-20 RPE scale, and active recovery was set at RPE = 7. Work rates were increased to maintain the proper intensities as fitness improved during training. Measures of aerobic fitness were not assessed in this study, but significant, 20%, improvements were noted for isometric knee extensor strength and timed sit-to-stand transitions. No changes in body composition or serum or muscle insulin-like growth factor-I (IGF-I) or IGF binding protein-3 (IGFBP3) were observed. The study was well tolerated and was deemed safe and clinically feasible.

Although high intensity exercise has been shown to be effective and safe in some patient groups, whether it is either appropriate, feasible, or effective for patients with advanced CKD remains to be demonstrated. It is prudent to require that individuals who are at risk for cardiovascular or orthopedic complications during exercise should avoid high intensity training until they undergo a careful evaluation of their condition. This examination must include cardiac stress tests, ideally with an imaging or ultrasonic evaluation of cardiac perfusion or function during exercise conditions. The evaluation must indicate that patients can safely undergo intensity training. As patients accommodate to regular exercise training, the careful introduction of interval training can provide variety and a greater stimulus for improvement. Much more systematic study with interval training in patients with advanced CKD is needed before it can be universally recommended.

Rest Interval

During the initial phases of the endurance training program, patients may need periodic rest so that they can accommodate to the exercise even though it may be at low intensity. No fixed time can be recommended; however the practitioner should encourage the patient to resume the exercise as tolerated while maintaining the recommended training intensity. Also, either no or only light exercise may be prudent during the recovery days in the early training phases. With adaptation, more consecutive days of moderate intensity activity can be added to the target.

Progression

For patients with CKD, increases in the duration of continuous exercise to target should be considered first. Afterwards, increased frequency to target (ideally ≥5 d/week) is recommended followed by gradual increases in intensity. Exercise prescription is part science and part art. The well trained practitioner should carefully monitor patient adaptations and provide guidance on when and how much to change exercise volume.

Guidelines for Progressive Resistance Exercise Training (PRT)

Type

There are several forms of resistance that can be used for progressive resistance exercise training (PRT). Simple elastic resistance (bands or tubes), weighted vests and ankle/wrist weights, dumbbell and barbell free weights, and various machine weights are available. Newer resistance exercise equipment makes use of weighted bars and balls, weighted rubber tubes and more. These forms of resistance can provide graduated resistance exercise starting at less than 1 pound.

Resistance exercises should be performed for the large major muscle groups or body parts including quadriceps and hamstrings, gastrocnemius/soleus, pectorals and latissimus dorsi, deltoids, abdominals, biceps, and triceps.

Carrying out PRT in the dialysis chair may be advantageous. Cheema et al. have described simple methods for implementing resistance training at the dialysis chair for all the major muscle groups [148]. Relatively inexpensive equipment, including dumbbells, ankle weights, and elastic bands/tubing, can be placed on a mobile cart and wheeled among patients [148]. Bennett et al have suggested that a specially built stack weight machine could be used at the dialysis chair for conducting lower extremity resistance exercise [183]. Another approach includes the use of weight machines before starting the dialysis procedure, although limitations of space in the dialysis unit and the cost of this equipment may preclude this option. On the positive side, the visibility of exercise equipment may be motivating to the dialysis patients. These types of equipment can also be used for interdialytic PRT, but the approach described by Cheema et al. could also be easily and inexpensively adapted for home use.

Frequency

Most existing guidelines suggest PRT on two nonconsecutive days per week with the assumption that all major muscle groups are exercised on each of the two days. When possible, a more equal distribution of days such as Monday and Friday or Tuesday and Saturday will allow more recovery time between sessions compared with typical Monday–Wednesday, Tuesday–Thursday, or Wednesday–Friday combinations. If PRT is carried out before or during dialysis, when such treatment is provided on three alternating days per week, i.e., Monday–Wednesday–Friday or Tuesday–Thursday–Saturday, exercise sessions could be conducted on these days three times per week.

An alternative to the two day per week regimen is splitting the body parts that are exercised so that half are performed on two days while the other half is exercised on two other days. This may be more difficult when PRT is performed exclusively at the dialysis unit, but patients might be empowered to execute the fourth day at home.

Duration (Sets and Repetitions)

As with most guidelines for healthy older adults and patient groups, starting with a single set and with 10–15 repetitions per set is recommended. Assuming one minute to correctly execute a set of 10–15 repetitions and 2 minutes for rest between sets, one exercise for each major muscle group can be completed in 25–30 minutes. With adaptation, a second set can be added. See below for additional progression guidelines.

Intensity (Resistance)

The recommended level of effort for resistance training for patient groups and healthy older adults is often based on subjective assessments of perceived exertion (Table 45.8). In this context, guidelines for initial conditioning suggest that moderate exertion is equivalent to 5–6 on a 0–10 scale [72]. This is not the Borg RPE scale (6–20) [143] or the Borg category-ratio scale (0–10) [144]. Presumably these Borg scales could be used if the patient constrained the level of effort to "moderate", which is identified as approximately 12–13 ("somewhat hard") on the Borg 6–20 scale or 3 (moderate) on the 0–10 scale. Neither of these Borg scales has been validated in maintenance HD patients for determination of resistance training intensity.

Although the intensity used in many PRT programs for individuals not undergoing maintenance hemodialysis is based on a percentage of the 1-RM, this may not be appropriate in the HD population. The risk of injury with the high loads required in the 1-RM test suggests that lower intensities, such as 3-RM or 5-RM, should be used. As with the 1-RM, these tests are effort dependent and can clearly be affected by motivation. Alternatively, for training prescription purposes, recommending a range of repetitions that leads to "substantial effort" or inability to successfully complete a repetition in good form (i.e., 10—15 RM), may be considered after the patient has undergone basic conditioning for at least 4-6 weeks.

Progression

Progression is the sine qua non in resistance training and can be achieved in many ways by providing overload in the form of increasing sets, resistance, and number of training days per body part. After adaptation, increasing the number of sets from one to two may be the first choice for HD patients. If time is available, a third day of PRT could be added. Since increases in muscle size and muscle strength are desirable outcomes in advanced CKD, increasing the load so that some or all of the training sets reach a high level of effort is desirable. For example, high levels of effort would be represented by 7—8 on the 0-10 scale, [61] 15—17, ("hard to very hard") on the Borg 6—20 scale, or 5—7 ("strong" to "very strong") on the Borg 0—10 scale. Finally, specific muscle groups might be targeted for additional emphasis. Since the muscles of ambulation are important for upright physical activity, including gait speed, and other lower extremity functions, additional PRT for quadriceps, hamstrings, hip abductors and adductors and triceps surae could be considered.

Guidelines for Enhancing Flexibility

Joint flexibility tends to decrease with age, but research shows that improvement in flexibility at any age can occur after as little as 3—4 sessions of regular 2—3 days/wk stretching [204,205]. Improving range of motion of joints through regular stretching is a useful adjunct to PRT for improving postural stability and balance [140,141]. Despite commonly held views, current evidence suggests that stretching is unlikely to be effective in reducing or preventing injuries, low back pain or delayed muscle soreness [140]. One RCT in HD patients examined the possible benefits of a modified yoga-based exercise program [69]. After twenty-four 15—30 minute yoga sessions distributed over 12 weeks, patients exhibited significant improvements, as compared to controls, in pain intensity, fatigue, sleep disturbance, grip strength, and plasma levels of urea, alkaline phosphatase and total cholesterol and blood erythrocytes, and hematocrit. Compliance was reported to be good. Although yoga exercise in this study included breathing and relaxation activities, six of the seven postures were essentially stretching exercises. Additional studies on the potential benefits of yoga or possibly stretching exercises as another form of flexibility training are needed to confirm the findings of this single study.

Type

Flexibility can be improved through a variety of stretching methods including static, dynamic, ballistic, and proprioceptive neuromuscular facilitation (PNF). Static stretching is generally preferred for its simplicity, effectiveness, and low injury risk. Greater increases in range of motion have been shown using PNF, a method that incorporates an isometric contraction of the muscle to be stretched followed by relaxation of that muscle and simultaneous passive stretch. However, for maximal effectiveness, PNF stretching requires a knowledgeable partner or practitioner and has a greater potential for injury than static stretching.

Frequency

Stretching is a low intensity activity; thus conducting stretching activity more than 2—3 days/wk is not likely to bring about negative consequences [77]. Daily stretching for those patients who could benefit from additional stretching sessions is acceptable and brings about greater gains. Stretching can be included in the warm-up and/or cool down phases of the training session. But providing dedicated time just for stretching is more likely to allow time to focus on this activity and to properly complete at least one stretch for each of the major muscle-tendon groups.

Duration

As with healthy individuals, holding a static stretch either actively or passively for 10—60 seconds is recommended. A target of 60 seconds of total stretching time for each major muscle-tendon group should be eventually achieved.

Intensity

The intensity of the stretch is determined by whether the final position achieved during the stretch is painful. It is recommended that the final stretching position should feel "tight" or slightly uncomfortable but no actual pain should be experienced.

Progression

Progression in stretching includes increasing the duration of each stretch, adding additional stretching postures to individual muscle-tendon groups, and increasing frequency. Increasing intensity is not appropriate.

Guidelines for Improving Balance and Stability

Patients undergoing hemodialysis have a higher rate of falling and greater morbidity from falls than the general population [206,207]. Risk factors for falls include fatigue and muscle weakness, both of which are exacerbated following the dialysis session [208].

Only recently included in guidelines for exercise and physical activity in healthy adults [77], neuromuscular training that includes balance and stability exercises are particularly beneficial in older persons to improve their balance, agility and strength and to reduce their risk of and fear of falling [141]. As such, it is reasonable to consider balance activities such as semi-tandem and tandem stands, one-legged stands, and more dynamic balance, coordination, and agility activities such as Tai-Chi. Tai Chi has been extensively investigated with several studies reporting the beneficial effects of improving balance, reducing falls [209–211], and improving motor control and quality of life [212,213].

RISKS OF EXERCISE IN THE ADVANCED CKD PATIENT

There is a lack of specific reporting of adverse events associated with exercise training in advanced CKD patients [37]. However, both intra- and interdialytic exercise training are generally thought to be safe as reported in three recent systematic reviews [24,35,37]. In healthy exercising individuals, the most common injuries experienced are musculoskeletal [214], and the most consistent association exists between greater total amounts of exercise performed over time and higher risks of injury. This is not surprising, since the total amount of exercise (volume) is the product of the intensity, duration and frequency of exercise. For healthy and patient populations alike, injuries can be effectively mitigated by appropriate screening, warm-up, and progression in the components of the exercise prescription. In most HD patients, the risk–benefit ratio generally favors exercise [24,35]. Instruction in proper technique, breathing, adherence to the recommended program, and reporting untoward responses to members of the healthcare team are important preventative strategies.

As with healthy individuals, musculoskeletal injuries are most common in exercising CKD patients, but other risks, particularly of cardiac origin are most serious and are most often seen with high intensity exercise [37,215]. Patients with CKD often have underlying cardiac disease, thus increasing their vulnerability to exercise-induced adverse events. However, no negative hemodynamic effects have been reported with exercise during HD, and in fact, systolic blood pressure stabilizes during such exercise and patients typically experience less cramping [23]. The greatest exposure to exercise-induced cardiopulmonary stress occurs at peak exercise, but to date, there are no studies that have reported adverse cardiovascular events associated with exercise

testing or training in HD patients [216]. Nonetheless, it is not uncommon for HD patients who have no history of coronary artery disease or ischemic heart disease and who volunteer for exercise training to be found to have electrocardiographic evidence of ischemic heart disease on stress testing. Thus, advanced CKD patients must be evaluated carefully for ischemic heart disease both before they are allowed into an exercise training program and while they participate in such a program.

About 45% of HD patients are diabetic [2]. Consequently, serum glucose control during exercise may be of concern. Exercise during dialysis may prevent large decreases in serum glucose since the dialysate glucose will serve as a form of a glycemic clamp, with serum glucose levels drifting toward the dialysate glucose concentration, which is usually about 100–200 mg glucose monohydrate/dL [216]. Nevertheless, monitoring of serum glucose levels may be appropriate if the HD patient is diabetic and is taking hypoglycemic medications, and these patients should learn their balance between quality and quantity of food intake, insulin, and exercise intensity and duration.

Advanced CKD is often associated with decreased bone mass and changes in bone architecture. Consequently, fracture risk is higher than in healthy individuals [104]. These changes worsen as CKD progresses. At least 50% of patients are reported to have had a fracture by the time they begin dialysis therapy [104]. Jamal et al. reported that increased fracture risk was associated with impaired muscle performance [102]. Although this could be interpreted to indicate that ESRD patients should not exercise, it is more likely that the appropriate inauguration, progression, and type of exercise training will help avoid fracture risk and perhaps improve it. Huang et al have suggested that increased exercise time is positively associated with femoral neck and lumbar spine bone mineral density, and that exercise training is positively correlated with these measures, although these relationships did not reach statistical significance [217]. Spontaneous tendon ruptures have been reported in HD patients [103] and tend to be associated with hyperparathyroidism and not with exercise. Only one trial has specifically studied exercise-induced injuries or adverse events [100] with no statistically significant differences between the resistance trained group and inactive controls seen over the 12 week study. One elderly female HD patient experienced a partial tear of the supraspinatus muscle in week 6 of exercise training, but she continued to train with lower extremity exercises. Studies specifically examining the injury vs. exercise dose-response relationship for various modes of exercise training in HD are needed. As recommended in Heiwe's systematic review, future RCT should specifically examine the frequency and nature of injuries and adverse events with special consideration for the dose and type of exercise [37].

URGENT NEED FOR DEVELOPMENT OF RENAL REHABILITATION PROGRAMS

Over 35 years of research in exercise training and of systematic reviews of these studies have reported compelling evidence for the substantial benefits available to advanced CKD patients who participate in systematic, comprehensive, regular exercise (Table 1). Despite these encouraging data, which include improved health related quality of life and, in epidemiological reports, greater survival (in non-interventional studies), exercise is an uncommon feature in the lifestyles of most HD patients. Indeed, two recent surveys of ESRD patients reported that only 13% [187] and 17% [184] of respondents achieved the commonly recommended guideline of 150 minutes per week of moderate intensity exercise. [33,72,138] It has been suggested that the downward spiral of decreasing physical ability consequent to ESRD, and possibly to chronic dialysis treatment itself, may lead to marked increases in a sedentary life style that lead to further decrements in physical performance and physical abilities. Unless broken, the spiral continues downward toward disability. Clearly, we must do more to remove barriers to exercise and encourage greater participation at target levels. There have been several calls to action [36,38,190,216, 218–220] to increase the participation of HD patients in regular exercise and the time for formal "renal rehabilitation" is upon us.

Implications for Practice

The 2005 Clinical Practice Guidelines for Cardiovascular Disease in Dialysis Patients [138], provide limited guidance to nephrologists for developing exercise training and physical activity patterns for their patients, but they do give the following important guidelines:

> "All dialysis patients should be counseled and regularly encouraged by nephrology and dialysis staff to increase their level of physical activity." (guideline 14.2)

> "The goal for activity should be for cardiovascular exercise at a moderate intensity for 30 minutes on most, if not all, days per week. Patients who are not currently physically active should start at very low levels and durations, and gradually progress to this recommended level." (Guideline 14.2.4.a.i)

> "Physical functioning assessment and encouragement for participation in physical activity should be part of the routine patient care plan. Regular review should include assessment of changes in activity and physical functioning." (Guideline 14.4.b.i)

These guidelines provide a basic framework for increasing participation in exercise and increased physical activity but more detailed and comprehensive guidance is lacking. Tables 45.7 and 45.8 contain details of program design for aerobic and resistance exercise training, respectively, that have been largely successful in improving aerobic and muscle performance and physical function in young and elderly healthy people and individuals with various chronic diseases, including advanced CKD. It is also important to note that these studies have essentially followed templates for published evidence-based medicine guidelines summarized in these tables. Given the low exercise tolerance of the CKD patient, almost any increase in physical activity will be beneficial and lead to progression in frequency, duration, and intensity of training and enhanced benefit. The idea that low training loads and volumes, such as those used in these studies, are capable of stimulating these improvements suggests a large adaptation window because of the significant debility of ESRD patients. Thus, the renal disease healthcare practitioner may draw from these guidelines, withindividual adjustments based on disease history, co-morbidities, exercise tolerance, clinical and patient-important outcomes, with the overarching goal of maximizing participation and adherence. Use of the AIDES method [221] shown in Table 45.9 may facilitate participant adherence to the exercise intervention.

Of clear importance is the need to remove barriers to participation in exercise training and physical activity as noted above. There is a need to improve the nephrologists' willingness to educate their patients regarding the evidence that regular exercise training may improve their walking capacity, physical fitness and possibly overall health. Physicians should determine the activity level of patients and encourage them to reach the targets for type, frequency, duration and intensity of exercise outlined in this chapter. Real and perceived barriers to participation in regular exercise and physical activity should be investigated and addressed. Since

TABLE 45.9 Adaptation of the AIDES Method [221] for Improving Adherence to Exercise Training and Physical Activity

A:	Assessment (see Table 45.4)	Assess All Components of Health Related Fitness and Physical Performance
I:	Individualization	Individualize the exercise training regimen
D:	Documentation	Provide written guidelines and progress monitoring
E:	Education	Provide accurate and continuing education tailored to the needs of the individual
S:	Supervision	Provide continuing supervision of the regimen

maintaining an in-center exercise program falls largely on the clinical staff, their training and support are vital [184]. Engagement in regular exercise for the HD patient might be better facilitated at the dialysis center which has the potential advantages of equipment, supervision, and monitoring but regular exercise training can also be successful in outpatient supervised settings or in community-based programs [216]; home exercise, including simple walking, is also useful.

These are difficult tasks for many physicians who may not have time, training, or desire to advise and monitor effective exercise training for their patients [184]. However, Painter has suggested [216] that even within the constraints of short patient-visits physicians can:

- ask about physical activity participation and help identify barriers;
- recommend increasing activity if levels are low by recommending walking when feasible and appropriate;
- provide educational materials (e.g., "Exercise for the Dialysis Patient" available free from www. lifeoptions.org);
- refer to a trained healthcare professional who is qualified to work with exercise patients with chronic disease, such as physical/occupational therapists, cardiac rehabilitation specialists, or clinical exercise physiologists.
- referrals can then be regularly followed up during the routine clinic visits to assess participation and progress and provide encouragement.

For the interested physician or healthcare provider, help is available in the form of a national initiative sponsored by the American College of Sports Medicine called Exercise is Medicine®. Shared with the American Medical Association, the guiding principles of Exercise is Medicine® are designed to help improve the health and well-being of the nation through a regular physical activity prescription from doctors and other health care providers. Many resources for physicians and health care workers are available through Exercise is Medicine® and include Exercise is Medicine Health Care Providers' Action Guide, Exercise is Medicine Action and Promotion Guide, Billing and Coding for Physical Activity Counseling, ACSM's Exercise is Medicine: A Clinician's Guide to Exercise, and National Center on Physical Activity and Disability brochure for Health Care Providers. Detailed information is available at http://exerciseismedicine.org/physicians.htm.

SUMMARY

This chapter has sought to provide physicians and other related healthcare providers with a summary of current evidence for the value of comprehensive exercise training and increased physical activity for the patient with advanced CKD. Basic principles underlying exercise training are reviewed, and specific methods for assessing health related fitness and physical function in patients with CKD are presented. The common elements that guide exercise training program design for endurance and resistance exercise, flexibility, and balance and stability are presented along with specific applications for patients with CKD with enough detail to guide practitioners toward implementing exercise training programs for their patients. Some of the predominant barriers to participation are identified along with risks and safety for exercise training in advanced CKD. Finally a renewed call for action is expressed in conjunction with implications for implementation of exercise training programs for patients with advanced CKD. There is an urgent need for physicians and associated staff who work with chronic kidney disease patients to inform them of the value of physical activity, assess current physical activity status and moderate barriers to participation, encourage regular exercise and increased physical activity, and ensure that appropriate intensity, duration, and frequency of exercise is added to the treatment plan. Resources for physicians and healthcare practitioners for increasing knowledge and skills in exercise prescription and training for patients are provided.

There are clear-cut benefits for improved performance and physical function awaiting patients who regularly exercise. A sea-change is needed in the manner in which patients with CKD engage in physical activity, and evidence suggests that the nephrologist and related staff are the individuals who are best positioned to effect this change.

References

[1] U.S. Department of Health and Human Services. Centers for Disease Control: National Chronic Kidney Disease Fact Sheet 2010. In, Altlanta, 2012, p Fact Sheet.

[2] USRDS 2011 Annual Data Report: Atlas of Chronic Kidney Disease and End-Stage Renal Disease in the United States. In: National Institutes of Health, National Institute of Diabetes and Digestive and Kidney Diseases, Bethesda, MD: 2011.

[3] National Institutes of Health, Diseases NIoDaDaK. In: U.S. Renal Data System, USRDS 2009 Annual Data Report: Atlas of Chronic Kidney Disease and End-Stage Renal Disease in the United States. Bethesda, MD: 2009.

[4] Collins AJ, Foley RN, Herzog C, et al. Excerpts from the US Renal Data System 2009 Annual Data Report. Am J Kidney Dis 2010;55:S1—420. A426—427.

[5] Cheung AK, Sarnak MJ, Yan G, et al. Cardiac diseases in maintenance hemodialysis patients: results of the HEMO Study. Kidney Int 2004;65:2380—9.

[6] Athyros VG, Katsiki N, Karagiannis A, et al. Editorial: should chronic kidney disease be considered as a coronary heart disease equivalent? Curr Vasc Pharmacol 2012;10:374—7.

[7] Parikh NI, Hwang SJ, Larson MG, et al. Chronic kidney disease as a predictor of cardiovascular disease (from the Framingham Heart Study). Am J Cardiol 2008;102:47—53.

[8] Weiner DE, Tighiouart H, Stark PC, et al. Kidney disease as a risk factor for recurrent cardiovascular disease and mortality. Am J Kidney Dis 2004;44:198—206.

[9] Port FK, Ashby VB, Dhingra RK, et al. Dialysis dose and body mass index are strongly associated with survival in hemodialysis patients. J Am Soc Nephrol 2002;13:1061—6.

[10] Argyropoulos C, Chang CC, Plantinga L, et al. Considerations in the statistical analysis of hemodialysis patient survival. J Am Soc Nephrol 2009;20:2034—43.

[11] Caspersen CJ, Powell KE, Christenson GM. Physical activity, exercise, and physical fitness: definitions and distinctions for health-related research. Public Health Rep 1985;100:126—31.

[12] Heiwe S, Clyne N, Dahlgren MA. Living with chronic renal failure: patients' experiences of their physical and functional capacity. Physiother Res Int 2003;8:167—77.

[13] Kettner-Melsheimer A, Weiss M, Huber W. Physical work capacity in chronic renal disease. Int J Artif Organs 1987;10:23—30.

[14] Kutner NG, Cardenas DD, Bower JD. Rehabilitation, aging and chronic renal disease. Am J Phys Med Rehabil 1992;71:97—101.

[15] Adams GR, Vaziri ND. Skeletal muscle dysfunction in chronic renal failure: effects of exercise. Am J Physiol Renal Physiol 2006;290:F753—761.

[16] Johansen KL. Physical functioning and exercise capacity in patients on dialysis. Adv Ren Replace Ther 1999;6:141—8.

[17] Johansen KL, Shubert T, Doyle J, et al. Muscle atrophy in patients receiving hemodialysis: effects on muscle strength, muscle quality, and physical function. Kidney Int 2003;63:291—7.

[18] Kopple JD, Storer T, Casburi R. Impaired exercise capacity and exercise training in maintenance hemodialysis patients. J Ren Nutr 2005;15:44—8.

[19] Kouidi E, Albani M, Natsis K, et al. The effects of exercise training on muscle atrophy in haemodialysis patients. Nephrol Dial Transplant 1998;13:685—99.

[20] Diesel W, Noakes T, Swanepoel C, et al. Isokinetic muscle strength predicts maximum exercise tolerance in renal patients on chronic hemodialysis. Am J Kidney Dis 1990;16:109—14.

[21] Fahal IH, Bell GM, Bone JM, et al. Physiological abnormalities of skeletal muscle in dialysis patients. Nephrol Dial Transplant 1997;12:119—27.

[22] Johansen KL, Mulligan K, Schambelan M. Anabolic effects of nandrolone decanoate in patients receiving dialysis: a randomized controlled trial. JAMA 1999;281:1275—81.

[23] Painter P. Physical functioning in end-stage renal disease patients: update 2005. Hemodial Int 2005;9:218—35.

[24] Smart N, Steele M. Exercise training in haemodialysis patients: a systematic review and meta-analysis. Nephrology (Carlton) 2011;16:626—32.

[25] Painter P, Nelson-Worel J, Hill M, et al. Effects of exercise training during hemodialysis. Nephron 1986;43:87—92.

[26] Storer TW, Casaburi R, Sawelson S, et al. Endurance exercise training during haemodialysis improves strength, power, fatigability and physical performance in maintenance haemodialysis patients. Nephrol Dial Transplant 2005;20:1429—37.

[27] Stack AG, Murthy B. Exercise and limitations in physical activity levels among new dialysis patients in the United States: an epidemiologic study. Ann Epidemiol 2008;18:880—8.

[28] Painter P. Exercise in chronic disease: physiological research needed. Exerc Sport Sci Rev 2008;36:83—90.

[29] Bhasin S, Storer TW. Anabolic applications of androgens for functional limitations associated with aging and chronic illness. Front Horm Res 2009;37:163—82.

[30] Desmeules S, Levesque R, Jaussent I, et al. Creatinine index and lean body mass are excellent predictors of long-term survival in haemodiafiltration patients. Nephrol Dial Transplant 2004;19:1182—9.

[31] Stack AG, Molony DA, Rives T, et al. Association of physical activity with mortality in the US dialysis population. Am J Kidney Dis 2005;45:690—701.

[32] Haskell WL, Lee IM, Pate RR, et al. Physical activity and public health: updated recommendation for adults from the American College of Sports Medicine and the American Heart Association. Med Sci Sports Exerc 2007;39:1423—34.

[33] U.S. Department of Health and Human Services. In: 2008 Physical Activity Guidelines for Americans. Washington, DC: 2008.

[34] Jette M, Posen G, Cardarelli C. Effects of an exercise programme in a patient undergoing hemodialysis treatment. J Sports Med Phys Fitness 1977;17:181—6.

[35] Brenner I. Exercise performance by hemodialysis patients: a review of the literature. Phys Sportsmed 2009;37:84—96.

[36] Cheema BS, Singh MA. Exercise training in patients receiving maintenance hemodialysis: a systematic review of clinical trials. Am J Nephrol 2005;25:352—64.

[37] Heiwe S, Jacobson SH. Exercise training for adults with chronic kidney disease. Cochrane Database Syst Rev 2011. CD003236.

[38] Johansen KL. Exercise in the end-stage renal disease population. J Am Soc Nephrol 2007;18:1845—54.

[39] Storer TW. Anabolic interventions in ESRD. Adv Chronic Kidney Dis 2009;16:511—28.

[40] Cooper CB, Storer TW. Exercise Testing and Interpretation: A Practical Approach. New York: Cambridge University Press; 2001.

[41] Taylor HL, Buskirk E, Henschel A. Maximal oxygen intake as an objective measure of cardio-respiratory performance. J Appl Physiol 1955;8:73—80.

[42] Wasserman K, Hansen JE, Sue DY, et al. Principles of exercise testing and prescription. 1st ed. Philadelphia: Lea & Febiger; 1987.

[43] Bohm CJ, Ho J, Duhamel TA. Regular physical activity and exercise therapy in end-stage renal disease: how should we move forward? J Nephrol 2010;23:235—43.

[44] Carmack CL, Amaral-Melendez M, Boudreaux E, et al. Exercise as a component in the physical and psychological rehabilitation of hemodialysis patients. International Journal of Rehabilitation & Health 1995;1:13—23.

[45] van Vilsteren MC, de Greef MH, Huisman RM. The effects of a low-to-moderate intensity pre-conditioning exercise programme linked with exercise counselling for sedentary haemodialysis patients in The Netherlands: results of a randomized clinical trial. Nephrol Dial Transplant 2005;20:141—6.

[46] Aspenes ST, Nilsen TI, Skaug EA, et al. Peak oxygen uptake and cardiovascular risk factors in 4631 healthy women and men. Med Sci Sports Exerc 2011;43:1465—73.

[47] Blair SN, Kohl 3rd HW, Paffenbarger Jr RS, et al. Physical fitness and all-cause mortality. A prospective study of healthy men and women. JAMA 1989;262:2395—401.

[48] Franklin BA. Fitness: the ultimate marker for risk stratification and health outcomes? Prev Cardiol 2007;10:42—5. quiz 46.

[49] Gulati M, Pandey DK, Arnsdorf MF, et al. Exercise capacity and the risk of death in women: the St James Women Take Heart Project. Circulation 2003;108:1554—9.

[50] Hsich E, Gorodeski EZ, Starling RC, et al. Importance of treadmill exercise time as an initial prognostic screening tool in patients with systolic left ventricular dysfunction. Circulation 2009;119:3189—97.

[51] Kokkinos P, Myers J, Kokkinos JP, et al. Exercise capacity and mortality in black and white men. Circulation 2008;117:614—22.

[52] Mark DB, Lauer MS. Exercise capacity: the prognostic variable that doesn't get enough respect. Circulation 2003;108: 1534—6.

[53] Mora S, Redberg RF, Cui Y, et al. Ability of exercise testing to predict cardiovascular and all-cause death in asymptomatic women: a 20-year follow-up of the lipid research clinics prevalence study. JAMA 2003;290:1600—7.

[54] Myers J, Gullestad L, Vagelos R, et al. Clinical, hemodynamic, and cardiopulmonary exercise test determinants of survival in patients referred for evaluation of heart failure. Ann Intern Med 1998;129:286—93.

[55] Myers J, Prakash M, Froelicher V, et al. Exercise capacity and mortality among men referred for exercise testing. N Engl J Med 2002;346:793—801.

[56] Myers J. Physical activity: the missing prescription. Eur J Cardiovasc Prev Rehabil 2005;12:85—6.

[57] Myers J, Kaykha A, George S, et al. Fitness versus physical activity patterns in predicting mortality in men. Am J Med 2004;117:912—8.

[58] Parsons TL, King-Vanvlack CE. Exercise and end-stage kidney disease: functional exercise capacity and cardiovascular outcomes. Adv Chronic Kidney Dis 2009;16:459—81.

[59] Sietsema KE, Amato A, Adler SG, et al. Exercise capacity as a predictor of survival among ambulatory patients with end-stage renal disease. Kidney Int 2004;65:719—24.

[60] Galvao DA, Newton RU, Taaffe DR. Anabolic responses to resistance training in older men and women: a brief review. J Aging Phys Act 2005;13:343—58.

[61] Kraemer WJ. Adaptations to resistance training. In: Ehrman JK, editor. ACSM's Resource Manual for Exercise Testing and Prescription. 6th ed. Philadelphia: Wolters Kluwer — Lippincott Williams & Wilkins; 2009. p. 489—508.

[62] Fiatarone MA, Marks EC, Ryan ND, et al. High-intensity strength training in nonagenarians. Effects on skeletal muscle. JAMA 1990;263:3029—34.

[63] Panton LB, Golden J, Broeder CE, et al. The effects of resistance training on functional outcomes in patients with chronic obstructive pulmonary disease. Eur J Appl Physiol 2004;91:443—9.

[64] Bhasin S, Storer TW, Javanbakht M, et al. Testosterone replacement and resistance exercise in HIV-infected men with weight loss and low testosterone levels. JAMA 2000;283: 763—70.

[65] Johansen KL, Painter PL, Sakkas GK, et al. Effects of resistance exercise training and nandrolone decanoate on body composition and muscle function among patients who receive hemodialysis: A randomized, controlled trial. J Am Soc Nephrol 2006;17:2307—14.

[66] Kopple JD, Wang H, Casaburi R, et al. Exercise in maintenance hemodialysis patients induces transcriptional changes in genes favoring anabolic muscle. J Am Soc Nephrol 2007;18:2975—86.

[67] Castaneda C, Gordon P, Uhlin K, et al. Resistance training to counteract the catabolism of a low-protein diet in patients with chronic renal insufficiency. A randomized, controlled trial. Ann Intern Med 2001;135:965—76.

[68] Chen JL, Godfrey S, Ng TT, et al. Effect of intra-dialytic, low-intensity strength training on functional capacity in adult haemodialysis patients: a randomized pilot trial. Nephrol Dial Transplant 2010;25:1936—43.

[69] Yurtkuran M, Alp A, Dilek K. A modified yoga-based exercise program in hemodialysis patients: a randomized controlled study. Complement Ther Med 2007;15:164—71.

[70] Johansen KL, Chertow GM, Ng AV, et al. Physical activity levels in patients on hemodialysis and healthy sedentary controls. Kidney Int 2000;57:2564—70.

[71] O'Hare AM, Tawney K, Bacchetti P, et al. Decreased survival among sedentary patients undergoing dialysis: results from the dialysis morbidity and mortality study wave 2. Am J Kidney Dis 2003;41:447—54.

[72] Nelson ME, Rejeski WJ, Blair SN, et al. Physical activity and public health in older adults: recommendation from the American College of Sports Medicine and the American Heart Association. Circulation 2007;116:1094—105.

[73] AACVPR. Guidelines for Pulmonary Rehabilitation Programs. 4th ed. Champaign, IL: Human Kinetics; 2004.

[74] AACVPR. Guidelines for Cardiac Rehabilitation and Secondary Prevention Programs-4th Edition. Champaign, IL: Human Kinetics; 2004.

[75] Langer D, Hendriks E, Burtin C, et al. A clinical practice guideline for physiotherapists treating patients with chronic obstructive pulmonary disease based on a systematic review of available evidence. Clin Rehabil 2009;23: 445—62.

[76] Ries AL, Bauldoff GS, Carlin BW, et al. Pulmonary Rehabilitation: Joint ACCP/AACVPR Evidence-Based Clinical Practice Guidelines. Chest 2007;131:4S—42S.

[77] Garber CE, Blissmer B, Deschenes MR, et al. American College of Sports Medicine position stand. Quantity and quality of exercise for developing and maintaining cardiorespiratory, musculoskeletal, and neuromotor fitness in apparently healthy adults: guidance for prescribing exercise. Med Sci Sports Exerc 2011;43:1334—59.

[78] Singh MA. Exercise comes of age: rationale and recommendations for a geriatric exercise prescription. J Gerontol A Biol Sci Med Sci 2002;57:M262—282.

[79] DeLorme TL, Watkins AL. Progressive resistance exercise: technic and medical application. New York: Appleton-Century-Crofts; 1951.

[80] Barnard RJ, Gardner GW, Diaco NV, et al. Cardiovascular responses to sudden strenuous exercise—heart rate, blood pressure, and ECG. J Appl Physiol 1973;34:833—7.

[81] Stewart D, Macaluso A, De Vito G. The effect of an active warm-up on surface EMG and muscle performance in healthy humans. Eur J Appl Physiol 2003;89:509—13.

[82] Thompson WR, editor. ACSM's Guidelines for Exercise Testing and Prescription. Philadelphia: Wolters Kluwer/Lippincott Williams & Wilkins; 2010.

[83] Wasserman K, Hansen JE, Sue DY, et al. Principles of Exercise Testing and Interpretation Including Pathophysiology and Clinical Applications. 5th edn. Philadelphia, PA: Lippincott Williams & Wilkins; 2011.

[84] American Thoracic Society and American College of Chest Physicians. ATS/ACCP Statement on cardiopulmonary exercise testing. Am J Respir Crit Care Med 2003;167:211—77.

[85] Granata S, Zaza G, Simone S, et al. Mitochondrial dysregulation and oxidative stress in patients with chronic kidney disease. BMC Genomics 2009;10:388.

[86] Painter P, Moore G, Carlson L, et al. Effects of exercise training plus normalization of hematocrit n exercise capacity and health-related quality of life. Am J Kidney Dis 2002;39: 257—65.

[87] Casaburi R, Porszasz J. Constant work rate exercise testing: a tricky measure of exercise tolerance. COPD 2009; 6:317—9.

[88] Crapo RO, Casaburi R, Coates AL, et al. ATS statement: guidelines for the six-minute walk test. Am J Respir Crit Care Med 2002:166.

[89] Fitts SS, Guthrie MR. Six-minute walk by people with chronic renal failure. Assessment of effort by perceived exertion. Am J Phys Med Rehabil 1995;74:54—8.

[90] Greenwood SA, Lindup H, Taylor K, et al. Evaluation of a pragmatic exercise rehabilitation programme in chronic kidney disease. Nephrol Dial Transplant 2012.

[91] Singh SJ, Morgan MD, Hardman AE, et al. Comparison of oxygen uptake during a conventional treadmill test and the shuttle walking test in chronic airflow limitation. Eur Respir J 1994;7:2016–20.

[92] Singh SJ, Morgan MD, Scott S, et al. Development of a shuttle walking test of disability in patients with chronic airways obstruction. Thorax 1992;47:1019–24.

[93] Cooper CB, Storer TW. Exercise prescription in patients with pulmonary disease. In: Swain DP, Ehrman JK, editors. ACSM's Resource Manual for Guidelines for Exercise Testing and Prescription. 6th edn. Philadelphia, PA: Wolters Kluwer/Lippicott Willams & Wilkins; 2010. p. 575–99.

[94] Baechle T, Earle R, Wathen D. Resistance Training. In: Baechle T, Earle R, editors. Essentials of Strength and Conditioning. 3rd ed. Champaign, IL: Human Kinetics; 2008. p. 381–411.

[95] Kaelin ME, Swank AM, Adams KJ, et al. Cardiopulmonary responses, muscle soreness, and injury during the one repetition maximum assessment in pulmonary rehabilitation patients. J Cardiopulm Rehabil 1999;19:366–72.

[96] Vilaro J, Rabinovich R, Gonzalez-deSuso JM, et al. Clinical assessment of peripheral muscle function in patients with chronic obstructive pulmonary disease. Am J Phys Med Rehabil 2009;88:39–46.

[97] Edelmann F, Gelbrich G, Dungen HD, et al. Exercise training improves exercise capacity and diastolic function in patients with heart failure with preserved ejection fraction: results of the Ex-DHF (Exercise training in Diastolic Heart Failure) pilot study. J Am Coll Cardiol 2011;58:1780–91.

[98] Williams MA, Haskell WL, Ades PA, et al. Resistance exercise in individuals with and without cardiovascular disease: 2007 update: a scientific statement from the American Heart Association Council on Clinical Cardiology and Council on Nutrition, Physical Activity, and Metabolism. Circulation 2007;116:572–84.

[99] Wise FM, Patrick JM. Resistance exercise in cardiac rehabilitation. Clin Rehabil 2011;25:1059–65.

[100] Cheema B, Abas H, Smith B, et al. Progressive exercise for anabolism in kidney disease (PEAK): a randomized, controlled trial of resistance training during hemodialysis. J Am Soc Nephrol 2007;18:1594–601.

[101] Oh-Park M, Fast A, Gopal S, et al. Exercise for the dialyzed: aerobic and strength training during hemodialysis. Am J Phys Med Rehabil 2002;81:814–21.

[102] Jamal SA, Leiter RE, Jassal V, et al. Impaired muscle strength is associated with fractures in hemodialysis patients. Osteoporos Int 2006;17:1390–7.

[103] Ryuzaki M, Konishi K, Kasuga A, et al. Spontaneous rupture of the quadriceps tendon in patients on maintenance hemodialysis—report of three cases with clinicopathological observations. Clin Nephrol 1989;32:144–8.

[104] West SL, Lok CE, Jamal SA. Fracture Risk Assessment in Chronic Kidney Disease, Prospective Testing Under Real World Environments (FRACTURE): a prospective study. BMC Nephrol 2010;11:17.

[105] Brechue WF, Mayhew JL. Upper-body work capacity and 1RM prediction are unaltered by increasing muscular strength in college football players. J Strength Cond Res 2009;23:2477–86.

[106] Desgorces FD, Berthelot G, Dietrich G, et al. Local muscular endurance and prediction of 1 repetition maximum for bench in 4 athletic populations. J Strength Cond Res 2010;24:394–400.

[107] Reynolds JM, Gordon TJ, Robergs RA. Prediction of one repetition maximum strength from multiple repetition maximum testing and anthropometry. J Strength Cond Res 2006;20:584–92.

[108] Bassey EJ, Fiatarone MA, O'Neill EF, et al. Leg extensor power and functional performance in very old men and women. Clin Sci (Colch) 1992;82:321–7.

[109] Bassey EJ, Short AH. A new method for measuring power output in a single leg extension: feasibility, reliability and validity. Eur J Appl Physiol Occup Physiol 1990;60:385–90.

[110] Bean JF, Kiely DK, Herman S, et al. The relationship between leg power and physical performance in mobility-limited older people. J Am Geriatr Soc 2002;50:461–7.

[111] Cuoco A, Callahan DM, Sayers S, et al. Impact of muscle power and force on gait speed in disabled older men and women. J Gerontol A Biol Sci Med Sci 2004;59:1200–6.

[112] Storer TW, Magliano L, Woodhouse L, et al. Testosterone dose-dependently increases maximal voluntary strength and leg power, but does not affect fatigability or specific tension. J Clin Endocrinol Metab 2003;88:1478–85.

[113] Takai Y, Ohta M, Akagi R, et al. Sit-to-stand test to evaluate knee extensor muscle size and strength in the elderly: a novel approach. J Physiol Anthropol 2009;28:123–8.

[114] Nelson ME, Layne JE, Bernstein MJ, et al. The effects of multidimensional home-based exercise on functional performance in elderly people. J Gerontol A Biol Sci Med Sci 2004;59:54–60.

[115] Shephard RJ, Berridge M, Montelpare W. On the generality of the "sit and reach" test: an analysis of flexibility data for an aging population. Res Q Exerc Sports 1990;62:326–30.

[116] Hoeger WW, Hopkins DR. A comparison of the sit and reach and the modified sit and reach in the measurement of flexibility in women. Res Q Exerc Sports 1992;63:191–5.

[117] Alaranta H, Hurri H, Heliovaara M, et al. Flexibility of the spine: normative values of goniometric and tape measurements. Scand J Rehabil Med 1994;26:147–54.

[118] Hoeger WK, Hoeger SA. Principles and Labs for Fitness and Wellness. 10th ed. Belmont, CA: Wadsworth; 2010.

[119] Frekany GA, Leslie DK. Effects of an exercise program on selected flexibility measurements of senior citizens. Gerontologist 1975;15:182–3.

[120] Cesari M, Onder G, Russo A, et al. Comorbidity and physical function: results from the aging and longevity study in the Sirente geographic area (ilSIRENTE study). Gerontology 2006;52:24–32.

[121] Fried LP, Guralnik JM. Disability in older adults: evidence regarding significance, etiology, and risk. J Am Geriatr Soc 1997;45:92–100.

[122] Guralnik JM, Ferrucci L, Pieper CF, et al. Lower extremity function and subsequent disability: consistency across studies, predictive models, and value of gait speed alone compared with the short physical performance battery. J Gerontol A Biol Sci Med Sci 2000;55:M221–231.

[123] Guralnik JM, Leveille SG, Hirsch R, et al. The impact of disability in older women. J Am Med Womens Assoc 1997;52:113–20.

[124] Onder G, Penninx BW, Ferrucci L, et al. Measures of physical performance and risk for progressive and catastrophic disability: results from the Women's Health and Aging Study. J Gerontol A Biol Sci Med Sci 2005;60:74–9.

[125] Reuben DB, Seeman TE, Keeler E, et al. The effect of self-reported and performance-based functional impairment on future hospital costs of community-dwelling older persons. Gerontologist 2004;44:401–7.

[126] Guralnik JM, Ferrucci L, Simonsick EM, et al. Lower-extremity function in persons over the age of 70 years as a predictor of subsequent disability. N Engl J Med 1995;332:556—61.

[127] Bean JF, Kiely DK, Leveille SG, et al. The 6-minute walk test in mobility-limited elders: what is being measured? J Gerontol A Biol Sci Med Sci 2002;57:M751—756.

[128] Newman AB, Haggerty CL, Kritchevsky SB, et al. Walking performance and cardiovascular response: associations with age and morbidity — the Health, Aging and Body Composition Study. J Gerontol A Biol Sci Med Sci 2003;58:715—20.

[129] Newman AB, Simonsick EM, Naydeck BL, et al. Association of long-distance corridor walk performance with mortality, cardiovascular disease, mobility limitation, and disability. JAMA 2006;295:2018—26.

[130] Studenski S, Perera S, Patel K, et al. Gait speed and survival in older adults. JAMA 2011;305:50—8.

[131] Studenski S, Perera S, Wallace D, et al. Physical performance measures in the clinical setting. J Am Geriatr Soc 2003;51:314—22.

[132] LeBrasseur NK, Bhasin S, Miciek R, et al. Tests of muscle strength and physical function: reliability and discrimination of performance in younger and older men and older men with mobility limitations. J Am Geriatr Soc 2008;56:2118—23.

[133] Storer TW, Woodhouse L, Magliano L, et al. Changes in muscle mass, muscle strength, and power but not physical function are related to testosterone dose in healthy older men. J Am Geriatr Soc 2008;56:1991—9.

[134] Travison TG, Basaria S, Storer TW, et al. Clinical meaningfulness of the changes in muscle performance and physical function associated with testosterone administration in older men with mobility limitation. J Gerontol A Biol Sci Med Sci 2011;66:1090—9.

[135] Overend T, Anderson C, Sawant A, et al. Relative and absolute reliability of physical function measures in people with end-stage renal disease. Physiother Can 2010;62:122—8.

[136] Knight EL, Ofsthun N, Teng M, et al. The association between mental health, physical function, and hemodialysis mortality. Kidney Int 2003;63:1843—51.

[137] Medicine ACoS. Guidelines for Graded Exercise Testing and Exercise Prescription. 1st ed. Philadelphia PA: Lea and Febiger; 1975.

[138] Workgroup KD. K/DOQI clinical practice guidelines for cardiovascular disease in dialysis patients. Am J Kidney Dis 2005;45:S1—153.

[139] Painter PL. Renal Failure. In: Durstine L, Moore G, Painter P, Roberts S, editors. ACSM's exercise management for persons with chronic diseases and disabilities. Champaign IL: Human Kinetics; 2009.

[140] Shrier I. Stretching before exercise does not reduce the risk of local muscle injury: a critical review of the clinical and basic science literature. Clin J Sport Med 1999;9:221—7.

[141] Bird M, Hill KD, Ball M, et al. The long-term benefits of a multi-component exercise intervention to balance and mobility in healthy older adults. Arch Gerontol Geriatr 2011;52:211—6.

[142] Costa PB, Graves BS, Whitehurst M, et al. The acute effects of different durations of static stretching on dynamic balance performance. J Strength Cond Res 2009;23:141—7.

[143] Borg GA. Psychophysical bases of perceived exertion. Med Sci Sports Exerc 1982;14:377—81.

[144] Borg G. Borg's perceived exertion and pain scales. Champaign, IL: Human Kinetics; 1998.

[145] Robertson RJ, Goss FL, Dube J, et al. Validation of the adult OMNI scale of perceived exertion for cycle ergometer exercise. Med Sci Sports Exerc 2004;36:102—8.

[146] Utter AC, Robertson RJ, Green JM, et al. Validation of the Adult OMNI Scale of perceived exertion for walking/running exercise. Med Sci Sports Exerc 2004;36:1776—80.

[147] Scherr J, Wolfarth B, Christle JW, et al. Associations between Borg's rating of perceived exertion and physiological measures of exercise intensity. Eur J Appl Physiol 2012. DOI: 10.1007/s00421-012-2421-x.

[148] Bouchard C. Physical activity, fitness, and health: overview of the consensus symposium. In: Quinney H, Gauvin L, Wall A, editors. Toward active living: Proceedings of the International Conference on Physical Activity, Fitness, and Health. Champaign: Human Kinetics; 1994. p 36.

[149] Beauchamp MK, Nonoyama M, Goldstein RS, et al. Interval versus continuous training in individuals with chronic obstructive pulmonary disease—a systematic review. Thorax 2010;65:157—64.

[150] Kortianou EA, Nasis IG, Spetsioti ST, et al. Effectiveness of Interval Exercise Training in Patients with COPD. Cardiopulm Phys Ther J 2010;21:12—9.

[151] Mador MJ, Krawza M, Alhajhusian A, et al. Interval training versus continuous training in patients with chronic obstructive pulmonary disease. J Cardiopulm Rehabil Prev 2009;29:126—32.

[152] Vogiatzis I, Nanas S, Roussos C. Interval training as an alternative modality to continuous exercise in patients with COPD. Eur Respir J 2002;20:12—9.

[153] Freyssin C, Verkindt C, Prieur F, et al. Cardiac Rehabilitation in Chronic Heart Failure: Effect of an 8-Week, High-Intensity Interval Training Versus Continuous Training. Arch Phys Med Rehabil 2012;93:1359—64.

[154] Fu TC, Wang CH, Lin PS, et al. Aerobic interval training improves oxygen uptake efficiency by enhancing cerebral and muscular hemodynamics in patients with heart failure. Int J Cardiol 2011. DOI: 10.1016/j.ijcard.2011.11.086.

[155] Moholdt T, Aamot IL, Granoien I, et al. Aerobic interval training increases peak oxygen uptake more than usual care exercise training in myocardial infarction patients: a randomized controlled study. Clin Rehabil 2012;26:33—44.

[156] Moholdt T, Aamot IL, Granoien I, et al. Long-term follow-up after cardiac rehabilitation: a randomized study of usual care exercise training versus aerobic interval training after myocardial infarction. Int J Cardiol 2011;152:388—90.

[157] Hwang CL, Wu YT, Chou CH. Effect of aerobic interval training on exercise capacity and metabolic risk factors in people with cardiometabolic disorders: a meta-analysis. J Cardiopulm Rehabil Prev 2011;31:378—85.

[158] Little JP, Gillen JB, Percival ME, et al. Low-volume high-intensity interval training reduces hyperglycemia and increases muscle mitochondrial capacity in patients with type 2 diabetes. J Appl Physiol 2011;111:1554—60.

[159] Burgomaster KA, Hughes SC, Heigenhauser GJ, et al. Six sessions of sprint interval training increases muscle oxidative potential and cycle endurance capacity in humans. J Appl Physiol 2005;98:1985—90.

[160] Gordon NF, Kohl 3rd HW, Pollock ML, et al. Cardiovascular safety of maximal strength testing in healthy adults. Am J Cardiol 1995;76:851—3.

[161] Hoeger WWK, Barette SL, Hale DF, et al. Relationship between repetitions and selected percentages of one repetition maximum. J Appl Sports Sci Res 1987;1:11—3.

[162] Hoeger WWK, Hopkins DR, Barette SL, et al. Relationship between repetitions and selected percentages of one repetition maximum: a comparison between untrained and trained males and females. J Appl Sports Sci Res 1990:47—54.

[163] Schairer JR, Jarvis RA, Keteyian SJ. Exercise prescription in patients with cardiovascular disease. In: Swain DP, Ehrman JK, editors. ACSM's Resource Manual for Guidelines

for Exercise Testing and Prescription. 6th ed. Philadelphia, PA: Wolters Kluwer/Lippicott Willams & Wilkins; 2010. p. 559—74.

[164] Cheema BS, O'Sullivan AJ, Chan M, et al. Progressive resistance training during hemodialysis: rationale and method of a randomized-controlled trial. Hemodial Int 2006;10:303—10.

[165] Goldberg AP, Geltman EM, Hagberg JM, et al. Therapeutic benefits of exercise training for hemodialysis patients. Kidney Int Suppl 1983;16:S303—309.

[166] Koh KP, Fassett RG, Sharman JE, et al. Effect of intradialytic versus home-based aerobic exercise training on physical function and vascular parameters in hemodialysis patients: a randomized pilot study. Am J Kidney Dis 2010;55:88—99.

[167] Konstantinidou E, Koukouvou G, Kouidi E, et al. Exercise training in patients with end-stage renal disease on hemodialysis: comparison of three rehabilitation programs. J Rehabil Med 2002;34:40—5.

[168] Kouidi EJ, Grekas DM, Deligiannis AP. Effects of exercise training on noninvasive cardiac measures in patients undergoing long-term hemodialysis: a randomized controlled trial. Am J Kidney Dis 2009;54:511—21.

[169] Ouzouni S, Kouidi E, Sioulis A, et al. Effects of intradialytic exercise training on health-related quality of life indices in haemodialysis patients. Clin Rehabil 2009;23:53—63.

[170] Parsons TL, Toffelmire EB, King-VanVlack CE. The effect of an exercise program during hemodialysis on dialysis efficacy, blood pressure and quality of life in end-stage renal disease (ESRD) patients. Clin Nephrol 2004;61:261—74.

[171] Segura-Orti E, Kouidi E, Lison JF. Effect of resistance exercise during hemodialysis on physical function and quality of life: randomized controlled trial. Clin Nephrol 2009;71:527—37.

[172] Akiba T, Matsui N, Shinohara S, et al. Effects of recombinant human erythropoietin and exercise training on exercise capacity in hemodialysis patients. Artif Organs 1995;19:1262—8.

[173] Carney R, Templeton B, Hong B, et al. Exercise training reduces depression and increases the performance of pleasant activities in hemodialysis patients. Nephron 1987;47:194—8.

[174] Deligiannis A, Kouidi E, Tourkantonis A. Effects of physical training on heart rate variability in patients on hemodialysis. Am J Cardiol 1999;84:197—202.

[175] Headley S, Germain M, Mailloux P, et al. Resistance training improves strength and functional measures in patients with end-stage renal disease. Am J Kidney Dis 2002;40: 355—64.

[176] Kouidi E, Grekas D, Deligiannis A, et al. Outcomes of long-term exercise training in dialysis patients: comparison of two training programs. Clin Nephrol 2004;61(Suppl. 1):S31—38.

[177] Molsted S, Eidemak I, Sorensen H, et al. Five months of physical exercise in hemodialysis patients: effects on aerobic capacity, physical function and self-rated health. Nephron Clin Pract 2004;96:c76—81.

[178] Tsuyuki K, Kimura Y, Chiashi K, et al. Oxygen uptake efficiency slope as monitoring tool for physical training in chronic hemodialysis patients. Ther Apher Dial 2003;7:461—7.

[179] Sakkas GK, Hadjigeorgiou GM, Karatzaferi C, et al. Intradialytic aerobic exercise training ameliorates symptoms of restless legs syndrome and improves functional capacity in patients on hemodialysis: a pilot study. ASAIO J 2008;54:185—90.

[180] Afshar R, Shegarfy L, Shavandi N, et al. Effects of aerobic exercise and resistance training on lipid profiles and inflammation status in patients on maintenance hemodialysis. Indian J Nephrol 2010;20:185—9.

[181] Parsons TL, Toffelmire EB, King-VanVlack CE. Exercise training during hemodialysis improves dialysis efficacy and physical performance. Arch Phys Med Rehabil 2006;87:680—7.

[182] Zaluska A, Zaluska WT, Bednarek-Skublewska A, et al. Nutrition and hydration status improve with exercise training using stationary cycling during hemodialysis (HD) in patients with end-stage renal disease (ESRD). Ann Univ Mariae Curie Sklodowska Med 2002;57:342—6.

[183] Delgado C, Johansen KL. Deficient counseling on physical activity among nephrologists. Nephron Clin Pract 2010;116: c330—336.

[184] Delgado C, Johansen KL. Barriers to exercise participation among dialysis patients. Nephrol Dial Transplant 2012;27: 1152—7.

[185] Kontos PC, Miller KL, Brooks D, et al. Factors influencing exercise participation by older adults requiring chronic hemodialysis: a qualitative study. Int Urol Nephrol 2007;39: 1303—11.

[186] Kutner NG. Rehabilitation in the renal population: barriers to access. Semin Nephrol 2010;30:59—65.

[187] Painter P, Ward K, Nelson RD. Self-reported physical activity in patients with end stage renal disease. Nephrol Nurs J 2011;38:139—47. quiz 148.

[188] Goodman ED, Ballou MB. Perceived barriers and motivators to exercise in hemodialysis patients. Nephrol Nurs J 2004;31: 23—9.

[189] Kutner NG. How can exercise be incorporated into the routine care of patients on dialysis? Int Urol Nephrol 2007;39:1281—5.

[190] Johansen KL, Sakkas GK, Doyle J, et al. Exercise counseling practices among nephrologists caring for patients on dialysis. Am J Kidney Dis 2003;41:171—8.

[191] Cheema BS, Smith BC, Singh MA. A rationale for intradialytic exercise training as standard clinical practice in ESRD. Am J Kidney Dis 2005;45:912—6.

[192] Bennett PN, Breugelmans L, Agius M, et al. A haemodialysis exercise programme using novel exercise equipment: a pilot study. J Ren Care 2007;33:153—8.

[193] Franklin BA, Swain DP. New insights on the threshold intensity for improving cardiorespiratory fitness. Prev Cardiol 2003;6: 118—21.

[194] Swain DP. Moderate or vigorous intensity exercise: which is better for improving aerobic fitness? Prev Cardiol 2005;8: 55—8.

[195] Swain DP, Franklin BA. Is there a threshold intensity for aerobic training in cardiac patients? Med Sci Sports Exerc 2002;34: 1071—5.

[196] Malik S, Winney RJ, Ewing DJ. Chronic renal failure and cardiovascular autonomic function. Nephron 1986;43:191—5.

[197] Floyd M, Ayyar D, Barwick D, et al. Myopathy in chronic renal failure. Q J Med 1974;43:509—24.

[198] Moore G, Parsons D, Stray-Gundersen J, et al. Uremic myopathy limits aerobic capacity in hemodialysis patients. Am J Kidney Dis 1993;22:277—87.

[199] Bruce RA, Kusumi F, Hosmer D. Maximal oxygen intake and nomographic assessment of functional aerobic impairment in cardiovascular disease. Am Heart J 1973;85:546—62.

[200] Fox III SM, Naughton JP, Haskell WL. Physical activity and the prevention of coronary heart disease. Ann Clin Res 1971;3: 404—32.

[201] Robergs RA, Landwher R. Commentary: The surprizing history of the "HRmax = 220—age" equation. Journal of Exercise Physiologyonline 2002:5.

[202] Robertson RJ, Goss FL, Rutkowski J, et al. Concurrent validation of the OMNI perceived exertion scale for resistance exercise. Med Sci Sports Exerc 2003;35:333—41.

[203] Macdonald JH, Marcora SM, Jibani M, et al. Intradialytic exercise as anabolic therapy in haemodialysis patients — a pilot study. Clin Physiol Funct Imaging 2005;25:113—8.

[204] Decoster LC, Cleland J, Altieri C, et al. The effects of hamstring stretching on range of motion: a systematic literature review. J Orthop Sports Phys Ther 2005;35:377—87.

[205] Kokkonen J, Nelson AG, Eldredge C, et al. Chronic static stretching improves exercise performance. Med Sci Sports Exerc 2007;39:1825—31.

[206] Cook WL, Tomlinson G, Donaldson M, et al. Falls and fall-related injuries in older dialysis patients. Clin J Am Soc Nephrol 2006;1:1197—204.

[207] Lockhart TE, Barth AT, Zhang X, et al. Portable, non-invasive fall risk assessment in end stage renal disease patients on hemodialysis. ACM Trans Comput Hum Interact 2010:84—93.

[208] Roberts R, Jeffrey C, Carlisle G, et al. Prospective investigation of the incidence of falls, dizziness and syncope in haemodialysis patients. Int Urol Nephrol 2007;39:275—9.

[209] Gatts S. Neural mechanisms underlying balance control in Tai Chi. Med Sport Sci 2008;52:87—103.

[210] Jahnke R, Larkey L, Rogers C, et al. A comprehensive review of health benefits of qigong and tai chi. Am J Health Promot 2010;24:e1—e25.

[211] Wang C, Collet JP, Lau J. The effect of Tai Chi on health outcomes in patients with chronic conditions: a systematic review. Arch Intern Med 2004;164:493—501.

[212] Leung DP, Chan CK, Tsang HW, et al. Tai chi as an intervention to improve balance and reduce falls in older adults: A systematic and meta-analytical review. Altern Ther Health Med 2011;17:40—8.

[213] Wolf SL, Barnhart HX, Kutner NG, et al. Selected as the best paper in the 1990s: Reducing frailty and falls in older persons: an investigation of tai chi and computerized balance training. J Am Geriatr Soc 2003;51:1794—803.

[214] Jones BH, Cowan DN, Knapik JJ. Exercise, training and injuries. Sports Med 1994;18:202—14.

[215] Copley JB, Lindberg JS. The risks of exercise. Adv Ren Replace Ther 1999;6:165—71.

[216] Painter P. Implementing exercise: what do we know? Where do we go? Adv Chronic Kidney Dis 2009;16:536—44.

[217] Huang GS, Chu TS, Lou MF, et al. Factors associated with low bone mass in the hemodialysis patients—a cross-sectional correlation study. BMC Musculoskelet Disord 2009;10:60.

[218] Cheema BS. Review article: Tackling the survival issue in end-stage renal disease: time to get physical on haemodialysis. Nephrology (Carlton) 2008;13:560—9.

[219] Painter P. The importance of exercise training in rehabilitation of patients with end-stage renal disease. Am J Kidney Dis 1994;24:S2—9.

[220] Painter P, Johansen K. Physical functioning in end-stage renal disease. Introduction: a call to activity. Adv Ren Replace Ther 1999;6:107—9.

[221] Bergman-Evans B. AIDES to improving medication adherence in older adults. Geriatr Nurs 2006;27:174—82. quiz 183.

[222] Deligiannis A, Kouidi E, Tassoulas E, et al. Cardiac effects of exercise rehabilitation in hemodialysis patients. Int J Cardiol 1999;70:253—66.

[223] Koufaki P, Mercer T, Naish P. Effects of exercise training on aerobic and functional capacity of end-stage renal disease patients. Clin Physiol Funct Imaging 2002;22:115—24.

[224] Kouidi E, Iacovides A, Iordanidis P, et al. Exercise renal rehabilitation program: psychosocial effects. Nephron 1997;77:152—8.

[225] DePaul V, Moreland J, Eager T, et al. The effectiveness of aerobic and muscle strength training in patients receiving hemodialysis and EPO: a randomized controlled trial. Am J Kidney Dis 2002;40:1219—29.

[226] Bohannon RW. Reference values for extremity muscle strength obtained by hand-held dynamometry from adults aged 20 to 79 years. Arch Phys Med Rehabil 1997;78:26—32.

[227] Bohannon RW. Intertester reliability of hand-held dynamometry: a concise summary of published research. Percept Mot Skills 1999;88:899—902.

[228] Bohannon RW, Smith J, Barnhard R. Grip strength in end stage renal disease. Percept Mot Skills 1994;79:1523—6.

[229] Mathiowetz V, Weber K, Volland G, et al. Reliability and validity of grip and pinch strength evaluations. J Hand Surg Am 1984;9:222—6.

[230] Mercer TH, Naish PF, Gleeson NP, et al. Development of a walking test for the assessment of functional capacity in non-anaemic maintenance dialysis patients. Nephrol Dial Transplant 1998;13:2023—6.

[231] Enright PL, McBurnie MA, Bittner V, et al. The 6-min walk test: a quick measure of functional status in elderly adults. Chest 2003;123:387—98.

[232] Podsiadlo D, Richardson S. The timed "Up & Go": a test of basic functional mobility for frail elderly persons. J Am Geriatr Soc 1991;39:142—8.

[233] Berg K, Wood-Dauphinee S, Williams JI, et al. Measuring balance in the elderly: validation of an instrument. Can J Pub Health 1992:S7—11.

[234] Nowicki M, Murlikiewicz K, Jagodzinska M. Pedometers as a means to increase spontaneous physical activity in chronic hemodialysis patients. J Nephrol 2010;23:297—305.

[235] Crouter SE, Churilla JR, Bassett Jr DR. Estimating energy expenditure using accelerometers. Eur J Appl Physiol 2006;98: 601—12.

[236] Bohannon RW, DePasquale L. Physical Functioning Scale of the Short-Form (SF) 36: internal consistency and validity with older adults. J Geriatr Phys Ther 2010;33:16—8.

[237] Hays RD, Kallich JD, Mapes DL, et al. Development of the kidney disease quality of life (KDQOL) instrument. Qual Life Res 1994;3:329—38.

[238] Rao S, Carter WB, Mapes DL, et al. Development of subscales from the symptoms/problems and effects of kidney disease scales of the kidney disease quality of life instrument. Clin Ther 2000;22:1099—111.

[239] Ware Jr JE, Kosinski M, Bayliss MS, et al. Comparison of methods for the scoring and statistical analysis of SF-36 health profile and summary measures: summary of results from the Medical Outcomes Study. Med Care 1995;33: AS264—279.

46

Motivating the Kidney Disease Patient to Nutrition Adherence and Other Healthy Lifestyle Activities

Steve Martino[1], Lydia Chwastiak[2], Frederic Finkelstein[3]

[1]Yale University School of Medicine, VA Connecticut Healthcare System, West Haven, CT, USA
[2]Yale University School of Medicine, Connecticut Mental Health Center, New Haven, CT, USA
[3]Yale University School of Medicine, New Haven, CT, USA

INTRODUCTION

Patients with kidney disease are required to manage multiple nutritional and lifestyle changes and medical treatments in order to improve their health, including adherence to recommended diet and exercise routines, medications and health monitoring activities, medical appointments, and in some cases, dialysis treatment. As kidney disease progresses, these demands increase and patients' motivation to meet them typically wanes. This diminished motivation may contribute to the patients' non-adherence and disengagement from their healthcare providers. Helping kidney disease patients implement and sustain necessary dietary plans, other healthy lifestyle activities, and medical regimens in collaboration with their nephrology team is critical for improving their treatment outcomes and quality of life. While treatment adherence for chronic illness involves many factors, such as patient demographics, treatment complexity and side effects, and availability of social and environmental supports [1], an important strategy to promote self-management is to activate the patients' motivation to manage their kidney disease [2].

This chapter describes an approach for enhancing patients' motivation for change, called motivational interviewing (MI) [3]. MI increasingly is being used in healthcare settings to counsel patients with chronic diseases such as kidney disease [4]. The chapter reviews the basic principles and techniques of MI and the evidence to support the use of MI for improving kidney disease patients' self-management.

WHAT IS MOTIVATIONAL INTERVIEWING?

Miller and Rollnick have defined MI as "a collaborative, person-centered form of guiding [patients] to elicit and strengthen motivation for change" (p. 138) [5]. The approach is grounded in humanistic psychology, especially the work of Carl Rogers [6], in that it employs a very empathic, nonjudgmental style of interacting with patients and presumes that the potential for change lies within everyone. MI is distinct from nondirective approaches, however, in that providers intentionally attend to and selectively reinforce patients' motives that support change [3,5,7]. Over the course of the interview, providers help patients identify these change-oriented motives, elaborate upon them, and resolve ambivalence about change. If successful, patients become more likely to commit to changing their behaviors and initiating a change plan.

The process of enhancing motivation in MI can be thought of as having two different phases [3]. The first phase involves building motivation for change. In this phase providers work with patients to understand and resolve their resistance to change and develop their sense of the importance and perceived ability to change. When patients show signs of readiness to change (e.g., reasons for change are prominent, they ask for advice or direction, they state their intention to change), providers shift to the second phase of motivational enhancement in which they work toward strengthening commitment to change, most often through the development of a change plan (described below). This process

Nutritional Management of Renal Disease
http://dx.doi.org/10.1016/B978-0-12-391934-2.00046-1

activates or mobilizes patients' motivations in that they identify how they will try to change and begin to enact these steps to improve their kidney disease self-management.

Skilled healthcare providers try to match their use of MI strategies to the patients' level of motivation. For example, providers move more quickly to change planning with patients who are already motivated to change. Extensive exploration of their motives for change might frustrate patients who want to move forward. In contrast, attempting to develop change plans with patients who are not yet committed to change will likely increase resistance in that this strategy would put patients in a position in which they might assert in words or in actions how they are not yet ready. This latter interaction illustrates how motives to change (called "change talk") and motives to stay the same (called "sustain talk") can be thought of as opposite sides of the same coin, meaning that if providers give insufficient attention to addressing important issues that impede change, patients are likely to raise these issues again during the interview [3]. Concomitantly, providers expect patients who initially argue against change to have some intrinsic motivation for change within them. It is the responsibility of providers to look for opportunities to draw it out.

MI is best construed as a style of communication that informs the way in which providers interact with patients throughout the change process [3,7]. In this regard, MI often is discussed within the context of the Stages of Change model by James Prochaska and Carlo DiClemente [8]. The Stage of Change model posits that behavior change occurs sequentially across recurring stages. The earlier stages include precontemplation (patients are unaware or do not believe there is a problem or need to change it), contemplation (patients are ambivalent about recognizing a problem and shy away from changing it), and preparation (patients are ready to work toward behavior change in the near future and develop a plan for change). The later stages include action (patients consistently make specific changes) and maintenance (patients work to maintain and sustain long-lasting change). Tailoring treatment strategies to achieve stage-related tasks is a hallmark of this model (e.g., conducting a cost–benefit analysis for someone contemplating change).

MI naturally fits into the Stage of Change model in that it can be used to help move patients from one stage to another, especially in the early stages [9]. Patient-centered counseling skills may build rapport and engage patients who are less motivated to change. Eliciting additional change talk might lead ambivalent individuals to conclude it is relatively worth it for them to change rather than to not address areas critical to their health and quality of life. Working with patients to identify steps they are able to take might help them feel more prepared to initiate a change plan. In later stages, MI strategies are useful for attending to wavering motivation as patients take action or try to maintain changes in stressful situations. Finally, the Stages of Change model illustrates how MI integrates well with other treatment approaches that are more action-oriented. For example, MI might be used to engage patients in kidney disease education and skill building activities (e.g., meeting with a dietician to learn how to consume the right balance of protein) or in other treatments for co-morbid conditions (e.g., cognitive behavioral therapy for depression). Combining MI with more action-oriented interventions is becoming more prevalent [10].

MI emerged out of early efforts to establish brief interventions for alcohol problems [11]. These interventions shared a harm reduction approach in that they aimed to help patients move toward reduced drinking to lower risks rather than to automatically advocate for total abstinence as the only acceptable goal. Common components of these brief interventions, as represented in a FRAMES acronym, were: Feedback, emphasis on personal Responsibility, Advice, a Menu of options, an Empathic counseling style, and support for Self-efficacy. With FRAMES as a guidepost, William Miller and his colleagues developed the "drinker's check-up" in which patients received feedback about their drinking relative to population or clinical norms and then explored what it might suggest about their drinking and motivation for reducing or stopping it. Early studies found the drinker's check-up to be quite effective [12]. Given this success, MI with personalized assessment feedback then became adapted into a more structured and manualized format and termed motivational enhancement therapy or MET [13].

As applied to the management of kidney disease, the harm reduction stance of MI implies that the aim of MI is to help patients prepare themselves to make changes in any behaviors that might positively impact their kidney disease. Determining what areas matter most to them (e.g., diet, exercise, medication), which areas they believe they can change (e.g., limiting fluid intake, increasing activity level), and what goal to achieve (e.g., walking 15 minutes per day) is more important than pushing them to commit to something they may not want to or feel able to achieve, even if full adherence would have obviously better health outcomes.

Implied in the above discussion is that MI is behaviorally specific and has direction. This means that providers need to be clear about what it is that they are trying to motivate patients to do or to change. Motivation for change in one area does not guarantee motivation for change in another (e.g., a patient may commit to taking a phosphorus binder, but not agree to substantially limit foods high in sodium). Each behavior may require a separate motivational enhancement process. MI also requires that providers take a stance about the preferred direction for change. For many behaviors related to kidney disease, this decision is relatively clear in that most patients would agree that it is ethically sound to enhance motivation for changes that decrease morbidity and mortality, such as blood glucose control or smoking cessation. However, some behavioral issues involved in kidney disease care do not have a clear change direction. For example, decisions about whether to start end-stage renal disease therapy with peritoneal dialysis or hemodialysis or proceed with a pre-emptive kidney transplant likely would require a nondirective approach in which providers suspend their own values or goals and assume a position of "equipoise" (i.e., indifference or no clear attachment to a position or recommendation). In these situations, a patient-centered counseling approach, devoid of evocation, would allow patients to explore their ambivalence without intentional provider influence.

WHAT ISN'T MOTIVATIONAL INTERVIEWING?

For clarification purposes, it is helpful to consider what MI is not [5]. As noted above, MI is not based on the Stages of Change model, though it is complementary to it. Stages of Change is more of a comprehensive way of thinking about how patients change, whereas MI is a clinical method that helps patients prepare for change. Likewise, MI is not cognitive behavioral therapy. The latter approach supplies patients with education and coping skill development and encourages the repeated practicing of these skills to better manage their problems. MI is fundamentally humanistic, not behavioral, in origin in that it elicits the patients' motivations for change rather than putting in place what is missing (knowledge and skills). MI also is not a way of manipulating others or making them change when they don't want to. Behavior change in MI is born out of a person's intrinsic motivations. Healthcare providers can only call forth motivations that already exist within patients; they cannot impose the concerns or wishes of others when an individual does not see these issues as in his/her best interest. Finally, MI does not require that providers conduct a decisional balance or give personalized feedback. These are techniques that often are helpful for eliciting change talk, but they are not essential to the conduct of MI, and they often are used in other treatment approaches. In this regard, MI is not a series of techniques, but rather a way of being with patients in which principles organize the practice, as Miller and Rollnick put it, like music to words of a song [3].

PRINCIPLES

Four key principles, embodied in the REDS acronym, compose the manner in which providers interact with patients when using MI [3].

Roll with Resistance

In MI, resistance refers to a patient's statements about what sustains his problematic behaviors. These expressions may be about the reasons for the behaviors ("Eating a lot relaxes me") or the difficulties of trying to change them ("I can't resist the urge to smoke"). Resistance informs providers about dilemmas faced by individuals, thereby providing opportunities for addressing obstacles to change. In using MI, a provider would avoid adopting a confrontational, authoritative, warning, or threatening tone (all inconsistent with MI), which might cause the patient to become even less engaged in treatment [14].

Express Empathy

Healthcare providers should attempt to accurately understand patients' dilemmas without judgment or criticism. Being able to listen carefully to what patients mean and reflect this back to them is a critical skill. Patients are more likely to explore their motivations for change and speak candidly when they feel comfortable with and understood by their providers [14].

Develop Discrepancy

Motivation for change often depends on the existence of a discrepancy between an individual's important values or goals and his current behavior. For example, a kidney disease patient who hopes to attend her grandson's wedding might consider how continued poor dietary adherence might affect the probability of this occurrence. In MI, providers reflect these discrepancies and explore how behavior change might help patients feel they are acting in accord with their preferred self-perceptions or aims.

Support Self-Efficacy

Patients typically become more motivated when they believe they can change their behavior. When patients lack confidence, they often shy away from change. Providers look for opportunities to support patients' self-efficacy by helping them recognize their personal strengths and available resources. Likewise, they draw attention to patients' past successful change efforts, which might inform how these individuals approach their current dilemmas.

By embracing these principles, providers adopt a style of interaction that is (1) collaborative by demonstrating respect for patients' ideas and goals and seeing the patient as an equal partner in the therapeutic process; (2) evocative by intentionally searching for the patients' motives that favor change; and (3) supportive of patients' autonomy and capacity to make decisions and initiate change. These three components embody the spirit of how providers interact with patients (referred to as "MI spirit") [15].

While MI is a style of being with others rather than merely an application of techniques, MI does incorporate several techniques that operationalize how providers use MI. Two main sets of techniques include (1) fundamental strategies or microskills such as open questions, affirmations, reflections, and summaries (the OARS); and (2) direct methods for evoking change talk [3]. Fundamental strategies are a mainstay of MI in that they help providers understand the patients' perspective, convey empathy, and build a positive relationship with their patients. As the conversation unfolds, healthcare providers attend to the balance of statements made by patients that support or thwart behavior change (i.e., change vs. sustain talk) to gauge the patients' level of motivation and adjust their use of MI techniques accordingly. The capacities to recognize and elicit change talk and to reduce sustain talk, with the aim of strengthening patient commitment to change, are necessary elements of MI [3,7,16]. The continuous interplay of fundamental patient-centered strategies and direct methods to elicit and reinforce change talk is essential to proficiently conduct MI (see Figure 46.1).

Fundamental Strategies

Open questions encourage patients to talk more and may be used to strategically draw out motivations for change (e.g., "What would be good about quitting smoking?). They stand in contrast to closed questions, in which providers seek specific information (e.g., demographics, history, symptoms), often with questions that can be answered with a "yes" or a "no" response. For example, a patient's positive response to the closed-ended question, "Have you been sticking with the diet we discussed last time?" would provide some useful information. However, he or she would not have fully elaborated on adherence to various aspects of the dietary plan, which an open question (e.g., "What parts of your plan have you been able to stick with since we last met?") might have elicited.

Affirmations (i.e., acknowledgment of a person's strengths, attitudes, and efforts that promote behavior change) build collaboration between providers and patients and promote self-efficacy. Sometimes this entails reframing a behavior in a manner that helps patients see it in a more positive light. For example, a provider who has a patient who becomes dismayed by his series of self-monitored high blood glucose readings might say, "You're keeping a close eye on your blood sugar in an effort to get it under better control".

MI also relies heavily on the skilled use of reflective listening in which providers restate or paraphrase their understanding of what patients have said to express empathy, as well as to bring attention to ambivalence, highlight change talk, and explore and lessen resistance. In MI, reflections are "simple" when a provider essentially repeats what the patient has said and "complex" when the provider articulates new meaning implied by the patient's original statements. Complex reflections demonstrate a deeper understanding of the patient's experiences. As an example, a provider asks a kidney disease patient, "How have things been going with dialysis?" The patient responds by saying, "What difference does it make?" A provider could use a simple reflection to encourage more discussion about the patient's expressed skepticism ("You're not sure dialysis makes a difference"). A complex reflection would capture the patient's implied demoralization and show more empathy ("You seem pretty discouraged").

Summaries provide opportunities for providers to demonstrate fuller understanding of their patients' experiences and help them consider the bigger picture of their motivations for change. Summaries also allow providers to collect multiple change talk statements as a strategy to enhance motivation, link discrepant statements that capture ambivalence, and shift focus to other behavioral areas (e.g., move from discussing medication adherence to exercise). The following is a dialogue that ends in a summary statement. Use of fundamental strategies is italicized.

Provider: How have you been doing? (*open question*)
Patient: Not too well actually. I have been having several annoying problems.

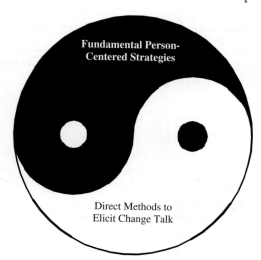

FIGURE 46.1 The continuous interplay of fundamental patient-centered strategies and direct methods to elicit and reinforce change talk.

Provider: You sound frustrated. (*complex reflection*)
Patient: I am really frustrated. [pause] Sometimes I feel like not even bothering with this treatment.
Provider: It is a lot to handle. (*complex reflection*) Tell me about the problems you've been having. (*open question/request*)
Patient: Well first of all, I've been having a lot of muscle cramps. They are mostly in my legs and they are quite painful. I get them especially when I sit around for awhile and sometimes when I am sleeping; they wake me up and I have to walk them off. The other thing is itching. It drives me crazy. I am scratching myself all the time. Between the cramps and the itching, I feel like I am being attacked from inside and outside. Is there anything we can do about it?
Provider: There are several things that are possible. Muscle cramps and itching are common for people with kidney disease. However, the causes may differ among people. We will have to talk a little more about it. I also will want to check your blood level of phosphorus and a hormone called PTH that can lead to itchy skin. (*patient-centered feedback*)
Patient: Alright. There is one more thing. I also feel tired most of the time. Sometimes I wonder if I am getting depressed.
Provider: You are not sure if you are tired because of the kidney disease or if it is due to being depressed over having to deal with the disease. (*complex reflection*)
Patient: Yeah. Sometimes it is hard to make sense of things. I guess I am hoping that you can help me figure things out.
Provider: It is confusing, and I certainly hope we can work together to figure it out. (*simple reflection that builds collaboration*) Thanks for telling me about what you're experiencing (*affirmation*).
Patient: Well, I really don't have anyone to talk to about what I am going through. Sometimes I want to forget all about it and give up. Other times, I try to be strong and positive and do everything I can to delay having dialysis. It's such a battle — one that I fear I might be losing.
Provider: And it might feel that way because there is a lot on the field. You've been having painful leg cramps, lots of itchiness, and you are beginning to feel depressed by it all. Nonetheless, you're still trying to work with us and find ways to address these problems. You haven't given up. (*summary; affirmation*)

Direct Methods

Direct methods for evoking change talk hinge on the capacity of healthcare providers to recognize how patients talk about change [7]. Providers' selection of direct methods for motivational enhancement depends on the type and strength of change talk provided by patients as the interview unfolds. Hence, a patient's statements continuously signal the provider about how to conduct the interview.

Change talk is embodied in the acronym DARN-CAT (see Table 46.1). DARN (desire, ability, reasons, and need) is sometimes referred to as preparatory language in that these statements represent the building of motivation that prepares patients to make a commitment to change (consistent with the first phase of motivational enhancement) [17]. Desire statements indicate a clear wish for change ("I don't want my kidney disease to get worse"). Ability statements indicate patients' beliefs that they can change, given their skills and available resources ("I used to swim, and there is a YMCA in my town that I could go to"). Reason statements note the benefits of change and the costs of not changing ("I will feel better" or "If I stop drinking soda, I might get my blood sugar under better control"). Need statements underscore how the problem behavior interferes with important areas of an individual's life and how changing the behavior would likely improve matters ("I don't want to be the next person in my family to die from kidney disease" or "I certainly want to teach my kids how to live a healthy life to prevent this from happening to them").

CAT (commitment, activation, taking steps) represents statements that suggest patients are mobilizing themselves for change (consistent with the second phase of motivational enhancement). Commitment statements convey the stated intention to change ("My quit date will be this Thursday"). Activation statements indicate how patients are getting ready to change ("I am going

TABLE 46.1 Change Talk Categories: DARN-CAT16

Category	Definition
Desire	Statements that indicate a clear wish for change
Ability	Statements that indicate patients' beliefs that they can change
Reason	Statements that note the benefits of change and the costs of not changing
Need	Statements that underscore how the problem behavior interferes with important areas of a patient's life and how changing the behavior would likely improve matters
Commitment	Statements that convey a patient's intention to change
Activation	Statements that indicate how patients are getting ready to change
Taking steps	Initial demonstration of behaviors that would support change

to fill the prescription at the pharmacy right after I leave here"). Statements about taking steps to change are the strongest demonstration of commitment in that the patients have put their words into action and are reporting these early efforts to the provider ("Instead of going out to drink after work, I went to the gym and exercised").

During the interview, providers identify the extent to which patients express motivation in each of these areas, use their fundamental skills to support and develop patients' change talk and have them elaborate further, and in a goal-oriented fashion, directly attempt to draw out more motivations for change. MI offers multiple techniques for these purposes. Some options are described below:

1. Evocative questions — directly asking patients for change talk (e.g., "In what ways do you think you can better manage your kidney disease?" "How would things be better for you if you followed the recommended diet?")
2. Personalized assessment feedback — providing patients information about their health status that affects how important it is to them to change their behavior (e.g., "Your test has come back and it shows further decrease in kidney functioning, meaning your kidneys continue to deteriorate in the absence of making changes in your diet and exercise. What do you make of that?")
3. Readiness rulers — asking patients to rate themselves from 0-10 about the importance of and their confidence in changing a specific behavior related to their kidney disease and following up with evocative questions designed to elicit change talk (e.g., "How come you said a 5 rather than a 0?" "What would it take for you to go from a 5 to a 6?")
4. Looking forward — asking patients to look to the future at some time interval (e.g., 5 years from now) and consider where their lives might be headed with and without healthy lifestyle changes (attempting to reveal potential reasons or need to change to enhance the importance of change).
5. Exploring goals and values — inquiring about what matters most to patients (e.g., being a good parent or available grandparent, independence) and how the targeted behavior fits with these goals or values (e.g., "How would being more physically active affect your level of independence?")
6. Past successes — exploring past periods when patients were successful in some areas and how they might import these experiences into their current circumstances ("You said you had a several year period when you had a healthy diet. How were you able to do that?" "Which of these things can you try again now?")

The following conversation between a provider and his patient demonstrates the use of direct methods for evoking change talk (italicized in text).

Provider: Last time we met, we reviewed some recommended changes to your diet because your blood pressure was elevated. Your blood pressure is still on the high side. Last time we talked about reducing salt in your food. How did it go?

Patient: Not that well. I tried to cut back on salt, but I don't like how things taste if they aren't seasoned.

Provider: Even though you like the taste of salt, you still tried to reduce how much you use. How come? (*evocative question*)

Patient: I was worried about my health, and I want to see my granddaughter graduate medical school. You said my blood pressure was high and that it increased my risk for all kinds of problems, especially heart problems. Did you say my blood pressure is still high?

Provider: Yes. It is 155 over 95, which is not good. The longer it remains high, the more risk you have for cardiovascular problems, like heart attack or stroke. (*personalized assessment feedback*)

Patient: It's just so hard to eat foods that taste bland and even more difficult figuring out what I can eat at a restaurant. I'm really upset with myself that I can't seem to control what I put in my body.

Provider: And you fear that if you don't begin to find ways to reduce how much salt you eat, you may even risk not being able to attend your granddaughter's graduation. (*exploring goals and values, looking forward*)

Patient: That's the worst of it. My granddaughter is working so hard to become a doctor, and I'm having trouble doing what the doctors tell me to do.

Provider: You'd like to better manage your health for yourself and your granddaughter. Finding ways to cut back on salt is very important to you. (*exploring goals and values*)

Patient: Yes. I just keep running into the same problems. Food just doesn't taste good without salt.

Provider: So how can you make food taste better without eating too much salt? (*evocative question*)

Patient: Well, I could cook with more spices and use more fresh food rather than canned foods or frozen dinners.

Provider: Would you be willing to meet with the dietician to help you discuss this matter some more? (*evocative question*) You have some good ideas and a few more suggestions might be helpful to you.

Patient: Sure. I thought I could just do it on my own, but I think I need some help learning how to cook in a different way.

Other Useful Techniques

Kidney disease management typically requires simultaneous attention to several behavioral issues (e.g., diet, exercise, medication adherence, adherence to the dialysis treatment regimen, blood glucose control, blood pressure control, phosphorus control, smoking cessation, co-morbid depression or anxiety), and this reality often is overwhelming to patients and their healthcare providers during any one appointment where time is limited. Providers can use a simple agenda setting chart in which they record the pertinent behavior change issues on paper and have patients indicate which of them they want to discuss during the interview [17]. It is important that these priorities be put in the context of the concerns the provider has about the patient's medical status. For example, if a patient is poorly compliant with the dialysis treatment regimen but wants to focus on his minimally elevated phosphorus level, the provider will need to organize the conversation appropriately.

Education, advice-giving, and direction are commonplace in the healthcare settings, particularly because providers' often have a natural tendency to try to fix patients' problems (referred to as the "righting reflex") [3]. When patients have not solicited professional input, however, they may not be receptive to it. Instead, providers ask permission to provide information or advice and employ an elicit-provide-elicit (or ask-tell-ask) technique in which providers (1) elicit from patients what they know about the topic being discussed; (2) provide information as needed; and (3) elicit patients' reactions to the shared information [4]. For example, a provider may wish to recommend that a patient meets with a dietician. Instead of providing the recommendation in an unsolicited manner, the provider would first ask the patient about his or her past experiences with dieticians and then, with permission, talk about how a dietician might be helpful to the patient and conclude by getting the patient's reaction. This technique promotes collaboration and reduces the chance that patients experience their providers as lecturing or telling them what to do.

Use of a decisional balance activity (i.e., exploring the costs and benefits of changing and not changing) is common in MI [3]. This activity provides a structured method for understanding the basis of a patient's ambivalence in that the benefits of change ("I'll delay the need for dialysis for many years") and the costs of not changing ("If I don't change how I eat and exercise, a heart attack may kill me before my kidney disease does") provide reasons to change, whereas the benefits of not changing ("A person has got to have some pleasure") and the costs of changing ("Healthy food is expensive") provide reasons to remain the same. By strategically eliciting more reasons for change and, to the extent possible, resolving reasons to remain the same (e.g., identify some healthy foods that taste good and are affordable), a provider might help the patient tip the balance toward change.

Another important skill is how to gauge patients' readiness to change and to transition from the first to second phase of motivational enhancement. Providers typically recapitulate what others have said, especially those statements that suggest how they are now ready to change. Following this summary, providers then pose a key question to solidify commitment to change ("What's your next step?" or "From what you've told me, how do you want to proceed?"). Miller and Rollnick have used the analogy of a person as a skier standing at the summit (assisted up the mountain by the provider) [3]. The key question provides a supportive nudge that helps the person go down the mountain.

Change planning is an overall strategy providers use to negotiate a plan with patients about how they will change their behavior [3]. Critical to this process is maintaining a patient-centered stance in which the plan is derived by the patient, with the assistance of the provider, rather than the provider becoming prescriptive at this point. Providers ask patients to set their targeted behavior change goal ("I am going to monitor my blood sugar once a day"), describe steps they will take to change ("I will test it in the morning before I eat my breakfast"; "I will record my level each day on my monitoring form"), identify who might support them and how ("I am going to ask my wife to review my sugar levels at the end of each week"), anticipate obstacles ("I travel once in awhile and need a way to not forget to take my glucometer with me"), and reaffirm their commitment to the plan. If during the process of mobilizing their commitment, patients become uncertain again (the cold-feet phenomenon), the provider reflects this ambivalence rather than trying to press through it and provides another opportunity to revisit the plan in the current meeting or at another time. Being in a hurry to complete the plan when patients are not ready is a common trap into which providers fall.

HANDLING RESISTANCE

Successfully managing kidney disease is difficult for several reasons. As described above, patients must continuously manage numerous medical treatments (scheduled appointments, dialysis regimens, prescribed medications, health monitoring activities) and address several nutritional and other lifestyle changes to treat their kidney disease and associated co-morbidities. These demands on patients increase as their kidney disease progresses, and their motivation to meet them typically fluctuates over time. Providers who use MI with patients understand resistance to change as an important communication by patients about what makes change hard for them rather than as a refusal to change or mere ignorance. The former perspective promotes empathic and supportive provider—patient interactions. The latter one might lead providers to label patients as "unmotivated" and confront, warn, or lecture them, thereby, risking putting patients in a position of defending themselves by arguing for their status quo behaviors [18].

Some strategies for skillfully handling resistance include: (1) simply reflecting the resistance to show empathy and better understand the issue ("You don't believe you should have to make any further changes in the way you eat when you feel you have made big changes elsewhere" in response to a patient who says, "I already take the meds, cut back on how much I drink, and started walking after work. I don't want to change my diet anymore"); (2) amplified reflections to determine the degree of commitment to a resistant statement ("Your wife has no basis to be concerned about your weight" in response to a person who complains how his wife needs to stop bothering him about his obesity); (3) double-sided reflections to pair the resistant statement with other things said that favor change, thereby introducing some ambivalence back into the conversation ("You feel like stopping the medication now that you have changed your diet and exercise, and you worry that if you do, you might develop hypertension again"); and emphasizing personal choice and control to assure the patients that it is they who determine what they will do, not others ("Dialysis is not easy, but it is manageable and you have a few options about how to do it. We will work with you to determine what the best way is to go about getting dialysis, but ultimately it really is your decision"). These strategies are delivered with an attitude of genuine interest, not sarcasm or manipulation and of seeing resistance as a natural part of the change process.

The dialogue below demonstrates the use of MI strategies for handling resistance (italicized in text) with a dialysis dependent patient who needs to lose weight to become eligible for a kidney transplant.

Provider: I'd like to talk with you about your weight if that's okay with you? (*emphasizing personal choice and control*)
Patient: Sure, but I already know what you are going to say.
Provider: You're concerned I'm going to give you a lecture rather than try to understand what makes losing weight difficult for you. (*reflection*)

Patient: Well I know what I have to do and I've tried it all before. It's just so hard now with all these adjustments to my diet, and I'm too tired to move around like I used to.
Provider: So having tried everything and being so exhausted, you feel like there is nothing you can do about your weight. (*amplified reflection*)
Patient: Well, it's not that I can't do anything. I just don't feel I can do it on my own. It's like I need a coach or something to help me, to point me in the right direction and keep me going. I'm worried about it because I want to get the kidney transplant.
Provider: So your diet is somewhat complicated and tiredness gets in your way. On the other hand, you want to go to the kidney transplant evaluation knowing you meet the criteria, which requires that you lose weight to be listed. You feel you might be able to lose weight if you had someone to coach you along the way. (*double-sided reflection*)
Patient: Yeah. Could I get someone like that to help me out?
Provider: Sure. There are a few options. You could meet with the dietician regularly, and she can serve as a coach. We also have a weight control program right here, which I can refer you to. Program counselors work closely with you to help you lose weight. Another option is for you to go to a program in the community, like Weight Watchers or others, if you don't want to come here. If these approaches don't work, then we can consider medication or surgical options, but it would be best to first try to improve your eating and exercising, especially since you will need to improve these areas anyway to increase the chance that kidney transplantation succeeds. What do you think? (*emphasizing personal choice and control*)
Patient: What's the program like here?

EMPIRICAL SUPPORT

Several meta-analyses [19—22] have examined the large body of MI research to determine if MI works across a wide range of problem areas (e.g., alcohol, tobacco, illicit drugs, diet/exercise, treatment adherence/engagement). A meta-analysis by Lundhal and colleagues [21] of 119 studies demonstrated that across problem areas MI exerted small yet clinically significant effects, consistent with effects produced by other behavior change interventions but in less time. MI also significantly increased patients' treatment engagement. The effects were durable, lasting up to one year.

Studies examining how MI works have supported the underlying theory of MI. Miller and Rose provide a helpful summary of this literature [7]. In brief, these studies have shown that providers who adhered to MI, in contrast to those who did not, were more likely to have patients who became more motivated to change and, in turn, had improved treatment outcomes (e.g., drinking, meeting dietary goals, increasing activity level) [16,23—30].

APPLICATIONS IN KIDNEY DISEASE MANAGEMENT

MI has been successfully adapted for use in healthcare settings to manage chronic disease, including diabetes. Several studies have shown that MI can be an effective method of working with teenagers and adults with diabetes, producing improvements in glycemic control, psychological wellbeing, and quality of life [31,32]. MI also has moderate to strong effect sizes for a variety of health related behaviors involved in the management of chronic kidney disease, such as healthier eating [33—36], increased physical activity [33,37,38], improved blood pressure control, weight loss [33], and better glucose self-monitoring [39]. A recent systematic review of 87 studies of behavior change strategies used in nutrition counseling demonstrated that motivational interviewing was a highly effective counseling strategy [40].

The nephrology literature has begun to report on applications of MI for kidney disease management. Fisher and colleagues [41] described efforts to improve fluid management among five hemodialysis adult patients. Their intervention combined MI with cognitive behavioral therapy for up to 12 sessions and found that three of the five patients reduced both the mean interdialytic weight gain and the frequency in which they gained in excess of 3% of their dry weight. Van Vilsteren et al. [42] randomly assigned 96 sedentary hemodialysis patients to a low-to-moderate 12-week renal rehabilitation exercise program with or without the addition of four MI sessions to improve exercise adherence. They showed that relative to the control condition, the addition of MI yielded significant increases in reaction time, lower extremity muscle strength, Kt/V, and three quality of life components. Others advocate for the use of MI as a method of engaging kidney disease patients to self-manage their own care [43]. A randomized trial of 793 kidney disease patients in nine Dutch hospitals is examining the extent to which the addition of a nurse provider trained to coach kidney disease patients with MI to adhere to treatment improves self-management over the course of 5 years and the impact this has on cardiovascular morbidity and mortality, all-cause

mortality, renal function, vascular damage markers, and quality of life [44].

LEARNING MOTIVATIONAL INTERVIEWING

A variety of training resources exist to learn MI. These resources include textbooks, treatment manuals, training videotapes, a supervision toolkit, and an international training group called the Motivational Interviewing Network of Trainers. Many of these resources are accessible at www.motivationinterview.org.

Literature on how to train providers in MI is emerging. The most popular approach has been the use of several day workshops. Research on the effectiveness of MI workshops (expert facilitated didactics and skill-building activities delivered in a group format) shows providers consistently improve their attitudes, knowledge, and confidence in MI, but immediate skill gains resulting from the training diminish within a few months [45,46].

Clinical supervision that includes direct observation of providers' sessions (via audio recordings), use of treatment integrity rating-based performance feedback, and individualized coaching has been shown to be more effective in improving providers' MI skills when it is used at least monthly for 3—4 months following workshop training [47,48]. Several provider performance rating scales are now available that can be used to reliably supervise MI practice in this manner [49—51]. This approach to supervision is particularly important given that providers typically evaluate their performance more positively than when the same sessions are reviewed by their supervisors or independent judges [52]. Moreover, in the absence of supervision in MI, providers may be more prone to initiate informal discussions (i.e., chat) about matters that are unrelated to their patients' treatment [53—55]. Careful training and supervision in MI may help providers better adhere to the approach.

Even with supervision, providers will vary in their capacity to learn MI. For example, Miller has speculated that a minimum level of pre-training empathic abilities might be necessary for providers to learn MI [56]. In addition, learning MI may require that providers sequentially build their skills in different stages. Miller and Moyers proposed eight stages (see Table 46.2) for learning MI [57]. First, providers need to develop openness to the spirit of MI such that they grasp the overriding philosophy of the approach (stage 1). Next, they must master the patient-centered counseling skills embodied in the OARS (stage 2), the foundation from which they then learn how to recognize and reinforce

TABLE 46.2 Eight Stages of Learning MI [57]

Stage	Definition
1	Developing an openness to interacting with patients with a spirit of collaboration, respect for autonomy, assumption of motives for change, and compassion
2	Developing proficiency in the use of patient-centered counseling skills such as open questions, affirmations, reflections, and summary statements.
3	Recognizing and differentially reinforcing change talk as it naturally occurs in conversation and in the context of a patient's ambivalence
4	Eliciting and strengthening change talk in a goal-oriented fashion using a variety of techniques
5	Rolling with resistance using various strategies to avoid provoking arguments
6	Developing a change plan once a patient has made a clear commitment to change
7	Consolidating commitment to the patient's specific change plan
8	Switching between MI and other counseling methods as one moves beyond MI or returns to it when motivation wanes

change talk (stage 3). Providers then learn strategies for evoking change talk (stage 4), rolling with resistance (stage 5), and developing a change plan (stage 6). Training in consolidating and strengthening commitment comes next (stage 7). If MI is to be used with other treatment approaches, learning how to switch between the methods or integrate MI into other practices is the last stage (stage 8). Providers may vary in the sequence and degree to which they learn the skills embedded within each stage. Nonetheless, the stages of learning MI imply a training progression that might be used to organize the design of training programs. Moreover, they suggest that MI involves a complex set of skills that providers must use flexibly and adaptively in response to what patients say during their healthcare appointments.

DISSEMINATION OF MOTIVATIONAL INTERVIEWING

MI has become very popular in the United States and internationally. Single State Authorities throughout the U.S. and their equivalent bodies in other countries frequently recommend MI as an empirically-supported clinical approach they want providers to learn [58–61]. The MI textbook has been translated into at least 22 languages, and there are now MI trainers in over

40 different countries. It may be that the person-centeredness of the approach and, hence, sensitivity to diverse cultural perspectives, make MI broadly attractive world-wide [20]. Moreover, the number of publications about MI has increased exponentially in the past two decades as well as funded research grants examining applications of MI to a variety of clinical problems and populations [7].

FUTURE RESEARCH DIRECTIONS IN KIDNEY DISEASE MANAGEMENT

Many questions remain about the use of MI for the management of kidney disease. First, the effectiveness of MI for improving self-management/health behaviors among patients with kidney disease remains an open question. Patients with kidney disease often have to deal with a complex variety of treatment regimens. This poses challenges for both patients and providers. Patients need to consider the consequences of their behaviors in a variety of domains. Providers must be trained to understand how patients process all the information provided to them so that there can be an effective collaboration established. The relative contributions to the effectiveness of MI of the person-centered strategies and the strategies for eliciting and reinforcing change talk remains unclear, including the role of personalized feedback as used in MET. In addition, more work is needed to identify effective strategies for training healthcare providers in MI, sustaining adequate provider performance over time, and linking these training efforts to improved patient outcomes. Strategies that have been found to work well in the addiction and mental health field (workshop plus clinical supervision) may not be as feasible in healthcare settings such as dialysis units or chronic kidney disease clinics. Finally, innovations in the delivery of MI might make the approach more feasible and acceptable for use in busy, multidisciplinary healthcare settings where it is increasingly being applied. The degree to which MI can be programmed for computer- or Web-based applications needs to be established.

CONCLUSIONS

MI is a recognized evidence-based practice for addressing behavioral problems that holds great promise for motivating patients with kidney disease to adhere to various aspects of the complex treatment regimens and other healthy lifestyle activities that are important for these patients. MI has a clear set of principles and techniques that guide implementation and substantial training resources to prepare providers to conduct MI proficiently. The popularity of MI is likely to grow and the healthcare field will be challenged to study if and how it works within its new applications, such as for the management of kidney disease, and to ensure that providers implement it with integrity in order to improve treatment outcomes. The nephrology community should learn how to apply MI techniques in chronic kidney disease clinics and dialysis facilities. Carefully done studies will then need to be done to document the impact of MI on a variety of patient outcomes.

Acknowledgement

National Institute on Drug Abuse grants (U10 DA13038, DA09241, DA023230) and National Institute of Mental Health grant (RMH0884772A, K23MH77824) supported this article. The views expressed within it are those of the authors and do not represent the views of NIDA or NIMH.

Conflicts of interest

None.

References

[1] Julius RJ, Novitsky MA, Dubin WR. Medication adherence: A review of the literature and implications for clinical practice. J Psychiat Pract 2009;15:34–44.

[2] Bodenheimer T, Wagner E, Grumbach K. Improving primary care for patients with chronic illness: the chronic care model, Part 2. JAMA 2002;288:1909–14.

[3] Miller WR, Rollnick S. Motivational interviewing: preparing people for change second edition. New York, New York, USA: Guilford Press; 2002.

[4] Rollnick S, Miller WR, Butler CC. helping patients change behavior, Motivational interviewing in healthcare. New York, New York, USA: Guilford Press; 2008.

[5] Miller WR, Rollnick S. Ten things that motivational interviewing is not. Beh Cog Psychoth 2009;37:129–40.

[6] Rogers CR. A theory of therapy, personality, and interpersonal relationships as developed in the client-centered framework. In: Koch S, editor. Psychology: the study of a science. formulations of the person and the social contexts, Vol 3. New York: New York, USA: McGraw-Hill; 1959. p. 184–256.

[7] Miller WR, Rose GS. Toward a theory of motivational interviewing. Am Psychol 2009;64:527–37.

[8] Prochaska JO, DiClemente CC. The transtheoretical approach: crossing traditional boundaries of therapy. Homewood, Illinois, USA: Dow Jones-Irwin; 1984.

[9] DiClemente CC, Velasquez MM. Motivational interviewing and the stages of change. In: Miller WR, Rollnick S, editors. Motivational interviewing preparing people for change second edition. New York, New York, USA: Guilford Press; 2002. p. 201–16.

[10] Arkowitz H, Westra HA, Miller WR, Rollnick S. Motivational Interviewing in the Treatment of Psychological Problems. New York, New York, USA: Guilford Press; 2008.

[11] Bien TH, Miller WR, Tonigan JS. Brief interventions for alcohol problems: a review. Addiction 1993;88:315–36.

[12] Miller WR, Sovereign RG, Krege B. Motivational interviewing with problem drinkers: II. The Drinker's Check-up as a preventive intervention. Beh Psychoth 1989;16:251–68.

[13] Miller WR, Zweben A, DiClemente CC, Rychtarik RG. Motivational Enhancement Therapy manual: A clinical research guide for therapists treating individuals with alcohol abuse and dependence. (Volume 2, Project MATCH Monograph Series). Rockville, Maryland, USA: National Institute on Alcohol Abuse and Alcoholism; 1992.

[14] Miller WR, Benefield RG, Tonigan JS. Enhancing motivation for change in problem drinking: a controlled comparison of two therapist styles. J Consult Clin Psychol 1993;61:455–61.

[15] Rollnick S, William WR. What is motivational interviewing? Beh Cog Psychoth 1995;23:325–34.

[16] Amhreim P, Miller WR, Yahne CE, Palmer M, Fulcher L. Client commitment language during motivational interviewing. J Consult Clin Psychol 2003;71:862–78.

[17] Rollnick S, Heather N. Negotiating behavior change in medical settings: the development of brief motivational interviewing. J Ment Health 1992;1:25–38.

[18] Brehm SS, Brehm JW. Psychological reactance: A theory of freedom and control. New York, New York, USA: Academic Press; 1981.

[19] Burke BL, Arkowitz H, Menchola M. The efficacy motivational interviewing: a meta-analysis of controlled trials. J Consult Clin Psychol 2003;71:843–61.

[20] Hettema J, Steele J, Miller WR. Motivational interviewing. Annual Rev Clin Psychol 2005;1:91–111.

[21] Lundahl BW, Kunz C, Brownell C, Tollefson D, Burke B. Meta-analysis of motivational interviewing: twenty Five years of empirical studies. Res Soc Work Pract 2010;20:137–60.

[22] Vasilaki E, Hosier S, Cox W. The efficacy of motivational interviewing as a brief intervention for excessive drinking: a meta-analytic review. Alcohol Alcoholism 2006;41:328–35.

[23] Moyers TB, Martin T. Therapist influence on client language during motivational interviewing sessions: support for a potential causal mechanism. J Subst Abuse Treat 2006;30:245–51.

[24] Moyers TB, Martin T, Christopher PJ, Houck JM, Tonigan JS, Amrhein PC. Client language as a mediator of motivational interviewing efficacy: where is the evidence? Alc Clin Exp Res 2007;31(Suppl. 3):40–7.

[25] Moyers TB, Martin T, Houck JM, Christopher PJ, Tonigan JS. From in-session behaviors to drinking outcomes: a causal chain for motivational interviewing. J Consult Clin Psychol 2009;77:1113–24.

[26] Apodaca TR, Longabaugh R. Mechanisms of change in motivational interviewing: a review and preliminary evaluation of the evidence: Addiction 2009;104:705–15.

[27] Baer JS, Beadnell B, Garrett SB, Hartzler B, Wells EA, Peterson PL. Adolescent change language within a brief motivational intervention and substance use outcomes. Psychol Addict Beh 2008;22:570–5.

[28] Gaume J, Gmel G, Faouzi M, Daeppen J. Counselor skill influences outcomes of brief motivation interventions. J Subst Abuse Treat 2009;37:151–9.

[29] Hodgins DC, Ching LE, McEwen J. Strength of commitment language in motivational interviewing and gambling outcomes. Psychol Addict Beh 2009;3:122–30.

[30] Strang J, McCambridge J. Can the Provider correctly predict outcome in motivational interviewing? J Subst Abuse Treat 2004;27:83–8.

[31] Channon SJ, Huws-Thomas MV, Rollnick S, Hood K, Cannings-John RL, Rogers C, et al. A multicenter randomized controlled trial of motivational interviewing in teenagers with diabetes. Diabetes Care 2007;30:1390—5.

[32] Ismail K, Thomas SM, Maissi E, Chalder T, Schmidt U, Bartlett J, et al. Motivational enhancement therapy with and without cognitive behavior therapy to treat type 1 diabetes: a randomized trial. Ann Intern Med 2008;149:708—19.

[33] Woollard J, Beilin L, Lord T, Puddey I, MacAdam D, Rouse I. A controlled trial of nursing counseling on lifestyle change for hypertensives treated in general practice: preliminary results. Clin Exp Pharm Phys 1995;22:466—8.

[34] Resincow K, Jackson A, Blissett D, Wang T, McCarty F, Rahotep S, et al. Results of the Healthy Body Healthy Spirit trial. Health Psychol 2005;24:339—48.

[35] Resnicow K, Jackson A, Wang T, Anindya K, De AK, McCarty F, et al. A motivational interviewing intervention to increase fruit and vegetable intake through black churches: results of the Eat for Life trial. Am J Public Health 2001;91: 1686—93.

[36] Bowen D, Ehret C, Pedersen M, Snetselaar L, Johnson M, et al. Results of an adjunct dietary intervention program in the Women's Health Initiative. J Am Diet Assoc 2002;102: 1631—7.

[37] Scales R, Miller JH. Motivational techniques for improving compliance with an exercise program: skills for primary care clinicians. Current Sports Med Reports 2003;2:166—72.

[38] Brodie DA, Inoue A. Motivational interviewing to promote physical activity for people with chronic heart failure. J Adv Nurs 2005;50:518—27.

[39] Smith DE, Heckemeyer DM, Kratt PP, Mason DA. Motivational interviewing to improve adherence to a behavioral weight-control program for older obese women with NIDDM: a pilot study. Diabetes Care 1997;20:52—4.

[40] Spahn JM, Reeves RS, Keim KS, Laquatra I, Kellogg M, Jortberg B, et al. State of the evidence regarding behavior change theories and strategies in nutrition counseling to facilitate health and food behavior change. J Am Diet Assoc 2010;110:879—91.

[41] Fisher L, Cairns HS, Amir-Ansari B, Scoble JE, Chalder T, Treasure J. Psychological intervention in fluid management. Palliat Support Care 2006;4:419—24.

[42] van Vilsteren MCBA, de Greef MHG, Huisman RM. The effects of a low-to-moderate intensity pre-conditioning exercise programme linked with exercise counseling for sedentary haemodialysis patient in The Netherlands: results of a randomized clinical trial. Nephrol Dial Transplant 2005;20: 141—6.

[43] McCarley P. Patient empowerment and motivational interviewing: engaging patients to self-manage their own care. Nephrol Nurse J 2009;36:409—13.

[44] van Zuilen AD, Wetzels JFM, Bots ML, Blankestijn PJ. MASTERPLAN: study of the role of nurse Providers in a multifactorial intervention to reduce cardiovascular risk in chronic kidney disease patients. J Nephrol 2008;21:261—7.

[45] Davis D. Does CME work? An analysis of the effect of educational activities on physician performance or healthcare outcomes. Int J Psychiatry Med 1998;28:21—39.

[46] Walters ST, Matson SA, Baer JS, Ziedonis DM. Effectiveness of workshop training for psychosocial addiction treatments: a systematic review. J Subst Abuse Treat 2005;29:283—93.

[47] Miller WR, Yahne CE, Moyers TB, Martinez J, Pirritano M. A randomized trial of methods to help clinicians learn motivational interviewing. J Consult Clin Psychol 2004;72:1052—62.

[48] Madson MB, Loignon AC, Lane C. Training in motivational interviewing: a systematic review. J Subst Abuse Treat 2009;31: 101—9.

[49] Martino S, Ball SA, Ball SA, Nich C, Frankforter TL, Carroll KM. Community program therapist adherence and competence in motivational enhancement therapy. Drug Alcohol Depend 2008;97:37—48.

[50] Moyers TB, Martin T, Manuel JK, Hendrickson SML, Miller WR. Assessing competence in the use of motivational interviewing. J Subst Abuse Treat 2005;28:19—26.

[51] Lane C, Huws-Thomas M, Hood K, Rollnick S, Edwards K, Robling M. Measuring adaptations of motivational interviewing: the development and validation of the Behavior Change Counseling Index (BECCI). Patient Educ Counsel 2005;56:166—73.

[52] Martino S, Ball SA, Nich C, Frankforter TL, Carroll KM. Correspondence of motivational enhancement treatment integrity ratings among therapists, supervisors, and observers. Psychoth Res 2009;19:181—93.

[53] Martino S, Ball SA, Nich C, Frankforter TL, Carroll KM. Informal discussions in substance abuse treatment sessions. J Subst Abuse Treat 2009;36:366—75.

[54] Bamatter W, Carroll KM, Añez LM, Paris M, Ball SA, Nich C, et al. Informal discussion in substance abuse treatment sessions with Spanish-speaking clients. J Subst Abuse Treat 2010;39: 353—63.

[55] McDaniel SH, Beckman HB, Morse DS, Silberman J, Seaburn DB, Epstein RM. Physician self-disclosure in primary care visits: enough about you, what about me? Archives Internal Med 2007;167:1321—6.

[56] Miller WR, Moyer TB, Arciniega L, Ernst D, Forcehimes A. Training, supervision and quality monitoring of the COMBINE study behavioral interventions. J Studies Alcohol 2005a;(Suppl. 15):188—95.

[57] Miller WR, Moyers TB. Eight stages in learning motivational interviewing. J Teach Addictions 2006;5:3—17.

[58] Miller WR, Sorensen JL, Selzer JA, Brigham GS. Disseminating evidence-based practices in substance abuse treatment: a review with suggestions. J Subst Abuse Treat 2006;31:25—39.

[59] Reickmann TR, Kovas AE, Fussell HE, Stettler NM. Implementation of evidence-based practices for treatment of alcohol and drug disorders: the role of the state authority. J Beh Health Ser Res. 2009;36:407—19.

[60] Giuseppe C, Clerici M. Dual diagnosis — policy and practice in Italy. Am J Addict 2006;15:125—30.

[61] Hintz T, Mann K. Co-occurring disorders: policy and practice in Germany. Am J Addict 2006;15:261—7.

Index

Note: Page numbers with "f" denote figures; "t" tables.

THE UBIQUITIN-PROTEASOME PATHWAY

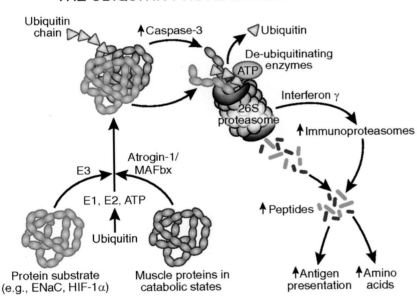

FIGURE 1.1 The UPS degrades protein. Proteins destined for degradation are conjugated to Ub by an ATP-dependent process involving three enzymes: E1, E2 and E3. Selectivity of the protein substrates for degradation principally depends on the E3 ubiquitin ligases. Once a chain of 5 Ubs is attached to the protein substrate, the complex can be recognized by the 26S proteasome. This particle releases Ubs, unfolds the substrate protein and injects it into the central pore of the 26S proteasome. In this channel, the protein is degraded to peptides which are released. Peptidases in the cytoplasm converted to amino acids. Under special conditions, peptides released are joined with the MCH class 1 molecules, becoming antigens. (Figure from Lecker, S.H. and Mitch, W.E. Proteolysis by the Ubiquitin-Proteasome System and Kidney Disease, Journal of the American Society of Nephrology, volume 22, pages 821–824, 2011.)

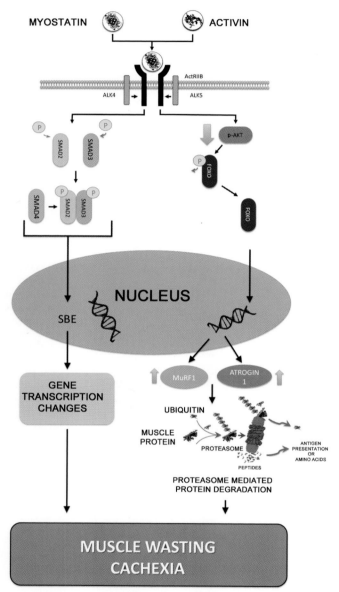

FIGURE 1.2 Myostatin and activin signaling in muscle. Myostatin or activin bind to type IIB activin receptor (ActRIIB) on muscle membranes and when it becomes a dimmer, there is recruitment and activation of the type I activin receptor transmembrane kinase (ALK4 or ALK5). The kinases initiate intracellular signaling cascades: Smad2 and Smad3 become phosphorylated to form a heterodimer and recruit Smad4 into a complex that translocates into the nucleus to bind Smad Binding Element which regulates transcription of downstream response genes. On the right, forkhead transcription factors (FoxO) are dephosphorylated, enter the nucleus and activate the transcription of atrophy-specific E3 ligases MuRF1 and Atrogin1. These E3 ubiquitin ligases provide the specificity that leads to degradation of muscle contractile proteins by the proteasome. (Figure from *Issues in Dialysis*, Edited by Stephen Z. Fadem, Nova Science Publishers, Inc., New York, 2012, page 157, Figure 2.)

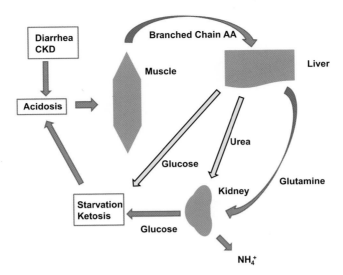

FIGURE 8.1 Starvation and acidemia alter gluconeogenesis from amino acids. In the fed state, excess amino acids are converted to glucose via the urea cycle (yellow). Urea formation has an energetic cost of ~35% of the energy equivalent in the glucose formed. In starvation (blue), ketone formation leads to a mild acidemia enhancing the release of branched chain amino acids from muscle. During acidemia, the liver preferentially converts branched chain amino acids to glutamine which is deaminated in the kidney to produce ammonium and glucose. Glucose production from glutamine is much more energetically favorable than the glucose generated during urea synthesis in the urea cycle making the former process more adaptive in starvation. Metabolic acidemia from other causes activates the same pathways leading to excretion of hydrogen ions via ammonium at the cost of losing amino acids and proteins.

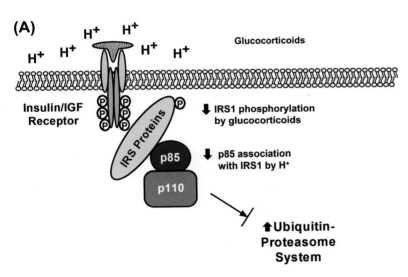

FIGURE 8.2 (A) Acidemia and glucocorticoids block insulin and/or insulin like growth factor-I (IGF-I) signaling to activate the ubiquitin-proteasome system in muscle. Signaling through the insulin or IGF-I receptors normally prevents muscle wasting. Acidemia and glucocorticoids work synergistically to impair signaling through the insulin receptor after the binding of insulin or IGF-I. Glucocorticoids partially reduce the phosphorylation of insulin receptor substrate-I induced by insulin binding, while acidemia blocks recruitment of the phosphoinositide 3-kinase p85 subunit to prevent downstream signaling. Impairing signaling allows activation of the ubiquitin proteasome system. (B) Acidemia stimulates the ubiquitin—proteasome system by affecting multiple steps. Proteins freed from the muscle fibers by caspase 3 are conjugated by ubiquitin. The ubiquitin presents these protein fragments to the proteasome where they are destroyed. Acidemia increases the amount of ubiquitin and proteasomes in cells and also increases the conjugation of protein with ubiquitin.

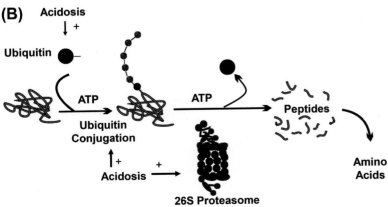

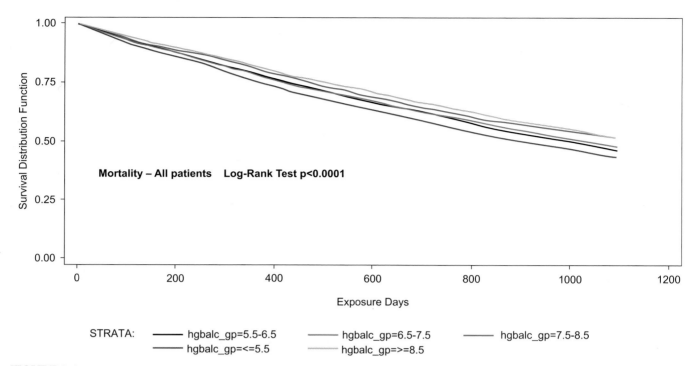

FIGURE 9.4 Kaplan–Meier survival curve. Shown are survival rates for baseline HgbA1c groups. *Reproduced with permission from Clin J Am Soc Nephrol. 2010;5(9):1595–601.*

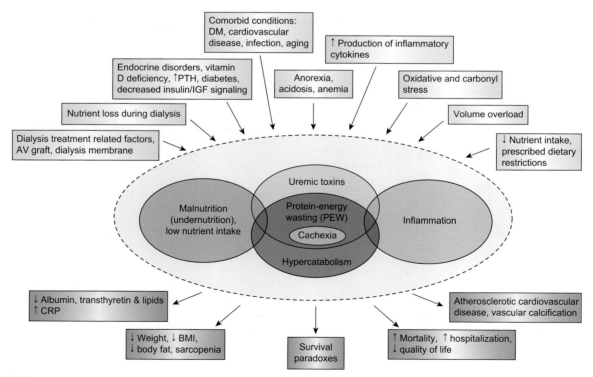

FIGURE 11.1 Schematic representation of the causes and manifestations of the protein–energy wasting syndrome in kidney disease. *Reprinted from reference [5].*

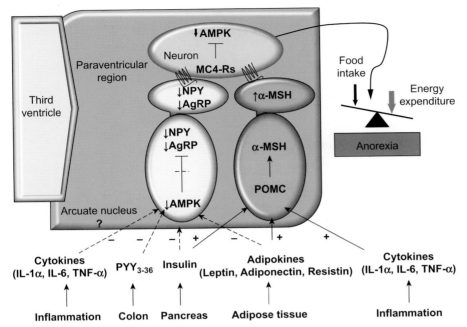

FIGURE 11.2 Orexigenic and anorexigenic mechanisms controlling energy homeostasis in CKD. Circulating hormones produced by the colon (PYY), pancreas (insulin) adipose tissue and cytokines all cause anorexia. Responses to these factors result in the modulation of the hypothalamic melanocortin signaling pathways with an increase in MC4-Rs which suppresses AMP activated protein kinase (AMPK) activity, leading to decreased food intake, increased energy expenditure, and weight loss. *Reprinted with permission from Mak et al. [99].*

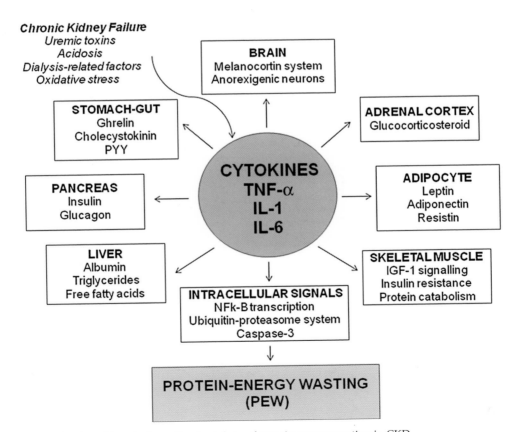

FIGURE 11.3   Central role of cytokines in the pathophysiology of protein energy wasting in CKD.

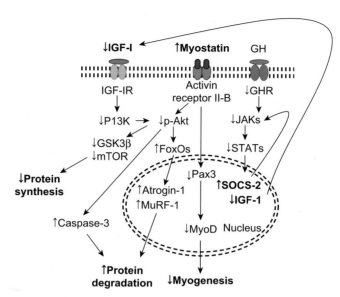

FIGURE 11.4 Pathophysiology of muscle wasting in CKD. Insulin-like growth factor (IGF)-I increases muscle mass while myostatin inhibits its development. Muscle wasting could be due to imbalance of this regulation. Phosphatidylinositol 3 kinase activity (PI3K) is key to activation of muscle proteolysis through regulation of caspase-3, and expression of atrogin-1/MAFbx. *Reprinted from Mak et al. [100].*

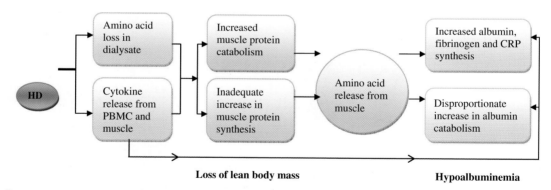

FIGURE 11.5 Integrating cytokine, amino acid kinetics and protein turnover in ESRD. Activation of cytokines during HD increases synthesis of acute phase protein, which is probably facilitated by constant delivery of amino acids derived from the muscle catabolism and intra-dialytic increase in IL-6 [101].

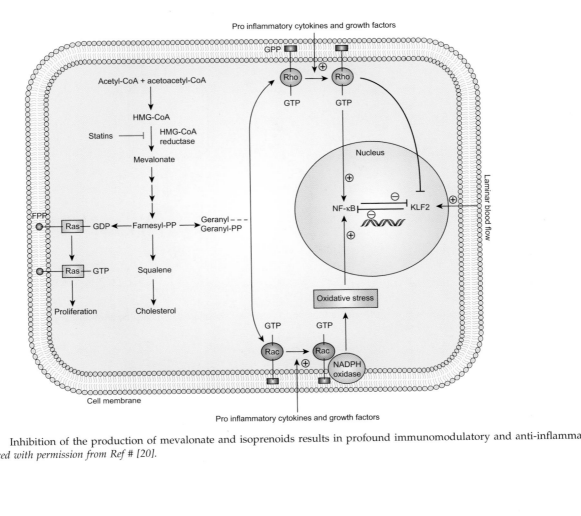

FIGURE 16.1 Inhibition of the production of mevalonate and isoprenoids results in profound immunomodulatory and anti-inflammatory effects. *Reproduced with permission from Ref # [20].*

Total Phosphate Distribution

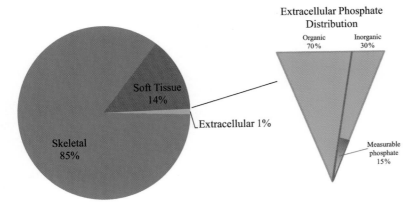

FIGURE 20.1 Total phosphate distribution. Sections of the pie chart indicate proportions of phosphate distribution throughout the body.

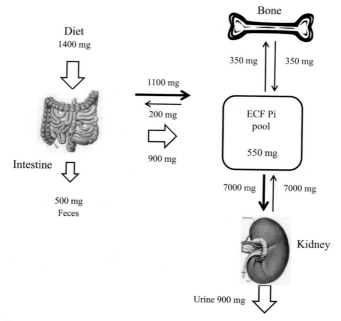

FIGURE 20.2 Phosphate metabolism in the bone, kidney and intestine. Phosphate regulation by three primary organs: kidney, bone and intestine. ECF Pi: extracellular fluid phosphorus.

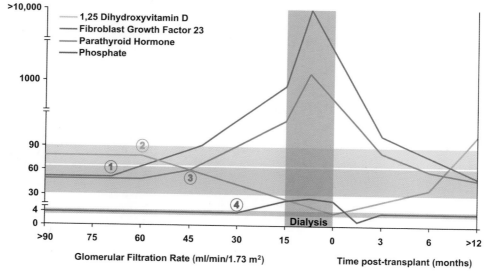

FIGURE 20.3 Temporal aspects of disordered phosphate metabolism in CKD. The x axis: represents the eGFR in the predialysis period (left); represents time after kidney transplantation in the postdialysis period (right). The y axis represents circulating concentrations of the individual analytes with the temporal changes in and normal ranges of individual analytes (C-terminal FGF-23 [RU/mL] − red; 1,25D [pg/mL] − yellow; PTH [pg/mL] − green; phosphate [mg/dL] − blue). Increased FGF-23 is the earliest abnormality in mineral metabolism in CKD and causes the subsequent decline in 1,25D levels that free PTH from feedback inhibition and lead to secondary hyperparathyroidism. All of these changes occur before serum phosphate levels increase. In early post-transplantation, FGF-23 and PTH levels rapidly decline and are variable thereafter. Tertiary FGF-23 excess contributes to post-transplantation hypophosphatemia and slow recovery of normal 1,25D production. *This figure is reproduced from Wolf [27], with permission from the American Society of Nephrology. Copyright © [2010] American Society of Nephrology. All rights reserved.*

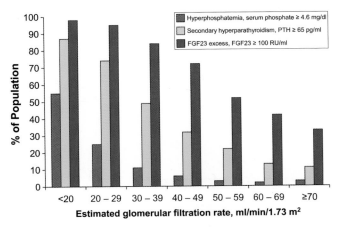

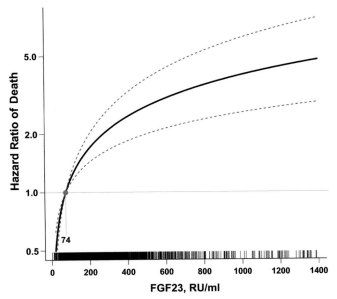

FIGURE 20.4 Prevalence of hyperphosphatemia, secondary hyperparathyroidism and elevated FGF-23 in CKD. Hyperphosphatemia was defined as serum phosphate ≥ 4.6 mg/dL, secondary hyperparathyroidism as parathyroid hormone (PTH) ≥ 65 pg/mL, and FGF-23 excess as FGF-23 ≥ 100 RU/mL. *This figure is reproduced from Isakova et al. [43], with permission from Macmillan Publishers Ltd: Kidney International. Copyright © [2011] Macmillan Publishers Ltd. All rights reserved.*

FIGURE 20.6 Multivariable-adjusted hazard function for death according to FGF-23. The median fibroblast growth factor 23 (FGF-23) level within the lowest FGF-23 quartile (74 RU/mL) served as the referent value (hazard = 1.0). The model was stratified by center and adjusted for age; sex; race; ethnicity; estimated glomerular filtration rate; natural log-transformed urine albumin-to-creatinine ratio; hemoglobin; serum albumin; systolic blood pressure; body mass index; diabetes; smoking status; low-density lipoprotein; history of coronary artery disease, congestive heart failure, stroke, and peripheral vascular disease; use of aspirin, β-blockers, statins, and angiotensin-converting enzyme inhibitors or angiotensin II receptor blockers; and serum calcium, phosphate, and natural log-transformed parathyroid hormone. Tick marks on the x-axis indicate individual observations at corresponding levels of FGF-23. The solid black line represents the multivariable-adjusted hazard of mortality as a function of the measured (nontransformed) FGF-23 level. The dashed lines indicate the 95% confidence intervals. *This figure is reproduced from Isakova et al. [43], with permission from the American Medical Association. Copyright © [2011] American Medical Association. All rights reserved.*

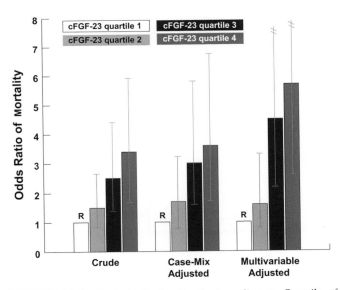

FIGURE 20.5 Odds Ratio for Death According to Quartile of FGF-23. Crude, case-mix adjusted, and multivariable adjusted odds ratios for death are shown according to quartile of cFGF-23 levels (quartile 1, <1090 reference units [RU] per milliliter; quartile 2, 1090 to 1750 RU per milliliter; quartile 3, 1751 to 4010 RU per milliliter; quartile 4, >4010 RU per milliliter). The case-mix adjusted analysis included the following variables: age, sex, race or ethnic group, blood pressure, body-mass index, facility-specific standardized mortality rate, vascular access at initiation of dialysis (fistula, graft, or catheter), cause of renal failure, urea reduction ratio, and coexisting conditions. The multivariable adjusted analysis included the case-mix variables plus phosphate, calcium, log parathyroid hormone, albumin, creatinine, and ferritin levels. Quartile 1 was the reference group in all models. I bars represent 95% confidence intervals. Asterisks indicate P < 0.05. R denotes reference. *This figure is reproduced from Gutiérrez et al. [56], with permission from the Massachusetts Medical Society. Copyright © [2008] Massachusetts Medical Society. All rights reserved.*

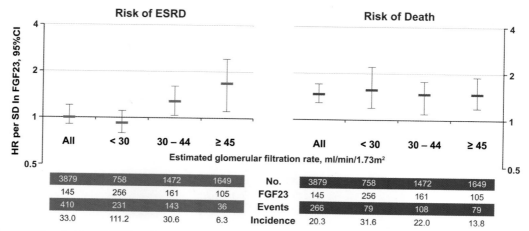

FIGURE 20.7 FGF-23 and risks of ESRD and death by baseline kidney function. Multivariable-adjusted risks of end-stage renal disease and death per unit increment in SD of natural log-transformed fibroblast growth factor 23 (FGF-23) in all participants and according to categories of baseline estimated glomerular filtration rate (GFR). See Figure 20.6 legend for adjusted variables. Error bars indicate 95% confidence intervals. HR indicates hazard ratio. *This figure is reproduced from Isakova et al. [43], with permission from the American Medical Association. Copyright © [2011] American Medical Association. All rights reserved.*

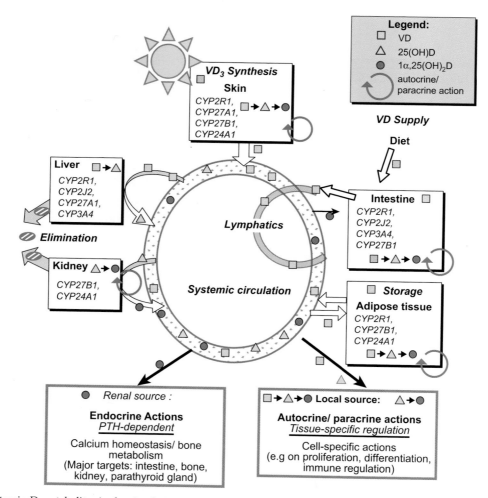

FIGURE 21.1 Vitamin D metabolites in the circulation and enzymes from the vitamin D synthetic pathway at major sites of endocrine and autocrine/paracrine functions of 1,25OH$_2$ D. Note that many locations can synthesize 1,25OH$_2$ D from its precursors. CYP2R1, CYP2J2, CYP27A1 and CYP3A4 can synthesize 25OH D. CYP27B1 synthesizes 1,25OH$_2$ D and CYP24A1 degrades both 25OH D and 1,25OH$_2$ D. Red arrows denote tissues that can respond to 1,25OH$_2$ D, red circles, 1,25OH$_2$ D and yellow triangles, 25OH D. *(Reprinted, with permission from Schuster, 2011.)*

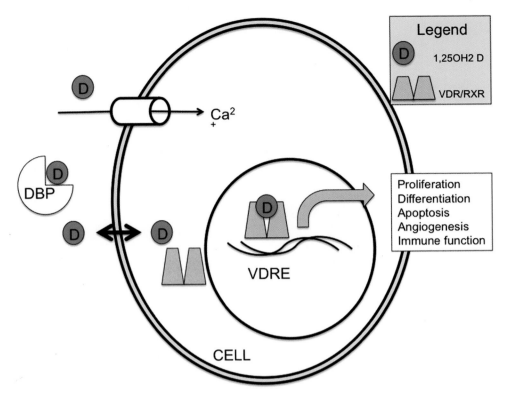

FIGURE 21.2 Cellular actions of 1,25OH$_2$ D, denoted with red circles. 1,25OH$_2$ D has classical gene-regulatory actions mediated by the VDR/RXR complex in the nucleus, which recruits transcriptional activators and remodeling factors upon 1,25OH$_2$ D binding. 1,25OH$_2$ D also acts as non-classical activator of calcium channels in a VDR-independent manner.

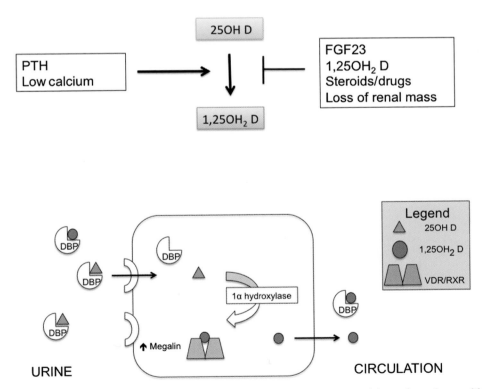

FIGURE 21.3 Factors affecting 1,25OH$_2$ D production. In CKD/ESRD, elevated FGF23 and loss of renal mass likely contribute to the decreased synthesis of 1,25OH$_2$ D. In the lower panel, reduction in 25OHD/DBP delivery to the proximal tubule cell, as well as decrease in the megalin receptor and the 1-α-hydroxylase amount contribute to reduced 1,25OH$_2$ D synthesis.

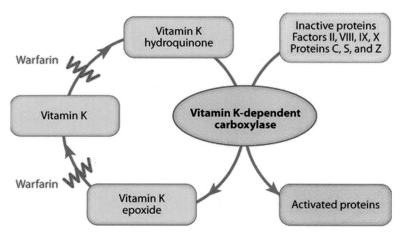

FIGURE 24.1 The vitamin K cycle from [235] with permission.

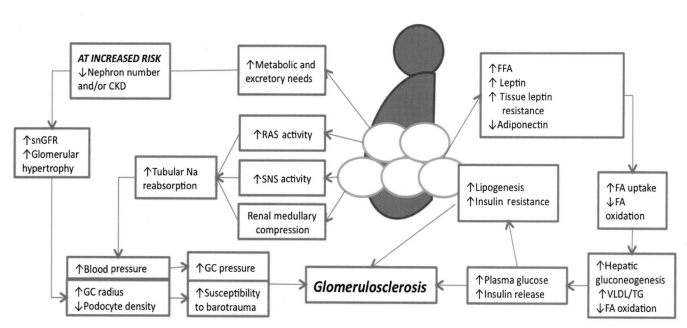

FIGURE 28.3 In obesity/the metabolic syndrome, free fatty acid delivery to the portal circulation is increased leading to increased synthesis of triglycerides TGs and atherogenic VLDLs. Leptin levels increase but tissue resistance develops. Adiponectin levels are reduced which increases hepatic gluconeogenesis and plasma glucose and insulin levels. Lipogenesis is thus augmented and cytosolic fatty acid levels increase resulting in insulin resistance. Blood pressure increases due to increased renal tubular sodium reabsorption. Autoregulation is impaired and higher blood pressures are transmitted to a glomerulus susceptible to barotrauma. Abbreviations: snGFR, single nephron glomerular filtration rate; GC, glomerulocapillary; RAS, renal-angiotensin system; SNS, sympathetic nervous system; FFA, free fatty acid; FA, fatty acid; VLDL, very-low-density lipoprotein; TG, triglycerides.

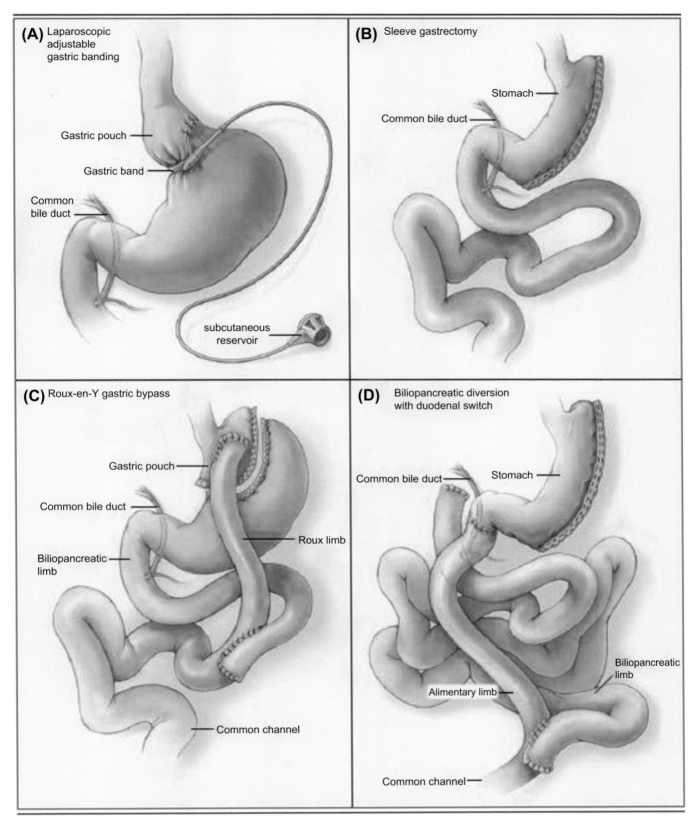

FIGURE 30.1 Bariatric procedures: (A) Adjustable gastric banding; (B) Sleeve gastrectomy; (C) Roux-n-Y gastric bypass; (D) Biliopancreatic diversion with duodenal switch.

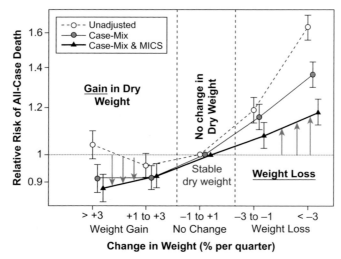

FIGURE 32.1 Association of change in dry weight over 6-months and 5-year mortality in 88,729 MHD patients. *Adapted from Kalantar-Zadeh et al., Mayo Clinic Proceedings, 2010 [16].*

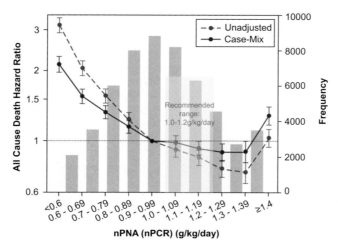

FIGURE 32.2 Association of estimated dietary protein intake (reflected by nPNA or nPCR) and 2-year mortality risk in 53,933 MHD Patients. *Adapted from Shinaberger et al., Am J Kidney Dis 2006; 48:37-49 [75].*

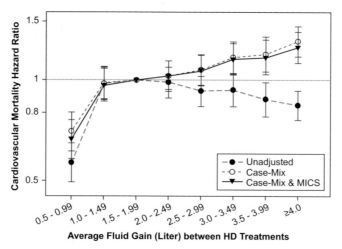

FIGURE 32.4 Association of fluid gain between two consecutive hemodialysis treatment sessions and 2-year cardiovascular mortality in 34,107 MHD patients. *Adapted from Kalantar-Zadeh et al., Circulation 2009 [231].*

(A) **CVVHD**

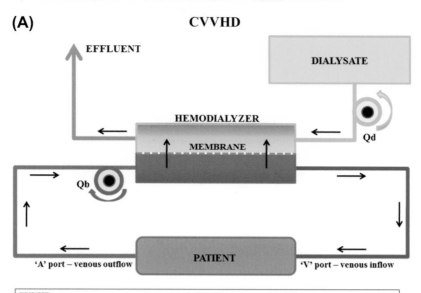

CVVHD: continuous venovenous hemodialysis; Qb: blood pump; Qd: dialysate pump

(B) **CVVH**

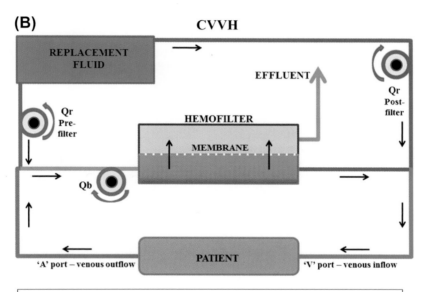

CVVH: continuous venovenous hemofiltration; Qb: blood pump; Qr: replacement fluid pump

(C) **CVVHDF**

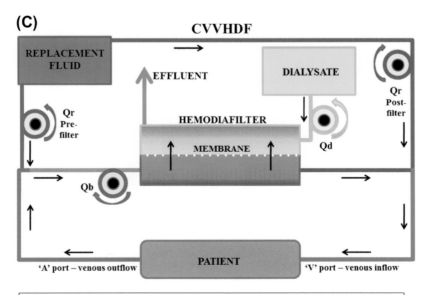

CVVHDF: continuous venovenous hemodiafiltration; Qb: blood pump; Qd: dialysate pump; Qr: replacement fluid pump

FIGURE 37.1 Modes of continuous renal replacement therapy.

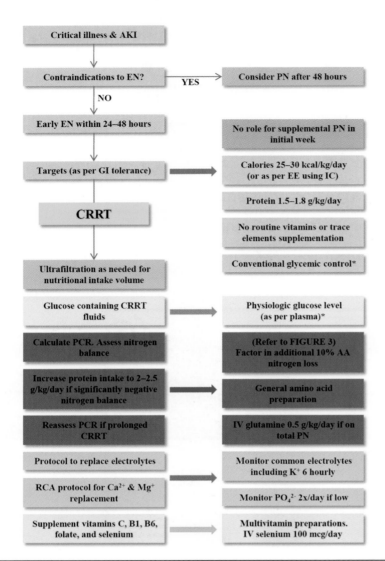

FIGURE 37.2 Algorithm for nutritional therapy.

AKI: acute kidney injury; EN: enteral nutrition; PN: parenteral nutrition; GI: gastro-intestinal; EE: energy expenditure; IC: indirect calorimetry; CRRT: continuous renal replacement therapy; PCR: protein catabolic rate; RCA: regional citrate anticoagulation.
*: target plasma glycemia of 144–180 mg/dL.

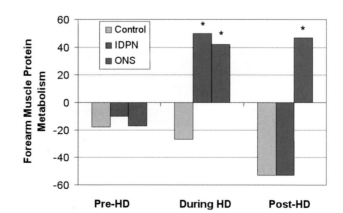

FIGURE 40.1 Effect of IDPN and Oral nutritional therapy on Forearm muscle homeostasis. *(Adapted from Pupim and coworkers [3]). HD, hemodialysis; ONS, oral nutritional supplement; IDPN, intradialytic parenteral nutrition.*